The Adult Hip - Master Case Series and Techniques

Eleftherios Tsiridis
Editor

The Adult Hip - Master Case Series and Techniques

Springer

Editor
Eleftherios Tsiridis
Aristotle University Medical School
Thessaloniki
Greece

ISBN 978-3-030-09710-3 ISBN 978-3-319-64177-5 (eBook)
https://doi.org/10.1007/978-3-319-64177-5

Softcover re-print of the Hardcover 1st edition 2018

This Springer imprint is published by Springer Nature, under the registered company Springer International Publishing AG
The registered company address is: Gewerbestrasse 11, 6330 Cham, Switzerland

To my wife Eva-Maria and my children Thea, Emile and Joanna for their unconditional love and support; for understanding the long hours of my absence from home and their lives.

To my late father Emile and my mother Alice, who inspired me endurance in life.

Preface

The Adult Hip—Master Case Series and Techniques is an essential textbook for those seeking to immerse themselves in the treatment methodologies of specific hip surgical problems. My vision was to create a "virtual travelling hip fellowship" around the world, inviting the reader to enter operating theatres with over 150 distinguished surgeons from every continent, to observe and discuss the crucial learning points of special hip surgical cases from beginning to end.

This book is written by international experts in a clinical and surgical perspective, which focuses specifically on the technical tips and tricks of hip surgery. It is an anthology of the invaluable experiences of world-renowned senior surgeons in a quest to promote and stratify a methodological approach to treating hip problems.

The top surgeons of our time, from Europe, USA, South America, Canada, Asia, Japan and Australia, who perform surgery based on evidence, present 173 unique surgical cases and 40 evidence-based literature reviews which amalgamate the current evidence and practice, with more than 650 illustrations over 730 pages.

Presented in a user-friendly manner, each case is displayed in the same format throughout, allowing the reader to easily find, learn from and compare cases, including crucial references. The reader is guided from the clinical evaluation and pre-operative planning, through to the decision-making process, the surgical procedure and the outcome. A set of critical questions to the surgeon are tackled at the end, further elucidating the essential points based on current evidence.

The Adult Hip—Master Case Series and Techniques is divided into six sections, namely conservative hip surgery, primary, complex primary, hip revision arthroplasty acetabulum and femur and Navigation and VR Software in Joint Reconstruction. It is an invaluable asset for any specialist hip surgeon as well as surgeons in training who are interested in the hip and require both a didactic reference and a complete review of the management of special hip pathologies.

My ambition is that this book will be the founding edition of a long-term publishing legacy to be delivered to the forthcoming generations of hip surgeons as a forum of international communication and exchange of knowledge in hip surgery.

Eleftherios Tsiridis, MD, MSc, PhD, FACS, FRCS
Professor of Orthopaedic Surgery, A.U.Th,
Hellas, Greece

Acknowledgments

I wish to cordially thank my trusted colleague Dr. Stathis Kenanidis, MD, MSc, PhD, Consultant Orthopaedic Surgeon and Academic Fellow of Orthopaedic Surgery; without his efforts and assistance this book would have never been materialized, my Editor Gabriele Schröder who supported this work for almost 2 years and my publisher Springer-Verlag Heidelberg for publishing my book.

Contents

Part III Complex Primary Hip Arthroplasty

Part I

Conservative Hip Surgery

1 Conservative Hip Surgery

Eustathios Kenanidis, Eleftherios Tsiridis, Michael Leunig, Reinhold Ganz, Aprato Alessandro, Massè Alessandro, Andrea M. Spiker, Ben-zion Rotter, Lazaros Poultsides, Bryan T. Kelly, Nicholas M. Desy, Rafael J. Sierra, Stig Storgaard Jakobsen, and Kjeld Søballe

1.1 Current Concepts

E. Kenanidis and E. Tsiridis

Joint preservation is an emerging field in orthopedics that evolved primarily due to the limitations in joint replacement technology. Hip preservation techniques aim to restore an optimal relationship between structure and joint kinematics, prevent or delay the onset of degenerative pathologic conditions, and provide a durable solution for pain and dysfunction [1]. The latter techniques avoid the limitations and disadvantages inherent to joint arthroplasty; however, they demand clear indications [2].

Hip-preserving techniques are usually dealing with acetabular dysplasia, alterations of proximal femoral alignment, and femoroacetabular impingement. The uncorrected acetabular dysplasia has been recognized as a risk factor for hip osteoarthritis development [3]. Joint incongruity resulting from abnormal version or inclination of the proximal femur may cause

E. Kenanidis, M.D., Ph.D., M.Sc. (✉)
Academic Orthopaedic Unit, Aristotle University Medical School, Thessaloniki, Greece

E. Tsiridis, M.D., Ph.D., F.A.C.S., F.R.C.S.
Academic Orthopaedic Unit, Papageorgiou General Hospital, Aristotle University Medical School, Thessaloniki, Greece
e-mail: etsiridis@doctors.org.uk

M. Leunig
Schulthess Clinic and ETH Zürich, Zürich, Switzerland
e-mail: leunig@me.com

R. Ganz, M.D., Dr. Hon, F.R.C.S.Ed.
University of Berne, Berne, Switzerland
e-mail: rd.ganz@bluewin.ch

A. Alessandro, M.D. · M. Alessandro
University of Turin, Turin, Italy

A.M. Spiker, M.D.
Department of Orthopaedic Surgery, University of Wisconsin—Madison, UW Health at The American Center, Madison, WI, USA

B.Z. Rotter, B.S. · B.T. Kelly, M.D.
Department of Orthopaedic Surgery, Center for Hip Preservation, Hospital for Special Surgery, New York, NY, USA

L. Poultsides, M.D., Ph.D., M.Sc.
New York University School of Medicine, New York, NY, USA

Division of Adult Reconstruction, Department of Orthopaedic Surgery, New York Langone Orthopaedic Hospital, New York Langone Medical Center, New York, NY, USA

N.M. Desy, M.D., F.R.C.S.C.
Section of Orthopaedic Surgery, University of Calgary, Calgary, AB, Canada

R.J. Sierra, M.D.
Mayo Clinic, College of Medicine, Rochester, MN, USA
e-mail: Sierra.Rafael@mayo.edu

S.S. Jakobsen, M.D., Ph.D. · K. Søballe, M.D., Ph.D., D.M.Sc.
Department of Orthopaedic Surgery, Aarhus University Hospital, Aarhus, Denmark
e-mail: STIG.JAKOBSEN@ki.au.dk; kjeld@soballe.com

E. Tsiridis (ed.), *The Adult Hip - Master Case Series and Techniques*,
https://doi.org/10.1007/978-3-319-64177-5_1

translational forces and accelerated degradation of the articular cartilage [4]. Impingement between the proximal femur and acetabulum leads to labral-chondral injury and has been considered as a significant causative factor of premature hip arthritis and resultant joint deterioration [5].

Hip joint preservation techniques include the periacetabular and proximal femoral osteotomy, surgical dislocation, and cartilage restoration techniques as well as arthroscopic treatment of labral and chondral abnormalities [1]. The Bernese periacetabular osteotomy otherwise known as the Ganz osteotomy [6] is a commonly used technique for large-scale correction of acetabular dysplasia and improvement of femoral head uncoverage or in the treatment of femoroacetabular impingement [7]. It can be used as an isolated procedure with exposure of the anterior hip via arthrotomy or in conjunction with hip arthroscopy for minimally invasive joint access or with surgical dislocation. The proximal femoral osteotomies are used to redirect rotational or angular deformities of the proximal femur, improve the mechanical environment of the joint, and delay total hip arthroplasty [8]. They are usually employed in conditions as Legg-Calve-Perthes and slipped capital femoral epiphysis or even femoroacetabular impingement [9].

Surgical dislocation offers circumferential access to the femoral head and permits unobstructed visualization of the central compartment of the hip for treatment of labral and chondral injuries. Comparable results have been reported between open and arthroscopic femoral osteoplasty techniques in bony correction; however, for global or superolateral and posterosuperior femoral head deformities, surgical dislocation seems to be preferred [9, 10]. Arthroscopic techniques are used to address intra-articular pathology as labral and chondral abnormalities and combined with reorientation techniques to treat acetabular dysplasia [11, 12]. Arthroscopic treatment is more controversial in patients with severe acetabular insufficiency, and careful patient selection regarding potential risks is recommended. Cartilage restoration techniques also have been applied to the hip with encouraging short-term clinical outcomes [13].

1.2 Case Title: Surgical Hip Dislocation Removal of Acetabular Rim Bony Fragment Repair of the Labrum and Removal of CAM Lesion

E. Kenanidis and E. Tsiridis

Intra-substance ossification and fracture of the ream of the acetabular roof with a cyst adjacent to the roof. Surgical dislocation of the hip using greater trochanteric osteotomy, removal of the fragment, and repair of the labrum using two suture anchors (visible at the roof of the socket). The CAM lesion has also been removed (Fig. 1.1).

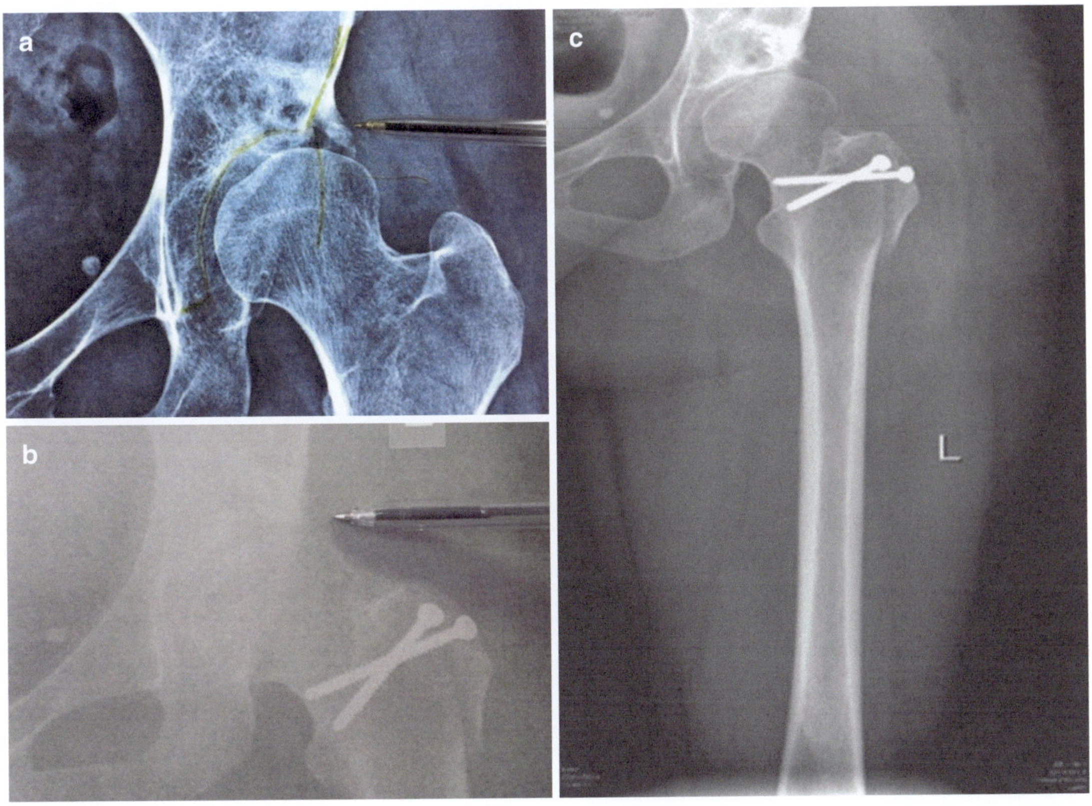

Fig. 1.1 (**a**) Preoperative x-ray of the left hip showing the fracture of the rim of the acetabular roof (pencil) (**b**) and (**c**) Postoperative hip and hip andfemur x-ray depicting the fixed trochanteric osteotomy and the removal of the fractured rim (pencil)

1.3 Case Title: Bernese Periacetabular Osteotomy for Residual Acetabular Dysplasia

M. Leunig and R. Ganz

1.3.1 Demographics

Age: 21 years
Sex: Female
BMI: 22

1.3.2 Relevant Past Medical History

Principal pathologies: Hip dysplasia with lateral uncoverage and labral tear

Previous surgical procedures: None

Medication: NSAR and physical therapy

Other: None

History of presenting complaint: Groin and trochanteric pain on and after activity. Unsuccessful nonsurgical treatment over twenty four months

1.3.3 Clinical Examination

Symptoms: Groin and trochanteric pain on activity

Range of motion: Normal range of motion which is painful at the end of motion

Specific tests: Positive impingement and apprehension tests

Main disability: Pain

Scoring if available: No preoperative scoring

Neurovascular evaluation: Normal

1.3.4 Preoperative Radiological Assessment/Imaging (Figs. 1.2, 1.3 and 1.4)

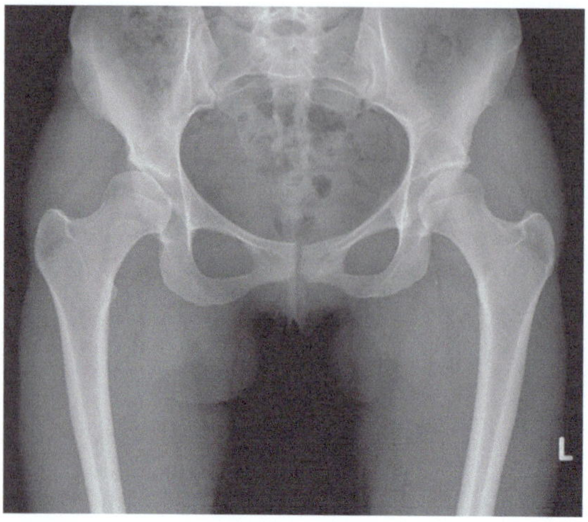

Fig. 1.2 Pelvic AP radiograph with a decreased anterolateral coverage of the femoral head, mild lateralization of the femoral head, and broken Shenton line

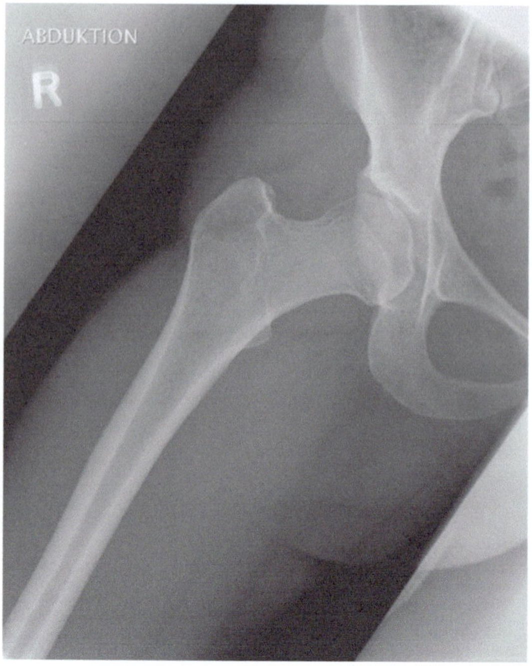

Fig. 1.4 Abduction view used to assess achievable congruency and congruity which is good in this case

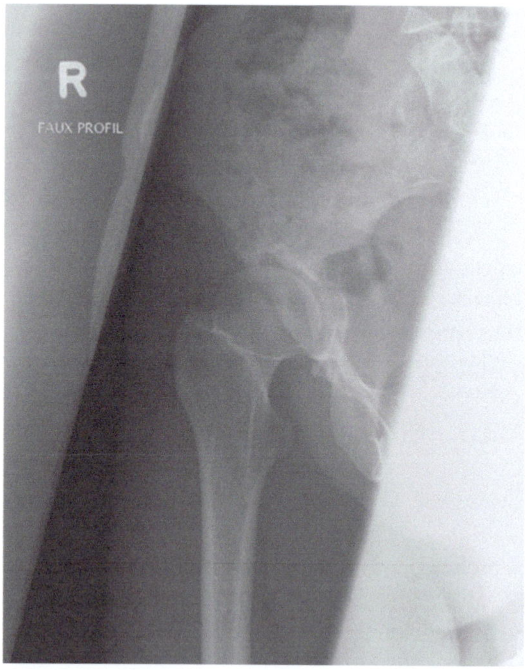

Fig. 1.3 False profile view demonstrating the insufficient anterior coverage

1.3.5 Preoperative Planning

Diagnosis: Severe acetabular dysplasia with lateral migration of the femoral head and ruptured labrum (Figs. 1.2, 1.3, and 1.4).

Possible treatment options: Femoral varus osteotomy, augmentation procedures (Chiari, shelf), reorientation procedures (innominate osteotomy (Salter), double innominate (Sutherland, Hopf), triple innominate (LeCoeur, Steel, Carlioz, Tönnis) spherical osteotomies (Eppright, Wagner, Nonomiya), Bernese periacetabular osteotomy (Ganz).

Chosen treatment method: Bernese periacetabular osteotomy.

Selection of implants if applicable and rational: 3.5 mm steel screws, 50–80 mm long [2] (removal of long titanium screws is extremely difficult!). Short 2 mm screws [14]. Eventually 4.5 mm screws for the large pelvic bone. Pelvic recon plate for 3.5 mm screws kept in reserve when extreme correction with large gaps or poor bone quality is to be expected.

Expected difficulties: (1) Penetration of the first ischial osteotomy maybe not deep enough which can impede the complete separation of the acetabular fragment after all osteotomy steps are completed. It can be the cause of a hinged correction with lateralization of the fragment and of limitation of versional correction. (2) Difficulties with the osteotomy of the pubis. (3) Difficulties with spatial correction of the acetabular fragment. (4) Prevention of nerve injuries during the procedure.

Strategies to overcome difficulties: (1) The first ischial osteotomy has to be repeated, eventually under fluoroscopic control. (2) Loss of purchase of the Hohmann retractor spiked medial to the osteotomy in the pubic bone will lead to a reduced visual control of this osteotomy. It may happen when the bone bridge between the osteotomy and retractor is too small leading to fissure lines and avulsion of the spike. (3) Resetting of the acetabular fragment and renewed radiographic control is necessary until the optimal position of the fragment is achieved. (4) Strict observance of details of surgical steps is imperative. Nerve lesions are not only the result of osteotomy; it can also be related to positioning of retractors and to the maneuvers for positioning of the fragment.

Templating: A preoperative radiography of the pelvis with the leg of the involved hip in abduction (without external rotation) gives sufficient information about amount and directions of the three-dimensional acetabular correction. To specify acetabular version, the pelvis radiography must show the tip of the coccyx pointing to the symphysis with a distance of 1–2 cm from its upper border.

1.3.6 Surgical Note

Patient's position: Supine decubitus on an image table; the iliac spines should be leveled before draping in order to get orthograde intraoperative radiographs of the pelvis.

Type of anesthesia: Conductive or general anesthesia.

Surgical approach: [14]

Main steps: A sequence of five osteotomies has to be performed. The space between the inferior capsule and psoas tendon is opened with scissors with spreading movements. Deep in this gap, the scissors should be kept proximal to the obturator externus muscle which is ensured by advancing the tip strictly in contact with the capsule. The tip of the closed scissors is used to feel the ischium. It is triangular in shape with the base posterior. Medially one should feel the tip of the scissors fall into the obturator foramen, and laterally the hamstring insertion protects the scissors from falling off the edge of the ischial bone. The space should be kept open to allow a curved bifid osteotome be placed onto the ischium. Proximally the subcotyloid groove should be felt with the osteotome which indicates the inferior border of the acetabulum. Start the *first* osteotomy at the tip of the triangle. Aim the osteotome toward the patient's opposite shoulder. Then the lateral part of the osteotomy should complete the osteotomy. Some abduction and extension of the hip and flexion of the knee is mandatory, especially when the osteotome is placed over the lateral border of the ischium in order to relax and bring the sciatic nerve more laterally; extension of the hip is the most effective move. Begin the osteotomy with steady blows onto the osteotome, and the surgeon's hand should be brought more perpendicular to the patient's body. Here it is important to listen to the change in sound and the feel of the bone. A solid sound indicates that the osteotome is in the bone. By side wiggling, feel that the osteotome is fully in the bone or exiting lateral or medial. Stop and slowly retrieve the osteotome palpating with the osteotome that the lateral aspect of the ischium is fully osteotomized. Commonly it is the lateral aspect of the ischium that still requires osteotomy. If so, translate carefully the osteotome laterally and repeat the osteotomy into the medial aspect of the ischium. Do not push the osteotome by hand; advancing the osteotome by careful hammer blows is safer. The ischial osteotomy is not a complete separation of the bone; it is sufficient with 2.5 cm of depth. It is more important to osteotomize the medial hard cortex. The lateral thinner cortex may eventually break at the end. The *second* osteotomy is a complete separation of the pubic bone. To visualize the pubis medial to the iliopectineal eminence, the periosteum must be split and elevated superiorly and inferiorly allowing to pass blunt retractors around the bone in order to protect the obturator neurovascular bundle from being injured during the osteotomy. To prepare the transverse osteotomy, a small sliver has to be excised from the cis-cortex, just medial to the eminence. The osteotome has to be positioned in 45° with an inferomedial direction, away from the joint. Secure protection is guaranteed with the blunt retractors placed just where the osteotome exits the posterior cortex. Completion of the osteotomy is verified with levering moves of the osteotome. Optimal overall view is kept by replacing the Hohmann retractor in the pubis with a blunt retractor in the osteotomy gap. Before performing the *third* osteotomy, the inner surface of the quadrilateral plate is cleared from the thick periosteal cover to place a so-called reverse Hohmann retractor deep on the base of the ischial spine. The outer table is freed from musculature over a 3–4 cm distance between the anterior inferior spine and the upper border of the osteotomy of the superior spine. Using straight and curved periosteal elevators, this tunnel reaches into the greater sciatic notch and allows insertion of a second reverse Hohmann retractor. Both retractors protect the musculature from being injured with the saw blade during this supraacetabular osteotomy. The starting point, direction, and end point of the osteotomy should be marked out with an osteotome before positioning the saw blade. The starting point is the distal border or the middle of the osteotomy surface of the superior spine. The end point is the corner with the fourth, the retroacetabular osteotomy. This point is usually 1–1.5 cm anterior to the pelvic brim. It should give an optimal bony bridge between osteotomy and joint to allow firm grip of a 5 mm Schanz' screw. When too close to the joint, the retroacetabular osteotomy may run into the joint; when too far, it may end in or fracture into the sciatic notch. An individual decision can be made safe with visual and palpatory control of the joint position relative to the planned osteotomy and with similar control of the direction of the retroacetabular osteotomy relative to the endpoint. The osteotomy is then performed with an oscillating saw under visual control on the inner side of the ileum. Care must be taken to finish the cut of the outer cortex at the same level as the inner endpoint. The *fourth* osteotomy is the retroacetabular continuation of the third osteotomy. Starting at the corner point at the inner side of the ilium, the first direction is given by the tip of the reverse retractor placed on the ischial spine. The correct placement is given by the fact that the retractor opens a wide gap. This would not be possible when placed more proximal or more distal, positions where the tip would fall into the greater or lesser sciatic notch; there it would not be able to produce a large space toward the quadrilateral plate. A 10-mm-straight osteotome is inserted into the corner point and directed toward the tip of the retractor. The palpating finger can give information whether this osteotomy direction leaves a 1–1.5 cm bone bridge posterior to the cut and whether it avoids penetration into the joint. When both questions can be affirmed, the osteotomy is performed. Only the inner cortex is cut which is secured by the edge of the osteotome staying visibly outside the bone. The osteotome should be advanced not more than 3–4 cm. At this moment, one may see a small step at the inner cortex of the third osteotomy. For the second part, a 15-mm-curved osteotome is used from medial to lateral to make the corner. It is advanced nearly perpendicular to the first osteotomy direction with the handle continuously pressed toward the patient's abdomen in order to create a rather short distance to the outer cortex. Hammer blows become a metallic sound, when reaching the outer cortex. The step in the third osteotomy increases when the osteotome comes closer to the outer cortex. With further hammer blows and under soft tissue protection with the second reverse retractor, separation of the outer cortex will be completed. If needed, the separation of the outer cortex in the third osteotomy down to the corner point can be completed with a straight osteotome. Caudad osteotomy propagation of the outer cortex is not recommended. It would cut the periosteal blood supply from superior and inferior gluteal vessels to the acetabulum, which remain intact when the cortex is broken. Further mobilization of the acetabular fragment is made by levering the acetabular fragment with a large straight osteotome placed in the proximal part of the retroacetabular osteotomy. With a 5 mm Schanz' screw inserted into the supraacetabular bone, the supraacetabular osteotomy gap can be opened to allow the placement of a large spreader for further widening of the gap. With this move, quite often the osteotomies propagate as an intentional fracture into the first, incomplete osteotomy of the ischium. In the majority of the cases, however, the *fifth* osteotomy has to be executed. It is a cut of the remaining bridge of the ischial bone. It is executed from medial to lateral under high tension produced by the spreader. A large bifid osteotome angulated 4 cm off the cutting edge, is placed against the posteroinferior border of the quadrilateral surface in such a way that the axilla is fitting to the pelvic brim. Opening of the handle to about 15–20° between the handle and quadrilateral surface allows to cut the bone posterior to the joint. Only the inner cortex must be cut. During this osteotomy, the hip should be somewhat extended and abducted, and at the same time, the knee should be flexed to allow relaxation of the sciatic nerve. After half way opening of the spreader, simultaneous and opposed rotation of Schanz' screw and spreader will break the remaining lateral cortex and allow free spatial positioning of the acetabular fragment.

Reconstruction techniques: Reorientation of the acetabular fragment has to be adjusted according to the individual deficiencies of femoral head coverage. Besides lateral deficiency of coverage as seen in most residual dysplasias after developmental dysplasia of the hip (DDH), there are hips with other deficiencies either isolated or in combination. Rather frequent are combinations with retroversion. Standard values of coverage do exist and most often reported is the CE angle in the frontal plane. However, deficiencies may not always be corrected to the normal value but rather to a balanced optimum of all values. In particular a normal CE angle should not be targeted when it is only attainable with a negative roof angle, a situation which is more critical in hips with a short roof. Schanz' screw and spreader are the principal instruments for positioning of the acetabular fragment. For extreme and for reverse corrections, a second Schanz' screw may be inserted into the supraacetabular bone from medial to lateral. Anterior rotation leads to an increase of anterior coverage, but at the same time, it increases lateral coverage. The achieved correction is preliminarily fixed with two or three K-wires. Intraoperative control radiography of the entire pelvis should be taken with neutral rotation and tilt of the pelvis. The following parameters are evaluated: The roof index should not be negative and is ideally 5–10°. Anterior and posterior border should meet at the lateral acetabular edge. The medial border of the femoral head should have the same distance to the ilioischial line as in the healthy opposite hip. If the opposite hip is also diseased, the distance should be 5–10 mm. Fluoroscopy is not as accurate as pelvic radiography. It is centered on the operated hip and not on the symphysis resulting in a different projection of the acetabular version; however, it may be used for repeated control when repositioning of the fragment was necessary. Before definitive fixation, joint mobility is checked. When internal rotation is clearly reduced, capsulotomy may reveal insufficient wasting of the anterior head-neck junction, leading to impingement after acetabular reorientation. This frequent finding can be addressed with osteochondroplasty. For definitive fixation, three 3.5 mm screws are used, two from the iliac crest into the fragment and one from the anteroinferior spine into the stable ilium near the sacroiliac joint. After capsular closure the rectus tendon is refixed with non-resorbable sutures, the fragment with the sartorius origin is refixed with one 2.0 mm screw, and further wound closure is performed layer by layer. Suction drainage is not necessary (Figs. 1.5 and 1.6).

1.3.7 Intraoperative Challenges

Challenges and solutions: Challenge related to periacetabular osteotomy is coupled with experience but can also be associated with primary morphological particularities or residuals of previous surgery. At the beginning of a learning curve, every step is challenging; the first and the fifth osteotomy remain somewhat challenging, even for an experienced surgeon. It always necessitates special attentiveness and strict adherence to a surgical step sequence. Undersized and oversized pelves require adaptation of the feel for dimensions. This is even more delicate when confronted with extreme morphological particularities of bone and soft tissues; revision surgery can turn out to be extremely difficult presenting intraoperative scaring and findings, which could hardly be anticipated. Many surgical mistakes, small or big, with or without consequences have to do with a wrong interpretation of anatomic structures. This is why it is so important to get steadily acquainted by doing repeated cadaver dissections including simulation of the potential course of mistakes. Not infrequently, acetabular dysplasia is combined with a primary or secondary short neck and high-riding greater trochanter, eventually limiting abduction after the acetabular correction. Severe deformities will not even allow sufficient acetabular correction. Other hips have a pathologically high or low version of the femoral neck. For both conditions, it is wise to address the femoral problem first with a relative lengthening of the femoral neck, advancement of the greater trochanter, and, where needed, a rotational osteotomy of the femur. The optimal level for such an osteotomy is the subtrochanteric area, where the necessary amount of correction can be established precisely with direct view on the proximal end of the femur. When starting the complex femoral and acetabular surgery on the femur, the first ischial cut of the periacetabular osteotomy can be executed via the femoral approach, allowing visual control and instrumental protection of the sciatic nerve.

Unanticipated problems and solution: [2]

Thorough description of decision making, including the reason for the final decision: Intraoperative complications which are detected only after surgery represent a particular challenge. For decision making, other factors like the age of the patient, the degree of the preexisting joint degeneration, and the expected result of revision surgery play an important role. The most frequent problem is acetabular retroversion either not addressed or increased with the correction. The consequence may be reduced internal rotation and anterior impacting impingement, while posterior subluxation or even dislocation is rare. Posterior instability can be clinically tested and often radiographically documented. When computer tomography confirms a posterior migration of the head, revision surgery is indicated. Re-intervention and correction of the version are easy when performed before consolidation of the osteotomies. After bone healing, a redo of the periacetabular osteotomy is more laborious than a primary procedure. When the head dislocates only in flexion, a posterior shelf osteoplasty may be sufficient. With the exception of severe retroversion, anterior impingement becomes typically symptomatic after a longer interval; the necessary evaluation should then include 3D simulation to understand better whether anterior osteochondroplasty may be sufficient or reorientation should be repeated. Persistent or newly developed lateral or anterior subluxation should be evaluated for an intra-articular obstacle, e.g., a femoral osteophyte; computer tomography gives the most relevant information. Such osteophytes are best removed with surgical dislocation. When functional views in abduction or flexion/abduction show good relocation of a subluxated head, it is obvious to redo an insufficient acetabular correction. Similar thoughts may be given to any other over- or under-correction. Additional femoral osteotomy is a rare alternative, mainly for undesired side effects. While intra-articular osteotomy cuts in the periphery of the acetabulum are often well tolerated, more central separations represent a substantial problem. Computer tomography is necessary to understand the pathomorphology of such a rare injury to the acetabulum and eventually the femoral head. When osteotomy or fracture gaps are relatively narrow without steps toward the head and when the head is not subluxating into a gap, one may wait and see in a patient late in his age spectrum for pelvic osteotomies; when the hip fails sooner or later, he may get a prosthesis. In a younger patient, it would be better to revise the hip by putting the acetabular fragment back into the preoperative position and perform a solid fixation. In some of these patients, a later approach for periacetabular osteotomy can be successful; others may not be prepared for a further trial. Surgical injury to nerves is a severe complication with a long healing period, and complete recovery may not be expected in every case. The incidence of sciatic and femoral injuries during periacetabular osteotomy among experienced surgeons is about 2%, the majority being sciatic lesions [15]. There is no evidence whether the use of fluoroscopy and/or nerve monitoring can decrease the incidence. The surgeon should make a thorough analysis of the procedure to eventually define the move which most probably has produced the nerve injury. A computer tomography may give further information. It is necessary to document the early neurological deficiencies as accurate as possible. Electromyographic evaluation is more conclusive after three weeks from surgery. The patient has to be informed about the status, realistic expectations, and the progress of recuperation. A patient with a femoral nerve lesion may need a splint to stabilize the knee during walking, while a patient with a sciatic lesion should be supplied with a frame against a drop foot. Complete nerve sectioning is rare and if considered may be an indication for surgical revision together with a specialized surgeon. Other indication for revision may be a bone fragment which may have pierced the nerve. In the majority of nerve lesions, one keeps a wait-and-see attitude. Other therapeutic measures? Time of nerve recuperation?

1.3.8 Postoperative Radiographs (Figs. 1.5 and 1.6)

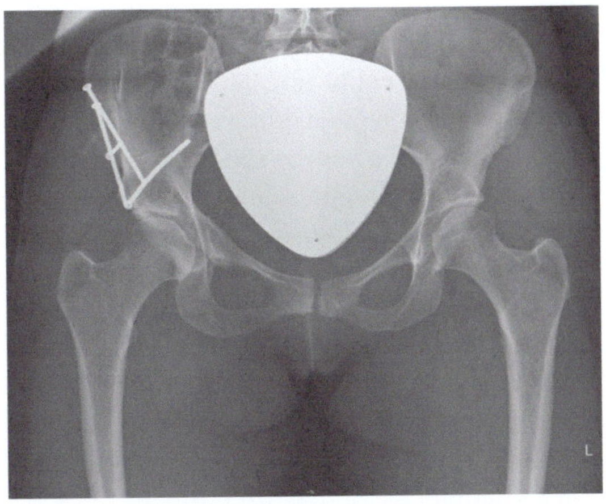

Fig. 1.5 AP pelvic radiograph five years postoperatively with a well-centered femoral head sufficiently covered by the acetabulum and no signs of OA

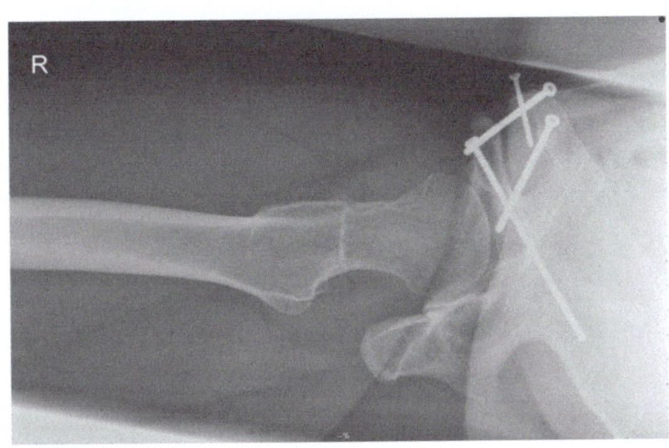

Fig. 1.6 Cross-table lateral radiograph demonstrating a well-recontoured femoral head-neck offset performed during the PAO procedure

1.3.9 Postoperative Management

Chemoprophylaxis and anticoagulant treatment period: Perioperative antibiosis was given for 24 h. Until full weight bearing, prophylaxis for DVT was given.

Gait/limb loading until full loading: Patients with a periacetabular osteotomy are young and can start with ambulation on elbow crutches at the second postoperative day. The amount of weight-bearing depends on the achieved stability of the fixation; this is normally about 15 kg, a value which the patient may test on a bathroom balance. To protect the refixation of the anterior superior spine, active lifting of the leg with extended knee should not be allowed until the first follow-up control at 6–8 weeks after surgery. At this time, an anteroposterior radiography is sufficient. When bridging callus at the pubis osteotomy and partial consolidation at the supraacetabular osteotomy becomes visible, loading of the hip can be increased stepwise, first with two crutches, going to one crutch in the opposite hand after two weeks. At this time, active raising of the extended leg is allowed as is full range of active motion. The patient is encouraged to do bicycling and swimming as well as exercises to reinforce the abductor musculature. Unrestricted loading is allowed 10–12 weeks after surgery provided a further radiography shows evidence of further consolidation. For walking free of crutches, the abductor musculature force should have reached an M5. Routine radiographs are performed at first year and every five years after surgery.

1.3.10 Follow-Up and Complications

Report of postoperative complications and their management (i.e., recurrent dislocation): Postoperative hematoma is a rare complication with this surgery and may be provoked by a deficient coagulation system either preexisting or drug induced. Large hematomas are best treated with surgical evacuation, when the hematoma is located close to a major nerve, or when new and substantial bleeding from a vessel is suspected, emergency evacuation has to be executed, and the bleeding vessel is ligated. When a nerve is compressed and shows deficits, there is no time left for a diagnostic MRI or for preparing an embolization. Accidental overload or a fall in the postoperative period may have created a loss of correction. This has to be controlled with a radiography or even with a computer tomography. An eventual decision for revision surgery may be balanced under consideration of the aspects discussed above. Our patient had no postoperative or later complication.

Scoring if available: The patient completely recovered. Since there has been no preoperative scoring, we did not ask her to fill a postoperative score.

1.3.11 Discussion

Advantages of the applied method: In terms of corrective potential, the Tönnis and to a lesser degree the Carlioz osteotomy are comparable with the Bernese periacetabular osteotomy, while the soft tissue attachment in triples more distant to the acetabulum may interfere with larger corrections. The Bernese osteotomy is performed without the need for repositioning the patient during execution of the different cuts and allows large capsulotomy without extending the approach. All triples have a potential to narrow the birth canal, which is not the case with the Bernese osteotomy, an important aspect when considering that the majority of patients with acetabular dysplasia are young females; it may become critical for a normal delivery in the pelvis with bilateral correction. The retroacetabular cut of the Bernese osteotomy crosses the posterior part of the triradiate cartilage, reason why it should be reserved for older children and adults. In double osteotomies the inferior cut runs either through the joint or through the parasymphyseal bone, both versions have not found general acceptance. Spherical osteotomies are performed rather close to the joint, which may have a negative influence on the perfusion of the acetabular fragment; this is the reason why the authors caution against additional capsulotomy. Furthermore, when correction of version has to be supplemented, the advantage of large cancellous contact will get lost. Femoral varus osteotomies have been performed in the past mainly with the idea to stabilize the femoral head. Today, such correction is abandoned. However, it is more and more recognized that dysplasia can be complex and the femoral side may necessitate additional surgery. Most frequent procedure is anterior osteochondroplasty for insufficient head-neck wasting, followed by relative neck lengthening to reestablish a sufficient femoro-pelvic clearance. Not infrequently a varus osteotomy at the neck or intertrochanteric level has to be added including correction of version.

Disadvantages of the method: The execution of the Bernese periacetabular osteotomy is rather demanding mainly because the ischial osteotomies have to be executed without direct visual control. Therefore, even experienced surgeons may prefer to do the cuts under fluoroscopic control, although there is no evidence that complications are less and precision of correction is higher.

Alternative evidence-based techniques for the case: The best alternative would be the Tönnis osteotomy.

Why is the chosen technique is better for this case? The general advantages are described above. However, the primary reason to choose the method is familiarity and experience with the technique.

Indications and contraindications for your technique: For this patient, there is no contraindication of the chosen technique relative to others (see also under "Advantages of the Applied Method"). The variety of hip morphologies, the amount of preexisting joint degeneration, and the age of the patient, offer a range of indications from optimal to borderline. An ideal indication comes with a patient in his twenties with a round femoral head, well centered in the socket. The center-edge angle should be between 10 and 20°, and the joint space is large without narrowing in the abduction. Any subtraction in these parameters moves the indication gradually to borderline. In a 15-year-old, one may still formulate an indication when the head contour is irregular, and the osteoarthritis is grade 2, provided the head can be covered and stabilized under the socket. In retrospect, deferring a prosthesis for even less than 10 years would justify the indication. However, a similar condition in a 35-year-old may represent a contraindication.

Learning curve and how to manage complications: Periacetabular osteotomy is a demanding procedure which can hardly be learned from reading books or looking to videos. A good way to get familiar is a fellowship in a center with a high volume of such surgeries. Surgical experience with acetabular fractures is a good precondition. Cadaver dissections help to internalize what has been learned. Mentorship during the first surgeries is a good safeguard to avoid complications or to get advice about how to manage it.

Level of evidence concerning the superiority of this method against others: The Bernese periacetabular osteotomy became a well-established method and is frequently used in Europe and North America. The reason may be a combination of its versatility as well as power and precision of correction. Several publications describe technique, complications, and up to 20 years of follow-up [2].

1.4 Case Title: Femoral Head Reduction Osteotomy

Aprato Alessandro and Ganz Reinhold

1.4.1 Demographics

Age: 15 years
Sex: Male
BMI: 20.5

1.4.2 Relevant Past Medical History

Principal pathologies: Complex deformity after Perthes disease

Previous surgical procedures: None

Medication: NSAR, physical therapy

Other: Non-weight bearing on crutches

History of presenting complaint: Pain with motion and during walking. Limitation of motion

1.4.3 Clinical Examination

Symptoms: Pain with passive motion

Range of motion: Limited abduction, limited internal rotation in flexion and extension

Specific tests: Positive impingement test

Main disability: Pain

Scoring if available: HHS 65.7

Neurovascular evaluation: Normal neurovascular status

1.4.4 Preoperative Radiological Assessment/Imaging (Figs. 1.7 and 1.8)

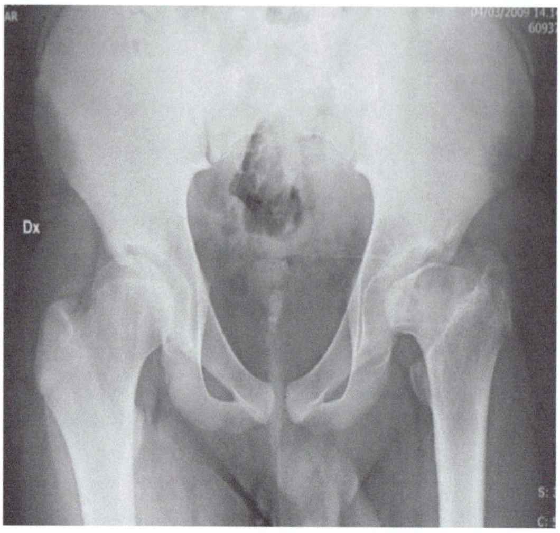

Fig. 1.7 AP pelvis radiograph with irregular flattening and extrusion of the epiphysis, no neck, high-riding trochanter, and leg shortening of 2 cm

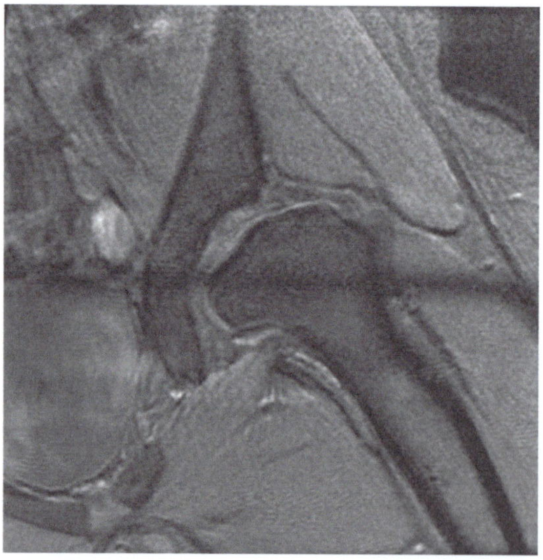

Fig. 1.8 MRA radial reconstruction slice showing the head deformation

1.4.5 Preoperative Planning

Diagnosis: Complex deformity after Perthes disease. (Figs. 1.7 and 1.8)

Possible treatment options: Advancement of the greater trochanter; varus osteotomy (together with trochanteric advancement); valgus femoral osteotomy; shelf acetabuloplasty, Chiari pelvic osteotomy, and periacetabular osteotomy, all with trochanteric advancement; and femoral head reduction osteotomy together with relative neck lengthening and trochanteric advancement.

Chosen treatment method: Femoral head reduction with relative neck lengthening and trochanteric advancement (Fig. 1.9).

Selection of implants if applicable and rational: 3.5 mm screws from 30 mm to 70 mm length.

Expected difficulties: Selection of shape and size of the head segment to be resected. A decision whether additional periacetabular osteotomy for joint stability is needed.

Strategies to overcome difficulties: Intraoperative drawing of the segment cuts on the cartilage surface. More recently, simulation of the cuts with 3D-CT models (Fig. 1.9).

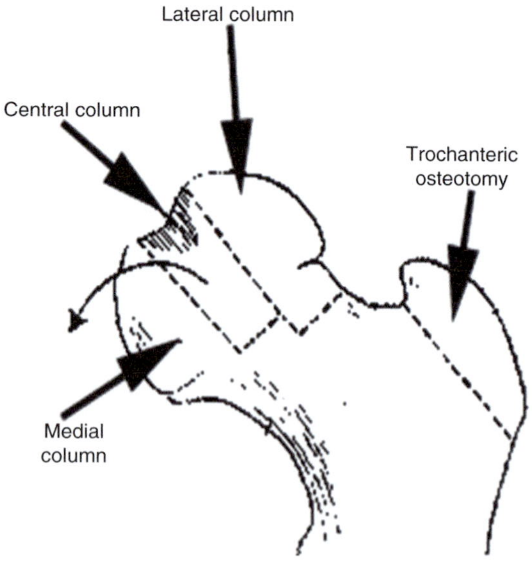

Fig. 1.9 Head reduction osteotomy plan

Templating: 3D-CT modeling is now possible, but was not available for this case.

1.4.6 Surgical Note

Patient's position: Lateral decubitus. Free leg draping. Skin preparation and draping should allow change to supine decubitus without the need for redraping.

Type of anesthesia: General anesthesia because repositioning may be necessary.

Surgical approach: Surgical dislocation approach as described in "Case Title: Surgical Hip Dislocation as the First Step for Revision of Instability from Arthroscopy" (Ganz R, Leunig M) (Chapter 1.5.).

Main steps: The surgical dislocation approach is extended by a subperiosteal dissection of the posterolateral retinaculum containing the necessary vessels for a sufficient perfusion of the epiphysis; the flap length from insertion at the head-neck junction to the level of the lesser trochanter is necessary to avoid overstretching of the vessels during manipulations for the osteotomy. The first step is a piece meal resection of the stable trochanter down to the level of the posterior neck applying a strictly subperiosteal execution. All external rotators are part of this flap. More proximally, the periosteum of the neck is longitudinally incised at the anterior border of the retinaculum. Both parts together are further dissected from the bone toward the posterior neck using a sharp periosteal elevator. Execution of the posteromedial flap is not necessary when dealing with a head reduction osteotomy because the medial 1/3 of the head remains connected with the femoral neck and shaft. Special care is taken to preserve Weitbrecht's ligament with the medial branch of the medial femoral circumflex artery, running on its surface and supplying this part of the epiphysis.

Reconstruction techniques: Based on MRI and CT, one gets already a conception of the central resection area. The stable medial part must have a neck column which is strong enough to resist adverse forces during manipulation and should allow refixation of the mobile lateral 1/3 of the head. The cuts are to be oriented in a way to keep the posterolateral retinaculum attached to the mobile fragment and to protect Weitbrecht's ligament with the blood supply to the medial portion of the head. Most frequently the middle part is resected with parallel cuts; however, the resected part can also be triangular with an anterior basis, always considering that the remaining cut surfaces become suitable. On the top view of the dislocated head, the cuts are mapped before executed. Execution is performed alternating with a small saw blade and straight osteotomes. The lateral fragment should include a neck portion allowing fixation against the stable part with 2–3 2.5 mm screws. Relative neck lengthening as needed in such cases is already the result of taking down the stable part of the greater trochanter; however, impingement-free motion may be tested again and optimized if needed. The stability of the joint is tested manually and with external rotation; it may lead to the decision for an additional periacetabular osteotomy. The posterolateral retinaculum is reattached only approximately and without creating tension; to allow it, the piriformis tendon may be released. Distal advancement of the greater trochanter is facilitated with a release of its long tendon along the anterior border of the fragment. Trochanteric fixation is performed with two 3.5 screws [16–18] (Figs. 1.10 and 1.11).

1.4.7 Intraoperative Challenges

Challenges and solutions: The first challenge is the decision about the size of the segment to be resected and the direction of the cuts. Mapping on top of the head is very helpful. Re-cutting can easily compensate a somewhat smaller segment. For optimal matching, the mobile lateral part may have to be advanced, rotated, and even angulated. Rarely fine - tuning of the cartilage contour is necessary. More recently, simulation with individual plastic models produced with 3D scan is available. In the majority of cases, secondary deformation of the acetabulum and the smaller head size necessitate an additional periacetabular osteotomy to restabilize the new head. In the presented case, however, this was not necessary.

Unanticipated problems and solution: Unexpected problems regarding this procedure may have to do with scarce experience. The operation should not be undertaken based on textbook knowledge or looking to videos only. Training is recommended in a center where such surgery is performed. Without optimal preoperative imaging, e.g., high-quality MRI focused on the diseased hip only and/or 3D computer tomography image decisions may not be based on realistic expectations. Nevertheless, occasionally intraoperative findings of cartilage quality or surface contour may not be as anticipated and compel to change to another procedure. For an intraoperative change of procedure, it is advantageous to have discussed such a possibility with patient and parents before surgery.

Thorough description of decision making, including the reason for the final decision: Occasionally, the medial contour of the head is deformed like a spike, and the lateral portion is large and round but extruded. In such a situation, resection of the medial spike, relative neck lengthening, and periacetabular osteotomy represent a better and less demanding operation. Similarly, when in a double-head deformity, the medial 2/3 are round and covered with good cartilage, and the lateral bump is small; it may be resected; again relative neck lengthening and periacetabular osteotomy may complete the correction. A relatively rare situation is when resection of a part of the head is not necessary, and periacetabular osteotomy together with relative neck lengthening is sufficient. Finally, it may happen that the lateral 2/3rds of the head are severely involved, but the medial contour is good. In such a condition, a valgus femoral osteotomy with or without periacetabular osteotomy may be considered, while an isolated varus femoral osteotomy is quite never indicated, and a simple debridement of the joint is a salvage procedure with very little chance for success.

1.4.8 Postoperative Radiographs (Figs. 1.10 and 1.11)

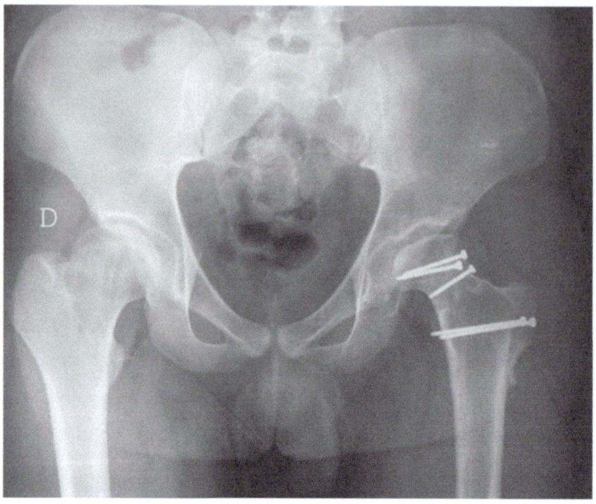

Fig. 1.10 AP radiograph of the pelvis five years after surgery with good containment and large joint space

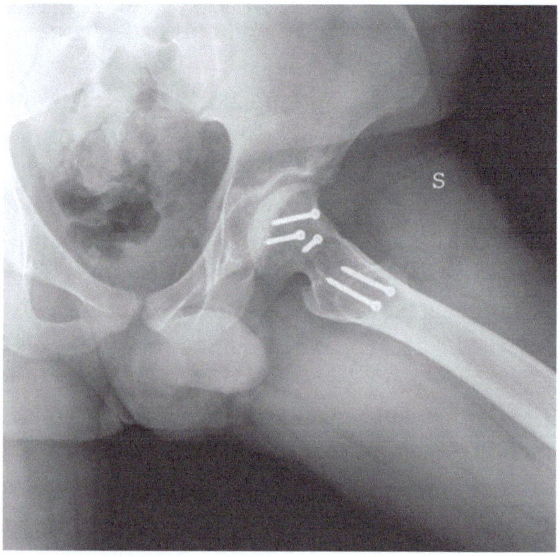

Fig. 1.11 Lateral view after five years with congruent joint lines and large joint space

1.4.9 Postoperative Management

Chemoprophylaxis and anticoagulant treatment period: Routine antibiosis is given for 24 h. Prophylaxis for DVT is not given up to the age of 18, provided there are no risk factors.

Gait/limb loading until full loading: Patients are starting ambulation the first or second day after surgery using elbow crutches. Allowed is toe-touch loading for six weeks when a first control radiography is performed. Thereafter, a stepwise increase of loading is allowed: first ten kg for two weeks and twenty kg for two weeks. After a second radiographic control at twelve weeks, walking on one crutch in the opposite hand is allowed and has to be kept until abductor force has regained an M5.

1.4.10 Follow-Up and Complications

Report of postoperative complications and their management (i.e., recurrent dislocation): Follow-up of the presented case was according to the abovementioned recommendations; no complications were recorded. At five years the patient had occasionally and little pain. Except for slight reduction of abduction, the range of motion was free and symmetrical. In our series of 37 cases since 2001, there is no necrosis but one fracture of the stable medial neck column which was successfully treated with screw fixation along the axis of the neck and a pelvic plaster for six weeks. Another paper about twenty hips reports one necrosis [19]. The 10-year results of our first eleven cases showed improved containment and sphericity and reduced pain [20].

Scoring if available: The presented case reached 92 HHS points at five years.

1.4.11 Discussion

Advantages of the applied method: Femoral head reduction osteotomy is a procedure to treat severe femoral head deformity, as seen in Perthes disease, at the level of deformity. It is often combined with relative neck lengthening and containment surgery of the acetabulum.

Disadvantages of the method: The technique is rather demanding and requires detailed knowledge of the blood supply and advanced experience with intracapsular hip surgery.

Alternative evidence-based techniques for the case: All alternative techniques have an indirect impact, be it reorientation of the proximal femur or augmentation and reorientation alone of the acetabulum.

Why is the chosen technique better for this case? Besides the direct approach to the femoral head deformity, it allows treating the secondary deformation like high-riding trochanter, absent femoral neck, and adaptive flattening of the acetabular fossa.

Indications and contraindications for your technique: The general indication for this technique is still under debate. So far the experience is best with patients between the age of nine and twenty years before. Before nine years of age, there is a concern of undesired effect on the growth plates; after the age of twenty years, joint degeneration may reduce the positive balance between expected result and expenditure of surgery.

Learning curve and how to manage complications: With a background of experience with the modern techniques of surgical hip preservation and with a strict period of supervision, the learning curve is steep regarding the technique and the management of complications.

Level of evidence concerning the superiority of this method against others: Although only 10-year results are available with a small number of cases and the combination of procedures was not homogeneous, a tendency becomes visible whereupon results are best when head reduction is combined with relative lengthening of the neck and periacetabular osteotomy; however, in selected cases additional periacetabular osteotomy may not be necessary. In general, it is obvious that congruency and containment of the hips are better with the proposed technique when compared with indirect approaches.

1.5 Case Title: Surgical Hip Dislocation as First Step for Revision of Instability from Arthroscopy

R. Ganz and M. Leunig

1.5.1 Demographics

Age: 33 years
Sex: female
BMI: 24

1.5.2 Relevant Past Medical History

Principal pathologies: Residual anterolateral acetabular dysplasia and high femoral anteversion. Anterolateral loss of the joint cartilage

Previous surgical procedures: Arthroscopic labrum resection

Medication: Pain medication after arthroscopy

History of presenting complaint: Occasional pain since many years in the left hip more frequent than right. A slight increase over time and during sports (synchronized swimming, skiing, general fitness). Increased pain after arthroscopy without improvement over a period of five months. Progredient limitation during ADL

1.5.3 Clinical Examination

Symptoms: Constant pain during ADL, aggravated when walking more than two blocks or sitting longer than 60 min. Feeling of instability when walking with an externally rotated foot

Range of motion: Normal ROM but painful toward full flexion and flexion/internal rotation

Specific tests: Positive impingement test. Positive apprehension in forced extension/external rotation

Main disability: Feeling of instability

Scoring if available: OHS 46 (of 48), EQ5D index 0.91, COMI 0.45, quality sat very satisfied, GOT operation helped

Neurovascular evaluation: Normal neurovascular status

1.5.4 Preoperative Radiological Assessment/Imaging (Figs. 1.12, 1.13, and 1.14)

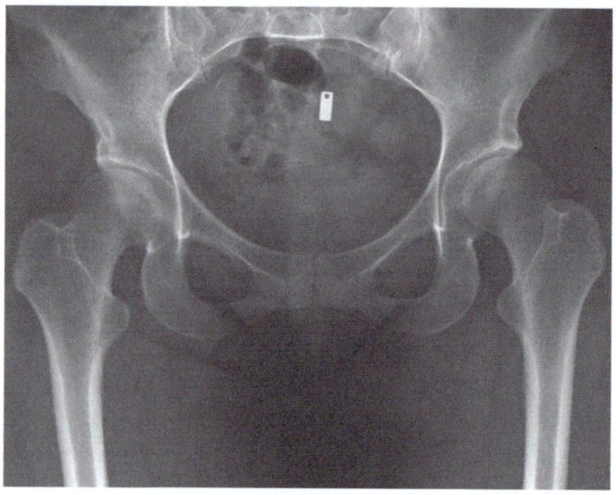

Fig. 1.12 AP pelvic radiography: right LCE angle 24°, left LCE 18°, roof inclination 20°

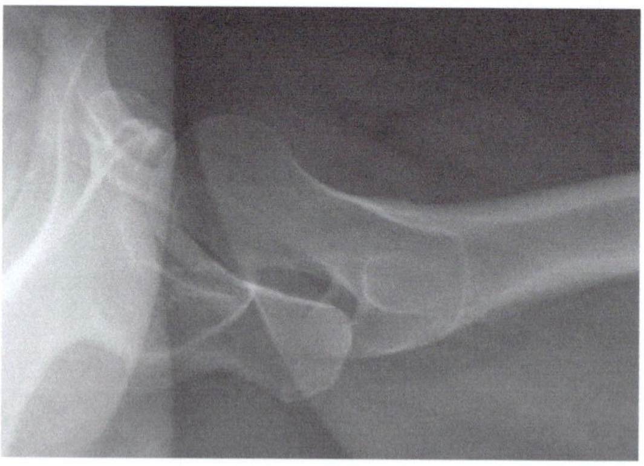

Fig. 1.13 Lateral view: high femoral anteversion (in MRI 36°)

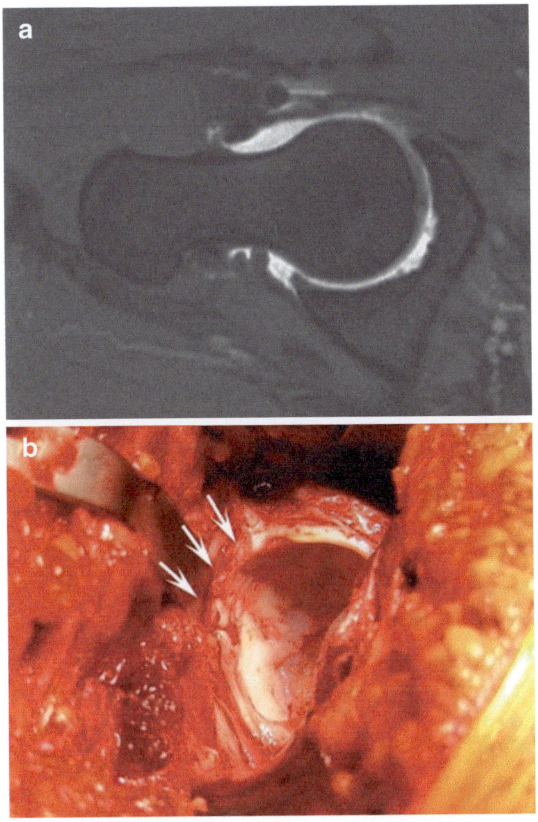

Fig. 1.14 (**a**) MRI showing the anterior migration of the femoral head and (**b**) intraoperative photograph demonstrating the severely altered acetabular cartilage and the absent labrum (*arrows*)

Other: Drawing of the surgical dislocation approach.

1.5.5 Preoperative Planning

Diagnosis: Multifactorial hip dysplasia (minor residual acetabular dysplasia, high femoral anteversion, joint instability after arthroscopy, and labrum resection) (Figs. 1.12, 1.13, and 1.14).

Possible treatment options: Intertrochanteric varus + derotation osteotomy. Surgical dislocation ± labrum reconstruction + derotation. Surgical dislocation ± labrum reconstruction, derotation, and periacetabular osteotomy.

Chosen treatment method: Surgical dislocation + labrum reconstruction + subtrochanteric derotation + periacetabular osteotomy.

Selection of implants if applicable and rational: Seven-hole straight narrow plate for 4.5 mm screws for derotation osteotomy. Metal anchors for labrum reconstruction. 5 × 3.5 mm screws, length 60–80 mm, for trochanter and acetabular fragment fixation.

Expected difficulties: Scarring around the joint capsule from the previous arthroscopy. Missing labrum and potential cartilage lesions. The decision whether the joint is sufficiently stabilized after the different reconstruction steps.

Strategies to overcome difficulties: The first aspect can only be overcome by careful and slowly advancing dissection. For the second aspect, the surgical dislocation approach offers the necessary information, and the presented case may show how it is processed: A first test revealed no pop signs indicating that there is no sufficient labral sealing and no intrinsic joint stability. It was clear that labrum reconstruction would not create sufficient stability, but it was thought to improve lubrication and joint physiology. After labrum reconstruction, retesting showed the reestablished pop phenomenon. Further testing the stability demonstrated (a) that the role of the high femoral anteversion could be reduced by 30° derotation and (b) that no additional varus correction would be necessary. Therefore, the derotation was performed at the subtrochanteric level where the execution is easier and the hardware less prominent. The stability was tested again, and the palpating finger revealed some bouncy stability with extreme external rotation in full extension. This impression together with the borderline acetabular coverage and the cartilage damage near the rim led to the definitive indication for a periacetabular osteotomy. The osteotomy was performed in the same anesthesia with the execution of the first ischial cut through the femoral approach.

Templating: Templating on transparent paper or with a computer program may be useful before an intertrochanteric osteotomy is executed but is not suitable for the surgical steps described here.

1.5.6 Surgical Note

Patient's position: The patient is kept in the lateral decubitus position. A holder is placed against the lower lumbar spine and the symphysis. Skin preparation and draping is performed for a free leg. In this case, draping should allow eventual subtrochanteric derotation as well as cushion periacetabular osteotomy (PAO) without redraping. The leg is positioned on a plastic foam bolster which is excavated on the undersurface to include the opposite leg. The primary incision is placed over the greater trochanter with a straight distal extension of about 10 cm from the trochanteric tip; the proximal extension is slightly curved toward the posterosuperior iliac spine. The leg to be operated should allow flexion/external rotation of the hip to bring the leg over the front of the table and place it into a sterile bag.

Type of anesthesia: General or conductive anesthesia. General anesthesia when an intraoperative change of decubitus is planned.

Surgical approach: Surgical hip dislocation is an anterior dislocation through a trochanteric flip osteotomy (1). All external rotators remain attached to the greater trochanter by which the blood supply to the head coming from the deep branch of the medial femoral circumflex artery and the anastomoses with the superior and inferior gluteal vessels is secured. The technique allows dislocating the head up to 10–12 cm from the acetabulum giving nearly 360° view to the head and 360° to the acetabulum. The approach can be extended distally to expose the entire femur (2). It is the workhorse for intra-articular surgery, e.g., labral and rim surgery, as well as for osteochondroplasty of the head-neck junction. Together with an extended retinacular flap, it is a safe approach for relative neck lengthening, subcapital realignment in SCFE, femoral neck osteotomy, and osteotomy to reduce the size of the femoral head. It is useful for difficult THR and acetabular and femoral head fracture fixation. When periacetabular osteotomy is a supplementary procedure, the first ischial cut can be executed via the surgical dislocation approach, allowing visual control of the sciatic nerve during execution of this osteotomy. Finally, intra-articular observations allowed to formulate and validate the impingement concept (3).

Main steps: After skin incision, the fascia lata is displayed over the anterior border of the gluteus maximus muscle; identification of perforans vessels helps to identify this level. The more proximal the fascia incision is extended, the easier becomes the mobilization and posterior retraction of the gluteus maximus. With an internal rotation of the leg, the posterior border of the gluteus medius is identified. The next step is the trochanteric osteotomy. It is first marked with the cautery knife from the posterosuperior tip of the trochanter extending distally to the posterior border of the vastus lateralis ridge before the osteotomy is executed using an oscillating saw. The fragment includes the insertion of the gluteus medius proximally, the origin of the vastus lateralis distally, and the long tendon of the gluteus minimus anteriorly; it has a maximal thickness of about 1.5 cm. At its proximal end, the osteotomy exits anteriorly to the most posterior insertion of the gluteus medius muscle; this helps to keep the majority of the piriformis tendon attached to the stable part of the trochanter. The trochanter fragment is mobilized anteriorly after releasing the vastus lateralis along its posterior border to about the middle of the tendon of the gluteus maximus muscle. The most posterior fibers of the gluteus medius are also released together with eventually remaining fibers of the piriformis tendon. With increasing flexion and external rotation of the leg, the vastus lateralis and intermedius are released from the lateral and anterior aspect of the proximal femur. Proximally, the tendon of the piriformis becomes visible in its fatty tissue layer after careful anterior retraction of the posterior border of the gluteus medius. The inferior border of the gluteus minimus is dissected and retracted from piriformis tendon and capsule, creating an interval which is safe for the blood supply to the femoral head. Care has to be taken to avoid injury to the sciatic nerve. The entire flap is then gradually retracted anteriorly and superiorly. Further flexion and external rotation of the leg facilitate a final visualization of the anterior, superior, and posterosuperior capsule. The capsular incision is Z shaped (right side) and is started anteriorly along the femoral neck; this avoids injury to the retinacular vessels. Elevation of the anterior flap is possible with an incision along the neck attachment and directed toward the anteroinferior border of the acetabulum. The first incision is then extended toward the acetabular rim, where it is turned posteriorly parallel to the labrum reaching the retracted piriformis tendon. Care must be taken not to injure the labrum. For dislocation the leg is flexed, externally rotated, and brought over the front of the table, where it is placed in a sterile bag. With a hook placed around the neck, the head can be subluxated allowing already some inspection of the acetabulum. For complete dislocation the round ligament is incised; the stump remaining on the head may be resected. Three retractors are used for optimal inspection of the acetabulum, while visualization of the femoral head is possible with lowering the knee and rotation of the leg. The retinaculum covering the terminal vessel branches to the head is visible on the posterosuperior circumference of the neck. During the inspection of the joint, the exposed cartilage is constantly irrigated to prevent drying. At the end of the procedure, the femoral head is easily reduced with axial pull on the slightly flexed femur and with the knee flexed. The capsule is readapted but not tightly sutured. For refixation of the greater trochanter two 3.5 mm, in large bones 4.5 mm cortical screws of 60–70 mm length are used. The wound is closed with running sutures layer by layer. Suction drainage is not routinely used (Figs. 1.15 and 1.16).

Reconstruction techniques: A surgical hip dislocation is an approach and not a procedure per se. It is, however, the door for a multitude of reconstruction procedures, some of which are demonstrated with this example. In a case where advancement of the trochanter is not planned as in this case, the osteotomy can be executed in a stepwise fashion which increases the intrinsic stability of the fixation. It may allow to reduce restrictions and start muscle rehabilitation and weight bearing earlier.

1.5.7 Intraoperative Challenges

Challenges and solutions: Very muscular hips may need a proximal and distal extension of the incision of the fascial lata followed by a release of gluteus maximus tendon to ease dislocation of the hip. In hips with fixed external rotation, the hip cannot be internally rotated sufficiently to perform the trochanteric osteotomy with the oscillating saw. In this situation, the osteotomy may be performed with an osteome from distal to proximal. In hips with protrusion but also in severe slips, the stable portion of the trochanter may impinge against the posterior acetabular wall, and dislocation may only be possible after trimming of the stable trochanter down to the level of the femoral neck. When soft tissue tension impedes the substantial distal advancement of the trochanter, the release of the long tendon of the gluteus minimus muscle along the anterior border of the trochanteric fragment is an effective measure.

Unanticipated problems and solution: Scarring from previous surgery or trauma may create difficulties to dissect the different structures. There is no special solution to offer but very careful dissection; advancing with small steps is the best strategy to succeed. Careful dissection and topographic identification of the sciatic nerve can be a very helpful step to avoid injury during further execution of the surgery, especially when preexisting scarring makes the procedure demanding. The best level to start this dissection is near the quadratus femoris muscle. After former intra-articular surgery, the joint capsule may be scarred near the distal circumference limiting mobilization of the femoral head. Presentation of head and acetabulum can be improved by step-by-step incision of the inferior capsule, eventually including the psoas tendon. The fracturing of the trochanteric fragment is a rare complication, and the result of insufficient thickness severely reduced mechanical quality or the result of levering the fragment before complete separation. The solution may be atypical screw fixation or wire cerclages, eventually combined with increased protection adding a plaster. Delayed or nonunion of the greater trochanter is an occasional problem in the early postoperative phase and is mainly initiated by overload and/or reduced bone quality. Refixation is performed with screw exchange. Local pain over the screw heads is a common problem in the later phase of rehabilitation. Screw removal can take place after six months postoperatively.

Thorough description of decision making, including the reason for the final decision: Visual and manual testing of the joint stability is the last step before closing the capsule. Warning signs may be anticipated and allow to get the necessary patient agreement for further surgical steps as demonstrated in the presented case. Occasionally joint instability is ascertained as a surprise, e.g., after rigorous trimming of the acetabular rim. Repeated testing before capsular suture should then lead to clarification: (1) about an audible pop indicating a good sealing function of the labrum which adds to joint stability, (2) about the direction and force of movements leading to subluxation/dislocation, and (3) about a possible fulcrum levering the femoral head out of the socket. When the head dislocates without audible sealing, labrum reconstruction may be executed. Using the round ligament, it may be executed even without a formal agreement of the patient. This also applies when only the posterosuperior aspect of the stable part of the greater trochanter serves as a fulcrum and has to be resected. Any other additional procedures like relative lengthening of the neck, derotation/angulation osteotomy, and periacetabular osteotomy have to be deferred until permission of the patient has been obtained.

1.5.8 Postoperative Radiographs

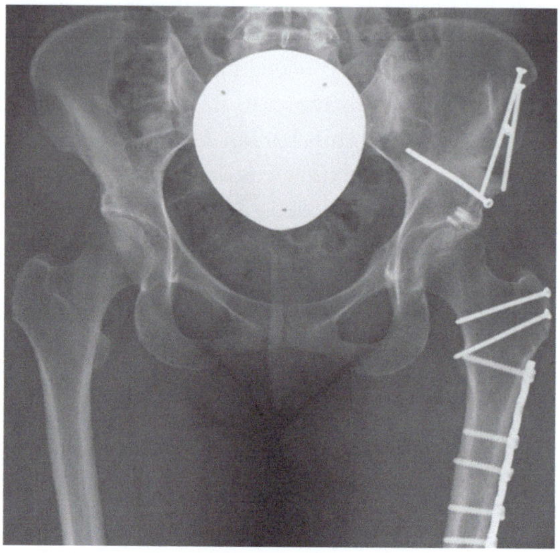

Fig. 1.15 Postoperative AP pelvic radiograph showing the different procedures undertaken by the surgical hip dislocation approach. All procedures were necessary step by step to finally guarantee joint stability without interfering with impingement-free motion: (1) reconstruction of the labrum fixed with metal anchors, (2) subtrochanteric derotation 30° to re-center the head into the socket, and (3) periacetabular osteotomy to overcome the rate of instability related to residual dysplasia + peripheral cartilage damage

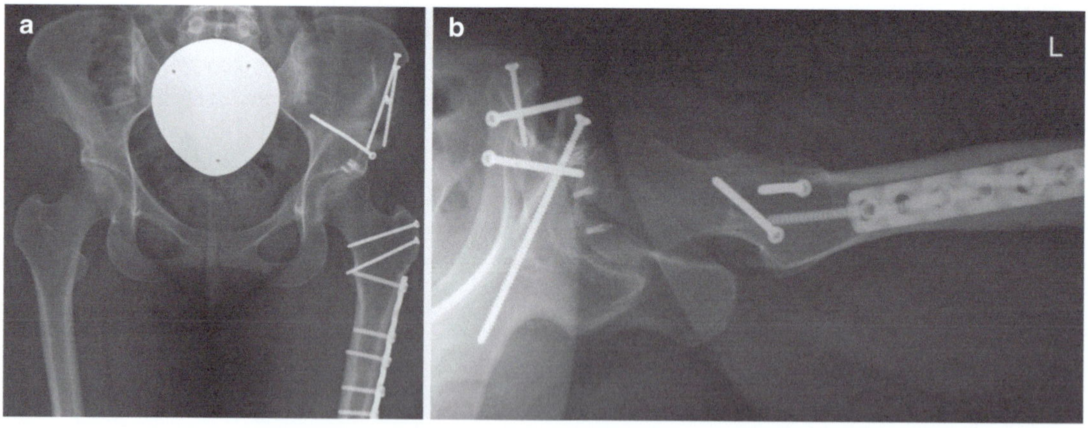

Fig. 1.16 1-year result with completely consolidated osteotomies in (**a**) the AP pelvic and (**b**) cross-table radiographs

1.5.9 Postoperative Management

Chemoprophylaxis and anticoagulant treatment period: Routine antibiosis is given for 24 h. Prophylaxis for DVT is maintained until full weight bearing.

Gait/limb loading until full loading: Patients with a surgical hip dislocation start ambulation on elbow crutches at the first or second postoperative day, depending on the complexity of additional procedures. Standard loading is 15 kp, to be controlled on a bathroom balance. The first clinical and radiographic follow-up control is normally fixed for six weeks after surgery; when a stepwise trochanteric osteotomy was performed, the first control date can be advanced to four weeks after surgery. At this time, rehabilitation measures for abductor training and joint mobility are started. When bridging callus becomes visible at the osteotomies, weight bearing can be gradually increased. Full and unrestricted weight bearing without crutches may be allowed after 10–12 weeks provided the force of the gluteus medius muscle has reached an M5 again.

1.5.10 Follow-Up and Complications

In our patient, no complication occurred during follow-up time; however, trochanteric pain radiating mainly to the lateral aspect of the knee persisted as did inguinal pain. Metal removal more than one year after surgery led to a marked improvement of her symptoms.

1.5.11 Discussion

Advantages of the applied method: Surgical hip dislocation is a versatile approach to the hip without the risk of avascular necrosis. It allows a 360° observation of the acetabulum and nearly 360° control of the femoral head. Besides surgery on the acetabular rim complex, joint cartilage, and head-neck junction, it is the workhorse for a number of new osteotomies only possible with this approach. Furthermore, it allows controlling impact and accuracy of extra-articular osteotomies, e.g., deroration.

Disadvantages of the method: Surgical hip dislocation as described here has no real disadvantages. From beginners it may be called an elaborate technique; however, it is not demanding in the proper sense. Failure of the trochanteric fixation is often mentioned as a major problem but has decreased with ongoing experience. Overall it is rated as a safe procedure with low morbidity [23].

Alternative evidence-based techniques for the case: Without the high pathological anteversion of the femur, straightforward periacetabular osteotomy could have been discussed as an alternative but would have made intra-articular surgery rather difficult. With the obvious indication for additional derotation, the best concept was to start on the femoral side. Doing so, additional surgical dislocation allowed optimal execution of intra-articular surgery and efficiency of the femoral procedures [22].

Why is the chosen technique better for this case? See above [23].

Indications and contraindications for your technique: The indication is given when intra-articular control and surgery are not possible with arthroscopy and vice versa.

Learning curve and how to manage complications: Under professional supervision, there is a rapid learning curve. For management of complications, see above.

Level of evidence concerning the superiority of this method against others: 15 years after the first publication [21], there is ongoing literature describing the unique benefit of this approach [24, 25].

1.6 Case Title: Subcapital Realignment in Unstable SCFE

Aprato Alessandro, Massè Alessandro, and Ganz Reinhold

1.6.1 Demographics

Age: 12 years
Sex: Female
BMI: 19

1.6.2 Relevant Past Medical History

Principal pathologies: Inconspicuous anamnesis

Previous surgical procedures: None

Medication: None

Other: None

History of presenting complaint: Left groin pain beginning during light physical activities such as running in the gym. The pain increased during the following hours to the extent that walking became impossible. Hospital admission on the same day, clinical findings looked like a hip fracture

1.6.3 Clinical Examination

Symptoms: Spontaneous leg position in the pronounced external rotation. Severe groin pain with any movement

Range of motion: Not tested because of pain

Specific tests: No specific tests

Main disability: Pain and inability to stand on the leg or walk

Neurovascular evaluation: No neurovascular abnormality

1.6.4 Preoperative Radiological Assessment/Imaging (Fig. 1.17)

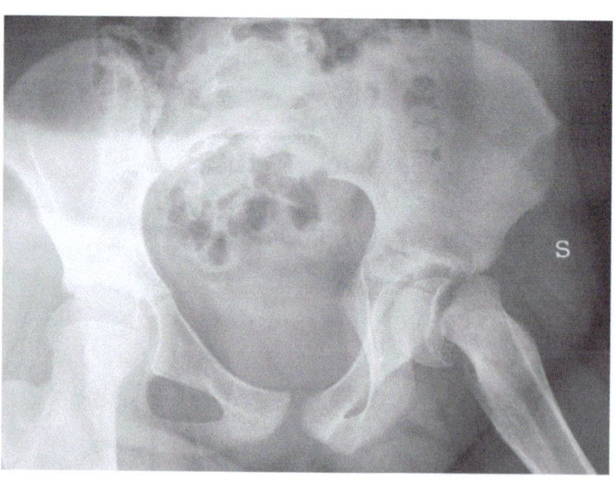

Fig. 1.17 The left hip with severe slip, diagnosed as unstable

1.6.5 Preoperative Planning

Diagnosis: Unstable SCFE (Fig. 1.17).

Possible treatment options: (1) Pinning in situ and Imhauser osteotomy later when needed. (2) Gentle closed reduction and pinning. (3) Subcapital realignment with Dunn technique. (4) Subcapital realignment with surgical dislocation and extended retinacular flap technique.

Chosen treatment method: Subcapital realignment with surgical dislocation and extended retinacular flap technique (Fig. 1.18).

Selection of implants if applicable and rational: 2–3 fully threaded 3 mm pins.

Expected difficulties: Difficulties to execute the trochanteric osteotomy due to the limited internal rotation. Disconnected epiphysis.

Strategies to overcome difficulties: When a fixed external rotation does not allow correct positioning of the saw plate, the osteotomy may have to be performed with an osteotome placed under the vastus lateralis and advanced proximally. With the diagnosis of an unstable slip, emergency surgery is indicated. If an experienced surgeon is not available, prophylactic in situ fixation of the epiphysis should be performed, and the definitive surgery be postponed.

Templating: Possibly measuring intraosseous pin length on the healthy opposite hip.

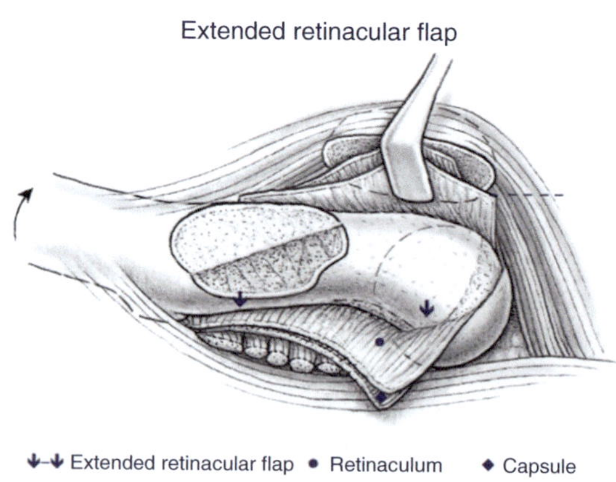

Fig. 1.18 Sketch of the extended retinacular flap

1.6.6 Surgical Note

Patient's position: Lateral decubitus position with holders placed against the lower lumbar spine and the symphysis. Skin preparation and draping for a free leg.

Type of anesthesia: General or conductive anesthesia.

Surgical approach: Surgical dislocation approach as described in "Case Title: Surgical Hip Dislocation as the First Step for Revision of Instability from Arthroscopy" (Ganz R, Leunig M) (Sect. 1.5).

Main steps: As mentioned above, in severe slips with limited internal rotation, placement of the oscillating saw for correct trochanteric osteotomy can be rather difficult; occasionally, the osteotomy has to be performed with an osteotome cutting from distal to proximal. The mobilized trochanter is then gradually retracted anteriorly and superiorly. Further flexion and external rotation of the leg facilitate visualization of the anterior, superior, and posterosuperior capsule. In the case of SCFE, a possible hemarthrosis is documented and also whether it is under pressure. After capsulotomy, the epi-metaphyseal stability is tested. When disconnection is obvious or even in doubt, 2–3 Kirschner wires are inserted from the trochanteric area to temporarily stabilize the head or to increase the stability. No attempt to reduce the epiphysis is made at this moment. Rupture of the anterior periosteum near the epiphysis is frequent; progression of the rupture into the retinaculum is rare and should be documented. When accessible, the epiphyseal cartilage is perforated with a 2 mm drill; bleeding from the drill hole indicates perfusion of the epiphysis. Only now the head is subluxated; the round ligament is cut with curved scissors and the head carefully and gradually dislocated placing the leg into a sterile bag on the opposite side of the table. Placing a large Hohmann retractor around the posteroinferior rim allows inspection of the entire acetabulum. Damage to the anterosuperior labrum and cartilage can come from impacting or inclusive impingement, which can be observed with flexion and internal rotation of the reduced head. The need for acetabular debridement or refixation of a ruptured labrum is rare. The next step is the subperiosteal dissection of the posterolateral retinaculum containing the necessary vessels for a sufficient perfusion of the epiphysis; the flap length from insertion at the head-neck junction to the level of the lesser trochanter is necessary to avoid overstretching of the vessels during manipulations for the osteotomy. It starts with piecemeal resection of the stable trochanter down to the level of the posterior neck applying a strictly subperiosteal execution. All external rotators are part of this flap. More proximally, the periosteum of the neck is longitudinally incised at the anterior border of the retinaculum. Both parts together are further dissected from the bone toward the posterior neck using a sharp periosteal elevator. While the preparation of the posterolateral retinaculum is best performed with the head reduced, dissection of the posteromedial retinaculum including Weitbrecht's ligament with the vessel providing perfusion of the inferomedial epiphysis is easier with the dislocated head. The end result is a posterior half tube of the periosteum allowing circumferential access to the neck without interfering with the perfusion of the epiphysis [16].

Reconstruction techniques: Before any attempt is made to reorient the epiphysis, a swab is placed into the acetabular socket, to avoid accidental reposition of the mobile epiphysis. It is only now that Kirschner wires fixing the epiphysis are removed. During this process, the epiphysis is manually preserved from being rotated. If necessary, further mobilization of the epiphysis is achieved with a curved osteotome introduced in the anteromedial metaphysis at the cartilage border and slightly propagated. Few parallel cuts may be necessary before levering attempts with the osteotome together with the careful external rotation of the leg result in increasing mobilization of the epiphysis. During this process, the complete posterior detachment of the periosteal tube from the neck must be secured. Further external rotation allows full presentation of the stump of the neck, while the epiphysis connected to the retinacular fold remains posteriorly. The posterior neck surface is now checked for callus formation. It has to be emphasized that such posterior bone apposition has been found even in cases of unstable slips without clinical warning signs, and it was also present in the case illustrated here. Such bone formation can be seen or palpated and has to be resected flash to the normal neck surface to prevent adverse tension in the retinaculum during anatomic epiphyseal alignment. Before attempting epiphyseal repositioning, debris of the growth plate has to be curetted, while the epiphysis is manually fixed to avoid adverse rotation. This is often resulting in visible bleeding from the epiphyseal bone. During manual positioning of the epiphysis on the metaphysis, the tension of the retinaculum is constantly tested, and if found too high, the neck has to be shortened millimeter by millimeter. Care has to be taken that the posterolateral retinaculum is unfolded before realignment of the epiphysis. While the position of the epiphysis is manually secured, an optimal offset all around the neck is visually examined. The first fixation is achieved with a retrograde wire inserted through the fovea capitis. Before reduction of the head into the socket, the swab has to be pulled from the acetabulum. The optimal spatial positioning of the epiphysis is controlled with fluoroscopy. Thereafter fixation is completed with two additional fully threaded wires, inserted from the subtrochanteric level of the lateral cortex and spaced out in the epiphysis. One may now repeat the drill holes to check the perfusion. Retinacula and joint capsule are readapted without any tension. The trochanteric fragment is refixed with two 3.5 mm screws, slightly distal to the original position. Before trochanteric fixation, a careful test for joint stability can give information about the amount of distal advancement of the trochanter (Figs. 1.19 and 1.20).

1.6.7 Intraoperative Challenges

Challenges and solutions: Many patients with SCFE are overweight; for sufficient exposure of the proximal femur, a marked distal and proximal extension of skin and subcutaneous tissue incision may become necessary. The gluteus maximus may act as a hammock limiting dislocation of the femoral head. Separation of the fibrous insertion on the femur can create the necessary muscle release to allow the dislocation. Dislocation may become impossible when external rotation is limited due to extra-articular impingement between the basis of the grater trochanter and posterior acetabular wall. Trimming of the posterior trochanteric bone being part of the execution of the retinacular flap may be brought forward to increase external rotation. Although the retinaculum was not damaged at direct visualization, one or several drill holes may not show discharge of blood. Nevertheless, surgery has to be continued as planned. The perfusion test may become positive after reduction of the epiphysis as seen in several cases [26]. Even when the perfusion test after reduction remains negative, surgery should be completed; the patient has to be informed about the increased risk of necrosis but also that uneventful outcome has been reported [26, 27].

Unanticipated problems and solution: (1) Rarely the posterolateral retinaculum is found to be almost completely disrupted. (2) Severe acetabular cartilage damage may become visible at dislocation and inspection of the joint, especially when a chronic slip becomes unstable. The head may migrate into the cartilage defect after anatomic correction. (3) Joint instability due to excessive shortening of the neck.

Thorough description of decision making, including the reason for the final decision: (1) One should omit to perform a dislocation in order to keep the ligamentum teres as additional blood supply intact. The posterior callus may be resected through the retinacular rupture although this is a delicate maneuver. An alternative would be to continue the procedure with in situ pinning and to wait for the further evolution of the case. (2) When such a cartilage damage was not anticipated, e.g., by a preoperative MRI, any surgery to re-center the head has to be discussed first with the patient. Further imaging including abduction/adduction views may help in the decision making. In the case of a high femoral anteversion, a subtrochanteric derotation would be in line, while an intertrochanteric correction is rather excluded in the presence of pins in the trochanteric area. A very powerful method to regain joint stability is a periacetabular osteotomy [28]. (3) To overcome this problem, the levering bone has to be removed and sufficient distal advancement of the greater trochanter be performed. Attempts to stabilize the joint with purse-string sutures of the capsule should be omitted. Additional fixation in a plaster may be discussed.

1.6.8 Postoperative Radiographs

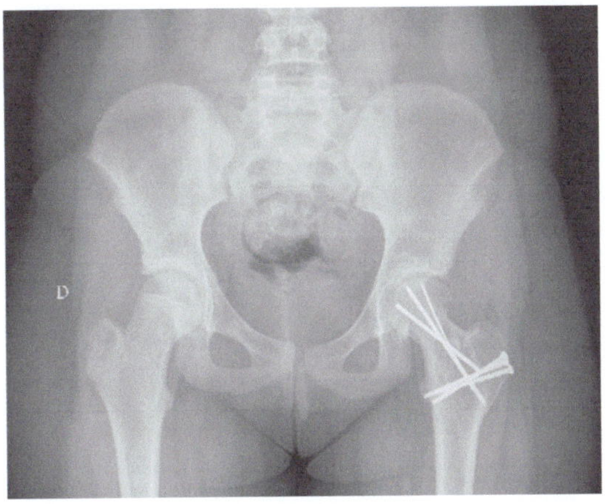

Fig. 1.19 Anteroposterior projection five years after surgery showing the anatomic alignment of the epiphysis without signs of necrosis

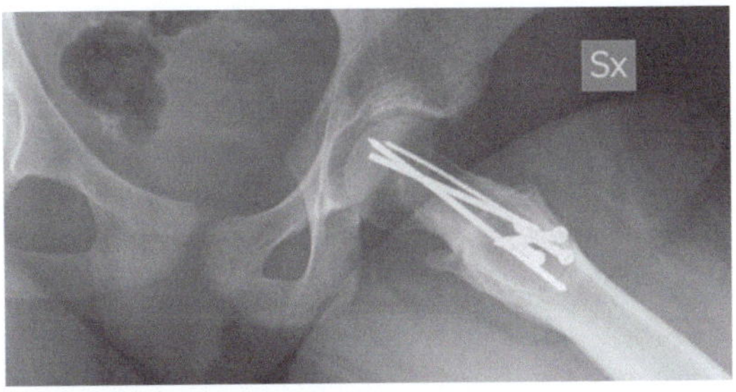

Fig. 1.20 Lateral view after five years with correct orientation of the vital epiphysis

1.6.9 Postoperative Management

Chemoprophylaxis and anticoagulant treatment period: The patient received routine antibiosis for 24 h. No anticoagulation treatment was given at this young age.

Gait/limb loading until full loading: Non-weight bearing with two elbow crutches for eight weeks followed by gradually increasing the load. Unrestricted walking after three months.

1.6.10 Follow-Up and Complications

The presented patient had no postoperative complications. In an earlier series, three patients needed revision surgery for metal failure (1); there was no head necrosis related to the surgery in stable and intraoperatively verified unstable slips (2).

Scoring if available: At 5-year follow-up, the HHS was 100.

1.6.11 Discussion

Advantages of the applied method: Anatomic realignment at the level of the deformity with low risk of surgically induced epiphyseal necrosis.

Disadvantages of the method: Dissection of the extended retinacular flap and execution of the subcapital realignment are technically demanding. It can hardly be learned from textbooks or video clips. The best way is to assist an expert on several occasions and do the first cases under his supervision.

Alternative evidence-based techniques for the case: The classic Dunn procedure can lead to similar results. However, it is less safe due to the limited subperiosteal exposure of the neck and the fact that the epiphysis remains in the socket during manipulations. Both aspects increase the risk of overstretching or rupture of the retinaculum.

Why is the chosen technique better for this case? In unstable SCFE, closed reduction has a high incidence of necrosis. The reason is the bone apposition in the posterior neck. Such bone formation may be present even in cases without warning signs [26], as it was seen in this case. The more the reduction will be anatomic, the more the retinaculum will be deviated and stretched over this bone, regardless whether the reduction was performed gently or not. With the open procedure as described, the incriminating bone can be removed before, and the retinacular tension can be controlled during epiphyseal reduction.

Indications and contraindications for your technique: The procedure is indicated for stable slips with an angle of 30° or more and all unstable slips. The procedure is not indicated when the physis is closing or already closed.

Learning curve and how to manage complications: As outlined above the learning curve is steep when the procedure is studied in a center with a reasonable volume of cases, and technique-related complications can be reduced when the first cases are executed under supervision.

Level of evidence concerning the superiority of this method against others: Despite the high technical demand, the procedure has gained increasing interest in the literature [29].

1.7 Case Title: Arthroscopic Excision of Intra-articular Osteoid Osteoma of the Femoral Neck

A.M. Spiker, B.Z. Rotter, L. Poultsides, and B.T. Kelly

1.7.1 Demographics

Age: 22
Sex: Male
BMI: 23.7

1.7.2 Relevant Past Medical History

Principal pathologies: Intra-articular osteoid osteoma

Previous surgical procedures: None

Medication: None

Other: No known drug allergies

History of presenting complaint: Z. F. is an otherwise healthy 22-year-old male who presented with sixteen months of insidious onset left groin pain. He described his pain as sharp and aggravated by weight-bearing activities, and he noted intermittent night pain as well. He was initially diagnosed with and treated for, a stress fracture of the femoral neck. He was given NSAIDs and instructed to be partial weight bearing. Three weeks after his initial presentation to an outside hospital, with a history of eight months of hip pain, a CT scan of the hip was performed. It was on CT that an osteoid osteoma was identified in the inferior femoral neck. At that time, the patient chose nonoperative management and eventually weaned off crutches. However, eight months later (a total of sixteen months after initial onset of hip pain), he continued to have persistent left hip pain and sought a second opinion at our institution for his symptoms.

1.7.3 Clinical Examination

Symptoms: Left anterior hip and groin pain, worse with activity as well as pain at night

Range of motion: Hip flexion to 85°; internal rotation at 90 degrees of flexion: −5°; and external rotation at 90 degrees of flexion: 15°

Specific tests: Positive FADIR (flexion, adduction, and internal rotation) and anterior pain with hip flexion

Main disability: Unable to perform sporting activities and forced to modify daily activities due to left hip pain

Scoring if available: Preoperative scores, Hip Outcome Score-Activities of Daily Living (HOS-ADL): 83.82; Modified Harris Hip Score (mHHS): 68.2

Neurovascular evaluation: Normal neurovascular exam

1.7.4 Preoperative Radiological Assessment/Imaging (Figs. 1.21, 1.22, and 1.23)

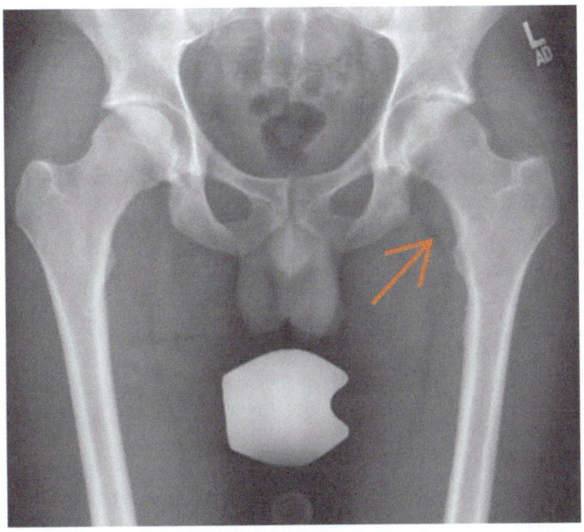

Fig. 1.21 Preoperative AP pelvis

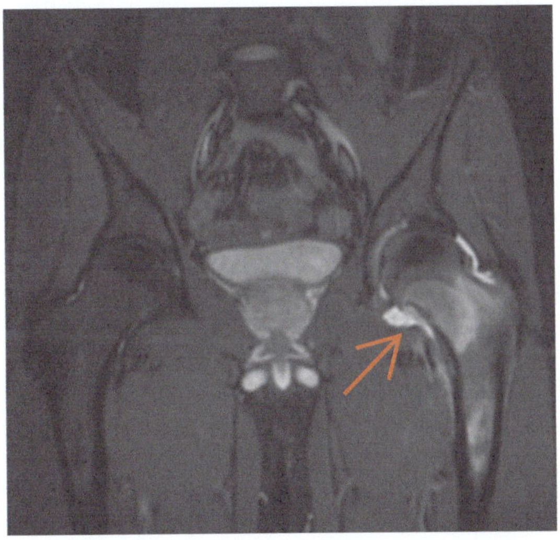

Fig. 1.22 Preoperative MRI demonstrating significant edema in the femoral neck surrounding the osteoid osteoma lesion

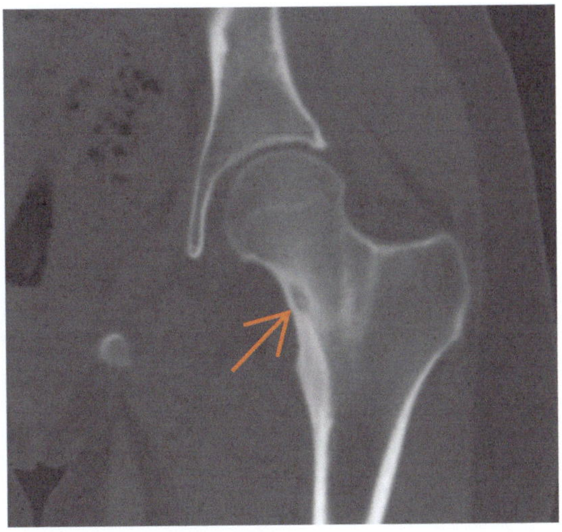

Fig. 1.23 Preoperative CT scan of characteristic CT findings of osteoid osteoma, demonstrating a nidus with the surrounding sclerotic bone

1.7.5 Preoperative Planning

Diagnosis: Labral tear with cam impingement, synovitis, osteoid osteoma of the femoral neck, and associated sclerosis (Figs. 1.21, 1.22, and 1.23).

Possible treatment options: Interventional radiology radiofrequency ablation, hip arthroscopy, or open surgical approach to address CAM impingement with excision of osteoid osteoma lesion.

Chosen treatment method: Hip arthroscopy with CAM decompression and excision of osteoid osteoma lesion.

Selection of implants if applicable and rational: Standard instrumentation for hip arthroscopy, including arthroscopic electrocautery/radiofrequency ablation device and arthroscopic burr.

Expected difficulties: The patient had symptoms consistent with both femoroacetabular impingement and painful osteoid osteoma. We chose to address his symptoms by repairing the labrum and decompressing his CAM-type femoroacetabular impingement, in addition to excising the osteoid osteoma lesion. The osteoid osteoma was located at the inferior femoral neck, which can be a difficult area to access via hip arthroscopy.

Strategies to overcome difficulties: Thorough preoperative discussion with the patient regarding our expected technical difficulties and the plan to first address the femoroacetabular impingement pathoanatomy with the goal to also remove the osteoid osteoma if technically possible with hip arthroscopy.

Templating: Careful examination of preoperative imaging allowed for optimal preoperative planning.

1.7.6 Surgical Note

Patient's position: Supine position on a traction table and approximately ten mm of distraction across the femoroacetabular joint.

Type of anesthesia: Spinal anesthetic and intravenous sedation.

Surgical approach: Standard lateral, mid-anterior, and distal anterolateral hip arthroscopy portals were utilized.

Main steps: Diagnostic hip arthroscopy was performed after traction was applied to the hip. An interportal capsulotomy was created between the mid-anterior and lateral portals to access the joint. A wide synovectomy was used to address synovitis in the joint, and a limited labral debridement was completed with a shaver to remove fibrillations of the labrum. The leg was then taken out of traction, and a T-capsulotomy was created to access the femoral head-neck junction, and a CAM decompression was performed with a shaver and burr. The osteoid osteoma lesion was identified, and an arthroscopic burr was used to shell out the lesion from the surrounding bone. The electrocautery device was used to heat this area and remove any residual soft tissue. At the completion of the case, a complete capsular closure was performed (Figs. 1.24 and 1.25).

Reconstruction techniques: Anatomical closure of T-capsulotomy and interportal capsulotomy with interrupted sutures and closure of arthroscopy portals with 3–0 nylon sutures. We used additional sutures to close the extensile T-capsulotomy created to allow for access to the osteoid osteoma lesion.

1.7.7 Intraoperative Challenges

Challenges and solutions: The location of the osteoid osteoma can present a challenge to arthroscopic access to the lesion. In this particular case, we created an extensile T-capsulotomy to gain access to the osteoid osteoma at the inferior femoral neck. The flexion angle of the hip, as well as external and internal rotation of the leg, can be adjusted using the leg slide of the traction table to allow for instruments to reach the osteoid osteoma.

Unanticipated problems and solution: Careful preoperative planning prevented any unanticipated problems.

Thorough description of decision making, including the reason for the final decision: This patient presented with hip pain symptoms that correlated with CAM-type femoroacetabular impingement but could also be related to a symptomatic osteoid osteoma lesion of his inferior femoral neck. While the location of his osteoid osteoma lesion was such that we might not have been able to reach it via an arthroscopic approach, we chose to first attempt hip arthroscopy, with the primary goal to address the bony morphology of his femoroacetabular impingement and the secondary goal to excise the osteoid osteoma lesion. We counseled the patient preoperatively that if we were not able to access the lesion via the arthroscopic technique and he continued to be symptomatic of his osteoid osteoma, other treatment options for this lesion (interventional radiology guidance radiofrequency ablation or open excision of the lesion) may be warranted.

1.7.8 Postoperative Radiographs

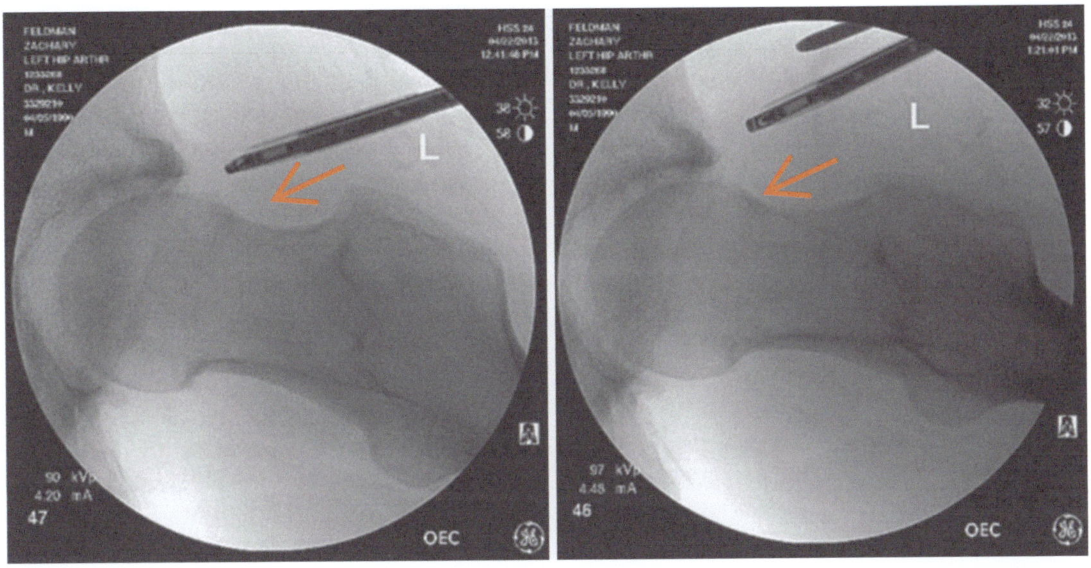

Fig. 1.24 Intraoperative radiographic images demonstrating the contour of the femoral head-neck junction prior to and after CAM decompression and osteoid osteoma excision

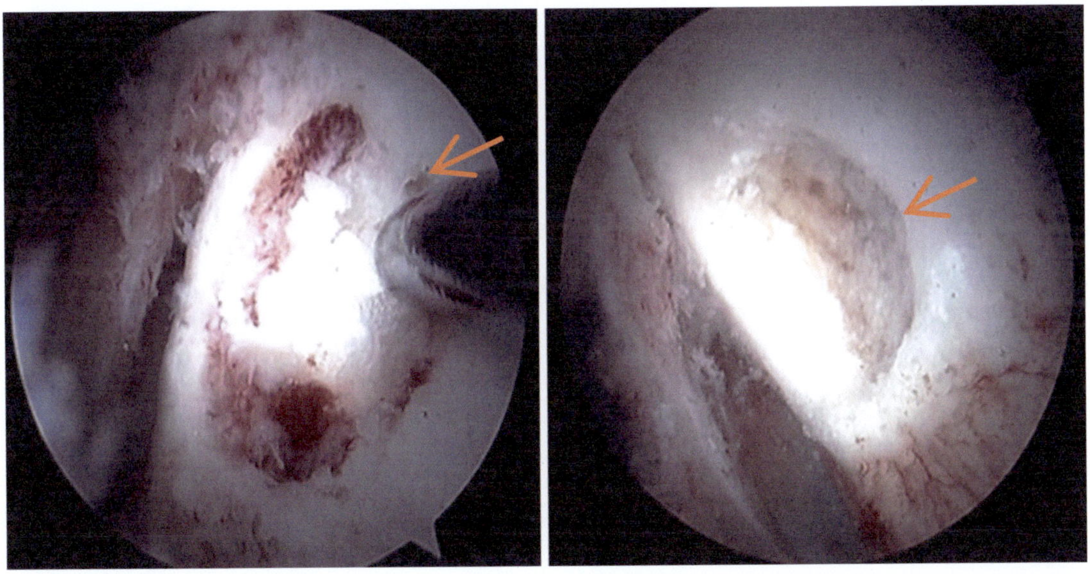

Fig. 1.25 Intraoperative arthroscopic images showing the osteoid osteoma prior to and after excision with an arthroscopic burr

1.7.9 Postoperative Management

Chemoprophylaxis and anticoagulant treatment period: a 4-day course of Indocin 75 mg daily for heterotopic ossification prophylaxis. No separate anticoagulant therapy was instituted per standard protocol.

Gait/limb loading until full loading: Initial toe-touch weight bearing on the operative leg, progressed to full weight bearing by six weeks postoperatively.

1.7.10 Follow-Up and Complications

Complication: None.

Scoring: 6-month Hip Outcome Score-Activities of Daily Living (HOS-ADL): 98.53; Hip Outcome Score-Sports Specific (HOS-SS):96.88; Modified Harris Hip Score (mHHS): 95.7; International Hip Outcome Tool-33 (iHot33):88.52; 1-year HOS-ADL: 100; HOS-SS: 100; mHHS:92.4; and iHot33:81.77.

1.7.11 Discussion

Advantages of the applied method: Hip arthroscopy is associated with less morbidity than a surgical hip dislocation or a mini-anterior open approach, yet it allows us to address any central compartment pathology as well as CAM bony morphology as well as the osteoid osteoma lesion. While there are no comparisons of open excision versus arthroscopic excision of intra-articular hip osteoid osteomas, we know that in the treatment of femoroacetabular impingement, hip arthroscopy and the prior standard treatment of open surgical dislocation have equivalent outcomes at medium-term follow-up based on hip-specific patient-reported outcomes [30, 31]. The advantages of hip arthroscopy include higher general health-related quality of life (HRQoL) score and smaller incisions and associated healing when compared to open procedures [30]. Hip arthroscopy has been described in multiple case reports to excision of osteoid osteoma of the intra-articular hip joint from both the acetabulum and the femoral neck [32–34].

Disadvantages of the method: Given the difficulty of accessing the osteoid osteoma, surgical skill and experience are required to appropriately excise the lesion in addition to addressing both the central and peripheral compartment pathology utilizing the arthroscopic technique.

Alternative evidence-based techniques for the case: Radiofrequency ablation (RFA) is traditionally the standard treatment of osteoid osteomas throughout the body once conservative management (including nonsteroidal anti-inflammatory medications) has failed. The concern with intra-articular osteoid osteomas is the close proximity of the articular cartilage, and the potential for damage due to the high temperatures associated with RFA, as well as skin and muscle burns and damage to nearby neurovascular structures. RFA of intra-articular hip osteoid osteomas has been reported to have a high clinical and technical success rate [35] and is a viable option for patients with this presentation. However, if the patient has concomitant intra-articular hip pathology, RFA alone will not address the entirety of their symptoms as well as hip arthroscopy.

Why is the chosen technique better for this case? Hip arthroscopy, if successful at addressing both the osteoid osteoma lesion and concomitant femoroacetabular impingement, allowed our patient to return to excellent function with a less invasive procedure, with one single procedure, and in a relatively short period of time.

Indications and contraindications for your technique: The location of the osteoid osteoma lesion will dictate whether it can be accessed arthroscopically. It can be technically very difficult to access the posterior and very inferior femoral neck with arthroscopic instruments. If the osteoid osteoma lesion is in one of these locations, a surgical hip dislocation may be indicated as a single procedure to address both the osteoid osteoma lesion and the femoroacetabular impingement.

Learning curve and how to manage complications: The learning curve for hip arthroscopy is substantial, and with lesions located in difficult-to-access regions of the hip joint, excision of osteoid osteomas can be technically very challenging. If hip arthroscopy is attempted and the surgeon is unable to access the osteoid osteoma with arthroscopic instruments, the patient may have to undergo a second procedure—either RFA or open excision. It is therefore important to counsel the patient on this possibility prior to the arthroscopic surgery.

Level of evidence concerning the superiority of this method against others: Expert opinion.

1.8 Case Title: Periacetabular Osteotomy

Nicholas M. Desy and Rafael J. Sierra

1.8.1 Demographics

Age: 28
Sex: Female
BMI: 29

1.8.2 Relevant Past Medical History

Principal pathologies: None

Previous surgical procedures: None

Medication: None

History of presenting complaint: A 28-year-old female presented with right hip pain for over 1 year. The pain was primarily located in the groin which was constant and worse at the end of the day. She had tried physical therapy and had a corticosteroid injection in her right hip that relieved 100% of her pain but only lasted approximately 25 min. She also complained of occasional left hip pain.

1.8.3 Clinical Examination

Symptoms: Right hip anterior groin pain with milder left hip groin pain

Range of motion: Extension-flexion: 0–125; internal-external rotation: 40–60; abduction-adduction: 45–30

Specific tests: Positive Stinchfield test, positive flexion-adduction-internal rotation test

Main disability: Anterior groin pain and difficulty with ambulating and physical activity

Neurovascular evaluation: Normal motor and sensory exams in the sciatic, femoral, and obturator nerves. Normal pulses in the posterior tibial and dorsalis pedis arteries

1.8.4 Preoperative Radiological Assessment/Imaging (Figs. 1.26, 1.27, and 1.28)

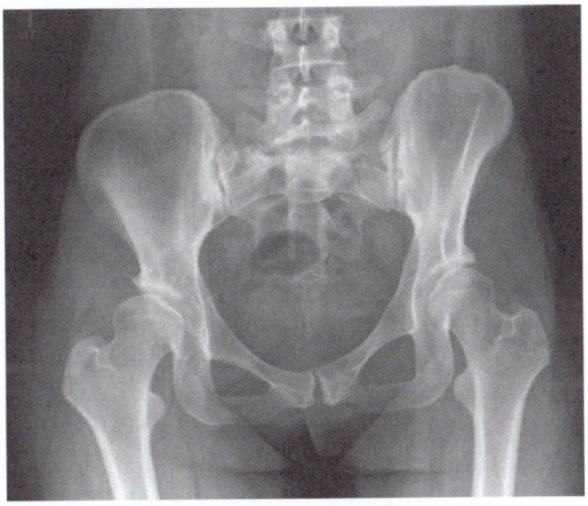

Fig. 1.26 Anteroposterior X-ray view of the pelvis demonstrates bilateral hip dysplasia. Note that the bilateral femoral head undercoverages laterally. The right hip lateral center-edge angle (CEA) measured 15-degrees, and the Tonnis angle was 17-degrees. The left hip lateral CEA and the Tonnis angle were 18 and 15 degrees, respectively

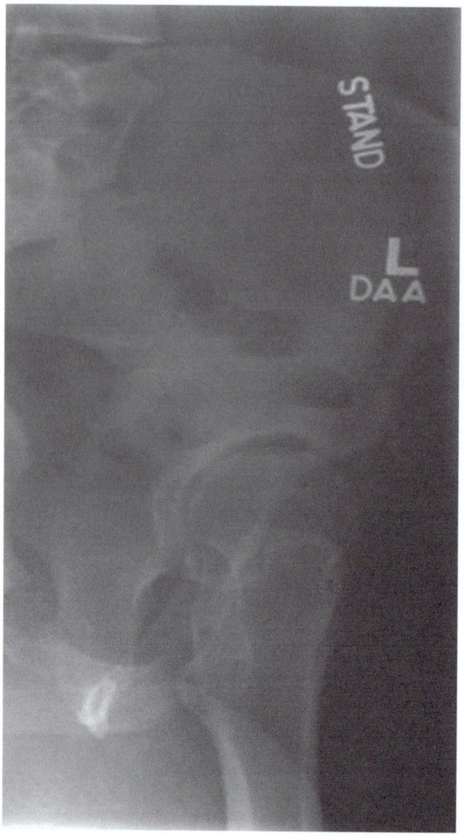

Fig. 1.27 Cross-table lateral X-ray view of the left hip demonstrates anteversion of the left acetabulum

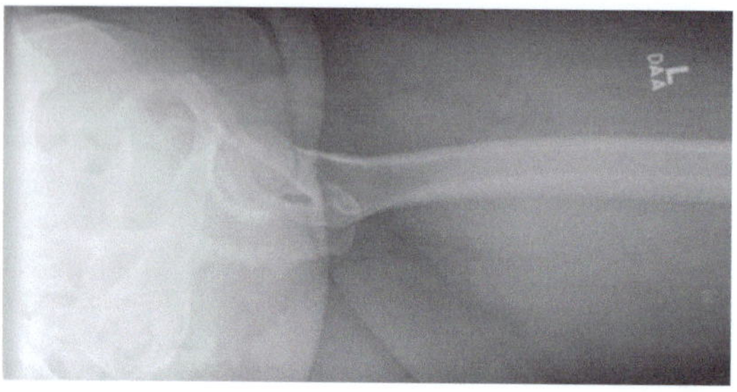

Fig. 1.28 False profile X-ray image of the left hip shows anterior undercoverage of the femoral head. The anterior CEA was 17- degrees. The right hip also had similar anterior undercoverage with a similar anterior CEA

1.8.5 Preoperative Planning

Diagnosis: Bilateral symptomatic mild hip dysplasia (Figs. 1.26, 1.27, and 1.28).

Possible treatment options: Continued nonoperative treatment, probable eventual total hip arthroplasty.

Chosen treatment method: Staged bilateral periacetabular osteotomies (PAOs). The right side was treated initially with a PAO and an open arthrotomy with anterior inferior iliac spine trimming. The left hip was then treated three years later with a combined hip arthroscopy to address a labral tear as well as acetabular and femoral chondroplasties and a PAO for correction of the dysplasia.

Selection of implants if applicable and rational: Large fragment 4.5 mm screws.

Expected difficulties: (1) Sufficient osteotomy to be able to completely mobilize the acetabular fragment in all planes. (2) Adequate deformity correction to address the anterior and lateral femoral head undercoverage. (3) Avoid acetabular overcorrection which would lead to anterior femoroacetabular impingement, and decrease the patient's flexion and internal rotation.

Strategies to overcome difficulties: (1) Ensure completely osteotomies of the ischium, pubis, and ilium. The acetabular fragment should be easily mobilized in all planes without much force. The most common location that requires extra attention is the junction of the ischial osteotomy with the posterior column. (2) The deformity correction is performed with a Schanz pin in the iliac portion of the acetabular fragment. A bone hook is also used at the pubic osteotomy to ensure complete release of the pubic segment without any tethering and allows the fragment to be rotated to increase lateral coverage without inadvertently causing retroversion. The fragment is then repositioned with slight extension, internal rotation, and medialization. Of note, it is important to understand that this deformity correction is different as compared to reverse PAOs for acetabular retroversion. The fragment is then temporarily stabilized with 3.2 mm Steinmann pins, and the correction is assessed carefully with intraoperative fluoroscopy. It is important to obtain an adequate anteroposterior view and modified false profile view. (3) Assess the patient's preoperative range of motion

(ROM) in flexion and internal rotation while the patient is under anesthesia and compare it to the patient's flexion and internal rotation following deformity correction and temporary fragment stabilization.

1.8.6 Surgical Note

Patient's position: Supine.

Type of anesthesia: General anesthetic as well as an epidural for postoperative pain management.

Surgical approach: Anterior approach with a curved skin incision centered just lateral to the anterior superior iliac spine (ASIS). The fascia over the tensor fascia lata (TFL) muscle is then seen and incised. The TFL is retracted laterally, and the sartorius is retracted medially. The direct and indirect heads of the rectus femoris are identified and protected. The anterior pelvic brim is then exposed by incising the fascia over the external oblique muscle just lateral to the iliac crest and elevating the iliacus muscle subperiosteally. The sartorius tendon is tagged with a suture and taken off the ASIS. Dissection is further developed along the anterior pelvic brim and superior pubic ramus. The dissection along the superior pubic ramus is advanced just medial to the iliopectineal eminence to ensure an adequate superior pubic ramus osteotomy. During this portion of the exposure, it is important to flex the ipsilateral hip and knee to protect the femoral nerve. Once the approach is complete, attention is then directed to completion of the osteotomies in a reproducible and sequential fashion.

Main steps:

1. Surgical exposure.
2. Identification of the ischial osteotomy which is found by following the medial edge of the rectus femoris tendon and the inferomedial capsule with large Metzenbaum scissors and a Cobb elevator. Fluoroscopic guidance is also utilized to ensure proper osteotomy placement within the infracotyloid groove at the superior edge of the ischium. This incomplete osteotomy is aimed toward the middle of the ischial spine.
3. Superior pubic osteotomy which is done under direct visualization. The osteotomy site is exposed with a sharp narrow Homan that is impacted into the superior pubic ramus just medial to the osteotomy site and blunt Homans placed around the superior and inferior aspects of the superior pubic ramus, respectively. This osteotomy is angled away from the hip joint starting medially to the pectineal eminence.
4. Iliac osteotomy which is usually started at the inferior edge of the ASIS and ends 1 cm from the pelvic brim. A large Homan is first placed into the greater sciatic notch to expose the inner table of the ilium, and fluoroscopy is used to identify the medial end point for the iliac osteotomy which also acts as a target. This site is marked with cautery and a burr. The osteotomy is then completed with an oscillating saw.
5. Posterior column osteotomy which is done with a combination of direct visualization and fluoroscopy. This osteotomy which is done with osteotome(s) is started at the medial edge of the iliac osteotomy and directed distally to join with the ischial cut. Fluoroscopy is used to ensure proper direction along the retroacetabular space. This helps to avoid osteotome penetration into the hip joint or completely osteotomizing the posterior column. The osteotomy usually propagates distally. As the osteotomy is nearing completion, a large laminar spreader can be placed into the iliac osteotomy to help with mobilization of the acetabular segment.
6. Placement of a Schanz pin into the superior aspect of the acetabular fragment in the ilium.
7. Determination of complete mobility of the fragment by moving the Schanz pin and fragment rotationally in a clockwise or counterclockwise fashion.
8. Reorientation of the fragment followed by temporary stabilization, fluoroscopic assessment of the correction, and assessment of the patient's hip range of motion, particularly in flexion and internal rotation.
9. Definitive fixation of the fragment.

Reconstruction techniques: Reorientation of the fragment to increase femoral head lateral and anterior acetabular coverage and to medialize the hip center of rotation. The fragment is stabilized with two to three 4.5 mm screws that are directed from superior to inferior from the iliac crest, across the iliac osteotomy site and into the fragment (Figs. 1.29 and 1.30).

1.8.7 Intraoperative Challenges

Challenges and solutions: Challenge: full mobilization of the acetabular fragment; solution: ensure complete osteotomies of the ischium, superior pubic ramus, ilium, and posterior column. This may require several passes with the osteotome(s). It is also beneficial to have several different types of osteotomes available that are different sizes and have varying amounts curvature that can help with osteotomy direction, especially with the posterior column osteotomy which is difficult in obese patients due to the large abdomen. Challenge: reorientation of the fragment to provide increased coverage anteriorly and laterally as well as medialization of the center of rotation; solution: make sure that the fragment is internally rotated, slightly extended, and medialized. This will likely require a bone hook into the superior pubic ramus osteotomy so that it is displaced and not hinged.

Unanticipated problems and solution: Problem: overcorrection that would cause anterior femoroacetabular impingement; solution: verify hip flexion and internal rotation perioperatively while the patient is under anesthesia and compare the patient's hip flexion and internal rotation after fragment reorientation. Overcorrection would be indicated by a significant change and limitation to flexion and internal rotation, which would necessitate an adjustment to the acetabular fragment's position. If the fragment is adequately positioned, it may be necessary to perform an arthrotomy and osteochondroplasty of the head-neck junction if needed.

Thorough description of decision making, including the reason for the final decision: Hip dysplasia can cause hip pain and is a known cause of early hip osteoarthritis. Given this patient's significant bilateral hip pain, labral tears, and hip dysplasia, the decision was made to undergo bilateral PAOs with the goals of improving the patient's symptoms, hip biomechanics, and longevity. The right hip, which was addressed first, was also treated with an open arthrotomy at the same time of the PAO. Three years later, a combined hip arthroscopy and PAO was performed to address the labral tear and dysplasia of the left hip. That is our treatment of choice today.

1.8.8 Postoperative Radiographs (Figs. 1.29 and 1.30)

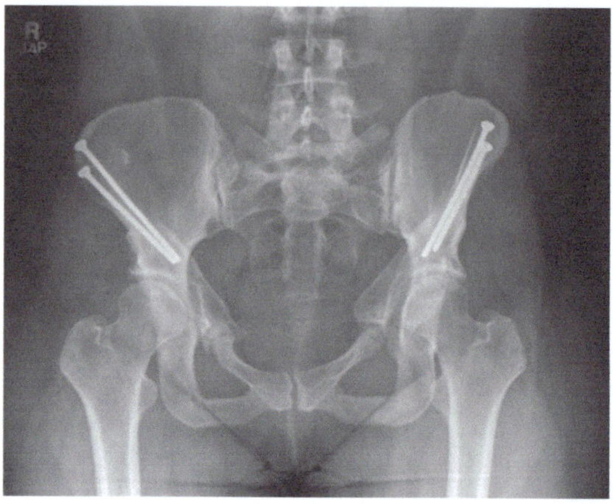

Fig. 1.29 Anteroposterior X-ray demonstrates bilateral periacetabular osteotomies, each stabilized with two 4.5 mm screws. Note increased lateral coverage of both femoral heads and medialization of both hip centers. Lack of anterior overcoverage was verified intraoperatively with ROM examination

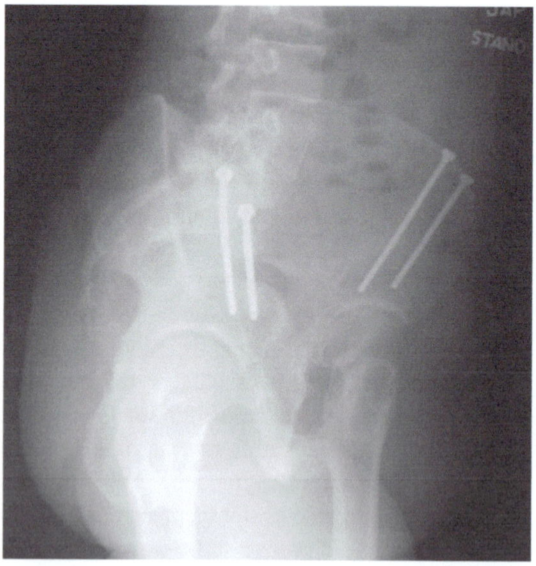

Fig. 1.30 False profile view of the left hip which demonstrates increased anterior coverage of the femoral head. The false profile view of the right hip demonstrated a similar correction

1.8.9 Postoperative Management

Chemoprophylaxis and anticoagulant treatment period: Sequential compression devices while in the hospital and compression stockings worn for six weeks. Aspirin 325 mg twice daily is also given for six weeks.

Gait/limb loading until full loading: Toe-touch weight bearing for four weeks with a maximum of 30 pounds on the operative limb. The patient was able to progress to weight bearing as tolerated four weeks postoperatively. She also used a continuous passive motion device for four weeks for the left hip from 0 to 90 degrees of knee flexion for 4–6 h per day because of the arthroscopic labral repair.

1.8.10 Follow-Up and Complications

None

1.8.11 Discussion

Advantages of the applied method: The periacetabular osteotomy has several advantages. First off, it is joint preserving and may extend or obviate the need for a total hip arthroplasty. The procedure allows for complete control of the fragment which provides a large degree of deformity correction in multiple directions. The posterior column also remains intact which provides acetabular stability and allows for partial weight bearing postoperatively. Furthermore, an anterior arthrotomy can be performed through the same approach at the same time to address any intra-articular pathology, such as a labral tear or a CAM lesion.

Disadvantages of the method: The PAO is a large surgical procedure that requires extensive rehabilitation, including a 4-week period of toe-touch weight bearing. It usually leads to injury to the lateral femoral cutaneous nerve causing a decreased sensation and occasionally can cause dysesthetic pain along the lateral aspect of the thigh. Symptomatic hardware is also not uncommon and often requires a second procedure for removal of hardware.

Alternative evidence-based techniques for the case: Total hip arthroplasty. No role of hip arthroscopy alone.

Why is the chosen technique better for this case? It is a hip preservation technique and allows for multidirectional reorientation of the acetabulum.

Indications and contraindications for your technique: Indications: hip dysplasia and isolated acetabular retroversion that causes impingement [36]. Contraindications, young pediatric patients with an open triradiate cartilage, patients with asymptomatic mild hip dysplasia or asymptomatic retroversion, and patients with radiographic evidence of osteoarthritis.

Learning curve and how to manage complications: The learning curve for performing a PAO is high, especially with patient selection. The most technically demanding portions of the surgery include fully mobilizing the acetabular fragment and performing an adequate deformity correction while avoiding under-correction or overcorrection. Proper patient selection and carefully determining the patient's preoperative radiographic undercoverage and ROM can help to avoid these pitfalls. Complications include superficial wound infection, wound dehiscence, deep infection, failed hardware, osteotomy delayed union or nonunion, intra-articular acetabular fracture, neurologic injury to the lateral femoral cutaneous nerve or sciatic or femoral nerve, and heterotopic ossification [37]. Recently, obesity was found to be a major independent risk factor for increased complication for a PAO [38]. Wound complications are typically treated with oral or intravenous antibiotics with or without an irrigation and debridement procedure. Established symptomatic aseptic nonunions are addressed with surgery for stabilization and bone grafting, but that is rarely required. Neurologic injuries, which are rare, are usually treated with observation as they are commonly neurapraxias. Symptomatic heterotopic ossification can be treated with heterotopic bone excision followed by prophylaxis with either indomethacin or radiation. Hardware failure may require revision of the fixation or removal of the hardware.

Level of evidence concerning the superiority of this method against others: Level IV [39].

1.9 Case Title: Open Surgical Dislocation of the Hip

Nicholas M. Desy and Rafael J. Sierra

1.9.1 Demographics

Age: 25
Sex: Female
BMI: 22

1.9.2 Relevant Past Medical History

Principal pathologies: Crohn's disease, obsessive-compulsive disorder

Previous surgical procedures: None

Medication: Celexa, Klaron, Remicade, Spironolactone

Other: N/A

History of presenting complaint: A 25-year-old female presented with an 8-month history of left hip pain located in the posterior trochanteric area. The pain started after running which then progressed to difficulty with sitting and walking. She denied any mechanical symptoms and a history of trauma. She did not get any relief with physical therapy or a steroid injection into the piriformis. She, did, however obtain 50% pain relief with an intra-articular hip injection.

1.9.3 Clinical Examination

Symptoms: Left hip posterior trochanteric pain

Range of motion: Extension-flexion: 0–110; internal-external rotation at 90 degrees of flexion: 45–45; abduction-adduction: 60–30. Decreased external rotation in extension

Specific tests: Negative flexion-adduction-internal rotation test (anterior impingement), positive extension-abduction-external rotation test (posterior impingement)

Main disability: Posterior hip pain and positive posterior impingement

Scoring if available: N/A

Neurovascular evaluation: Normal motor and sensory exams (sciatic and femoral nerve distributions). Normal dorsalis pedis and posterior tibial arterial pulses

1.9.4 Preoperative Radiological Assessment/Imaging (Figs. 1.31, 1.32, and 1.33)

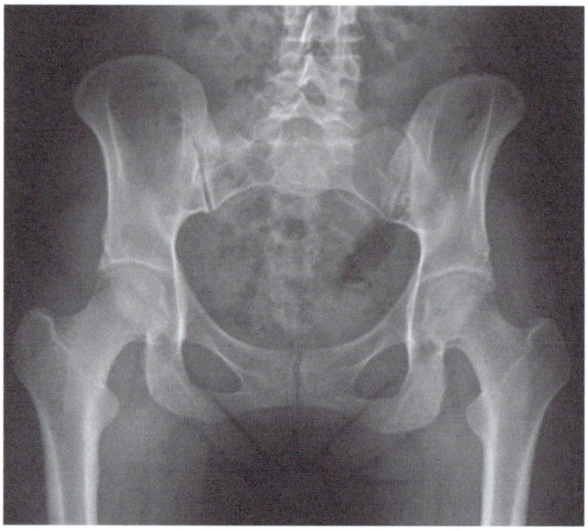

Fig. 1.31 Anteroposterior pelvic X-ray demonstrates a prominent left hip posterior acetabular wall. Note the posterior overcoverage (*arrows*) but normal anterior coverage as depicted by the anterior and posterior wall contours. Also, note the labral ossification posterosuperiorly

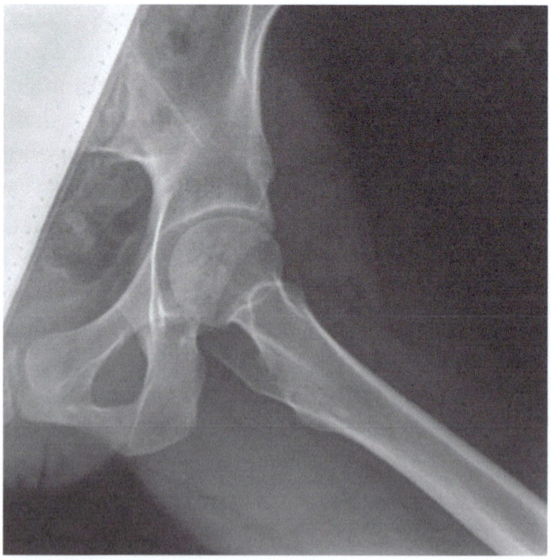

Fig. 1.32 Frog leg lateral radiograph demonstrates around the the femoral head with no CAM lesion present

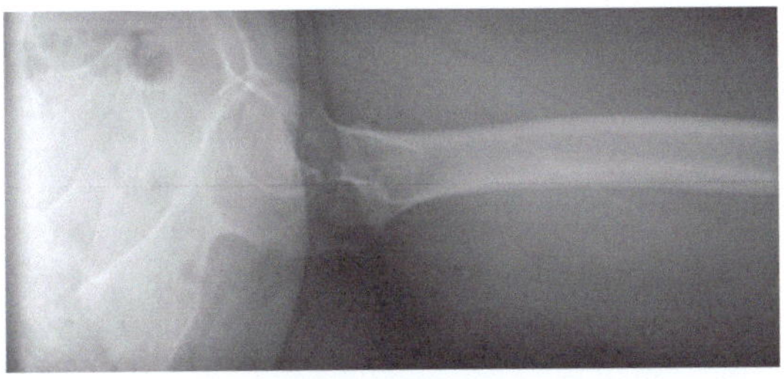

Fig. 1.33 Cross-table lateral X-ray that further shows the prominent posterior wall of the left acetabulum

1.9.5 Preoperative Planning

Diagnosis: Left hip posterior femoroacetabular impingement (Figs. 1.31, 1.32, and 1.33).

Possible treatment options: Open surgical hip dislocation with posterior wall trimming and offset procedure, arthroscopic posterior wall trimming.

Chosen treatment method: Left hip surgical hip dislocation with offset procedure, posterior wall rim trimming, and labral reconstruction with fascia lata.

Selection of implants if applicable and rational: 2 mm suture anchors for the labral reconstruction with fascia lata, two 3.5 mm cortical screws for the trochanteric fixation.

Expected difficulties: (1) Treatment of an ossified posterior labrum, (2) intraoperative finding of a CAM lesion.

Strategies to overcome difficulties: (1) Anticipate the possibility that after rim trimming has been achieved, the labral deficiency will either be accepted, or reconstruction could be performed. In this case, reported grafts include ipsilateral hamstring, allograft labrum, ipsilateral fascia lata autograft, or round ligament. The graft will need to be stabilized with suture anchors to reconstruct the posterior labrum; (2) prepare to inspect the femoral head-neck junction to make sure no CAM lesion is present; and (3) impingement-free range of motion (ROM) should be achieved.

1.9.6 Surgical Note

Patient's position: Right lateral decubitus.

Type of anesthesia: General anesthesia.

Surgical approach: Superficial dissection, skin incision similar to the Kocher-Langenbeck approach and associated split of the fascia lata; deep dissection, surgical hip dislocation with greater trochanteric flip osteotomy and Z-shaped capsulotomy.

Main steps:

1. Skin incision similar to a Kocher-Langenbeck approach to the hip.
2. Fascial split.
3. Internal rotation of the leg and identification of the posterior edge of the gluteus medius and the proximal portion of the vastus lateralis.
4. Greater trochanteric osteotomy is made along the posterior edge from the posterior border of the gluteus medius to the deep posterior portion of the vastus lateralis. The osteotomy is made through the trochanter and not under the trochanteric overhang to avoid injury to the femoral head blood supply.
5. The fragment is then retracted anteriorly with the attached gluteus medius and vastus lateralis.
6. Dissection of the interval between the gluteus minimus and piriformis tendons.
7. Z-shaped capsulotomy with careful dissection not to injure the labrum.
8. Dislocation with hip flexion and external rotation as well as adduction to deliver the femoral head superficially.
9. Inspection of the acetabulum. The patient had significant posterior overcoverage, a deep socket, and ossified labrum from the 5 to 11 o'clock position.
10. Posterior wall trimming using osteotomes and then a burr for final finishing touches (Figs. 1.34 and 1.35).
11. Fascia lata autograft harvest.
12. Attachment of the graft to the posterosuperior acetabulum with suture anchors.
13. Assessment of the femoral head and neck. This patient did not have a CAM lesion, and the cartilage was intact.
14. Testing of hip ROM.
15. Closure with fixation of the greater trochanteric osteotomy with two 3.5 mm cortical screws.

Reconstruction techniques: Posterior wall trimming, labrum reconstruction with ipsilateral fascia lata autograft and suture anchors, and greater trochanter fixation with two 3.5 mm cortical screws (Figs. 1.36 and 1.37).

1.9.7 Intraoperative Imaging

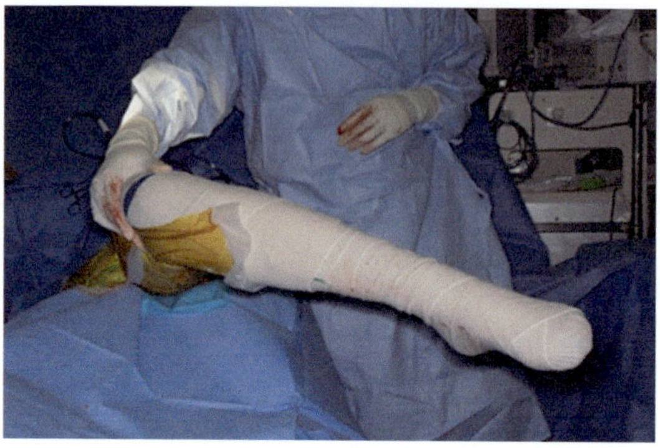

Fig. 1.34 Intraoperative photograph demonstrates the extent of the patient's hip external rotation prior to the acetabular rim trimming. The patient is currently in the lateral decubitus position

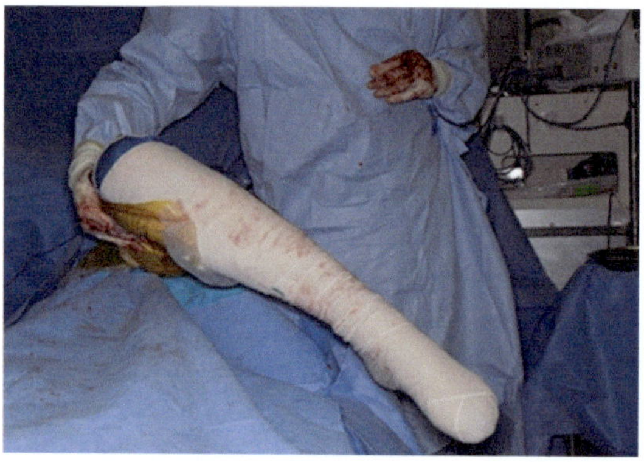

Fig. 1.35 Intraoperative image shows the increased amount of hip external rotation following rim trimming of the posterior wall of the acetabulum. Note the difference in hip rotation compared to the first image

1.9.8 Intraoperative Challenges

Challenges and solutions: Challenge: maintaining femoral head blood supply during surgical hip dislocation; solution: avoid injury to the deep branch of the medial femoral circumflex and the anastomosis in between this vessel and the inferior gluteal that runs distally to the piriformis. The use of a Z-shaped capsulotomy with careful dissection posteriorly at the acetabular rim to avoid injuring the labrum. Challenge: inspection of the posterior acetabulum and labrum; solution: elevation of the knee and the use of axial pressure to deliver the head posteriorly to access the posterior rim. Trochanteric reduction and stable fixation. Rehabilitation: toe-touch weight-bearing for four weeks and then weight bearing as tolerated. Challenge: the presence of an ossified labrum with a large area of deficient labrum; solution: the use of fascia lata autograft and suture anchors to reconstruct the deficient labrum.

Unanticipated problems and solution: Problem: inability to fully visualize the posterior acetabulum; solution: requires release of the anterior capsule, mobilization of the femur, and muscle relaxation helps. Problem: over- or undertrimming the acetabular rim; solution: progressive trimming of the rim with verification of improvements in ROM in extension and external rotation. Problem: fixation of the fascia lata autograft; solution, the graft is tubularized and fixed to the posterior and superior aspect of the acetabulum. The graft was performed as this was a young patient. Problem: trochanteric fixation if a soft bone is encountered; solution: the use of washers is recommended in situations with weak or soft bone.

Thorough description of decision making, including the reason for the final decision: Intra-articular hip pathology such as posterior femoroacetabular impingement can be very debilitating to patients. Hip arthroscopy has evolved significantly over the years, whereby several hip abnormalities can now be addressed arthroscopically. However, it requires a large learning curve and is unable to address all hip pathology. Among the deformities that are hard to address arthroscopically are those that involve the posterior aspect of the acetabulum. Surgical hip dislocation is an excellent approach to treat intra-articular hip disease both as a first-line surgical approach and when hip arthroscopy is insufficient. Surgical dislocation of the hip was chosen in this case because it was felt that hip arthroscopy would not be able to address precisely the large area of posterior acetabular overcoverage and potential labrum issues. A precise correction and check for persistent impingement should be carried out in cases with this degree of overcoverage (see intraoperative photographs).

1.9.9 Postoperative Radiographs (Figs. 1.36 and 1.37)

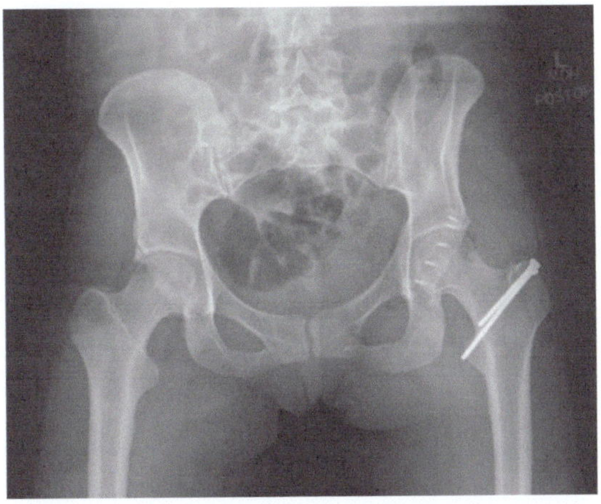

Fig. 1.36 Anteroposterior pelvic X-ray that shows the trimmed left posterior superior acetabular wall and superior and suture anchors for the labral reconstruction. Please note the distal extent of the rim trimming (*arrows*). The rim was trimmed down to the attachment of the posterior inferior attachment of the transverse ligament

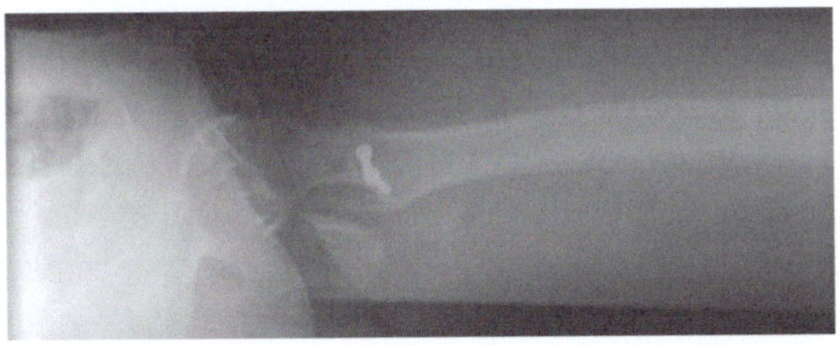

Fig. 1.37 Cross-table lateral radiograph further delineates the posterior acetabular wall trimming, suture anchor fixation for the labrum, and two screws for the trochanteric fixation

1.9.10 Postoperative Management

Chemoprophylaxis and anticoagulant treatment period: Thromboprophylaxis was provided with 5000 units of Fragmin daily for ten days followed by aspirin 325 mg twice a day for an additional four weeks as well as compression stockings. Spontaneous compression devices were also used while in hospital. Indomethacin 75 mg daily was given for five days to prevent heterotopic ossification.

Gait/limb loading until full loading: Heel to flat foot weight bearing for four weeks followed by progression to full weight bearing. A continuous passive motion device was also provided for six weeks for 4–6 h a day from 0 to 90 degrees of hip flexion.

1.9.11 Follow-Up and Complications

Report of postoperative complications and their management (i.e., recurrent dislocation): The patient complained of symptomatic hardware at the greater trochanter osteotomy site. Therefore, the two screws were removed four months after the index operation.

1.9.12 Discussion

Advantages of the applied method: Surgical hip dislocation is a reliable and versatile surgical option for several intra-articular, and extra-articular hip pathologies such as femoroacetabular impingement, labral tears, excision of benign tumors, unstable slipped capital femoral epiphyses, femoral head fractures, femoral head chondral defects, some acetabular fractures, and post-Perthes disease. There are several advantages to this approach which include the ability to visualize the entire femoral head and acetabulum as well as the ability to address both intra-articular and extra-articular pathologies at once. When compared to hip arthroscopy, it does not require a traction table which has its risks, and there may be a lower risk of chondral injury [40].

Disadvantages of the method: The biggest disadvantage to the surgical hip dislocation is likely the trochanteric osteotomy. Retained hardware can lead to pain postoperatively and require removal of hardware. There is also a larger dissection compared to hip arthroscopy and delays in the rehabilitation of the hip abductors. Its most common complication is heterotopic ossification [23]. The larger dissection may also be a cosmetic concern to patients. Furthermore, it may be more difficult to appreciate smaller labral tears as compared to hip arthroscopy.

Alternative evidence-based techniques for the case: Hip arthroscopy.

Why is the chosen technique better for this case? Surgical hip dislocation allowed for full visualization of the acetabulum and femoral head to precisely address the large area of posterior acetabular overcoverage. It also provided the ability to perform a labral reconstruction with a fascia lata autograft.

Indications and contraindications for your technique: Indications: intra-articular and extra-articular causes for femoroacetabular impingement, excision of benign tumors (synovial chondromatosis, pigmented villonodular synovitis, osteoid osteoma, exostosis, etc), some acetabulum fractures, femoral head fractures, femoral head osteochondral defects, unstable slipped capital femoral epiphyses, and post-Perthes disease. Contraindications: evidence of osteoarthritis in the setting of femoroacetabular impingement or post-Perthes disease and patients with a retroverted acetabulum and a deficient posterior wall. While not an absolute contraindication, it is becoming increasingly evident that patients over the age of 40 years have less predictable outcomes with surgical hip dislocations for femoroacetabular impingement [41].

Learning curve and how to manage complications: In experienced hands, the surgical hip dislocation is a safe procedure with a low complication rate. The learning curve for this procedure is high, but it may not be as long as that for hip arthroscopy. The most important component to learning the surgical hip dislocation is knowing and understanding femoral head vascularity. One of the most feared complications of this approach is femoral head osteonecrosis, but this is rare. Failure to understand and protect the ascending branch of the medial femoral circumflex artery as well as the posterosuperior retinacular vessels may lead to femoral head osteonecrosis. Therefore, it is paramount that the surgeon performs the osteotomy well and recognizes the need to protect the quadratus femoris muscle during dissection and master the Z-shaped capsulotomy. Other complications include neurologic injury to the sciatic nerve which is usually a neurapraxia and transient, heterotopic ossification, symptomatic hardware, and greater trochanteric nonunion. Sciatic nerve neurapraxia is usually treated with observation, foot drop splints, and physiotherapy. Heterotopic ossification can be prevented with the use of medical prophylaxis, such as indomethacin. Symptomatic hardware is treated with removal of hardware.

Level of evidence concerning the superiority of this method against others: Level IV.

There are currently no high-level studies comparing arthroscopy versus surgical hip dislocation in the treatment of hip pathology. A new systematic review on the mid- to long-term follow-up of arthroscopic versus open surgical treatment of femoroacetabular impingement did not find any high-level studies [30]. They concluded that both procedures maintained the same survival rates. Furthermore, both procedures had the same clinical outcomes scores except for the 12-Item Short-Form Survey (SF-12) which was superior with arthroscopy. A recent study demonstrated that 80% of patients treated for femoroacetabular impingement with a surgical hip dislocation at a minimum of 10 years of follow-up maintained good clinical outcomes and had no osteoarthritis progression [42].

1.10 Case Title: Bilateral Symptomatic Hip Dysplasia

Stig S. Jakobsen and Kjeld Søballe

1.10.1 Demographics

Age: 47 years
Sex: Female
BMI: 20.5

1.10.2 Relevant Past Medical History

Principal pathologies: Leiden Factor 5 thrombophilia, heterozygote

Previous surgical procedures: 2005, appendicitis acuta; 2001, 1998, and 1995, child birth; 1987, arthroscopy right knee, Osteochondritis Dissecans; 1986, re-arthroscopy left shoulder; 1985, re-arthroscopy right shoulder; 1985, z-plasty left iliotibial band; 1985, z-plasty right iliotibial band; 1984, arthroscopy left shoulder; 1984, arthroscopy right knee, osteochondritis dissecans; 1983, arthroscopy right shoulder; 1982, arthroscopy right knee, cartilage defects on the patella; 1973, fracture of the right patella

Medication: Tablet omega-3 1000 mg × 1, capsule morphine 10 mg × 2, tablet ibuprofen 600 mg × 3, capsule tramadol 50 mg PN, tablet paracetamol 1000 mg PN

History of presenting complaint: Increasing bilateral activity-related hip pain during several years. The pain is localized in the groin, pointed out with C-sign, and radiating down in the anterior aspect of the femur. Pain is described the same way on both sides, but it is worst on the left side. The patient rides bike 25 km every day without any significant worsening of the pain. Walking, standing, and running worsen the pain, and the patient scores VAS 8 (0–10) after 15 min walk. At rest she scores VAS 2 and often sleeping is impaired since falling asleep can be difficult, and she also often wakes up with pain in the groin because of rotational movements while sleeping.

1.10.3 Clinical Examination

Symptoms: Bilateral activity-related groin pain. Impaired sleeping

Range of motion: left hip: 0/140, 45/35, and 45/45; right hip: 0/140, 45/35, and 45/45

Specific tests: Left side, impingement test: positive; FABERS test: positive; Ober's test: negative; Lasegue test: negative; Trendelenburg test: positive. Right side: impingement test: positive; FABERS test: positive; Ober's test: negative; Lasegue test: negative; Trendelenburg test: negative.

Neurovascular evaluation: Sensation, force, and reflexes were found normal and equal on both sides. Pulses were felt in a. dorsalis pedis, a. popliteal, and a. femoralis.

1.10.4 Preoperative Radiological Assessment/Imaging (Figs. 1.38, 1.39, and 1.40)

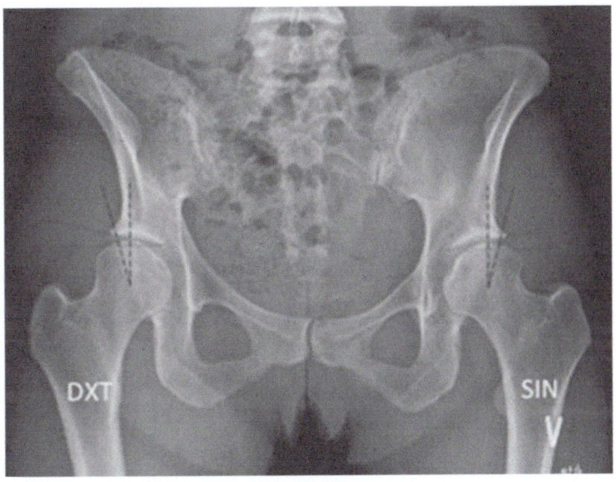

Fig. 1.38 Preoperative standing pelvis X-ray. CE angle left: 17. AI angle left: 12. CE angle right: 19. AI angle rigth: 11

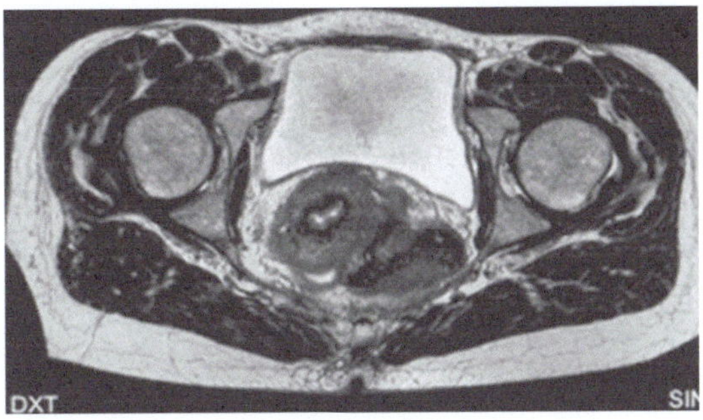

Fig. 1.39 Preoperative evaluation of the cartilage in a T2 MR scan shown in a transversal section

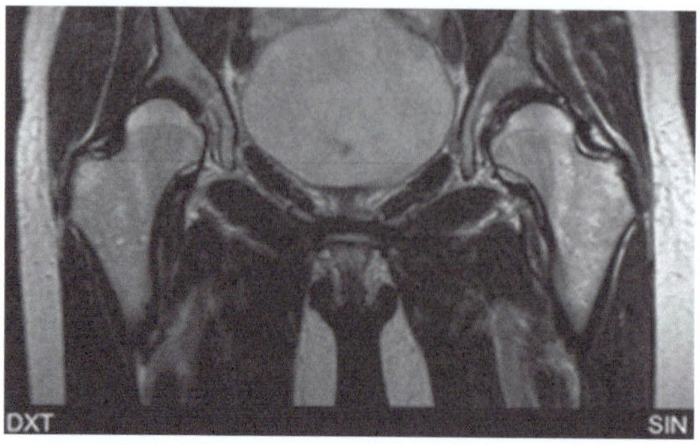

Fig. 1.40 Preoperative evaluation of the cartilage in a T2 MR scan shown in a coronal section

1.10.5 Preoperative Planning

Diagnosis: Developmental dysplasia of the hip (DDH) (Figs. 1.38, 1.39, and 1.40).

Possible treatment options: Total hip arthroplasty or periacetabular osteotomy.

Chosen treatment method: Periacetabular osteotomy.

1.10.6 Surgical Note

Patient's position: The patient is placed supine on a radiolucent table.

Type of anesthesia: Spinal anesthesia is induced at the L2–L3 levels with a dose of 3 mL bupivacaine (5 mg/mL).

Surgical approach: The minimally invasive transsartorial approach is used. The skin is incised from the anterior superior iliac spine and distally 7 cm along the sartorius muscle. The lateral cutaneous nerve is isolated and carefully retracted. The inguinal ligament is cut at the insertion of the anterior superior iliac spine. The ilium is approached subperiosteally with the iliacus and psoas major muscles protecting the femoral neurovascular bundle.

Main steps: The first of the five osteotomies is the ramus superior ossis pubis cut; then a 1 cm anterior-posterior cut is made in the ischium 1 cm distal the joint. The third cut is also in the ischium and is made from the inside of the pelvis and outward. The fourth cut is made on the ilium at the level of the spina iliaca anterior. The fifth and last cut is connecting the fourth ilial cut with the third ischial cut.

Reconstruction techniques: Redirection of the acetabular fragment is done primarily by medializing the ischial part but also lateralizing the ilium. Care should be taken not to unintendedly rotate the fragment which can be easily be observed with the nonparallel alignment of the ilium cut. Internal rotation of the fragment will antevert the acetabulum and external rotation will retrovert the acetabulum (Figs. 1.41 and 1.42).

1.10.7 Intraoperative Challenges

Challenges and solutions: Fluoroscopic evaluation is necessary throughout the operation, and therefore the pelvis is kept in a neutral position to avoid excessive tilting or rotation. The fluoroscopy equipment is positioned to facilitate the attainment of anteroposterior and 60 degrees (false profile) views. After the fifth cut, a pointy forceps is used to reorientate the fragment; sometimes this can be challenging but can be aided with a Schantz screw. Finally, inserting a 30 degree angled osteotome in the third ischial cut and apply rotating movements can further help the reorientation by ensuring that the fragment is entirely free of any bone or soft tissue adhesions.

1.10.8 Postoperative Radiographs (Figs. 1.41 and 1.42)

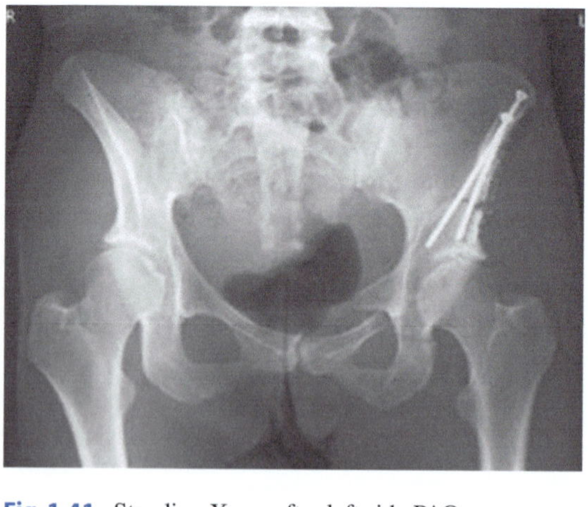

Fig. 1.41 Standing X-ray after left side PAO

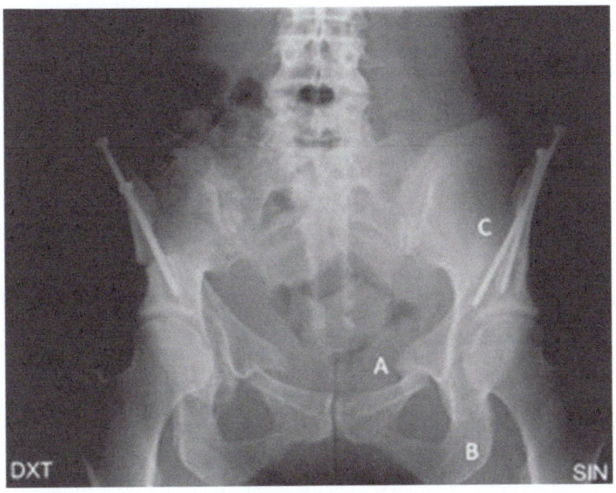

Fig. 1.42 Standing X-ray after right side PAO. A, B, and C marks solid bony healing of ramus superior os pubis, os ischium, and os ilium

1.10.9 Postoperative Management

Chemoprophylaxis and anticoagulant treatment period: Before anesthesia, 1.5 g of cefuroxime is administered, and to reduce blood loss, tranexamic acid is administered; 10 mg/kg is given at the beginning of the surgery. For thromboprophylaxis, a tablet of 10 mg rivaroxaban is administered 6 h postoperative and then every day until mobilized.

Gait/limb loading until full loading: 30 kg partial weight bearing for six weeks is recommended for patients <40 years and eight weeks for patients >40 years of age.

1.10.10 Follow-Up and Complications

Report of postoperative complications and their management (i.e., recurrent dislocation): femoral nerve palsy, peroneal nerve plasty, obturator nerve palsy, femoral artery and vein lesion/thrombosis, intra-articular osteotomy, secondary displacement, malposition of acetabulum, nonunion, infection, and DVT. Nerve palsy is due to neurapraxia and will normalize during 6 weeks to 3 month. Extremely rare permanent neurological deficiencies will reside. Damage to the vessels can also occur, and vascularization should always be evaluated immediately postoperative. Secondary displacement and malposition can be addressed by either re-PAO or a total hip replacement if contraindications exist. Nonunion of ramus superior is quite often seen and is correlated with large correction and age. It rarely causes any problems but is known to give rise to stress fractures in ramus inferior ossis pubis close to the symphyses. Infection is a very rare event and can often be handled with a simple soft tissue revision.

1.10.11 Discussion

Advantages of the applied method: The benefit of joint sparing procedure periacetabular osteotomy is obvious since it spares the joint but offers an everyday life with less pain and the chance of high-intensity sporting. Furthermore, the minimally invasive approach offers a surgical procedure with few complications, minimal surgical trauma, and no compromise in long-term results.

Disadvantages of the method: The risk of complications, reoperation with hip arthroscopy, or conversion to a total hip arthroplasty is present. Furthermore, using the minimal invasive approach offers no direct visualization of the ischial cut which some surgeons feel discomfortable.

Alternative evidence-based techniques for the case: Total hip replacement is also a validated treatment for acetabular dysplasia especially in this case with a patient above 45 years. The negative consequence of a total hip arthroplasty will diminish with increasing age when comparing with a periacetabular osteotomy.

Why is the chosen technique better for this case? This patient is very active with a desire for high-intensity sporting/recreation activity. No signs of arthrosis were present before surgery.

Indications and contraindications for your technique: If patients suffer from persistent hip pain (groin, C-sign) with a center-edge angle of Wiberg <25 degrees, pelvic bone maturity, internal rotation >15 degrees, and hip flexion <110 degrees without any signs of arthrosis, they can be considered for joint preserving surgery. Furthermore, we consider age > 45 years and BMI > 30 a relative contraindication. If any contraindications, we suggest surgery with an uncemented total hip replacement. We prefer to operative only one side at the time due to challenges with mobilization.

Learning curve and how to manage complications: The learning curve is steep, and a high volume is necessary to sustain expertise. Furthermore, to handle the potential complications safely, the surgeon must establish a collaboration with vascular surgeons and experienced pelvic surgeons [43–45].

Level of evidence concerning the superiority of this method against others: CEMB Oxford level 3-4.

References

1. Adler KL, Cook PC, Yen YM, Giordano BD. Current concepts in hip preservation surgery: part I. Sports Health. 2015;7(6):518–26.
2. Steppacher SD, Tannast M, Ganz R, Siebenrock KA. Mean 20-year follow-up of Bernese periacetabular osteotomy. Clin Orthop Relat Res. 2008;466:1633–44.
3. Goldstein RY, Kaye ID, Slover J, Feldman D. Hip dysplasia in the skeletally mature patient. Bull Hosp Joint Dis. 2014;72:28–42.
4. Ganz R, Leunig M, Leunig-Ganz K, Harris WH. The etiology of osteoarthritis of the hip: an integrated mechanical concept. Clin Orthop Relat Res. 2008;466:264–27.
5. Ganz R, Parvizi J, Beck M, Leunig M, Notzli H, Siebenrock KA. Femoroacetabular impingement: a cause for osteoarthritis of the hip. Clin Orthop Relat Res. 2003;417:112–20.
6. Ganz R, Klaue K, Vinh TS, Mast JW. A new periacetabular osteotomy for the treatment of hip dysplasias technique and preliminary results. Clin Orthop Relat Res. 1988;232:26–36.
7. Siebenrock KA, Steppacher SD, Tannast M, Büchler L. Anteverting periacetabular osteotomy for acetabular retroversion. JBJS Essent Surg Tech. 2015;5(1):e1.
8. Zweifel J, Hönle W, Schuh A. Long-term results of intertrochanteric varus osteotomy for dysplastic osteoarthritis of the hip. Int Orthop. 2011;35:9–12.
9. Leunig M, Ganz R. The evolution and concepts of joint-preserving surgery of the hip. Bone Joint J. 2014;96:5–18.
10. Botser IB, Smith TW Jr, Nasser R, Domb BG. Open surgical dislocation versus arthroscopy for femoroacetabular impingement: a comparison of clinical outcomes. Arthroscopy. 2011;27:270–8.
11. Domb BG, Philippon MJ, Giordano BD. Arthroscopic capsulotomy, capsular repair, and capsular plication of the hip: relation to atraumatic instability. Arthroscopy. 2013;29:162–17.
12. Parvizi J, Bican O, Bender B, et al. Arthroscopy for labral tears in patients with developmental dysplasia of the hip: a cautionary note. J Arthroplast. 2009;24:110–3.
13. Peterson L, Vasiliadis HS, Brittberg M, Lindahl A. Autologous chondrocyte implantation: a long-term follow-up. Am J Sports Med. 2010;38:1117–24.
14. Clohisy JC, Barrett SE, Gordon JE, Delgado ED, Schoenecker PL. Periacetabular osteotomy in the treatment of severe acetabular dysplasia. Surgical technique. J Bone Joint Surg Am. 2006;88(suppl 1 p+1):65–83.
15 Kalhor M, Gharehdaghi J, Schöniger R, Ganz R. Reducing the risk of nerve injury during Bernese periacetabular osteotomy: a cadaveric study. Bone Joint J. 2015;97:636–41.
16 Ganz R, Huff TW, Leunig M. Extended retinacular soft-tissue flap for intra-articular hip surgery: surgical technique, indications, and results of application. Instr Course Lect. 2009;58:241–55.
17 Leunig M, Ganz R. Relative neck lengthening and intracapital osteotomy for severe Perthes and Perthes-like deformities. Bull NYU Hosp Jt Dis. 2011;69(Suppl 1):S62–7.
18 Ganz R, Horowitz K, Leunig M. Algorithm for femoral and periacetabular osteotomies in complex hip deformities. Clin Orthop Relat Res. 2010;468:3168–80.
19 Paley D. The treatment of femoral head deformity and coxa magna by the Ganz femoral head reduction osteotomy. Orthop Clin North Am. 2011;42:389–99. viii
20 Siebenrock KA, Anwander H, Zurmühle CA, Tannast M, Slongo T, Steppacher SD. Head reduction osteotomy with additional containment surgery improves sphericity and containment and reduces pain in Legg-Calvé-Perthes disease. Clin Orthop Relat Res. 2015;473:1274–83.
21 Ganz R, Gill TJ, Gautier E, Ganz K, Krügel N, Berlemann U. Surgical dislocation of the adult hip. A technique with full access to the femoral head and acetabulum without the risk of avascular necrosis. J Bone Joint Surg Br. 2001;83-B:1119–24.
22 Kamath AF, Ganz R, Zhang H, Grappiolo G, Leunig M. Subtrochanteric osteotomy for femoral maltorsion through a surgical dislocation approach. J Hip Preserv Surg. 2015;2:65–79.
23 Sink EL, Beaulé PE, Sucato D, Kim YJ, Millis MB, Dayton M, Trousdale RT, Sierra RJ, Zaltz I, Schoenecker P, Monreal A, Clohisy J. Multicenter study of complications following surgical dislocation of the hip. J Bone Joint Surg Am. 2011;93:1132–6.
24 Ross JR, Schoenecker PL, Clohisy JC. Surgical dislocation of the hip: evolving indications. HSS J. 2013;9:60–9.
25 Masse A, Aprato A, Rollero L, Bersano A, Ganz R. Surgical dislocation technique for the treatment of acetabular fractures. Clin Orthop Relat Res. 2013;471:4056–64. CORR Multimedia Award 2013
26 Ziebarth K, Leunig M, Slongo T, Kim YJ, Ganz R. Slipped capital femoral epiphysis: relevant pathophysiological findings with open surgery. Clin Orthop Relat Res. 2013;471:2156–62.

27 Schöniger R, Kain MSH, Ziebarth K, Ganz R. Epiphyseal reperfusion after subcapital realignment of an unstable SCFE. Hip Int. 2010;20:273–9.

28 Ganz R, Aprato A, Mazziotta G, Pignatti G. Joint instability after anatomic reconstruction of severe chronic SCFE. Report of three cases with high femoral anteversion (1) and adaptive acetabular roof deformation (3). J Bone Joint Surg Am. Case Connector. Accepted for publication.

29 Novais EN, Hill MK, Carry PM, Heare TC, Sink EL. Modified Dunn procedure is superior to in situ pinning for short term clinical and radiographic improvement in severe stable SCFE. Clin Orthop Relat Res. 2015;473:2108–17.

30 Nwachukwu BU, Rebolledo BJ, McCormick F, Rosas S, Harris JD, Kelly BT. Arthroscopic versus open treatment of femoroacetabular impingement: a systematic review of medium- to long-term outcomes. Am J Sports Med. 2016;44(4):1062–8.

31 Sussmann PS, Ranawat AS, Lipman J, Lorich DG, Padgett DE, Kelly BT. Arthroscopic versus open osteoplasty of the head-neck junction: a cadaveric investigation. J Arthrosc Relat Surg. 2007;23(12):1257–64.

32 Marwan YA, Abatzoglou S, Esmaeel AA, et al. Hip arthroscopy for the management of osteoid osteoma of the acetabulum: a systematic review of the literature and case report. BMC Musculoskelet Disord. 2015;16:318.

33 Nehme AH, Bou Ghannam AG, Imad JP, Jabbour FC, Moucharafieh R, Wehbe J. Arthroscopic excision of intra-articular hip osteoid osteoma: a report of 2 cases. Case Rep Orthop. 2012;2012:820501.

34 Said HG, Abdulla Babaqi A, AbdelSalam E-AM. Hip arthroscopy for excision of osteoid osteoma of femoral neck. Arthrosc Tech. 2014;3(1):e145–8.

35 Papagelopoulos PJ, Mavrogenis AF, Kyriakopoulos CK, et al. Radiofrequency ablation of intra-articular osteoid osteoma of the hip. J Int Med Res. 2006;34(5):537–44.

36 Leunig M, Ganz R. Evolution of technique and indications for the Bernese periacetabular osteotomy. Bull NYU Hosp Jt Dis. 2011;69(Suppl 1):S42–6.

37 Zaltz I, Baca G, Kim YJ, Schoenecker P, Trousdale R, Sierra R, Sucato D, Sink E, Beaule P, Millis MB, Podeszwa D, Clohisy JC. Complications associated with the periacetabular osteotomy. J Bone Joint Surg Am. 2014;96:1967–74.

38 Novais EN, Potter GD, Clohisy JC, Millis MB, Kim YJ, Trousdale RT, Carry PM, Sierra RJ. Obesity is a major risk factor for the development of complications after peri-acetabular osteotomy. Bone Joint J. 2015;97B(1):29–34.

39 Clohisy JC, Schutz AL, St. John L, Schoenecker PL, Wright RW. Periacetabular osteotomy: a systematic literature review. Clin Orthop Relat Res. 2009;467:2041–52.

40 Tibor LM, Sink EL. Pros and cons of surgical hip dislocation for the treatment of femoroacetabular impingement. J Pediatr Orthop. 2013;33:S131–6.

41 Boone GR, Pagnotto MR, Walker JA, Trousdale RT, Sierra RJ. Caution should be taken in performing hip dislocation for the treatment of femoroacetabular impingement in patients over the age of 40. HSS J. 2012;8:230–4.

42 Steppacher SD, Anwander H, Zurmuhle CA, Tannast M, Siebenrock KA. Eighty percent of patients with surgical hip dislocation for femoroacetabular impingement have a good clinical result without osteoarthritis progression at 10 years. Clin Orthop Relat Res. 2015;473:1333–41.

43 Søballe K, Troelsen A. Approaches and perioperative management in periacetabular osteotomy surgery: the minimally invasive transartorial approach. Instr Course Lect. 2013;62:297–303. Review. PMID: 23395035

44 Troelsen A, Elmengaard B, Søballe K. A new minimally invasive transsartorial approach for periacetabular osteotomy. J Bone Joint Surg Am. 2008;90(3):493–8. doi:10.2106/JBJS.F.01399.

45 Klit J, Hartig-Andreasen C, Jacobsen S, Søballe K, Troelsen A. Periacetabular osteotomy: sporting, social and sexual activity 9–12 years post surgery. Hip Int. 2014;24(1):27–31. doi:10.5301/hipint.5000077. Epub 2013 Sep 20

Part II

Primary Hip Arthroplasty

Surgical Approaches of the Hip

2

Eustathios Kenanidis, Dimitrios Rigkos, Georgios Paparoidamis, Aristotelis Yfantis, Zakareya Gamie, Eleftherios Tsiridis, Michael J. Feldstein, and William Hozack

2.1 Current Concepts

E. Kenanidis, D. Rigkos, G. Paparoidamis, A. Yfantis, Z. Gamie, and E. Tsiridis

2.1.1 Lateral Approach

This approach exploits the intermuscular plane between the tensor fasciae latae (TFL) and the gluteus medius with the partial or complete detachment of the abductor mechanism from the greater trochanter [1]. There is no true internervous plane as both these muscles have a common nerve supply, the superior gluteal nerve [2]. The fascia lata is divided at the interval between the TFL and the gluteus maximus, and then the tendon and muscle fibers of the gluteus medius are split with various techniques leaving a cuff of gluteus medius tendon for repair following the procedure [2, 3]. The gluteus minimus and the joint capsule are split either in line with the neck of the femur or line with the tendinous part of the gluteus minimus [1].

The patient is placed in the supine or lateral decubitus position on a standard table [3]. The foot of the operated leg is wrapped in a sterile bag to permit intraoperative manoeuvers for the hip dislocation and the femur broaching [1].

2.1.1.1 Advantages

1. Adequate exposure of both the proximal femur and the acetabulum [2]. It can be extended to both the acetabulum and the femur, thus being suitable for primary and revision operations [3].
2. Low reported dislocation rate from 0.4 to 0.61% [1, 4].
3. In the supine position, the implant orientation might be better reproducible [3].

2.1.1.2 Disadvantages

1. The risk of the sciatic nerve irritation from retractors used to elevate the femur [3].

E. Kenanidis, M.D., Ph.D., M.Sc. (✉) · D. Rigkos, M.D.
G. Paparoidamis M.D. · A. Yfantis, M.D.
Academic Orthopaedic Unit, Aristotle University Medical School, Thessaloniki, Greece

Z. Gamie, B.Sc., M.B.Ch.B., M.R.C.S.
Northern Institute for Cancer Research, Paul O'Gorman Building, Medical School, Newcastle University, Newcastle upon Tyne, UK
e-mail: ugm1zg@doctors.org.uk

E. Tsiridis, M.D., Ph.D., F.A.C.S., F.R.C.S.
Academic Orthopaedic Unit, Papageorgiou General Hospital, Aristotle University Medical School, Thessaloniki, Greece
e-mail: etsiridis@doctors.org.uk

M.J. Feldstein, M.D., S.M.
Kaiser Permanante, Oakland, CA, USA
e-mail: Michael.Feldstein@rothmaninstitute.com

W. Hozack, M.D.
Sidney Kimmel Medical School at Thomas Jefferson University, Rothman Institute Orthopaedics, Philadelphia, PA, USA
e-mail: william.hozack@rothmaninstitute.com

E. Tsiridis (ed.), *The Adult Hip - Master Case Series and Techniques*,
https://doi.org/10.1007/978-3-319-64177-5_2

2. As in all other approaches, there is a risk of the femoral nerve and vessel damage when retractors are placed on the the anterior rim of the acetabulum (0.1–2.4%) [1, 3].
3. The jeopardy of the superior gluteal nerve damage from the extensive splitting of the gluteus medius muscle ranging from 2.2 to 42.5% in different studies [1, 5]. The nerve palsy can lead to abductor insufficiency, Trendelenburg sign, and poorer functional outcomes following THA. The majority of cases, however, improve spontaneously [6, 7].
4. The risk of the abductor insufficiency not only from the superior gluteal nerve palsy but also from a failure of the repaired tenotomy, chronic fatty degeneration of the gluteus medius and minimus tendon preoperatively, or irreparable tears in up to 20% of patients undergoing the procedure usually done from femoral reaming [8–10]. It causes abductor muscle weakness, inefficient gait mechanics, and peritrochanteric pain [11, 12].
5. Intraoperative fractures. There is a paucity of the literature for examining the incidence of intraoperative fractures. In a previous study of 372 primary THAs, Hendel et al. [13] revealed 4% intraoperative greater trochanter fractures with this approach.

2.1.2 Posterior Approach

The posterior approach also has no true internervous plane as it proceeds through the fibers of gluteus maximus; this muscle, however, is not significantly denervated as it receives its nerve supply well proximal to the split [2]. Following skin incision, the fascia lata overlying the gluteus maximus is incised, and the muscle fibers are bluntly divided down to the short external rotators. The gluteus medius is retracted, the sciatic nerve is protected, and the short external rotators are tenotomized at their insertion onto the greater trochanter to get access to the capsule [1, 3]. The short external rotators and the capsule are repaired at the end of the procedure to diminish the dislocation risk.

The patient is placed in the lateral position [1, 3], and the operated limb is wrapped to facilitate dislocating and other manoeuvers.

2.1.2.1 Advantages

1. Less damage to the abductor mechanism compared to the lateral approach [3].
2. Adequate visualization of both the acetabulum and femur. It can be extended to both acetabulum and femur and thus is suitable in primary and revision hip arthroplasty [1, 3].

2.1.2.2 Disadvantages

1. A higher reported dislocation rate versus the lateral and the anterior approach, ranging from 1 to 5% [1, 3]. The meticulous reconstruction of the capsule and short external rotators, however, decrease the risk of postoperative dislocation. The risk of dislocation is reported to be eight times less when the posterior soft tissue repair is performed [4]. The capsulorrhaphy and the transosseous bone tunnels in the greater trochanter for short external rotators repair are some proposed techniques [14, 15].
2. Nerve injuries: The risk of the sciatic nerve injury seems greater during the posterior approach. Previous studies have shown an incidence of isolated sciatic nerve palsy of 1.3% [16, 17].

2.1.3 Direct Anterior Approach

The anterior approach is a muscle-sparing approach that uses a true internervous, intermuscular plane between the tensor fascia latae and the sartorius muscles first and then between the rectus femoris and gluteus medius to expose the anterior joint capsule of the hip [1, 18]. Divisions of the ascending branch of the lateral femoral circumflex artery lie between these two muscles and must be carefully ligated [18].

The patient is placed in the supine position on a standard or a fracture table. The foot is firmly secured to boot that permits positioning and applying traction to the limb. The latter combined with intraoperative fluoroscopy, facilitates the exposure to optimize component placement [1, 3, 18].

2.1.3.1 Advantages

1. It is a muscle-sparing approach; however, damage of the tensor fasciae latae muscle has been reported [3, 19].
2. The early functional improvement and limited hospital stay and the earlier restoration of hip gait kinematics [3, 19].
3. The reported low dislocation rates from 0.61 to 1.5% [18–22].

2.1.3.2 Difficulties/Disadvantages

1. The need for the special operating table, the intraoperative fluoroscopy, and the special tools [18].
2. The difficult performance in patients with BMI > 40 or with a large abdominal panniculus [18].
3. It cannot be extended considerably to the femur and hardly performed in patients with a history of previous hip surgery or retained instrumentation and impossible for femoral revisions [3, 18].
4. The exposure is proximally extensile for acetabular revisions, but the posterior column cannot be reconstructed [3].
5. Moving the reamers in and out of the acetabulum can be challenging [18].
6. The femoral preparation can be difficult due to limited proximal femoral exposure [1]. Traction and elevation of the limb improve the accessibility of the proximal femur; however, a forceful external rotation can result in soft tissue injuries to the knee and ankle or an intraoperative fracture. In a recent meta-analysis, Geest et al. [20] found an evident but small intraoperative risk of 0.8% for trochanter and 0.5% for femoral fractures in patients undergoing THA with DAA.
7. A technically demanding procedure with precipitous learning curve [18, 20, 23, 24].
8. Nerve damage risk. As in all approaches, the femoral nerve and vessels are at risk from retractors placed on the anterior rim of the acetabulum and the lateral branches of the femoral nerve from caudal retractors [1, 3]. Damage to the lateral femoral cutaneous nerve and potential meralgia paresthetica is described especially following DAA. The unsteady course of the nerve around the anterior superior iliac spine as it crosses the surgical plane at the sartorial-TFL plane more distally plays a crucial role. The reported incidence of neurapraxia ranges 15–80% [1, 25–27]. Geest et al. [20] reported 0.9% risk for postoperative transient lateral cutaneous femoral nerve (LCFN) impairment. Most of them usually resolve without functional limitation; true meralgia paresthetica is extremely rare (1%).

2.1.4 Comparisons Between Different Approaches

There are not precise comparative results between different approaches that are attributed to the lack of high-quality comparative clinical studies in the literature. As each approach has its own advantages and disadvantages, the surgeons should choose the approach for each patient separately according to their preferences and experience and patient's characteristics.

2.1.4.1 Direct Anterior Approach vs. Lateral Approach (LA)

Several studies suggested that the DAA may be associated with greater early postoperative improvements in patient-reported outcomes than the direct LA [1, 19, 28]. In a prospective randomized study, Restrepo et al. [29] demonstrated no difference in the duration of surgery, the blood loss, the need for blood transfusions, or the hospital stay between groups of these two approaches. Interestingly the DAA group demonstrated significantly better improvement in both the mental and physical health dimensions of SF-36 and WOMAC Index compared with direct LA group till the first postoperative year but not later. In a retrospective study with several methodological concerns, Goebel et al. [30] supported that the patients undergone DAA are discharged earlier from the hospital than those experienced LA probably due to a better pain mitigation after surgery and differences in the anatomic pathology. In another study with methodological concerns, Bremer et al. [31] recorded significantly greater number of abductor tears or detachments, trochanteric fluid collections, gluteus medius tendinosis, and fatty atrophy of the abductor muscles in the direct LA group compared to DAA on the MRI at one year postoperatively. Other studies, however, supported that there are no differences between these two approaches concerning the muscle damage and the functional outcome. In a randomized controlled prospective study, Anta Diaz et al. [32] found higher levels of serum markers of muscle damage up to the fourth postoperative day, more fatty atrophy in the gluteal muscles at six months in the LA group, and lower mean thickness of the tensor fasciae latae at the DAA group. As the functional outcome was similar between groups at three and twelve postoperative months, the authors concluded that both approaches for THA are similarly safe and feasible, and the choice depends only on the preference and experience of the surgeon. A recent meta-analysis supported that the available evidence is still insufficient; DAA, however, was associated with significantly shorter hospitalization, greater functional rehabilitation, lower perceived pain during the early postoperative period, and with longer surgery time than the LA approach [33]. Both approaches were associated with a similar rate of perioperative surgical complications (dislocation, intraoperative fracture, nerve palsy, superficial infection, deep infection, postoperative hematoma).

2.1.4.2 Direct Anterior Approach vs. Posterior Approach (PA)

The quality and quantity of the available comparative information in the literature between these two approaches are also insufficient to make any firm conclusion on the optimum choice of surgical approach in patients undergoing primary THA. Additional high-level comparative studies are certainly needed. There are currently active trials comparing the DAA approach with the PA approach to THA listed on ClinicalTrials.gov that will probably help us to decide.

In a recent meta-analysis, Higgins et al. [34] studied 2302 patients undergoing primary THA performed via the DAA or the PA. The DAA was related with benefits in the early patient-reported pain and functional outcomes, hospital stay, dislocations, and postoperative narcotic consumption. The PA was associated with lower but nonsignificant estimated blood loss and operative time. There was no difference in the rate of intraoperative fractures or postoperative recovery of gait function. In a prospective randomized study comparing both approaches, Barret et al. [35] demonstrated that the total duration of surgery was on average 23.8 min longer in the DAA than the PA group. The DAA was related to a lower hospital stay and provided earlier restoration of the function after THA at six weeks postoperatively; this difference dissipated at three months and became insignificant at one year. Bergin et al. [36] compared acute-phase reactants proteins among patients undergone DAA or PA. CK was significantly increased after PA till the second postoperative day, but no difference was found then. TNF-a, IL-6, IL-1β, CRP, and myoglobin levels were similar between groups.

2.1.4.3 Lateral Approach vs. Posterior Approach

There is a paucity of evidence comparing PA and LA. In a recent meta-analysis performed according to Cochrane guidelines, Berstock et al. [37] studied 517 patients from six prospective studies (including three RCTs). The PA conferred a significant reduction in the risk of Trendelenburg gait (OR, 0.31; $p = 0.0002$) and stem malposition (OR, 0.24; $p = 0.02$) and a nonsignificant reduction in the risk of dislocation (OR, 0.37; $p = 0.16$) and heterotopic ossification (OR, 0.41; $p = 0.13$). There was no difference between these two approaches in the functional results. In a previous systematic review form the Cochrane database, Jolles et al. [38] demonstrated no significant difference between these two approaches regarding Trendelenburg sign and dislocation and a general higher risk of nerve injury for lateral approaches but not for the sciatic nerve. The mean internal rotation in extension was also greater for posterior approaches. Again, data were considered as insufficient. Mukka et al. [39] supported the use of the PA for lower mortality in patients undergone THA and the LA for lower dislocation rate in patients undergone hip fracture treatment. Other studies, however, reported no difference in pain and dislocation rate [40, 41].

2.2 Case Title: Direct Superior Approach

E. Kenanidis and E. Tsiridis

The skin incision is made 45° backward and upward from the tip of the greater trochanter (Fig. 2.1a). The tip area is divided into thirds, and the incision is made between the 2nd and 3rd thirds (Fig. 2.1b, c).

The short rotators are tagged with Ethibond suture size 5 and detached from their base for reattachment after the end of surgery (Fig. 2.1d, e). The capsule is also tagged and will be reattached in layers at the end. The gluteus medius and minimus are protected using the ring retractor (Fig. 2.1f). The sciatic nerve is protected by the tagged sort rotators and capsule, and the acetabular fossa is exposed easily.

Compare the size of the femoral head to the size of the incision (the head occupies nearly the 2/3 of the incision) (Fig. 2.1f, g). Observe the size of the THA ceramic head and neck in comparison to the incision before closure (Fig. 2.1h).

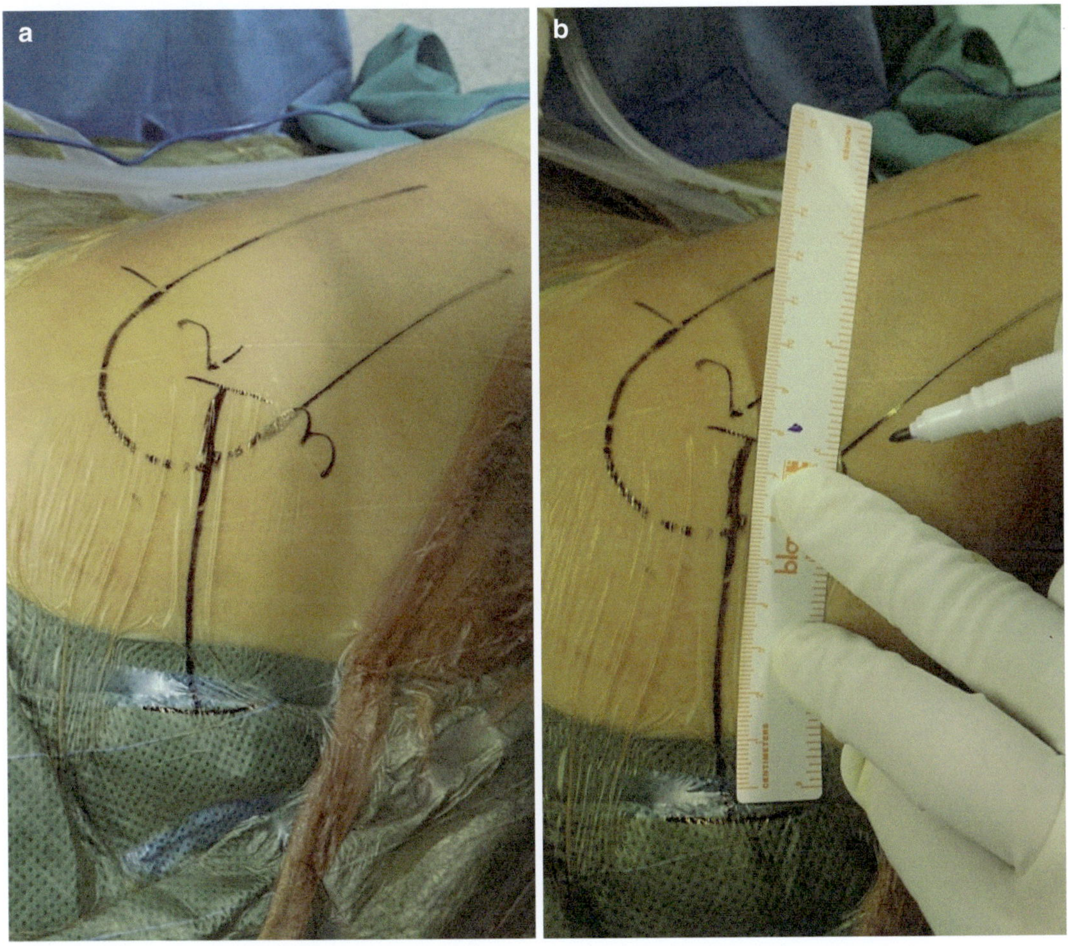

Fig. 2.1 (**a–h**) Direct Superior Hip Approach. The pictures (**a–h**) depict different crucial steps of the procedure

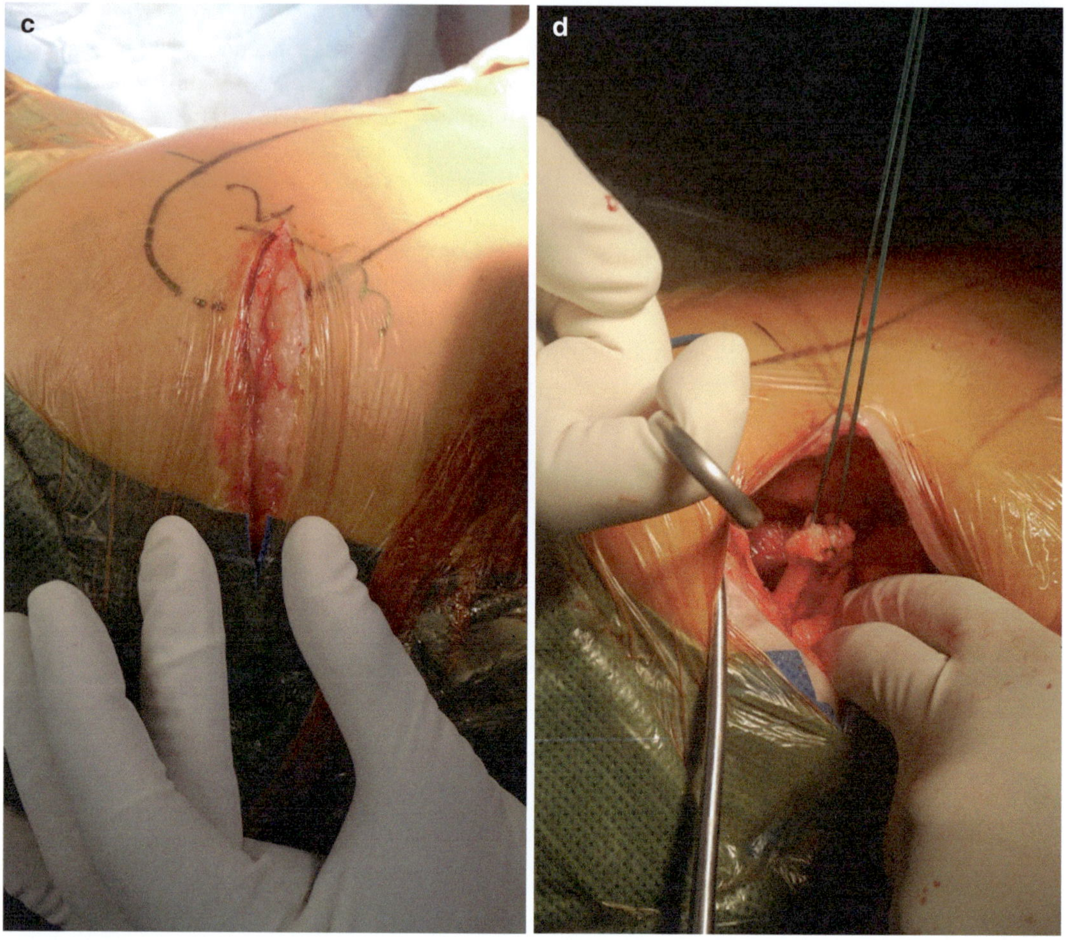

Fig. 2.1 (continued)

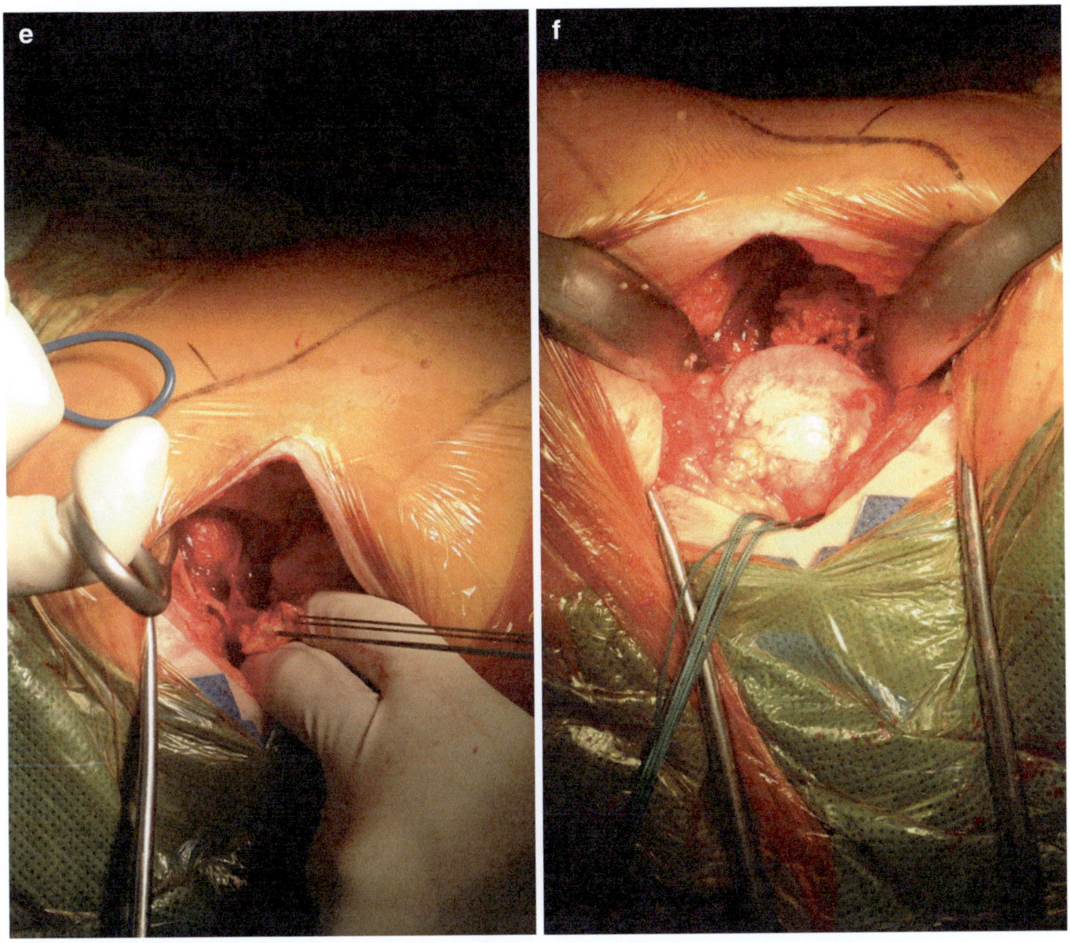

Fig. 2.1 (continued)

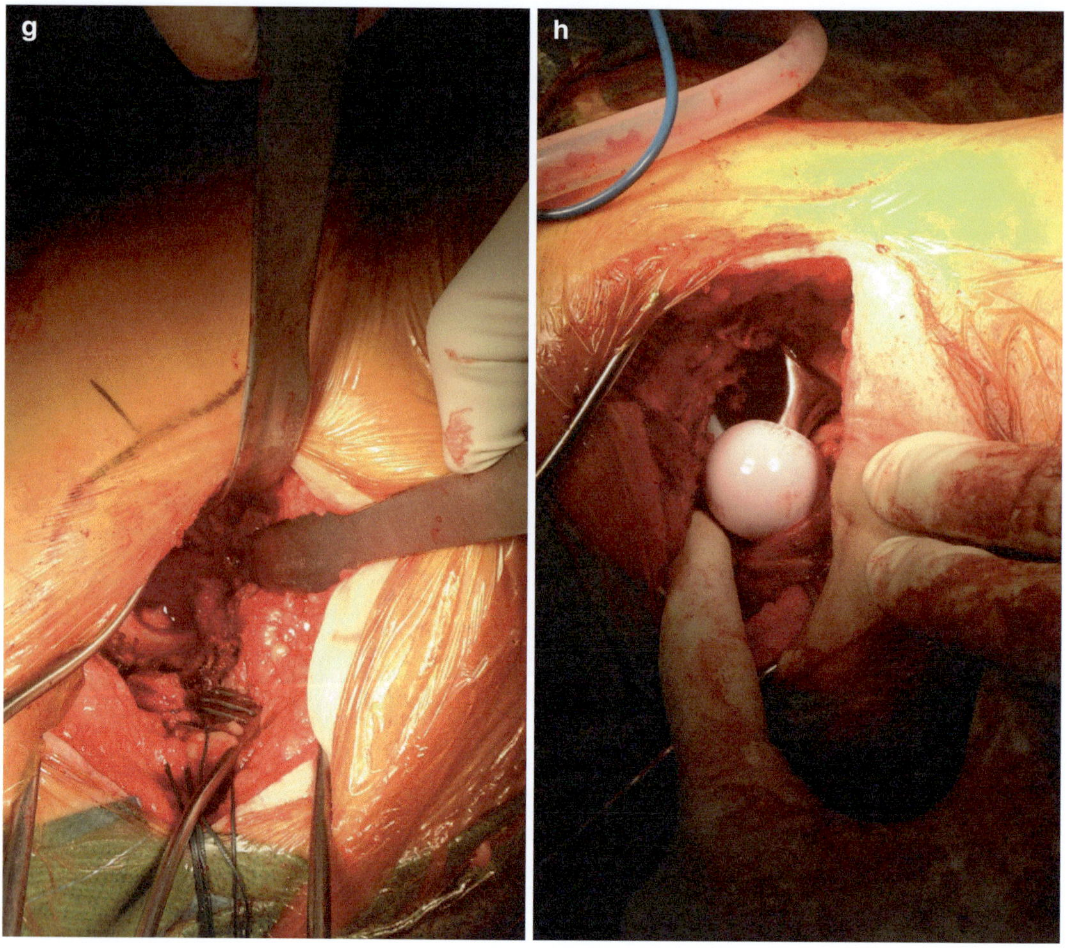

Fig. 2.1 (continued)

2.3 Case Title: Primary Hip Arthroplasty Using Direct Anterior Approach Without a Traction Table

Michael Feldstein and William Hozack

2.3.1 Demographics

Age: 74
Sex: Female
BMI: 30

2.3.2 Relevant Past Medical History

Principal pathologies: Gout, HTN, HLD, and osteoporosis.

Previous surgical procedures: Bilateral TKA, total shoulder, appendectomy.

Medication: Allopurinol, furosemide, irbesartan, oxycodone, raloxifene.

History of presenting complaint: This 74-year-old woman has had several years of progressive right hip pain that is refractory to conservative management including NSAIDs, injections, physical therapy, and activity modification. Her quality of life was severely impacted by her arthritis, and her pain is now severe and constant. She is currently dependent on a walker for ambulation.

2.3.3 Clinical Examination

Symptoms: Severe, constant pain localized to the groin. Exacerbated by motion and weight bearing

Range of motion: 0–100 flexion, 50/40 Abd/Add, 20/0 ER/IR

Specific tests: Stinchfield test positive, Trendelenburg negative

Main disability: Severe pain is causing inability to ambulate without a walker

Neurovascular evaluation: Distal sensation and pulses intact

2.3.4 Preoperative Radiological Assessment/Imaging (Figs. 2.2, 2.3, and 2.4)

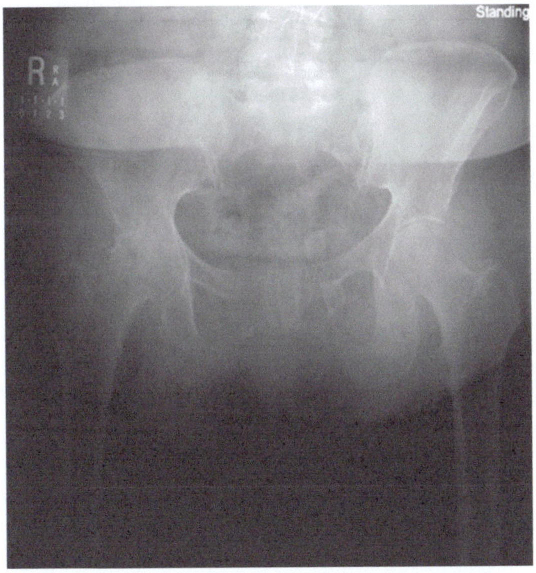

Fig. 2.2 AP pelvis preop demonstrating severe right hip osteoarthritis

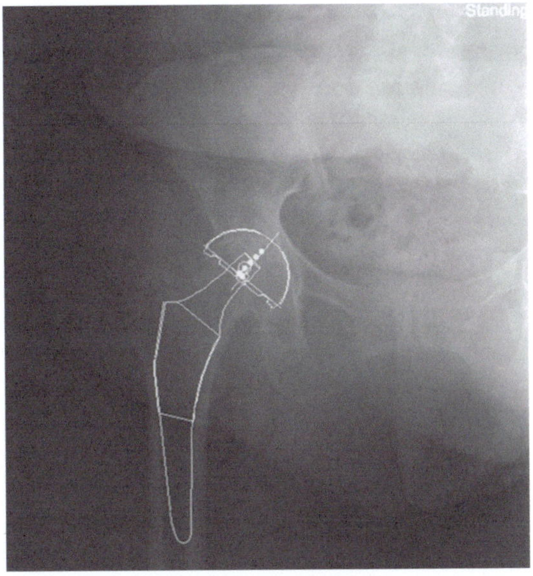

Fig. 2.3 Templated AP of the right hip preop

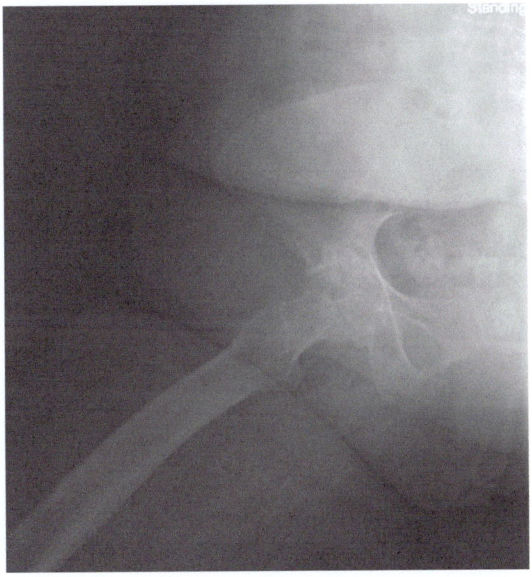

Fig. 2.4 Lateral preop

2.3.5 Preoperative Planning

Diagnosis: Right hip degenerative joint disease (Figs. 2.2 and 2.4).

Possible treatment options: Total hip arthroplasty via posterior, direct lateral, anterolateral, direct anterior with special table, or direct anterior with regular table.

Chosen treatment method: Total hip arthroplasty via direct anterior approach with a regular table.

Selection of implants if applicable and rational: A non-cemented hemispherical cup with UHMWPE liner combined with a taper-wedge titanium stem and a ceramic head were chosen.

Expected difficulties: As with all approaches to the hip joint, the direct anterior approach can present difficulties on exposure, but these can be overcome with proper technique. Potential complications include damage to the lateral femoral cutaneous nerve, bleeding and hematoma, femoral fracture, femoral nerve palsy, prolonged surgical time, and wound complications. Only LFC neurapraxia is a complication specific to the DAA.

Strategies to overcome difficulties: As with all approaches to the hip, a detailed knowledge of the vascular, neural, and muscular anatomy of the direct anterior approach is crucial to avoiding problems.

Templating: Templating was performed using built-in software of our PACs system (Fig. 2.3).

2.3.6 Surgical Note

Patient's position: Supine on a regular table with the patient's pelvis elevated on a gel bump.

Type of anesthesia: Spinal.

Surgical approach: Direct anterior.

**Main steps*: The ASIS and groin crease are marked along with hash marks during preparation. An 8–10 cm incision is made approximately 2 cm lateral and distal to the ASIS. This incision should be extended as needed to improve exposure. Subcutaneous fat is cleared manually with a lap sponge. The sartorius/TFL border is identified by the red/purple appearance of the TFL lateral to the sartorius and the small perforating vessels of the TFL. The TFL fascia is incised 5 mm lateral to the sartorius border and care is taken to avoid the LFCN by minimizing medial dissection. A blunt Hohmann retractor is placed over the superior femoral neck. A sharp Hohmann retractor is placed over the vastus lateralis and lateral femur distally in the wound. The fascia of the quadriceps is incised and a Hibbs retractor placed within the fascia to hold tension. The interval between the quadriceps and TFL is carefully dissected using a Bovie with care to identify and cauterize the ascending branches of the lateral femoral circumflex vessels. The area between the rectus femoris and vastus is cleared with a Cobb, and a blunt retractor is placed along the capsule of the inferior femoral neck. The Cobb is then used to develop the interval over the anterior acetabulum under direct visualization and in the direction of the contralateral kidney. A lighted Hohmann is placed in this interval under direct visualization. An anterior partial capsulectomy is then performed. We prefer capsulectomy because it facilitates proper exposure of the hip. The femoral neck is cut sub-capitally first and then distally to form a napkin ring of bone, which is then removed. The femoral head is removed with a corkscrew. The lateral retractor is then placed carefully under the posterior acetabulum. All bleeding is controlled (the area of the inferior capsule is carefully evaluated as it is often a source of bleeding at this stage). The acetabulum is prepped and reamed to the appropriate size, in this case for a 48 mm cup. The cup is press fit into place with the appropriate zero degree liner. Attention is then turned to the femur. The leg is placed in figure four to facilitate elevation of the femur. A lateral retractor is placed to retract the TFL. A long-tooth double-footed retractor is placed at the superior lateral greater trochanter to expose the superior capsule. A triangle of superior capsule is then removed. The double-footed retractor is then placed over the top of the greater trochanter between the trochanter and the insertion of the gluteus medius, thus minimizing the potential for damage to the gluteus medius muscle. A vertical incision in the superior capsule is then made and carried over the superior-posterior trochanter. Once done, the femur is elevated with a bone hook. The lighted anterior acetabular retractor is then removed, and a double-footed retractor is placed over the lesser trochanter.

Access to the femur is now accomplished by repositioning the leg (still in external rotation) into adduction with the knee fully extended. Of importance, *no* extension of the limb is required for full exposure of the proximal femur with this technique. An angled curette is used to sound the femoral canal, and then the femur is broached to the appropriate size component, in this case a size 6. The femoral head and neck are trialed and full stability and equal leg lengths are confirmed. This represents an important advantage of performing the surgical procedure without encumbering the leg using a special table. Small adjustments in offset and neck length can substantially improve stability and leg length with this technique, something that is not possible to assess using fluoroscopy of the hip as is done when a special table is used. The final femoral components (stem and ceramic head) are inserted and the hip is reduced. The wound is again checked for bleeding—vessels previously identified during the exposure and cauterized may resume bleeding because of the manipulations of the operation. The wound is then closed in layers with absorbable suture (monocryl in the superficial layers) and glue on the skin. A silicone-based dressing was placed.

2.3.7 Intraoperative Challenges

Challenges and solutions: Correct identification of the surgical interval is crucial to avoid damage to the LFCN and the femoral nerve and to avoid muscle damage by remaining within the true internervous plane. The ASIS is easily identified in most patients and is the origin of the sartorius and the anterior border of the TFL. Making the incision distal and lateral to this landmark and avoiding medial dissection minimize risk to the LFCN. For larger patients, the location of the ASIS can be confirmed after initial skin dissection by palpation through the subcutaneous fat and adjust the dissection accordingly.

- Correct identification of the TFL can be confirmed by noting the purple hue of the muscle belly and the perforating vessels that are notably absent from the medially located sartorius. Knowledge of muscular anatomy in relation to the femoral neck and capsule are key to ensure that muscles are handled carefully and not violated.
- Careful retractor placement ensures the protection of muscles and nervous structures. The femoral nerve is medial to the anterior acetabulum, and care should be taken that retractors inserted over the anterior rim of the acetabulum are directed toward the opposite kidney and always placed under direct visualization. Retraction of the anterior retractor should be done carefully.
- Identification and cauterization of the circumflex vessels with re-inspection prior to closure minimizes the risk of postoperative hematoma.
- During exposure of the femur, it is important to release the superior and superomedial capsule to allow elevation of the femur out of the wound. The positioning of the leg in figure four helps with exposure of the superior capsule for excision. As the femur is elevated, further release of the superior and posterior capsule can be performed as needed. To complete elevation of the femur, a double-footed retractor is placed over the greater trochanter, while the entire thigh and leg are externally rotated and adducted with the knee straight.
- Intraoperative fracture of the femur is prevented by inserting the femoral component by hand (no attached mechanical inserter) and then impacted into place using a gentle force directed distally and laterally.
- After placement of components, the wound should again be thoroughly checked for bleeding before closure.
- We recommend closure with absorbable suture and subcutaneous skin suture with skin glue and a silicon base dressing to help prevent wound complications. This dressing is kept in place for 1 week to limit external contamination of the wound.

Unanticipated problems and solution: An unanticipated problem that occurred postoperatively was the loosening of the acetabular component (Fig. 2.5). This was addressed with a revision of the acetabular component through the direct anterior approach on a regular table (Fig. 2.6).

Thorough description of decision-making, including the reason for the final decision: The direct anterior approach can be used for revising components, and the identical setup on a regular table can be used for the revision. In this case, only the acetabular component needed revision, for which the direct anterior approach gives excellent exposure. In cases needing femoral component revision, especially those requiring ETO, an extended incision may be used that tracks posterior and lateral at the distal aspect of the standard DA incision. The acetabular bone was inspected to determine that there was NO acetabular fracture responsible for the early loosening. A larger cup with screws to augment fixation was used during the revision because the original press fit had not adequately stabilized the component.

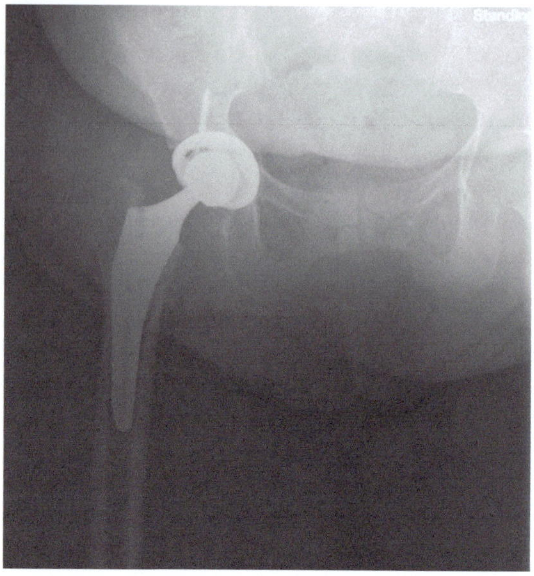

Fig. 2.6 The cup was revised through a DA approach, and a larger cup with screws was placed

2.3.8 Postoperative Radiographs

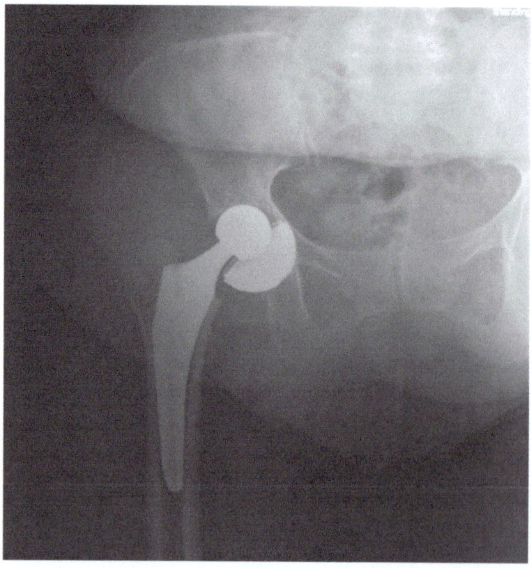

Fig. 2.5 Postoperatively, the cup came loose

2.3.9 Postoperative Management

Chemoprophylaxis and anticoagulant treatment period: ASA 81 mg for 1 month

Gait/limb loading until full loading: WBAT, no restrictions, even after the revision surgery

2.3.10 Follow-Up and Complications

The acetabular cup came loose postoperatively. This was treated with revision to a larger cup with screws through a DA approach.

2.3.11 Discussion [18, 35, 42, 43]

Advantages of the applied method: The DA approach in an internervous plane with minimal muscle disruption. It can be performed on a regular table with the patient supine so that stability and leg length can be easily checked. For the vast majority of patients, a porous-coated acetabular component can be placed without screws. Screws can be used at the discretion of the surgeon to supplement fixation but should not be relied upon for primary fixation of the component. Screws may put neurovascular and pelvic structures at risk, and as such, they should be used judiciously in primary total hip surgery only when supplemental fixation is required [43].

Disadvantages of the method: The lateral femoral cutaneous nerve is at risk if the approach is not performed correctly. As for all approaches, the femoral and sciatic nerve is at risk as well.

Alternative evidence-based techniques for the case: There are multiple papers describing alternative approaches for total hip arthroplasty.

Why is the chosen technique better for this case? The senior author is very experienced in direct anterior approach and can perform the operation efficiently with minimal complications.

Indications and contraindications for your technique: Indications are the need for a total hip replacement. There are no strict contraindications.

Learning curve and how to manage complications: The learning curve for this approach is estimated to be 40–100 cases.

Level of evidence concerning the superiority of this method against others: Level IV.

References

1. Petis S, Howard JL, Lanting BL, Vasarhelyi EM. Surgical approach in primary total hip arthroplasty: anatomy, technique and clinical outcomes. Can J Surg. 2015;58(2):128–39.
2. Hoppenfeld S, DeBoer P, Buckley R. Surgical exposures in orthopaedics: the anatomic approach. Philidelphia, PA: Lippincott Williams & Wilkins; 2009.
3. Ilchmann T. Approaches for primary total hip replacement. Hip Int. 2014;24(10):S2–6.
4. Kwon MS, Kuskowski M, Mulhall K, et al. Does surgical approach affect total hip arthroplasty dislocation rates? Clin Orthop Relat Res. 2006;447:34–8.
5. Ramesh M, O'Byrne JM, McCarthy N, Jarvis A, Mahalingham K, Cashman WF. Damage to the superior gluteal nerve after the Hardinge approach to the hip. J Bone Joint Surg Br. 1996;78(6):903–6.
6. Khan T, Knowles D. Damage to the superior gluteal nerve during the direct lateral approach to the hip: a cadaveric study. J Arthroplast. 2007;22:1198–200.
7. Picado CH, Garcia F, Marques W. Damage to the superior gluteal nerve after direct lateral approach to the hip. Clin Orthop Relat Res. 2007;455:209–11.
8. Lachiewicz PF. Abductor tendon tears of the hip: evaluation and management. J Am Acad Orthop Surg. 2011;19:385–91.
9. Miozzari HH, Dora C, Clark J, et al. Late repair of abductor avulsion after the transgluteal approach for hip arthroplasty. J Arthroplasty. 2010;25:450–7.e1.
10. Howell GE, Biggs R, Bourne R. Prevalence of abductor mechanism tears of the hips in patients with osteoarthritis. J Arthroplast. 2001;16:121–3.
11. Iorio R, Healy W, Warren P, et al. Lateral trochanteric pain following primary total hip arthroplasty. J Arthroplast. 2006;21:233–6.
12. Valente G, Taddei F, Jonkers I. Influence of weak hip abductor muscles on joint contact forces during normal walking: probabilistic modeling analysis. J Biomech. 2013;46:2186–93.
13. Hendel D, Yasin M, Garti A, et al. Fracture of the great trochanter during hip replacement: a retrospective analysis of 21/372 cases. Acta Orthop Scand. 2002;73:295–7.
14. Pellicci PM, Potter H, Foo L, et al. MRI shows biologic restoration of posterior soft tissue repairs after THA. Clin Orthop Relat Res. 2009;467:940–5.
15. Chiu FY, Chen C, Chung T, et al. The effect of posterior capsulorrhaphy in primary total hip arthroplasty: a prospective randomized study. J Arthroplast. 2000;15:194–9.
16. Farrell CM, Springer B, Haidukewych G, et al. Motor nerve palsy following primary total hip arthroplasty. J Bone Joint Surg Am. 2005;87:2619–25.
17. Schmalzried TP, Amstutz H, Dorey F. Nerve palsy associated with total hip replacement: risk factors and prognosis. J Bone Joint Surg Am. 1991;73:1074–80.
18. Post ZD, Orozco F, Diaz-Ledezma C, Hozack WJ, Ong A. Direct anterior approach for total hip arthroplasty: indications, technique, and results. J Am Acad Orthop Surg. 2014;22:595–603.
19. Matta JM, Shahrdar C, Ferguson T. Single-incision anterior approach for total hip arthroplasty on an orthopaedic table. Clin Orthop Relat Res. 2005;441(441):115–24.
20. De Geest T, Fennema P, Lenaerts G, De Loore G. Adverse effects associated with the direct anterior approach for total hip arthroplasty: a Bayesian meta-analysis. Arch Orthop Trauma Surg. 2015;135(8):1183–92.
21. Siguier T, Siguier M, Brumpt B. Mini- incision anterior approach does not increase dislocation rate: a study of 1037 total hip replacements. Clin Orthop Relat Res. 2004;426:164–73.
22. Sariali E, Leonard P, Mamoudy P. Dislocation after total hip arthroplasty using Hueter anterior approach. J Arthroplast. 2008;23(2):266–72.

23. Bhandari M, Matta JM, Dodgin D, et al. Anterior total hip arthroplasty collaborative investigators: outcomes following the single-incision anterior approach to total hip arthroplasty: a multicenter observational study. Orthop Clin North Am. 2009;40(3):329–42.
24. Seng BE, Berend KR, Ajluni AF, Lombardi AV Jr. Anterior-supine minimally invasive total hip arthroplasty: defining the learning curve. Orthop Clin North Am. 2009;40(3):343–50.
25. Goulding K, Beaulé PE, Kim PR, Fazekas A. Incidence of lateral femoral cutaneous nerve neuropraxia after anterior approach hip arthroplasty. Clin Orthop Relat Res. 2010;468(9):2397–404.
26. Bhargava T, Goytia RN, Jones LC, Hungerford MW. Lateral femoral cutaneous nerve impairment after direct anterior approach for total hip arthroplasty. Orthopedics. 2010;33(7):472.
27. Jewett BA, Collis DK. High complication rate with anterior total hip arthroplasties on a fracture table. Clin Orthop Relat Res. 2011;469(2):503–7.
28. Alecci V, Valente M, Crucil M, et al. Comparison of primary total hip replacements performed with a direct anterior versus the standard lateral approach: perioperative findings. J Orthop Traumatol. 2011;12:123–9.
29. Restrepo C, Parvizi J, Pour A, et al. Prospective randomized study of two surgical approaches for total hip arthroplasty. J Arthroplasty. 2010;25:671–9.e1.
30. Goebel S, Steinert A, Schillinger J, et al. Reduced post-operative pain in total hip arthroplasty after minimal-invasive anterior approach. Int Orthop. 2012;36:491–8.
31. Bremer AK, Kalberer F, Pfirrmann CW, Dora C. Soft-tissue changes in hip abductor muscles and tendons after total hip replacement: comparison between the direct anterior and the transgluteal approaches. J Bone Joint Surg Br. 2011;93:886–9.
32. De Anta-Díaz B, Serralta-Gomis J, Lizaur-Utrilla A, Benavidez E, López-Prats FA. No differences between direct anterior and lateral approach for primary total hip arthroplasty related to muscle damage or functional outcome. Int Orthop. 2016;40(10):2025–30.
33. Yue C, Kang P, Pei F. Comparison of direct anterior and lateral approaches in total hip arthroplasty: a systematic review and meta-analysis (PRISMA). Medicine (Baltimore). 2015;94(50):e2126.
34. Higgins BT, Barlow DR, Heagerty NE, Lin TJ. Anterior vs. posterior approach for total hip arthroplasty, a systematic review and meta-analysis. J Arthroplast. 2015;30(3):419–34.
35. Barrett WP, Turner S, Leopold J. Prospective randomized study of direct anterior vs posterolateral approach for total hip arthroplasty. J Arthroplast. 2013;28:1634–8.
36. Bergin PF, Doppelt J, Kephart C, et al. Comparison of minimally invasive direct damage markers. J Bone Joint Surg Am. 2011;93:1392–8.
37. Berstock JR, Blom AW, Beswick AD. A systematic review and meta-analysis of complications following the posterior and lateral surgical approaches to total hip arthroplasty. Ann R Coll Surg Engl. 2015;97(1):11–6.
38. Jolles BM, Bogoch ER. Posterior versus lateral surgical approach for total hip arthroplasty in adults with osteoarthritis. Cochrane Database Syst Rev. 2006;3:CD003828.
39. Mukka SS, Sayed-Noor AS. An update on surgical approaches in hip arthoplasty: lateral versus posterior approach. Hip Int. 2014;24(Suppl 10):S7–S11.
40. Barber TC, Roger D, Goodman S, et al. Early outcome of total hip arthroplasty using the direct lateral vs the posterior surgical approach. Orthopedics. 1996;19:873–5.
41. Witzleb WC, Stephan L, Krummenauer F et al. Short-term outcome after posterior versus lateral surgical approach for total hip arthro- plasty: a randomized clinical trial. Eur J Med Res. 2009;14:256–63.
42 Martin CT, Pugely AJ, Gao Y, Clark CR. A comparison of hospital length of stay and short-term morbidity between the anterior and the posterior approaches to total hip arthroplasty. J Arthroplasty. 2013;28:849–54. doi:10.1016/j.arth.2012.10.029.
43 Tabata T, Kaku N, Hara K, Tsumura H. Initial stability of cementless acetabular cups: press-fit and screw fixation interaction—an in vitro biomechanical study. Eur J Orthop Surg Traumatol. 2015;25:497–502. doi:10.1007/s00590-014-1571-4.

3 Implant Fixation

Eustathios Kenanidis, Theodosios H. Stamatopoulos, Georgios Kynigopoulos, Zakareya Gamie, Eleftherios Tsiridis, Nicholas M. Desy, Rafael J. Sierra, Richard L. Purcell, Charles A. Engh Jr, Albert Wee Tun Ngu, Vaibhav Punjabi, and Fares S. Haddad

3.1 Current Concepts

E. Kenanidis, T.H. Stamatopoulos, G. Kynigopoulos, Z. Gamie, and E. Tsiridis

There are available long-term survival data of primary THA coming from single referral centres or surgeons, large national population-based registry studies or unpublished registry data. Long-term studies from single centres or surgeons that usually referred to a particular type of implant [1–5] have reported survival free of revision greater than 90% at ten years and 80% at twenty five years [1–3, 6–9]. Studies from experts do not support just one technique, and excellent implant survivorship has been reported for cemented and uncemented THAs [1, 10–12].

Large national and regional samples have usually higher revision rates than referral centres due to the heterogeneity of the patients and hospital factors and multiple doctors involved. It is supported that large population-based studies from national registries provide results that can be more easily generalized to the group receiving THA

E. Kenanidis, M.D., Ph.D., M.Sc. (✉)
T.H. Stamatopoulos, M.D.
G. Kynigopoulos, M.D.
Academic Orthopaedic Unit, Aristotle University Medical School, Thessaloniki, Greece

Z. Gamie, B.Sc., M.B.Ch.B., M.R.C.S.
Northern Institute for Cancer Research, Paul O'Gorman Building, Medical School, Newcastle University, Newcastle upon Tyne, UK
e-mail: ugm1zg@doctors.org.uk

E. Tsiridis, M.D., Ph.D., F.A.C.S., F.R.C.S. (✉)
Academic Orthopaedic Unit, Papageorgiou General Hospital, Aristotle University Medical School, Thessaloniki, Greece
e-mail: etsiridis@doctors.org.uk

N.M. Desy, M.D., F.R.C.S.C.
Section of Orthopaedic Surgery, University of Calgary, Calgary, AB, Canada
e-mail: Desy.Nicholas@mayo.edu

R.J. Sierra, M.D.
Mayo Clinic, College of Medicine, Rochester, MN, USA
e-mail: Sierra.Rafael@mayo.edu

R.L. Purcell, M.D.
Anderson Orthopaedic Research Institute, Alexandria, VA, USA

Walter Reed Military Medical Center, Bethesda, MD, USA
e-mail: rhopper@aori.org

C.A. Engh Jr, M.D.
Anderson Orthopaedic Research Institute, Alexandria, VA, USA

Inova Mount Vernon Joint Replacement Center, Alexandria, VA, USA
e-mail: andy@andersonclinic.com

A.W.T. Ngu, B.M., M.R.C.S. · F.S. Haddad, B.Sc., M.D., M.Ch., F.R.C.S.
University College London Hospital, London, UK
e-mail: fsh@fareshaddad.net

V. Punjabi, M.B.B.S., M.S., F.R.A.C.S., F.A.A.
Wollongong Hospital, Wollongong, Australia

E. Tsiridis (ed.), *The Adult Hip - Master Case Series and Techniques*,
https://doi.org/10.1007/978-3-319-64177-5_3

[13]. Population-based studies from Finland [8, 9, 14–17], Sweden [18–20], Norway [21–23] or England [24] evaluating the 10-year revision risk following THA reported revision-free survival for cemented prostheses from 88 to 95% and for uncemented prostheses from 80 to 85%. A recent meta-analysis of reports with more than ten years of follow-up from national registry-based studies demonstrated that older patients who live for ten years following THA experience a 10-year revision risk of about 10%, while younger patients have a slightly greater risk of revision [13]. Survival of hybrid implants was only reported in Swedish registry, reaching a 10-year survival of 92.7% [13].

Taking into account the methodological complexity of implant failure studies, one should also consider possible confounding factors as the age, activity level, preoperative diagnosis, etc. Both implant fixation and patient age influence the prosthesis revision rates in the large population or community-based samples. The uncemented implants are usually used in younger patients with a greater activity that possibly may have an impact on the survival. Corbett et al. [13] reported that patients less than sixty years old had a 10-year survival ranging from 72% in Finland to 86% in Swedish registry and for older patients from 90% in Finland to 97% in Swedish registry. The majority of patients suffered preoperatively from osteoarthritis [13]. The cemented implants had a lower revision risk than the uncemented implants both in younger and in older patients. It is likely, however, that this finding is due to residual confounding factors as the age and activity level. Another confounding factor when someone tries to interpret implant revision data is the number of patients still at risk for revision THA at long-term follow-up. What the sample at long-term follow-up is usually small due to loss to follow-up, revision or death of patients; thus, revision-free survival estimates may be based on a minority of the entire sample. Furnes et al. [22] reported that of 37,215 THAs in Norway for OA, just 2384 hips were still at risk at ten years, which means the estimated survival rate of 88.8% was based upon the data from just 6% of the original sample.

There are also valuable unpublished data from several other registries in countries outside Scandinavia and England [23, 24]. The Australian registry demonstrated higher survival rates compared to others [23]; the estimated 10-year survival rate of the Australian registry was 94.1% and for New Zealand 93.5% [23, 24]. The Australian registry also reported similar survival for cemented and uncemented implants [23]. The disparity of the published results between various national registries may reflect differences across countries in technique, materials or indications, control for potential confounders or different prosthesis survival experience.

Although the reported survival of uncemented implants seems to be lower than cemented, paradoxically the prevalence of uncemented THA is steadily increasing in many countries worldwide during the last years [25]. There is a wide variability in the type of fixation used in different countries. It is estimated that 86% of all THAs performed in the USA are uncemented; the majority of the remaining are hybrid, and only 1% of all THAs are cemented [26]. Fixation strategies are different in Scandinavian countries and especially Sweden where the majority of THAs performed, are cemented, and only 15% are uncemented. Sweden and Norway have the lowest prevalence of uncemented implants, whereas Denmark and Canada the greatest [25]. The largest absolute increase in uncemented fixation use was reported by the Danish (from 47 to 68%) and England-Wales (from 25 to 43%) registries [25].

In a recent systematic review of fixation methods and results from registries, Troelsen et al. [25] showed that cemented fixation resulted in statistically significantly lower revision rates than uncemented fixation in the age groups greater than 65 years old of all registries surveyed (Australian, New Zealand, England and Wales and Denmark) except in Australian in age groups between 65 and 75 years. There was no difference also in revision rate between fixation types for age groups lower than 50 years except New Zealand where cemented had worse results than uncemented. Cemented fixation resulted in lower revision rates than hybrid (cemented femur) fixation in the age group greater than 65 years for England and Wales and Denmark greater than 60 [25]. Australian registry demonstrated higher risk for revision of cemented versus hybrid in the age group of 60–74 years. Although no difference was found in age groups lower than 60 years in New Zealand registry, hybrid implants had better survival in age groups lower than 60 years [25]. The comparison between hybrid (cemented femur) and uncemented implants is less clear, and only the Australian and New Zealand registries reported significantly reduced revision risks when fixation was hybrid (cemented femur) compared with an uncemented fixation for the oldest age group. In Denmark registry, there was higher risk for revision after hybrid versus uncemented THA for all age groups lower than 75 years old [25]. On the contrary, in Australian registry, the reported risk was similar between hybrid and uncemented THA in age groups lower than 75 years.

In a previous meta-analysis, Morshed et al. [27] found superiority of cemented fixation over uncemented fixation not just in the older age groups. The authors however recognized that the performance of uncemented implants improved with time. Hailer et al. [20] studied 170,000 cemented or uncemented THAs from the Swedish arthroplasty registry and showed superiority for ten years' survival of cemented in all groups. They found a poorer performance of uncemented cups and an increased risk of revision resulting from periprosthetic fractures in uncemented stems. However, they recognized continuous improvement of uncemented cups by the introduction of new developments. In a recent register-based cohort study reporting the outcome of 275,000 cemented and uncemented THAs, McMinn et al. [28] reported a small but significantly lower risk of revision for cemented THAs but significant lower mortality rate in uncemented THAs. Possible confounding factors, however, were not excluded. In another systematic review, van der Veen et al. [29] supported that a higher annual wear rate may be encountered in uncemented acetabular components as compared to cemented components.

3.2 Case Title: Bilateral Simultaneous THAs Using Uncemented Monobloc All HXLP Acetabular Components

E. Kenanidis and E. Tsiridis

Advanced osteoarthritis bilaterally. Osteonecrosis and complete obliteration of the joint space on both sides. Bilateral simultaneous THA using monobloc acetabular all poly components (Mathys Vitamys) and ceramic heads (Fig. 3.1)

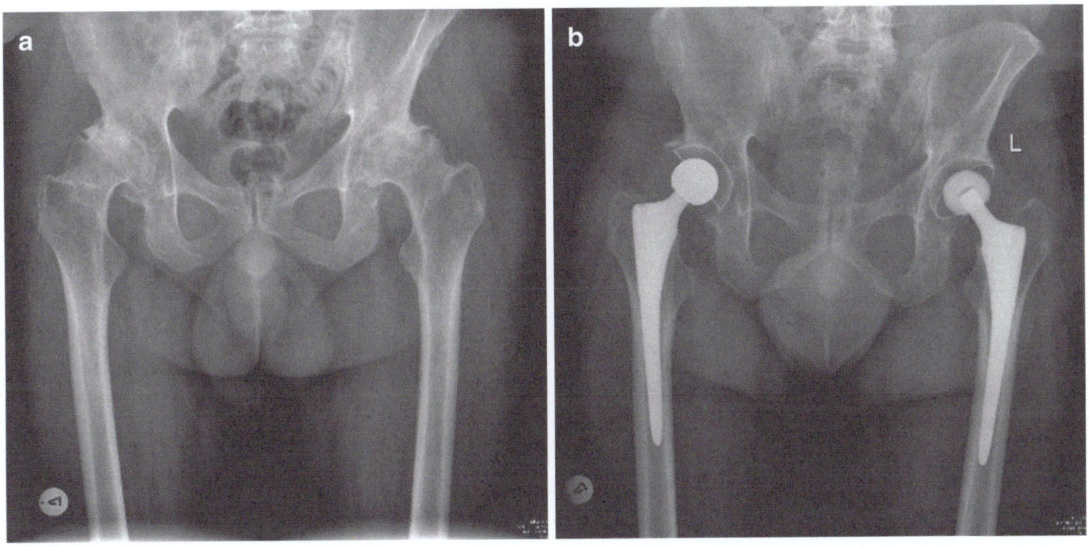

Fig. 3.1 (**a**) Preoperative pelvic x-ray (**b**) Postoperative pelvic x-ray demonstrating bilateral uncemented monoblock THAs

3.3 Case Title: Primary Cemented Total Hip Arthroplasty

E. Kenanidis and E. Tsiridis

3.3.1 Demographics

Age: 43
Sex: Male, retired army officer (for medical reasons)
BMI: 30

3.3.2 Relevant Past Medical History

Principal pathologies: Rheumatoid arthritis, osteoporosis and pulmonary fibrosis.

Medication: Injection of etanercept, methotrexate, alendronate, calcium carbonate, prednisolone and sulfasalazine.

History of presenting complaint: Pain of the left hip.

3.3.3 Preoperative Radiological Assessment/Imaging (Fig. 3.2)

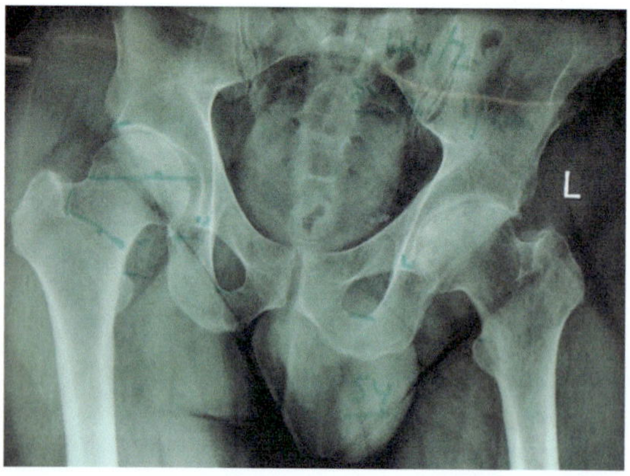

Fig. 3.2 This is a typical rheumatoid arthritis radiograph demonstrating the global destruction of the articular cartilage of the left hip joint and evident osteoporosis from disuse osteopenia and long-term use of corticosteroids

3.3.4 Preoperative Planning

Diagnosis: Osteoarthritis of the left hip (RA) (Fig. 3.2).

Possible treatment options: For those people who have severe rheumatoid arthritis, cemented implants performing very well compared to uncemented implants. Although there is some conflicting evidence for the latter, in our opinion and experience, cement allows for early rehabilitation and better long-term results and survival of the prosthesis.

Chosen treatment method: Cemented cup Depuy 43 mm/28 mm Monobloc, cemented hip stem Stryker Exeter 44–2, 150 mm and ceramic femoral head Stryker 28 mm, 0 mm.

3.3.5 Surgical Note

This is a box standard cemented Exeter triple hip arthroplasty including both sides. The third-generation cementing technique was employed using bone aspirators for blood and intensive drying of the cancellous bone before pressurizing the cement in. A minimum of 2 mm of cement mantle was necessary for better interlocking with the deficient cancellous bone (Fig. 3.3).
Patient's position: Lateral decubitus.
Type of anaesthesia: General.
Surgical approach: Direct Superior.

3.3.6 Postoperative Radiographs (Fig. 3.3)

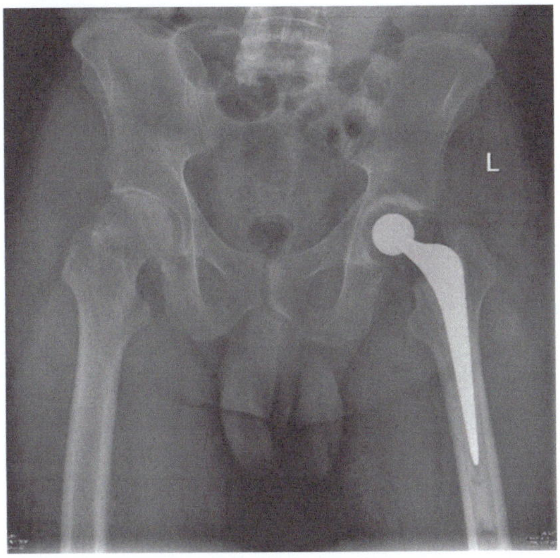

Fig. 3.3 The leg length has been recovered compared to the preoperative radiograph; the cement mantle is adequate on both sides, and the orientation of the implant is satisfactory

3.3.7 Postoperative Management

Chemoprophylaxis and anticoagulant treatment period: Cefuroxime 750 mg 1 × 3 for one day and ciprofloxacin 400 mg 1 × 2 for two days, vancomycin 500 mg 1 × 2 for two days, tinzaparin 1 × 1 for the days of hospitalization and then rivaroxaban for thirty days.

Gait/limb loading until full loading: Partial weight-bearing for four weeks. At six weeks, full weight-bearing and without an assistive device.

3.3.8 Follow-Up and Complications

It is usually expected to wait a minimum of two weeks after surgery before starting the medication again for the treatment of rheumatoid arthritis. The reason is to protect wound healing and prevent joint infection. Although there is no significant evidence to suggest extensive perioperative antibiotic prophylaxis, in our experience, we advise extending the prophylaxis to five days instead of 24 h postoperatively. In this particular case, obesity was an additional reason for doing so.

3.4 Case Title: Uncemented Primary Total Hip Arthroplasty Metal Back Socket

E. Kenanidis and E. Tsiridis

3.4.1 Demographics

Age: 69
Sex: Female

3.4.2 Relevant Past Medical History

Principal pathologies: None.

History of presenting complaint: Pain of the right hip worsen in the last months.

3.4.3 Preoperative Radiological Assessment/Imaging (Fig. 3.4)

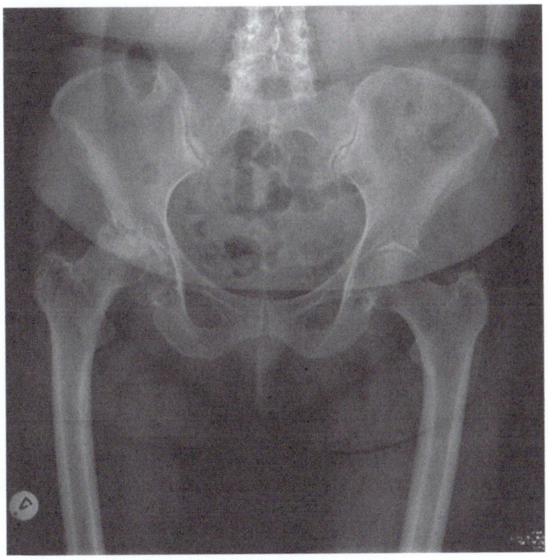

Fig. 3.4 Osteoarthritis of the right hip

3.4.4 Preoperative Planning

Diagnosis: Osteoarthritis of the right hip (Fig. 3.4).

Chosen treatment method: Uncemented acetabular shell Depuy PINNACLE POROCOAT 50 mm, polyethylene Depuy PINNACLE MARATHON 32 mm, uncemented hip stem Depuy, size 1, STD, 125 mm and ceramic femoral head Depuy 32 mm, + 9 mm.

3.4.5 Surgical Note

Patient's position: Lateral decubitus

Type of anaesthesia: General

Surgical approach: Direct Superior

3.4.6 Postoperative Radiographs (Figs. 3.5 and 3.6)

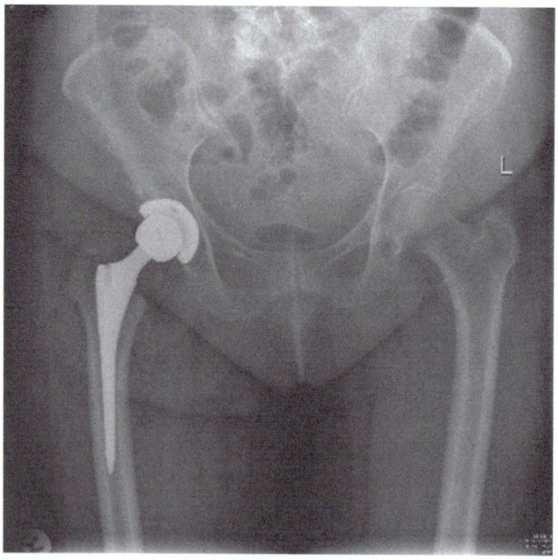

Fig. 3.5 AP of the right hip, first day

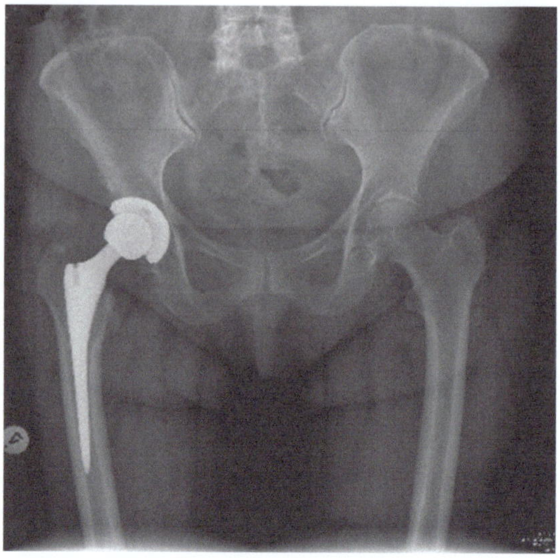

Fig. 3.6 AP of the right hip, first month

3.4.7 Postoperative Management

Chemoprophylaxis and anticoagulant treatment period: Vancomycin 500 mg 1 × 2 for two days, cefuroxime 750 mg 1 × 3 for two days, enoxaparin 1 × 1 for two days and then rivaroxaban 10 mg for thirty days.

Gait/limb loading until full loading: Partial weight-bearing for four weeks. At six weeks, full weight-bearing.

3.5 Case Title: Ceramic on Monobloc Vitamin E Enhanced HXLP Titanium Spray Coated: THA with Impaction Autografting of the Acetabulum

E. Kenanidis and E. Tsiridis

3.5.1 Demographics

Age: 69
Sex: Male
BMI: 28

3.5.2 Relevant Past Medical History

Principal pathologies: Hyperuricemia.

Previous surgical procedures: Appendectomy 40 years ago.

Medication: Allopurinol.

History of presenting complaint: Pain due to arthritis as potential contribution of high uric acid arthritis.

3.5.3 Clinical Examination

Symptoms: Pain, inability to walk and night pain.

Range of motion: 0–90°, limited internal/external rotation and the joint was locked in a protrusion type of deformity due to extensive erosions. Unable to abduct and adduct.

Specific tests: Thomas positive in 25°.

Main disability: Pain all day long and inability to walk.

Scoring if available: HHS 65.

Neurovascular evaluation: Intact.

3.5.4 Preoperative Radiological Assessment/Imaging (Fig. 3.7)

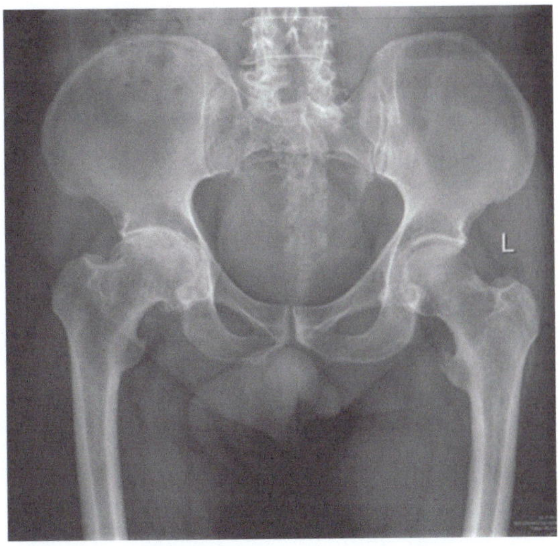

Fig. 3.7 Significant erosions of the right hip. Protrusion deformity with deepening of the inner plate with sclerotic margins. Loss of cancellous bone in the periphery of the socket. Bone quality in general reasonable for the age of the patient

3.5.5 Preoperative Planning

Diagnosis: Osteoarthritis of the right hip (Fig. 3.7).

Possible treatment options: Cemented or uncemented THA.

Chosen treatment method: Uncemented acetabular cup, vitamin E HXLP Mathys 56 mm/36 mm, uncemented femoral stem Mathys 10 STD and femoral head Mathys 36 L.

Selection of implants if applicable and rationale: Sufficient bone stock for uncemented implantation. A decision to enhance the acetabular cancellous bone stock using impaction autografting.

3.5.6 Surgical Note

Acetabular preparation: With the patient in lateral decubitus position, a direct superior approach was used to approach the hip. The acetabulum was easily exposed in a standard way, and the sequential reaming allowed a trial 56 × 36 mm acetabular component to be inserted. Reaming was difficult in places due to sclerosis. Smaller reamers are used to remove the sclerotic surface along with curved osteotomes. Eventually, a bleeding cancellous bone was exposed; however, the lack of cancellous bone stock and the medialization of the reaming were not acceptable. The decision was made to impaction autograft the acetabular bed using the large available patient's femoral head. The cartilage and the osteophytes were removed using the saw and then the head was divided into several rounded segments before creating 1 cm cartilaginous bone chips. Tight impaction grafting using special impactors was then performed until the new bed was created. Trial socket insertion achieved better position and less medialization with good ream fit of the implant. The real implant was then inserted tightly to the proper direction. The design of this implant is hemispherical thus allowing a better fit to the periphery of the acetabular ream. There is no need for supporting screws.

Femoral preparation: The femur was prepared using the appropriate rasps that compact the bone into an anatomical shape to fit the stem. The stem is collarless, double tapered, anatomic without shoulder and fully coated with hydroxyapatite. Easy rasping and trial reduction are used for assessing the leg length and the offset. A 36 mm ceramic head was used to achieve the final reduction (Fig. 3.8).

3.5.7 Postoperative Radiographs (Fig. 3.8)

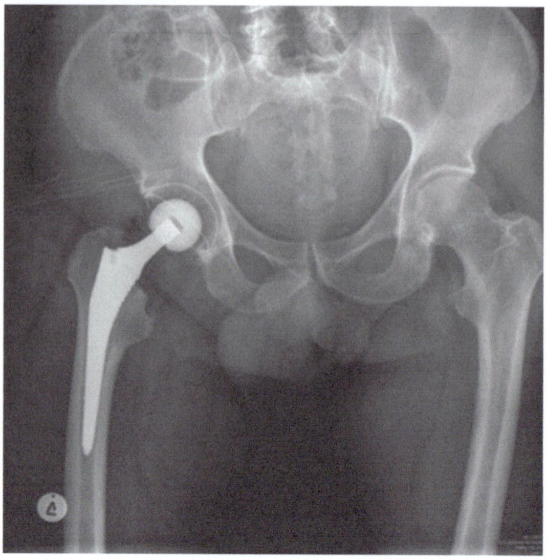

Fig. 3.8 Evident impaction autografting of the acetabular bed bringing the floor more lateral compared to the preoperative radiograph. Proper fit of the socket and the stem and right orientation

3.5.8 Postoperative Management

- *Chemoprophylaxis and anticoagulant treatment period*: Vancomycin 500 mg (one dose preoperatively, two doses postoperatively), cefuroxime 750 mg (one dose preoperatively, two doses postoperatively), enoxaparin 1 × 1 for the days of hospitalization and then rivaroxaban 10 mg 1 × 1 for thirty days.
- *Gait/limb loading until full loading*: Partial weight-bearing for four weeks and then as tolerated.

3.6 Case Title: Hybrid Primary Hip Arthroplasty

Nicholas M. Desy and Rafael J. Sierra

3.6.1 Demographics

Age: 76
Sex: Female.
BMI: 26

3.6.2 Relevant Past Medical History

Principal pathologies: Mild cognitive impairment, osteoporosis and hypercholesterolemia.

Previous surgical procedures: Bilateral total knee arthroplasties, appendectomy and hysterectomy.

Medication: Citalopram, donepezil and acetaminophen.

History of presenting complaint: 76-year-old female presented with bilateral hip and thigh pain which limited her daily activities for the past 2–3 years. She had failed nonoperative treatment methods which included anti-inflammatory medication and steroid injections.

3.6.3 Clinical Examination

Symptoms: Bilateral hip and thigh pain.

Range of motion: Extension-flexion, 0–100°; limited internal rotation due to pain.

Main disability: Pain and difficulty with ambulation.

Scoring: Harris Hip Score = 45.

Neurovascular evaluation: Normal motor and sensory exams of both her feet. She also had palpable pulses which included the dorsalis pedis and posterior tibial arteries.

3.6.4 Preoperative Radiological Assessment/Imaging (Figs. 3.9, 3.10 and 3.11)

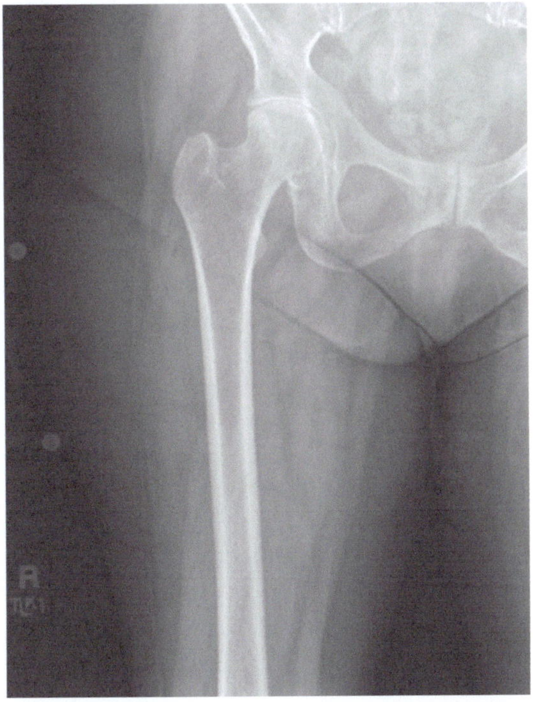

Fig. 3.9 Anteroposterior pelvic X-ray demonstrates significant osteoarthritis in both hips

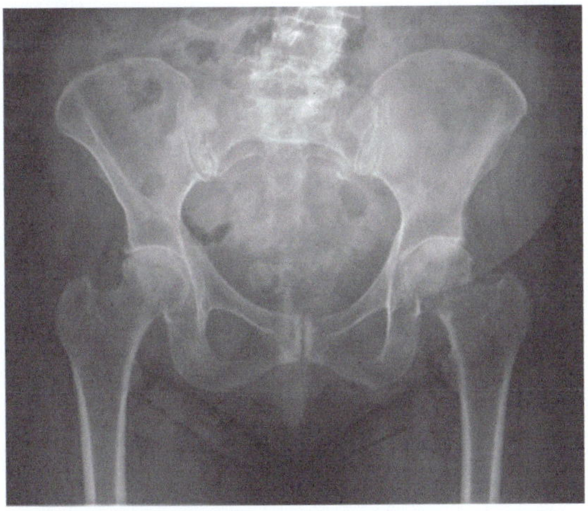

Fig. 3.10 Anteroposterior view of the right hip shows prominent osteoarthritis of the right hip

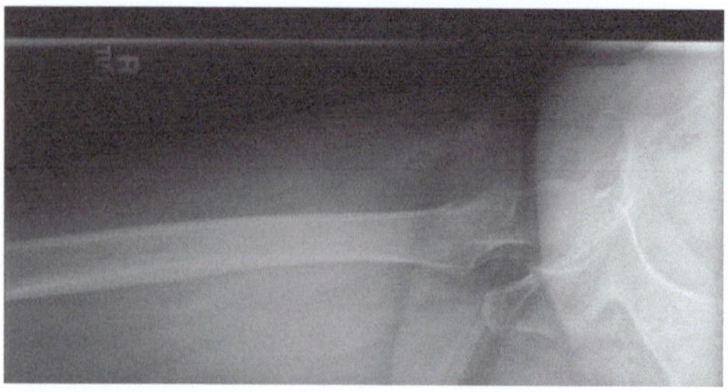

Fig. 3.11 Cross-table lateral X-ray further demonstrates the significant osteoarthritis, especially anteriorly

3.6.5 Preoperative Planning

Diagnosis: Bilateral hip osteoarthritis (Figs. 3.9, 3.10 and 3.11).

Possible treatment options: Staged total hip arthroplasty (THA), cemented versus uncemented femoral stem.

Chosen treatment method: Staged THA beginning with the right side which was more symptomatic.

Selection of implants if applicable and rational: Press-fit uncemented acetabular component and a cemented femoral stem. A cemented femoral stem was chosen as the patient's bone quality was deemed to better fit a cemented stem. In addition, the risk of periprosthetic fractures is lower when compared to press-fit stems [30]. The cemented femoral stem of choice was the Exeter cemented femoral stem (Stryker Howmedica, Kalamazoo, MI, USA).

Expected difficulties: Femoral bone preparation should be meticulous trying to avoid removing cancellous bone that is required for proper cement/bone interdigitation. Obtaining good cement mantle/bone interdigitation.

Strategies to overcome difficulties: Hand reaming and broaching, leaving 3 mm of cancellous bone in zone 1. Removing soft tissue from zone 7. Maintenance of pressurization within the femur during the cementing process which is important for cement penetration into the surrounding cancellous bone.

Templating: This patient was templated for a 52 mm uncemented acetabular shell and a 37.5, 0 cemented Exeter femoral component.

3.6.6 Surgical Note

Patient's position: Lateral decubitus position

Type of anaesthesia: Regional anaesthesia

Surgical approach: Standard posterior approach

Main steps:

1. Exposure and dislocation of the hip joint.
2. Femoral neck resection according to a preoperatively templated neck length.
3. Exposure and preparation of the acetabulum underreaming by 1 mm.
4. Implantation of a press-fit uncemented acetabular shell and screws as needed.
5. Preparation of the proximal femur with hand reamers and broaches.
6. Placement of an appropriately sized cement plug.
7. Irrigation of the femoral canal with a pulsatile lavage.
8. Insertion of a plastic suction catheter deep into the femoral canal.
9. Epinephrine-soaked swabs are placed into the femoral canal followed by dry swabs.
10. The proximal femur is then filled with cement in a retrograde fashion using a cement gun and long nozzle.
11. The plastic suction catheter is removed early as the cement is being placed.
12. Once the proximal femur is completely filled, it is pressurized with an excellent seal for a few seconds.
13. The dried 60-degree preheated stem is placed with one hand on the stem and the thumb from the opposite hand over the medial neck to increase the pressure during stem insertion.
14. Excess cement is removed and a horse collar is placed around the neck of the stem until the cement fully cures.

15. A trial of range of motion and stability is completed with a trial femoral head.
16. The final femoral head is placed.

Reconstruction techniques: Uncemented acetabular shell and maintenance of pressure within the femoral canal during cementing of the femoral component (Figs. 3.12 and 3.13).

3.6.7 Intraoperative Challenges

Challenges and solutions: Challenge: poor bone quality from conditions such as osteoporosis. Solution: Utilize a cemented femoral component to minimize iatrogenic intraoperative proximal femur fractures. Challenge: Maintenance of constant pressure during cemented stem insertion. Solution: Placement of the contralateral thumb over the medial neck throughout stem insertion.

Unanticipated problems and solutions: Challenge: Iatrogenic fracture of the proximal femur calcar during preparation. Solution: Increase exposure to identify the extent of the fracture. Place wires or cables around the fracture for stability as needed.

Thorough description of decision-making, including the reason for the final decision: Total hip arthroplasties in patients with poor bone quality can be challenging. Press-fit stems in these situations pose a risk for iatrogenic intraoperative fractures [30]. For that reason, we prefer to implant cemented femoral stems in female patients over the age of 70 years and male patients over the age of 80 years given the increased frequency of osteoporotic bone. The patient described was female and over 70 years old with the comorbidity of osteoporosis, which is why we felt a cemented femoral stem would be appropriate.

3.6.8 Postoperative Radiographs (Figs. 3.12 and 3.13)

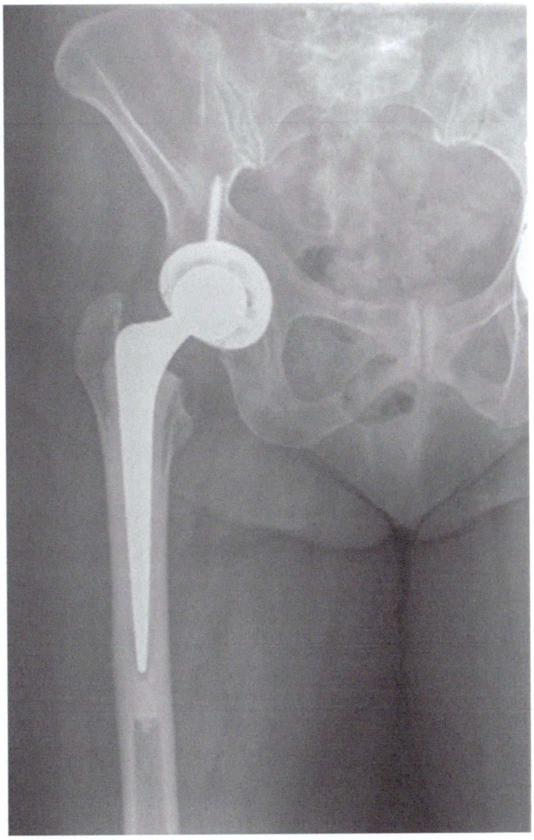

Fig. 3.12 Anteroposterior X-ray of the right hip demonstrates an uncemented acetabular component with screws for additional fixation and a cemented femoral component. Note the adequate cement mantle

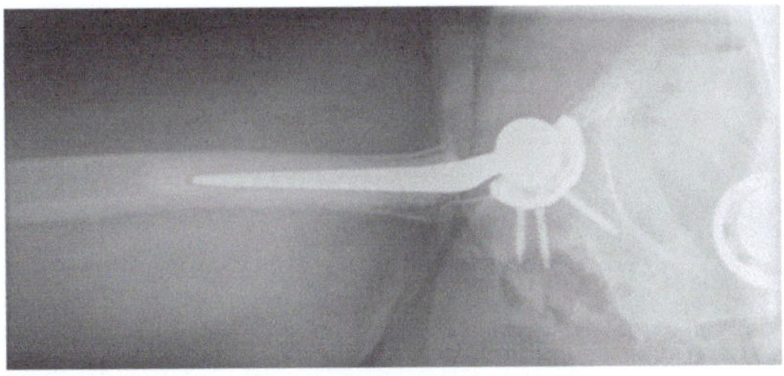

Fig. 3.13 Lateral X-ray shows the acetabular component with the correct version and the placement of three screws. The cement mantle for the femoral stem can again be seen surrounding the entire portion of the stem within the proximal femur

3.6.9 Postoperative Management

Chemoprophylaxis and anticoagulant treatment period: Aspirin 325 mg twice a day and compression stockings for six weeks. The patient also receives omeprazole while on aspirin. Sequential compression devices are also worn during the hospitalization period.

Gait/limb loading until full loading: Weight-bearing as tolerated immediately after surgery with no restrictions.

3.6.10 Follow-Up and Complications

No postoperative complications. Harris Hip Score = 85.

3.6.11 Discussion

Advantages of the applied method: Primary THA has been a successful operation for most patients. The debate between the superiority of uncemented and cemented femoral stems continues within the literature with no clear answer. There are several advantages to cemented femoral stems which include the decreased risk of iatrogenic proximal femur fractures in weaker bone as they do not rely on a press fit for initial stability and the ability to adjust version as the stem is implanted into the cement mantle. The positive long-term results of the cemented Exeter polished femoral component has been extensively documented [31]. Furthermore, the UK has demonstrated increased survivorship for cemented THAs as compared to uncemented hips [32].

Disadvantages of the method: The main disadvantage with cemented femoral stems is the risk of sudden death during pressurization of the cement within the femoral canal. This is thought to be caused by cement debris, fat and blood that embolizes to the lungs during cement pressurization and stem insertion which leads to cardiopulmonary collapse. The act of judicious lavage and suctioning of the femoral canal prior to pressurization has been credited with a decreased risk of sudden death [33]. Furthermore, in a recent study, cemented stems were found to have a higher revision rate for any reason at a mean follow-up of 6.5 years in patients less than 70 years old [34].

Alternative evidence-based techniques for the case: An uncemented femoral stem.

Why is the chosen technique better for this case? Press-fit femoral stems pose a higher risk of intraoperative fracture of the proximal femur in patients with weaker bone quality. A cemented femoral stem minimizes this risk because a press fit is not required for initial mechanical stability which is provided by the cement mantle.

Indications and contraindications for your technique: Indications: Any patient with weaker bone quality caused by conditions such as osteoporosis, female patients older than 70 years old and male patients older than 80 years old. Contraindications: Patients with an active infection or with comorbidities that make it unsafe for surgery.

Learning curve and how to manage complications: The most critical part of the learning curve with this technique is adequately preparing the proximal femur with lavage and suction followed by retrograde cement filling and pressurization. This will allow for an excellent cement mantle that interdigitates with the surrounding cancellous bone. Complications include those that are inherent to any primary THA such as acute and chronic infection, dislocation and nerve injury. The most feared complication associated with cemented femoral stems is sudden death during cement pressurization. To prevent this complication, it is crucial to aggressively lavage and suction the femoral canal prior to instrumentation and place a small suction tube into the femoral canal just prior to cementation. It is also advisable to inform the anaesthesiology team during pressurization and involve them early to monitor the cardiac and respiratory status.

Level of evidence concerning the superiority of this method against others: Level II [35].

3.7 Case Title: Uncemented Primary Total Hip Arthroplasty (Using an Extensively Porous-Coated [Anatomic Medullary Locking, AML] Stem)

Richard L. Purcell and C. Anderson Engh Jr

3.7.1 Demographics

Age: 61
Sex: Female
BMI: 34.1

3.7.2 Relevant Past Medical History

Principal pathologies: Hypertension, hyperlipidaemia and coronary artery disease with previous myocardial infarction.

Previous surgical procedures: Tonsillectomy and adenoidectomy.

Medication: Lisinopril 10 mg daily and Crestor 4 mg nightly.

History of presenting complaint: Our patient was a 61-year-old woman with right hip pain for the past year, predominately located in the groin precipitated by walking. She has difficulty with daily activities such as putting on shoes and socks. She has tried Tylenol with some relief, has received an intra-articular hip injection which only lasted one day and has also performed physical therapy with limited benefit.

3.7.3 Clinical Examination

Symptoms: Right groin pain with walking and daily activities.

Range of motion: Extension: 0°; flexion: 70°; abduction: 20°; adduction: 10°; external rotation: 20°; and internal rotation: 10°.

Specific tests: Antalgic gait.

Main disability: Ability to ambulate.

Neurovascular evaluation: 5/5 DF, PF, EHL and FHL with 2+ DP/PT pulses.

3.7.4 Preoperative Radiological Assessment/Imaging (Figs. 3.14, 3.15, and 3.16)

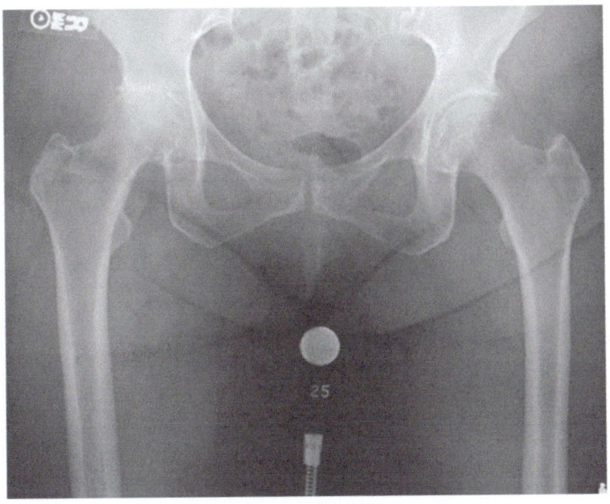

Fig. 3.14 Preoperative AP radiograph demonstrating severe osteoarthritis of the right hip with significant loss of joint space, osteophyte formation and subchondral sclerosis

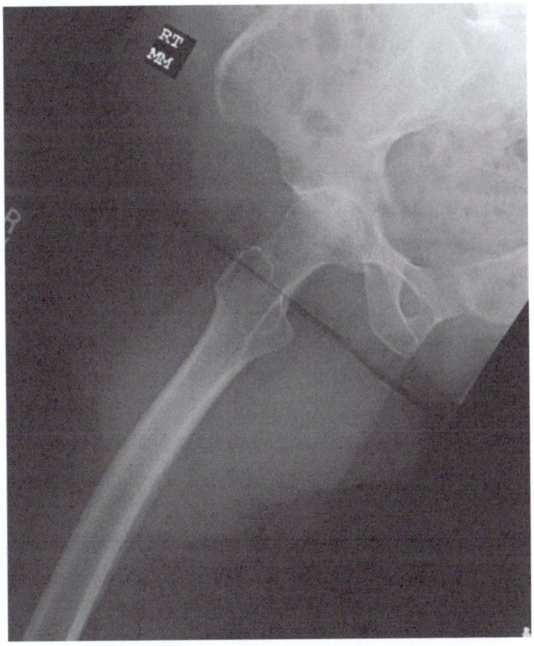

Fig. 3.15 Preoperative lateral radiograph demonstrating the same as above

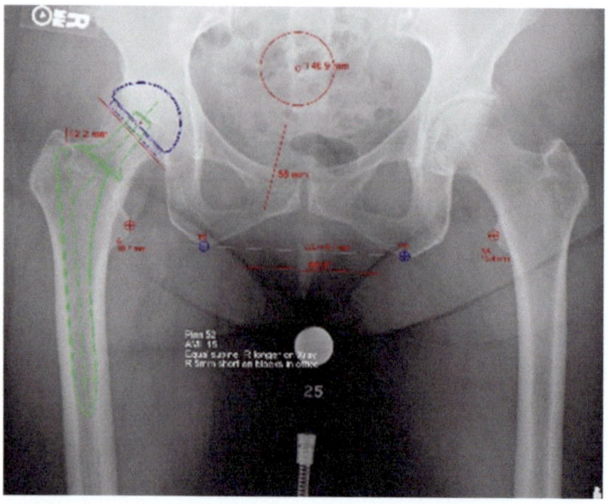

Fig. 3.16 Preoperative AP radiograph with template imaging overlaid. Preoperatively we templated a standard offset femoral stem with a 15 mm distal diameter and an acetabular cup with a 52 mm diameter. The patient was also noted to have a 4.7 mm leg length discrepancy

3.7.5 Preoperative Planning

Diagnosis: Osteoarthritis of the right hip (Figs. 3.14 and 3.15).

Possible treatment options: Nonoperative, however the patient already has exhausted all non-surgical treatment options to include activity modification, physical therapy, oral pain medications and intra-articular injections, and her pain has continued to affect her basic activities of daily living.

Chosen treatment method: Primary cementless total hip arthroplasty with an extensively porous-coated femoral stem featuring a cylindrical distal geometry.

Selection of implants if applicable and rational: At the time of the surgery, our institution predominately used an uncemented extensively porous-coated stem for femoral fixation as they achieve immediate diaphyseal cortical fixation and have been shown to have 98% survivorship at 20 years. A fully porous-coated implant allows for the greatest surface area for cortical bone-implant apposition and the best potential for ingrowth into the prosthesis.

Expected difficulties: Due to the importance of achieving adequate distal scratch fit between the prosthesis and the femur, it is imperative that the direction of the femoral reamer is controlled by the diaphysis and not by more proximal structures such as the greater trochanter or femoral neck. To the surgeon less experienced with implanting a fully porous-coated stem, this may be easily overlooked and risks malpositioning or undersizing the component.

Strategies to overcome difficulties: To help avoid a malpositioned or undersized component, in addition to an adequate exposure and soft tissue releases, it may be helpful to use a high-speed burr to create the starting pilot hole for femoral reaming. This helps to remove potential proximal impingement structures such as a portion of the overhanging greater trochanter.

Templating: The leg lengths were measured on the preoperative AP radiograph, and the right lower extremity was found to be 4.7 mm shorter (Fig. 3.16). The next step in templating is to identify the correct location of the true acetabulum, the correct size and the inclination and evaluate the extent of bony contact between the implant and host bone. We templated to have the inferior border of the cup at the inferior aspect of the teardrop and the medial aspect of the cup adjacent to the medial wall of the acetabulum with approximately 45 degrees inclination. With the chosen location and size of the cup, we felt comfortable that there was adequate bony contact between the host bone and the superior lateral aspect of the cup implant. With the cup centre established, the location of the femoral neck cut and size and offset of the femoral implant are determined. The location of the neck cut is much more critical for a cementless stem compared to a cemented stem because cutting the neck too long or too short will not allow the implant to sit properly within the medullary cavity and result in unintentionally lengthening or shortening of the limb. With this implant, we template to have the lateral aspect of the stem approximately 12 mm below the tip of the greater trochanter. In this case, we templated a femoral stem with a standard offset neck and a 15 mm distal diameter that appeared to fill the diaphyseal canal, restore the native offset and allow for at least 5 cm of distal scratch fit.

3.7.6 Surgical Note

Patient's position: Lateral decubitus position with the left hip down.

Type of anaesthesia: Spinal anaesthesia with conscious sedation.

Surgical approach: Posterior approach with posterior capsule and external rotator repair.

Main steps: For implantation of a fully porous-coated cementless prosthesis, any surgical approach may be utilized. However, the direct anterior approach is difficult with a long straight stem such as this. In the lateral position for a posterior approach, the surgeon must ensure the pelvis is tightly secured to the table and perpendicular to the floor to allow for easier intraoperative determination of leg lengths and acetabular version. After the surgical approach and adequate visualization of the head/neck and acetabulum, the femoral neck osteotomy is made at the level of the templated cut. Once the femoral osteotomy has been made, attention is turned to preparing and implanting the acetabulum. However, for the purposes of this chapter, we will continue discussing the femoral side of the arthroplasty. The first step in preparing the femoral canal is locating the correct starting point for canal reaming. It is imperative that the pilot hole is in the correct location, which is just slightly anterior to the piriformis fossa and right off the medial wall of the greater trochanter, in order to prevent reamer deflection off the trochanter resulting in a varus stem position. Start with a small size reamer and ream incrementally up by 1 mm until cortical contact is encountered, and at which time, sequentially increase the size of the reamer by 0.5 mm. Continue to ream until a cutting resistance in the proximal femoral diaphysis is encountered for approximately 5–7 cm. There should be visible cortical bone between the flutes of the last reamer. The final reamer should be 0.5 mm smaller than the implant size in order to achieve maximal diaphyseal scratch fit. The final step in canal preparation is incremental broaching of the proximal femur to accept the triangular geometry of the AML stem. Once the final broach size is achieved and proper stability is confirmed, trialling may proceed as indicated by the leg lengths and offset (Figs. 3.17 and 3.18).

Reconstruction techniques: Reconstruction using a fully porous-coated implant follows the general principles of primary total joint arthroplasty for osteoarthritis, and the specific steps for achieving proper component size and position are described elsewhere in this chapter.

3.7.7 Intraoperative Challenges

Challenges and solutions: Intraoperative femoral fractures during stem insertion can occur with cylindrical, extensively porous-coated stems. These fractures can be proximal, around the stem or distal to the stem tip. Proximal femur fractures typically occur as a result of a geometric mismatch between the triangular pattern of the implant and the femoral metaphysis. Risk factors that may predispose one to this are patients of smaller stature, female gender, a low femoral neck cut and femoral coxa vara. If there is a sudden 'jump' in stem position during impaction or the stem begins to advance more rapidly with successive blows, this should alert the surgeon to the possibility of a fracture that can be evaluated with intraoperative X-ray. A non-displaced distal femur fracture noted intraoperatively can be treated using a cerclage wire with protected weight-bearing postoperatively. In the rare event of a distal displaced fracture, the surgeon must be prepared to extend the approach distally, expose the fracture site and perform standard internal fixation principles with plates, screws and cables. Fractures noted on postoperative radiographs that are distal to the stem tip and non-displaced can be treated with or protected from weight-bearing and typically heal uneventfully. These hairline fractures are only apparent on either the AP or lateral radiograph just distal to the tip of the stem.

Unanticipated problems and solutions: Femur insertional fractures are an unanticipated problem but have been reported to occur approximately 3% of the time when using an AML-type prosthesis.

Thorough description of decision-making, including the reason for the final decision: Extensively porous-coated femoral stems, were pioneered at our institution. Because of the ability to achieve immediate distal cortical fixation with a reproducible surgical technique, these stems became our implant of choice for primary total hip arthroplasty. The long-term durability of the fixation has also been demonstrated with a stem survivorship rate of 97.8% at twenty years using revision for any reason as an endpoint.

3.7.8 Postoperative Radiographs (Figs. 3.17 and 3.18)

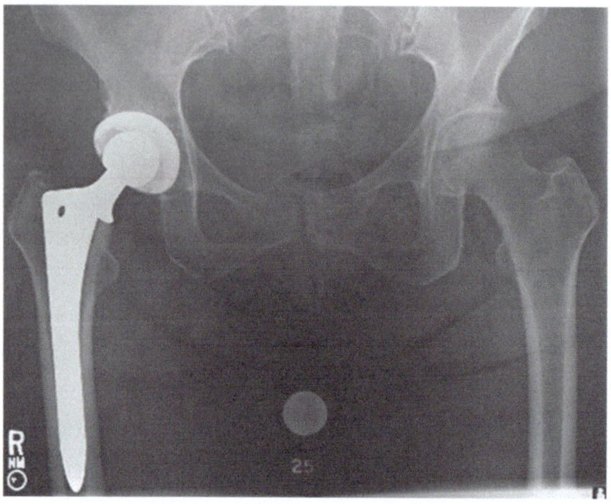

Fig. 3.17 Immediate postoperative AP radiograph demonstrating adequate sizing of the femoral component with 5 cm of canal filling, diaphyseal cortical fit, restoration of leg lengths and appropriate cup orientation

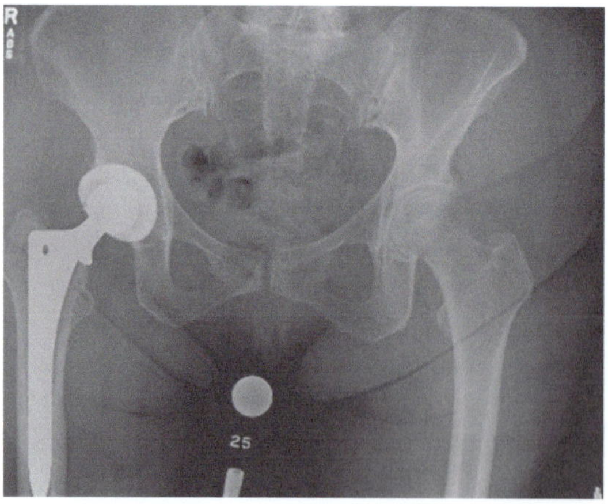

Fig. 3.18 1-year postoperative AP radiograph demonstrating stable component position without evidence of osteolysis or loosening and adequate distal stem osseous ingrowth

3.7.9 Postoperative Management

Chemoprophylaxis and anticoagulant treatment period: For deep venous thrombosis prophylaxis, the patient was started on low-dose warfarin therapy with a goal INR of 1.5–2 for a period of thirty days.

Gait/limb loading until full loading: The patient was allowed 50% weight-bearing on the right lower extremity for three weeks postoperatively and then transitioned to full weight-bearing as tolerated.

3.7.10 Follow-Up and Complications

There were no complications related to the management of this patient.

3.7.11 Discussion [36–39]

Advantages of the applied method: The two main advantages of performing an uncemented primary hip arthroplasty with an extensively porous-coated stem such as the AML are the cementless design and immediate distal cortical fixation. Cementless arthroplasty was popularized in the 1980s, and although there is no consensus about the optimal technique for femoral fixation, cementless stems were preferred in younger patients with adequate bone stock without abnormal morphologic features of the femur. Twenty-year results of this stem have demonstrated proven success across a spectrum of diseases. Although other designs of cementless stems have 20-year results, the AML was one of the first successful cementless stems implanted. Successful cementless fixation requires rigid interface fit to the host bone strong enough to support body weight. By reaming until cortical chatter is encountered, and then press fitting a 0.5 mm larger stem into the canal, the surgeon achieves instant distal cortical fixation that is stable for immediate postoperative weight-bearing. Retrieval studies have demonstrated intimate cortical ingrowth into these stems that can be seen on postoperative radiographs as thick, dense, hypertrophied cortices distally around the implant.

Disadvantages of the method: The same features that contribute to the advantages of extensively porous-coated cylindrical stems like the AML are also associated with some potential drawbacks. The distal cortical bony ingrowth and the transfer of stresses that occurs from the implant to the bone at this point can result in proximal stress shielding and bone density loss in the intertrochanteric region. While proponents for proximally coated stems contend that stress shielding results in greater incidences of thigh pain, the potential for fracture of the femur, loss of implant fixation and increase in the severity of osteolysis and can cause difficulties during revision, there is currently no literature that definitively substantiates these theoretical disadvantages. Countering these concerns, long-term follow-up data has shown durable fixation for these implants with ~98% survivorship at twenty years, and studies have shown no correlation between the degree of radiographic stress shielding and incidence of thigh pain. Bone mineral density studies have also shown no correlation between hip and pain scores and bone density changes. Additionally, retrieval analysis studies have shown no correlation between stress shielding and radiographic evidence of osteolysis or clinical evidence of stem loosening. Due to the extensive cortical ingrowth that occurs with this type of stem, in the event of a revision surgery where the stem needs to be removed, an extensile approach such as an extended trochanteric osteotomy is typically necessary in order to safely remove the stem that has a cortical bone grown into it. A more detailed discussion of these revision approaches is discussed elsewhere.

Alternative evidence-based techniques for the case: For cementless total hip arthroplasty, the other more commonly used implant is a proximally porous-coated stem. Proponents of these implants cite a decreased incidence of postoperative thigh pain and proximal stress shielding compared to extensively porous-coated implants. Contraindications to using a proximally porous-coated stem are few if any.

Why is the chosen technique better for this case? As discussed previously, we believe that the extensively porous-coated stem allows for immediate distal cortical fixation, and complications such as thigh pain can be limited by following our steps to ensure proper component positioning and sizing.

Indications and contraindications for your technique: Indications for the use of this extensively porous-coated cementless stem include primary total hip arthroplasty for osteoarthritis, rheumatoid arthritis, avascular necrosis of the femoral head, post-traumatic arthritis and intracapsular femoral neck fractures. These stems may also be utilized in revision surgery for treatment of a periprosthetic fracture with adequate proximal bone stock or revision for reasons other than fracture where the patient has a proximal bone loss that would not support a proximally porous-coated press-fit stem. The only absolute contraindication for the use of this stem, or any cementless stem for that matter, is an active infection. Relative contraindications include patients with femoral diameters of less than 10 mm or larger than 21 mm or patients with significant preoperative femoral anteversion, such as the case in a hip dysplasia patient, where retroverting the stem to a normal version would not allow for adequate canal filling distally. In this instance, the surgeon may want to consider a cemented or a modular design stem.

Learning curve and how to manage complications: As previously discussed, the incidence of thigh pain following implantation of extensively porous-coated stems has been shown to be 3–8%. Controversy exists regarding the true aetiology of thigh pain, as historically it has been associated with a loose femoral component. An inexperienced surgeon implanting this type of stem may encounter the initial cortical chatter and presume that this is the final size for the stem, inadvertently undersizing the component. In actuality, once the initial chatter is heard, the surgeon must continue incrementally reaming 0.5 mm size at a time until cortical bone is noticed between the reamer flutes on the final one or two reamers. Once the surgeon believes that the last reamer has been used, a method to check and determine the amount of distal scratch fit present is to use the same size reamer as the final femoral stem and insert it until it comes into contact with the diaphysis.

The proximally exposed portion of the reamer estimates the distance of the diaphyseal cortical contact. It is important to note that proximal bone loss secondary to stress shielding is not a complication, but rather a sign of success. Only bone ingrown implants demonstrate stress shielding related to bone loss.

Level of evidence concerning the superiority of this method against others: The highest level of evidence reporting on the use of these extensively porous-coated femoral stems is level IV.

3.8 Case Title: Hybrid Primary Total Hip Arthroplasty

Albert Ngu, Vaibhav Punjabi, and Fares Haddad

3.8.1 Demographics

Age: 86
Sex: Female
BMI: 25

3.8.2 Relevant Past Medical History

Principal pathologies: Gorham's 'vanishing bone' disease, osteoarthritis, hypertension, asthma, type 2 diabetes mellitus, psoriasis and gastro-oesophageal reflux disease.

Previous surgical procedures: Left hybrid total hip replacement in May 2006 and a hysterectomy in 1988.

Medication: Ciclosporin, metformin 500 mg BD, lansoprazole 15 mg OM, felodipine 2.5 mg OD, perindopril 8 mg OM, alendronic acid 70 mg weekly, adcal-D3 1.25 g OM, QVAR 50 mcg BD, rivaroxaban 10 mg OD, salbutamol 200 mcg prn, tramadol 50 mg BD and paracetamol 1 gm QDS.

History of presenting complaint: Right-sided groin and buttock pain with radiation up to the knee. She has night pain and rest pain. The pain is worse on weight-bearing, and her walking distance is now limited to a few yards. She takes paracetamol and tramadol. Over the last 3 months, her pain has become significantly worse. She has difficulty putting on socks and shoes. She struggles to get in and out of bed and to get up from a chair. She has had a left hybrid total hip arthroplasty nine years ago and is extremely happy with the outcome of the surgery.

3.8.3 Clinical Examination

Symptoms: The patient has a significant pain from the movement of her right hip and mobilizes with an antalgic and Trendelenburg gait.

Range of motion: The patient's range of motion of her right hip joint is hip flexion 80°, abduction 10°, adduction 5°, internal rotation 0° and external rotation 5°.

Specific tests: Thomas test demonstrates 20° fixed flexion deformity as well as positive Trendelenburg test.

Main disability: Patient could only mobilize a few yards (even so with great difficulty).

Neurovascular evaluation: The right lower limb was neurovascularly intact.

3.8.4 Preoperative Radiological Assessment/Imaging (Figs. 3.19, 3.20, and 3.21)

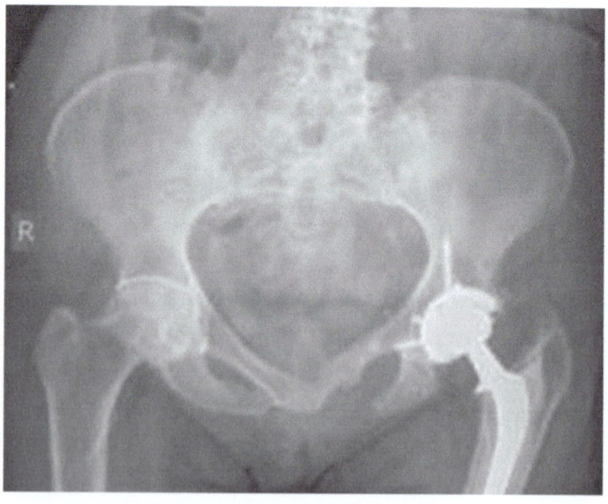

Fig. 3.19 Anteroposterior pelvis radiograph showing osteoarthritis of the right hip with Gorham's 'vanishing bone' disease affecting the left ischium

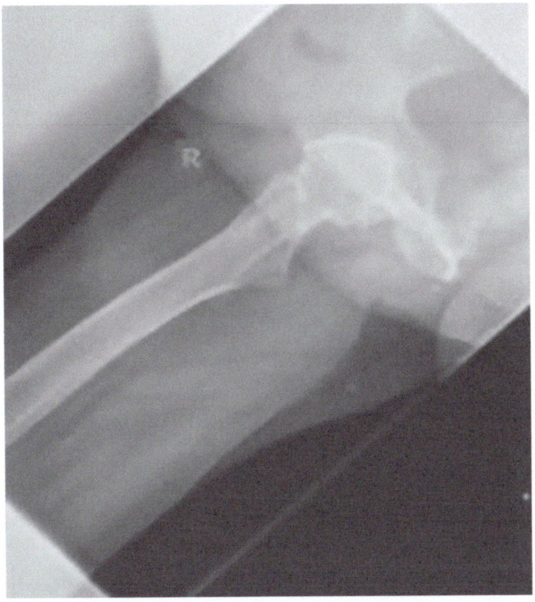

Fig. 3.20 Lateral radiograph of the right hip

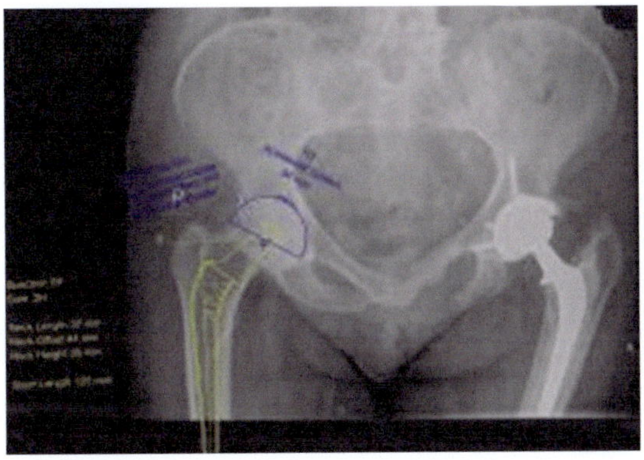

Fig. 3.21 Templating of the right hip with hybrid arthroplasty

3.8.5 Preoperative Planning

Diagnosis: Osteoarthritis of the right hip (Figs. 3.19 and 3.20).

Possible treatment options: (1) Hybrid primary total hip arthroplasty. (2) Cemented primary total hip arthroplasty. (3) Uncemented primary total hip arthroplasty.

Chosen treatment method: Hybrid primary total hip arthroplasty.

Selection of implants if applicable and rational: Uncemented porous-coated acetabular component, cross-linked polyethylene (XLPE) liner, oxidized zirconium femoral head and cemented femoral component.

Expected difficulties: (1) Osteoporotic bone with a risk of intraoperative fracture. (2) Varus neck-shaft angle predisposing to leg length discrepancy.

Strategies to overcome difficulties: (1) Gentle controlled hip dislocation after adequate capsular release. (2) Low neck cut and use of high-offset femoral component.

Templating: Templated as shown in Fig. 3.21.

3.8.6 Surgical Note

Patient's position: Lateral decubitus.

Type of anaesthesia: Spinal anaesthetic.

Surgical approach: Posterior approach.

Main steps: A standard posterior approach to the hip. Incision through fascia lata. Gluteus maximus fibres were split proximally. Gluteus medius and minimus are retracted superomedially to expose short external rotators. The sciatic nerve was identified and protected throughout. The leg was internally rotated to place the short external rotators on a stretch. Short external rotators were detached close to femoral insertion. Capsule and short external rotators were detached as one layer. The hip was dislocated gently with internal rotation. Using the osteotomy guide, the femoral neck was osteotomized, and the femoral head was excised. Then, the acetabulum was exposed circumferentially. The transverse acetabulum ligament was identified. The acetabulum was reamed to its true floor. A trial acetabular cup was inserted. Following this, a definitive porous-coated acetabular component was inserted with good anterior coverage and 5° more closure than her native anatomy, and in her own anteversion, parallel to the transverse acetabular ligament. Two posterosuperior screws were inserted. The acetabular osteophytes were removed. XLPE liner was inserted. With the knee flexed at 90°, the medullary canal was opened at the transected neck with a box chisel, aiming posteriorly and laterally. A blunt medullary reamer was then inserted to open up the canal. The femur was broached to the appropriate stem size, and following which the broach handle was removed, leaving the broach within the medullary canal, and a calcar reamer was used to ream the calcar level with the broach. A high-offset trial neck and appropriate femoral head were then used, and the hip was reduced. The hip was assessed for soft tissue tension, leg length as well as stability. The femoral component was cemented using fourth-generation cementing technique. The definitive femoral head was inserted after retrialling. The hip joint was reduced. The joint was lavaged. The short external rotators and the capsule were repaired with transosseous sutures to the greater trochanter. A layered closure was performed and a sterile dressing was applied to the wound (Figs. 3.22 and 3.23).

3.8.7 Intraoperative Challenges

Challenges and solutions: As described in preoperative planning and surgical note.

Unanticipated problems and solutions: No unanticipated problems were identified in this case.

Thorough description of decision-making, including the reason for the final decision: As described in the discussion below.

3.8.8 Postoperative Radiographs (Figs. 3.22 and 3.23)

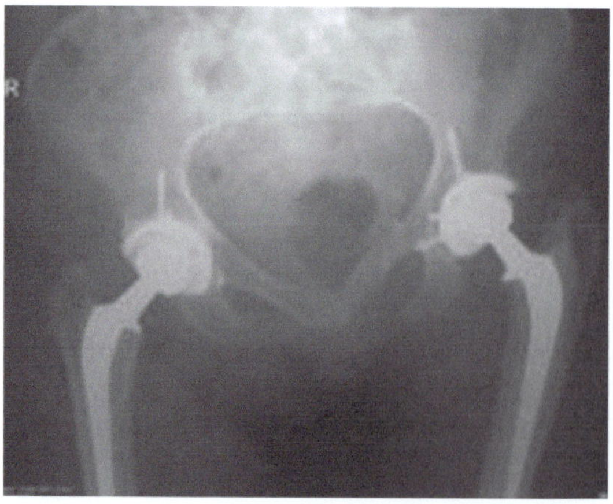

Fig. 3.22 Postoperative anteroposterior pelvis radiograph

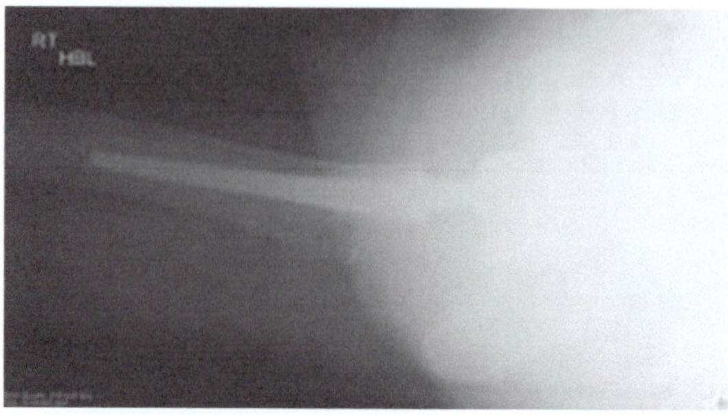

Fig. 3.23 Postoperative lateral right hip radiograph

3.8.9 Postoperative Management

Chemoprophylaxis and anticoagulant treatment period: T.E.D anti-embolism stockings, foot pumps and dalteparin 5000 IU for 35 days.

Gait/limb loading until full loading: Early mobilization to achieve full weight-bearing status as soon as possible.

3.8.10 Follow-Up and Complications

There have been no complications with both her hybrid total hip replacements. The left total hip arthroplasty was performed nine years ago, and the right total hip arthroplasty was performed 2 months ago.

3.8.11 Discussion

Advantages of the applied method: Gorham's disease, otherwise known as 'vanishing bone' disease, is characterized by destruction of osseous matrix and proliferation of vascular structure, resulting in bone absorption and destruction. There have only been approximately 200 reported cases since it was first described by Gorham in 1838 [40]. Due to its rarity, there has not been a clear consensus on the treatment and management of this disease as it is often individualized [40]. Apart from this case, we have been aware of nine other reports of total or partial hip arthroplasty in Gorham's disease [40]. From the literature, aseptic loosening of cemented acetabular components remains a significant complication resulting in revision surgery [41]. For the same reason, we opted to use an uncemented porous-coated acetabular component to promote osteointegration. The advantage of a cemented femoral stem, in this case, was to achieve adequate fixation in osteoporotic bone, allowing the patient to start full weight-bearing immediately. Additionally, with modern cementing techniques, outcomes of cemented femoral stems have improved [42].

Disadvantages of the method: Disadvantage of using an uncemented acetabular component is the risk of intraoperative acetabular fracture on insertion [43]. Disadvantages of the cemented femoral stem are potential aseptic loosening and cement-related embolism [44].

Alternative evidence-based techniques for the case: An alternative technique for this case, as described in other case reports, is cemented primary total hip arthroplasty.

Why is the chosen technique better for this case? The patient had a successful outcome with the same technique on the opposite hip and hence the decision to reproduce it on the current symptomatic side.

Indications and contraindications for your technique: Indications for hybrid total hip replacement, in this case, are the osteoporotic femur, patient's age and comorbidities. Contraindications are young, fit and active patients with adequate bone stock.

Learning curve and how to manage complications: Standard routine and reproducible technique used to minimize complications.

Level of evidence concerning the superiority of this method against others: As discussed above.

References

1. Berry DJ, Harmsen WS, Cabanela ME, Morrey BF. Twenty-five-year survivorship of two thousand consecutive primary Charnley total hip replacements: factors affecting survivorship of acetabular and femoral components. J Bone Joint Surg Am. 2002;84-A:171–7.
2. Kavanagh BF, Wallrichs S, Dewitz M, Berry D, Currier B, et al. Charnley low-friction arthroplasty of the hip. Twenty-year results with cement. J Arthroplasty. 1994;9:229–34.
3. Wroblewski BM, Siney PD, Fleming PA. Charnley low-frictional torque arthroplasty in patients under the age of 51 years. Follow-up to 33 years. J Bone Joint Surg Br. 2002;84:540–3.
4. Aldinger PR, Thomsen M, Mau H, Ewerbeck V, Breusch SJ. Cementless Spotorno tapered titanium stems: excellent 10–15-year survival in 141 young patients. Acta Orthop Scand. 2003;74:253–8.
5. McLaughlin JR, Lee KR. Total hip arthroplasty in young patients. 8- to 13-year results using an uncemented stem. Clin Orthop Relat Res. 2000;373:153–63.
6. Callaghan JJ, Templeton JE, Liu SS, Pedersen DR, Goetz DD, et al. Results of Charnley total hip arthroplasty at a minimum of thirty years. A concise follow-up of a previous report. J Bone Joint Surg Am. 2004;86-A:690–5.
7. Eskelinen A, Remes V, Helenius I, Pulkkinen P, Nevalainen J, et al. Total hip arthroplasty for primary osteoarthrosis in younger patients in the Finnish arthroplasty register. 4,661 primary replacements followed for 0–22 years. Acta Orthop. 2005;76: 28–41.
8. Makela K, Eskelinen A, Pulkkinen P, Paavolainen P, Remes V. Cemented total hip replacement for primary osteoarthritis in patients aged 55 years or older: results of the 12 most common cemented implants followed for 25 years in the Finnish Arthroplasty register. J Bone Joint Surg Br. 2008;90:1562–9.
9. Makela KT, Eskelinen A, Paavolainen P, Pulkkinen P, Remes V. Cementless total hip arthroplasty for primary osteoarthritis in patients aged 55 years and older. Acta Orthop. 2010;81:42–52.
10. Callaghan JJ, Bracha P, Liu SS, Piyaworakhun S, Goetz DD, Johnston RC. Survivorship of a Charnley total hip arthroplasty: a concise follow-up, at a minimum of thirty-five years, of previous reports. J Bone Joint Surg Am. 2009;91:2617–21.
11. Corten K, Bourne RB, Charron KD, Au K, Rorabeck CH. Comparison of total hip arthroplasty performed with and without cement: a randomized trial. A concise follow-up, at twenty years, of previous reports. J Bone Joint Surg Am. 2011;93:1335–8.
12. Della Valle CJ, Mesko NW, Quigley L, Rosenberg AG, Jacobs JJ, Galante JO. Primary total hip arthroplasty with a porous-coated acetabular component: a concise follow-up, at a minimum of twenty years, of previous reports. J Bone Joint Surg Am. 2009;91:1130–5.
13. Corbett KL, Losina E, Nti AA, Prokopetz JJ, Katz JN. Population-based rates of revision of primary total hip arthroplasty: a systematic review. PLoS One. 2010;5(10):e13520.
14. Eskelinen A, Remes V, Helenius I, Pulkkinen P, Nevalainen J, et al. Uncemented total hip arthroplasty for primary osteoarthritis in young patients: a mid-to long-term follow-up study from the Finnish Arthroplasty register. Acta Orthop. 2006;77:57–70.
15. Makela KT, Eskelinen A, Pulkkinen P, Paavolainen P, Remes V. Total hip arthroplasty for primary osteoarthritis in patients fifty-five years of age or older. An analysis of the Finnish arthroplasty registry. J Bone Joint Surg Am. 2008;90:2160–70.
16. Ogino D, Kawaji H, Konttinen L, Lehto M, Rantanen P, et al. Total hip replacement in patients eighty years

of age and older. J Bone Joint Surg Am. 2008;90: 1884–90.
17. Puolakka TJ, Pajamaki KJ, Halonen PJ, Pulkkinen PO, Paavolainen P, et al. The Finnish arthroplasty register: report of the hip register. Acta Orthop Scand. 2001;72:433–41.
18. Malchau H, Herberts P, Eisler T, Garellick G, Soderman P. The Swedish total hip replacement register. J Bone Joint Surg Am. 2002;84-A(Suppl 2):2–20.
19. Herberts P, Malchau H. Long-term registration has improved the quality of hip replacement: a review of the Swedish THR register comparing 160,000 cases. Acta Orthop Scand. 2000;71:111–21.
20. Hailer NP, Garellick G, Karrholm J. Uncemented and cemented primary total hip arthroplasty in the Swedish hip arthroplasty register. Acta Orthop. 2010;81:34–41.
21. Espehaug B, Furnes O, Engesæter LB, Havelin LI. 18 years of results with cemented primary hip prostheses in the Norwegian arthroplasty register. Acta Orthop. 2009;80:402–12.
22. Furnes O, Lie SA, Espehaug B, Vollset SE, Engesaeter LB, et al. Hip disease and the prognosis of total hip replacements. A review of 53,698 primary total hip replacements reported to the Norwegian Arthroplasty Register 1987–99. J Bone Joint Surg Br. 2001;83:579–86.
23. Australian Orthopaedic Association National Joint Replacement Registry Annual Report 2009. http://www.dmac.adelaide.edu.au/aoanjrr/publications.jsp?section=reports2009; 2010.
24. The New Zealand Joint Registry Ten Year Report. http://www.cdhb.govt.nz/njr/; 2010.
25. Troelsen A, Malchau E, Sillesen N, Malchau H. A review of current fixation use and registry outcomes in total hip arthroplasty: the uncemented paradox. Clin Orthop Relat Res. 2013;471:2052–9.
26. Huo MH, Dumont GD, Knight JR, Mont MA. What's new in total hip arthroplasty. J Bone Joint Surg Am. 2011;93:1944–50.
27. Morshed S, Bozic KJ, Ries MD, Malchau H, Colford JM Jr. Comparison of cemented and uncemented fixation in total hip replacement: a meta-analysis. Acta Orthop. 2007;78:315–26.
28. McMinn DJ, Snell KI, Daniel J, Treacy RB, Pynsent PB, Riley RD. Mortality and implant revision rates of hip arthroplasty in patients with osteoarthritis: registry based cohort study. BMJ. 2012;344:e3319.
29. van der Veen HC, van Jonbergen H-PW, Poolman RW, Bulstra SK, van Raay JJAM. Is there evidence for accelerated polyethylene wear in uncemented compared to cemented acetabular components? A systematic review of the literature. Int Orthopaed (SICOT). 2013;37:9–14.
30. Taunton MJ, Dorr LD, Long WT, Dastane MR, Berry DJ. Early postoperative femur fracture after uncemented collarless primary total hip arthroplasty: characterization and results of treatment. J Arthroplasty. 2015;30(11):2008–11.
31. Ling RS, Charity J, Lee AJ, Whitehouse SL, Timperley AJ, Gie GA. The long-term results of the original exeter polished cemented femoral component. J Arthroplasty. 2009;24(4):511–7.
32. Bolland BJ, Whitehouse SL, Timperley AJ. Indications for early hip revision surgery in the UK—a re-analysis of NJR data. Hip Int. 2012;22(2):145–52.
33. Sierra RJ, Timperley JA, Gie GA. Contemporary cementing technique and mortality during and after exeter total hip arthroplasty. J Arthroplasty. 2009;24(3):325–32.
34. Wechter J, Comfort TK, Tatman P, Mehle S, Gioe TJ. Improved survival of uncemented versus cemented femoral stems in patients aged <70 years in a community total joint registry. Clin Orthop Relat Res. 2013;471:3588–95.
35. Abdulkarim A, Ellanti P, Motterlini N, Fahey T, O'Byrne JM. Cemented versus uncemented fixation in total hip replacement: a systematic review and meta-analysis or randomized controlled trials. Orthop Rev. 2013;5(1):e8.34–44.
36. Belmont PJ Jr, Powers CC, Beykirch SE, et al. Results of the anatomic medullary locking total hip arthroplasty at minimum of twenty years. J Bone Joint Surg Am. 2008;90(7):1524–39.
37. Engh CA Jr, Mohan V, Nagowski JP, et al. Influence of stem size on clinical outcome of primary total hip arthroplasty with cementless extensively porous-coated femoral components. J Arthroplasty. 2009;24(4): 554–9.
38. Kwon DG, Lee TJ, Kang JS, et al. Correlation between stress shielding and clinical outcomes after total hip arthroplasty with extensively porous coated stems. J Arthroplasty. 2013;28(10):1728–30.
39. Engh CA Jr, Young AM, Engh CA Sr, et al. Clinical consequences of stress shielding after porous-coated total hip arthroplasty. Clin Ortho Relat Res. 2003;417: 157–63.
40. Browne JA, Shives TC, Trousdale RT. Thirty-year follow-up of patient with Gorham disease (massive osteolysis) treated with hip arthroplasty. J Arthroplasty. 2011;26(2):339.e7–10.
41. Crites BM, Berend ME, Ritter MA. Technical consideration of cemented acetabular components. A 30-year evaluation. Clin Orthop. 2000;381:114–9. doi:10.1097/00003086-200012000-00014.
42. Oishi CS, Walker RH, Colwell CW Jr. The femoral component in total hip arthroplasty. Six to eight-year follow-up of one hundred consecutive patients after use of a third-generation cementing technique. J Bone Joint Surg Am. 1994;76(8):1130–6.
43. Squire M, Griffin WL, Mason JB, Peindl RD, Odum S. Acetabular component deformation with press-fit fixation. J Arthroplasty. 2006;21(Suppl 2): 72–7.
44. Yli-Kyyny T, Ojanpera J, Venesmaa P, et al. Perioperative complications after cemented or uncemented hemiarthroplasty in hip fracture patients. Scand J Surg. 2013;102(2):124–8.

4 Hip Resurfacing Arthroplasty (HRA)

Eustathios Kenanidis, Alexandros Stamatopoulos, Michail E. Klontzas, Andreas Leonidou, Eleftherios Tsiridis, Lafayette de Azevedo Lage, Yusuf Mirza, Sujith Konan, and Fares S. Haddad

E. Kenanidis, M.D., Ph.D., M.Sc. (✉) · A. Stamatopoulos, M.D.
Academic Orthopaedic Unit, Aristotle University Medical School, Thessaloniki, Greece
e-mail: stathiskenanidis@gmail.com

M.E. Klontzas, M.D.
Imperial College London, Biological Systems Engineering Lab, London, UK
e-mail: miklontzas@gmail.com

A. Leonidou, P.G.Dip., M.Sc., F.R.C.S.
Reading Shoulder Unit, Hospital & Health Care, Tonbridge, UK
e-mail: leonidou@doctors.org.uk

E. Tsiridis, M.D., Ph.D., F.A.C.S., F.R.C.S. (✉)
Academic Orthopaedic Unit, Papageorgiou General Hospital, Aristotle University Medical School, Thessaloniki, Greece
e-mail: etsiridis@doctors.org.uk

L. de Azevedo Lage, M.D.
University of São Paulo, São Paulo, Brazil
e-mail: lafayettelage@gmail.com

Y. Mirza, Mu.Dr., M.R.C.S., M.Sc.
Wales Deanery, Cardiff, UK
e-mail: mirzyusuf@gmail.com

S. Konan, M.B.B.S., M.D.(Res.), F.R.C.S.
Department of Trauma & Orthopaedics, University College Hospital, London, UK
e-mail: docsujith@yahoo.co.uk

F.S. Haddad, B.Sc., M.D., M.Ch., F.R.C.S.
University College Hospital, London, UK
e-mail: fsh@fareshaddad.net

4.1 Current Concepts

E. Kenanidis, A. Stamatopoulos, M.E. Klontzas, A. Leonidou, and E. Tsiridis

- HRA is an alternative type of hip arthroplasty that is mainly used to young, active, male patients with end-stage joint arthritis with sufficient bone quality and minimal mechanical deformity.
- The head of the femur is partially removed and reconstructed to accept a new metal head that fits a metal acetabular component [1].
- There have been different types of the prosthesis (cemented, uncemented, and hybrid), various types of the surface-bearing materials (MoP, CoP, MoM, and CoC), and different generations of HRAs (first generation, MoP; modern hip resurfacing systems, MoM) used.
- The first-generation MoP HRA failed mainly due to wear and wear-induced complications. During the mid-1990s, the introduction of the third-generation MoM HRA was promising as to decrease complications [2].
- The third generation of HRA implant has a cementless, porous-coated, press-fit monoblock acetabular and a cemented femoral component and a metal-on-metal bearing articulation [3, 4].
- Following an initial popular period during the past decade with promising results [5–7], the indications of use are rather decreasing fol-

E. Tsiridis (ed.), *The Adult Hip - Master Case Series and Techniques*, https://doi.org/10.1007/978-3-319-64177-5_4

lowing concerns with regard to the long-term consequences of the presence of metal ions in the blood and the plethora of questions for the reported series of adverse local tissue reactions (ALTRs) [8].

- The excellent however published results from high-volume centres at 10–15 years in selected patient populations [9–13], the unfavorable results of the majority of registries [14], the heterogeneity the studies, and inconsistent outcome definitions dispute our ability to compare arthroplasty outcome studies and have a definite point of view [1].

4.1.1 Advantages

- The preservation of the proximal femoral bone and the retention of the femoral neck that facilitates revision to a THA [15–17].
- The increase of the prosthetic joint stability and the improvement of ROM due to the use of a large bearing surface [1, 18].
- The decrease in wear rates due to the use of larger bearing surfaces [19].
- The easier replication of better hip biomechanics and limb length [20, 21].
- An improved function as a consequence of the retention of the femoral head.
- More precise biomechanical restoration.
- The regular load transmission that reduces stress shielding.
- It has been suggested that the approximation of the native femoral head-to-neck ratio enables a higher range of motion before impingement and an upgrated function over conventional THA [22, 23]. However, this needs further evaluation [2, 17].
- Permits return to moderate- to high-impact activities due to the physiological loading of the proximal femur [20]:
  - Girard et al. [24]: 82% of patients responded to high-impact activities as tennis.
  - Fouilleron et al. [25]: 91.6% of the patients returned to competitive running.
  - Le Duff et al. [26]: high-impact activities increase the risk of revision of a HRA.
- The absence of tapered connections between the modular components [20].
- The less embolization risk due to the lack of femoral reamin g or cementation.
- Decreased thigh pain associated with the femoral stem in conventional THA.

4.1.2 Disadvantages

- The risk of femoral neck fracture [27]:
  - Relatively rare complication. The reported rate averages 1.69% (range 0–9.2%) [27–29].
  - Usually at the initial postoperative period [27, 30].
  - Recognized risk factors: notching of the superior cortical bone of femoral neck, prosthesis malpositioning (varus position), inappropriate patient selection (poor bone quality) [31], inadequate surgical technique [31], surgeon's learning curve [32] (other reasons not uniformly accepted are reduced vascularization inherent to the posterior approach [33], or a possible injury to the femoral neck during reaming [34, 35]).
- Avascular necrosis of the femur head.
- Technically demanding procedure [7, 36, 37].
- Need for a more extensive exposure because the non-resected femoral head must be retracted [7].
- Long learning curve [17].
- Better results from high-volume centres with appropriately trained surgeons.
- Suitable only for selected patients (especially young active men).
- Adverse biological reactions (local soft tissue toxicity, delayed-type hypersensitivity reactions, osteolysis, risk of carcinogenesis).
- Adverse reaction to metal debris (ARMD), adverse local tissue reactions (ALTR), and pseudotumors are the most commonly used terms for the local reactions [8, 38–42]:
  - The actual cause of these reactions is uncertain.
- Increased peripheral metal ion levels (cobalt and chrome):
  - These are strongly associated with wear production [43, 44], positioning of the acetabular component (abduction and anteversion) [45], different designs of HRA devices [46], and component size [47].

- Raise in plasma levels about 2–13 times for chromium and 4–7 times for cobalt [48].
- The relationship of metal ion plasma levels and the failure of arthroplasty is not linear. There is some agreement that cobalt levels above 7 ppb is more likely to be associated with ALTR and can be used as a rough "screening tool."
- In a systematic review and meta-analysis of trials comparing hip resurfacing to metal-on-metal total hip arthroplasty, there was not a difference in serum metal ion levels, although there was a tendency for lower serum cobalt ion levels in patients receiving HRA. The dominant theory is that fretting and crevice corrosion occurs between the femoral neck and the head of metal-on-metal THA implants, while this source of metal ion production is not present in hip resurfacing implants [49].

• Pseudotumors
  - The incidence varies between series. It was usually 1–2%. There was a lower incidence in short-lasting series with a limited number of patients [41].
  - The risk of developing a pseudotumor is related to the patient and surgical and implant factors. The patient-related factor includes female gender, small component size, and hip dysplasia [41].
  - Women are shorter than men; they have higher head-neck ratios and a higher incidence of dysplasia, which predisposes to a high combined anteversion, all of which increase the risk.
  - One of the most critical surgical factors is the acetabular component orientation [50]. The optimal orientation is 40–45° inclination and 20–25° anteversion [50].
  - Mal-orientation increases the risk of edge loading, either directly if the joint contact force passes near the edge of the socket or indirectly if there are impingement and minor subluxation [51]. This is also attributed to an abnormal femoral anatomy as dysplasia and unfavorable head-neck ratio [52].
  - The design of the implant has a profound effect on wear mainly due to the internal geometry and the thickness of the socket, the design of the socket rim, the clearance, and the metallurgy [53].
  - The MoM bearing is more sensitive to ball coverage by the socket than metal-on-polyethylene bearings and on a parallel with ceramic-on-ceramic bearings. Maximum functional coverage of the head by the acetabular component avoids edge loading and abnormal wear patterns. This can be achieved by choosing a design with large coverage, sufficient clearance, and optimal implant orientation.
  - The best assessment of functional coverage can be made by calculating the contact patch to rim (CPR) distance [54]. There is considerable agreement that a CPR of 10 mm is consistently associated with minimal risk of edge wear [54].
  - Asymptomatic pseudotumors have been recognised on ultrasound and MRI scanning in 27–32% of patients with MoM hip replacements [55].
  - The Australian National Joint Registry data highlight that female patient and those under the age of 40 had significantly increased risk of revision due to pseudotumor. The number of HRAs performed on female patients were dramatically reduced since 2007, to the point where only 1% of hip resurfacing operations were performed on women in 2013 [55].

4.1.3 Indications

- Male sex, age less than 60 years, and larger patient size.
- The ideal patient for HR is a young, active male affected by primary hip osteoarthritis and with a femoral head larger than 50 mm [36, 37].
- Studies vary in defining "young" patients, ranging from 55 to 65 [36].
- Good bone quality and shape that allow resurfacing of the femoral head without causing damage to the femoral neck.
- Osteoarthritis, posttraumatic arthritis, osteonecrosis of the femoral head with femoral neck cysts <1 cm that does not significantly extend into the neck or areas of implant fixation, and moderate degenerative sequelae associated with childhood hip disease such as chondrolysis or Crowe type I and II developmental dysplasia.

- Patients with osteoarthritis have been shown to have better results than those with other diagnoses, particularly developmental dysplasia [56].

4.1.4 Contraindications

- DDH:
  - Limited acetabular bone stock to permit secure implantation of the cup.
  - The femoral anteversion deformity in DDH cannot be corrected with HR [37].
  - Amstutz et al. reported excellent results in Crowe type I/II DDH but this is not the rule [57].
- Osteonecrosis with a large area >50% of femoral head involvement or collapse [7]:
  - Some good results have been reported [58].
- Marked alteration in hip mechanics (severe slipped capital femoral epiphysis, coxa vara, Crowe type III and IV dysplasia).
- Inadequate bone stock in the femoral head, femoral neck, or acetabulum.
- A diameter of the femoral head that is smaller than the diameter of the neck (some patients with Legg-Calve-Perthes disease).
- Unknown sensitivity to metal, women of child-bearing age due to the unexplored effects on the fetus of the metal ion release, and renal insufficiency [7, 55].
- Rheumatoid arthritis (relative contraindication):
  - Some good results have been reported [59].
- Older adults with osteoporosis. DEXA screening might be necessary for assessment [7].
- Obesity is not an absolute contraindication. For severely overweight people, however, HRA is a containdication:
  - The lower likelihood that obese patients will engage in high levels of activity.
  - Significantly a greater number of obese [BMI $\geq$ of 30 kg/m^2] patients suffer from femoral neck fractures particularly if the components are improperly implanted [60].
- Presence of active or suspected infection.
- Skeletal immaturity.
- Multiple cysts of the femoral head (greater than 1 cm).
- Immunosuppression.

4.1.5 Surgery

4.1.5.1 Preoperative Planning

- Select the proper patient [37].
- Choose a well-established prosthetic model (tribology or implant design) [37].
- Preoperative X-ray planning of cup positioning [20].

4.1.5.2 Intraoperatively

- The selection of surgical approach seems not to affect the risk of avascular necrosis:
  - Some information exists that the blood supply is preserved with an anterolateral approach or trochanteric flip approach [61].
  - Equal however results are possible with a posterior approach. McBryde et al. reported no different outcomes between the posterolateral and anterolateral approaches [62].
- Use more extensive exposure to overcome the retracted and non-resected femoral head and efficiently identify the bony acetabular landmarks for reaming and socket insertion [7, 20].
- Implant the components correctly:
  - Avoid varus placement of the femoral component. The valgus position is preferred by many surgeons to reduce tension and shear stresses [63] and complications [36] and to resemble the standard physiologic strain patterns [63].
  - Avoid an excessive valgus positioning as it can lead to notching in the femoral neck and increase the risk for femoral neck fracture [63].
  - Cover entirely and maximize the size of the femoral component to reduce the overall complication rate from 13.4 to 2.1% and the femoral neck fracture rate from 7.2 to 0.8% [32].
  - Ensure the proper positioning of the cup including inclination and version of the shell [37]. Remember that the initial stability of the cup in the pelvis may be challenging based on the size of the implant and the limited availability of anchoring devices such as screws [7].

  - Avoid the notching of the femoral neck [37].
- A hybrid method of cementation is recommended, uncemented socket and cemented femur:
  - Cup cementation resulted in higher failure rates [32].
  - Proper cementation of the femoral component requires correct cement viscosity, cement application, and mantle thickness.
  - Use lower viscosity cement and manually pack it to penetrate deeply and interdigitate the cancellous bone [64], approximately 2–3 mm but not so deep as to cause bone necrosis [64].
  - Avoid excess cement as it is considered a potential cause for implant failure; thick cement mantles (1.5 mm) cause higher temperatures at the cement-femoral bone interface [65].
  - Drill holes made in the femoral head to maximize the cement fixation area to achieve enduring fixation [66].
  - Clean thoroughly the femoral head after reaming to remove all cystic or necrotic material, dry the bone, and keep it dry during cement application with intertrochanteric hole suctions [20].

4.1.6 Published Results

The reported results of MoM HRA have differences between national registries and clinical cohorts [67, 68]. The average survival rate of clinical cohorts was significantly higher than the national registries. Possible explanations are that these studies are often held by a single-operator experienced surgeon and usually from design centers, which probably introduces a confounding factor [67, 69]. There are also many confounding factors and bias that can lead to misinterpretation of the results of national registries. The missing essential information as the history of patient and radiography, the non-guaranteed completeness of records, the failure to estimate the exact reason for failure, and that the records do not account for the learning curve associated with the use of new implants are some of them [67].

Initial short- to -mid-term clinical follow-up reports of 4–7 years mainly from the designer centres suggest survival rates varying between 94% and 100% [5, 6, 19, 56, 70–76]. The reported complications ranged from 0 to 18%. Femoral neck fractures and aseptic loosening were the most frequent causes of failure [4].

There are several however clinical cohort studies presenting long-term follow-up of HRAs [9–12, 77–84]. The sample size of these studies ranged from 54 to 1000 HRAs. The main arthroplasty used was BHR (Birmingham). The mean follow-up ranges from 8 to 13.7 years. The survival rate of HRAs at a 10-year follow-up was between 88 and 97%. In the longest follow-up, Daniel et al. [10] reported that the survival rate of 1000 BHRs at 15 years was 95.8%. Survival rate of men (93–98%) was consistently better in all these studies compared to women (74–96%).

The annual reports of registries have demonstrated the following:

1. HRA had a higher revision rate compared to THA [4]:
   - The majority of national registries reported higher revision rates for MoM HRA compared with THAs. Data from NARA database supported that HRA had an almost threefold increased revision risk compared to THA at two years (RR = 2.7, 95% CI, 1.9–3.7) [16]. Data from the Australian registry supported that the cumulative percent revision of HRA at eight years was 5.3, as compared to 4.0 for THA [14].
   - Sepannen et al. [85] reported data from NARA and the National Joint Register of England and Wales and supported that there was no statistically significant difference in revision risk between HRAs and THAs at 3.5 years (RR = 0.93, 95% CI, 0.78– 1.10) [85].
   - In a systematic review of the English literature after 1996, Marshal et al. [1] with only 7.2% randomized controlled trials MoM HRA demonstrated sooner average time to revision (3.0 vs. 7.8 years) and more fre-

quent revisions and reoperations (10.7 vs. 7.1, $p = 0.068$) compared to THA. When discontinued devices were removed from the analysis, the early revisions were still more frequent for HRA compared with THA, however, at nonsignificant level. The reoperations were more frequent in MoM HRA (7.9 vs. 1.8 per 1000 person-years) than THA devices ($p = 0.084$). The most common reasons reported for reoperation in MoM HRA were the fracture (femoral neck, greater trochanter, subtrochanteric femur fracture), heterotopic ossification, and component mismatch whether for THAs were heterotopic ossification, osteolysis, excessive polyethylene wear, and infection. Dislocations were more frequent with THA than HRA (4.4 vs. 0.9, $p = 0.008$) per 1000 person-years, respectively. Adverse event rates changed when discontinued devices were included.

2. HRA provides equivalent, if not better, functional outcomes in well-selected patients [86]:
   - In a literature review, van Gerwen et al. [2] with only one RCT have shown better functional outcomes than THA. The need however for high-level evidence studies was demonstrated.
   - In a meta-analysis, T. Smith et al. [87] reported that functional outcomes for patients following HRA were better than or the same as for patients with a THA; there were however significantly greater incidences of heterotopic ossification, aseptic loosening, and revision surgery with HRA compared to THA.
   - Longer-term studies are necessary to determine whether the potential functional benefits of HRA in younger, active patients persist for the lifetime of the prosthesis [86].
3. The implant design had an influence on revision rates:
   - There are two extreme examples of this. ASR (DePuy, Warsaw, IN) that recalled due to abnormally increased failure rates reaching 13% during the first years.
   - The Birmingham Hip Resurfacing (BHR) (Smith & Nephew, Memphis, TN) was the most commonly used device with the longest follow-up [4]. Several studies and registries have demonstrated that this HRA has the lowest revision rate [4, 16, 85, 88, 89].
   - Corten et al. [4] supported that the number of revisions per 100 observed component years for the BHR was 0.8 compared to 2.6 and 2.3 for the ASR (DePuy, Warsaw, IN) and Durom (Zimmer, Warsaw, IN), respectively [4].
   - Using data from NARA database, the risk of non-septic revision was reduced with the use of BHR than the other designs as a group (RR = 0.3, CI, 0.1–0.7) [16]. ASR had inferior outcome with higher revision risk than the BHR (RR = 1.8, CI, 1.2–2.7) [85].
   - Different brands of prosthesis have different revision probabilities at ten years. The 10-year revision probability of the ASR is reported at 30.36%, compared to the Birmingham Hip Resurfacing (BHR) at 9.04% [55].
4. Gender, age, and surgical indication are considered as prognostic factors between HRA and THA [4]:
   - The majority of studies demonstrated that male had better results than females [4, 16, 85, 90]. This was more pronounced for the younger male. The effect however of sex on HRA failure rates was questioned as the head size was considered as a confounding factor [14].
   - Corten et al. [4] supported that females had 2.5 higher revision risk than males irrespective of age, but this difference disappeared after adjustment for femoral component sizes 50 mm or greater. Males younger than 64 years of age did best with HRA [4]. Female patients had about double the revision risk of male patients (RR = 2.0, CI, 1.4–2.7) in Nordic Arthroplasty Register Association (NARA) and the National Joint Register of England and Wales [85].
   - National Joint Registry for England and Wales (NJR) does not recommend HRA in women but only in men with preoperative measurement that is used to assess suitability. Predicted 5-year revision rates in 55-year-old women were 8.3% with a

42 mm resurfacing head, 6.1% with a 46 mm resurfacing head, and 1.5% with a 28 mm cemented metal-on-poly stemmed THR. Predicted 5-year revision rates in 55-year-old men were 4.1% with a 46 mm resurfacing head, 2.6% with a 54 mm resurfacing head, and 1.9% with a 28 mm cemented metal-on-poly stemmed THR [90].
   - Prosser et al., using data from the Australian registry, stated that on adjusting for femoral head size, female sex no longer remained as an independent risk factor [14].
   - In a systematic review, Bryan D. Haughom et al. [91] also reported that women demonstrated a significantly increased odds of developing ALTR (OR, 5.70), dislocation (OR, 3.04), aseptic loosening (OR, 3.18), and revision (OR, 2.50) after primary MoM HRA.
   - Age has an opposite effect on the risk of HRA compared with THA; the younger the patients undergoing HRA, the lower the failure risk [4].
   - Primary osteoarthritis (OA) as an indication for HRA is reported to have lower revision risk than DDH and AVN.
   - Corten et al. [4] reported that the 5-year CRR of SRA for OA was 1% higher than that of THA, whereas for DDH it was four times higher than that of THA (3%).
5. The effect of femoral head size and especially of component sizes 50 mm or greater in diameter on the survival of HRA is debated:
   - Johanson et al. [16] and Sepannen et al. [85] did not supported that increased femoral head diameter had affected the risk of revision.
   - The Australian Orthopaedic Association National Joint Replacement Registry reported that prostheses with head sizes <50 mm had a higher revision rate than those with head sizes ≥50 mm [14].
6. Low hospital procedure volume worsened the outcome of HRA:
   - NARA database: Within the HRA group, the risk of non-septic revision was reduced in hospitals performing ≥70 HRAs annually (RR = 0.3, CI, 0.1–0.7) [16].
   - Nordic Arthroplasty Register Association (NARA) and the National Joint Register of England and Wales: Hospitals that had performed 100 or more HRA procedures had a lower revision risk than those with less than 100 HRAs (RR = 0.6, CI, 0.4–0.9) [85].
   - Aseptic loosening (31%) and periprosthetic fracture (31%) accounted for 66% of revisions of HRA followed by pain and instability and osteolysis. In THA, aseptic loosening (46%) and dislocation (19%) represented 66% of the indications for revision [4].

4.1.7 Complications

- In a systematic review, Paile et al. [67] reported that the most frequent complications of HRA were aseptic loosening 33.5%, followed by femoral neck fractures. Other complications were ALVAL, infection, malpositioning, persistent pain, avascular necrosis, etc.
- Aseptic loosening (0–1.3% with a 5-year follow-up):
  - The rate of femoral aseptic loosening after HRA is low, typically ranging from 1 to 3% at a minimum of 10 years [9–11], and it was reduced with improvement of the surgical technique.
  - The reported acetabular aseptic loosening from the same studies reported less than 2% at 7–12 years.
- Femoral neck fractures (0–9.2%, most common complication).
- Pseudoarthrotic features.
- Notching.
- Refractive groin pain (6%).
- Adverse local tissue reactions to wear products (adverse periprosthetic tissue reactions, metal allergy, metallosis, pseudotumors) (1%) [42] .
- Dislocation and impingement (0–1%).
- Heterotopic ossification (Brooker grades I–IV).
- Femoral nerve palsy (0–1.6%).
- Thromboembolic phenomena (less than 1%).

4.2 Case Title: Hemiresurfacing for Hip Osteonecrosis in Active Young Patients

Lafayette de Azevedo Lage

4.2.1 Demographics

Age: 32
Sex: Male
BMI: 29.1

4.2.2 Relevant Past Medical History

Principal pathologies: Bilateral osteonecrosis of the femoral head.

Previous surgical procedures: None.

Medication: None.

Other: Important alcohol abuse—the patient drinks beer every day for many years.

History of presenting complaint: Right hip pain since December 2013 after a subchondral fracture of the femoral head. On December 12, 2014, he was submitted to hemiresurfacing arthroplasty with a cemented ReCap 50 mm from Biomet, since the chondral damage of acetabular cartilage was minimal and the labrum was intact (Figs. 4.1, 4.2 and 4.3). The postoperative course was very good and he returned to the horse riding with no pain. He works as a cowboy in the interlands of Brazil. After eight months, he started having pain in the left hip, and a CT demonstrated a subchondral fracture. On December 11, 2015, he was submitted to left hip hemiresurfacing arthroplasty with cemented ReCap 50 mm, and the acetabular cartilage and labrum were perfect. In both surgeries, he stayed in the hospital only for 48 h and started full weight bearing on the first day with a pair of crutches since the posterolateral approach was utilized.

4.2.3 Clinical Examination

Symptoms: Important right (and later left) hip pain when walking and limping was visible.

Range of motion: Internal rotation = zero, flexion, external rotation, abduction, adduction, and extension with no abnormalities within normal range of motion.

Specific tests: Negative Trendelenburg.

Main disability: Minimal limping when walking.

Scoring if available: Analog pain rating scale = 4.

Neurovascular evaluation: Normal.

4.2.4 Preoperative Radiological Assessment/Imaging

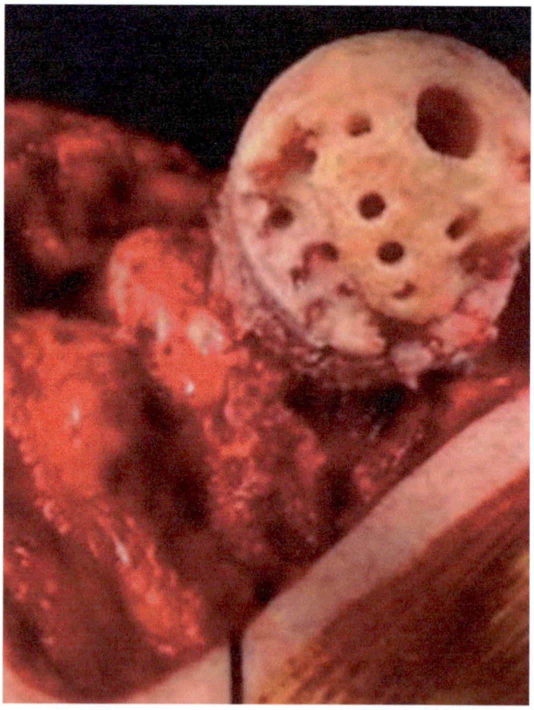

Fig 4.1 Right femoral head with big cysts which were filled with Biomet cement from Switzerland

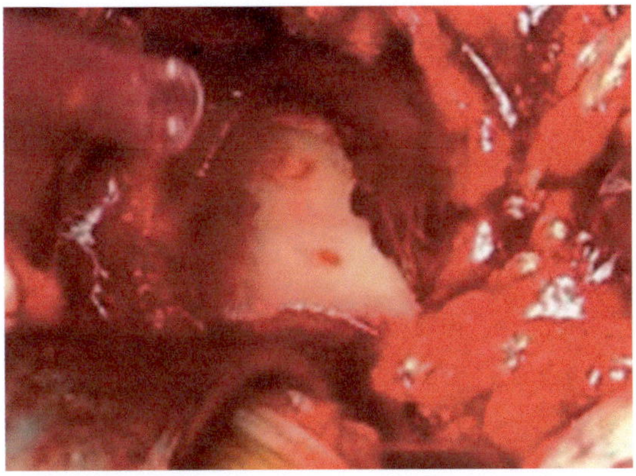

Fig. 4.2 Minimal erosions on acetabular cartilage due to the subchondral fracture

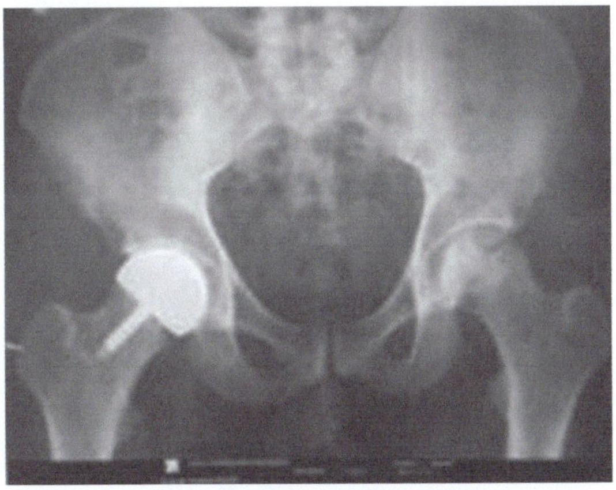

Fig. 4.3 Pelvis X-ray of second postoperative day for hemiresurfacing arthroplasty of the right hip

4.2.5 Preoperative Planning

Diagnosis: Our first thought was to implant a total hip arthroplasty, but, in exceptional cases of patients having a good acetabulum and no labral tear or labral detachment, we still prefer hemiresurfacing; although the outcomes of this type of arthroplasty are reported to be unpredictable, we still prefer to use this in certain cases with satisfactory results.

Possible treatment options: Hemiresurfacing or conventional total hip arthroplasty.

Chosen treatment method: Following consultation of the patient we choose the hemiresurfacing solution.

Selection of implants if applicable and rational: We have used Biomet and Conserve Plus femoral components which could be converted to total, so we do not use the original Conserve component since it cannot be converted to total in case of failure.

Expected difficulties: We start surgery by inserting the metal pin guide using an image intensifier without allowing the pin to cross the femoral head which can damage the acetabular cartilage. This surgery has to be done very carefully mainly when opening the capsule taking care not to damage the labrum. Never remove the fat pad, even if it is very inflamed, as it is usually seen in osteonecrosis. The severe synovitis of the foveal pad should be preserved and never be removed since we noticed that it works as a cushion or shock absorber and the patient has only a minimal discomfort.

Strategies to overcome difficulties: Patient selection is crucial. It is very important to explain to the patient that the duration of pain-free joint might not be long. If this is the case and when the patient is not satisfied, revision and conversion to a total resurfacing or a conventional total hip arthroplasty doing the osteotomy of the femoral neck are possible.

Templating: As we do not have resurfacings with increments of 1 mm anymore, always choose the smaller size, that is, in this case, we measure a 51 mm head and implant a 50 mm head in order to fit the acetabulum!

4.2.6 Surgical Note

Patient's position: Lateral.

Type of anesthesia: General.

Surgical approach: Posterolateral (MIS -maximum incision surgery) with incision varying between 15 and 25 centimeters depending on the BMI).

Main steps: During the initial step we pass the guide pin through the skin with the aid of image intensifier trying to be in the middle of the femoral neck not allowing it to penetrate the femoral cartilage. Only after this start the skin incision;

this saves you time during surgery, less blood loss, and increase the precision of surgery.

Reconstruction techniques: It is important, if you can close the capsule, but sometimes we need to retrieve part of it and leave it open. It is very important to check if the labrum is not unturned when you reduce the femoral head back in the acetabulum. Check the total range of motion and feel in your fingers if there is no "entrapment of soft tissues"!

4.2.7 Intraoperative Challenges

Challenges and solutions: Whether performing hemiresurfacing or total resurfacing is an intraoperative decision depending on the local conditions. It is always necessary to have a conventional prosthesis in case you do not have a good femoral head or you do not achieve a stable acetabulum resurfacing fixation since you cannot put screws, except in dysplastic hips. Although MRI and CT can give us explicit images, sometimes we are surprised with severe acetabular cartilage erosions which are not seen in these exams. In these cases we take a picture and show the patient later that hemiresurfacing was not possible.

Unanticipated problems and solution: As explained above, never start operation without having a conventional prosthesis available. It only happened once in our hands but it can happen, and we cannot ream the acetabulum more to insert a bigger resurfacing acetabulum.

Thorough description of decision-making, including the reason for the final decision: Young active patients with necrosis of the femoral head are ideal candidates for hemiresurfacing if well selected and prepared to live with eventual minimal pain after hemiresurfacing (some patients have some minimal discomfort but are satisfied with hemiresurfacing). This patient was so happy that we operated the other hip 1 year later. Note at 1-year post-op X-ray that there was new bone formation on medial calcar after 1 year (Figs. 4.4 and 4.5). The left hip had a substantial lateral cyst and was filled with cement which we believe will support the horse riding with no problems since the medial column was ok (Fig. 4.5).

4.2.8 Postoperative Radiographs (Figs. 4.3, 4.4, and 4.5)

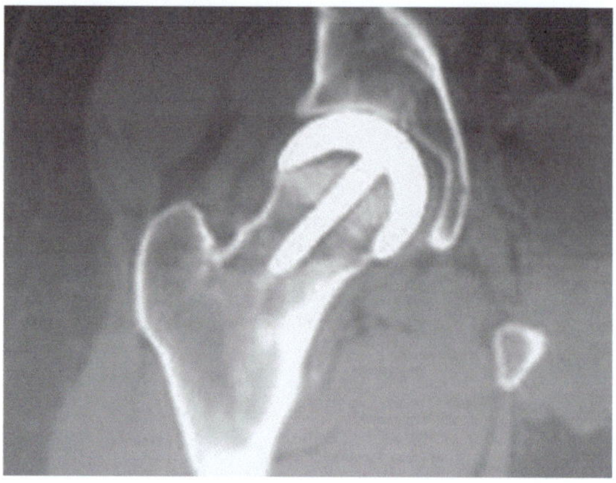

Fig. 4.4 Seven-month post-op right hip CT

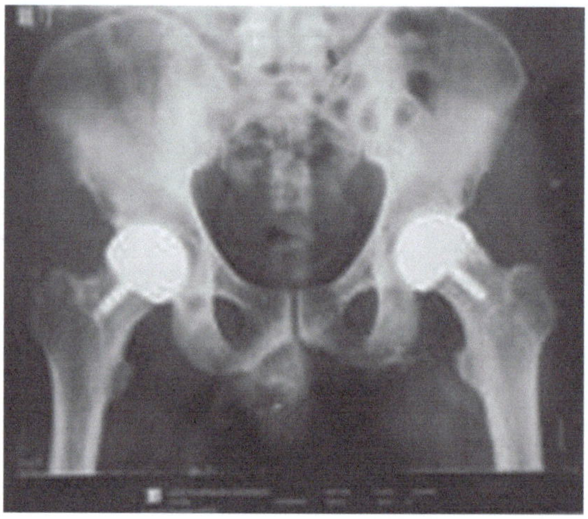

Fig. 4.5 One-year post-op right hip and one-day post-op left hip (which had a substantial lateral cyst)

4.2.9 Postoperative Management

Chemoprophylaxis and anticoagulant treatment period: Aspirin 100 mg for 20 days, use of cefuroxime for 48 h, use of drain which was removed at 24 h, no blood transfusion necessary

Gait/limb loading until full loading: Use of a pair of crutches with full weigh bearing for 2–3 weeks maximum and one crutch contralateral side until limping stops

4.2.10 Follow-Up and Complications

Report of postoperative complications and their management (i.e., recurrent dislocation): We needed to convert to a total hip resurfacing only a case of us since this 28-year-old young active male surfer refered considerable pain after walking more than two km. This patient had a lot of pain in the immediate postoperative period and is allergic to several anti-inflammatory drugs (usually our patients have no pain at all after total hip replacement using posterolateral approach with big incision—maximum incision surgery). We usually infiltrate the trauma with a topical anesthetic solution made of 30 mg of Ketorolac and 1 mg of adrenaline in the muscles immediately before closure when using general anesthesia. If we use intradural anesthesia with morphine, we do not infiltrate locally the muscles with the above mentioned solution since anesthesia lasts for 24 h.

Scoring if available: Analog pain rating scale = 1.

4.2.11 Discussion [92–94]

Advantages of the applied method: Hip resurfacing (HR) arthroplasty is a procedure that preserves bone and allows patients to return to a higher level of function with a longer prosthesis life compared with patients who receive a total hip arthroplasty (THA). It's considered an alternative to THA in a selected group of patients who might potentially outlive a THA. During HR, the femoral neck is preserved, and the femoral head is shaped and capped with a metal device and short stem. The acetabulum is also lined with a specific metal device. We had the opportunity to visit professor Harlan Amstutz in 1993, 1995, and 1996 to see the wonderful lasting results of the hemiresurfacing prosthesis in young active athletes who continue to be active with hemiresurfacing.

Disadvantages of the method: Some patients may feel a certain discomfort, but it is acceptable. Close follow-up with annual X-rays is important.

Alternative evidence-based techniques for the case: Easy to revise if necessary.

Why is the chosen technique better for this case? The ideal patient is the one that withstands well pain (unfortunately there is no method to confirm if the patient will accept metal well on cartilage). Even for overweight patients or in the presence of an important subchondral fracture, the patient does not refer VAS score pain greater than 4, so we explained it was worthwhile to try.

Indications and contraindications for your technique: A very careful surgical technique is mandatory in this surgery, retrieving the dead bone with arthroscopic curette, careful meticulous pulse lavage, placing a 3 mm hole in the femoral neck to aspirate the saline from pulse lavage which helps drying the bone before cementing is very important, and filling all cysts with finger pressuring cementation is recommended.

Learning curve and how to manage complications: Do not remove fat from the fovea and leave the ligamentum teres (unless there is much ligamentum teres)—*they act as shock absorbers. Never damage the labrum!*

Level of evidence concerning the superiority of this method against others: We think it is a very good time saving method which can last more than 15 years as we were able to see many cases in the Joint Replacement Institute operated by professor Harlan Amstutz. People could not reproduce his results, probably because they are not being so meticulous, careful, and skilled as he was (he used to take 3 h to do a hemiresurfacing). We think hemiresurfacing has a place when a careful surgical technique is applied and the right patient selected.

4.3 Case Title: Resurfacing Primary Hip Arthroplasty

Yusuf Mirza, Sujith Konan, and Fares Haddad

4.3.1 Demographics

Age: 52 years old
Sex: Male
BMI: 24.7

4.3.2 Relevant Past Medical History

Principal pathologies: Hypercholesterolemia.

Previous surgical procedures: Ankle fracture in 1985, managed nonoperatively.

Medication: Simvastatin 40 mg once daily.

Other: Lives on the third floor flat without a lift and freely mobile.

History of presenting complaint: A 10-year history of worsening bilateral hip pain. Pain is worse on the left side than the right. Unable to walk for time periods greater than 30 min due to groin pain and can no longer play squash.

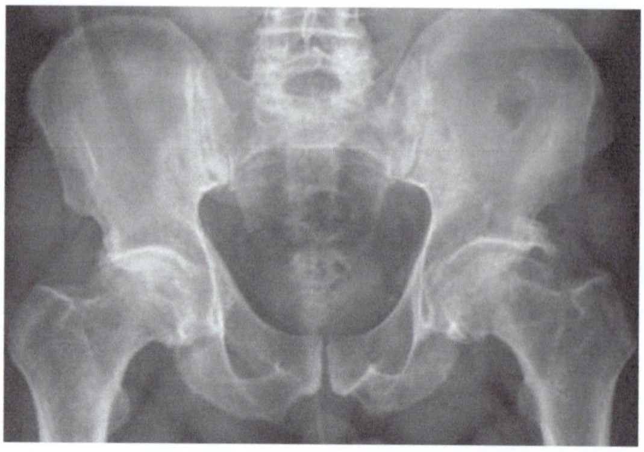

Fig. 4.6 AP pelvis

4.3.3 Clinical Examination

Symptoms: Left groin pain with pain traveling down to thighs.

Range of motion: Hip flexion to 95° with internal rotation limited to less than 15°. No external rotation of the hip with hip flexing into fixed internal rotation.

Specific tests: Leg length discrepancy of 1.5 cm.

Main Disability: Prior to hip pain was unable to play squash.

Scoring if available: Harris Hip Score of 44 and WOMAC 46.7.

Neurovascular Evaluation: Normal sensation in all lower limb dermatomes and pulses palpable at dorsalis pedis and posterior tibial arteries.

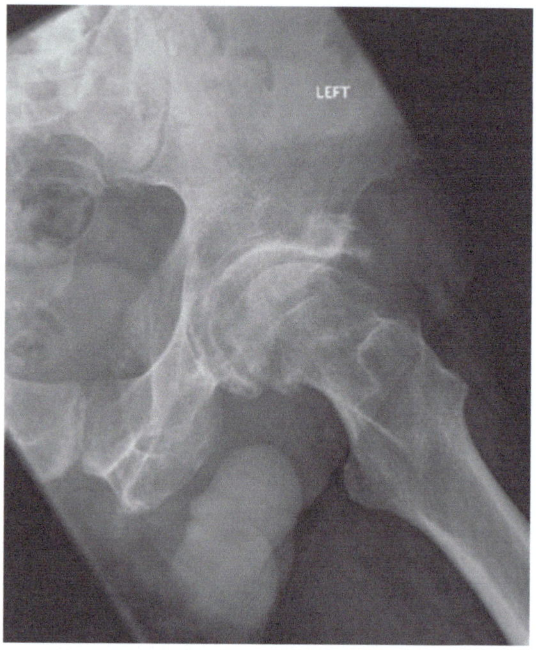

Fig. 4.7 Lateral left hip

4.3.4 Preoperative Radiological Assessment/and Imaging (Figs. 4.6 and 4.7)

4.3.5 Preoperative Planning

Diagnosis: Osteoarthritis (Figs. 4.6 and 4.7)

Possible treatment options: (1) Birmingham Hip Resurfacing (Smith & Nephew, Andover, MA, USA), (2) uncemented total hip arthroplasty, and (3) cemented total hip arthroplasty

Chosen treatment method: Hip resurfacing

Selection of implant if applicable and rational: Birmingham Hip Resurfacing because it is the best performing hip resurfacing implant on the UK National Joint Registry

Expected difficulties: Femoral head bone stock deficiency due to severe osteoarthritis

Strategies to overcome difficulties: Possibility of conversion to total hip arthroplasty if femoral head bone stock deficiency is present

4.3.6 **Templating** (Fig. 4.8)

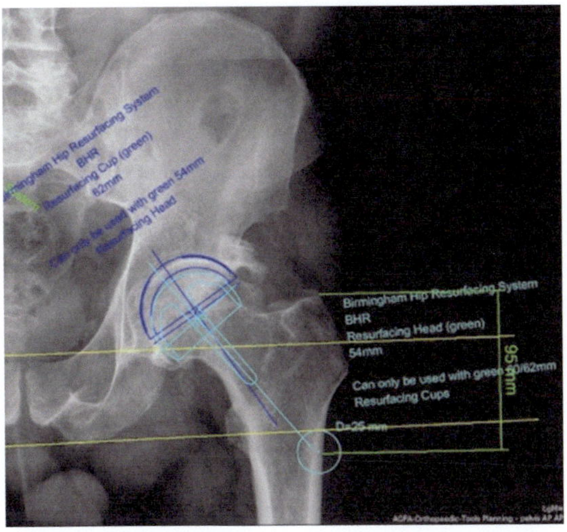

Fig. 4.8 Legend for image—templating of left hip with use of TraumaCad software (Brainlab, Munich, Germany). A 62 mm cup with a 54 mm head was recommended. Note the avoidance of varus positioning

4.3.7 **Surgical Note**

Patient's position: Lateral decubitus.

Type of anesthesia: Spinal with sedation. Local periarticular injection.

Surgical approach: Posterior approach.

Main steps: A 15 cm incision made over the posterior aspect of the greater trochanter through the skin and fat. Fascia lata cut with the hip in slight abduction. Gluteus maximus was bluntly dissected. The sciatic nerve was identified and protected throughout. The piriformis tendon was identified and gluteus minimus and medius retracted anterosuperiorly using sharp Hohmann retractor. Piriformis tendon, short external rotators, and quadratus muscle with underlying capsule raised as a single flap posteriorly. Femoral head dislocated and delivered into the wound. Limited anterior capsulotomy may be necessary to achieve this. Centre line of implant template is determined as distance from the lesser trochanter by jig ruler, according to preoperative templating. The area of the posterior femur marked and collared alignment pin inserted with a drill, perpendicular to the neck of the femur. Long alignment jig set up, and stylus used to check femoral component positioning avoiding varus and neck impingement. When judged to be satisfactory regarding the lateral and coronal alignment, the guidewire is inserted. Guidewire overdrilled. Guide bar insertion over the guidewire. Recheck femoral component impingement. Sleeve cutter stop device placed over guide bar with corresponding head-neck template to prevent shoot through the sleeve cutter. Identify medial head-neck junction and summit of head marked. Plain cutter used to resect down to the identified level. Chamfer cutter used to shape the femoral head. Head trial placed over prepared bone and head subluxated anteriorly. This along with postero-inferior retractor allows wide exposure of the acetabulum.

Acetabular preparation: Labrum resected and excised. Osteophytes are in the floor of the acetabulum and ligamentum teres resected. True acetabular floor identified. Reaming commenced at 46 mm, increasing in 2 mm increments. When sure of reaching the true acetabular floor, reaming increases in 1 mm, until press -fit fell is achieved by the reamer. Measurement is confirmed by trial cup size and also to confirm anterior coverage. Acetabular component positioned in the acetabular rim, at correct orientation to ensure splines are adjacent to the ischium and pubis and impacted onto the position. Osteophytes removed. A gauze swab is placed into the acetabulum, and the femur is prepared for cementation.

The drill is used to form cement keyholes in the femoral head. Use of a taper drill to overream the central hole. Guide rod reinserted to recheck head-neck junction and mark depth of advancement of the femoral component. Pulse lavage and careful drying of the femoral head in preparation for cementing. Femoral component checked. Low viscosity cement prepared and poured into femoral component till 1/3 full and wet cement in contact with implant surface. Femoral component impacted onto head at 1 min. Excess cement removed. Rongeur used to resect any further osteophytes. Hip reduced with traction. The range of motion and the leg length equality confirmed on table (Figs. 4.9 and 4.10).

Reconstruction technique: As described.

4.3.8 Intraoperative Challenges

Challenges and solutions: Careful assessment of the suitability of the patient for resurfacing. Larger incision utilized to ensure satisfactory placement of the implant. Careful dissection of the capsule to preserve retinacular blood supply of the femoral head. In the presence of small defects, cysts should be curetted to allow adequate cement interdigitation.

Unanticipated problems and solutions: Notching of the femoral neck prevented by careful pre-op planning and meticulous operative technique. Varus position of acetabular component should be avoided.

4.3.9 Postoperative Radiographs (Figs. 4.9 and 4.10)

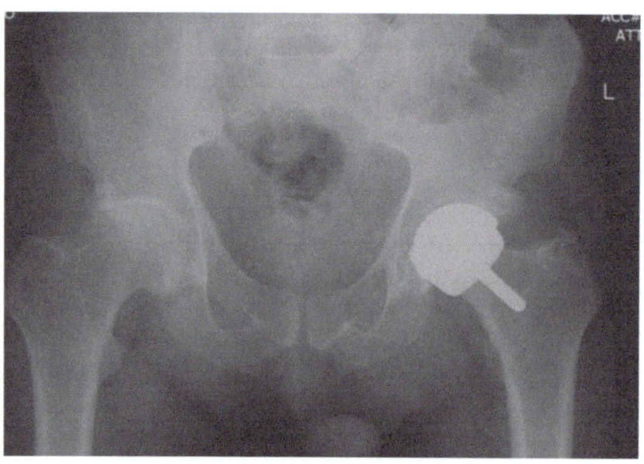

Fig. 4.9 AP pelvis. Left Birmingham Hip Resurfacing

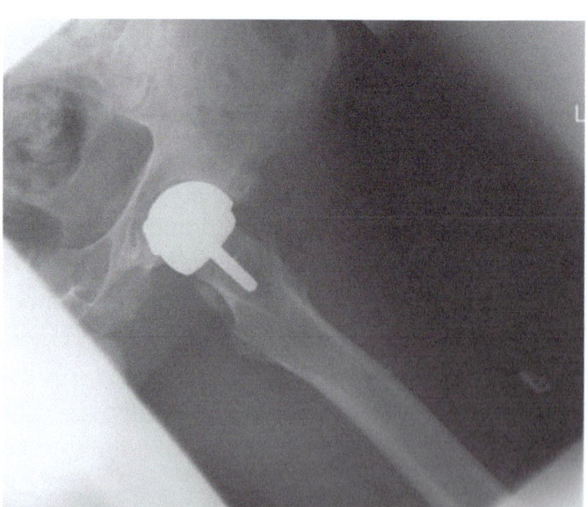

Fig. 4.10 Lateral left hip, Birmingham Hip Resurfacing in situ

4.3.10 Postoperative Management

Chemoprophylaxis and anticoagulant treatment period: The patient was placed on dalteparin, 5000 units subcutaneous, administered once daily. The thromboprophylaxis was given for 28 days. The patient was additionally given three doses of antibiotics in the immediate 24 h perioperatively.

Gait/limb loading until full loading: The patient was permitted to fully weight bear postoperatively.

4.3.11 Follow-Up and Complications

No postoperative complications

Scoring if available: Harris Hip Score of 96 and WOMAC 3.24

4.3.12 Discussion

Advantages of the applied method: Hip resurfacing is a treatment option for the active younger patient, seeking surgery intending to returning to sport participation. Technically, the procedure offers the surgeon an opportunity to conserve proximal femoral bone stock. Other benefits include a lower rate of dislocation, owing to a larger diameter of the femoral head. Hip resurfacing arthroplasty was previously thought to offer improved proprioception but has been recently refuted according to Larkin [95]. There is also a proposed ease of revision. From the viewpoint of the patient, hip resurfacing has been demonstrated, by Daniel and colleagues [10], to permit those working in physically demanding occupations to return to work as well as a high proportion, 87% or greater, to return to "leisure time" sporting activities.

Disadvantages of the method: Drawbacks of the method include that it may be limited to a narrow cohort of patients, namely, male patients with larger femoral heads as suggested by registry data from both the Australian and UK registries. Female patients may be more at risk of fracture of the femoral neck secondary to osteoporosis. More recently, the disease of ARMD (adverse reaction to metal debris) has come to light. ARMD is a spectrum of soft tissue reactions about the implant, which can cause local destruction of tissue, deep vein thrombosis, pain, and swelling. The incidence of this is unknown, but Pandit and colleagues estimate that this may occur in approximately 1% of all patients receiving metal-on-metal hip resurfacing within five years [96]. Risk factors for this include female sex and small component size [8]. Achieving accurate implant position is also essential to avoid failure as well as the risk of avascular necrosis of the femoral head and a limited inability of the technique to alter the patients offset or length.

Alternative evidence-based techniques for the case: Other techniques for this would be the use of an uncemented total hip arthroplasty using cross-linked polyethylene and ceramic or Oxinium head.

Why is the chosen technique better for this case? The patient is young and the keen sportsman. The technique will allow him to return to an active lifestyle.

Indications and contraindications for your technique: Indications include the younger, active patient with a larger femoral head.

Contraindications: Female patient with a smaller femoral head. Severely dysplastic hip secondary to DDH.

Learning curve and how to manage complications: A majority consensus (81%) from an international meeting in Ghent of notable surgeons suggested that surgeons ought to have 200 orthodox total hip replacements prior to embarking on hip resurfacing.

Level of evidence concerning the superiority of this method against others: Haddad and colleagues conducted a prospective cohort study comparing hip resurfacing to total hip arthroplasty [97]. The results are long-term findings (at ten years), and there was no loss to follow up. The study suggests improved function secondary to hip resurfacing. Other authors mirror the finding, but the follow-up is not as extensive.

References

1. Marshall DA, Pykerman K, Werle J, Lorenzetti D, Wasylak T, Noseworthy T, Dick DA, O'Connor G, Sundaram A, Heintzbergen S, Frank C. Hip resurfacing versus total hip arthroplasty: a systematic review comparing standardized outcomes. Clin Orthop Relat Res. 2014;472:2217–30.
2. van Gerwen M, Shaerf DA, Veen RM. Hip resurfacing arthroplasty: a systematic review of functional outcome. Acta Orthop. 2010;81(4):680–3.
3. Grigoris P, Roberts P, Panousis K, Bosch H. The evolution of hip resurfacing arthroplasty. Orthop Clin North Am. 2005;36(2):125–34.
4. Corten K, SJ MD. Hip resurfacing Data from National Joint Registries What do They Tell us? What do they not tell us? Clin Orthop Relat Res. 2010;468:351–7.
5. Treacy RB, McBryde CW, Pynsent PB. Birmingham hip resurfacing arthroplasty. A minimum follow-up of five years. J Bone Joint Surg Br. 2005;87(2):167–70.
6. Back D, Dalziel R, Young D, Shimmin A. Early results of primary Birmingham hip resurfacings. An independent prospective study of the first 230 hips. J Bone Joint Surg Br. 2005;87(3):324–9.
7. Buergi ML, M. William L. Walter. Hip Resurfacing Arthroplasty The Australian Experience The Journal of Arthroplasty. 2007;22(7 Suppl):3.
8. Pandit H, Glyn-Jones S, Mc Lardy-Smith P, et al. Pseudotumours associated with metal-on-metal hip resurfacings. J Bone Joint Surg Br. 2008;90(7):847–51.
9. Coulter G, Young DA, Dalziel RE, Shimmin AJ. Birmingham hip resurfacing at a mean of ten years: results from an independent centre. J Bone Joint Surg Br. 2012;94(3):315–21.
10. Daniel J, Pradhan C, Ziaee H, Pynsent PB, McMinn DJ. Results of Birmingham hip resurfacing at 12 to 15 years: a single-surgeon series. Bone Joint J. 2014;96-B(10):1298–306.
11. Holland JP, Langton DJ, Hashmi M. Ten-year clinical, radiological and metal ion analysis of the Birmingham hip resurfacing: from a single, non-designer surgeon. J Bone Joint Surg Br. 2012;94(4):471–6.
12. Murray DW, Grammatopoulos G, Pandit H, Gundle R, Gill HS, Mc L-SP. The ten-year survival of the Birmingham hip resurfacing: an independent series. J Bone Joint Surg Br. 2012;94(9):1180–6.
13. Amstutz HC, Takamura KM, Le Duff MJ. The effect of patient selection and surgical technique on the results of conserve® plus hip resurfacing—3.5- to 14-year follow-up. Orthop Clin North Am. 2011;42(2):133–42.
14. Gareth H. Prosser, Piers J yates, David J wood, Stephen E graves, Richard N de Steiger, and Lisa N miller. Outcome of primary resurfacing hip replacement: evaluation of risk factors for early revision 12,093 replacements from the Australian joint registry. Acta Orthop. 2010;81(1):66–71.
15. Shimmin A, Beaulé PE, Campbell P. Metal-on-metal hip resurfacing arthroplasty. J Bone Joint SurgAm. 2008;90(3):637–54.
16. Johanson P-E, Fenstad AM, Furnes O, Garellick G, Leif I Havelin, Sören Overgaard, Alma B Pedersen, and Johan Kärrholm. Inferior outcome after hip resurfacing arthroplasty than after conventional arthroplasty Evidence from the Nordic Arthroplasty Register Association (NARA) database. to 2007Acta. Orthopaedica 2010. 1995;81(5):535–41.

17. Malviya A, Ng L, Hashmi M, Rawlings D, Holland JP. Patterns of changes in femoral bone mineral density up to five years after hip resurfacing. J Arthroplast. 2013;28(6):1025–30.
18. Hing CB, Young DA, Dalziel RE, et al. Narrowing of the neck in resurfacing arthroplasty of the hip. A radiological study. J Bone Joint Surg (Br). 2007;89(8):1019–24.
19. Steffen RT, Pandit HP, Palan J, et al. The five-year results of the Birmingham hip resurfacing arthroplasty: an independent series. J Bone Joint Surg (Br). 2008;90(4):436–41.
20. Amstutz HC, Le Duff MJ. Hip resurfacing: history, current status, and future. Hip Int. 2015;25(4):330–8.
21. Aqil A, Drabu R, Bergmann JH, et al. The gait of patients with one resurfacing and one replacement hip: a single blinded controlled study. Int Orthop. 2013;37(5):795–801.
22. Alberton GM, High WA, Morrey BF. Dislocation after revision total hip replacement: an analysis of risk factors and treatment opinions. J Bone Joint Surg Am. 2002;84(10):314–21.
23. Barrack RL. Dislocation after total hip arthroplasty: implant design and orientation. J Am Acad Orthop Surg. 2003;11(2):89–99.
24. Girard J, Miletic B, Deny A, Migaud H, Fouilleron N. Can patients return to high-impact physical activities after hip resurfacing? A prospectivestudy Int Orthop. 2013;37(6):1019–24.
25. Fouilleron N, Wavreille G, Endjah N, Girard J. Running activity after hip resurfacing arthroplasty: a prospective study. Am J Sports Med. 2012;40(4):889–94.
26. Le Duff MJ, Amstutz HC. The relationship of sporting activity and implant survivorship after hip resurfacing. J Bone Joint SurgAm. 2012;94(10):911–8.
27. Shimmin AJ, Back D. Femoral neck fractures following Birmingham hip resurfacing: a national review of 50 cases. J Bone Joint SurgBr. 2005;87(4):463–4.
28. Amstutz HC, Le Duff MJ, Campbell PA, Wisk LE, Takamura KM. Complications after metal-on-metal hip resurfacing arthroplasty. Orthop Clin North Am. 2011;42(2):207–30.
29. Cossey AJ, Back DL, Shimmin A, et al. The nonoperative management of periprosthetic fractures associated with the Birmingham hip resurfacing procedure. J Arthroplast. 2005;20:358.
30. Marker DR, Seyler TM, Jinnah RH, Delanois RE, Ulrich SD, Mont MA. Femoral neck fractures after metal-on-metal total hip resurfacing: a prospective cohort study. J Arthroplasty. 2007;22(7(Suppl 3)):66–71.
31. Zustin J, Krause M, Breer S, et al. Morphologic analysis of periprosthetic fractures after hip resurfacing arthroplasty. J Bone Joint Surg Am. 2010;92(2):404–10.
32. Mont MA, Seyler TM, Ulrich SD, et al. Effect of changing indications and techniques on total hip resurfacing. Clin Orthop RelatRes. 2007;465(465):63–70.
33. Khan A, Yates P, Lovering A, Bannister GC, Spencer RF. The effect of surgical approach on blood flow to the femoral head during resurfacing. J Bone Joint Surg Br. 2007;89(1):21–5.
34. Beaulé PE, Campbell P, Shim P. Femoral head blood flow during hip resurfacing. Clin Orthop Relat Res. 2006;456:148–52.
35. Ullmark G, Sundgren K, Milbrink J, Nilsson O, Sörensen J. Osteonecrosis following resurfacing arthroplasty. Acta Orthop. 2009;80(6):670–4.
36. Cara M. Maguire, Thorsten M. Seyler, Harold S. Boyd, Lawrence P. Lai, Ronald E. Delanois, Riyaz H. Jinnah. Hip Resurfacing—Keys to Success Bulletin of the NYU Hospital for Joint Diseases. 2009;67(2):142–5.
37. Cadossi M, Tedesco G, Sambri A, Mazzotti A, Giannini S. Hip resurfacing implants. Orthopaedics. 2015;38(8):504–9.
38. Smith AJ, Dieppe P, Vernon K, Porter M, Blom AW. National Joint Registry of England and Wales. Failure rates of stemmed metal-on-metal hip replacements: analysis of data from the National Joint Registry of England and Wales. Lancet. 2012;379(9822):1199–204.
39. de Souza RM, Parsons NR, Oni T, Dalton P, Costa M, Krikler S. Metal ion levels following resurfacing arthroplasty of the hip: serial results over a ten-year period. J Bone Joint Surg Br. 2010;92(12):1642–7.
40. Williams DH, Greidanus NV, Masri BA, Duncan CP, Garbuz DS. Prevalence of pseudotumor in asymptomatic patients after metal-on-metal hip arthroplasty. J Bone Joint SurgAm. 2011;93(23):2164–71.
41. Glyn-Jones S, Pandit H, Kwon YM, Doll H, Gill HS, Murray DW. Risk factors for inflammatory pseudotumour formation following hip resurfacing. J Bone Joint Surg Br. 2009;91:1566–74.
42. Ollivere B, Darrah C, Barker T, Nolan J, Porteous MJ. Early clinical failure of the Birmingham metal-on-metal hip resurfacing is associated with metallosis and soft-tissue necrosis. J Bone Joint Surg (Br). 2009;91(8):1025–30.
43. Van Der Straeten C, Grammatopoulos G, Gill HS, Calistri A, Campbell P, De Smet KA. The 2012 Otto Aufranc award: the interpretation of metal ion levels in unilateral and bilateral hip resurfacing. Clin Orthop RelatRes. 2013;471(2):377–85.
44. Sidaginamale RP, Joyce TJ, Lord JK, et al. Blood metal ion testing is an effective screening tool to identify poorly performing metal-on-metal bearing surfaces. Bone Joint Res. 2013;2(5):84–95.
45. De Haan R, Pattyn C, Gill HS, Murray DW, Campbell PA, De Smet K. Correlation between inclination of the acetabular component and metal ion levels in metal-on-metal hip resurfacing replacement. J Bone Joint Surg Br. 2008;90(10):1291–7.
46. Underwood R, Matthies A, Cann P, Skinner JA, Hart AJ. A comparison of explanted articular surface replacement and Birmingham hip resurfacing components. J Bone Joint Surg Br. 2011;93(9):1169–77.

47. Shimmin AJ, Walter WL, Esposito C. The influence of the size of the component on the outcome of resurfacing arthroplasty of the hip: a review of the literature. J Bone Joint Surg Br. 2010;92(4):469–76.
48. Vendittoli PA, Mottard S, Roy AG, Dupont C, Lavigne M. Chromium and cobalt ion release following the Durom high carbon content, forged metal-on-metal surface replacement of the hip. J Bone Joint Surg Br. 2007;89(4):441–8. Review
49. PRT Kuzyk, Sellan M, Olsen M, Schemitsch EH. Hip resurfacing versus metal-on-metal total hip Arthroplasty. Are metal ion levels different? Bull NYU Hosp Jt Dis. 2011;69(Suppl 1):S5–11.
50. Langton DJ, Jameson SS, Joyce TJ, Webb J, Nargol AV. The effect of component size and orientation on the concentrations of metal ions after resurfacing arthroplasty of the hip. J Bone Joint Surg Br. 2008;90:1143–51.
51. David W. Murray, George Grammatopoulos, Roger Gundle, C. L. max H. Gibbons, Duncan Whitwell, Adrian Taylor, Sion Glyn-Jones, Hemant G. Pandit, Simon Ostlere, Harinderjit S. Gill, Nick Athanasou, Peter McLardy-smith. Hip resurfacing and pseudotumour Hip Int. 2011;21(03):279–83.
52. Kluess D, Zietz C, Lindner T, Mittelmeier W, Schmitz KP, Bader R. Limited range of motion of hip resurfacing arthroplasty due to unfavorable ratio of prosthetic head size and femoral neck diameter. Acta Orthop. 2008;79:748–54.
53. Langton DJ, Sprowson AP, Joyce TJ, et al. Blood metal ion concentrations after hip resurfacing arthroplasty: a comparative study of articular surface replacement and Birmingham hip resurfacing arthroplasties. J Bone Joint Surg Br. 2009;91:1287–95.
54. Yoon JP, Le Duff MJ, Johnson AJ, Takamura KM, Ebramzadeh E, Amstutz HC. Contact patch to rim distance predicts metal ion levels in hip resurfacing. Clin Orthop Relat Res. 2013;471(5):1615–21.
55. Drummond J, Tran P, Fary C. Metal-on-metal hip arthroplasty: a review of adverse reactions and patient management. J Funct Biomater. 2015;6(3):486.
56. McBryde CW, Shears E, O'Hara JN, Pynsent PB. Metal-on-metal hip resurfacing in developmental dysplasia: a case-control study. J Bone Joint Surg Br. 2008;90(6):708–14.
57. Amstutz HC, Le Duff MJ, Harvey N, Hoberg M. Improved survivorship of hybrid metal-on-metal hip resurfacing with second-generation techniques for Crowe-I and II developmental dysplasia of the hip. J Bone Joint SurgAm. 2008;90(suppl 3):12–20.
58. Madadi F, Eajazi A, Kazemi SM, Aalami Harandi A, Madadi F, Sharifzadeh SR. Total hip arthroplasty in advanced osteonecrosis: the short-term results by metal-on-metal hip resurfacing. Med Sci Monit. 2011;17(2):CR78–82.
59. Aulakh TS, Kuiper JH, Dixey J, Richardson JB. Hip resurfacing for rheumatoid arthritis: independent assessment of 11-year results from an international register. Int Orthop. 2011;35(6):803–8.
60. Nunley RM, Della Valle CJ, Barrack RL. Is patient selection important for hip resurfacing? Clin Orthop Relat Res. 2009;467:56–65.
61. Amarasekera HW, Ml C. Foguet P, et al. The blood flow to the femoral head/neck junction during resurfacing arthroplasty: a comparison of two approaches using laser Doppler flowmetry. J Bone Joint Surg Br. 2008;90:442–5.
62. McBryde CW, Revell MP, Thomas AM, et al. The influence of surgical approach on outcome in Birmingham hip resurfacing. Clin Orthop Relat Res. 2008;466:920–6.
63. Radcliffe IAJ, Taylor M. Investigation into the effect of varus-valgus orientation on load transfer in the resurfaced femoral head: a multi-femur finite element analysis. Clin Biomech. 2007;22:780–6.
64. Beckmann J, Goldapp C, Ringleff K, Schaumburger J, Grifka J, Perlick L. Cementing technique in femoral resurfacing. Arch Orthop Trauma Surg. 2009;129(10):1317–25.
65. Little JP, Gray HA, Murray DW, et al. Thermal effects of cement mantle thickness for hip resurfacing. J Arthroplast. 2008;23:454–8.
66. Amstutz HC, Le Duff MJ. Cementing the metaphyseal stem in metal-on-metal resurfacing: when and why. Clin Orthop Relat Res. 2009;467:79–83.
67. Pailhé R, Sharma A, Reina N, Cavaignac E, Chiron P, Laffosse J-M. Hip resurfacing: a systematic review of literature. International Orthopaedics (SICOT). 2012;36:2399–410.
68. Sedrakyan A. Hip resurfacing: a complex challenge for device regulation. Lancet. 2012;380:1720.
69. Pabinger C, Bridgens A, Berghold A, Wurzer P, Boehler N, Labek G. Quality of outcome data in total hip arthroplasty: comparison of registry data and worldwide non-registry studies from 5 decades. Hip Int. 2015;25(5):394–401.
70. Amstutz HC, Beaulé PE, Dorey FJ, Le Duff MJ, Campbell PA, Gruen TA. Metal-on-metal hybrid surface arthroplasty: two to six-year follow-up study. J Bone Joint Surg Am. 2004;86:28–39.
71. Daniel J, Pynsent PB, McMinn DJ. Metal-on-metal resurfacing of the hip in patients under the age of 55 years with osteoarthritis. J Bone Joint Surg Br. 2004;86:177–84.
72. Stulberg BN, Trier KK, Naughton M, Zadzilka JD. Results and lessons learned from a United States hip resurfacing investigational device exemption trial. J Bone Joint Surg Am. 2008;90:21–6.
73. Jacobs MA, Goytia RN, Bhargava T. Hip resurfacing through an anterolateral approach. J Bone Joint Surg Am. 2008;90:38–44.
74. Heilpern GN, Shah NN, Fordyce MJ. Birmingham hip resurfacing arthroplasty: a series of 110 consecutive hips with a minimum five-year clinical and radiological follow-up. J Bone Joint Surg Am. 2008;90:1137–1142.15.
75. Hing CB, Back DL, Bailey M, Young DA, Dalziel RE, Shimmin AJ. The results of primary Birmingham hip resurfacings at a mean of five years: an indepen-

dent prospective review of the first 230 hips. J Bone Joint Surg Br. 2007;89:1431–8.
76. Pollard TC, Baker RP, Eastaugh-Waring SJ, Bannister GC. Treatment of the young active patient with osteoarthritis of the hip. A five- to seven-year comparison of hybrid total hip arthroplasty and metal-on-metal resurfacing. J Bone Joint Surg Br. 2006;88:592–600.
77. Daniel J, Ziaee H, Kamali A, Pradhan C, Band T, McMinn DJ. Ten-year results of a double-heat-treated metal-on-metal hip resurfacing. J Bone Joint Surg Br. 2010;92(1):20–7.
78. Treacy RB, McBryde CW, Shears E, Pynsent PB. Birmingham hip resurfacing: a minimum follow-up of ten years. J Bone Joint Surg Br. 2011;93(1):27–33.
79. Matharu GS, McBryde CW, Pynsent WB, Pynsent PB, Treacy RB. The outcome of the Birmingham hip resurfacing in patients aged < 50 years up to 14 years post-operatively. Bone Joint J. 2013;95-B(9):1172–7.
80. Mehra A, Berryman F, Matharu GS, Pynsent PB, Isbister ES. Birmingham hip resurfacing: a single surgeon series reported at a minimum of 10 years follow-up. J Arthroplast. 2015;30(7):1160–6.
81. Azam MQ, McMahon S, Hawdon G, Sankineani SR. Survivorship and clinical outcome of Birmingham hip resurfacing: a minimum ten years' follow-up. Int Orthop. 2016;40(1):1–7.
82. Amstutz HC, Le Duff MJ, Campbell PA, Gruen TA, Wisk LE. Clinical and radiographic results of metal-on-metal hip resurfacing with a minimum ten-year follow-up. J Bone Joint Surg Am. 2010;92(16):2663–71.
83. Baker RP, Pollard TC, Eastaugh-Waring SJ. Bannister GCA medium-term comparison of hybrid hip replacement and Birmingham hip resurfacing in active young patients. J Bone Joint Surg Br. 2011;93(2):158–63.
84. Hartmann A, Lutzner J, Kirschner S, Witzleb WC, Günther KP. Do survival rate and serum ion concentrations 10 years after metal-on-metal hip resurfacing provide evidence for continued use? Clin Orthop RelatRes. 2012;470:3118–26.
85. Seppänen M, Mäkelä K, Virolainen P, Remes V, Pulkkinen P, Eskelinen A. Hip resurfacing arthroplasty: short-term survivorship of 4,401 hips from the Finnish Arthroplasty Register. Acta Orthopaed. 2012;83(3):207–3.
86. Shimmin AJ, Baré JV. Comparison of functional results of hip resurfacing and total hip replacement: a review of the literature. Orthop Clin North Am. 2011;42(2):143–51.
87. Smith TO, Nichols R, Donell ST, Hing CB. The clinical and radiological outcomes of hip resurfacing versus total hip arthroplasty: a meta-analysis and systematic review. Acta Orthop. 2010;81(6):684–95.
88. McMinn DJW, Snell KIE, Daniel J, Treacy RBC, Pynsent PB, Riley RD. Mortality and implant revision rates of hip arthroplasty in patients with osteoarthritis: registry based cohort study. BMJ. 2012;344:e3319.
89. Junnila M, Kostensalo I, Virolainen P, Remes V, Matilainen M, Vahlberg T, Pulkkinen P, Eskelinen A, Itälä A, Mäkelä K. Hip resurfacing arthroplasty versus large diameter head metal-on-metal total hip arthroplasty: comparison of three designs from the Finnish arthroplasty register. Scand J Surg. 2013;103:54–9.
90. Alison J. Smith, Paul Dieppe, Peter W Howard, Ashley W Blom, on behalf of the National Joint Registry for England and Wales failure rates of metal-on-metal hip resurfacings: analysis of data from the National Joint Registry for England and Wales. Lancet. 2012;380:1759–66.
91. Haughom BD, Erickson BJ, Hellman MD, Jacobs JJ. Do complication rates differ by gender after metal-on-metal hip resurfacing arthroplasty? A systematic review. Clin Orthop Relat Res. 2015;473:2521–9.
92. Beaulé P, Le Duff M, Amstutz H. Hemiresurfacing arthroplasty of the hip for failed free-vascularized fibular graft. J Arthroplasty. 2003;18:519–23.
93. Beaulé P, Amstutz H, Le Duff M, Dorey F. Surface arthroplasty for osteonecrosis of the hip: hemiresurfacing versus metal-on-metal hybrid resurfacing. J Arthroplasty. 2004;19:54–5.
94. Beaulé P, Schmalzried T, Campbell P, Dorey F, Amstutz H. Duration of symptom and outcome of hemiresurfacing for hip osteonecrosis. Clin Orthop. 2001;385:104–17.
95. Larkin B, Nyazee H, Motley J, Nunley RM, Clohisy JC, Barrack RL. Hip resurfacing does not improve proprioception compared with THA. Clin Orthopaed Relat Res. 2014;472(2):555–61. http://doi.org/10.1007/s11999-013-3082-8
96. Langton DJ, Jameson SS, Joyce TJ, Hallab NJ, Natu S, Nargol AV. Early failure of metal-on- metal bearings in hip resurfacing and large-diameter total hip replacement: a consequence of excess wear. J Bone Joint Surg Br. 2010;92(1):38–46.
97. Haddad FS, Konan S, Tahmassebi J. A prospective comparative study of cementless total hip arthroplasty and hip resurfacing in patients under the age of 55 years: a ten-year follow-up. Bone Joint J. 2015;97-B(5):617–22. http://doi.org/10.1302/0301-620X.97B5.34537

Part III

Complex Primary Hip Arthroplasty

Acetabular Dysplasia

5

Eustathios Kenanidis, Panagiotis Kakoulidis, Eleftherios Tsiridis, Bülent Atilla, Goran Bicanic, Zoran Sulje, Domagoj Delimar, Stanislav Bondarenko, Volodymyr Filippenko, Mandus Akonjom, Zoltán Csernátony, Gergely Huszanyik, László Kiss, Richard L. Purcell, Charles A. Engh Jr, Hiroshi Fujita, John B. Meding, E. Michael Keating, Tatsuya Sueyoshi, Per Wretenberg, Sebastian Mukka, Ahmad S. Khaled, Sujith Konan, Fares S. Haddad, Gyula Győrfi, Lei Zhang, Chitranjan S. Ranawat, Michael Gaudiani, Ibrahim Azboy, Antonia F. Chen, Richard Rothman, Volker Otten, Arkan S. Sayed-Noor, Alberto V. Carli, Lazaros Poultsides, Seth A. Jerabek, Kalliopi Lampropoulou-Adamidou, and George Hartofilakidis

E. Kenanidis, M.D., Ph.D., M.Sc. (✉) · P. Kakoulidis, M.D.
Academic Orthopaedic Unit, Aristotle University Medical School, Thessaloniki, Greece

E. Tsiridis, M.D., Ph.D., F.A.C.S., F.R.C.S. (✉)
Academic Orthopaedic Unit, Papageorgiou General Hospital, Aristotle University Medical School, Thessaloniki, Greece
e-mail: etsiridis@doctors.org.uk

B. Atilla, M.D.
Faculty of Medicine, Hacettepe University, Ankara, Turkey

G. Bicanic, M.D., Ph.D.
Al Zahra Hospital Dubai, Dubai, UAE
e-mail: goran@bicanic.eu

Z. Sulje, M.D.
Department of Orthopaedic Surgery and Traumatology, University Hospital Centre Zagreb, Zagreb, Croatia

D. Delimar, M.D., Ph.D.
University of Zagreb, School of Medicine, Zagreb, Croatia

Department of Orthopaedic Surgery, University Hospital Centre Zagreb, Zagreb, Croatia
e-mail: domagoj.delimar@kbc-zagreb.hr

S. Bondarenko, M.D., Ph.D. · V. Filippenko, M.D. · M. Akonjom, M.B.B.Ch., M.D., F.I.C.S.
Department of Joint Pathology, Sytenko Institute of Spine and Joint Pathology, Kharkiv, Ukraine

Z. Csernátony, D.Sc. · L. Kiss, M.D. · G. Győrfi, M.D. · L. Zhang, M.D.
Department of Orthopaedic Surgery, University of Debrecen, Debrecen, Hungary
e-mail: csz@med.unideb.hu

G. Huszanyik, M.D.
Department of Traumatology, University of Debrecen, Debrecen, Hungary

E. Tsiridis (ed.), *The Adult Hip - Master Case Series and Techniques*,
https://doi.org/10.1007/978-3-319-64177-5_5

R. L. Purcell, M.D.
Anderson Orthopaedic Research Institute,
Alexandria, VA, USA

Walter Reed Military, Medical Center, Bethesda, MD, USA
e-mail: rhopper@aori.org

Charles A. Engh Jr, M.D.
Anderson Orthopaedic Research Institute,
Alexandria, VA, USA

Inova Mount Vernon Joint Replacement Center,
Alexandria, VA, USA
e-mail: andy@andersonclinic.com

H. Fujita, M.D.
Department of Orthopaedic Surgery, Institute of Joint Replacement, Kyoto Katsuta Hospital, Kyoto, Japan

John B. Meding, M.D. · E. Michael Keating, M.D.
The Center for Hip and Knee Surgery, St. Francis Hospital, Mooresville, IN, USA

T. Sueyoshi, M.D., Ph.D.
Kobe City Medical Center General Hospital, Kobe, Japan

P. Wretenberg, M.D., Ph.D.
University Hospital Örebro, Örebro, Sweden
e-mail: per.wretenberg@regionorebrolan.se

S. Mukka, M.D., Ph.D. · V. Otten, M.D. · A. S. Sayed-Noor, M.D., Ph.D., F.R.C.S.
Department of Surgical and Perioperative Sciences, Umeå University, Umeå, Sweden

A. S. Khaled, M.B.Ch.B., M.R.C.S. ·
F. S. Haddad, B.Sc., M.D., M.Ch., F.R.C.S.
University College London Hospital, London, UK
e-mail: ahmad.khaled@nhs.net; fsh@fareshaddad.net

S. Konan, M.B.B.S., M.D.(Res.), F.R.C.S.
Department of Trauma & Orthopaedics, University College Hospital, London, UK

C. S. Ranawat, M.D. · A. V. Carli, M.D., M.Sc., F.R.C.S.C.
Hospital for Special Surgery, New York, NY, USA
e-mail: alberto.carli@mail.mcgill.ca

M. Gaudiani, M.D.
Department of Orthopedic Surgery, Hospital for Special Surgery, New York, NY, USA

I. Azboy, M.D.
Department of Orthopaedic and Traumatology, Koşuyolu Medipol Hospital, İstanbul Medipol University, İstanbul, Turkey

A. F. Chen, M.D., M.B.A.
Department of Orthopaedics, Harvard Medical School, Boston, MA, USA

Brigham and Women's Hospital, Boston, MA, USA
e-mail: Antonia.Chen@rothmaninstitute.com

R. Rothman, M.D., Ph.D.
Rothman Institute, Philadelphia, PA, USA

L. Poultsides, M.D., M.Sc., Ph.D.
New York University School of Medicine, New York, NY, USA

Department of Orthopaedic Surgery, Division of Adult Reconstruction, New York Langone Orthopaedic Hospital, New York Langone Medical Center, New York, NY, USA

S. A. Jerabek, M.D.
Hospital for Special Surgery, New York, NY, USA

Orthopaedic Surgery, Weill Cornell Medical College, New York, NY, USA
e-mail: JerabekS@hss.edu

K. Lampropoulou-Adamidou, M.D., M.Sc., Ph.D. ·
G. Hartofilakidis M.D., F.A.C.S.
Laboratory for the Research of Musculoskeletal System "Th. Garofalidis", Medical School, University of Athens, General Hospital of Athens KAT, Athens, Greece

5.1 Current Concepts

E. Kenanidis, P. Kakoulidis, and E. Tsiridis

Developmental dysplasia of the hip (DDH) is the most common childhood hip disorder [1]; its prevalence, however, shows remarkable ethnic changes [2, 3]. The anatomical and biomechanical alterations of the acetabulum, femur and pelvis in DDH predispose to hip OA development [4]. Possible deformities encountered in different types of the disease are:

1. The true acetabulum may be shallow with full contact with the femoral head or partly connected with a false acetabulum or severely small, shallow and triangular with complete loss of congruency with the femoral head [5].
2. Limited bone stock and anterior acetabular segmental wall defects. The bone stock is usually rearranged posteriorly related to acetabulum [6, 7].
3. Version deformities of the acetabulum; up to 1/3 are retroverted [6, 8, 9].
4. Insufficient coverage of the femoral head from the acetabulum.
5. Anteversion of the iliac rim [6].

6. Femoral hypoplasia with loss of the metaphyseal flare [10].
7. Narrow and straight femoral intramedullary canal [11, 12].
8. Marked femoral anteversion and torsion and short neck [10, 13].
9. Coxavalga and lower offset [6].
10. Posterior position of the greater trochanter [6, 13].
11. Proximal femoral deformity from the previous osteotomies [10, 13].
12. Distorted hip biomechanics with shortening and deficiency of the abductors, flexors and extensors due to the persistent dislocation [6].
13. Abundant soft tissue (capsule and ligaments) [6].
14. Unilateral limping and LLD.

There are many proposed classifications of the OA following DDH. The most popular are the Hartofylakidis [5, 14] and Crowe classifications [15]; both of them have excellent reliability [17, 18]. The Hartofylakidis classification [5] is a qualitative classification that explains the underlying pathology and anatomic variations. There are some difficulties, however, to categorize borderline cases. It recognizes three types:

(a) Type A/mild dysplasia
 The femoral head is contained within the original shallow acetabulum. There is a small degree of subluxation and segmental deficiency of the superior wall.
(b) Type B/low dislocation
 A false acetabulum articulates with the femoral head. It is continuous and partially covers the true acetabulum that has a narrow opening and inadequate depth. There is the complete absence of the superior wall and anterior and posterior segmental deficiency. It is further divided into two subtypes with extended or little coverage of the two acetabuli [18].
(c) Type C/high dislocation
 – A false acetabulum (neoacetabulum) not continuous with the true acetabulum exists. The true acetabulum has a narrow opening, inadequate depth and excessive anteversion. The bone stock is abnormally distributed mainly superoposteriorly. The femoral head is completely out of the true acetabulum and migrated superiorly and posteriorly to a varying degree. There are two subtypes: C1 where the false acetabulum is found at the iliac wing and in C2 where the femoral head is in the abductors. C2 is related to higher revision rate than C1 [18].
 The Crowe classification [15] classifies DDH in four types based on the quotient of the vertical distance between intertear drop line and the line of head-neck junction (A) and the vertical distance between the line connecting the ischial tuberosities and the line connecting the iliac crest (B). In type I the quotient $A/B < 0.10$, in type II between 0.10 and 0.15, in type III between 0.16 and 0.20 and in type >0.20. This quantitative classification needs the whole pelvic radiograph, has some difficulties to define landmarks and to explain the underlying pathology and it is not helpful in preoperative planning.

5.1.1 Preoperative Planning

- Take full standard anteroposterior and lateral radiographs [19] for templating; the mean mediolateral diaphyseal diameter of femoral canal is smaller than the anteroposterior in all types, and generally small diameter implants are needed [6].
- Evaluate the acetabular indexes used for the diagnosis and treatment planning as the lateral centre-edge Wiberg angle, the Tonnis angle and the Lequesne's acetabular index [4].
- Perform CT with 3D reconstruction to evaluate wall deficiencies, socket size and medial bone stock at true acetabulum [4].
- Classify the deformity. Be aware, however, that not all anatomic abnormalities get worse as the classification progress [1, 15]. Robertson et al. [12] showed that the advancing disease is poorly related to the increasing femoral anteversion and decreasing femoral offset and

neck-shaft angle. In addition, the anteroposterior acetabular dimension and the mean acetabular volume that is crucial in cup size selection are very similar across Crowe types [6]. The LLD [6] and decreased acetabular anteversion [20] however correlate with the advancing disease.

- Be aware that there are ethnic variations that affect the preoperative evaluation [1].
- Decide the surgical approach [19] and the need for trochanteric osteotomy that provides superior access to the hip joint and also the capability to restore abductor biomechanics by advancing the trochanter distally [19].
- Template to decide the type and implant size [19].
- Be prepared to solve the technical difficulties as the loss of bone stock, increased neck-shaft angle, valgus orientation, increased anteversion, muscle contracture, LLD, etc. [19].

5.1.2 Acetabular Reconstruction

- Restore the hip centre as close as possible to the normal. Ideally, place the cup in the true acetabulum that restores anatomy and hip biomechanics [21].
- Identify the native acetabulum using as landmarks the distal cotyloid notch or transverse acetabular ligament.
- Clear the fovea from the residual soft tissue.
- Start reaming at the level of the true acetabulum with a small reamer and expand it to the anterior and posterior columns. Optimally medialize the cup and achieve proximal coverage of at least 80%; this may be difficult as the surgeon tries to save the bone and to avoid fractures [1, 19].
- Ream till approximately 3–4 mm from the inner cortex remains to leave sufficient bone stock for future revision surgery.
- Try to achieve 75–80% coverage of the cup [22] (mainly anteroposteriorly); a small cup is usually used that however, reduces the head-neck ratio and has inferior wear properties [19].
- If the cup is not covered to a minimum of 70%, then consider other methods as the use of structural bone allografts, metal augments or newer porous metal backing components, bone cement augmentation and reinforcement rings that may reduce the amount of uncoverage [1, 19, 23, 24].
- The inclination of the cup >45°, lateral placement of the cup >25 mm from the true floor and vertical placement of the cup >25 mm from the tear-drop were predictors of increased wear rate at ten years following implantation of uncemented cups in dysplastic hips [25].

The acetabular bone deficiency can be substituted by any of the following methods:

(a) High hip centre

The placement of the cup in a higher position is a technically easier method with limited need for a bone graft that usually achieves full coverage from native bone and provides increased initial stability. Previous reports supported that a high but not lateral cup position may be acceptable [26–29]. Russoti et al. [28] reported 83% excellent and good results in 37 patients with cemented THA in a high but not lateral hip centre. Kaneuji et al. [29] also showed no loosening in 29 dysplastic hips treated with porous-coated acetabular components implanted at more than 20 mm above the tear drop at a mean of 10-year follow-up.

The persistent limping, high dislocation rate, excessive shear stresses and high rate of loosening are the main disadvantages [30–34]. Bicanic et al. [30] supported that for every mm of proximalization, the acetabular load increases by 0.1%. Cup lateralization, lack of lateral support, high distance from the true acetabulum and incidence of preoperative dislocation are the main predictors of loosening [19]. The high hip centre also makes difficult the leg lengthening and revision due to loss of bone stock [19].

(b) Augmentation of the uncovered part with cemented or uncemented THA.

This technique augments the uncovered part of the uncemented cup with bone grafting or metal augments. Bone graft may be bulk allograft, free or vascularized autograft from the iliac bone or fibula [35]. Bone autograft has osteoinductive action with the potential for enhanced bone stock for revision surgery; however, it should not cover more than 50% of the cup [19]. Bone particle grafting has been proposed to improve small uncovered areas in patients with DDH [36]. Autografts or structural allografts are used for larger defects of the supero-anterolateral aspect of the acetabulum to support the cup (Fig. 5.1). The graft is fixed with 4.5 mm cancellous screws to the pelvis and then is reamed of the residual graft to accommodate the cup. Optionally morselized autograft is placed at the graft-host junction [19].

Several studies reported good long-term survival rates for free or vascularized grafts in uncemented or cemented THAs for DDH. Kim et al. [42] reported 94% survival rate of 70 uncemented THAs combined with autologous femoral bone graft in patients with DDH at ten years. Kobayashi et al. [40] demonstrated no loosening for 37 patients with DDH treated with cemented THA and bulk femoral head autograft at a mean of nineteen years. The graft did not cover more than 50% of the cup. Others also supported that the greater the extent of the coverage of the acetabular component by the graft, the greater the rate of late failure [44]. The graft resorption and secondary instability of the cup are reported as the disadvantages of the technique [45, 46].

(c) Porous metal cups or porous metal augments.

The characteristics of the trabecular metal are usually helpful for revisions [47]. They can be used for dysplastic hips to enhance stability [48, 49]. The use of TM cups for 45 dysplastic hips provided satisfactory 10-year clinical and radiographic results [48].

(d) Cotyloplasty

This technique advances the cup medially and subsequently decreases the hip load. It is supported that for every mm of lateral displacement of the cup relative to the ideal centre of rotation, the hip load increases by 0.7% [30]. It was first introduced by Dunn [50] with cemented cup and later modified by Hartofylakidis who named it cotyloplasty. This method perforates the medial acetabular wall making a controlled fracture of it, protects the wall with autogenous femoral allograft and inserts the cup with the medial aspect of its dome beyond the Kohler line. It restores the hip biomechanics and leg length, increases the lateral coverage of the cup and decreases the chance for impingement [3, 5]. The main disadvantages are the loss of

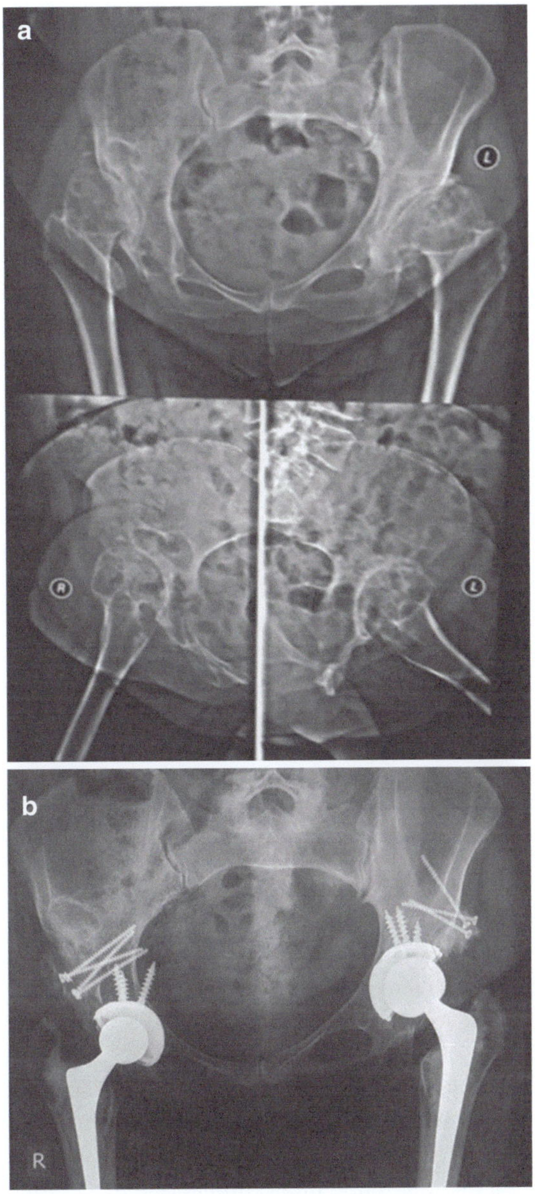

Fig. 5.1 (**a**) AP and lateral pelvic x-ray demonstrating bilateral hip OA Hartofylakidis type II (**b**) Posteoperative AP x-ray showing hybrid THAs with roof reinforcement with autograft

medial bone stock and the possibility of progression of the fracture at the medial wall increasing the risk of early catastrophic acetabular component migration in the pelvis [3] Dorr et al. reported good results with cotyloplasty and porous-coated implants in patients with acetabular dysplasia [51].

(e) Reinforcement rings

Reinforcement rings have been used with success in dysplastic hips. The reinforcement rings in combination with autologous graft augmentation help to reconstruct of the anatomic hip centre and protect the graft for osseointegration. Good results have been reported for reconstruction with reinforcement ring with a hook and autologous graft [52–54]. Seibenrock et al. [52] evaluated retrospectively 33 THAs using an acetabular reinforcement ring with a hook for osteoarthritis associated with developmental dysplasia, mainly Crowe II and III. There was revision rate of 9% for aseptic loosening at a mean of 10.8 years.

In patients with dysplasia of the acetabulum (Crowe types I and II), placement of the cup in the true acetabulum and medialization is usually possible. Cementless press-fit cup is often the treatment option [4]. In low dislocation (Crowe III), medialization and use of smaller cups are usually necessary to achieve better coverage. Autologous grafts or allografts, small uncemented or cemented cups, porous metal cups or augments and reinforcement rings are further options. Supplement screw fixation is often needed. Ceramic on ceramic implants may be used for younger patients [55]. In high dislocation (Crowe IV), the acetabular defects are somewhat easier to manage than femoral where an osteotomy is always required. The anatomic acetabulum has minimal proximal erosion as the femoral head was not located within the true acetabulum [1].Placement of a small acetabular cup (38–44 mm) in the true acetabulum is the usual option. Uncemented cups are preferred, when possible, due to the younger age of patients [56, 57]. Cemented cups showed worse results especially for high dislocations [56, 57].

The surgeon has to choose the correct combined orientation of the acetabular cup and femoral stem that will yield a maximized, stable range of motion and will reduce the risk for dislocation [58, 59]. The technique of combined cup and stem anteversion in THA is a visual judgement that has been suggested as a method to compensate for the abnormal femoral anteversion [58]. The femoral neck and head have to be aligned coplanar to the acetabular cup periphery. Dorr et al. [59] demonstrated that the anatomic stem anteversion is better to be compensated with altering cup anteversion than changing stem anteversion to avoid postoperative rotational deformities of the leg and foot.

5.1.3 Femoral Reconstruction

- Keep the knee flexed throughout the procedure to minimize the risk of nerve palsy [21].
- Retain 15–20 mm of the medial neck above the lesser trochanter to maximize the proximal contact and stability of the femoral component [1].
- Identify and ream the femoral canal to obtain diaphyseal contact [1].
- Introduce a femoral trial stem and try to reduce the hip.
- If the reduction is not possible, then perform complete capsulectomy to improve exposure and allow lengthening [1]. The release of tendons as the iliopsoas tendon, the rectus femoris and gluteus maximus tendon from bony attachments; an adductor tenotomy could further help [21].
- If the hip is reducible, then check possible sites of impingement and risk of dislocation (e.g. the greater trochanter on the posterior acetabulum or ischium). Treatment options include the increasing the offset or performing a femoral rotational osteotomy [1, 10, 13].
- If the hip is still irreducible, think about a shortening femoral osteotomy [1].
- It is better first to prepare the femur and then perform the osteotomy [60, 61].
- The osteotomy is secured with cerclage wires, and then the trial reduction is done.

(a) Stem options

The choice of implant depends on the extent of deformity [19]. In case of mild dysplasia, small-sized conventional stems or proximally coated monolithic stems may be used. For severe dysplasia, a straight and narrow stem with limited medial curvature is beneficial, since there is frequently little remaining calcar following the femoral neck osteotomy [19].In case of more marked deformity, a modular tapered stem or custom implant with or without a corrective osteotomy may be needed [60, 61]. Deformities with anteversion >40° need for reconstruction a custom or modular implant with derotational osteotomy [62]. When a subtrochanteric osteotomy is done, uncemented stems are predominantly used to avoid nonunion at osteotomy site from cement. Charity et al. [63], however, reported the results of eighteen hips with Crowe IV dysplasia that were treated with shortening and derotational osteotomy and cemented Exeter stem; only one osteotomy failed to unite. Intramedullary autograft was used to prevent cement interposition at the osteotomy site and promoted healing [63].

It is difficult to press fit an uncemented when there is a severe metaphyseal mismatch [1]. A small cemented stem is easier to control the anteversion; however, it is difficult to have rotational control in the distal segment. Modular cementless stems make the procedure easier as these can deal separately with the LLD, offset, anteversion and also with the torsional stability [1].

(b) Femoral osteotomy:

- Osteotomy may be performed in each DDH type as a variety of deformities may be present. More frequently, however, in types III and IV [3].
- There are different types of osteotomies as shortening [61] or rotational osteotomies; proximal [64], shaft and distal osteotomies; and transverse [64], oblique, double-chevron [65] and step-cut osteotomies.
- Their main goal is to restore the leg length, the function of the abductor mechanism and femoral anteversion. The shortening osteotomy is also done to protect the sciatic nerve from palsy [3, 66]. The risk for sciatic nerve palsy is greater with the placement of the cup in the true acetabulum and especially with lengthening >4 cm [3, 66].
- In Crowe II a rotational osteotomy may be required whether in Crowe III and IV a shortening and rotational osteotomy. Occasionally, in case of femoral bowing even at Crowe I, an osteotomy may be needed [1].
- An osteotomy needs a detailed preoperative planning [67]. The amount of bone resected will be determined pro- and intraoperatively [68].
- The main problem is the nonunion of the osteotomy.
- Use a transverse osteotomy if the stem has a good diaphyseal stability; if not, better perform an oblique osteotomy from lateral proximal to distal medial [1].

The majority of osteotomies are done in the proximal femur. These are trochanteric and subtrochanteric osteotomies.

1. Greater trochanter osteotomy

   There are several modifications used in complex primary THAs (as DDH) or complex revision THAs. It offers excellent exposure of the femur and acetabulum, helps in lowering the femur, protects the abductor mechanism and allows reposition in its original position [68]. Pseudarthrosis has been reported at 6% in some studies [69, 70]. Paavilainen method includes placement of the cup in the original acetabulum and an extended trochanteric osteotomy with distal advancement of the trochanter. A cementless stem is used. Thorup et al. [71] reported good results with low complication rate for nineteen hips treated with this method and followed up for a mean of 4–8 years.
2. Lesser trochanter osteotomy

   It involves a progressive femoral shortening, while the head neck and part or whole lesser trochanter are removed without the greater trochanter. The complication rate is lesser. Bao et al. evaluated 28 cases of Crowe IV DDH where a shortening osteotomy of the lesser trochanter was used [72]. At a mean follow-up of 55 months, there was improvement of patient scores and no loosening. There were two sciatic nerve palsies.

3. Subtrochanteric osteotomy

   This is an osteotomy done on the femoral metaphysis that is used for shortening and derotational procedures. It is the most frequently used procedure for femoral shortening. There are however several modifications. Becker et al. [65] described a double-chevron shortening derotational osteotomy for DDH patients. Cementless THA using a modified double-chevron subtrochanteric osteotomy provided good short- to midterm results in twenty two Crowe type IV hip dislocations at a mean follow-up of 5.6 years [73].

   Different techniques of transverse subtrochanteric osteotomies have been reported [10, 61, 74–76]. Yasgur et al. [10] described a modified technique of a transverse subtrochanteric and derotational osteotomy with enhanced torsional stability with allograft struts and cables and uncemented fully porous-coated stems, press fit into the diaphysis. Bruce et al. [76] also demonstrated a new technique with the prosthesis in situ and minimal complications. In his series of nine patients, there were three complications, namely, a recurrent dislocation, a breach of the femoral branch and a split of the proximal part of the osteotomy.

4. Shaft osteotomies

   Proximal and distal shaft osteotomies have also been reported with excellent results [60, 77–79]. Sener et al. [60] used a proximal diaphyseal step-cut shortening osteotomy stabilized with two to three cerclage wires and bone grafting in 28 DDH hips; he demonstrated almost 90% good results at 4-year follow-up.

5.1.4 Complications

1. The complication rate is higher for dysplastic than non-dysplastic hips [19].
2. The increased reported risk of femoral or sciatic nerve palsy ranging from 0.8–4.5% [66, 80, 81]. It is frequently the result of traction, haematoma [66], multiple previous procedures [81] or the restoring of the centre of rotation in Crowe III–V hips. Length elongation <2 cm is considered safe [1, 22]; elongation of >4 cm increases the risk substantially [1, 82]. The intraoperative evaluation with electromyography or wake-up test is used for protection.
3. The increased rate of instability [1, 19]. Possible causes are the frequent use of small heads (usual in DDH), decreased offset (medialization of the cup) [1], trochanteric nonunion and impingement due to short neck or retroverted greater trochanter to the posterior acetabulum [1].
4. The increased rate of femoral fractures [19]. This is mainly attributed to the increased incidence of femoral deformities (narrow canal/loss of medial calcar flare) [1]. The risk is increased with conventional stems compared with straight or modular [1]. In case of penetration, the femoral component must bypass the perforation by at least two cortical diameters.
5. The higher rate of infection [19]. This is probably multifactorial in the cause. THAs in patients with DDH are time-consuming, complex procedures usually done through extensile exposures with a stripping of muscles and use of bone graft [83].
6. An increased early rate of loosening especially with cemented implants [84–86]:
   - DiFiazio (43% at a mean of 13 years)[84]
   - Hartofylakidis (32% at 15–32 years)[85]
   - Woolson (15% at 5 years) [86]
7. The early polyethylene wear

This is attributed to the small components and thinner inlays used and to the young age of patients.

5.2 Case Title: Primary THA for DDH Hartofylakidis 1

E. Kenanidis and E. Tsiridis

5.2.1 Demographics

Age: 49
Sex: Female
BMI: 28

5.2.2 Relevant Past Medical History

Principal pathologies: Osteoarthritis due to DDH

Previous surgical procedures: None

Medication: None

History of Presenting Complaint: Pain, instability sense of subluxation

5.2.3 Clinical Examination

Symptoms: Pain, instability, sense of subluxation

Range of motion: Full ROM, painful internal rotation

Specific tests: All normal

Main disability: Pain

Scoring if available: HHS < 70 due to pain

Neurovascular evaluation: Intact

5.2.4 Preoperative Radiological Assessment/Imaging (Fig. 5.2)

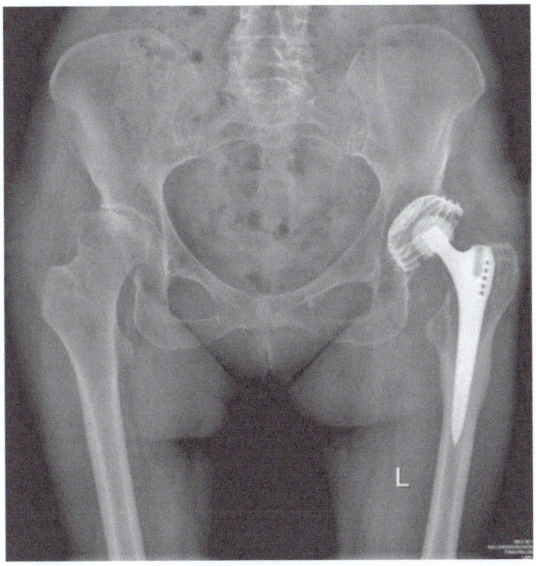

Fig. 5.2 DDH Hartofylakidis type 1 of the right hip with shallow socket and uncovered head with mild subluxation. Femoral canal Dorr A

5.2.5 Preoperative Planning

Diagnosis: Femoral head osteonecrosis (Fig. 5.2).

Possible treatment options: Short offset requires special stem design, i.e. DDH series of cemented or uncemented implants.

Chosen treatment method: Exeter hybrid stem 33.5 mm offset, ceramic head and uncemented 48 × 32 mm socket.

Selection of implants if applicable and rational: 33.5 mm offset available in Exeter series was templated and fitting the needs of the femoral replacement.

Expected difficulties: Shape the socket to achieve better roof coverage and medialization. Maintaining the leg length.

Strategies to overcome difficulties: Deepen the socket inwards and upwards to shape a new roof, and cut the neck low to keep the leg length equal.

Templating: Done.

5.2.6 Surgical Note

With the patient in lateral decubitus position and under general anaesthesia, the hip was approached using a mini-posterior approach. Easy access to the hip joint but the relation to the sciatic nerve was too close thus careful tagging, and release freed the nerve and allowed good inspection during surgery. The neck was osteotomized low to compensate for the lengthening of the leg. The acetabulum was easily approached, and the reaming aimed upwards and inwards to shape a roof for the shell medialization and coverage thus achieved. Attention was then turned to the femur. Preparation of the canal and third-generation cementing of a DDH Exeter stem 35.5 mm offset was inserted. The leg length was equal to the contralateral side and the stability good (Fig. 5.3).

5.2.7 Postoperative Radiographs (Fig. 5.3)

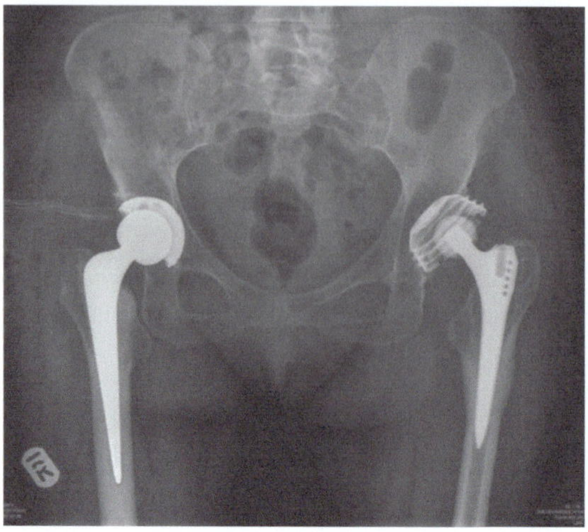

Fig. 5.3 AP pelvic X-ray of the postoperative first day showing the hybrid right THA

5.2.8 Postoperative Management

Chemoprophylaxis and anticoagulant treatment period: Vancomycin 500 mg 1 × 2 for two days, cefuroxime 750 mg 1 × 3 for two days, tinzaparin 1 × 1 for 35 days

Gait/limb loading until full loading: Partial weight bearing for four weeks and then as tolerated

5.3 Case Title: Acetabular Dysplasia Hartofilakidis Type 1 and Femoral Head Osteonecrosis Secondary to Osteoarthritis

E. Kenanidis and E. Tsiridis

5.3.1 Demographics

Age: 54
Sex: Female

5.3.2 Relevant Past Medical History

Principal pathologies: Hypothyroidism

Medication: Laevothyroxine

History of Presenting Complaint: Pain of right hip the last 5–7 years, worsen the last months

5.3.3 Preoperative Radiological Assessment/Imaging (Fig. 5.4)

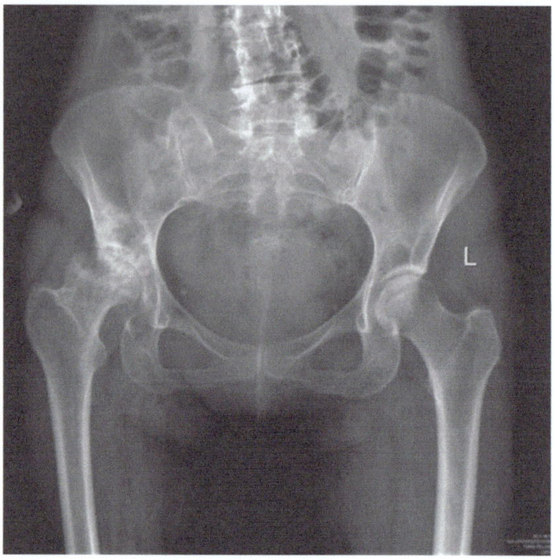

Fig. 5.4 AP X-ray of the right hip demonstrates acetabular dysplasia and iliac osteolysis

5.3.4 Operative Planning

Diagnosis: Osteoarthritis of right hip, acetabular dysplasia (Fig. 5.4)

Possible treatment options: The challenge, in this case, remains the reconstruction and replacement of the acetabular side. In our opinion, in this case, this can be achieved using an uncemented component. For the femoral side, an uncemented implant could work well, though the long-term disability and disuse secondary to dysplasia and arthritis may have led to the early osteoporosis of the proximal femur, in which case a cemented implant was elected.

Chosen treatment method: Uncemented acetabula shell Stryker Trident 50 mm, cancellous bone screws 6.5 mm (2 × 20 mm, 1 × 25 mm), cemented hip stem STRYKER EXETER 44–0, 150 mm, ceramic femoral head 36 mm, + 7.5 mm.

5.3.5 Surgical Note

Due to the hip migration of a nearly two cm cranially, a lull neck cut was elected to bring the leg down to the true socket and the tear-drop level without lengthening the whole lower limb. The acetabular preparation with significant deepening towards the medial plate was sufficient in this case for the insertion and full coverage of the socket around the roof. Due to the previous sclerosis of the roof bone, regardless the exposure of the cancellous bone after reaming, two screws were added to stabilize the acetabular component. After that the operation was standard, with third-generation cementing technique and insertion of the appropriate offset Exeter stem (Figs. 5.5 and 5.6).

Patient's position: Lateral decubitus
Type of anaesthesia: General
Surgical approach: Mini-posterior

5.3.6 Postoperative Radiographs (Figs. 5.5 and 5.6)

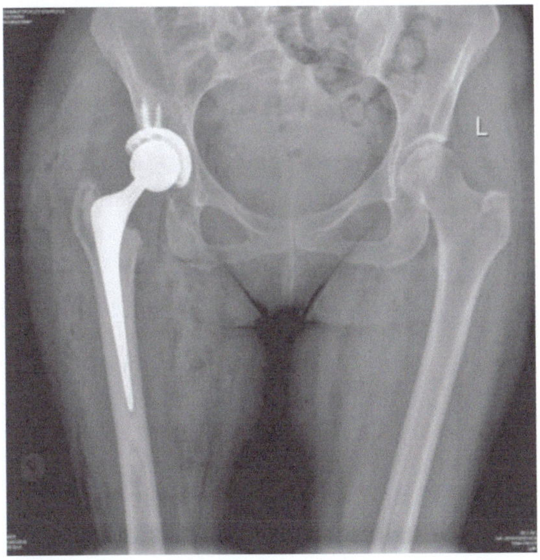

Fig. 5.5 AP x-ray of the right hip first day showing the cup reconstruction with bone autograft from the femoral head

5.3.7 Postoperative Management

Chemoprophylaxis and anticoagulant treatment period: Vancomycin 500 mg 1 × 2 for two days, cefuroxime 750 mg 1 × 3 for the days of hospitalization, enoxaparin 1 × 1 for the days of hospitalization and then rivaroxaban 10 mg 1 × 1 for thirty days

Gait/limb loading until full loading: Partial weight bearing for four weeks and then as tolerated

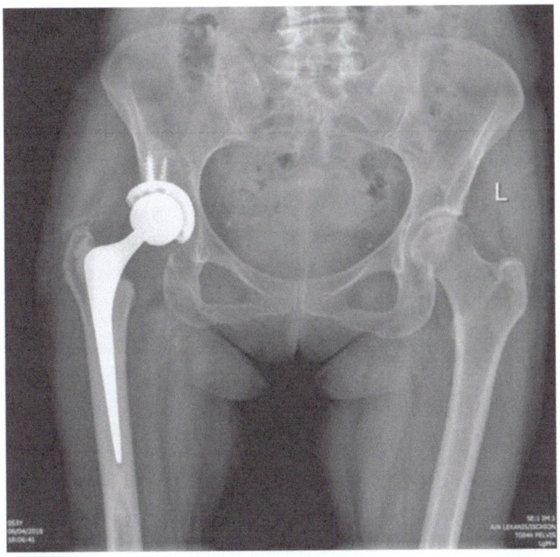

Fig. 5.6 AP x-ray of the right hip at the third postoperative month with total osseointegration of the autograft

5.4 Case Title: Bilateral Hartofilakidis Type II Hip DDHs Following Previous Proximal Femoral Varus Osteotomies Without Removing the Hardware. Bilateral Hybrid Cemented Exeter THAs with Constrained Liners and Hardware Removal at One Stage

E. Kenanidis and E. Tsiridis

5.4.1 Demographics

Age: 29
Sex: Female
BMI: 20

5.4.2 Relevant Past Medical History

Principal pathologies: Unsuccessfully treated early hip dislocation on both sides leading to the formation of false acetabulum adjacent to the roof of the true acetabulum. Proximal femoral deformity following previous varus osteotomies. Early osteoarthritis as expected. Global pelvic dysplasia with hypoplasia of the pelvis and positive Trendelenburg on both sides.

Previous surgical procedures: Varus osteotomies bilaterally at childhood.

Medication: None.

History of Presenting Complaint: Pain, inability to walk, Trendelenburg gait.

5.4.3 Clinical Examination

Symptoms: Pain

Range of motion: Right, flexion: 60°, extension: −10°, rotation: 45°/25°, abd/add: 20°/20°; Left hip, flexion: 70°, extension: 0°, rotation: 25°/25°, abd/add: 20°/20°

Specific tests: Trendelenburg positive RT and LT

Main disability: Pain

Scoring if available: Right HHS < 70, left HHS < 70

Neurovascular evaluation: Intact

5.4.4 Preoperative Radiological Assessment/Imaging (Fig. 5.7)

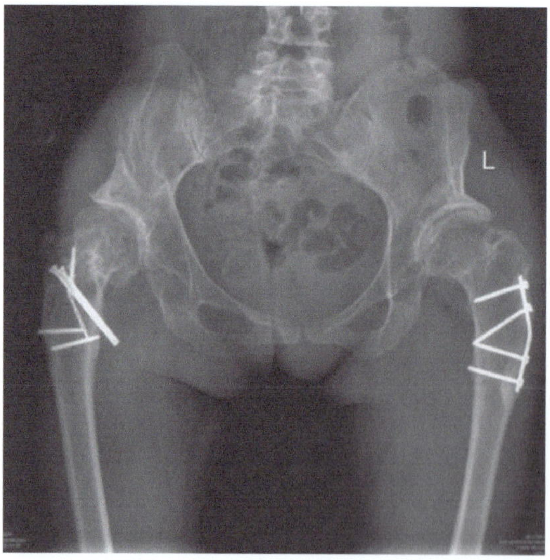

Fig. 5.7 Bilateral hip DDHs Hartofylakidis type II. Post varus osteotomies bilaterally, single procedure on the left; double procedure on the right. Broken drill bit inside the femoral canal on the right and broken screw heads

5.4.5 Preoperative Planning

Diagnosis: DDH Hartofylakidis type II right and left post varus osteotomies bilaterally (Fig. 5.7).

Possible treatment options: *First option*: Uncemented small modular or monolithic tapered fluted Wagner-type stem. The latter stem is straight and may not be suitable for our case as insertion of such stem may require subtrochanderic corrective valgus osteotomy. Should we select this surgical avenue, then a longer stem should be considered to bypass the osteotomy site two femoral diameters for stability. *Second option*: cemented Exeter short stem with a short offset to accommodate for the short distance between the neck and the acetabulum. For the acetabular site, roof reinforcement with autograft is deemed necessary to reconstruct and support the roof. An uncemented shell would have been an option; however, the lack of abductors necessitates a stable construct using either large head or dual mobility that was not possible either considering the small diameter of the socket or a cemented constrained liner that was selected as the reaming of the socket went only up 44 mm.

Chosen treatment method: Right and left THA, cemented constrained acetabular insert 44 mm (Stryker) femoral head 22, cemented hip stem Exeter 33 mm offset (Stryker).

Selection of implants if applicable and rational: Cemented implant acetabulum constrained unable us to use metal shell due to size. Cemented Exeter hip 33 mm to accommodate the short offset and to bypass easily the varus femoral deformity.

Expected difficulties: Removing metal work, acetabular reaming and stem insertion with reasonable cement mantle around it.

Strategies to overcome difficulties: Careful removal of the screws plate and ready for treating an intraoperative periprosthetic femoral fracture.

Templating: Bilateral hip templating in a 100% magnification radiograph.

5.4.6 Surgical Note

With the patient in lateral decubitus position and a mini-posterior approach, the hip was exposed easily. Identification of the sciatic nerve in a close proximity to the femoral neck. Careful tagging of the sciatic nerve and release of the surrounding adhesions to be able to observe its track up and down. Easy dislocation of the femoral head from the false acetabulum, removal of the thickened and excess anterior capsule reaching the level of the lesser trochanter which was very difficult to identify due to the previous osteotomy. Attention was then turned to the removal of the hardware from the femur that appeared to be very challenging. Unscrewing the screws was impossible, therefore, cutting out the screw heads and drilling out the screw shaft from the femur perpendicular to the longitudinal axis using screw removing cutting tubes. The screw fixation in the medial cortex was occasionally a challenge, therefore externally rotating the femur and hammering the screw from medial to lateral was necessary to remove it from the lateral cortex. The femur was then placed anteriorly and attention was turned to the acetabular side. The true acetabular fossa was identified, the size of which was as small as a thumbnail. The anterior and posterior wall was then exposed. The posterior wall was well developed therefore reaming relied entirely onto it protecting the anterior wall that was very weak. The reaming was directed downwards towards the tear-drop and inwards towards the inner plate to create the new acetabular fossa. The limited bone stock restricted our ability to deepen the socket enough to achieve good roof coverage. The femoral head was then shaped to be fixed onto the false acetabulum, adjacent to the roof of the socket. The false acetabulum was large enough to accommodate a 44 mm reamer in order to remove the existing pseudocartilage and to expose the cancellous bone underneath it. Grafting of the false acetabulum was achieved bone to bone using two fully threaded 4.5-mm-long cancellous screws. These were inserted until the heads were buried underneath the graft surface. Reaming of the true acetabulum was then revisited shaping the inferior part of the graft to the shape of the expected roof to cover the shoulder of the socket. Final reaming of the socket was achieved using a 44 mm reamer. The smallest constraint liner (Stryker) was trialled on using the original implant, to make sure that the socket is properly covered all around. Thereafter cementation using third-generation technique was applied, and the acetabular component was put in place. Attention thereafter was turned again to the femur. Preparation was challenging as the subtrochanteric osteotomy has created an uneven endosteum with malalignment in varus. Extensive rasping using the small 33 mm offset Exeter rasp failed to go through proximally; thus diamond-tipped speed burr was necessary to enlarge the proximal femur to accommodate the rasp and to allow for adequate cement mantle. Cement plug size nine was then inserted as the canal was very narrow. The stem was then inserted after preparation and drying of the canal in a neutral position to avoid proximal undertortion and varus deformity. The reduction was successful and the joint stable without impingement (Figs. 5.8 and 5.9).

5.4.7 Intraoperative Challenges

Challenges and solutions: The proximal femoral deformity was bypassed by using cemented implants in a reasonable position, however, in both cases a mild varus. Subsequently, the medial cement mantle (Gruen zones 1,2) is not adequately thick, due to varus positioning of the stem. A subtrochanteric corrective osteotomy would have been a solution, however, considering the small size of the femur; the narrow canal, the undertortion and the many screw holes would have compromised the integrity of the proximal bone stock risking a periprosthetic fracture. In the latter case, a longer stem would have been necessary which however not available with a short offset, i.e. 33 mm in the market.

Unanticipated problems and solution: Treating Hartofylakidis type II DDH is very challenging, as one needs to graft the roof of the socket and sometimes to medialize the socket by breaking the medial wall to achieve inclination and coverage. Should one use uncemented shells, one must always use screws for early stability. A considerable disadvantage using constrained liners in young individuals can be overcomed by using dual mobility implants, but not however always available in small sizes like in our case.

Thorough description of decision making, including the reason for the final decision: Major decisions were first to use the smallest size constrained liner to prevent dislocation and to widen the proximal femoral canal with a speed burr to accommodate the smallest stem available.

5.4.8 Postoperative Radiographs (Figs. 5.8 and 5.9)

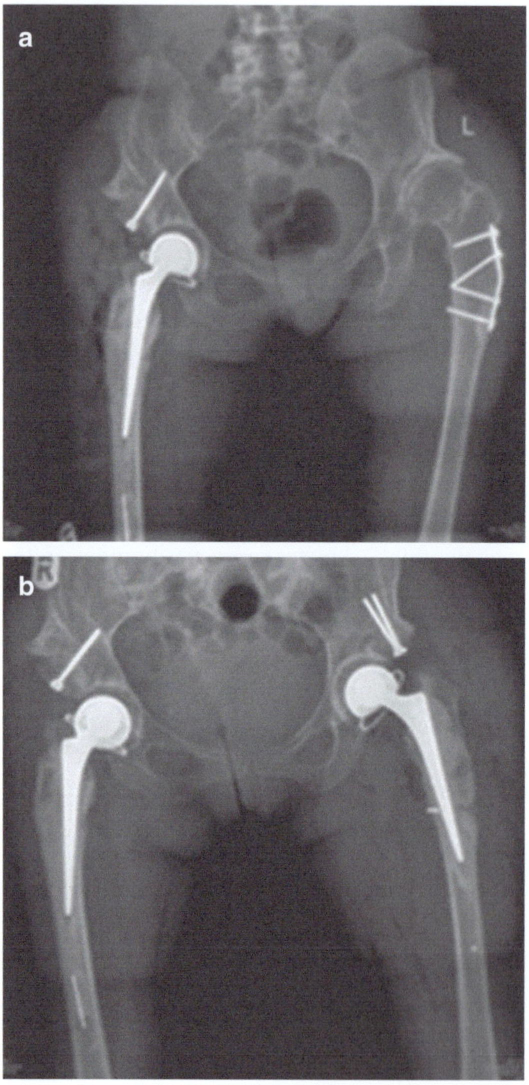

Fig. 5.8 (**a**, **b**) Good roof reconstruction on both sides using autograft and good orientation of the constrained liners. The stems are in reasonable position, and the cement mantles though slim medially are more than adequate laterally

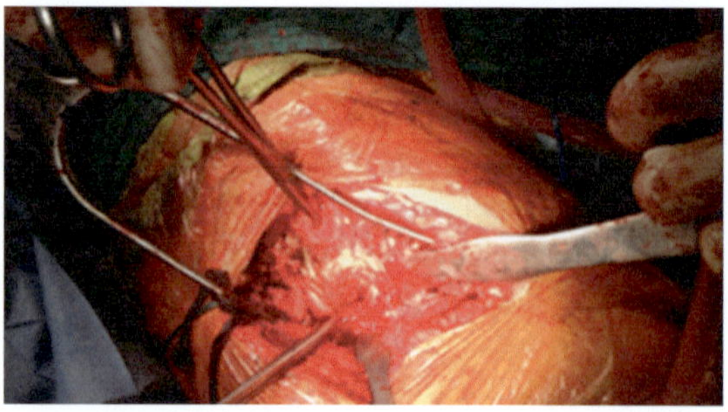

Fig. 5.9 Intraoperative view of the left hip reconstruction through a standard posterior approach. The needle holder points out the false socket while the scissors the true socket. The Hohmman retractors are placed to the front of the anterior wall and below the remnants of the transverse ligament at the tear drop

5.4.9 Postoperative Management

Chemoprophylaxis and anticoagulant treatment period: Vancomycin 500 mg 1 × 2 for two days, cefuroxime 750 mg 1 × 3 for two days, tinzaparin 1 × 1 for 35 days.

Gait/limb loading until full loading: Partial weight bearing for four weeks and then as tolerated

5.4.10 Follow-Up and Complications

There was no complication in this case. HHS improved to 90 bilaterally.

5.5 Case Title: Developmental Dysplasia of the Hip. DDH Hartofylakidis II. Acetabular Reconstruction Using the Femoral Head

E. Kenanidis and E. Tsiridis

5.5.1 Demographics

Age: 50
Sex: Female
BMI: 25

Relevant Past Medical History: No relevant medical history. The patient was fit and well otherwise
Principal pathologies: None
Previous surgical procedures: None
History of Presenting Complaint: Pain, night pain, inability to walk due to pain and instability, short limb gate and back pain

5.5.2 Clinical Examination

Symptoms: Pain, walking and standing pain, leg length discrepancy shortening three cm and instability

Range of motion: Hip flexion of 70 degress, internal and external rotation normal, abduction and adduction limited

Specific tests: Thomas test positive at 30 degrees

Main disability: Pain instability and short limb

Scoring if available: HHS 60

Neurovascular evaluation: Intact

5.5.3 Preoperative Radiological Assessment/Imaging (Fig. 5.10)

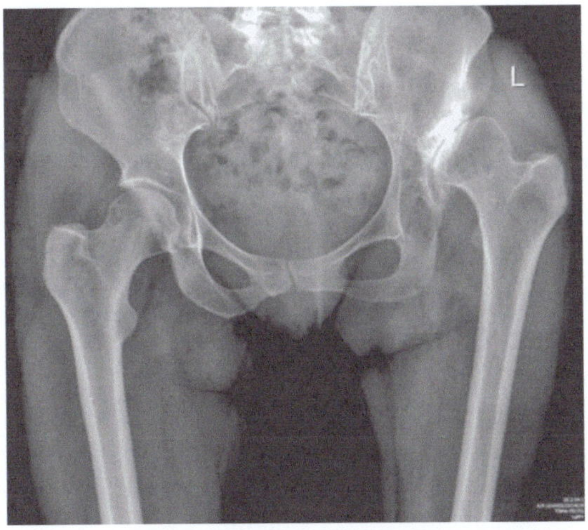

Fig. 5.10 Typical Hartofylakidis type II dysplasia of the left hip. The false socket is halfway up the true socket damaging the roof. The rest of the femur is well developed with moderate anteversion of the femoral neck. The true socket is visible radiologically just beneath the lower end of the false socket. Leg length discrepancy is evident up to three cm

5.5.4 Preoperative Planning

Diagnosis: Congenital hip dysplasia, osteoarthritis of left hip (Fig. 5.10)

Possible treatment options: Cemented or uncemented or hybrid THA but necessary grafting of the roof

Chosen treatment method: Cemented hip stem Exeter 44–0, 150 mm, femoral head Stryker 28 mm, acetabular shell uncemented Trident 44 mm, three cancellous bone screws (2 × 20 mm, 1 × 25 mm), two cortical screws 4.5 mm for the fixation of the graft

5.5.5 Surgical Note

With the patient in lateral decubitus position, a posterior approach was performed to expose the hip. The orientation of the approach was slightly more vertical to find the false socket and the elevated femoral head easier. The hip was found and easily dislocated from the false socket. Osteotomy of the femoral neck as low as possible to the extent that the upper 1/3 of the lesser trochanter was divided just preserving the iliopsoas tendon. The femur was then mobilized, and the redundant anterior capsule was removed to allow more motion. The femur was then retracted forward behind the anterior retractor, and the false socket was widely exposed. The sciatic nerve was found and tagged up and down to be protected and monitored during the phase of reduction.

Acetabular reconstruction: The false socket was found shallow and sclerotic as expected. A small reamer 38 mm was used in a circumferential reaming manner to remove the pseudocartilage and to expose the cancellous bone. That was easily achieved deepening the false socket and inevitably exposing the deficient roof. It is important to realize that one cannot rely on the false socket for reconstruction of the true socket unless grafting is performed. Hartofylakidis II is the most challenging DDH reconstruction category.

Attention was then turned to the true socket. The tear drop and the remnants of transverse ligament were found at the bottom of the true socket.

The opening was as small as a nailbed and reaming started small using 38 mm reamer. It went up to 44 mm and we stopped as we reached the inner plate and the anterior wall started thinning. The posterior as expected was strong and robust. We need up having shaped the false and the true socket into subsequent cavities one over the top of the other. The femoral head was then shaped to fit the cavity of the false socket and was stabilized using two 4.5 mm fully threaded cortical screws of at least 40 mm long. The rood was such way reconstructed, and the trial 44 mm socket was trialled underneath if into the true acetabulum. Snag fitting was achieved, and the real shell was introduced reinforced with three screws through the shell (Fig. 5.11).

Femoral preparation: Standard 37.5 mm Exeter hip was inserted using the third-generation cementing technique described elsewhere. The stem was deepened enough to compensate for the leg length. Checking the sciatic nerve all the way through the process protected it from stretching or direct trauma.

5.5.6 Postoperative Radiographs (Fig. 5.11)

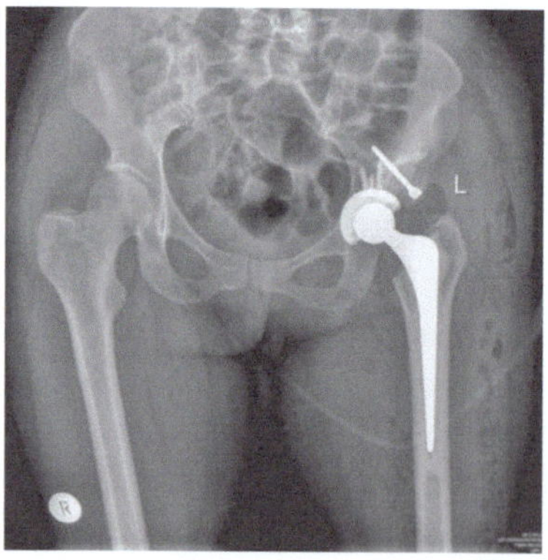

Fig. 5.11 Low cut of the neck and deepening of the stem to allow leg length equality. Femoral head screwed into the false socket

5.5.7 Postoperative Management

Chemoprophylaxis and anticoagulant treatment period: Vancomycin 1 × 2 for two days, cefuroxime 750 mg 1 × 3 for two days, enoxaparin 1 × 1 for 35 days

Gait/limb loading until full loading: Partial weight bearing for four weeks and then as tolerated

5.6 Case Title: DDH Hartofylakidis III Shortening Neck Osteotomy and Grafting of the False Socket

E. Kenanidis and E. Tsiridis

5.6.1 Demographics

Age: 59
Sex: Female
BMI: 23

5.6.2 Relevant Past Medical History

Principal pathologies: DDH, pain, osteoarthritis and instability of the right hip

Previous surgical procedures: None

Medication: Enalapril, metformin

History of Presenting Complaint: Pain and instability

5.6.3 Clinical Examination

Symptoms: Pain

Range of motion: Full ROM flexion: 90°, extension: 0°, internal/external rotation: 25°–35°, adduction: 25°, abduction: 35°

Specific tests: Trendelenburg functional test positive

Main disability: Pain and instability

Scoring: HHS: 70

Neurovascular evaluation: Intact

5.6.4 Preoperative Radiological Assessment/Imaging (Fig. 5.12)

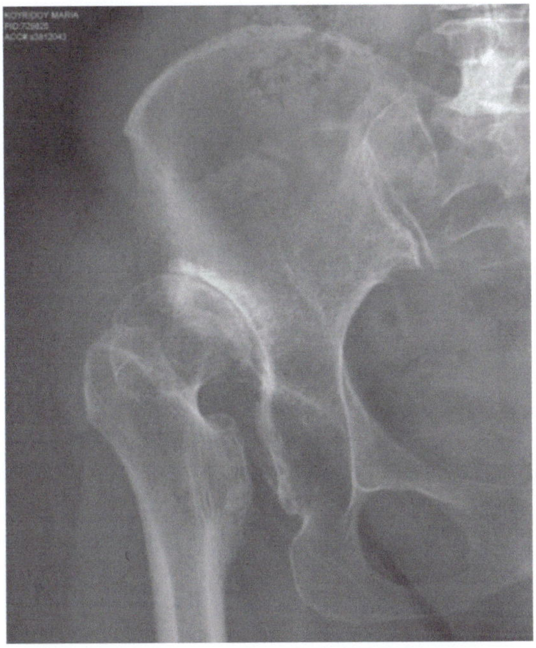

Fig. 5.12 Hartofylakidis type III right hip DDH false acetabulum with osteoarthritis causing pain and instability. The femur is dysplastic as well with narrow canal antetorsion of the proximal femur; thus, the lesser trochanter is facing anteriorly, and the greater trochanter is sitting at the back, anteversion of the femoral neck and short neck offset. The true socket is intact with a reasonable roof but small. The lesser trochanter is elongated and deformed possibly by the chronic traction of iliopsoas tendon which is attached to it. Should the latter be attached low enough, then we could shorten the neck to the upper limit of the tendon to compensate for the lengthening of the limp when we will bring the femur down to the true socket

5.6.5 Preoperative Planning

Diagnosis: DDH Hartofylakidis type III osteoarthritis of the false joint (Fig. 5.12)

Possible treatment options: THA hybrid or uncemented

Chosen treatment method: Uncemented acetabular cup 40 mm/22 mm (Stryker), Exeter hip stem 35.5 mm offset

Selection of implants if applicable and rational: DDH Exeter hybrid system viable solution for dysplastic hips

Expected difficulties: Adjusting leg length and reconstructing the socket

Strategies to overcome difficulties: Autografting the false socket and shortening the neck to adjust the leg length

Templating: Done

5.6.6 Surgical Note

With the patient in lateral decubitus position and under general anaesthesia, the hip was approached using a posterior approach. The approach was directed slightly more vertical to the usual landmarks to get closer to the false socket and hip. The false joint was identified easily, and the hip dislocated exposing the false socket. Immediate attention was turned to find the true socket beneath it. The opening was as expected too small but eventually after removing the redundant capsule anteriorly and posteriorly of the hip, the true columns were identified as well as the remnants of the transverse ligament. Having identified the true socket attention was then turned again to the femur. Low neck osteotomy performed just above the iliopsoas tendon preserving it. After that, the anterior capsule was also excised extensively, and the femur was freely mobilized downwards and anteriorly. The false socket was exposed and denuded from the false cartilage using consecutive reamers until bleeding bone was exposed, and then the half femoral head autograft was screwed in to fill the gap and reinforce the roof of the true socket. Attention was then turned to the true floor. The anterior and inferior retractors allowed good visualization of the entry point, and then using a curved osteotome, the bone was removed until the inner plate was apparent. The posterior wall was thick as expected, and reaming was safely directed backwards and downwards to start shaping the socket. The socket was reamed up to 40 mm, and a shell 40 (Stryker) was inserted tightly with two screws. Attention was then turned again to the femur. The canal was identified in a somewhat neutral position from the piriformis fossa to compensate for the neck anteversion. This is usual for the dysplastic hip reconstruction as if one gives more anteversion to the existing neck version, then there is an increased risk of anterior dislocation. A rasp 35.5 mm was used to prepare the canal, and the hip was trialled to the socket. Easy reduction was achieved and the hip was tested for lengthening. It was then decided to take another slice of at least one cm from the top of the neck above the lesser trochanter, and the rasp was inserted deeper to reduce the length. Trial reduction again showed good leg length and stable reduction with a 22 mm head. Third-generation cementing technique and insertion of the stem in the appropriate depth followed. Final reduction stable and leg length equal. The sciatic nerve was tested all the way through the procedure also in flexion and extension of the hip and was found properly tensioned without stretching or impinging to the joint (Fig. 5.13).

5.6.7 Intraoperative Challenges

Challenges and solutions: Socket reaming, false socket reconstruction to support the roof, shortening neck osteotomy to keep leg length equal.

Unanticipated problems and solution: Adjustments of the neck cut to the limp length.

Thorough description of decision making, including the reason for the final decision: Leg length and sciatic nerve tensioning is important to reconstruct the joint. A well-established technique is the subtrochanteric shortening osteotomy; however, if the sciatic nerve tension allows the neck shortening, it is an easier alternative up to the limit of the iliopsoas tendon.

5.6.8 Postoperative Radiographs (Fig. 5.13)

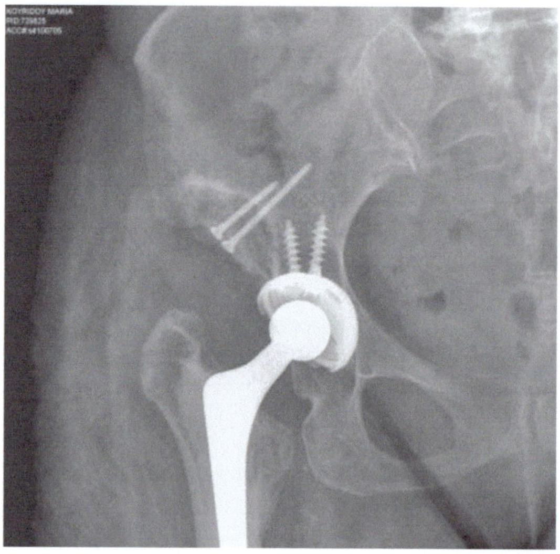

Fig. 5.13 Reconstruction of the false socket with autograft head. Low neck resection and insertion of a short offset 35.5 mm stem to adjust the hip to the true socket

5.6.9 Postoperative Management

Chemoprophylaxis and anticoagulant treatment period: Vancomycin 500 mg 1 × 2 for two days, cefuroxime 750 mg 1 × 3 for two days, tinzaparin 1 × 1 for 35 days

Gait/limb loading until full loading: Partial weight bearing for four weeks and then as tolerated

5.6.10 Follow-Up and Complications

There was no complication. Postoperative score HHS, 90

5.7 Case Title: Achondroplastic Dwarfism with Bilateral DDH Hartofylakidis I and Post-bilateral Varus Subtrochanteric Corrective Osteotomy. Proximal Femoral Deformity and Dysplasia both Acetabulum and Femur. Staged Bilateral THAs

E. Kenanidis and E. Tsiridis

5.7.1 Demographics

Age: 44
Sex: Female
BMI: 25

5.7.2 Relevant Past Medical History

Principal pathologies: DDH post osteotomy, proximal femoral deformity and small size

Previous surgical procedures: Bilateral varus osteotomies during childhood

Medication: None

History of Presenting Complaint: Pain, instability and Trendelenburg walking bilaterally

5.7.3 Clinical Examination

Symptoms: Pain, LLD 4 cm, Trendelenburg walking

Range of motion: Limited ROM

Specific tests: Thomas test positive bilateral in 30 degrees

Main disability: LLD and pain instability

Scoring: HHS: 70

Neurovascular evaluation: Trendelenburg positive test bilateral

5.7.4 Preoperative Radiological Assessment/Imaging (Fig. 5.14)

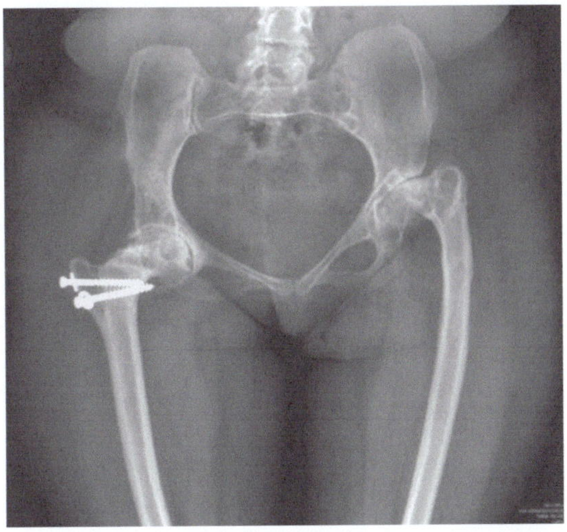

Fig. 5.14 Right hip varus osteotomy with greater trochanter transfer with two partially threaded screws and advanced osteoarthritis. Left hip subtrochanteric varus osteotomy, proximal femoral deformity incompatible with stem insertion without corrective valgus osteotomy and advanced osteoarthritis

5.7.5 Preoperative Planning

Diagnosis: DDH post varus osteotomies (Fig. 5.14).

Possible treatment options: Cemented or uncemented THA for the treatment of instability and abductor insufficiency possible use of constrained liner.

Chosen treatment method: Right hip: uncemented acetabular Shell Stryker Trident PSL 46 mm, cancellous bone screw 6.5 mm (1 × 20 mm), cemented hip stem Styker Exeter offset 30 mm, constrained acetabular insert Stryker Trident size D, femoral head 22 mm. Left hip: same but cemented constrained liner for the socket and subtrochanteric valgus corrective osteotomy to allow stem insertion.

Selection of implants if applicable and rational: DDH Exeter stem 30 mm offset is the only stem measured that could fit the canal; most importantly, the offset is so small that a standard stem even small in length and diameter cannot simulate the small offset of this patient.

Expected difficulties: Right side removal of screws/left side subtrochanteric osteotomy.

Templating: Done.

5.7.6 Surgical Note

Right THA: With the patient in lateral decubitus position, a posterior approach was employed to enter the right hip joint. The anatomical structures were too close to the bone due to previous osteotomies, and care was taken to tag the sciatic nerve to avoid injury. Another crucial point was the previous skin incisions scar tissue and the subcuticular adhesions that threatened with skin necrosis. The abductors were founded wasted with extensive fatty degeneration and poor blood supply. Dislocation was easy as the hip joint was shallow and relatively superficial. The acetabulum was found easily; the dimensions were too small and careful evaluation of the anterior and the posterior wall was made to prevent intraoperative acetabular fracture. The hip osteotomy left a somewhat ossified top end at the site of the osteotomy just above the insertion of the screws. Removing the screws from the intertrochanteric region was challenging as the putsches to the medial wall were well ossified. Medial wall approach through extreme external rotation of the hip that eventually lead to screw removal. The femur was then displaced anteriorly behind the anterior retractor, and the acetabulum was prepared carefully. Reaming up to 45 mm and insertion of an uncemented HA coated shell and a constrained liner in neutral position. Attention was then turned to the femoral side. The canal was occluded proximally with sclerotic bone around the osteotomy site. Reaming was difficult as penetration of the canal was not possible. A speed diamond-tipped burr was used to open the sclerotic canal to a size capable of accommodating a reamer with 30 mm offset. The canal was widened, and a cemented 30 mm stem was inserted using the third-generation cemented technique. Easy reduction with a 22 mm head good length and stability with full ROM. The greater trochanter was thinned out too much thus was elected to be reinforced with a cerclage wire in a figure of eight tension banding to prevent breakage (Fig. 5.15).

Left THA: The patient in lateral decubitus position and a posterior approach to the hip lead to an easy dislocation and assessment of the abductors. Dysfunctional wasted and degenerative muscles were also found on that side. The acetabulum was prepared again to accommodate a cemented constrained liner as the dimensions were too small to accept a metallic shell. The smallest cemented constrained liner was inserted using third-generation cementing technique.

Attention was then turned to the femoral side. The canal was bowed laterally, and the canal was occluded by sclerotic bone at the osteotomy site. A subtrochanteric straightening shortening and valgus osteotomy at the tip of the bowing executed to allow reaming and stem insertion. The osteotomy was stabilized with a five-hole 3.5 mm small fragment plate and screws that penetrated the posterior cortex of the proximal femur leaving the canal free for the stem. Following straightening of the proximal femur, the reaming of the canal was easily completed to accommodate a 33 mm offset cemented Exeter DDH stem. The proximal femur was reinforced with cerclage wired to avoid fractures caused by hoop stressed during reaming. Third-generation cementing technique followed by stem insertion and a 22 mm head to reduce the THA. Easy reduction full ROM and equal leg length compared to the contralateral side (Fig. 5.16).

5.7.7 Postoperative Radiographs (Figs. 5.15 and 5.16)

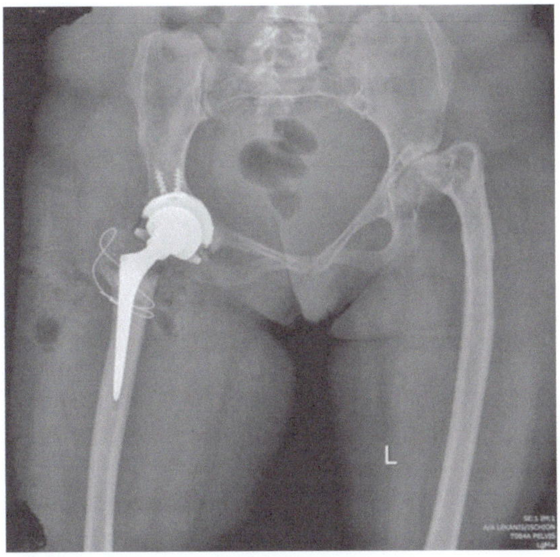

Fig. 5.15 AP x-ray of the right hip first day

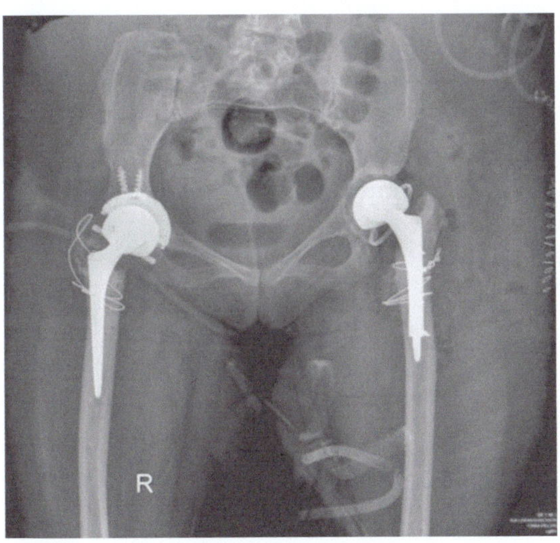

Fig. 5.16 AP x-ray of the left hip first day

5.7.8 Postoperative Management

Chemoprophylaxis and anticoagulant treatment period: Vancomycin 500 mg 1 × 2 for two days, cefuroxime 750 mg 1 × 3 for two days, enoxaparin 1 × 1 for the days of hospitalization and then rivaroxaban 10 mg 1 × 1 for 30 days

Gait/limb loading until full loading: Partial weight bearing for eight weeks and then as tolerated

5.8 Case Title: Staged Bilateral Hybrid THAs for DDH Left Harftofylakidis III, Right Hartofylakidis II. Shortening Subtrochanteric Derotational Osteotomy Technique and Acetabular Roof Autografting

E. Kenanidis and E. Tsiridis

5.8.1 Demographics

Age: 52
Sex: Female
BMI: 27

5.8.2 Relevant Past Medical History

Principal pathologies: Pain, bilateral Trendelenburg gate, leg length discrepancy

Previous surgical procedures: None

Medication: None

History of Presenting Complaint: Pain, instability, Trendelenburg gate

5.8.3 Clinical Examination

Symptoms: Pain

Range of motion: Hip flexion right 70°, left 65° limited ROM otherwise

Specific tests: Thomas positive bilateral at 25 degrees

Main disability: Instability and pain

Scoring: HHS: 70

Neurovascular evaluation: Intact

5.8.4 Preoperative Radiological Assessment/Imaging

Figure 5.17a Right hip Hartofylakidis type II, acetabular roof deficiency, central acetabular osteophyte pushing the femoral head laterally.

5.8.5 Preoperative Planning

Diagnosis: Bilateral hip DDH (Fig. 5.17a).

Possible treatment options: Cemented or uncemented THA left side will need shortening osteotomy to avoid excess lengthening and injury to the sciatic nerve.

Chosen treatment method: Left hip: acetabular shell (trident) 44 mm with 3 × 6.5 mm (2 × 25 mm, 1 × 20 mm), cemented Exeter stem offset 35.5, 125 mm, ceramic femoral head 28 mm–2.7 mm, small fragment 3.5 mm DCP plate 7 holes. Right hip: cemented Exeter hybrid 37.7 mm offset, 32 mm head.

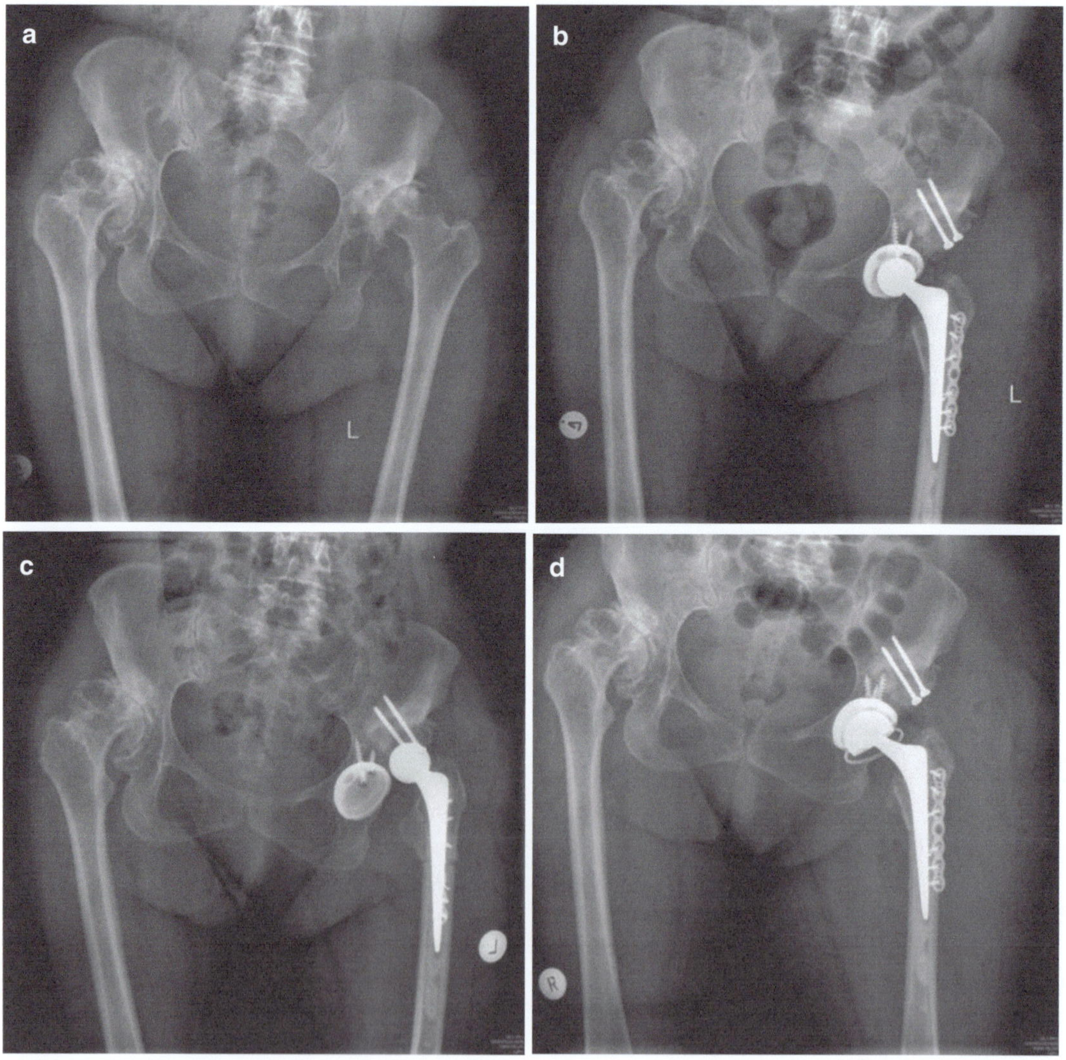

Fig. 5.17 (**a**) Left hip Hartofylakidis type III false acetabulum with advanced osteoarthritis and visible subchondral cysts rood of the true acetabulum deficient (**b**, **c**). The case was complicated by an early dislocation due to deficient abductors (**d**). It was revised to a constrained liner fitting the metal shell for long-term stability

Selection of implants if applicable and rational: Exeter system for small offsets and slim implants to accommodate for the hip dysplasia.

Expected difficulties: Acetabular preparation and femoral shortening.

Templating: Done.

5.8.6 Surgical Note

Left hip:

With the patient in lateral decubitus position, a posterior approach was used to expose the hip. The incision was directed slightly superior parallel to the gluteus maximus muscle fibres. The hip was found high riding at the false acetabular site. The exposure was relatively easy due to capsular laxity and muscular degeneration from the chronic disuse. The false acetabulum was exposed, and the hip was dislocated easily due to its superficial position. The anterior capsule was then excised extensively from the anterior aspect of the hip allowing easy displacement of the femur to the front of the acetabulum. The neck was cut as low as possible adjacent to the intertrochanteric line. Attention was then turned to the false acetabular fossa. Its surface was denuded by the cartilage using small reamers until the cancellous bone was exposed. The true socket was then more apparent below. The true acetabulum was very small and reaming started using 35 mm reamers. The posterior wall was strong with significant bone stock thus reaming began against the posterior wall and downwards above the transverse ligament. Consecutive reaming reached 42 mm diameter. Attention was then turned again to the false acetabulum. The roof of the true acetabulum was deficient and the false socket was autografted using part of the femoral head stabilized with two partially threaded cancellous screws. The roof was strongly reinforced and the true socket now appeared solidly concentric. A shell of 44 mm was inserted and stabilized with three screws. Attention again was turned to the femur. The reduction was not possible as lengthening was excessive. The decision was made to shorten the hip. Prior to shortening, reaming of the canal initiated and a rasp was inserted to check for the length of the osteotomy site. It was estimated that taking down 3 cm would have been sufficient to accommodate a 35.5 mm offset Exeter stem and reach the acetabular implant without stretching the sciatic nerve too much. The segment was excised, and then the two ends were reapproached and fixed together with a 3.5 mm small fragment seven-hole plate. The rasp was left in situ the two-end reduced over, and the hip was reduced for trial easily with a standard 22 mm head. The 3–5 mm plate was then secured using screws at the back of the femur to allow stem insertion. The small gaps were filled with bone graft in and outside the osteotomy. A third-generation cementing technique followed by stem insertion. The cement was not stopped from extruding outside the osteotomy site; it was only after setting that was detached using an osteotomy from the bony ends and the gap again was filed with autograft again. Reduction was achieved easily and stability was checked ok (Fig. 5.17b).

Complication: Three weeks down the line following the procedure, the patient had a dislocation with minimal effort (Fig. 5.17c). The hip was reduced easily under anaesthesia and discussed with the patient the possibility of the revision to improve stability or to constrain the liner. The decision was made to proceed, and the liner was revised to constrain as the orientation of the stem and the socket were found adequate though the quality of the ipsilateral abductors was inadequate for long-term stability (Fig. 5.17d).

Right THA: With the patient in lateral decubitus position and using a mini-posterior approach, the right hip was exposed and found ridding higher into the deformed socket. The neck osteotomy was as low as possible to avoid lengthening the leg compared to the contralateral. The acetabulum cleared for the surrounding osteophytes and the anterior/posterior margins were identified. The femur was then first prepared with the adequate rasps to accommodate a rasp size 37.5 mm finally. The hip was then assessed with the rasp in situ for the reduction ability to the socket taking into consideration the leg length. It was found that a slightly higher position of the acetabular component would allow easy reduction and equal leg length compared to the contralateral side. The position was marked using the diathermy, and the femur was displaced anteriorly to start the acetabular preparation. The predetermined position elected for the reaming starting with small reamers to go deep and superiorly under the roof to achieve good coverage. To achieve that, we elected to stay small in size as priority was given to position and coverage. Final reaming reached size 46 mm and a socket 46 mm inserted with a liner accepted a 32 mm ceramic head. The reduction was easy and stability adequate (Fig. 5.18).

5.8.7 Intraoperative Challenges

Challenges and solutions: Maintaining leg length equality.

Unanticipated problems and solution: Dislocation after shortening osteotomy.

Thorough description of decision making, including the reason for the final decision: We elected to do the left hip first and to adjust the length of the right to its position. Technically is always preferable to our opinion to the worst first.

5.8.8 Postoperative Radiographs (Fig. 5.18)

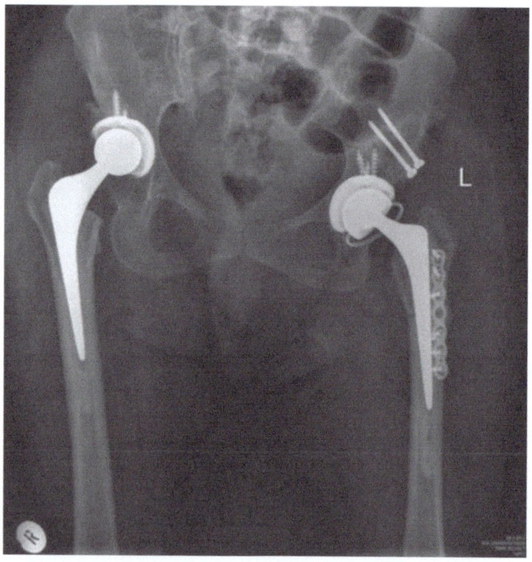

Fig. 5.18 Right hip: Hybrid Exeter cemented hip, high ridding socket to adjust the leg length to the left hip. The position is about two cm above the tear drop but within the substance of the iliac wing and the roof of the socket. It is an acceptable position from the biomechanical point of view, and the coverage of the shell has been achieved by digging deep inside the acetabular fossa but towards the roof and leaving the shell small enough to have coverage all around

5.8.9 Postoperative Management

Chemoprophylaxis and anticoagulant treatment period: Vancomycin 1 × 2 for two days, cefuroxime 750 mg 1 × 3 for two days, enoxaparin 1 × 1 for 1 day after rivaroxaban 10 mg 1 × 1 for 35 days

Gait/limb loading until full loading: Partial weight bearing for four weeks

5.8.10 Follow-Up and Complications

Dislocation to the left revised to a constrained liner (see above).

Improved score to HHS 95 on both sides.

5.9 Case Title: Total Hip Arthroplasty with Acetabular Graft Augmentation in Patients with Hartofylakidis Type II Neglected Developmental Hip Dysplasia

Bülent Atilla

5.9.1 Demographics

Age: 41
Sex: Female
BMI: 27.5

5.9.2 Relevant Past Medical History

Principal pathologies: Bilateral hip dysplasia diagnosed at the age of two. She had two previous operations at the age of 4 and 5.

Previous surgical procedures: Radical hip reduction at the age 4 comprising of subtrochanteric femoral shortening and innominate osteotomy for femoral head coverage according to Çakırgil technique via the Klisic approach. Removal of implants at the age of 5.

History of Presenting Complaint: Right hip pain, limping, limb length inequality.

5.9.3 Clinical Examination

Symptoms: Overt limping, 2 cm short right leg, groin pain.

Range of motion: Flexion: 50 degrees, Flexion contracture 10 degrees, ABD 10, ER 5 with 10 degrees ER contracture.

Specific tests: Trendelenburg test, Thomas test, Stinchfield test; abductor strength test revealed relatively weak abductors of musculoskeletal scale grade IV.

Main disability: Pain in the groin, incapacity to walk more than 300 meters, unable to sequential climbing up and going downstairs. Marked limping, unable to put on socks and foot nail trimming due to the limitation of motion.

Neurovascular evaluation: Clinical examination revealed intact lower extremity pulses, no neurologic impairment.

5.9.4 Preoperative Radiological Assessment/Imaging (Figs. 5.19 and 5.20)

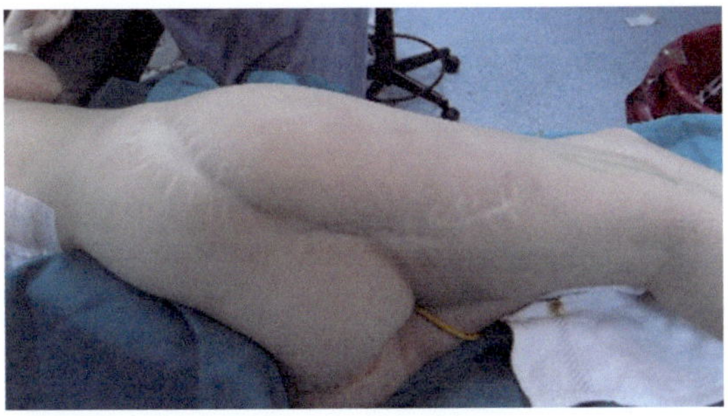

Fig. 5.19 The preoperative positioning of the patient on operating table. Lateral decubitus position with posterolateral approach allows for easy access to both the acetabulum and femur for adequate exposure and soft tissue release

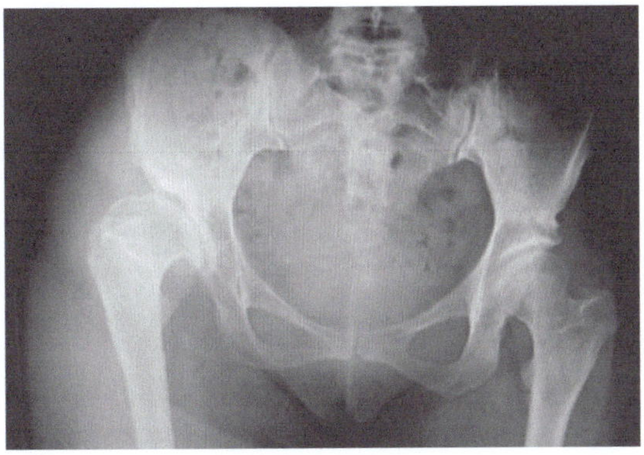

Fig. 5.20 Preoperative AP pelvic x-ray of the patient demonstrating bilateral hip dysplasia. The patient had previous pelvic osteotomy on both sides. Residual dysplasia with head subluxation is visible on the right hip

5.9.5 Preoperative Planning

Diagnosis: Developmental dysplasia of right hip. Previously operated (Figs. 5.19 and 5.20).

Possible treatment options: Regarding the evolved arthritis and incongruency of the femoroacetabular surfaces, joint restoration by pelvic or proximal femoral osteotomies is not feasible. Total hip arthroplasty is the only option. Concern arises on acetabular component coverage and fixation due to the existent residual dysplasia. There are several options for secure fixation. Accepting the presenting deformity and implantation of an acetabular component where superior coverage is available in a high hip centre is one option. The other is the anatomic reconstruction by respecting the normal anatomy with regards to hip joint rotation centre and offset. The third option may be medialization of the acetabulum using a controlled medial wall osteotomy as described by Hartofylakidis 'cotyloplasty' technique.

Chosen treatment method: Anatomic acetabular reconstruction at the level of the true acetabulum with an uncemented implant is chosen, as a reproducible method for better joint kinematics. Regarding the superior coverage defect, this technique requires autograft augmentation for cup support. Autografting is preferred over the superior placement of the acetabular component (high hip centre) to achieve better cup coverage and limb length equalization and to avoid lateralization and risk of bony impingement.

Selection of implants if applicable and rational: Although good results are also published on cemented reconstructions, there is an increased tendency to perform uncemented techniques in the recent literature. A multihole acetabular component with hydroxyapatite coating is used and secured with at least two screws. On the femoral side, a cementless stem with proximal metaphyseal fill is selected owing to its superiority on long-term survival and bone stock preservation through proximal load distribution. In previously operated patients where the proximal femoral anatomy is distorted, the cementless fixation is more forgiving compared to cemented for subtle varus position of the stem. At this young age group, both ceramic and metal head data against highly cross-linked polyethylene is encouraging, and cross-linked poly inserts are appeared to be relatively insensitive to wear regarding the head size and component positioning where component positioning is more critical for ceramic on ceramic bearings.

Expected difficulties: In Hartofylakidis type II dislocations, acetabular reconstruction is particularly difficult. Usually, the acetabulum is enlarged in superior-inferior diameter over a large head, and the anterior wall is insufficient. To find the anatomic centre of rotation and take advantage of using the best available bone stock, reaming should be directed posteriorly. Initially, the superior defect is neglected, and acetabular size is adjusted according to its AP diameter. After achieving an AP contact, the superior defect is addressed by fixation of the autologous head. The head should be trimmed in L-shape where neck portion goes upward towards the iliac bone, and relatively softer head lies within the acetabulum. Two screw fixations are usually enough for a secure fixation. The excessive portion of the graft within the acetabulum will then be removed with acetabular reamers to previously chosen AP size. Superior placement of graft fixing screws is critical to avoid impingement of the acetabular cup after reaming. Cementless cup with screw fixation is preferred.

Strategies to overcome difficulties: Obtain a good exposure on the posterior side of the acetabulum and ischium, identify sciatic nerve and carefully retract. The junction between the ischium, pubis and obturator foramen is a good indicat or of the inferior edge of acetabular component. Transverse ligament delineates this bottom line. Reaming should be done to posteriorwise. Prefer almost full-sized head autograft. Cutting the graft into halves usually makes them insufficiently small. Fine contouring and removing the excessive parts after fixation are always possible after fixation. Tightening of the fixation screws should be done in an alternative manner; overtightening one risks graft fracture. Avoiding grafting procedure and trying to achieve superior contact will usually bring in excessive high inclination of the acetabular component.

Templating: On femoral templating, careful preoperative templating with more than one prosthesis design is essential to determine which design gives the best. In unilateral cases, the contralateral site is used to define the anatomic hip rotation centre; in bilateral cases, we use Ranawat's triangle to determine the centre of rotation and to determine the size of existing superior bone defect.

5.9.6 Surgical Note

Patient's position: Lateral decubitus. Secured with hip supports from symphysis pubis anteriorly and sacrum posteriorly.

Type of anaesthesia: Epidural anaesthesia is preferred with numerous benefits compared to general anaesthesia. Regional anaesthesia can offer both surgical anaesthesia and effective postoperative analgesia. Periarticular injection of Ranawatt's solution is included for multimodal analgesia.

Surgical approach: After the skin incision, the gluteus maximus tendon and the intermuscular septum should be released from their insertion on the linea aspera exposing the sciatic nerve under visual control as a routine part of the exposure. Visualization of the posterior bony structures including a good part of the ischium down to tuberosity is preferred. When lengthening is a part of the procedure, release of the iliopsoas is done to avoid later painful impingement.

Main steps: After the soft tissue release and joint dislocation, the femoral neck cut is made and the head autograft is secured. Femoral canal preparation is made first. Before broaching, preparing the canal with flexible reamers is helpful both in sizing and carefully regularizing the deforming medullary canal. Over-reaming is not advised. On the acetabular side medialization is important; for this purpose usually visualization of the subchondral bone is aimed. The fixation of the graft should be secure enough to bear secondary acetabular reaming. After acetabular fixation, intraoperative X-ray control with trial components is recommended (Figs. 5.21 and 5.22).

5.9.7 Intraoperative Challenges

Challenges and solutions: Avoid minimal invasive surgery, an exposure large enough to visualize critical structures is mandatory. Soft tissue releases are recommended; stiffness due to insufficient releases is painful and does not resolve over time. The appropriate fit of the head graft into the existing defect may become challenging. Trimming the superior osteophytes, carefully reaming the defect and impacting cancellous graft into unfit surfaces are helpful. On trimming the head, always try to preserve the neck portion where the hard cortical bone is available; femoral head is usually weak, cystic and fragile. Use washers for screw fixation towards the head. On femoral side, anteversion problems are critical; undersizing the femoral component helps to achieve correct version but should not risk component fixation.

Unanticipated problems and solution: In the case when autografting fails for technical reasons and not enough graft material is available, the next step should be application of a reinforcement cage. Augmentation with allograft has inferior results. Sometimes after reconstruction, the operated side is longer. Never accept this; patients prefer shorter legs on the previous short side. Elongations about a centimetre can be overcomed by femoral downsizing and shorter neck cut. More than a centimetre requires femoral shortening osteotomy.

Thorough description of decision making, including the reason for the final decision: Anatomic reconstruction is preferred to achieve better joint kinematics which is important both for functional status including leg length equalization and long-term wear performance.

5.9.8 Postoperative Radiographs (Figs. 5.21 and 5.22)

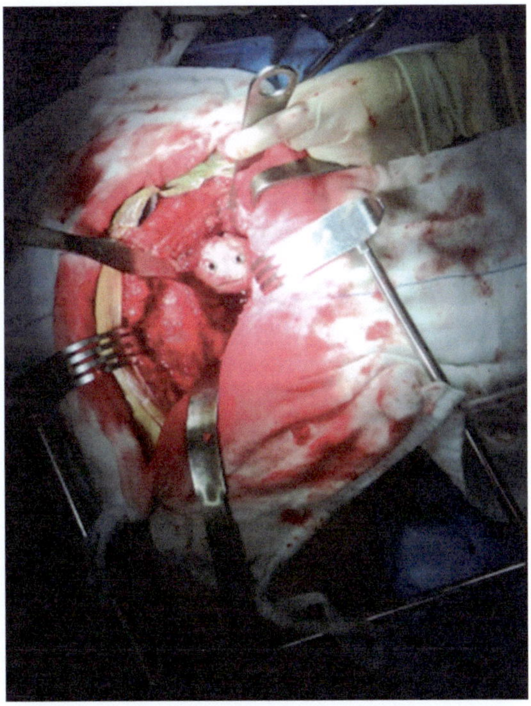

Fig. 5.21 Intraoperative photo demonstrating the application of the autologous femoral 'head' graft. After L-shaped cut, the femoral head is fixed at the anterosuperior acetabulum into the defect created by subluxation. Heads of two cannulated screws and below the cut for the excessive portion of the graft gave the appearance of a ghost head within the wound. After trimming the graft is ready to support a cementless acetabular component

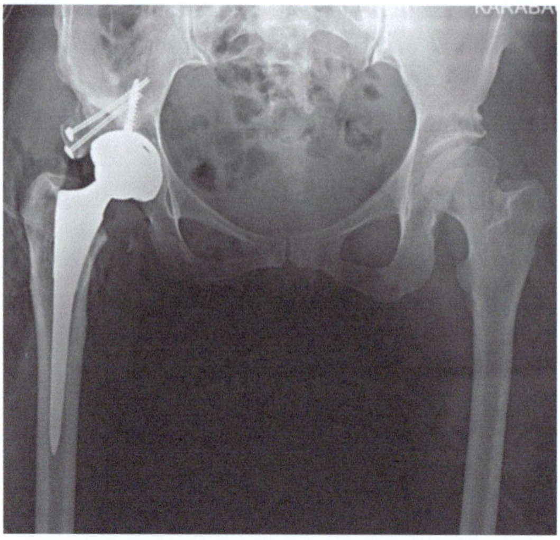

Fig. 5.22 Postoperative AP pelvis view. Anatomical reconstruction of the right hip, leg length equalization, the hip level and support provided by graft augmentation are noted. Subtle varus deformity of the femoral component is due to altered proximal femoral anatomy on previous operations and well tolerated by the cementless implant

5.9.9 Postoperative Management

Chemoprophylaxis and anticoagulant treatment period: Chemoprophylaxis is routinely done according to MSIS consensus statement, and 2 grams of cephalosporins were given ten min before anaesthesia induction at OR. Anticoagulation is started eight h after the operation by 4 mL enoxaparin daily for a month as an extended prophylaxis regimen.

Gait/limb loading until full loading: Patient kept on crutches for six weeks. In the first 2-week period only toe-touch weight bearing is allowed to protect the femoral head graft, and then for four weeks partial weight bearing as tolerated is encouraged. At the end of this period, full weight bearing is allowed. During the initial rehabilitation period, hip abductor and flexor strengthening are specifically implemented.

5.9.10 Discussion [87–89]

Advantages of the applied method: Developmental hip dysplasia presents considerable technical challenges to the primary arthroplasty surgeon. Autogenous bulk grafting with the native femoral head is a reliable and reproducible method to achieve anatomic cup placement and superolateral bone coverage. Reported outcomes of this technique have been controversial on graft consolidation and loosening in the long term. Careful investigation of this reports demonstrates that many of them have used hip implants with conventional poly inserts with a proven wear problem on long-term; therefore deterioration of the graft after seven years more probably attributed to the poly wear and not the healing of the graft. In some series, primary cases were mixed with revisions and allograft augmentation. In more recent series with homogenous autograft, reconstruction in primary hip arthroplasty outcome results over 10 years is more encouraging.

Disadvantages of the method: It is a technically challenging technique that requires identification of hip rotation centre. Wide exposure and soft tissue releases are necessary. It is time-consuming with regards to the straightforward technique of implanting a cup into the false acetabulum. Rehabilitation period is longer than other techniques due to autograft protection until healing.

Alternative evidence-based techniques for the case: High hip centre is the alternative technique to restore the hip joint. In this technique, acetabular component is placed where the actual dislocated head lies. False acetabulum has been the joint and receiving the loads for over the years plus osteophyte regeneration makes this part of ilium dense and usually provides sufficient bone stock for adequate primary stability. Disadvantages are the altered joint mechanics mainly due to the lateralization of the hip centre and risk for bony impingement. To achieve a good long-term result, the lateralization of the component should be avoided. To obtain superior coverage at the anatomical hip centre, another alternative is to medialize the centre of rotation by carefully produced medial acetabular wall osteotomy. The technique is called as 'medial protrusion technique' or 'cotyloplasty' and realized by careful chiselling of the medial cortex, pushing it mediaward and grafting the defect with cancellous bone. Medialization brings the advantage of better peripheral support including the superior dome and reducing joint contact stresses while increasing the abductor lever arm.

Why is the chosen technique better for this case? In this young age group, lowering the contact stress at the joint is important to achieve long-term survival of the artificial hip.

Indications and contraindications for your technique: This technique is indicated in low hip dislocations presenting with advanced hip arthritis and when the acetabular component remains unsupported after adequate reaming at its anterosuperior portion by 30% or more of its surface area. Contraindications are inappropriate technique, inability to achieve primary stability after grafting or to use other graft materials such as allo, xeno or synthetic graft for augmentation.

Learning curve and how to manage complications: Learning curve requires adequate knowledge on arthroplasty exposures, soft tissue release, fixation and small bone fragment techniques and careful application.

Level of evidence concerning the superiority of this method against others: In the literature, there is still ongoing controversy regarding the long-term outcome of grafted reconstruction where some previous series reports deterioration with graft loosening after 7-year follow-up. However, in recent series eliminating the methodological errors such and mixing primary cases with revisions and avoiding inappropriate graft material (allografts), large case series reports favourable outcome with anatomic reconstruction and bone grafting. Almost all of them were retrospective consecutive case series without a control group, and the patient selection were nonrandomized.

5.10 Case Title: Total Hip Arthroplasty using Subtrochanteric Shortening Osteotomy in Hartofilakidis Type III Dysplasia

Bülent Atilla

5.10.1 Demographics

Age: 47
Sex: Female
BMI: 29

5.10.2 Relevant Past Medical History

Principal pathologies: Bilateral hip dysplasia diagnosed at the age of 5.

Previous surgical procedures: No previous surgical intervention.

Medication: The patient was on Coumadin due to a deep vein thrombosis attack on her right leg. She is diagnosed with factor V Leiden thrombophilia.

History of Presenting Complaint: Right hip pain, limping, limb length inequality. Patellar instability in the right knee, callosities under right foot.

5.10.3 Clinical Examination

Symptoms: Patient is complaining about limb length inequality and pain on both hips, worse on the right side. Valgus deformity with mild medial instability and pain at the knee joint, callosity of the metatarsal heads on right foot due to tiptoe walking to compensate short limb.

Range of motion: There is a limitation on internal rotation on left hip. Right hip is unstable with excessive internal rotation over 90 degrees, pistoning on leg traction.

Specific tests: Trendelenburg test is positive on both sides.

Main disability: Main disability is walking disturbance, limping and hip pain.

Neurovascular evaluation: Neurovascular evaluation revealed intact extremity pulses and no signs of neurologic impairment. However, the patient has abductor muscle weakness at the right hip.

5.10.4 Preoperative Radiological Assessment/Imaging (Figs. 5.23 and 5.24)

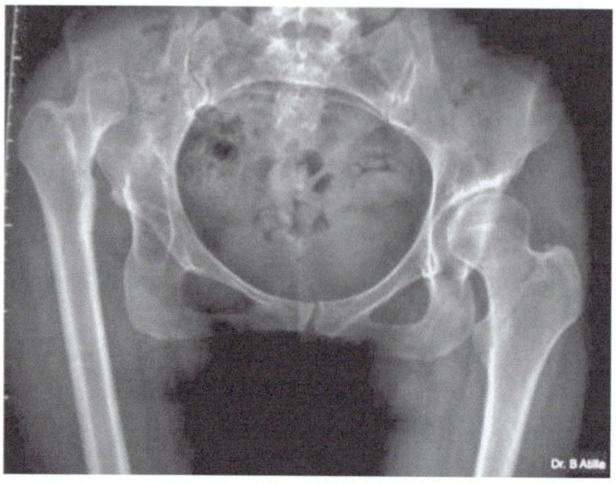

Fig. 5.23 AP pelvis view of the patient demonstrates Hartofylakidis type III high hip dislocation on the right hip and acetabular dysplasia on the left side. There is seven cm of limb length inequality

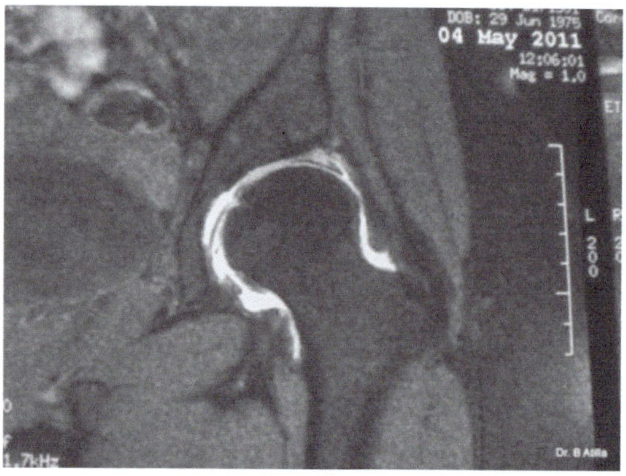

Fig. 5.24 On arthro-MRI examination of the left hip anterosuperior labral tear is visible

5.10.5 Preoperative Planning

Diagnosis: Neglected developmental dislocation of the hip joint. Hartofylakidis type III (Fig. 5.23).

Possible treatment options: After the age of 4–6 years, anatomic reduction of the dislocated hip is not recommended due to the poor function, the risk of avascular head necrosis and consequent stiff and painful hip joint. Available reconstruction methods are completely dislocating the joint using a subtrochanteric valgus osteotomy or reconstructing the hip joint mechanics by total hip arthroplasty. Valgus extension osteotomy of the hip provides dislocation of the femoral head from arthritic false acetabulum thereby eliminating hip pain and increasing available hip motion by correcting flexion contracture with extension component. Subtrochanteric lever facing the ischium provides some hip stability. However, subtrochanteric valgus changes the axial alignment of the lower limb and creates knee valgus. This has to be dealt with a corrective osteotomy at supracondylar level.

Chosen treatment method: Total hip arthroplasty has several advantages. It is the only option for near-complete restoration of the native joint biomechanics, dramatically eliminates arthritic pain. Allows for contracture correction by a series of muscle and soft tissue releases, and it is durable with the recent available technique and implants.

Selection of implants if applicable and rational: Although good results are also published on cemented reconstructions there is an increased tendency to perform uncemented techniques in the recent literature. A multihole acetabular component with hydroxyapatite coating and securing with two screws is recommended. Our preferred femoral implant has two different distal stem diameters for each proximal metaphyseal size, providing better adjustment and fixation distal to the osteotomy. Rotational stability is further enhanced with the oblique osteotomy surfaces and unicortical fixation of a small fragment (3.5 mm) AO plate. Bearing options should be judged according to the currently available evidence; ceramics have favourable wear properties and are excellent choices for young patients. But component fracture and squeaking are reported related to the component position. Researchers found that patients with squeaking and fracture were more likely to have acetabular components placed outside the optimum range of anteversion and abduction. Highly cross-linked polyethylene bearing surface data is more promising and appeared to be relatively insensitive to head size and component positioning.

Expected difficulties: The femoral head is typically hypoplastic and in valgus above a short neck with a smaller offset. Head is usually in excessive anteversion, but this is reported as highly variable. The metaphyseal femur is hypoplastic, and its diameter in AP plane may be smaller than lateral, presenting difficulty to use large metaphyseal fit and fill type femoral stems. Medullary canal is stenotic over a large isthmic segment, frequently presents rotational deformity. Limb length inequality and small offset are responsible for anatomic changes on lower extremity both in AP and rotational planes with substantial shortening of the affected limb. Equalization of more than three cm is associated with nerve injury due to excessive traction. A shortening osteotomy is required, but the optimum technique is not defined yet.

Strategies to overcome difficulties: Anatomic restoration of the hip joint. Adequate exposure via posterolateral approach. Proper soft tissue releases. Subtrochanteric shortening to avoid nerve damage and excessive soft tissue tension. Rotational alignment through the osteotomy to achieve stable hip.

Templating: On femoral templating, careful preoperative templating with more than one prosthesis design is essential to determine which design gives the best fit. The level of subtrochanteric osteotomy is planned just below the trochanter minor, preserves the strength of the proximal fragment while allowing enough stem length on the distal fragment for stability. Lateral templating is also essential since proximal femur deformity may prevent straightforward insertion of a stem. In unilateral cases, the contralateral site is used to define the anatomic hip rotation centre; in bilateral cases, we use Ranawat's triangle to determine the centre of rotation. Then, required shortening is to be determined. Limb length equalization is critical, trochanter minor is a valuable reference point for comparison but is not flawless because dislocated femurs tend to be longer in overall length; all measurements should be judged against the clinical picture regarding pelvic and lumbar deformities, and remaining femoral segment below trochanter minor may deteriorate radiographic measuring from a short pelvic view. Various authors have suggested routine CT imaging as a part of preoperative evaluation.

5.10.6 Surgical Note

Patient's position: Patient is positioned in the lateral decubitus position. This position allows for easy manipulation of the affected hip in every direction, use of any surgical approach with extensile alternatives, providing better visualization of both the acetabulum and the femur, access for soft tissue releases and allows for better visualization for assisting surgeons. Cons are decreased pelvic rotation; sometimes complicating acetabular orientation, and pelvic tilt may be confusing on limb length adjustment.

Type of anaesthesia: Epidural anaesthesia is preferred. Regional anaesthesia and epidural catheterization can offer both surgical anaesthesia and effective postoperative analgesia. Periarticular injection of Ranawatt cocktail is recommended for multimodal analgesia.

Surgical approach: The presented patient was operated in the lateral decubitus position with a posterolateral approach. A percutaneous adductor tenotomy was performed in supine position before the patient was turned into lateral decubitus. After the skin incision, gluteus maximus tendon and intermuscular septum were released from their insertion at linea aspera. Following the release of short external rotators, the joint capsule is exposed, capsulotomy is made, and the capsule is released from the entire proximal femur. To locate the true acetabulum, elongated capsule is followed down to iliac bone.

Main steps: Femoral preparation is done first; a relatively longer neck cut is preferred to obtain a strong bone collar to avoid fracture of the soft proximal femoral segment during stem insertion. The canal is reamed with a flexible reamer first to avoid perforations. A trial stem is inserted before shortening osteotomy, because once the osteotomy is done handling of the proximal fragment becomes more difficult. Acetabulum has a minimal entry and deficient at anterior margin. Preserving the superior rim is crucial, and removal of bone should be directed posterior wise where sufficient structural bone stock is available. Medial wall is fragile and reaming should proceed with care. Seating of the component is realized on between superior and posterior walls, and regarding the oval shape of the existing acetabulum and the hemispheric component, the deficient anterior wall may be further sacrificed. The acetabular component is fixed with screws. A trial reduction is attempted to estimate the required femoral shortening. A subtrochanteric osteotomy is done, and the original stem is inserted while attention is directed towards anteversion adjustment. A small fragment plate is then fixed prior to reduction of the hip maintaining the desired anteversion. After reduction and stability control, minor adjustments can be done by releasing the distal screws from the plate (Fig. 5.25).

Reconstruction techniques: A multihole small-sized acetabular component is inserted with great care and secured with at least two screws. Autograft bone available from the head or acetabular reaming can be placed as a bone paste on the medial wall before component insertion.

5.10.7 Intraoperative Challenges

Challenges and solutions: On the acetabular side, reconstruction the high-riding hip is a demanding procedure that requires extensive soft tissue release, visualization of both the false and the true acetabulum which is usually obscured by osteophytic bone. The hourglass-shaped capsule is followed down to the bone. Careful dissection by tracking the joint capsule is suggested for identification of the true acetabulum. Preparation of the femoral canal is helpful prior to osteotomy for easy handling. Required shortening can be estimated by inserting the trail components first then attempting for a trial reduction. Short oblique osteotomy is more stable than a transverse one.

Unanticipated problems and solution: Acetabular fixation is tricky and sometimes superior coverage is not sufficient, the femoral head should be preserved for a graft augmentation in such cases. If a concern arises on the stability of the acetabular component, a reconstruction cage and cemented acetabular component can solve the problem. Following reduction of the hip joint excessive tension on the iliotibial tract and lateral structures occasionally may dislocate the patella. A lateral release may be indicated.

Thorough description of decision making, including the reason for the final decision: Anatomic reconstruction is preferred to achieve better joint kinematics which is important both for functional status including leg length equalization and durability of the prosthetic joint. A subtrochanteric osteotomy is therefore required for avoiding excessive stretching of the sciatic nerve.

5.10.8 Postoperative Radiographs (Figs. 5.25 and 5.26)

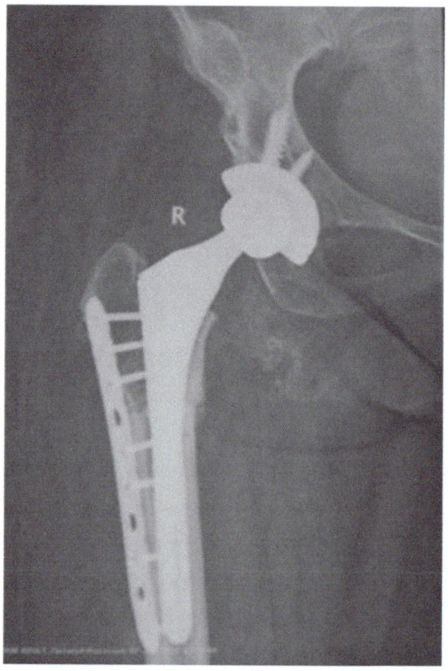

Fig. 5.25 Right hip x-ray of the patient following THA and subtrochanteric shortening

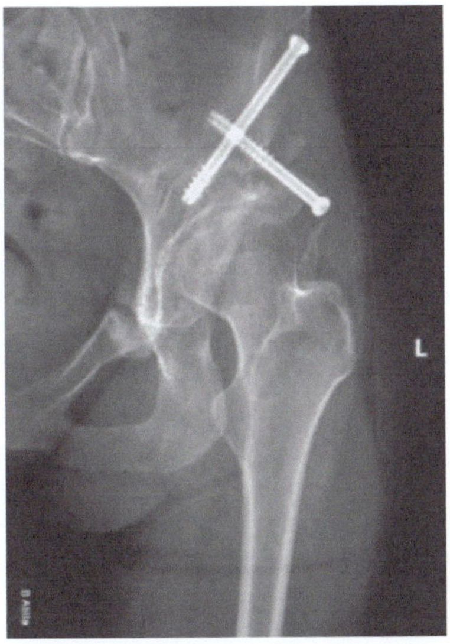

Fig. 5.26 She had a previous PAO and labral repair prior to right hip replacement

5.10.9 Postoperative Management

Chemoprophylaxis and anticoagulant treatment period: Infection prophylaxis was done by 24 h administration of a first-generation cephalosporin. Prior to her operation, the patient was bridged from warfarin to SC enoxaparin for thromboprophylaxis, and warfarin was readministered at the second post-op week.

5.10.10 Follow-Up and Complications

Postoperative period was uneventful.

5.10.11 Discussion [63, 90, 91]

Advantages of the applied method: Allows for anatomic reconstruction of the hip joint, uses best available bone stock on the acetabular side and restores kinematics of the native hip. Allows for limb length adjustment.

Disadvantages of the method: There are some difficulties and shortcomings attributed to this particular technique. It is a technically challenging technique that requires identification of the exact location of true acetabulum. Wide exposure is necessary to identify the intersection of the pubic and ischial rami to locate the true acetabulum. Rehabilitation period is longer than other techniques due to autograft protection until healing.

Alternative evidence-based techniques for the case: Existing alternatives to the presented technique are subtrochanteric valgus osteotomy for the very young and adolescents. When decision is made on arthroplasty reconstruction, available alternatives are on implant type and regarding the osteotomy technique. Various femoral stems have been reported with success including cone type distal fixation stems, modular S-ROM type stems and Zweymuller type stems; osteotomy alternatives are step-cut osteotomy, transverse osteotomy, double-chevron osteotomy, major trochanteric osteotomy and osteotomy with intramedullary bone-peg fixation.

Why is the chosen technique better for this case? The presented technique allows for better kinematics and function. Cementless fixation has proven better long-term track record. Short oblique osteotomy allows for adequate tensioning, leg length and rotational control. Plate fixation secures the osteotomy by allowing rotational control on the fragments.

Indications and contraindications for your technique: Subtrochanteric osteotomy is indicated when leg lengthening of more than three cm is anticipated on preoperative plans. Previous sepsis is the only contraindication.

Learning curve and how to manage complications: The learning curve is steep, and the technique is demanding considering the difficulty associated with locating the true acetabulum, fixation of the acetabulum and adequate positioning. Femoral shortening requires expertise on arthroplasty as well as fracture fixation.

Level of evidence concerning the superiority of this method against others: Subtrochanteric osteotomy is superior to great trochanteric osteotomy and sequential resection of proximal femur regarding the nonunion of the greater trochanter and femoral component fixation. The results of different types of subtrochanteric osteotomies have been reported in several case series with midterm follow-up. Significant improvement in clinical function was noted with a high rate of implant fixation and osteotomy union.

5.11 Case Title: Total hip Arthroplasty in Crowe 3 Hip Dysplasia

Goran Bicanic, Zoran Sulje, and Domagoj Delimar

5.11.1 Demographics

Age: 51
Sex: Female
BMI: 28.8

5.11.2 Relevant Past Medical History

Principal pathologies: Arterial hypertension.

Previous surgical procedures: None.

Medication: Lisinopril, alprazolam, ketoprofen, pantoprazole.

History of Presenting Complaint: The patient was complaining because of pain and the decreased range of motion in the left hip for past 20 years. She never visited an orthopaedic surgeon until 50 years of age when symptoms became stronger, and she started limping. After clinical examination and X-rays of pelvis, the diagnosis of hip osteoarthritis due to hip dysplasia was made.

5.11.3 Clinical Examination

Symptoms: Pain during walking, decreased range of motion and three cm shortening of the left leg

Range of motion: Decreased range of all motions in the left hip

Main disability: Pain on walking, limping and shortening of the left leg

Neurovascular evaluation: Without pathology

5.11.4 Preoperative Radiological Assessment/Imaging (Figs. 5.27 and 5.28)

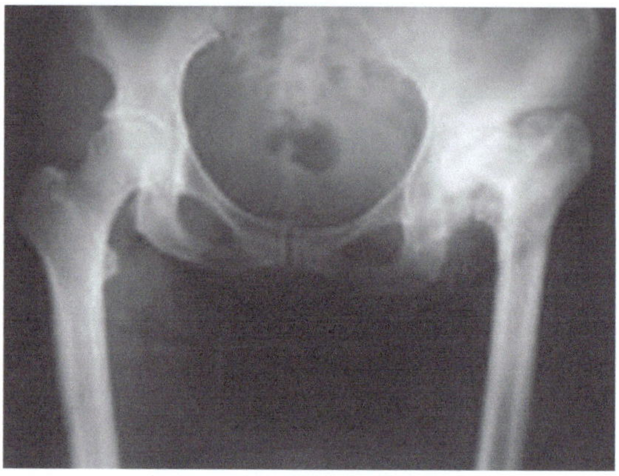

Fig. 5.27 Preoperative pelvic X-ray (AP)

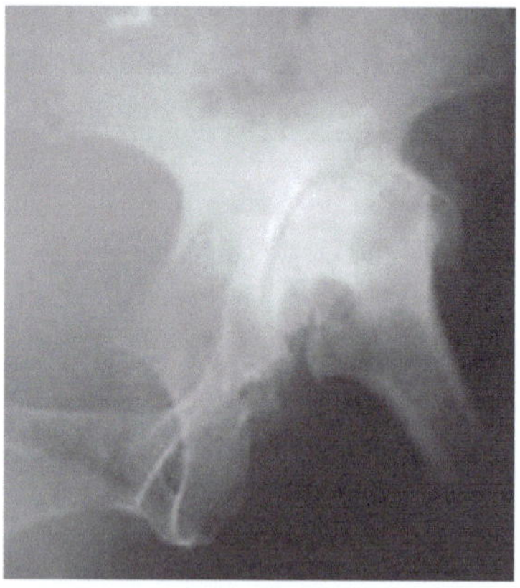

Fig. 5.28 Preoperative hip X-ray (Lowenstein)

5.11.5 Preoperative Planning

Diagnosis: Secondary hip osteoarthritis, dysplastic left hip (Crowe type III) (Figs. 5.27 and 5.28).

Possible treatment options: Physical therapy or hip arthroplasty.

Chosen treatment method: Hip arthroplasty.

Selection of implants if applicable and rational: Cementless hip endoprosthesis. Trabecular metal acetabular cup with X-crossed poly. Usually, in dysplastic hips, there is lack of bone stock on the superior rim. This is seen especially in Crowe type III hip dysplasia. For cotyloplasty technique usually, cups of 44 or 46 mm are used. This leaves space for a 28 mm head and small and thin liner. Since the liner is thin, it should be either ceramic or X-crossed poly. On the femoral side, various options are available, but the major problem is the small diameter of the diaphysis and deformities of the proximal femur. For this, we need small-sized standard endoprosthesis (Zweimuller or cylindrical or any other option with a small diameter of the endoprosthesis.).

Expected difficulties: Problem with scares bone stock on superior edge and sometimes lack of posterior acetabular wall. Obtaining the ideal centre of rotation is difficult. Shortening of the femur is also difficult.

Strategies to overcome difficulties: Detailed preoperative planning. For the acetabular side usually controlled medialization of the acetabular cup is sufficient (cotyloplasty). For the femoral side, some kind of femoral shortening is necessary.

Templating: Yes, standard templating (usually small-sized acetabulum, 44 mm or 46 mm, on femoral side small femoral stems are used).

5.11.6 Surgical Note

Patient's position: Supine position.

Type of anaesthesia: Spinal anaesthesia.

Surgical approach: Direct lateral.

Main steps: First, the standard direct lateral approach is used. The level of the true acetabulum is identified and exposed. Acetabular preparation is then accomplished with 2 mm underreaming. During placement of the acetabular cup (trabecular metal), the cup is on purpose medialized (controlled fracture of the medial wall) and secured additionally with screws. Then the approach continues with the femoral side in the standard way. But if there is a need for femoral shortening, then a modified lateral approach is used. The modification consists of subperiosteal peeling off of the bone flake with the posterior part of the abductors completely from the greater trochanter so that the greater trochanter is completely exposed and stripped of the abductors. Additionally the proximal femur can be shortened as much as needed. When the appropriate femoral length is achieved, then final endoprothesis is inserted and operation is finished. Abductor sleeve is reattached. Postoperative physical therapy is then continued in standard manner (Fig. 5.29).

Reconstruction techniques: If the proximal femoral canal is grossly deformed, a corrective osteotomy can be performed. On the acetabular side, if there is a significant bone loss on the superior acetabular rim then it is mandatory to achieve primary stability with screws (sometimes leaving the lateral rim of the metal acetabular cup without bone support more than 30% and up to 50% of diameter). Only then bone grafting from the head is applied on superolateral acetabular cup rim to give allow bone remodelling for possible future revision and to make better cup coverage through remodelling.

5.11.7 Intraoperative Challenges

Challenges and solutions: The major challenge is to place the acetabular cup in the ideal centre of rotation with sufficient primary stability. The technique on how to achieve that is already described. On the femoral side, the major challenge is the proper leg length which can be achieved with various femoral shortening osteotomies. The authors' preferred technique is described above.

Unanticipated problems and solution: Inability to obtain good primary stability of the acetabular cup. Care should be taken during preoperative planning (MSCT can be useful to allow visualization of the posterior wall and measuring the depth of the superior acetabular rim). Also, some kind of bone grafting technique could be useful, but the literature shows that the majority of the structural bone graft is resorbed after ten years. Also, one should be familiar with at least one technique for femoral shortening.

Thorough description of decision making, including the reason for the final decision: First, the decision about the placement of the acetabular cup should be made (ideal centre of rotation or neoacetabulum?). For the level of the ideal centre of rotation, usually some medialization should be made; therefore proper acetabular sizing and templating should be performed. Also templating and sizing should be performed for femoral side.

5.11.8 Postoperative Radiographs (Fig. 5.29)

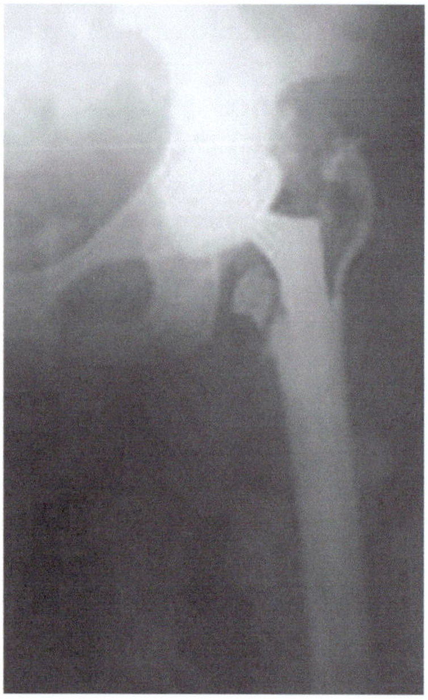

Fig. 5.29 Postoperative X-ray of the left hip

5.11.9 Postoperative Management

Chemoprophylaxis and anticoagulant treatment period: Preoperative chemoprophylaxis with cephalosporines, anticoagulant treatment for six weeks

Gait/limb loading until full loading: Weight bearing as tolerated (with crutches)

5.11.10 Follow-Up and Complications

None.

5.11.11 Discussion [3, 30, 43]

Advantages of the applied method: Relatively easy, no need for special equipment, 10–15 min additional to the standard operative time, same postoperative protocol as for any primary THA, good postoperative results.

Disadvantages of the method: Not for inexperienced orthopaedic surgeons. If there is an uncontrolled fracture of the medial wall then usually there is a need for additional bone grafting from a bone bank.

Alternative evidence-based techniques for the case: Reconstruction of the acetabular rim with structural grafts (poor long-term follow-up results). Different femoral shortening osteotomies.

Why is the chosen technique better for this case? This is the authors' preferred method, but other techniques can be used.

Indications and contraindications for your technique: Any Crowe type III or type IV hip dysplasia with secondary hip osteoarthritis.

Learning curve and how to manage complications: Learning curve is moderate.

Level of evidence concerning the superiority of this method against others: Level 4, case controls.

5.12 Case Title: Total Hip Arthroplasty in Crowe 4 hip Dysplasia

Goran Bicanic, Zoran Sulje, and Domagoj Delimar

5.12.1 Demographics

Age: 60
Sex: Female
BMI: 27.5

5.12.2 Relevant Past Medical History

Principal pathologies: Supraventricular tachycardia.

Previous surgical procedures: None.

Medication: Bisoprolol.

History of Presenting Complaint: The patient was complaining because of pain in both hips and decreased the range of motion in right hip for past ten years. She never visited an orthopaedic surgeon until 59 years of age when symptoms became stronger, and she started limping. After clinical examination and X-ray, bilateral hip dysplasia is found.

5.12.3 Clinical Examination

Symptoms: Pain during walking, decreased the range of motion in the right hip and five cm shortening of the left leg.

Range of motion: Decreased range of all motions in right hip, increased ROM in left hip (increased internal and external rotation).

Main disability: Pain and shortening of the left leg.

Neurovascular evaluation: Without pathology.

5.12.4 Preoperative Radiological Assessment/Imaging (Figs. 5.30 and 5.31)

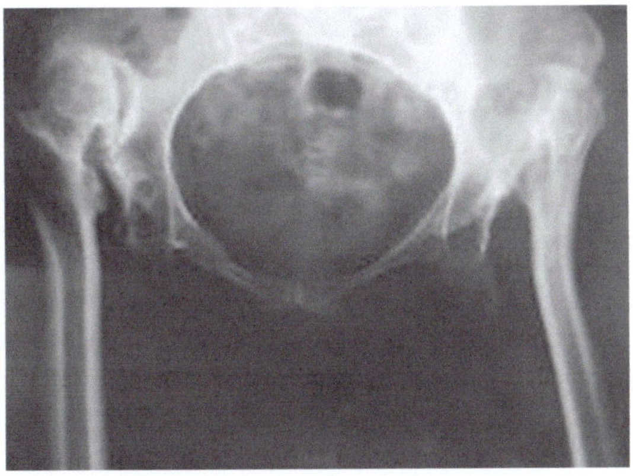

Fig. 5.30 Preoperative X-ray (AP) of the pelvis

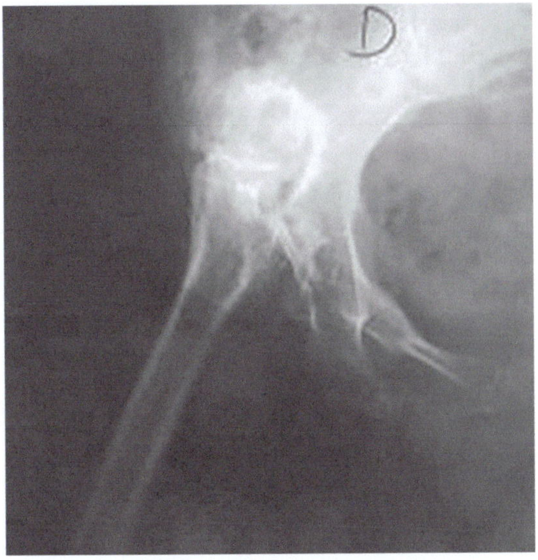

Fig. 5.31 Preoperative X-ray (Lowenstein)

5.12.5 Preoperative Planning

Diagnosis: Secondary hip arthritis, bilateral dysplastic hip (Crowe 4) (Figs. 5.30 and 5.31).

Possible treatment options: Physical therapy and hip arthroplasty.

Chosen treatment method: Hip arthroplasty.

Selection of implants if applicable and rational: Cementless hip endoprosthesis. Trabecular metal acetabular cup with X-crossed poly. Usually, in dysplastic hips, there is a lack of bone stock on the superior rim. For the cotyloplasty technique, usually, cups of 44 or 46 mm are used. This leaves space for a 28 mm head and small and thin liner. Since the liner is thin, it should be either ceramic or X-crossed poly. On the femoral side, various options are available, but the major problem is the small diameter of the diaphysis and deformities of the proximal femur. For this we need small-sized standard endoprosthesis (Zweimuller or cylindrical or any other option with small diameter of the endoprosthesis).

Expected difficulties: Problem with scares bone stock on the superior edge and sometimes lack of posterior acetabular wall. Obtaining the ideal centre of rotation is difficult. Shortening of the femur is also difficult.

Strategies to overcome difficulties: Detailed preoperative planning. For the acetabular side, usually controlled medicalization of the acetabular cup is sufficient (cotyloplasty). For the femoral side, some kind of femoral shortening is necessary.

Templating: Yes, standard templating (usually small-sized acetabulum, 44 mm or 46 mm, on the femoral side small femoral stems are used).

5.12.6 Surgical Note

Patient's position: Supine position.

Type of anaesthesia: Spinal anaesthesia.

Surgical approach: Direct lateral (modified direct lateral according to the authors).

Main steps: First, the standard direct lateral approach is used. The level of the true acetabulum is identified and exposed. The acetabular preparation is then accomplished with two mm underreaming. During placement of the acetabular cup (trabecular metal), the cup is on purpose medialized (controlled fracture of the medial wall) and secured additionally with screws. Then the approach continues with the femoral side in standard way. But if there is a need for femoral shortening, then the modified lateral approach is used. The modification consists of subperiosteal peeling off of the bone flake with the posterior part of the abductors completely from the greater trochanter so that the greater trochanter is completely exposed and striped of the abductors. Additionally, proximal femur can be shortened as much as needed. When the appropriate femoral length is achieved, then final endoprothesis is inserted and operation is finished (Fig. 5.32). Abductor sleeve is reattached. Postoperative physical therapy is then continued in standard manner.

Reconstruction techniques: If the proximal femoral canal is grossly deformed, a corrective osteotomy can be performed. On the acetabular side if there is significant bone loss on the superior acetabular rim, then it is mandatory to achieve primary stability with screws (sometimes leaving the lateral rim of the metal acetabular cup without bone support more than 30% and up to 50% of diameter). Only then bone grafting from the head is applied on the superolateral acetabular cup rim to allow bone remodelling for possible future revision and to make better cup coverage through remodelling.

5.12.7 Intraoperative Challenges

Challenges and solutions: The major challenge is to place the acetabular cup in the ideal centre of rotation with sufficient primary stability. The technique on how to achieve that is already described. On the femoral side the major challenge is the proper leg length which can be achieved with various femoral shortening osteotomies. The authors' preferred technique is described above.

Unanticipated problems and solution: Inability to obtain a good primary stability of the acetabular cup. Care should be taken during preoperative planning (MSCT can be useful to allow visualization of the posterior wall and measuring the depth of the superior acetabular rim). Also, some kind of bone grafting technique could be useful, but the literature shows that the majority of structural bone graft is resorbed after ten years. Also, one should be familiar with at least one technique for femoral shortening.

Thorough description of decision making, including the reason for the final decision: First, a decision about the placement of the acetabular cup should be made (ideal centre of rotation or neoacetabulum?). For the level of the ideal centre of rotation, usually some medialization should be made; therefore proper acetabular sizing and templating should be performed. Also, templating and sizing should be performed for femoral side.

5.12.8 Postoperative Radiographs (Fig. 5.32)

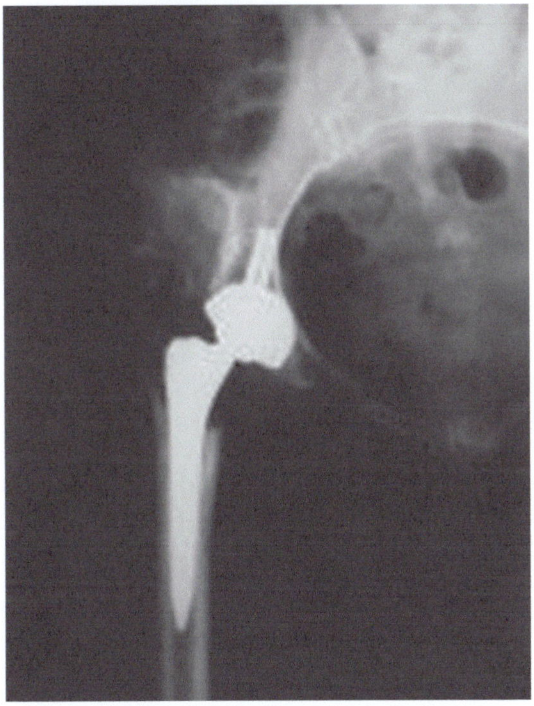

Fig. 5.32 Postoperative hip X-ray

5.12.9 Postoperative Management

Chemoprophylaxis and anticoagulant treatment period: Preoperative chemoprophylaxis with cephalosporines, anticoagulant treatment for six weeks

Gait/limb loading until full loading: Weight bearing as tolerated (with crutches)

Follow-up and Complications

No complications.

5.12.10 Discussion [3, 30, 43]

Advantages of the applied method: Relatively easy, no need for special equipment, 10–15 minutes additional to the standard operative time, same postoperative protocol as for any primary THA, good postoperative results.

Disadvantages of the method: Not for inexperienced orthopaedic surgeons. If there is an uncontrolled fracture of the medial wall, then usually there is a need for additional bone grafting from a bone bank.

Alternative evidence-based techniques for the case: Reconstruction of the acetabular rim with structural grafts (poor long-term follow-up results). Different femoral shortening osteotomies.

Why is the chosen technique better for this case? This is the authors' preferred method but other techniques can be used.

Indications and contraindications for your technique: Any Crowe type III or type IV hip dysplasia with secondary hip osteoarthritis.

Learning curve and how to manage complications: Learning curve is moderate.

Level of evidence concerning the superiority of this method against others: Level 4, case controls.

5.13 Case Title: Primary Complex Hip Arthroplasty 'Congenital Hip Dislocation and Illizarov Destruction'

Stanislav Bondarenko, Voldymyr Filippenko, and Mandus Akonjom

5.13.1 Demographics

Age: 45
Sex: Female
BMI: 26.6

5.13.2 Relevant Past Medical History

Principal pathologies: Crowe Type IV developmental dysplasia of the left hip.

Previous surgical procedures: None.

Medication: Analgesics and NSAID's, antibiotics and anticoagulants

Other: No medical comorbidity.

History of Presenting Complaint: Left groin and lumbar pain, left leg shorting and limping for ten years. The patient was apparently in good health until ten years before the presentation when she complained of severe left groin pain, intermittent, worst when climbing the stairs or when undertaking activity that increases hip flexion and relieved at rest. The patient also noticed limitation of movement. She had been on pain medications which temporarily relieved her symptoms. There was associated left lumbar decompensation with pain.

5.13.3 Clinical Examination

Symptoms: Leg length discrepancy of 65 mm, VAS pain scale was 7, Harris Hip Score was 35. Trendelenburg gait, pelvic obliquity, lumbar scoliosis, quadriceps muscle hypertrophy and abductor muscles weakness.

Range of motion: Extension/flexion: 10/0/0; abduction/adduction: 10/0/0; internal rotation: 10; external rotation: 5

Specific tests: ESR: 7 mm/hr; CRP: negative; CBC, T/D normal; serum electrolyte, urea and creatinine,within normal limit; ECG,symptoms suggestive of CAD; Doppler USS: normal.

Main disability: Pain and limping.

Scoring if available: VAS pain scale 7, HHS 35.

Neurovascular evaluation: All major lower limb nerves, (sciatic, femoral, obturator and superior gluteal nerves), were intact.

5.13.4 Preoperative Radiological Assessment/Imaging (Figs. 5.33, 5.34, and 5.35)

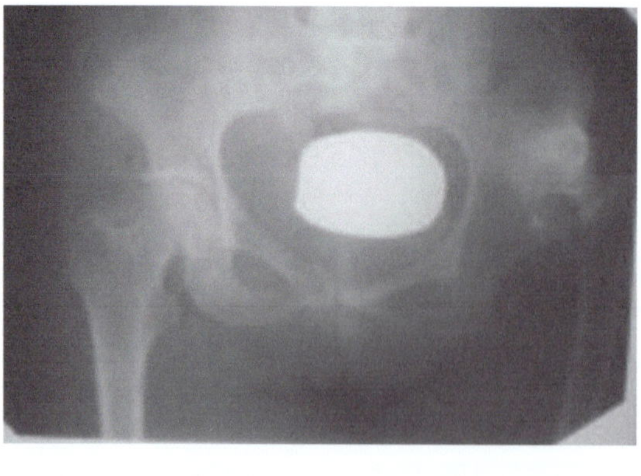

Fig. 5.33 AP pelvic X-ray view showing Crowe Type IV DDH of the left hip with false acetabulum and pelvic obliquity

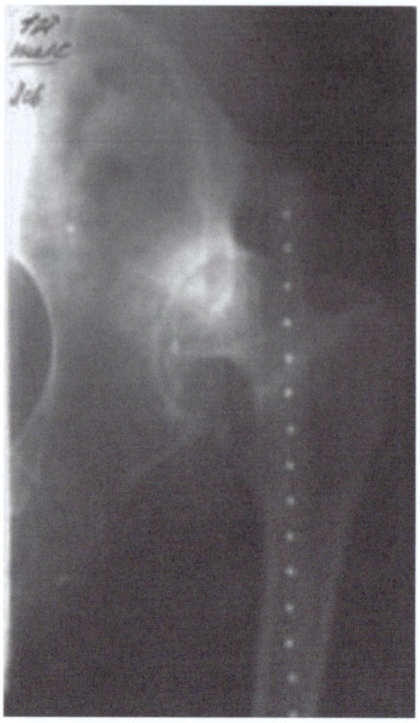

Fig. 5.34 AP left hip X-ray showing stage IV osteoarthritis at the false hip joint, femoral head deformity, osteoporosis at the level of false acetabulum, deficiency of the superior and anterior walls of the acetabulum

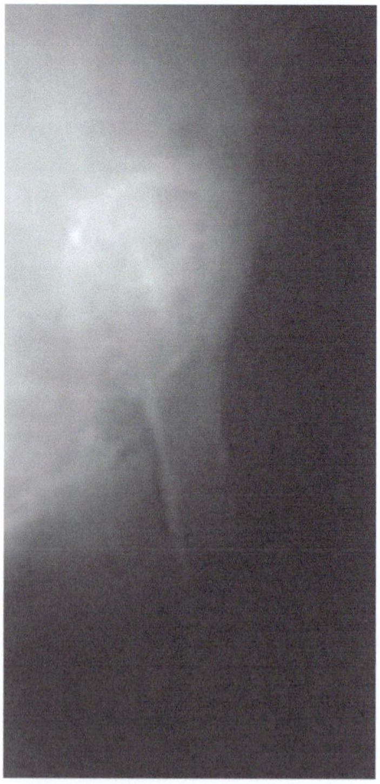

Fig. 5.35 Left lateral Hip X-ray showing the femoral head in the false acetabulum, excess femoral neck anteversion, osteoporosis at the level of false acetabulum, deficiency of the superior and anterior walls of the acetabulum

5.13.5 Preoperative Planning

Diagnosis: Crowe Type IV DDH of the left hip (Figs. 5.33, 5.34, and 5.35)

Possible treatment options: 1. Total hip arthroplasty after iliofemoral distraction of high hip dislocation. 2. THA with femoral shortening osteotomy.

Chosen treatment method: Total hip arthroplasty after iliofemoral distraction of high hip dislocation.

Expected difficulties: The technical difficulties of THA with Crowe Type IV DDH are due to deformities and defects of the acetabulum which require reconstruction, the difficulty of insertion of the cup in the true acetabulum, difficulty with reducing the prosthetic head into the true acetabulum.

Strategies to overcome difficulties: Prior to THA, the iliofemoral distraction for about seven weeks at the rate of 1–2 mm per day is carried out to accommodate the rate of nerve regeneration. Part of the femoral head and capsule is resected; adductor and subspinal tenotomy are carried out.

Templating: Manual templating was done using AP and lateral radiographs. This is supplied by the implant manufacturers.

5.13.6 Surgical Note

Patient's position: Lateral position.

Type of anaesthesia: Spinal.

Surgical approach: Direct lateral for THA.

Main steps: The first step in this two-stage approach is the arthrotomy with resection of the capsule and part of the femoral head. Next are the adductor and subspinal tenotomy, total soft tissue release, and insertion of two pins in the ilium in parallel fashion and two pins in the femur parallel to the screws in the ilium. Rods are attached to the pins and distracted 1–2 mm per day until the femoral head reaches the level of the true acetabulum. After seven weeks, the pins were removed, and the wounds from pin track insertion were observed for healing within seven days. During this period the patient is put on skin traction to prevent femoral migration and loss of correction. The second stage is THA: After incision of the skin, subcutaneous tissue and fat, the fascia lata is identified and incised longitudinally along the femur. The gluteus medius is incised at its tendinous insertion at the lateral portion of the greater trochanter. Dislocation of the remaining portion of the femoral head and osteotomy of the femoral neck. We proceed to remove soft tissues from the level of the true acetabulum. Identifying the true acetabulum was challenging due to the rudimentary nature of the ligamentum teres. We had to rely on the transverse acetabular ligament as a landmark to determine the true acetabulum. The next step is reaming of the acetabulum with hand reamer, correction of acetabular defects with autografts, insertion of the cemented acetabular cup. The reaming of the femoral canal and insertion of femoral stem was uneventful. A trial reduction of the head into the acetabular cup was done, and range of movements was tested in all directions with leg length measurement. We then proceed to insert the head of the implant into the femoral neck, reduced it into the cup, insert drainage, and wound closure in layers (Figs. 5.36 and 5.37).

Reconstruction techniques: We impacted the osteoporotic bone of the acetabulum with granules of calcium phosphate ceramics due to its osteoporotic nature following non-weight bearing and to protect medial protrusion of the cup into the pelvis postoperatively. We performed reconstruction of the superior and anterior wall of the acetabulum using autograft from the resected femoral head and neck which was held in place with two screws. This gave us the opportunity to insert the acetabular cup with the full coverage and correct inclination. For the index case, we used a cerclage in the proximal femur as to osteosynthesize a nondisplaced fracture.

5.13.7 Intraoperative Challenges

Challenges and solutions: The challenges we encountered which are common to this procedure were difficulties in locating the paleo-acetabulum; this was overcome by finding the ligamentum transversum. The other challenge which was preempted was difficult and reducing the femoral head into the paleo-acetabulum due to the muscular tone of the thigh muscles. This challenge was overcome by giving the patient muscle relaxant drugs for two weeks during the period of distraction to relax muscles. The third challenge was the defects of the superior and anterior acetabular wall which was reconstructed using the bone graft.

Unanticipated problems and solution: The bone defect of the acetabular wall was more severe than it was anticipated from the radiograph. We impacted the osteoporotic bone of the acetabulum with granules of calcium phosphate ceramics due to its osteoporotic nature from the prolonged no weight bearing. For the index case, we used a cerclage in the proximal femur to hold the nondisplaced fracture of the femoral bone.

Thorough description of decision making, including the reason for the final decision: Due to the marked osteoporotic nature of the acetabular bone, it was difficult to receive press-fit effect for uncemented cup, and any attempt to impact uncemented cup might fracture the acetabulum wall or even weakens it leading to future protrusion during weight bearing. That is why we decided to use cemented cup. Also, because the patient was young, we decided to use short proximal fixation stem sparing significant part of the femoral bone.

5.13.8 Postoperative Radiographs (Figs. 5.36 and 5.37)

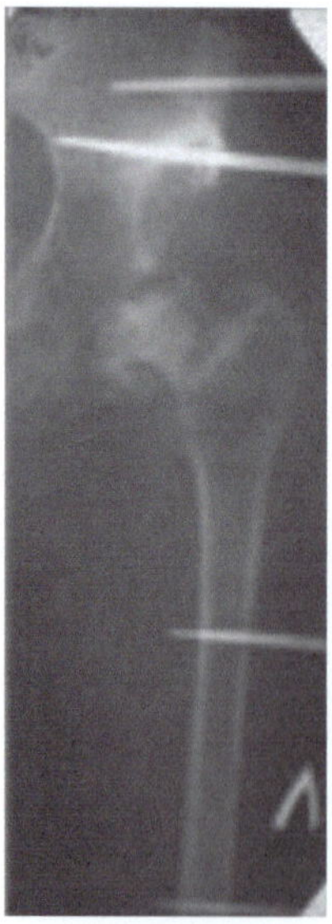

Fig. 5.36 Distraction to the level of the true acetabulum after partial resection of femoral head and soft tissue dissection

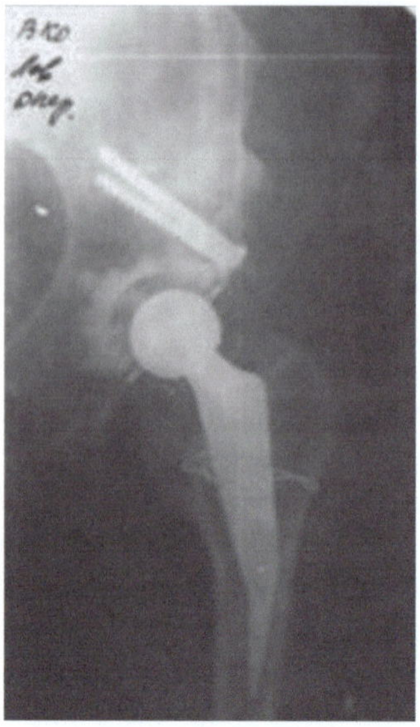

Fig. 5.37 AP left hip x-ray showing THA with acetabular reconstruction

5.13.9 Postoperative Management

Chemoprophylaxis and anticoagulant treatment period: Cefuroxime 750 mg twice daily for three days, Clexane 40 mg once daily for 35 days postoperative, Celecoxib 200 mg once daily for seven days.

Gait/limb loading until full loading: Patient was on restricted weight bearing with crutches for three months before commencing full weight bearing. During this period, there was limited hip flexion and adduction until full weight bearing.

5.13.10 Follow-Up and Complications

For this index case, there were no postoperative complications. But the possible complications of this procedure and their management are pin track infection which can be prevented by strict aseptic techniques and meticulous pin care. Also, nerve palsy is a possible complication.

5.13.11 Discussion [3, 92, 93]

Advantages of the applied method: Iliofemoral distraction is indicated to restore limb length without nerve palsy and to reduce the technical difficulties associated with the operation. There is no need for femoral shortening osteotomy which carries the risk of prolonged operation time, delayed union or nonunion, increased metabolic demand for healing and functional recovery. This method is very important in cases of unilateral high hip dislocation to restore leg length.

Disadvantages of the method: Because it is a two-stage procedure, it requires longer treatment time, more expensive for the patient and labour intensive for the surgeons.

Alternative evidence-based techniques for the case: One stage procedure with femoral shortening osteotomy. Femoral shortening, either by metaphyseal resection or subtrochanteric osteotomy, trochanteric osteotomy with distal advancement and soft tissue release has been advocated. These procedures are technically demanding and need careful study of the anatomy. The high rates of complications include loosening of the acetabular component, femoral or sciatic nerve palsy, dislocation, wound infection and nonunion. However, most osteotomies of the femur leave the leg significantly shortened.

Why is the chosen technique better for this case? Restoration of leg length is more probable with this two-stage method than one-staged femoral shortening osteotomy. Prevention of muscles imbalance is easily achieved with this method.

Indications and contraindications for your technique: Indications: Dislocation of the proximal femur more than six cm due to different aetiologies which could be dysplastic or post-traumatic, non-reduced acetabular fracture with the migration of the femoral head into the pelvis with pelvic discontinuity. Contraindications: Contraindications for iliofemoral distraction include severe aortic or proximal ipsilateral common iliac artery occlusive disease.

Learning curve and how to manage complications: This procedure has a steep learning curve and should only be undertaken by experienced surgeons. In cases of pin-track infection which is an unfortunate complication, the pins should be extracted to manage the infection, and then the pins can be reinserted in different sites.

5.14 Case Title: Total Hip Replacement of High Hip Dislocation with Off-Label Use of an Expander for Stretching the Gluteal Region

Zoltan Csernátony, Gergely Huszanyik, and László Kiss

5.14.1 Demographics

Age: 30
Sex: Female
BMI: 25.1

5.14.2 Relevant Past Medical History

Principal pathologies: Untreated bilateral congenital high hip dislocation

Previous surgical procedures: None

Medication: Nonsteroid anti-inflammatory drugs

Other: complex physiotherapy (extension treatment)

History of Presenting Complaint: Hip pain on walking and at rest. Impaired quality of life

5.14.3 Clinical Examination

Symptoms: Hip pain

Range of motion: Right side: Flexion 90°, extension 0°, abduction 20°, adduction 20°, external rotation 20° and internal rotation 30°. Left side: Flexion 95°, extension 0°, abduction 20°, adduction 30°, external rotation 20° and internal rotation 30°

Specific tests: Trendelenburg and Duchenne walking, centaur standing position

Main disability: Pain on walking

Neurovascular evaluation: No neurovascular disorder

5.14.4 Preoperative Radiological Assessment/Imaging (Figs. 5.38, 5.39, and 5.40)

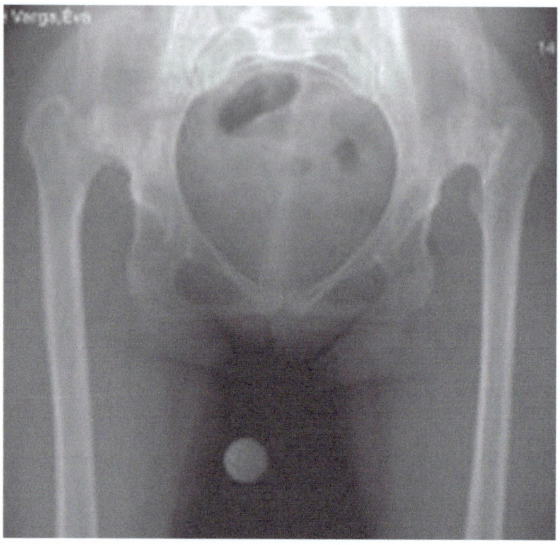

Fig. 5.38 Preoperative pelvic X-ray showing the bilateral high hip dislocation

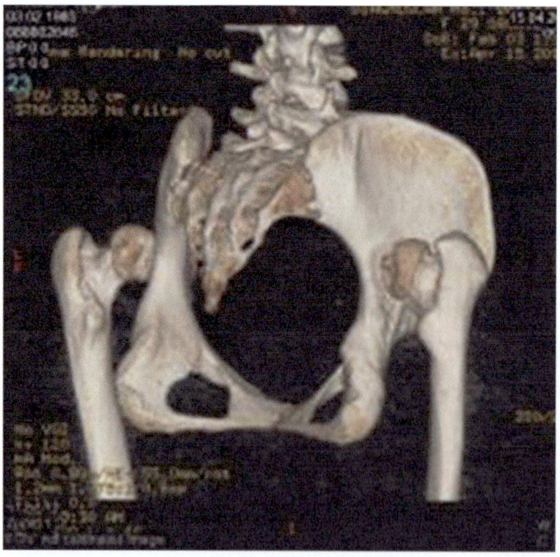

Fig. 5.39 CT 3D reconstruction of the pelvis (posterior view)

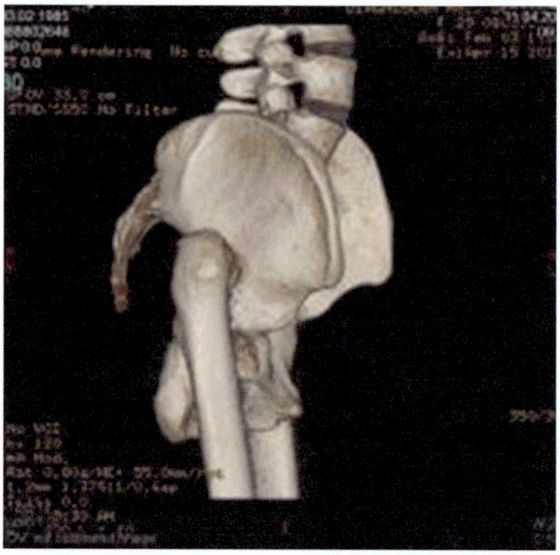

Fig. 5.40 CT 3D reconstruction of the right hip (lateral view)

5.14.5 Preoperative Planning

Diagnosis: X-ray, CT and physical examination (Figs. 5.38, 5.39 and 5.40).

Possible treatment options: Conservative treatment or surgical treatment with a trochanteric slide or femoral osteotomy or hip replacement in the secondary acetabulum.

Chosen treatment method: In the first step, subgluteal expander implantation for stretching the gluteal region, initial infiltration with radiopaque fluid. Then percutaneous regular filling of the expander with normal saline to gradually stretch the muscles. Twelve weeks later expander removal and total hip replacement in the primary acetabulum.

Selection of implants if applicable and rational: Expander used in plastic surgery in this case Polytech 200 mL (Dieburg, Germany). Small acetabular cup, and dysplastic stem, in this case, Aesculap (Tuttlingen, Germany).

Expected difficulties: Even with the expander implantation, femoral osteotomy might be necessary. Care must be taken during reposition to avoid jerking the extremity as this can lead to neurological damage.

Strategies to overcome difficulties: Careful reduction as the extremity is lengthened quite a bit, in this case, five cm.

Templating: Preoperative digital templating was used. It is extremely important, to have the right size implant before proceeding with the surgery.

5.14.6 Surgical Note

Patient's position: Supine position with the operated hip slightly elevated.

Type of anaesthesia: Spinal anaesthesia for the expander implantation, and periodical percutaneous filling of the expander with magnetic guidance. Narcosis for the total hip replacement.

Surgical approach: Anterolateral approach according to Watson-Jones, but the procedure can also be done from a lateral approach (Harding, Bauer).

Main steps: First surgery, exposure of the space between the medial gluteal muscle and the joint capsule, without damaging the capsule. Implantation of the expander in the space and intraoperative filling with 50 ml of saline containing radiopaque fluid. Twice before the definitive surgery, percutaneous filling with 50–50 ml of fluid was performed using a magnetic guide (Fig. 5.40). Twelve weeks after the primary operation, expander removal and total hip replacement. After exposing the primary acetabulum, a 40 mm cementless cup was implanted, with a dysplastic cementless stem, and reduced with a 22 mm medium head (Fig. 5.41).

Reconstruction techniques: The supra-acetabular region was grafted (according to Harris) using the bone from the femoral head attached with two screws, and a metal net was needed as the graft bone was very fragile. During the implantation of the smallest available stem, a controlled osteotomy of the medial neck region was necessary, which was stabilized with cerclage wires.

5.14.7 Intraoperative Challenges

Challenges and solutions: Narrow and steep primary acetabulum, which required bone grafting for the smallest cup to fit. As an alternative augmentation can also be used.

Unanticipated problems and solution: The broach of the smallest available femoral stem just fit the femoral canal, but during the implantation of the final stem, the canal seemed narrow; therefore, a controlled medial femoral neck osteotomy was required.

Thorough description of decision making, including the reason for the final decision: During the first surgery, the right hip was exposed according to Watson-Jones at the proximal part. With blunt preparation, the virtual space between the attachment of the gluteus medius muscle and the hip capsule was exposed. A Polytech 200 mL expander was implanted in the prepared space and filled with 50 mL saline containing radiopaque fluid. The wound was closed in the usual manner. Twice, four and eight weeks after the operation, the expander was percutaneously filled with 50–50 mL saline using a magnetic guide and image intensifier control. Twelve weeks after the operation, the right hip was exposed again using the previous incision, and the expander was removed. The anterior third of the medial gluteal muscle is sharply detached from its insertion. The joint capsule was incised, and the hip dislocated from the high secondary acetabulum. After femoral neck osteotomy, the original acetabulum was exposed and reamed to fit a 40 mm Aesculap acetabular cementless cup. The anterior-posterior diameter of the primary acetabulum was measured preoperatively on the CT scan. The proximal part of the cup was uncovered; therefore, a trapezoid-shaped graft was made from the removed femoral head. After decortication of the proximal part of the acetabulum, the graft was fixed to the pelvis with two screws and washers. As the graft was unexpectedly fragile, a metal net was also used to hold the graft in place. The two screws were placed bicortical, and the screw ends were checked manually by reaching over the anterior rim of the acetabulum, to make sure they are safely under the illiacus muscle. Then the acetabular cup was impacted, although it had good primary stability, a screw was placed in the cup to enhance it further. The proximal femur was mobilized, with the stretched gluteus medius muscle. Following broaching, an Aesculap size 9 dysplastic SD stem was implanted. During implantation, the final stem would not sit as proud as the broach; therefore, a controlled osteotomy of the medial neck region of the femur was required which was stabilized by two cerclage wires following proper implantation of the stem. The plastic insert with a 10 degree anteromedially placed augmentation was impacted into the cup. The reduction was done with a 22 mm medium (M) femoral head. Care was taken during the reduction process as the extremity was lengthened by five cm. The anterior detached gluteal muscle could be reinserted to the greater trochanter, and the wound was closed in the usual manner.

5.14.8 Postoperative Radiographs (Figs. 5.41 and 5.42)

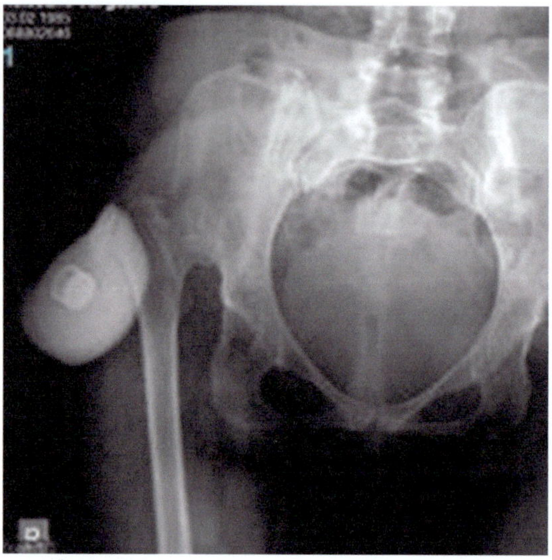

Fig. 5.41 Pelvic X-ray after expander implantation

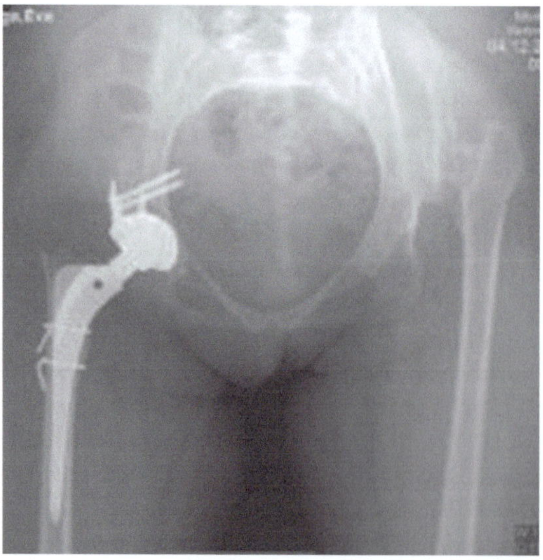

Fig. 5.42 Postoperative X-ray

5.14.9 Postoperative Management

Chemoprophylaxis and anticoagulant treatment period: 10 mg of per os rivaroxaban (Xarelto) for 30 days. A single dose of 1.5 gram of cefuroxime (Zinacef) was given as antibiotic prophylaxis.

Gait/limb loading until full loading: For eight weeks weight bearing was only allowed with the weight of the extremity, and after gradual weight bearing until the full load was achieved by the 12th week.

5.14.10 Follow-Up and Complications

No postoperative complications occurred.

5.14.11 Discussion

Advantages of the applied method: Trochanteric osteotomy is not required; the hip is reduced to the primary acetabulum.

Disadvantages of the method: Two surgeries are required.

Alternative evidence-based techniques for the case: Trochanteric slide osteotomies, or subtrochanteric femur osteotomy [71, 94–95].

Why is the chosen technique better for this case? The hip can be reduced to the primary acetabulum without using trochanteric slide osteotomy.

Indications and contraindications for your technique: Indications, congenital high hip dislocation. Contraindications, older age, as the muscles are not as stretchable.

Learning curve and how to manage complications: The technique requires high experience in hip surgery; complications should be managed with alternative techniques used for congenital dysplastic hip surgery (e.g. trochanteric slide osteotomies).

Level of evidence concerning the superiority of this method against others: Level of evidence 4.

5.15 Case Title: Primary Total Hip Arthroplasty in Developmental Dysplasia of the Hip with a High Dislocation Utilizing a Modular Femoral Component (S-ROM) with a Shortening Subtrochanteric Osteotomy

Richard L. Purcell and C. Anderson Engh Jr

5.15.1 Demographics

Age: 52
Sex: Female
BMI: 31.9

5.15.2 Relevant Past Medical History

Principal pathologies: Hypertension, depression, asthma

Previous surgical procedures: Bilateral tubal ligation, breast biopsy

Medication: Hydrochlorothiazide 25 mg daily, Singulair 10 mg daily

History of Presenting Complaint: A 52-year-old female with a chief complaint of right leg length inequality and chronic activity-related buttock pain. She reports this as being a lifelong issue, however, has progressively gotten worse and is essentially confined indoors as she can only walk 2–10 minutes before she experiences severe pain in her buttock and entire right leg.

5.15.3 Clinical Examination

Symptoms: Activity-related right buttock and right hip/leg pain

Range of motion: Approximately four cm shortening of her right lower extremity on the clinical exam with full active flexion and extension, however, she did have internal rotation limited to 10 degrees

Main disability: Ability to ambulate longer than 2–10 minutes, essentially confined indoors

Neurovascular evaluation: 5/5 DF, PF, EHL, FHL. 2+ DP/PT pulses

5.15.4 Preoperative Radiological Assessment/Imaging (Figs. 5.43, and 5.44)

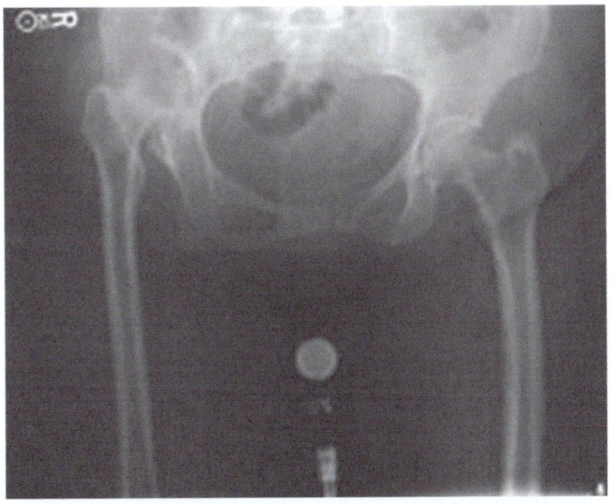

Fig. 5.43 Preoperative AP radiograph demonstrating complete congenital dislocation of the right hip with formation of a pseudoacetabulum consistent with Crowe 4 or Hartofylakidis type C

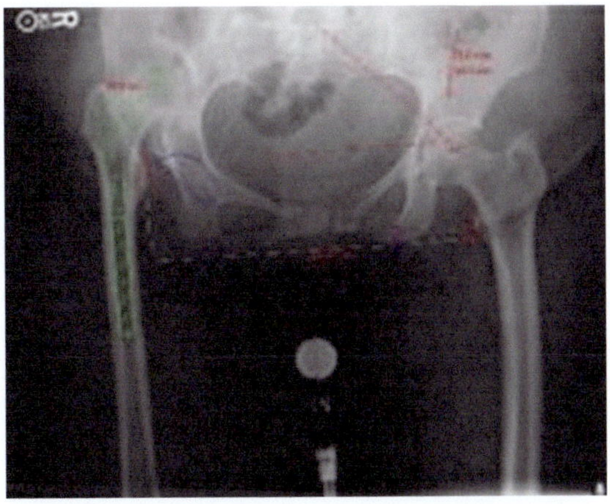

Fig. 5.44 Preoperative AP radiograph with template overlay. This patient had a 47.7 mm leg length discrepancy as well as significant femoral anteversion and a narrow medullary canal, all characteristics of hip dysplasia

5.15.5 Preoperative Planning

Diagnosis: Developmental dysplasia of the hip with complete hip dislocation and high-riding femoral head, classified as a Hartofylakidis type C (Figs. 5.43 and 5.44).

Possible treatment options: Nonoperative treatment with a shoe lift, cane and anti- inflammatory pain medication; however, it was discussed with the patient that none of these had been successful.

Chosen treatment method: Cementless total hip arthroplasty using a modular femoral stem with a subtrochanteric shortening osteotomy.

Selection of implants if applicable and rational: For the cup, we used a cementless press-fit designed implant; however, due to anatomic abnormalities in patients with hip dysplasia, we planned for a smaller acetabular component than we would typically implant to prevent leaving the implant unsupported by native bone. Due to the excessive femoral anteversion typically encountered with hip dysplasia cases, we opted to use a modular femoral system (S-ROM, DePuy Warsaw, IN) in order to correct for this anteversion and prevent the potential for post-operative instability. Modular systems also aide in the metaphyseal-diaphyseal mismatch commonly encountered in dysplastic hips and give the surgeon the ability to independently size the component to the canal and the metaphysis according to the patient's specific anatomy. The flutes on the stem allow for control of distal femoral rotation while the metaphyseal segment controls proximal rotation. These aspects of the implant allow for excellent osteotomy fixation.

Expected difficulties: The two most obvious and important difficulties in reconstructing a hip with such degree of dysplasia and dislocation are proper identification of the true acetabulum and hip centre and at the same time being cognizant of the amount of limb lengthening it will require to anatomically reduce the hip while avoiding undue tension on the sciatic nerve.

Strategies to overcome difficulties: Intraoperative identification of the true acetabulum is typically best achieved by identifying the hip capsule upon entering the hip joint and using it as an important landmark for orientation. This hourglass-shaped structure can be used to guide the surgeon into the true acetabulum, which can prove quite difficult to identify. By placing a finger in the capsule, a pathway can be tracked inferiorly to the acetabulum. Secondly, identification of the obturator foramen ensures that the cup is placed at the proper level. In cases such as this one where a shortening osteotomy is needed to prevent over lengthening and causing a sciatic nerve injury, we prefer to make the subtrochanteric osteotomy immediately after identifying and releasing the gluteus maximus insertion on the femur and tracing the nerve proximally to the sciatic notch, completing the neurolysis. We planned on making the osteotomy approximately four cm distal to the lesser trochanter and by doing so prior to cup or canal reaming, ensured that the bulk of the procedure could be performed without any tension on the nerve.

Templating: Several strategies have been described for acetabular reconstruction in dysplastic hips; however, we prefer to place the reconstructed acetabulum at the location of the true acetabulum. In doing so, one must be aware that planning for a typical sized 50–54 mm acetabular component in the true location will be too large. Being aware of this, we templated for a size 44 mm acetabular component which maintained superior-lateral acetabular bone. When choosing smaller cups, the surgeon will also likely have to use a smaller diameter femoral head than typically used to preserve polyethylene thickness. The femoral component was templated with an S-ROM stem with a standard offset neck and size 11 mm stem. Determining the amount of femoral bone resection needed to prevent sciatic nerve injury is done intraoperatively by overlapping the diaphyseal aspect of the femur over the metaphyseal fragment in the reduced position. This is further described in detail later in the chapter.

5.15.6 Surgical Note

Patient's position: Lateral decubitus position with left hip down.

Type of anaesthesia: Spinal anaesthesia with conscious sedation.

Surgical approach: We utilized a posterior approach; however, because of the high-riding dislocation, we extended the incision more proximal than usual and also extended it distally two thirds down the femur because of the need to perform a subtrochanteric shortening osteotomy. The gluteus maximus insertion on the femur was released to allow for adequate mobilization of the femur and visualization of the sciatic nerve.

Main steps: The critical steps, in this case, were as follows: adequate exposure, creating the osteotomy, identification and preparation of the true acetabulum, preparation of the femur, determining the amount of femoral resection and finally trial reduction.

Reconstruction techniques: As previously discussed, there are several ways to reconstruct the acetabulum in dysplastic hips, either by creating a high hip centre, augmentation with bone grafting or by medialization of the cup. Due to the biomechanics of the hip joint and studies demonstrating optimal implant survival rates with this technique, we placed the cup in the true location for the acetabulum. The 44 mm cup was determined by the intraoperative AP dimension of the pelvis. Taking care not to disrupt the anterior or posterior walls, the cup is medialized until there is adequate coverage and stability. In some cases, this requires the creation of a medial wall defect. This is acceptable as long as there is an intact acetabular ring. We reamed the acetabulum to a size 43 and press fit a 44 m shell into place. Due to diminished bone stock and quality in these cases, we chose to augment our initial acetabular fixation with a single dome screw into the ilium. Reconstructing the femur in the setting of a subtrochanteric shortening osteotomy can be challenging. We prefer to create the osteotomy prior to canal preparation to ensure that tension is taken off the sciatic nerve during the majority of the case. With the osteotomy completed, we reamed the distal femoral fragment up to the desired size and then retrograde reamed the proximal fragment to the same size. We then we able to securely hold the proximal fragment with clamps and ream the metaphysis to accommodate the proximal sleeve portion of the implant. After the sleeve was implanted, we confirmed the patient's native hip could be reduced into this new acetabulum, and that the abductors were not unduly tensioned. In cases where the abductors are noted to be over-tensioned, a release of the iliopsoas tendon may be done with little overall dysfunction. After confirmation that the abductors were appropriately tensioned, we were able to assemble a trial and reduce the proximal fragment to the acetabulum without placing the sciatic nerve in tension as the distal leg was not attached. With the hip reduced, and longitudinal traction placed on the leg, while ensuring the safety of the sciatic nerve, we were able to overlap the two femoral fragments and measure for the amount of diaphyseal femur to resect (Figs. 5.45 and 5.46).

5.15.7 Intraoperative Challenges

Challenges and solutions: Several difficulties and solutions to reconstructing a dysplastic hip have already been discussed; however, the importance of identifying and creating the true location of the acetabulum in high hip dislocations deserves further discussion. Once located by following the hip capsule, the acetabulum can be exposed with retractor placement over the anteroinferior acetabular rim and another placed in the obturator foramen. In dysplastic hips, the femoral nerve and femoral artery may have an atypical course, and anterior retractors should be placed under direct visualization. Prior to reaming, the amount of available bone stock should be determined by palpating the anterior and posterior columns and aiming to preferentially ream towards the area of thickest bone. The reaming of the acetabulum in cases of high dislocations varies considerably from that of a standard acetabulum with osteoarthritis. As in our case, the sizes of the reamers are typically much smaller than traditionally used. The surgeon usually has less familiarity with these sizes, and they are usually quite sharp as they are infrequently used. In addition, the true hip centre bone is osteoporotic as this bone has never been loaded during weight bearing. This combination of factors will require that acetabular reaming progresses with far greater caution than a standard reconstruction case.

Unanticipated problems and solution: A small nondisplaced hairline fracture was noted in the shaft of the proximal femoral fragment during removal of the trial. The fracture did not propagate and was not unstable, so we were able to place a single cable around the distal aspect of the proximal femoral fragment prior to final component insertion.

Thorough description of decision making, including the reason for the final decision: Due to the patient's debilitating pain with basic daily activities in the setting of her dysplastic hip with a high dislocation and failure of nonoperative management, we believed performing a reconstruction was her best option for the optimal long-term outcome. Given the patient's relatively young age with significantly distorted proximal femoral anatomy, we felt that the use of a cementless modular implant system would provide the best option for long-term implant survival while providing for optimal function and hip stability.

5.15.8 Postoperative Radiographs (Figs. 5.45 and 5.46)

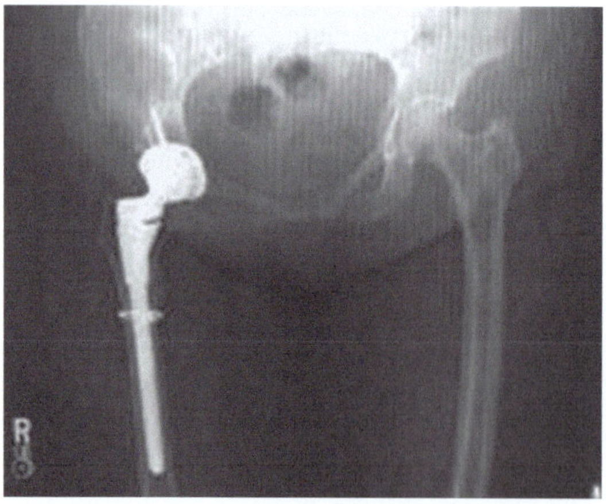

Fig. 5.45 Immediate postoperative AP radiograph demonstrating placement of the acetabular component within the true location with appropriate bony coverage and inclination as well as adequate canal fit of the stem and position of the proximal body

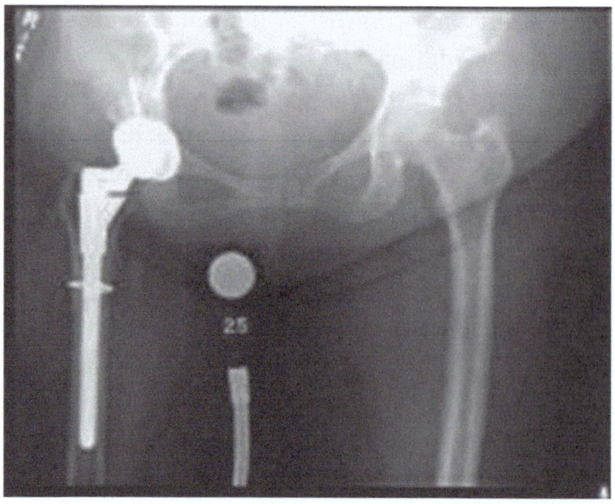

Fig. 5.46 1-year follow-up radiograph demonstrating stable components without evidence of lysis or loosening with a well-healed subtrochanteric osteotomy

5.15.9 Postoperative Management

Chemoprophylaxis and anticoagulant treatment period: For deep venous thrombosis prophylaxis, the patient received low-dose warfarin therapy with a goal INR of 1.5–2.

Gait/limb loading until full loading: The patient was made 10% weight bearing on the right lower extremity for four weeks postoperatively, followed by 50% weight bearing for four additional weeks and was allowed full weight bearing as tolerated eight weeks after surgery to allow for the subtrochanteric osteotomy to fully heal.

5.15.10 Follow-Up and Complications

To date, there have been no major postoperative complications. The patient did report some mild intermittent drainage from the incision three weeks postoperatively but was evaluated and diagnosed with a suture reaction that resolved without any further intervention.

5.15.11 Discussion [96–98]

Advantages of the applied method: In young patients presenting for total hip arthroplasty, some degree of dysplasia is common. The unique anatomic characteristics of these patients, including excessive femoral anteversion, small canal diameters with metaphyseal-diaphyseal mismatch, coxa valga and limb length discrepancies, make the use of modular systems very attractive. Prior to the development of modular implants, various advanced reconstructive techniques were required to restore the anatomy of a dysplastic hip. These included cementing a smaller prosthesis in retroversion, performing a derotational femoral osteotomy, using a custom prosthesis with a retroverted neck or reaming the canal to modify the shape to accommodate an implant placed in retroversion. Development of modular components such as the S-ROM allows the surgeon to customize the implant to the patient to maximize implant stability and decrease the additional morbidity of aforementioned procedures. In cases such as ours where a shortening osteotomy is necessary, these system designs allow for independent proximal and distal sizing of the component and various options to achieve the optimal offset and leg length.

Disadvantages of the method: The most commonly discussed disadvantages to using a modular system are related to the junctions and the material properties of the implant. Concerns have been raised about fretting and corrosion at the modular junction, however recent literature with reports of revision following modular implants have not shown signs of gross metallic debris or discolouration of surrounding tissues. The main disadvantage of a subtrochanteric osteotomy is the possibility of nonunion. Although we did not require supplemental fixation, options include using the resected portion of the femur as a structural autograft at the osteotomy site. In cases where rotational control of the osteotomy site becomes an issue, the surgeon can use a step-cut to gain rotational control of the osteotomy.

Alternative evidence-based techniques for the case: For high dislocations such as our patient, along with the severely distorted anatomy of the proximal femur and acetabulum, minimal controversy exists in the literature regarding successful alternative options for reconstruction. One alternative to cementless stems would be the use of cemented components. However, due to the young age of most patients presenting with dysplastic hips, mid- and long-term survival studies have shown relatively poor outcomes when compared to their cementless counterparts. Multiple studies have reported rates of loosening of cemented acetabular cups on the order of 37–50% at 14–16 years. While this may be an option in cases where modular cementless options are not available, we do not routinely recommend the use of cemented implants for dysplastic hips.

Why is the chosen technique better for this case? As discussed previously, the ability to use a modular stem prosthesis for reconstructing a dysplastic hip negates the need for more advanced surgical procedures such as a derotational osteotomy or using a cemented stem.

Indications and contraindications for your technique: The indications for the reconstruction of a dysplastic hip are similar to those of a primary osteoarthritic process and typically include pain not relieved by nonoperative modalities. A patient whose primary complaint is a limb length discrepancy or a limp must be extensively counselled preoperatively, as this may or may not be corrected with surgical intervention, especially in the setting of a shortening osteotomy. As in our patient, patients with high dislocations typically present with pain localized to regions other than the groin such as the buttock or lower back. Pain and dysfunction that affect the patient's ability to perform basic tasks of living and quality of life remain the principal indications for surgical intervention.

Learning curve and how to manage complications: As one would anticipate, complications following the reconstruction of a dysplastic hip are increased as compared to a standard hip arthroplasty for osteoarthritis. As in our case where a significant limb lengthening is required to restore reasonable function and stability, the surgeon must be aware of the potential for traction injury to the sciatic nerve. It has been shown that lengthening more than 2–4 cm during arthroplasty is associated with increased rates of neural injury. If more lengthening is needed, use of a shortening osteotomy is required to prevent such complications from occurring. The rates of dislocation have been reported to be as high as 10% following arthroplasty of the dysplastic hip, and the explanation for this is typically multifactorial with prior surgeries and distorted anatomy accounting for a majority of cases. Abductor dysfunction postoperatively can lead to patient dissatisfaction. This is more common in patients who have had prior surgery and when it is difficult to reduce the hip joint. In addition to monitoring sciatic function postoperatively, be sure to also monitor abductor function.

Level of evidence concerning the superiority of this method against others: To our knowledge, there have not been any studies prospectively comparing modularly designed implants with other reconstructive options and most of the literature consists of level 4 studies.

5.16 Case Title: Bilateral Crowe 4 Dysplastic Hip

Hiroshi Fujita

5.16.1 Demographics

Age: 73
Sex: Woman
BMI: 21.1 kg/m^2 (height, 146 cm; body weight, 45 kg)

5.16.2 Relevant Past Medical History

Principal pathologies: Bilateral developmental dysplasia of hip.

Previous surgical procedures: None.

Medication: None.

History of Presenting Complaint: Bilateral developmental dysplasia of hip has been symptomatic at initial gait. No preventative or therapeutic method has been applied because of slight pain. In her 60s, bilateral hip and low back pain increased. Since three years ago, due to severe pain and loss of range of motion especially at right hip joint, she has been suffering gait disturbance.

5.16.3 Clinical Examination

Symptoms: Bilateral hip pain and gait disturbance

Range of motion: Flexion, abduction, adduction, external rotation, internal rotation, extension Right (70°, 10°, 15°, 15°, 5–3), Left (95°, 30°, 20°, 60°, 50–5)

Main disability: Gait disturbance and bilateral hip pain.

Scoring if available: Merle D'Aubigné-Postel score Right; 2 + 3 + 4 = 9 Left; 5 + 3 + 6 = 14

Neurovascular evaluation: Nothing particular

5.16.4 Preoperative Radiological Assessment/Imaging (Figs 5.47, 5.48, and 5.49)

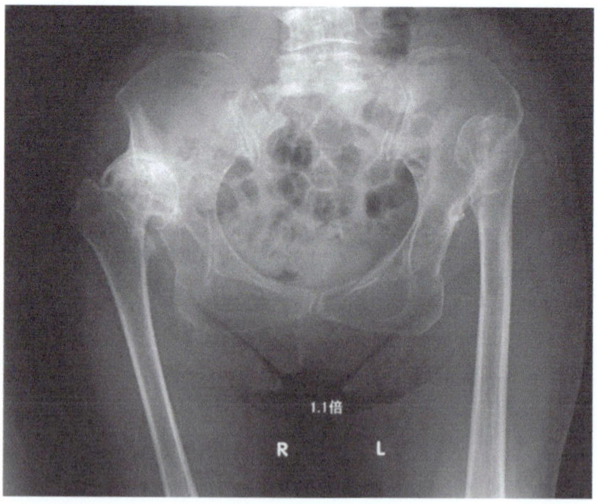

Fig. 5.47 Preoperative plain radiograph (supine position)

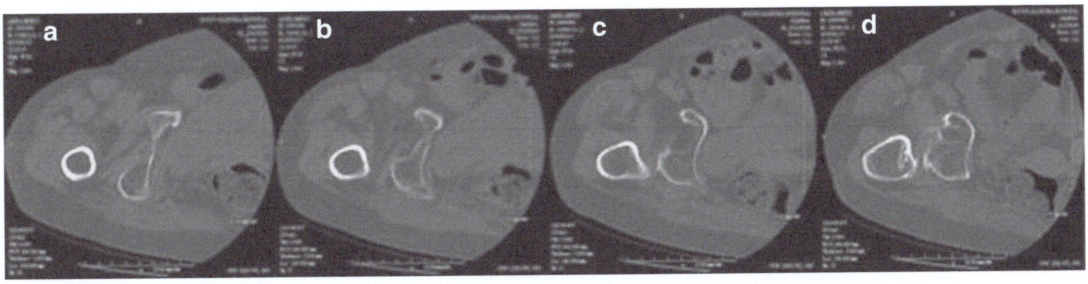

Fig. 5.48 Preoperative CT images of the right hip (**a**) level of the teardrop, (**b**) level 1 cm above the teardrop, (**c**) level 2 cm above the tear drop, (**d**) level 3 cm above the teardrop

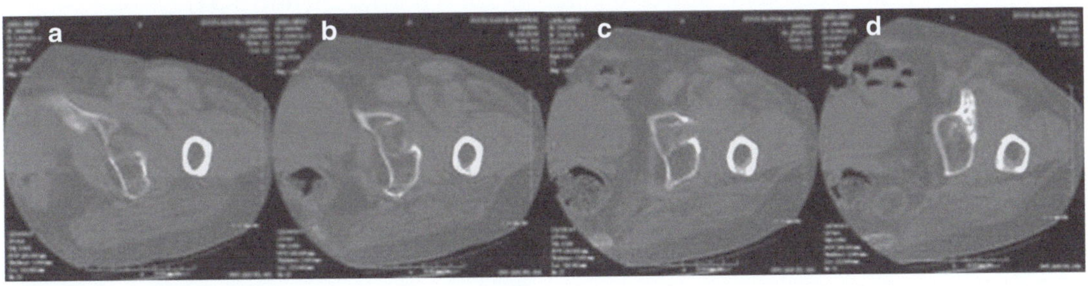

Fig. 5.49 Preoperative CT images of the left hip (**a**) level of the teardrop, (**b**) level 1 cm above the teardrop, (**c**) level 2 cm above the teardrop, (**d**) level 3 cm above the teardrop

5.16.5 Preoperative Planning

Diagnosis: Bilateral Crowe 4 dysplastic hip (Crowe %; 106% for right hip and 212% for left hip) (Figs. 5.47, 5.48 and 5.49).

Possible treatment options: Bilateral Total hip arthroplasty, right hip first.

Chosen treatment method: Bilateral total hip arthroplasty on same day.

Selection of implants if applicable and rational: Highly cross-linked polyethylene cup (X3) fixed with interface bioactive bone cement technique (IBBC) for the acetabular side [99], Exeter stem fixed with IBBC technique for the femoral side [100].

Expected difficulties: 1. Small-sized patient 2. Right, shortening of gluteus medius, high hip centre was mandatory. 3. Left, anteroposterior distance of the acetabulum was very small, and longest distance existed at 2 cm above tear drop. So, normal hip centre was a single candidate for fixing the cup.

Strategies to overcome difficulties: Right, high hip centre was mandatory. Left, normal hip centre and shortening osteotomy of the femur.

5.16.6 Surgical Note

Patient's position: Lateral position.

Type of anaesthesia: General anaesthesia.

Surgical approach: Modified Dall approach.

Main steps: Under general anaesthesia, and while the patient was in the lateral position, THA was performed via Dall's anterolateral approach [101]. An intentional hypotension during the operation was not performed. On the acetabular side, complete containment had been achieved through bulk bone grafting taken from the femoral head and fixed with PLLA screws. Then pulsatile lavage followed by gauze packing was performed to obtain a dry bony surface during the cement mixing. When the polymethyl methacrylate (PMMA) cement reached the dough stage, the gauze was removed, and then HA granules were smeared onto the acetabulum (interface bioactive bone cement technique, IBBC) [99]. Finally, the PMMA bone cement was pressurized, and then a highly cross-linked all-polyethylene cup (sized 40 mm, X3, Stryker Orthopaedics, Mahwah, New Jersey) was fixed in place. On the femoral side, complete containment had been achieved via distal bone grafting using several bone chips taken from the femoral head. Then pulsatile lavage followed by gauze packing was performed to obtain a dry bony surface during the cement mixing. After HA granules had been smeared into the femoral canal, the PMMA bone cement was pressurized, and then an Exeter stem (Offset 35.5, Stryker Orthopaedics, Mahwah, New Jersey) was fixed in place. In the left side, subtrochanteric shortening osteotomy of four cm was combined with above technique [63]. Onlay bone grafting using allograft (tibia plateau) was applied on osteotomized site after cementing. A combination of the IBBC technique and modern cementing techniques was used in both sides. The IBBC technique involves the smearing of HA granules onto the target bone just before the cementing procedure. The HA granules were manufactured by sintering at 1200 °C and then sieved to obtain granules with diameters of 300–600 μm (Boneceram P13 G-2, Olympus Terumo Biomaterials Corp., Tokyo, Japan). Two grams of HA granules were smeared onto the inner surface of the prepared acetabular surface and femoral canal just before the application of cement. Surgical Simplex P radiopaque bone cement (Stryker Orthopaedics, Mahwah, New Jersey) was used in every case (Figs. 5.50 and 5.51).

5.16.7 Intraoperative Challenges

Challenges and solutions: For the right hip, the high hip centre had to be selected because of shortening of the gluteus medius. Otherwise, gluteus medius had to be disrupted. For the left hip, the original hip centre was mandatory because maximum anteroposterior bony coverage could be obtained at that level, and the cup size was 40 mm. Subtrochanteric shortening osteotomy had to be selected, and resected femur was four cm in length. Stabilizing osteotomized femoral bones was achieved by three bone forceps during cement polymerization. A small leak of the cement through the gap between both fragments was tolerated.

Unanticipated problems and solution: Preparation was perfect, and no unanticipated problems had occurred.

5.16.8 Postoperative Radiographs (Figs. 5.50 and 5.51)

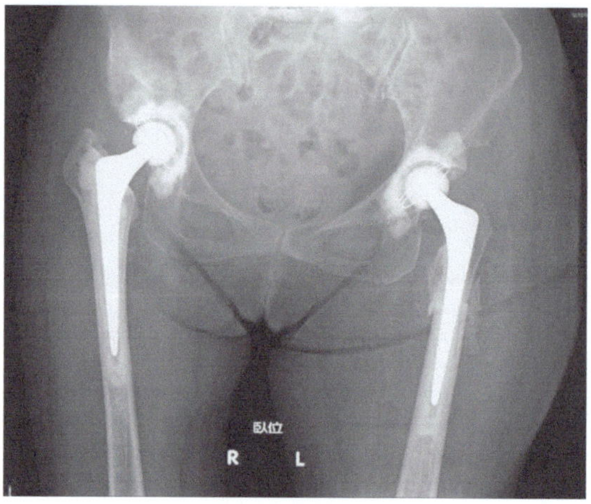

Fig. 5.50 Postoperative radiograph (one month) at supine position cup centre was located at 3.5 cm above the tear drop for the right side and 2.6 cm above the tear drop for the left side

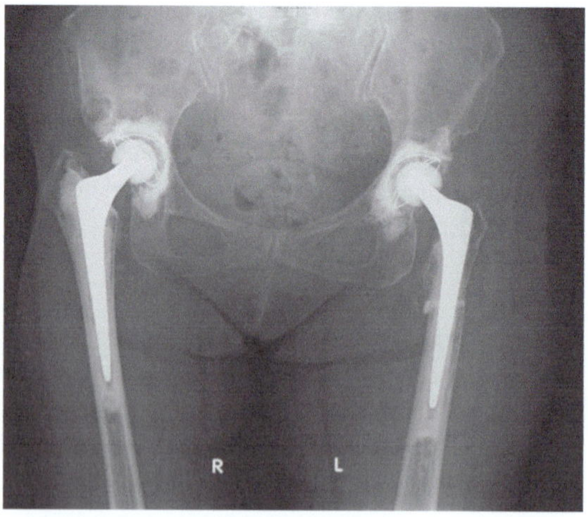

Fig. 5.51 Postoperative radiograph (one year and six months) at the supine position. No radiolucent line at bone cement interface was observed. The implanted bulk bone of both sides was remodelled, and the osteotomized femur was united for the left side

5.16.9 Postoperative Management

Chemoprophylaxis and anticoagulant treatment period: Edoxaban (an oral anticoagulant drug which acts as a direct factor Xa inhibitor) of 15 mg was administered for ten days

Gait/limb loading until full loading: The patient was allowed to walk with full weight bearing at postoperative day one and discharged at postoperative day fifty three

5.16.10 Follow-Up and Complications

None: complication

Scoring if available: Merle D'Aubigné-Postel score at 1.5 year postoperative right, 6 + 5 + 4 = 15; left, 6 + 5 + 4 = 15 flexion, abduction, adduction, external rotation, internal rotation, extension right (70°, 15°, 15°, 10°, 15°, 5°), left (80°, 25°, 15°, 15°, 20°, 1°)

5.16.11 Discussion

Advantages of the applied method: Secure initial fixation, rapid rehabilitation.

Disadvantages of the method: Longer operative time and possibility of higher complication rate.

Alternative evidence-based techniques for the case: Cementless implants, staged operation.

Why is the chosen technique better for this case? Small-sized dysplastic hips have several challenges for the surgeon. 1. Smallest size, for example, 40 mm for the acetabular side and relatively thin femoral component, 35.5 mm offset Exeter stem, was necessary. 2. The superolateral bony defect of the acetabular side must be reconstructed by bulk bone grafting for the establishment of complete coverage. 3. Stiff soft tissue must be released for a better range of motion and to prevent fracture of the greater trochanter. 4. Sophisticated modern cementing and IBBC technique is necessary for the longevity of the implants. 5. In case of revision, the cement-in-cement technique can be used which facilitates less invasive revision. 6. Bilateral simultaneous THA is useful for rapid rehabilitation which facilitates earlier discharge and functional recovery.

Indications and contraindications for your technique: The technique described in this paper can be indicated for every primary case. No contraindications as far I know.

Learning curve and how to manage complications: To know and master cementing technique, studying, visiting a dedicated hospital and complete preparation of the surgical tools and materials are mandatory.

Level of evidence concerning the superiority of this method against others: Many manuscripts had been proved the superiority of all-polyethylene cup and Exeter stem fixed with modern cementing technique combined with IBBC technique.

5.17 Case Title: Total Hip Arthroplasty with DDH (Crowe IV)

John B. Meding, E. Michael Keating, and Tatsuya Sueyoshi

5.17.1 Demographics

Age: 81 years
Sex: Female
BMI: 24 kg/sq.m

5.17.2 Relevant Past Medical History

Principal pathologies: Crowe IV DDH right hip.

Previous surgical procedures: None.

Medication: OTC analgesics.

Other: Lumbar Disc Disease.

History of Presenting Complaint: Leg length inequality since birth. Progressive right hip pain for over five years.

5.17.3 Clinical Examination

Symptoms: Pain with ambulation. Pain at rest

Range of motion: 85 degrees flexion. 10 degrees contracture. 20 degrees of ER. -10 degrees of IR. Adduction 10 degrees. Abduction 10 degrees

Specific tests: Pain with flexion and IR of the hip

Main disability: Pain and activity limitation

Scoring if available: Harris Hip Score, 47 points

Neurovascular evaluation: No focal motor or sensory loss

5.17.4 Preoperative Radiological Assessment/Imaging (Figs. 5.52, 5.53, and 5.54)

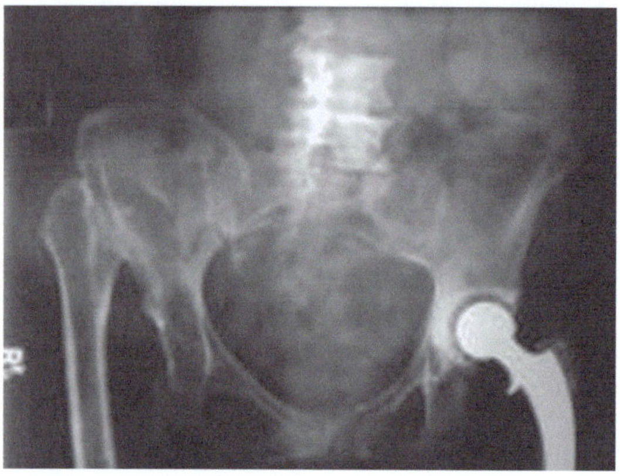

Fig. 5.52 Preoperative AP view

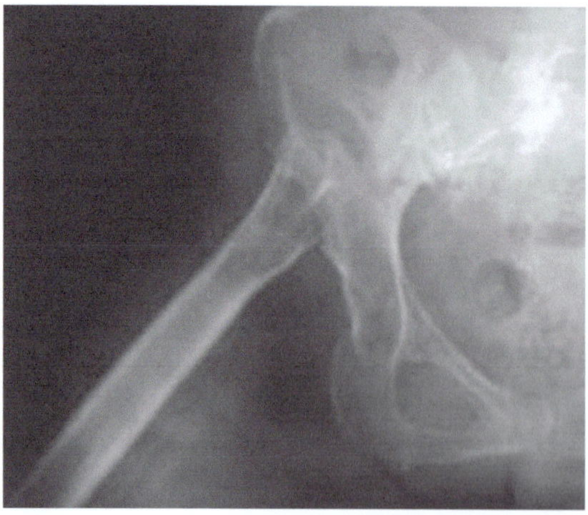

Fig. 5.53 Preoperative frog leg view

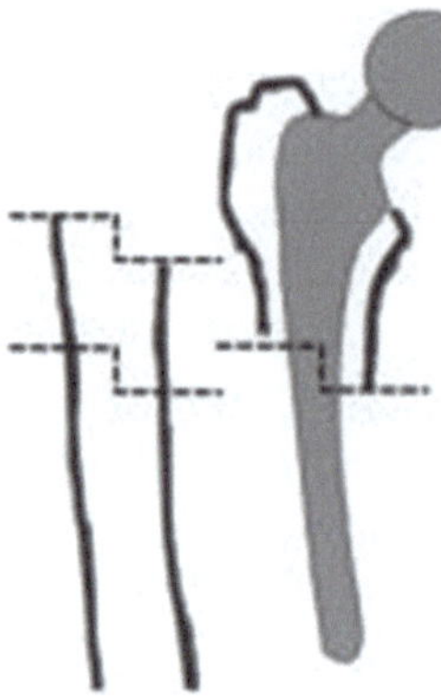

Fig. 5.54 How to gauge the shortening of the proximal femur

5.17.5 Preoperative Planning

Diagnosis: Hip arthritis secondary to DDH (Crowe type IV) (Figs. 5.52 and 5.53).

Possible treatment options: Total hip arthroplasty, fusion, resection arthroplasty.

Chosen treatment method: Total hip arthroplasty.

Selection of implants if applicable and rational: Cementless implants are preferred for both acetabular and femoral sides. For the case suggested, we used S-ROM Hip system (Depuy. Inc, IN, USA). The prosthesis is a cementless modular type and applicable for deformed hip and narrow femoral canal with option to determine femoral anteversion at surgery.

Expected difficulties: There may be altered anatomical structures. The gluteal musculature is often contracted. The bony acetabulum is hypoplastic superiorly. In order to re-establish the acetabulum, a femoral shortening osteotomy is planned.

Strategies to overcome difficulties: An extensile approach should be performed to get a better view of the surgical field via anterolateral approach or posterior approach. We recommend using a transtrochanteric approach, a trochanteric slide or a subtrochanteric osteotomy. Femoral shortening osteotomy is usually necessary.

Templating: The importance of preoperative planning cannot be overemphasized. X-ray evaluation should include not only typical AP and lateral views of the hip but also standing full leg AP and lateral views to check out a limb length discrepancy, an inclination of the pelvis and a posture. Computed tomography (CT) images are more accurate in evaluating the bony deformity or deficiencies of the femur and the acetabulum. Template the planned implant for femoral and acetabular sides, and gauge an estimated femoral resection.

5.17.6 Surgical Note

Patient's position: Lateral decubitus position.

Type of anaesthesia: General anaesthesia with epidural anaesthesia.

Surgical approach: Anterolateral approach with a subtrochanteric osteotomy.

Main steps: After an anterolateral approach, a subtrochanteric osteotomy should be done to get a better view of the hip joint. Without the osteotomy, the perspective of the acetabulum is limited and an extensive muscle or ligament detachment would be needed. Identify the true hip socket where the cup should be seated. After reaming with care, place a cementless cup. For a femoral side, a shortening of the proximal femoral shaft is necessary for highly dislocated DDH. After reaming and rasping of a proximal femur and a distal femur, cut out the femoral shaft accordingly and place a cementless stem in the jointed femur. Make some cerclage wires to reinforce the stability of femoral shaft. Reposition the femur to the cup carefully and gently. Make a flexion/extension/abduction/adduction of the hip joint and check out if there is any tightness or impingement. Illigation and wound closure (Figs. 5.55 and 5.56).

Reconstruction techniques: Reconstructing the hip at the original joint level is a key for this surgery. The first step is to identify the anatomical landmarks, which are often severely compromised. To set a true cup position, identify a transverse ligament, a round ligament of the acetabulum and an edge of the obturator foramen. Do not over-ream the acetabulum because the wall should not be thick or solid, especially an anterior wall is fragile. Place a small cementless acetabular cup (average outer diameter 38–44 mm). For the femoral side, how to measure the shortening intraoperatively and cutting off the proximal femur is the key. In our group, parallel the proximal femur and distal femur as side by side and mark the cutting line as shown above (see attached figure). In order to facilitate bone union, we cut a ladder shape. Three to four cerclage wiring around the femoral stem should be recommended with some local bone graft. We usually use a small monoblock or modular cementless implant.

5.17.7 Intraoperative Challenges

Challenges and solutions: There are three challenges with this surgery. The first one is the approach. The periarticular anatomy would be changed, and the muscles have degeneration or contracture, which would make the surgery more difficult. We suggest doing a subtrochanteric osteotomy in the first place at the approach. The second challenge is the shortening of the femoral shaft. When the centre of the hip is reduced to its original position, the limb lengthening would be too much, which will often lead to a nerve palsy. Surgeons can estimate the amount of bone cut in preoperative planning, but things do not always go along with it. We suggest gauging the amount of femoral shaft cut paralleling the proximal and the distal femur after subtrochanteric osteotomy (Fig. 5.54). The last tip is the release of hamstrings from ischial tuberosity. Some surgeons suggest an adductor muscle release from a pubic bone to make the limb lengthening and take a balance of the hip joint, but we suggest the hamstring release would be more efficient than the adductor release.

Unanticipated problems and solution: Inability to reduce hip. Revision of femoral osteotomy may be required after soft tissue releases.

Thorough description of decision making, including the reason for the final decision: Medialization of the cup allowed adequate superior coverage and screw placement. Step-cut osteotomy according to pre-op planning to restore hip joint. Fusion was not an option because of age. Resection arthroplasty only as a last resort.

5.17.8 Postoperative Radiographs (Figs. 5.55 and 5.56)

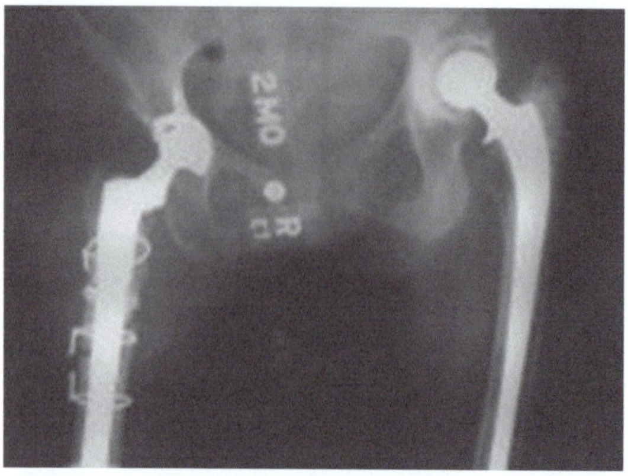

Fig. 5.55 Postoperative pelvic x-ray at two months. Femoral shaft osteotomy is not healed

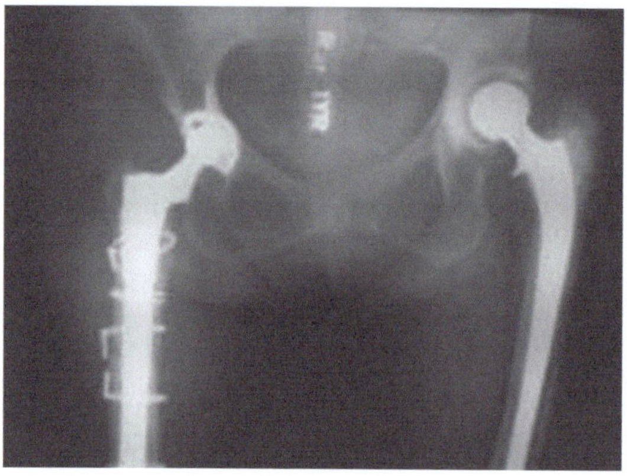

Fig. 5.56 Postoperative pelvic x-ray at the first year. Femoral shaft osteotomy has achieved union

5.17.9 Postoperative Management

Chemoprophylaxis and anticoagulant treatment period: 1500 units of heparin sodium intraoperatively and ECASA 325 mg q day for six weeks.

Gait/limb loading until full loading: TTWB until bony union

5.17.10 Follow-Up and Complications

There was a superficial infection, which was treated with superficial debridement with intravenous and oral antibiotics. There was no dislocation.

Scoring: Harris Hip Score at ten years (age 91 years) of 88 points

5.17.11 Discussion

Advantages of the applied method: Allows restoration of hip centre and maintains the ability to ambulate.

Disadvantages of the method: Technically demanding due to subtrochanteric osteotomy.

Alternative evidence-based techniques for the case: The poor function of fusion and resection arthroplasty.

Why is the chosen technique better for this case? Restoration of gait.

Indications and contraindications for your technique: Subtrochanteric osteotomy not needed if hip can be reduced. Generally, not possible for Crowe IV high hip centre.

Learning curve and how to manage complications: Meticulous pre-op planning and templating. Reoperation/bone grafting if nonunion is present. Surgeons should have a very low threshold for reoperating if sciatic nerve function is compromised.

Level of evidence concerning the superiority of this method against others: See references [4, 102, 103].

5.18 Case Title: Hip Dysplasia in an Adult Patient with Developmental Dislocation of the Hip

Per Wretenberg and Sebastian Mukka

5.18.1 Demographics

Age: 27 years
Sex: Female
BMI: 29

5.18.2 Relevant Past Medical History

Principle pathologies: The patient has, since the age of five years, been complaining of pain and instability of her right hip. Otherwise healthy and without any known medical conditions.

Previous surgical procedures: None.

Medication: Analgesic for the hip pain with different types of nonsteroidal anti-inflammatory drugs and paracetamol.

History of present complaint: The patient came as a refugee to Sweden from Syria in 2013. She had developed problems with her hip since the age of five years complaining of increasing leg length discrepancy and the feeling of instability in the left hip. She also had muscle weakness and a severe Trendelenburg sign. In Syria, she had only visited local doctors and was never offered any consultation by an orthopaedic surgeon. During the last year, she suffered severe pain and difficulties in walking without a walking aid. Maximum walking distance with crutches is 300 m. The diagnosis was therefore not identified, however in the absence of previous hip trauma and according to the radiographs (Fig. 5.57), the most likely diagnosis is hip dysplasia secondary to congenital dislocation of the hip (CDH).

5.18.3 Clinical Examination

Symptom: Severe pain in the right hip during weight bearing. Limping problems due to the prominent leg length discrepancy.

Range of motion: 70 degrees of flexion, extension deficit of 10 degrees, complete restriction of internal rotation, external rotation 20 degrees, abduction 20 degrees, adduction 10 degrees.

Specific tests: Clinical leg length discrepancy of 4.0 cm.

Scores: Harris Hip Score: 31. Even though this is not a CDH, the corresponding Crowe classification is four with a complete dislocation of the hip.

Neurovascular evaluation: No nerve disorders and good circulation in the lower extremities.

5.18.4 Preoperative Radiological Assessment/Imaging (Fig. 5.57)

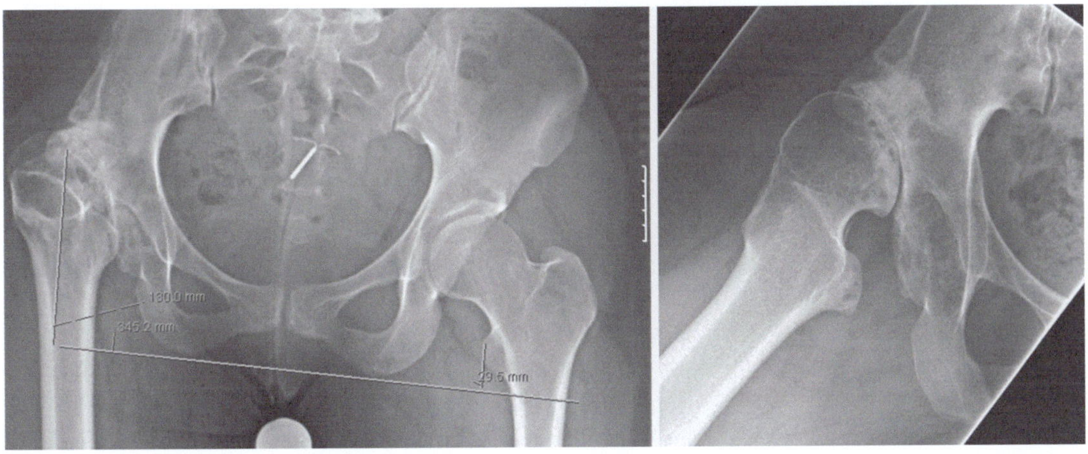

Fig. 5.57 Preoperative radiographs of the pelvis and right hip, showing severe hip dysplasia (Crowe grade III) with the absence of superior acetabular coverage

5.18.5 Preoperative Planning

Diagnosis: Congenital dislocation of the right hip comparable to Crowe grade III with secondary osteoarthritis (Fig. 5.57).

Possible treatment options: 1. Girdlestone operation with the extraction of caput femoris. Simple operation with possible pain reduction but an increased problem with biomechanical function and leg length discrepancy. 2. Arthrodesis of the hip with the option of a future implantation of a total hip arthroplasty (THA). 3. Prosthesis with a high hip centre. Technically less demanding to put the cup high and easier to reduce the system but only minor correction of the leg length and an increased risk of dislocation. 4. A prosthesis in anatomical hip centre and reposition with or without shortening osteotomy of the femur. Good anatomical reconstruction with biomechanical advantages but technically demanding and poor coverage of the cup that demands augments or bone transplantation. The cup could either be cemented or uncemented.

Chosen treatment option: THA at the anatomical hip centre, no femoral shortening to maximize the reconstruction of leg length, bone block transplantation with screws to the acetabular roof.

Selection of implants: Marathon cup, DePuy, size 46 mm, cross-linked polyethylene for 28 mm head. Biolox head 28 mm with standard neck, cone stem, Zimmer, size 14 with 125 degrees CCD (Fig. 5.58).

Expected difficulties: Deranged anatomy and need for meticulous initial dissection especially concerning the sciatic nerve. Soft tissue release to be able to move the femur distally and hopefully get close to the anatomical position. More than four cm lengthening is not recommended due to the sciatic nerve. Poor and thin bone in the acetabulum and minimal coverage of the cup. Careful reaming of the acetabulum to avoid penetration of the acetabulum. It might also be difficult to get the bone transplant in a good and solid position to be able to ream without loosening the transplant. The patient is informed that postoperative leg length will still not be totally equal.

Templating: The cone stem is available in 11 mm proximal width, and the templating showed that the 13 mm was likely to be used. The radiograph indicated no abnormality in the sagittal plane, and therefore no specific problem regarding stem position was expected. Templating of cup position was focused on restoring adequate biomechanics of the hip regarding centre of rotation. In these cases, with severe derangements of the anatomy, it is essential to focus on anatomical landmarks that can be identified during surgery. In this case, it should be possible to identify the dysplastic acetabulum, and the centre of rotation was templated close to its centre. This indicated that the position of the cup during surgery should not be too difficult. The cup size was hard to estimate during templating but it should be possible to implant at least a 44 mm cup. With the cup in this position, the lengthening of the sciatic nerve should not exceed four cm. A plan for a step osteotomy of the femur was also performed in case the tension in the sciatic nerve was judged to be extensive and in case reposition of trial components was not possible.

5.18.6 Surgical Notes

Patient's position: Lateral decubitus position.

Type of anaesthesia: Spinal anaesthesia with sedation.

Surgical approach: Posterolateral approach.

Main steps: Sharp dissection of the skin, subcutaneous fatty layer and fascia lata. Blunt dissection of the fibres of gluteus maximus. Good and careful exposure is essential, especially to find the sciatic nerve. The anatomy was severely deranged, and the gluteus medius muscle was very hypotrophic. The short rotator muscles could not be identified. The pseudo capsule was, on the other hand, thick and very tight. The sciatic nerve was found more dorsally located than expected. On the other hand, the tension in the nerve was low which suggested the possibility of no need for osteotomy of the femur. Osteotomy of the collum femoris was performed in situ. After that, a complete capsulotomy was performed. The gluteus minimus muscle was cut to be able to mobilize the femur distally. Soft tissue resection was performed gradually from the edge, and after that, the centre of the dysplastic acetabulum could be identified. To be able to expose the acetabulum fully, the gluteus maximus tendon was cut. It was possible, due to step incisions in the thin gluteus medius, to leave its attachment in place. When the position of the acetabulum and full exposure of the rim was established, careful reaming was performed. A 2.5 mm drill was used to control for bone thickness. The quality of the bone was good, but the possible reaming depth was measured to around six mm. As expected the coverage of the acetabulum was poor. The bone cranial to the acetabulum was exposed without difficulties, and a big part of the caput and collum femoris was cut and adapted to the decorticated host bone. The graft was held in place with a pelvic fracture clamp and after that secured with two screws. It is important that the graft bone hangs over the pre-reamed shallow acetabulum so that the finished reaming now includes the graft and thereby an even surface for the cup is created. Six 2.5 mm drill holes were made in the acetabular wall and four in the acetabular graft. The cup was cemented with gentamycin-loaded Refobacin cement (Biomet) with pre-compression of the cement for three minutes and then full compression on the cup for up to twelve minutes. The cup was cemented in about 45 degrees of inclination and 15 degrees anteversion. The preparation of the femur was done according to a standard procedure, and the trial components were put in their preferred position with an estimated 15 degrees of anteversion. The trial reposition was done with force but still in a slow and controlled fashion. Since the capsule was removed, the gluteus maximus tendon was cut, and the gluteus medius was lengthened with stab incisions until it was possible to reduce the hip without severe tension to the nerve (which was unexpected).The permanent femoral component was then implanted with a common technique. During the closure, there was no capsule to restore. The gluteus medius tendon was reattached to the femur more proximally with osteo-sutures. The fascia was resutured in a standard fashion using Stratafix suture (Ethicon) (Fig. 5.58).

5.18.7 Postoperative Radiographs (Fig. 5.58)

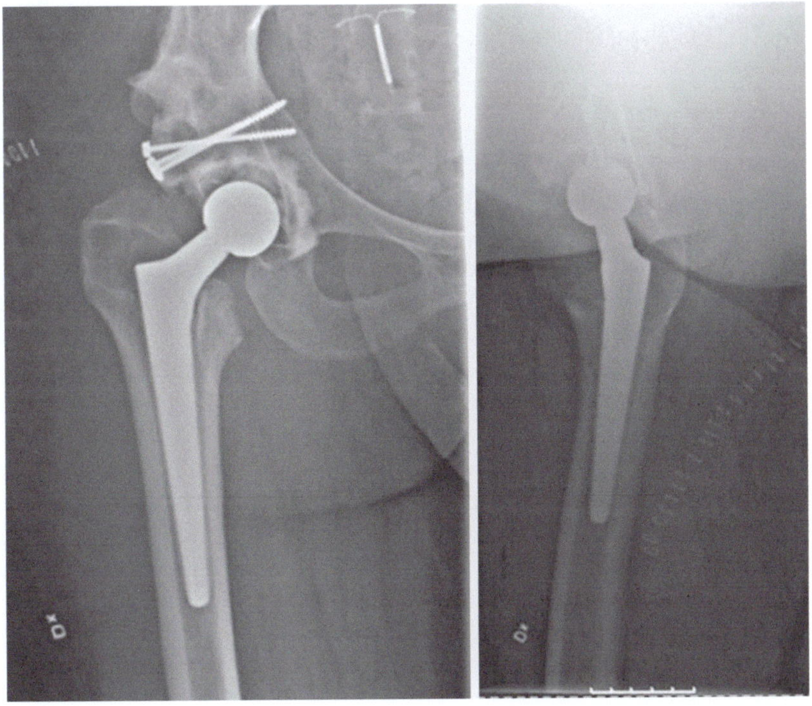

Fig. 5.58 Postoperative radiograph showing the implantation of the hip prosthesis without femoral shortening

5.18.8 Postoperative Management

Chemoprophylaxis and anticoagulant treatment period: Low-molecular-weight heparin (5000 IE dalteparin/day) during four weeks after the operation as anticoagulant treatment. Oxycodone and paracetamol as analgesics during the first week postoperatively

Gait/limb loading until full loading: Weight bearing as soon as tolerated postoperatively. Crutches for six weeks

5.18.9 Follow-Up and Complications

On the second postoperative day, affection to the sciatic nerve was noticed with a weakness in dorsiflexion of the foot. It was however not a complete motoric dysfunction since exposure of the nerve during surgery was very accurate; we did not believe it to be a major injury to the nerve. No neurophysiological investigation was performed, and at the 3-month evaluation, the function was completely restored.

Scores: Three month postoperatively the patient had a maximal flexion of 90 degrees and full extension, internal rotation 10 degrees and external 25 degrees. She had slight pain during walking but almost no limping.

5.18.10 Discussion

Advantages of the applied method: If possible it is an advantage to restore the hip to an anatomic centre of rotation. Such a reconstruction of the hip provides good long-term results regarding function, dislocation rate and loosening of the prosthesis. In a case like this, it is also possible with this technique to restore much of the leg length. The use of a bone graft to get acceptable coverage of the cup is quite an easy technique with a possibility of biological reconstruction. It demands a good fit of the graft to host bone with compression.

Disadvantages of the method: It is always a risk to aim for a leg-lengthening of this magnitude. During surgery attention to the sciatic nerve must be kept in mind. It is of great importance to judge the tension in the nerve and be prepared to perform a shortening of the femur. The bone graft might not create the same stability as trabecular metal wedges that of course can also be used.

Alternative evidence-based techniques for the case: There is no evidence that a high hip centre operation should be better than restoring the hip in its normal position. The surgery, when placing the cup high, is usually easier but the risk of a dislocation is increased. The use of TMT wedges to reinforce and create a deeper acetabulum is well-established and can be used as an alternative to the bone graft technique.

Why is the chosen technique favourable for this case? The posterolateral approach gives the best possible exposure of the sciatic nerve. It also exposes the cranial aspects of the acetabulum thereby optimizing the fixation of the bone graft. In anticipation that should it be necessary to cut the gluteus maximus tendon, then this is easy with the posterolateral approach. The use of bone graft instead of wedges has not been shown to be better but is more a matter of surgeon's preference. In this case, we also had wedges available.

Indications and contraindications for your technique: For patients with developmental deformity of the hip as well as late discovered congenital dislocation of the hip where the dislocation is severe (Crowe 3–4). We recommend to aim at restoring the anatomy of the hip, but the opt-out alternative during the procedure is to place the centre of rotation higher than the anatomical position. In our opinion the use of bone graft for a biological reconstruction should not be forgotten but should only be used if the fixation of the graft can be done optimally.

Learning curve and how to manage complications: These operations are technically challenging. The learning can be expected to be long, and there are only a few patients in our region with congenital deformities in adulthood. A transition of knowledge should be done over a long period where an experienced hip surgeon operates together with a colleague under advanced hip surgery training. We also believe that to achieve as good results as possible, two surgeons should perform these procedures.

5.19 Case Title: Management of Leg Length Discrepancy in Primary Complex Hip Arthroplasty

A. Khaled, S. Konan, and F.S. Haddad

5.19.1 Demographics

Age: 26
Sex: Female
BMI: 27.5

5.19.2 Relevant Past Medical History

Principal pathologies: Bilateral developmental dysplasia of the hips (DDH) with high dislocations.

Previous Surgical procedures: Bilateral femoral heads excision and Schanz osteotomies at the age of seventeen.

Medication: Paracetamol, dihydrocodeine and morphine patches.

Other: No childhood treatment for DDH.

History of Presenting Complaint: A 26-year-old female who was born through normal spontaneous vaginal delivery and was diagnosed with bilateral DDH at the age of four. She was treated nonoperatively at that point. She was able to walk long distances as a child but was unable to take part in physical exercises. At the age of seven, she noticed worsening bilateral hips pain and radiating knee pain. There was severe deterioration in mobility impacting her school education. She became increasingly wheelchair bound. At the age of sixteen, she underwent bilateral sequential femoral head excision and Schanz osteotomy. This allowed her to mobilize pain-free on flat ground within the house, but she remained wheelchair bound outdoors. She was able to drive using a car with hands controls. At the age of twenty two she started developing bilateral groin pains (2/10). Her pain continued to progress affecting left side more than right. She also had lower back pain. Her pain score progressively worsened requiring higher doses of analgesia, and eventually, she was opioid dependent. She was unable to work part-time anymore as a nursery nurse. Her mobility deteriorated requiring two crutches indoors and wheelchair outdoors. She reported that the progressive symptoms (pain 8/10) and poor mobility had a significant impact on her overall wellbeing, psychology and ability to provide self-care. The patient was offered reconstructive surgery for pain relief and improvement in the quality of life.

5.19.3 Clinical Examination

Symptoms: Groin, buttock, lower back and lateral thigh pain exacerbated by movements and causing sleep disturbance.

Range of motion: Active movements restricted by pain. Passive range; flexion 100°, abduction 0–30°, adduction 0–25°, internal rotation 0–10°, external rotation 0–30°.

Specific tests: Positive Trendelenburg test implying weak abductors (pain and shortened lever arm from the osteotomy). Normal Thomas's test is implying the absence of fixed flexion deformity. Left-sided shortening of 10 mm.

Main Disability: Constant rest pain, walking distance restricted to 2–3 meters with two crutches. Inability to cope with simple daily life activities. Wheelchair-bound.

Scoring if available: Harris Hip Score [104] of 22.

Neurovascular evaluation: Normal vascular examination of the lower limbs. Intact sensory and motor supply of sciatic nerve.

5.19.4 Preoperative Radiological Assessment/Imaging (Figs. 5.59, 5.60, 5.61, and 5.62)

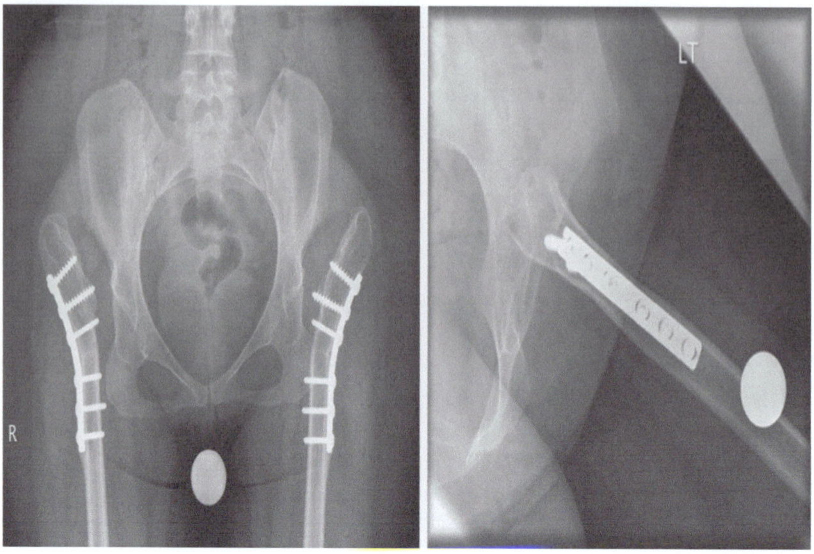

Fig. 5.59 AP pelvis and lateral left hip plain radiographs demonstrating previous Crowe IV dysplasia with excised femoral heads and Schanz osteotomy plates. Radiopaque marker ball aids calibration of plain radiograph image to correct for magnification

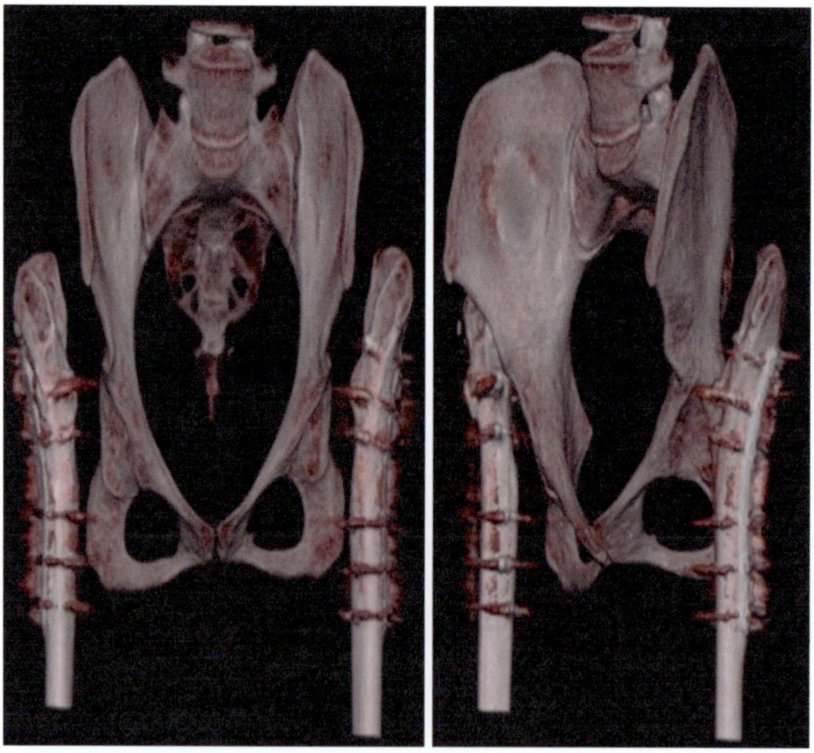

Fig. 5.60 AP and oblique 3D views of the pelvis to assess the acetabular bone stock and femoral anatomy. The CT images may also be used for calibration of the X-rays and correction of magnification

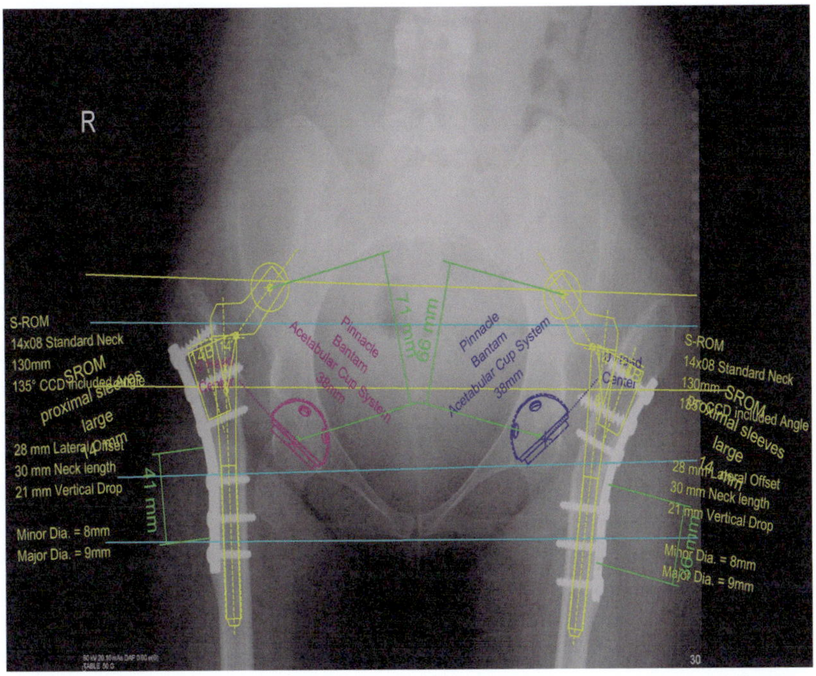

Fig. 5.61 Templating for the proposed sequential procedures for high and low hip centres

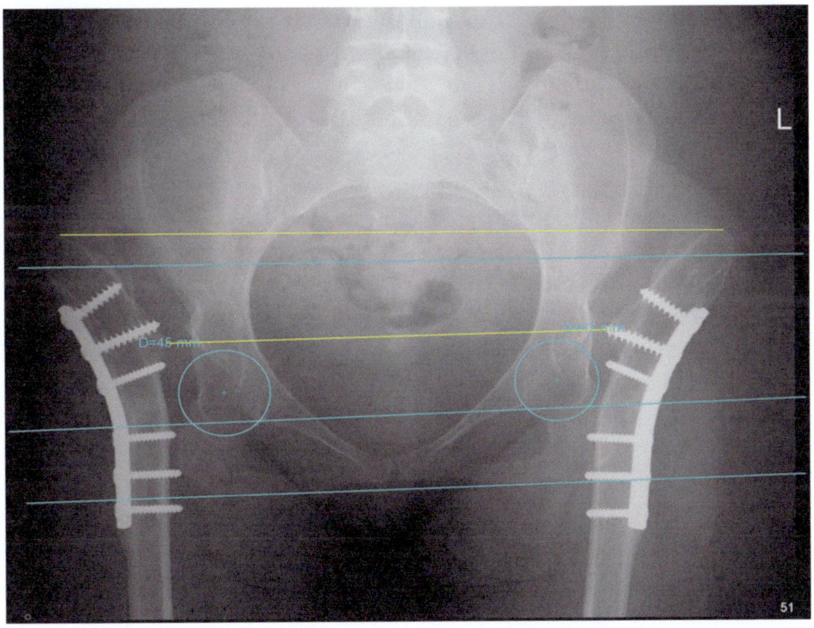

Fig. 5.62 Radiographic template to identify true hip centre as well as bony landmarks that can be identified on the operating table, such as greater trochanter, lesser trochanter, tear drop and previous osteotomy site

5.19.5 Preoperative Planning

Diagnosis: Bilateral dislocated dysplastic hips with excised femoral heads and Schanz osteotomies (Figs. 5.59 and 5.60)

Possible treatment options: Nonoperative focusing on management with analgesia, arthrodesis or operative (reconstruction arthroplasty)

Chosen treatment method: Removal of hardware, modified total hip arthroplasty with limb length correction and restoration of hip centres. Sequential surgery was planned to start with the most symptomatic side.

Selection of implants if applicable and rational: Modular hip system (S-ROM®), that has the following design features of significant benefits to this case, (1) multiple combinations of stems, sleeves and femoral heads allowing for customization to suite configuration of the patient's altered femoral anatomy and to achieve restoration of biomechanics. (2) Modular neck which helps in changing offset without consequences on leg length. Also allows flexibility in stem-to-cup alignment for the range of motion, hip stability and proximal fit allowing for version independent of stem position. (3) Reamer/Mill preparation of the femoral canal supporting fit of precisely sized components. (4) Coronal slots of distal stem helping in achieving rotational stability and preventing distal impingement. Distal flutes enhance rotational stability (5) ZTT® porous proximal sleeves which have steps helping prevention of subsidence. The sleeve has a conical and extended triangle parts. It is independent of the neck and allows its rotation to fit in best available bone. On the acetabular side, (Bantam®) shell was chosen. Its features provide the following benefits to this patient; (1) it provides a cementless porous-coated shell with three holes aiding to achieve stable fixation. (2) It is available in small sizes of 38–46 mm that are often needed to reconstruct a small acetabulum. (3) Highly X-linked polyethylene liners are available in different inner diameters (22–48 mm). (4) Variable stability options consisting of neutral or lipped liners.

Expected difficulties: (1) Altered soft tissue anatomy and scarring from previous surgery. (2) Removal of hardware that has been in situ for nine years with the risk of bone stock weakening and intraoperative fracture. (3) Available bone stock in the true acetabulum, whether to accept low or high hip centre, femoral shortening osteotomy if choosing true acetabulum to prevent overstretching the nerve. (4) Achieving optimal shell coverage. (5) Altered femoral anatomy from previous Schanz osteotomy. (6) Achieving desired leg length. (7) Achieving stable stem implantation.

Strategies to overcome difficulties: (1) Preoperative counselling, ideas, concerns and expectations of the patient were taken into consideration carefully. Details of procedure were explained to the patient at two clinic visits to ensure full understanding. Agreed aims were to relieve pain and improve mobility. (2) Surgical planning, this starts with the preoperative clinical evaluation of structural and functional leg lengths using a measuring tape, blocks and tests such as Thomas and Ober tests [105] to assess the level of fixed deformities. A further radiological evaluation was done using plain films and 3D Computed Tomography reconstruction images. This was followed by AP pelvis templating as shown above. Details of the osteosynthesis plate were identified, and appropriate-sized screwdrivers were ordered. Choice of implants and rationale is as discussed above. Reconstruction techniques were carefully planned (described in more details below). It is necessary to ensure that cabling systems as well as acetabular reconstruction devices (rings, cages, mesh, plates) were made available for the day. Finally, femoral heads were made available for potential need of bone stock augmentation.

Templating: This relies on having at least two reference points: in the pelvis and femur. Intertear drops (IT) line provides a reliable pelvic reference point but can be difficult to recognize in dysplastic hips. An alternative option would be the biischial line [106]. The reference point on the femoral side would be the centre of the hip when using intertear drop line and a line transecting the tips of lesser trochanters. Leg length correction was planned based on these estimates. As the plan was to perform sequential surgery, it was more crucial to get the second side equalized to the first hip (Figs. 5.61 and 5.62).

5.19.6 Surgical Note

Patient's position: Lateral decubitus with two-side supports to secure anterior superior iliac spines and sacrum ensuring shoulder and pelvis are in alignment and approximately perpendicular to the operating table.

Type of anaesthesia: General.

Surgical approach: Modified posterior approach.

Main steps:

1. Referencing true and apparent leg lengths in supine and lateral positions and leg-to-leg comparison with knees and hips in flexion.
2. Posterolateral incision utilizing the previous scar.
3. Fascia lata was incised in line with skin incision.
4. Gentle splitting of gluteus maximus fibres.
5. Charnley retractor was used to retract the fasica lata.
6. Sciatic nerve was visualized and protected.
7. Piriformis was identified, and deep abductors were protected.
8. The piriformis with short external rotators and quadratus muscle, and underlying capsule were raised as single flap posteriorly using diathermy.
9. The vastus was raised off the bone, and the AO plate over the femur was identified, and bony on growth over the plate was removed with osteotomes, followed by removal of the six screws and plate.
10. The true acetabulum was identified using the teardrop, and acetabular preparation started with hemispherical reaming to the true floor aiming for alignment in the desired position (40–45° abduction and 15–20° anteversion) while ensuring no changes have occurred to patient's positioning.
11. Acetabulum was sized to 38 mm.
12. Cementless three-hole Bantam® shell was implanted and augmented with a posterosuperior and an anterosuperior cancellous screw.
13. Pinnacle Marathon® highly cross-linked UHMW neutral liner with 22.225 mm internal diameter was impacted into the shell.
14. Proximal femur osteotomy was performed at the site of previous one to correct angulation and shorten the femur.
15. The bone from the osteotomy site was used to wrap over as bone struts and secured with two 2 mm Accord® cables.
16. A lateral runway was created into the femoral canal.
17. The osteotomized femur was prepared distally and then proximally to allow the S-ROM implant.
18. This was followed by calcar preparation.
19. Following trials and testing for range of movement and stability, shuck test, tissue tension, dropkick test [105] and leg-to-leg comparison were used to ascertain adequate restoration of leg length. A standard 150 mm long S-ROM stem with 16 mm proximal diameter and 11 mm distal diameter was implanted.
20. Size 14B proximal sleeve, 30 standard neck and +0 22.225 mm femoral head was implanted.
21. 40 ml of 0.25 % Marcain was injected into the capsule and soft tissues.
22. A transosseus repair of short external rotators and capsule was undertaken to the greater trochanter using no. 5 Ethibond® sutures.
23. It was confirmed that the sciatic nerve was intact at the end.
24. The fascia lata was closed with no. 2 Vicryl® suture.
25. The further closure was in layers with no. 1 Vicryl and clips to the skin.
26. Nonadhesive dressing and gauze were applied and all was covered with mepore.
27. Patient was carefully transferred off the table.

Reconstruction techniques: Cementless 38 mm cup without the need for bone grafting. Femoral osteotomy to correct the leg length discrepancy (LLD) from choosing to reconstruct the true acetabulum. A modular stem was used to achieve precise press-fit implantation and adjust for rotational deformity, offset and length (Figs. 5.63 and 5.64).

5.19.7 Intraoperative Challenges

Challenges and solutions: Adduction contractures present could have impacted the function of the prosthetic hip. More importantly, it can have a significant impact on leg length management as it can result in abduction of the pelvis and the limb can be measured too short when it is correct [107]. Therefore adductor and capsular release was done.

Unanticipated problems and solution: None.

Thorough description of decision making, including the reason for the final decision: The patient would not have coped with nonoperative management. Following the surgical approach, assessment confirmed that restoration of hip centre was possible. True acetabulum was identified from the teardrop and reconstructed to restore the hip centre. Implantation with a small-sized 38 mm shell provided more than 75% coverage, with some anterior and superior deficit. Excellent primary stability of shell was achieved, but as is our routine practice, additional fixation was achieved using one posterosuperior and one anterosuperior cancellous screws. On the femoral side, 3 cm shortening was achieved using an osteotomy. This was done at previous osteotomy site; however, the amount of shortening had to be precise enough to ensure stem stability without compromising desired leg length. The modularity of the S-ROM® stem was utilized to achieve a precise press-fit femoral implantation. Different trials of neck lengths, lateralized neck options, offsets and head sizes were tested. Intraoperative leg length checks were correlated with preoperative templating, and most appropriate neck length, offset, and head sizes were chosen by achieving the balance between the desired leg length, the range of movement and stability.

5.19.8 Postoperative Radiographs (Figs. 5.63 and 5.64)

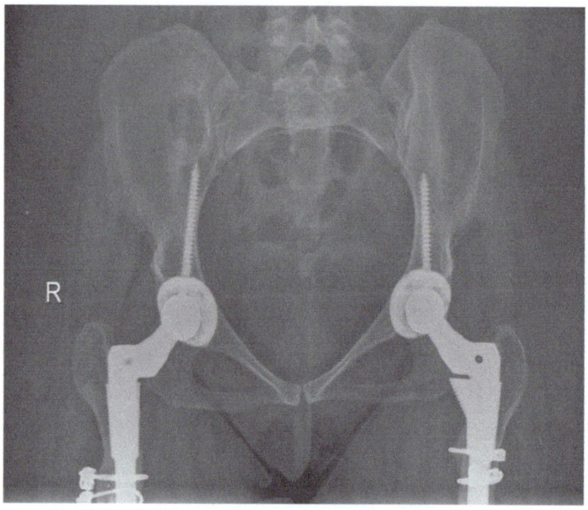

Fig. 5.63 AP pelvis plain film following sequential bilateral THR

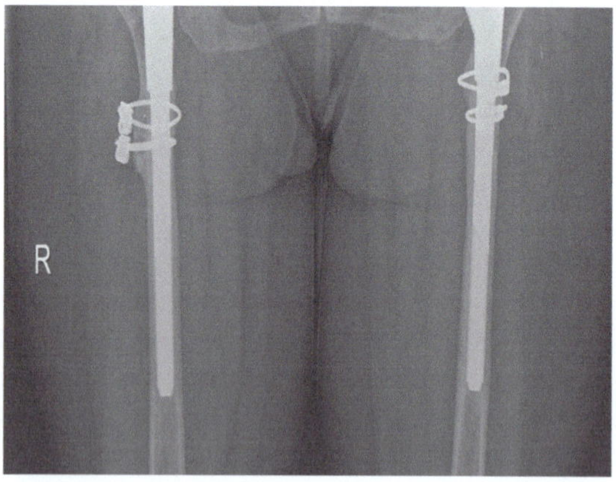

Fig. 5.64 Proximal femur AP view showing well-healed osteotomies and position of press-fit stems in relation to the osteotomy site

5.19.9 Postoperative Management

Chemoprophylaxis and anticoagulant treatment period: Total of 35 days of LMWH anticoagulation from day one post-op.

Gait/limb loading until full loading: Non-weight bearing for six weeks. The patient was reviewed in a clinic and allowed to 50% weight bear as able with crutches for six weeks. Full weight bearing was allowed at three months when pain resolved, and osteotomy looked healed.

5.19.10 Follow-Up and Complications

No complication.

Scoring: Harris Hip Score improved to 81 at twelve weeks post-op with the biggest improvement in pain score (10 to 44).

5.19.11 Discussion

Advantages of the applied method: We have discussed preoperative and intraoperative methods earlier. Clinical assessment is a paramount, especially in more complex cases. Being aware of fixed deformities and associated spinal, pelvic, femoral and tibial pathology makes the surgeon more likely to achieve the desirable leg length. The use of the validated radiographic templating [106] using bony landmarks is essential. This is a reproducible, simple and cheap tool that can apply to most patients. Standardization of how the images are taken and recalibration using a radiopaque ball with known size next to the patient, (Fig. 5.60) allow for intraobserver and interobserver reproducibility. Films should ideally be taken with both legs internally rotated to 20 degrees with a fixed pelvis. Careful attention has to be paid to patients with dysplastic hips and/or contralateral hip pathology as this can give inaccurate measurements. Another advantage is that surgeon can also plan for the other hip and get an estimate of how much to lengthen in the first surgery without imposing difficulties to the planned surgery on the contralateral side. The use of modular hip system provides many advantages as described earlier and allow for fine-tuning leg length and offset.

Disadvantages of the method: Patient has bilateral dysplastic hips with high dislocation making anatomical landmarks difficult to identify. Templating can be inaccurate in the presence of adduction, flexion or rotational deformities.

Alternative evidence-based techniques for the case: The basic principle for all alternative techniques is to measure the distance between a fixed pelvic reference point and a variable point on the femur prior to dislocation. This allows for measurements to be taken throughout the procedure and compared against initial measurement. The use of callipers, pins, sutures and rulers have all been described in the literature [105, 107]. In some centres, computer navigation has been used as a method for managing LLD [107].

Why is the chosen technique better for this case? Many of the above-mentioned techniques are cumbersome, expensive, lack interobserver reproducibility, time-consuming and lack of correlation with clinical and radiographic results. Although navigators can provide very accurate measurements, they are not well developed in hip surgery [105, 107].

Indications and contraindications for your technique: Techniques concerning leg length apply to any patient undergoing primary total hip arthroplasty. Lengthening is limited by the amount of stretching that the sciatic nerve will undergo. We aim for a maximum of 3 cm lengthening beyond which femoral osteotomy is necessary.

Learning curve and how to manage complications: Differences in leg length is the most common reason for litigation post total hip arthroplasty [105–107]. Equalization of the lengths should not be at the expense of stability, the range of movement or overstretching neurovascular bundles. In complex cases, combinations of preoperative, intraoperative and postoperative assessment of measurements are essential. When there are concerns regarding lengthening over 3 cm, the surgeon should consider shortening osteotomy as an option. Risk of sciatic nerve palsy is always a worry to the surgeon. Immediate and regular neurovascular checks postoperatively are mandatory. If there is evidence of nerve palsy, the surgeon has to consider this as being caused by either direct or indirect damage. Direct damage can occur during the surgical approach, removal of the hardware, osteotomy or using cabling systems. Indirect damage can occur as a result of overstretching the nerve by retraction or overlengthening. Immediate assessment of the possible underlying cause and liaison with peripheral nerve specialists to assess and possibly explore nerve is essential.

Failure to identify the true floor can result in a change in the desired leg length. Inadvertent malpositioning of the acetabular component can result in instability of the prosthetic hip. Attempting to achieve stability by increasing offset can result in overlengthening, stretch the sciatic nerve and cause trochanteric symptoms. Therefore careful attention to the positioning of implants is paramount. The use of the modular system can allow for adjustments to the offset by laterizing neck without consequences on leg length.

Delayed and nonunion at the osteotomy site are possible complications. The surgeon has to consider patients at risk prior to surgery (e.g. older patients, smokers, diabetics) and make a contingency plan accordingly. Devascularization of the bone should be avoided. At the time of primary surgery, utilizing the osteotomized bone and using this as a wrap around the site would act as an autograft.

Failed fixation is another possible risk. Stable fixation of implants should be achieved on the table.

Level of evidence concerning the superiority of this method against others: Level 1 diagnostic study [106] and level 4 therapeutic evidence [105, 107].

5.20 Case Title: Roof Step Cut—A Novel Technique for Bony Reconstruction in Acetabular Roof Deficiency

Zoltán Csernátony, Gyula Győrfi, and Lei Zhang

5.20.1 Demographics

Age: 41
Sex: Female
BMI: 28

5.20.2 Relevant Past Medical History

Principal pathologies: Developmental dysplasia of the right hip joint Crowe Type II

Previous surgical procedures: None

Medication: Nonsteroid anti-inflammatory and chondroprotective drugs

History of Presenting Complaint: Constant pain in the right hip joint, limping caused by limb length discrepancy, the affected hip joint is painful for fifteen years

5.20.3 Clinical Examination

Symptoms: Limping, painful active and passive movements, decreased movements of the right hip joint, right lower limb is four cm shorter than the left one

Range of motion: Flexion: 30°; full extension, abduction: 20°; adduction: 10°; external rotation: 20°; internal rotation: 0°

Specific tests: Positive Trendelenburg sign on both sides

Main disability: Decreased and painful movement

Neurovascular evaluation: Intact innervation and circulation

5.20.4 Preoperative Radiological Assessment/Imaging (Fig. 5.65)

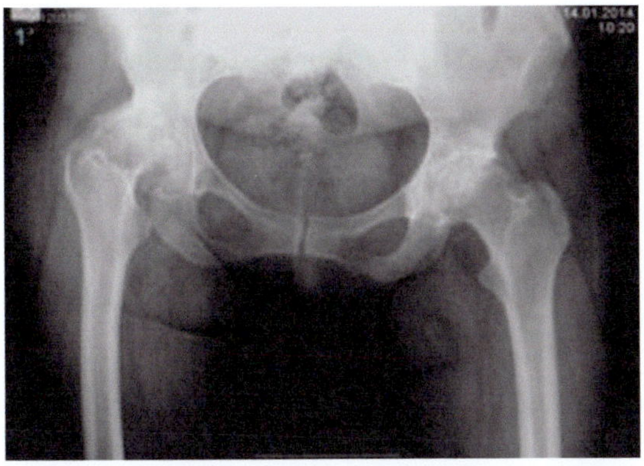

Fig. 5.65 Preoperative X-ray with Crowe Type II hip dysplasia on the right side, consecutive secondary osteoarthritis, moderate osteoarthritis on the left side

5.20.5 Preoperative Planning

Diagnosis: X-ray, physical examination (Fig. 5.65).

Possible treatment options: Total hip replacement with high hip centre, total hip replacement with bulk bone grafting using cementless or cemented implants, physiotherapy.

Chosen treatment method: Total hip replacement into the primary rotational hip centre with reconstruction of the acetabular roof, using the so-called roof step-cut technique.

Selection of implants if applicable and rational: Cementless acetabular cup (Sanatmetal, Hungary), cementless femoral stem (Sanatmetal, Hungary).

Expected difficulties: Possible bony defects on the acetabular rim, reconstruction of the acetabular roof, avoiding neurovascular complications, difficulty in reposition of the prosthesis because of limb length discrepancy.

Strategies to overcome difficulties: Reconstruction of the acetabular roof with the roof step-cut technique, cementless cup insertion, precaution to avoid neurovascular complications.

Templating: We use digital templating, EndoMap® software.

5.20.6 Surgical Note

Patient's position: The patient lies in the supine position with the operated hip slightly elevated.

Type of anaesthesia: We use subarachnoid anaesthesia.

Surgical approach: We usually use the standard anterolateral approach (Watson-Jones).

Main steps: Localizing the true medial wall in the primary acetabulum, reaming to the smallest diameter assuring good anterior and posterior coverage, determining the size of the uncovered area of the acetabular cup, preparing the host area on the inner and superolateral surface of the acetabulum, preparing an L-shaped graft from the femoral head and fixation of the graft with two special screws and washers.

Reconstruction techniques: We use a special technique for reconstruction of the acetabular roof. If the acetabulum is oval shaped, and we want to place the cup into the primary rotational centre, a triangle-shaped gap may remain on the inner superolateral surface of the acetabulum. After identifying the primary acetabulum, we ream it with the smallest diameter reamer, and we see the gap above the trial cup. We modify this gap with a chisel to achieve a plane horizontal superior wall inside the acetabulum. Then the superolateral cortical is cut perpendicular to the previous cut. Both cuts result in a bleeding surface. We use the oscillating saw to prepare an L-shaped graft from the femoral head, fitting to the previously carved surface, which is fixed with two screws and washers inserted in 45°. Once the graft is well fixed, we undermine the internal part of the graft, avoiding to harm its external edge. Finally, we insert the fitting cementless cup, which might be secured with an additional screw if needed. The rest of the operation doesn't differ from the ordinary way (Figs. 5.66 and 5.67).

5.20.7 Intraoperative Challenges

Challenges and solutions: The main challenge is that the acetabulum is oval and the acetabular cup is partially uncovered. In those cases, our solution is the roof step-cut technique. If there is any bony defect on the acetabular rim, we may place an extra screw into the acetabular cup to gain perfect stability. We take all precautions to avoid neurovascular injuries.

Unanticipated problems and solution: None.

Thorough description of decision making, including the reason for the final decision: The patient lies in the supine position. We expose the hip joint through the standard anterolateral (Watson-Jones) approach. We open anteriorly and partially remove the joint capsule. After dislocating the hip and removing the femoral head, we recognize that the original method for bulk bone autografting described by Harris wouldn't be eligible because the acetabulum is oval shaped and flat. If we would like to place the cup into the primary rotational centre, a gap would remain on the inner superolateral surface of the acetabulum. At first, we ream the acetabulum to the smallest size, then we determine the size of the gap, and gain an L-shaped graft from the femoral head with an oscillating saw. We prepare the host area by removal of the cartilage and cortical bone. We fix the graft temporary with one K-wire, and with maintaining the optimal position of the graft, we fix it with two screws (Sanatmetal, Hungary), inserted at 45° angle. We undermine the cranial surface of the acetabulum and the graft with a lower diameter reamer and then insert the acetabular cup; we use neutral or if necessary augmented polyethylene insert. We prepare the medullary canal of the femur, and after using trial components, we insert the final cementless stem. After using trial femoral heads, we choose the one with we can equalize limb length discrepancy with perfect stability and a good range of motion of the prosthesis. After reposition, we leave an intraarticular drain and close the wound with absorbable fascia, subcutaneous suture and with absorbable intracutaneous suture.

5.20.8 Postoperative Radiographs (Figs. 5.66 and 5.67)

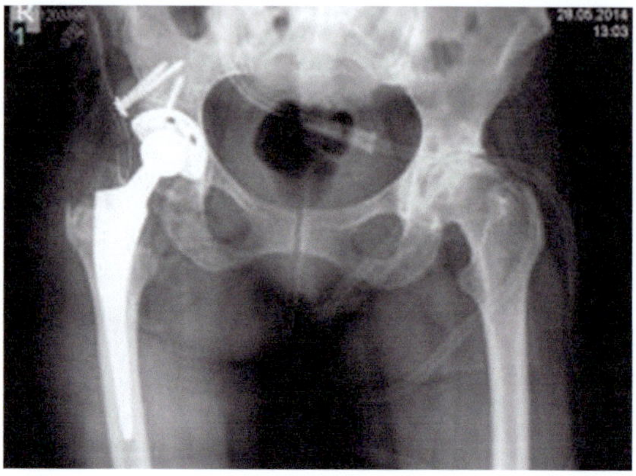

Fig. 5.66 The postoperative X-ray: cementless prosthesis implanted, the cup secured with one screw, the acetabular roof reconstructed with the L-shaped graft fixed with two screws

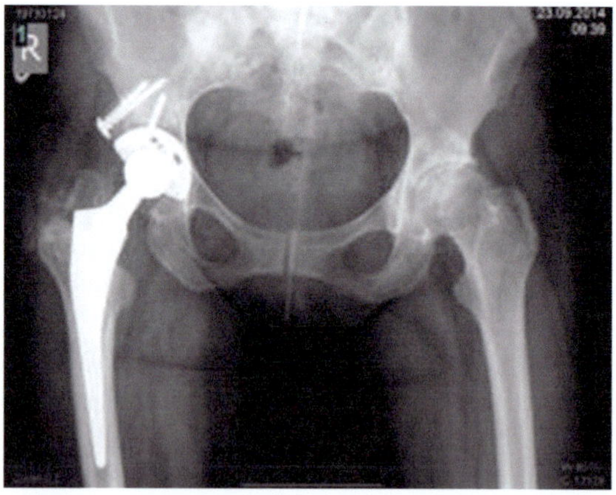

Fig. 5.67 Latest check-up, one year after the operation – the patient is free of complaints, there is no bone resorption in the host-graft junction area, the graft is united with the superolateral aspect of the acetabulum

5.20.9 Postoperative Management

Chemoprophylaxis and anticoagulant treatment period: Oral anticoagulation for six weeks postoperative period (rivaroxaban), antibiotic prophylaxis (single shot or for 2–3 days if necessary)

Gait/limb loading until full loading: six weeks partial weight bearing, full weight bearing after six weeks

5.20.10 Follow-Up and Complications

There were no complications.

5.20.11 Discussion [42, 108, 109]

Advantages of the applied method: Using autologous bulk bone graft decreases the chance of resorption. The L-shaped graft has greater contact surface than the grafts used during previously described techniques that provides a better environment for bony fusion. The screws fixing the grafts are positioned at a 45° angle, which is parallel to the impaction force of the acetabular cup.

Disadvantages of the method: The main problem might be malunion in the host-graft junction area. If the femoral head contains cysts, the graft cannot be prepared properly.

Alternative evidence-based techniques for the case: The acetabular roof reconstruction by tantalum is a much less cost-effective method. The bulk bone autograft technique described by Harris gains smaller contact surfaces, proving a less optimal environment for the host-graft fusion. The acetabular roof reconstruction described by Radojevič uses nearly the same L-shaped graft, but the fixation of the graft is less stable because it is fixed with one horizontal screw. Oblong acetabular cups didn't become widespread.

Why is the chosen technique better for this case? This method provides an optimal environment for the autologous graft and bony fusion; resorption hasn't occurred yet. The technique creates the possibility to place the acetabular cup in the primary rotational centre. It's cost-effective.

Indications and contraindications for your technique: Main indications are Crowe type I and II hip dysplasia when bony reconstruction of the acetabular roof is needed. There is no absolute contraindication, in some cases the technique cannot be performed because of the poor bone quality and cysts of the femoral head, or because of extremely increased acetabular angle.

Learning curve and how to manage complications: The technique demands a highly experienced surgeon. One severe complication can be the fracture of the graft; in this case, we may use allografts.

Level of evidence concerning the superiority of this method against others: The level of evidence is level 4.

5.21 Case Title: Primary Complex Hip Arthroplasty 'Crowe Type 4'

Chitranjan S. Ranawat and Michael Gaudiani

5.21.1 Demographics

Age: Born in 1947
Sex: Female
BMI: 26.6

5.21.2 Relevant Past Medical History

Principal pathologies: Hip dysplasia

Previous surgical procedures: Cholecystectomy

Medication: NSAIDS for pain

History of Presenting Complaint: Pain in the hip region and limp

5.21.3 Clinical Examination

Symptoms: Pain in the right hip

Range of motion: Limited flexion and rotation

Specific tests: Telescopic test positive

Main disability: difficulty in walking

Neurovascular evaluation: Intact

5.21.4 Preoperative Radiological Assessment/Imaging (Fig. 5.68)

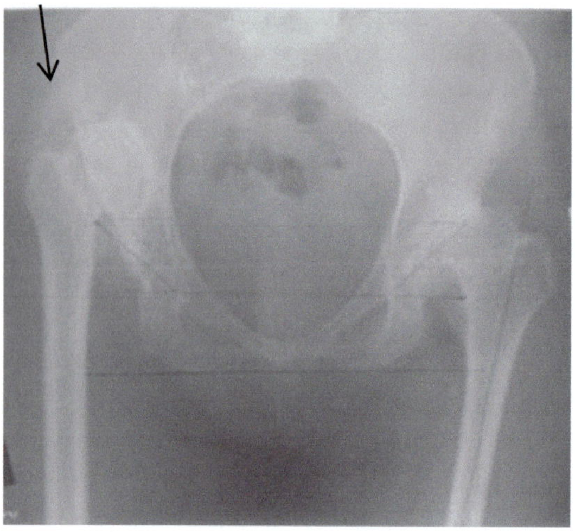

Fig. 5.68 AP x-ray of the pelvis. Crowe IV right hip dysplasia

5.21.5 Preoperative Planning

Diagnosis: Hip dysplasia (Fig. 5.68)

Possible treatment options: Surgical reconstruction

Chosen treatment method: Surgical reconstruction, total hip replacement

Selection of implants if applicable and rational: S-ROM Stem, PSL cup. For achieving stable hip with properly combined anteversion

Expected difficulties: Exposure, shortening of the femur, avoid sciatic nerve palsy

Strategies to overcome difficulties: Proper execution of surgical procedure

Templating: Acetabulum and femur for size

5.21.6 Surgical Note

Patient's position: Lateral

Type of anaesthesia: Epidural

Surgical approach: Posterior lateral

Main steps: Anatomic location of the cup, shortening osteotomy of femur (Fig. 5.69)

Reconstruction techniques: Release of all tight soft tissue structure, capsular iliopsoas rotators, part of gluteus maximus, preserve gluteus minimus

5.21.7 Intraoperative Challenges

Challenges and solutions: Identifying the original acetabulum and appropriate shortening. Solution, identifying inferior aspect of the acetabulum and anterior-posterior wall of the acetabulum.

Unanticipated problems and solution: Injury to branches of femoral vessels to femoral nerve and sciatic nerve. Solution, be aware of anatomic location of structures.

Thorough description of decision making, including the reason for the final decision: (1) Location and placement after appropriate reaming of the acetabulum without compromising anterior-posterior column (2) reaming and broaching of the femur to accurately size the S-ROM sleeve and stem.

5.21.8 Postoperative Radiographs (Fig. 5.69)

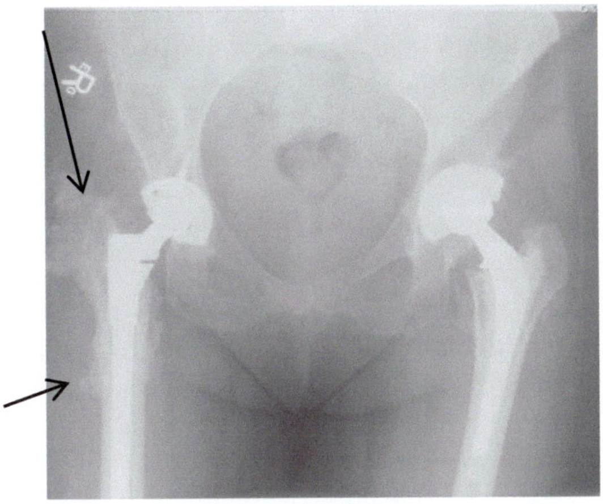

Fig. 5.69 AP x-ray of the Pelvis. Note: Anatomic location of acetabulum and heel osteotomy of the femur. Heterotopic bone around the trochanter

5.21.9 Postoperative Management

Chemoprophylaxis and anticoagulant treatment period: Aspirin, one BID for six weeks

Gait/limb loading until full loading: Partial to full load bearing for ambulation, precaution for dislocation

5.21.10 Follow-Up and Complications

No complication

5.21.11 Discussion [15, 103, 110, 111]

Advantages of the applied method: Restoration of the mechanics of the hip in terms of centre of rotation, offset and small residual shortening of 3⁄4 centimetres.

Disadvantages of the method: Technically demanding.

Alternative evidence-based techniques for the case: Reconstruction without shortening.

Why is the chosen technique better for this case? More effective with reduced or no complication especially neurovascular.

Indications and contraindications for your technique: Indication: Crowe IV hip dyslasia, contraindications: in experience.

Learning curve and how to manage complications: The surgeon should observe and assist several Crowe IV cases reconstructive surgery before undertaking such a procedure by himself.

Level of evidence concerning the superiority of this method against others: IV.

5.22 Case Title: Primary Complex Hip Arthroplasty—Hip Dysplasia Crowe Type 4

Ibrahim Azboy, Antonia F. Chen, and Richard H. Rothman

5.22.1 Demographics

Age: 38
Sex: Female
BMI: 23 kg/m^2

5.22.2 Relevant Past Medical History

Principal pathologies: Limping, pain.

Previous surgical procedures: None.

Medication: Nonsteroidal anti-inflammatory drugs (NSAIDs).

Other: No known drug allergies.

History of Presenting Complaint: This is a 38-year-old female who presented with limping and pain in her bilateral hips. She complained of pain when walking three blocks and climbing up and downstairs. She tried mitigating her pain with NSAIDs and using a cane. She had no complaints of numbness and tingling. She failed conservative management.

5.22.3 Clinical Examination

Symptoms: Pain with bilateral hip range of motion, with the right being worse than the left.

Range of motion: Left hip flexion was 95°, internal rotation was 30°, external rotation was 20°, abduction was 20°, adduction was 15° and extension was 20°.

Specific tests: Trendelenburg test was positive.

Main disability: Limping.

Scoring if available: Harris Hip Score was 42.

Neurovascular evaluation: Normal.

5.22.4 Preoperative Radiological Assessment/Imaging (Fig. 5.70)

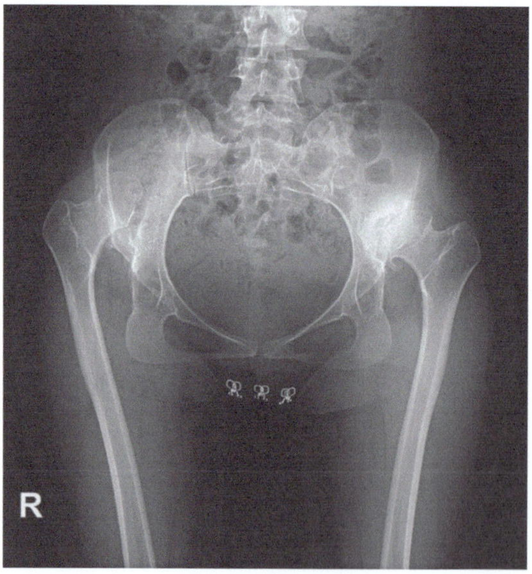

Fig. 5.70 AP radiograph of the pelvis of a 38-year-old woman with bilateral developmental dysplasia of the hip (DDH) and high dislocations of the hips

5.22.5 Preoperative Planning

Diagnosis: Crowe Type IV developmental dysplasia of the hip (DDH) (Fig. 5.70).

Possible treatment options: Nonoperative treatment, femoral transverse shortening subtrochanteric osteotomy, total hip arthroplasty (THA).

Chosen treatment method: Cementless THA with transverse shortening subtrochanteric osteotomy.

Selection of implants if applicable and rational: We preferred to use a cementless right total hip arthroplasty with a subtrochanteric femoral shortening osteotomy that provided anatomic restoration of the hip rotation centre and correction of excessive femoral anteversion.

Expected difficulties: THA in the presence of severe DDH is technically demanding and presents many challenges to the surgeon. Restoration of the proximal femoral anatomy is important to allow enhanced abductor function [95]. During the acetabular reconstruction of the dysplastic adult hip, it is acknowledged that the anatomic centre of hip rotation should be restored. The high-riding femoral head must be reduced into the original acetabulum, as this decreases hip joint reaction forces and improves the abductor lever arm, prolonging the survival of the acetabular component. If the cup is inserted into the false acetabulum, the abductor muscles remain relaxed, and one cannot correct Trendelenburg gait and limb length discrepancy. When the acetabular cup is placed in the true acetabulum, reduction of the hip is nearly impossible, and there is a risk of nerve injury if there is greater than four cm of limb lengthening. Furthermore, there are difficulties in identifying and preparing the true acetabulum and achieving stable fixation of the acetabular component. On the femoral side, there are further technical challenges, including marked hypoplasia of the femur with a frequently narrow medullary canal which leads to difficulty of obtaining stable implantation of an adequately sized femoral component. Finally, the presence of excessive femoral neck anteversion may be difficult to correct and may result in posterior positioning of the greater trochanter and chronic shortening of soft tissue structures.

Strategies to overcome difficulties: Using a subtrochanteric femoral shortening osteotomy technique, femoral length, abductor impairment, femoral version and greater trochanter position can be addressed concurrently. However, obtaining good fit and fill in the small and straight femoral canal of a hip with DDH is sometimes difficult. Using fluoroscopy to identify the medullary canal can be beneficial. In addition, the subtrochanteric shortening osteotomy itself requires stable fixation of the metaphyseal and diaphyseal fragments. A plate should be available to provide fixation. Additionally, one must be prepared to use cables in case of fracture or fixation of femoral autograft around the osteotomy site. Finally, one must prepare appropriate components for fixation. Patients with DDH often require small acetabular components for a hypoplastic acetabulum, 22 mm femoral heads should be available for small acetabular components, and femoral components where the version can be adjusted may be beneficial.

Templating: Templating was used to determine the length of the subtrochanteric femoral osteotomy and to identify the approximate implant size of the acetabulum and femur.

5.22.6 Surgical Note

Patient's position: Lateral decubitus position.

Type of anaesthesia: General anaesthesia.

Surgical approach: Posterolateral approach.

Main steps: A posterolateral approach to the left hip was used with distal extension to access the proximal femoral shaft. The sciatic nerve was identified and protected. A total capsulectomy was performed.

Reconstruction techniques: The femoral head was resected. Reaming and rasping of the femoral canal were performed before acetabular preparation and femoral osteotomy. A transverse osteotomy was performed just distal to the lesser trochanter and perpendicular to the femoral shaft. After the subtrochanteric transverse osteotomy was performed, the proximal fragment of the femur was retracted lateral and cephalad for adequate exposure of the acetabulum. The acetabulum was identified and prepared. The true acetabular fossa was deepened in a posterior and medial direction using reamers. Medialization allowed for increased coverage of the acetabular component. The 44 mm acetabular component was implanted and fixed with three dome screws. Then, the trial insert was inserted. The proximal femur fragment was reduced. Traction was applied to the distal fragment, and the amount of overlap between the proximal and distal femur segments was noted. A distal, transverse osteotomy was carried out, and the osteotomized fragment was used as bone graft around the osteotomy site after cutting it down the midline. Using distal femoral broaching, the distal fragment was prepared until secure fixation was obtained. Femoral anteversion was adjusted, while the osteotomy fragments were secured with bone clamps. The rotational position was indicated by marking both osteotomy fragments. The femoral component was then inserted while holding the osteotomy fragments in place to ensure appropriate rotational alignment and anteversion. The hip was reduced, and trial components were stable. Then a fibre metal taper cementless femoral stem, a ceramic insert and a ceramic head were inserted in the same manner, and the resected bone segments were used as strut grafts to augment fixation of the osteotomy site. The soft tissue connections of resected bone segments were preserved to maintain the blood supply. The short external rotators were reattached to the greater trochanter, and the wound was closed in layers (Figs. 5.71 and 5.72).

Implants: A modular femoral stem and 44 mm acetabular cup (VerSys Fiber metal taper stem and Trilogy cup, Zimmer, USA) were used for the left hip.

5.22.7 Intraoperative Challenges

Challenges and solutions: There was no need to cut the iliopsoas or perform an adductor tenotomy. The tension of the sciatic nerve was controlled manually to avoid excessive stretching. Limb length discrepancy was measured by preoperative standing radiographs and intraoperatively by comparing the levels of the patellae. Placement of the acetabular cup in the true acetabular fossa and superior-lateral coverage of the acetabular component was another challenge. The true acetabular fossa was deepened in a posterior and medial direction using reamers. Medialization allowed increased coverage of the acetabular shell.

Unanticipated problems and solution: None.

Thorough description of decision making, including the reason for the final decision: The stability of the hip, soft tissue tension, limb length discrepancy, secure component fixation and reposition of osteotomy sites were the main issues for the final decision of implant and bony fixation.

5.22.8 Postoperative Radiographs (Figs. 5.71 and 5.72)

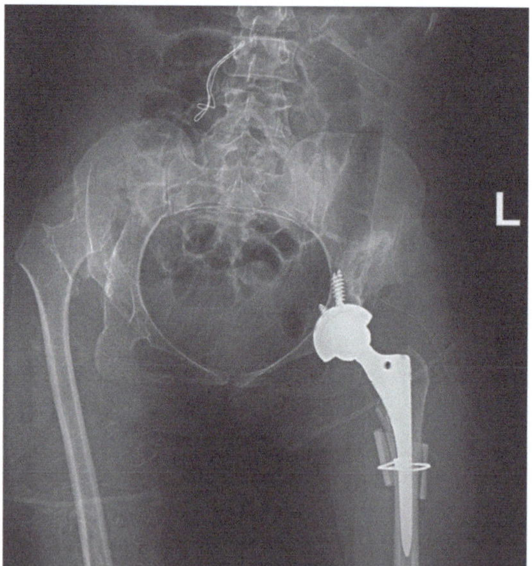

Fig. 5.71 AP radiograph of the pelvis at early postoperative follow-up

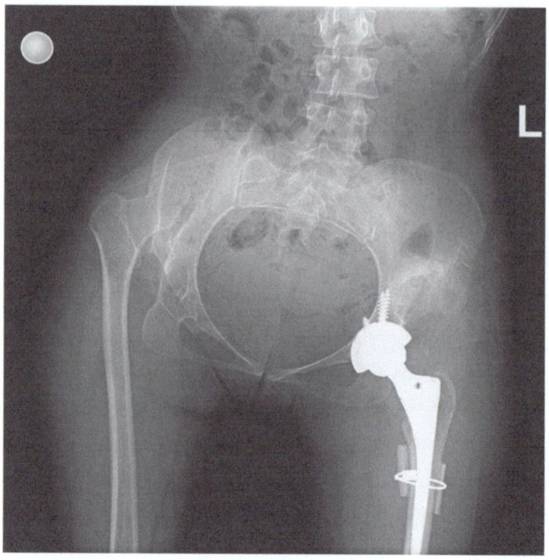

Fig. 5.72 AP radiograph of the pelvis at 4-month follow-up. The right total hip arthroplasty was completed six months after the left total hip arthroplasty

5.22.9 Postoperative Management

Chemoprophylaxis and anticoagulant treatment period: The patient was administered 2 g of a first-generation cephalosporin 30 min preoperatively as a prophylactic measure, which was continued for 24 h. For venous thromboembolism prophylaxis, 2850 IU of nadroparin (a low-molecular-weight heparin) was administered daily to all patients for 21 days.

Gait/limb loading until full loading: On the second postoperative day, patients were allowed to walk a few steps with ten kg partial weight bearing. At six weeks after the operation, partial weight bearing of twenty kg was allowed. Weight bearing was increased depending on the consolidation of the osteotomy site. When the patient demonstrated radiographic signs of union at the osteotomy site, the patient was allowed to bear full weight. The left hip underwent reconstruction six months after the right side was completed.

5.22.10 Follow-Up and Complications

No complications.

Scoring: Harris Hip Score was 90

5.22.11 Discussion

Advantages of the applied method: Using the subtrochanteric shortening technique, limb length discrepancy, abductor impairment, excessive femoral anteversion, and the greater trochanter position could be addressed concurrently. Subtrochanteric shortening osteotomy itself requires stable fixation of the metaphyseal and diaphyseal fragments. This concern has lead surgeons to address this problem using a step-cut osteotomy, which is more difficult and time-consuming and may require additional fixation with plates. We preferred a tapered stem for left hip. We obtained excellent primary fixation. We achieved union in four months.

Disadvantages of the method: The transverse-cut osteotomy is easier to perform; however, this osteotomy may result in a poor torsional stability because it is thought that there is a greater possibility of the nonunion or delayed union at the osteotomy site.

Alternative evidence-based techniques for the case: An oblique-cut osteotomy and step-cut osteotomy are alternative techniques [95, 112]. However, the step-cut osteotomy is difficult to perform and is time-consuming. The oblique osteotomy was introduced to improve healing at the osteotomy site. However, in cases of excessive femoral anteversion, these procedures are more complex for correcting anteversion.

Why is the chosen technique better for this case? This case of a Crowe IV high-riding DDH, a subtrochanteric shortening osteotomy was required to maintain the anatomic centre of hip rotation. At the same time, it allowed for correction of excessive femoral anteversion.

Indications and contraindications for your technique: The indication for this technique is Crowe Group IV developmental dysplasia of the hip. In cases with severe femoral deformity, a transverse osteotomy may not be enough, and other surgical considerations should be made.

Learning curve and how to manage complications: This technique is highly demanding and should not be done early in a surgeon's learning curve. The surgeon should prepare the patient carefully. Preoperative radiological assessment is crucial. The acetabular component should be placed in the true acetabulum, and small acetabular components should be available.

Every step of surgery is challenging, and potential complication should be addressed properly. Soft tissue tension and hip stability should be considered as the main part of the operation to prevent dislocation. Thus, it may be beneficial to place a larger femoral head in these patients. The osteotomy site should be reopposed and grafted to prevent delayed union or nonunion. Finally, nerve injuries are more common in this patient population, and preventing excessive stretching of the nerve will be beneficial for reducing complications. If a traction injury does occur, it is first treated conservatively by flexing the knee and extending the hip. If sciatic nerve injury persists, the patient is fitted with an ankle-foot orthosis for drop foot, and further nerve testing can be done at a later point in time.

Level of evidence concerning the superiority of this method against others: The use of cementless total hip arthroplasty with a subtrochanteric femoral shortening osteotomy provides high rates of successful implant fixation and facilitates osteotomy union [98, 112].

5.23 Case Title: Developmental Dysplasia of the Hip in an Adult Patient

Volker Otten and Arkan S. Sayed-Noor

5.23.1 Demographics

Age: 30 years
Sex: Female
BMI: 30

5.23.2 Relevant Past Medical History

Principle pathologies: Developmental dysplasia of the hip (DDH) bilaterally with shortening of the left leg. The patient had no other health problems.

Previous surgical procedures: None.

Medication: Analgesics for hip pain with different types of nonsteroidal anti-inflammatory drugs and paracetamol.

5.23.3 History of Present Complaint

This 30-year-old female complained of severe pain in the left hip during and after walking during the last year. Her maximum walking distance without crutches was 400 m. She had suffered from problems with both hips since childhood and complained about leg length discrepancy and the feeling of instability in her left hip. There was muscle weakness and pain on both sides when walking.

5.23.4 Clinical Examination

Symptom: Severe pain in the left hip during weight bearing.

Range of motion: On physical examination, the left hip had a range of motion of 80 degrees in flexion and full extension. Internal rotation was not possible without severe pain, and external rotation was 20 degrees. Abduction and adduction were restricted to about ten degrees because of the pain.

Specific tests: There was a clinical leg length discrepancy of 6.5 cm with the left leg shorter.

Scores: The Harris Hip Score was 33, the CE angle was 5 degrees on the right hip and 170 degrees on left. The Crowe classification was type II on the right hip and type IV on the left.

Neurovascular evaluation: There were no nerve disorders and circulation in the lower extremities was good.

5.23.5 Preoperative Radiological Assessment/Imaging (Figs. 5.73 and 5.74)

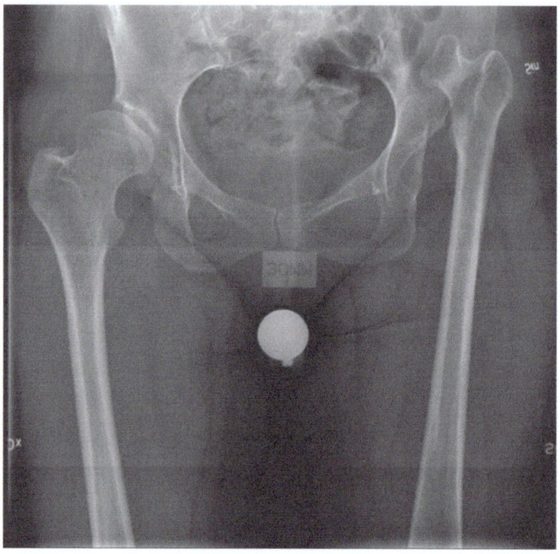

Fig. 5.73 Preoperative X-ray showing a DDH of Crowe type IV on the left side and type II on the right side

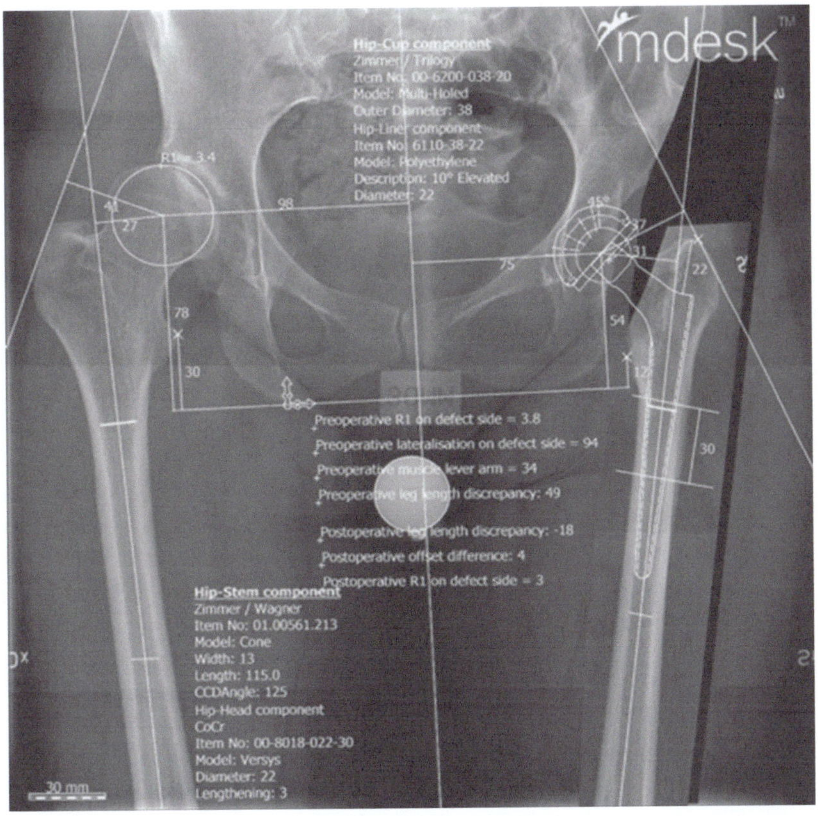

Fig. 5.74 Preoperative digital templating using the Mdesk™ system

5.23.6 Preoperative Planning

Diagnosis: DDH of Crowe type IV on the left side with secondary osteoarthritis (Fig. 5.73).

Possible treatment options: Extraction of the caput femoris to reduce the pressure on the ilium. Prosthesis with a high hip centre. Prosthesis with the normal hip centre and femoral shortening osteotomy.

Chosen treatment method: THA with the anatomical hip centre and femoral shortening osteotomy.

Selection of implants: Cup continuum, Zimmer, size 44 mm, cross-linked PE liner for 28 mm head, Biolox head 28 mm with the neck length of +3.5, cone stem, Zimmer, size 13 with 125 degrees CCD.

Expected difficulties: Anticipate weak bone in the acetabulum, a small femur canal, rotational instability in the femur osteotomy and tension to the sciatic nerve. Very careful reaming of both the acetabulum and femur is required and step osteotomy to give maximum rotational stability. There should be good exposure of the sciatic nerve and preparedness to shorten the femur more than that preoperatively planned on X-ray. The patient was informed that her leg lengths would still not be equal postoperatively.

Templating: Preoperative templating was crucial to be prepared for a small prosthesis size (Fig. 5.74). In some cases, with an extremely small joint, a custom-made prosthesis might be necessary and this has to be decided during the planning of the operation. The templating gave a size of 38 mm for the acetabulum component and a size 13 for the stem, which is the smallest standard prosthesis for this implant type. The shortening of the femur was planned to be three cm giving a lengthening of the leg of about 3.5 cm with the centre of rotation in the anatomical place.

5.23.7 Surgical Notes

Patient's position: Lateral decubitus position.

Type of anaesthesia: Spinal anaesthesia with sedation.

Surgical approach: Posterolateral approach combined with an anterior capsulotomy through a window between the gluteus medius muscle and the tensor fascia lata.

Main steps: Good exposure was essential, especially for the sciatic nerve to avoid overtension when lengthening the leg. First, the femur was prepared with osteotomy of the collum femoris and then reaming of the femur shaft. When the proximal part of the femur gives a good fit to the planned stem, the step osteotomy is performed, and the planned portion is extracted. Subsequently, the anterior and posterior wall of the anatomical acetabulum is identified. With the help of the incisura acetabuli as the third point, the centre of the true acetabulum can be identified and a 2.5 mm hole was drilled through the medial wall. The reaming is straightforward leaving at least five mm of medial wall. Care should be taken because the bone is mostly very soft. Most often extra screws are necessary to give good initial stability in the soft bone. The step of osteotomy was held together and the femur diaphysis was reamed to fit the planned stem. A trial stem in the femur, holding together the femur osteotomy is used to test the tension on the sciatic nerve with the joint in place. The tension should be evaluated in both flexion and extension of both the hip and the knee. After that, the stability of the hip in flexion, internal rotation, extension and external rotation is checked. The trial stem was replaced with the actual implant, and the osteotomy is secured with cerclage wires. If the stability of the osteotomy is doubtful, the resected part of the femur can be used as a structural graft around the osteotomy (Figs. 5.75 and 5.76).

Intraoperative challenges: The main challenges in these patients are to get the implants in an anatomically correct position, to prevent fractures during operation despite the weak bone, to pay attention to the tension of the sciatic nerve carefully and to assure the good primary stability of the implant and the osteotomy.

Unanticipated problems and solution: In this specific case, the weak bone in the acetabulum did not give sufficient stability together with the planed cup size. First, a several mm larger cup gave a good press fit. This has led to a more medialized cup than planned but with a still intact medial wall. During trial reduction, it became clear that the planned shortening of the femur gave too much tension on the sciatic nerve. When the femur was shortened by 4 cm instead of the preoperatively planned 2.5 cm, the tension of the nerve was acceptable. This resulted in a bigger postoperative leg length discrepancy but a much lower risk for nerve palsy.

Thorough description of decision making, including the reason for the final decision: A thicker medial acetabular wall is preferable with potential future revisions in mind, but the primary stability of the cup is most important for long-term results.

5.23.8 Postoperative Radiographs (Figs. 5.75 and 5.76)

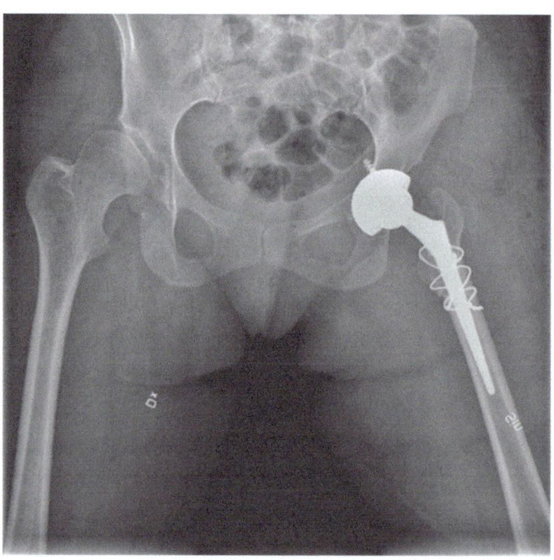

Fig. 5.75 Postoperative X-ray on the 1st postoperative day

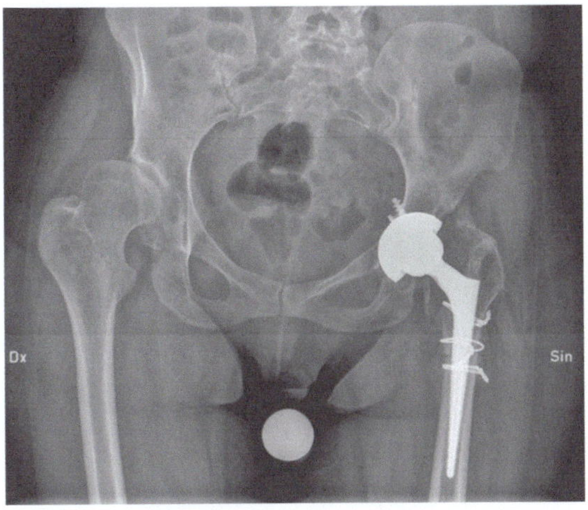

Fig. 5.76 Postoperative x-ray at 4 months. Note the heterotopic ossification between the tip of the greater trochanter and acetabulum. The prosthetic components are well placed

5.23.9 Postoperative Management

Chemoprophylaxis and anticoagulant treatment period: Low-molecular-weight heparin (5000 IE dalteparin/day) was administered for five weeks postoperatively as anticoagulant treatment. Oxycodone and paracetamol as pain treatment during the first weeks as needed.

Gait/limb loading until full loading: Rehabilitation consisted of partial weight bearing during the first eight weeks and crutches for twelve weeks.

5.23.10 Follow-Up and Complications

Report of postoperative complications and their management: During the first two weeks, the patient could not adduct the leg fully because of tension in the abductor muscles. During the first month, there was pain in the back of the leg when flexing the hip in combination with an extended knee. Both problems have disappeared without further treatment. No dislocations, fractures or nerve palsy occurred after the operation.

Scores: Four months postoperatively the patient had a maximal flexion of 100° and full extension. Both internal and external rotations were about 15°. There was no pain in the hip but a slight limp when walking.

5.23.11 Discussion

Advantages of the applied method: The reconstruction of the DDH with an anatomical placed centre of rotation provides good long-term results regarding function, dislocation rate and loosening of the prosthesis [19]. Leg lengthening to some degree is possible with the tension of the sciatic nerve as the limit. An anatomical lever arm for the abductor muscles reduces, after rehabilitation, limping to the minimum. The use of a subtrochanteric osteotomy allows both the possibility of leg shortening and if necessary angular and rotational correction of the proximal femur for optimal function and minimization of dislocation risk [113]. Step-cut osteotomy is technically more difficult to perform compared to transverse osteotomies but enhances the rotational stability. The healing rate of subtrochanteric osteotomies is very good. A posterior approach in combination with a subtrochanteric osteotomy gives good access to the acetabulum, the femur and the sciatic nerve. At the same time, this approach does allow to preserve the main part of the soft tissue and vascularity to the metaphysis and thereby reduces the risk for nonunion. Uncemented components provide good results with low revision rate because of loosening. Cemented femoral components in combination with osteotomy might raise the risk for the nonunion of the osteotomy [114].

Disadvantages of the method: The operation is technically more challenging compared to the possible alternatives; subtrochanteric osteotomy comes with a risk of nonunion and fracture. When doubtful of the initial stability of the osteotomy, additional stabilization using the resected part of the femur as autologous graft around the osteotomy should be used. Generally, in patients with normal anatomy, the posteralateral approach has been shown to give a higher risk for dislocation compared to direct lateral or anterolateral approach.

Alternative evidence-based techniques for this case: In mild dysplasia (as in the right hip of this patient) a joint preserving alternative like a periacetabular osteotomy should be considered, especially in younger patients. Some preserved cartilage is needed to give good results after these operations. In the case of THA in severe DDH, slide osteotomies for the shortening osteotomy can be an alternative. A trochanteric slide osteotomy is technically easier to perform, provides good access to the acetabulum, allows for the shortening of the femur and can be used even when earlier osteotomies have been performed. Nevertheless, this osteotomy type doesn't give the same degree for rotational and angular corrections. Furthermore, when shortening the femur several centimetres, the trochanter minor and the psoas tendon might be lost, and the hip flexion strength is compromised [114].

Why is the chosen technique better for this case? The patient had no additional neuromuscular disorders besides the DDH and therefore had good chance to reach a good functional outcome with a THA. Preoperative X-rays revealed an existing osteoarthritis of the caput femoris and nonexisting acetabulum. Consequently, a joint-preserving operation was not possible. Because of the patient's young age and good health, a high level of activity for many decades is anticipated. THA with a small head and with the anatomical centre of rotation gives good long-term functional results. The posterolateral approach gives the best exposure to the sciatic nerve and good access to the subtrochanteric region. For the shortening of the femur, a subtrochanteric step osteotomy was chosen to provide good rotational stability, the possibility for rotation correction and a minimal impact on the abductor muscles.

Indications and contraindications for your technique: A shortening osteotomy should only be performed if necessary due to the risk of nonunion. In milder degree of DDH (Crowe grade I to III) and older patients, even in some cases with high dislocations, shortening of the femur can be avoided. In patients who have had previous anterior hip operations, it can be beneficial to use the same approach again to handle the scar tissue.

Learning curve and how to manage complications: These operations are technically challenging. A good experience in the procedure of THA and detailed knowledge of the anatomy of the hip is mandatory. The surgeon should also be familiar with the handling of periprosthetic fractures in both acetabulum and femur. It is difficult to know the maximum tolerated tension for the neurovascular structures or what is the optimal force when impacting the implant in the soft bone; experience does certainly help. There is definitively a learning curve, which can be shortened by earlier experience with hip surgery in normal anatomy.

5.24 Case Title: Management of Crowe III Acetabular Dysplasia Using Robot-Assisted Surgery

Alberto Carli, Lazaros Poultsides, and Seth Jerabek

5.24.1 Demographics

Age: 63
Sex: Female
BMI: 28.2 (Height = 147 cm)

5.24.2 Relevant Past Medical History

Principal pathologies: Hypertension, hyperlipidaemia, major depression

Previous surgical procedures: Hysterectomy

Medication: Duloxetine, pregabalin, rosuvastatin

Other: 30 pack-year history of smoking

History of Presenting Complaint: This patient reports chronic left hip pain that has been steadily increasing over the past twenty years. She currently requires a walker to ambulate one city block and uses a motorized scooter to perform outdoor activities.

5.24.3 Clinical Examination

Symptoms: (1) Left groin pain, (2) leg length inequality

Range of motion: 70° flexion, 0° extension, 45° external rotation, 0° internal rotation

Specific tests: Positive Stinchfield test (resisted hip flexion), perceived leg length discrepancy felt corrected when patient stood on a 2 cm block

Main disability: Pain and leg length discrepancy arising from the left hip

Neurovascular evaluation: Normal

5.24.4 Preoperative Radiological Assessment/Imaging (Figs. 5.77, 5.78, and 5.79)

Other: CT scan confirmed leg length discrepancy of 21 cm as measured by comparing left and right distances of the anterior superior iliac spine (ASIS) to the greater trochanter.

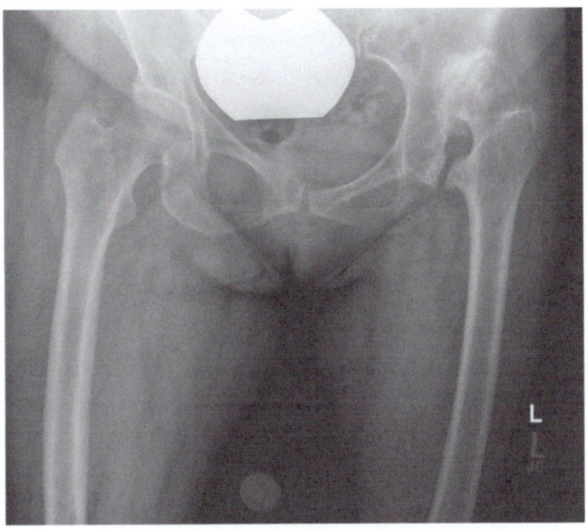

Fig. 5.77 Anteroposterior view of pelvis demonstrating left Crowe III acetabular dysplasia with associated degenerative changes, valgus femoral neck, externally rotated (and potentially excessively anteverted) femur and suspected impingement of the lesser trochanter

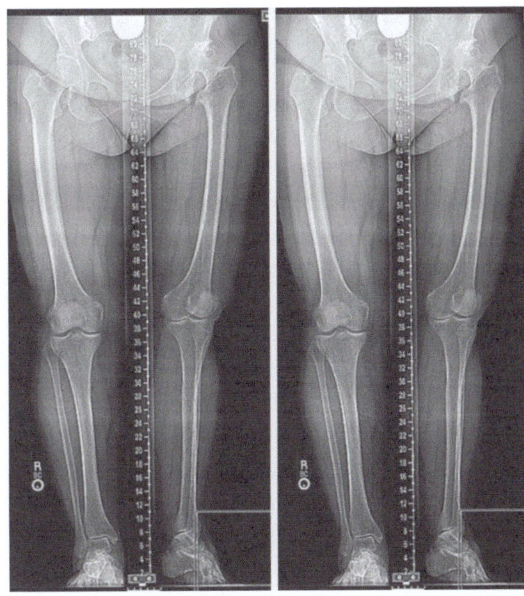

Fig. 5.78 Standing lower extremity view demonstrating leg length discrepancy

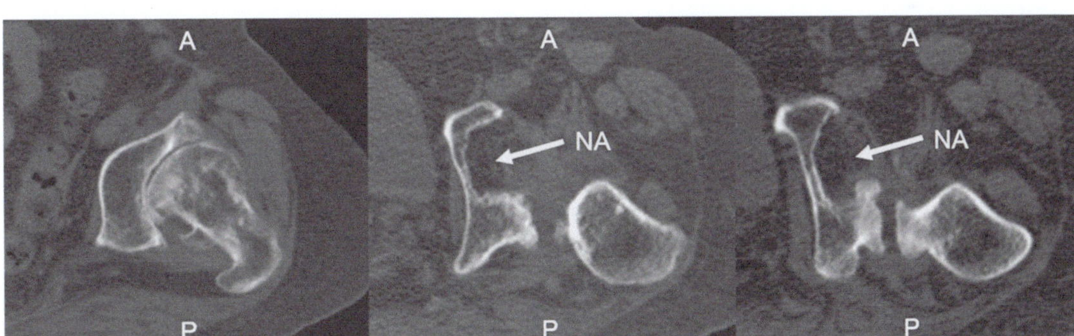

Fig. 5.79 Consecutive axial CT images showing (from left to right): Retroverted pseudoacetabulum and femoral neck with 45° anteversion; native acetabulum (NA) with thin medial and anterior walls; inferiorly, the native acetabulum (NA) is shallow and has excessive anteversion. Note also degenerative changes along the lesser trochanter

5.24.5 Preoperative Planning

Diagnosis: Crowe III acetabular dysplasia with associated superolateral bone deficiency, excessively anteverted femoral neck (Figs. 5.77 and 5.78).

Possible treatment options: Robotic-assisted, navigated or non-navigated total hip arthroplasty with superolateral bone grafting ± femoral shortening osteotomy.

Chosen treatment method: Robotic-assisted total hip arthroplasty.

Selection of implants if applicable and rational: See expected difficulties (below).

Expected difficulties: (1) Identification and protection of sciatic nerve, (2) locating the native acetabulum, (3) reaming concentrically and placing cup at native hip centre, (4) achieving lateral cup coverage with bone and (5) sestoring normal femoral anteversion and leg length and offset.

Strategies to overcome difficulties: (1) Meticulous exposure, place hip in extension when placing Charnley retractor; (2) carefully examining preoperative CT scan, following the ligamentum teres, identifying the transverse acetabular ligament; (3) proper registration of acetabular bone with the robotic software, confirmation with anatomic landmarks; (4) fill acetabular defect with the autologous femoral head structural bone graft and fix it with large fragment screws; (5) use a proximally modular femoral component to restore anteversion, use robotically-assisted intraoperative leg length and offset measurements to fine tune implant placement. Can also consider intraoperative X-ray.

Templating: A preoperative CT scan was performed (Fig. 5.79), and Mako software was used to create a three-dimensional preoperative plan. A CAD model of the acetabular component was inserted. Its position and diameter were adjusted such that its centre of rotation would be located at the height more similar to the contralateral hip, balancing the restoration of hip centre and best available bone stock for reconstruction. It was positioned at 40 degrees of inclination and 20 degrees of anteversion. Bony landmarks for this position were noted. A two-dimensional anteroposterior representation of the planned cup position was then produced (Fig. 5.80). Using the anteroposterior view, the proximally modular femoral component size was templated, and the planned level of femoral neck resection was marked. The preoperative plan was to correct the leg length discrepancy of 2 cm as much as possible. A subtrochanteric femoral shortening osteotomy was tentatively planned as a contingency in case the proximal femur could not be sufficiently mobilized. The level of the osteotomy was templated to be located 2 cm below the level of the femoral sleeve, within the subtrochanteric region.

5.24.6 Templating Images

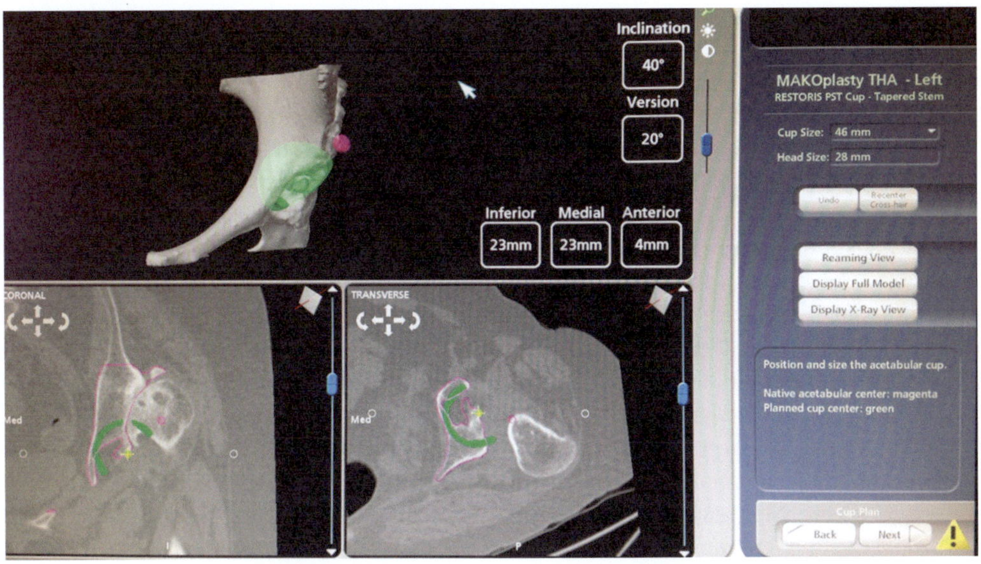

Fig. 5.80 Preoperative acetabular templating: The acetabular component is virtually placed in the true acetabulum through positioning it on coronal (*bottom left image*) and sagittal (*bottom right image*) CT sections. The AP implant view is provided (*top image*) with measures of implant abduction and anteversion

5.24.7 Surgical Note

Patient's position: Lateral, with pelvis secured by bolsters on the pubic symphysis and sacrum.

Type of anaesthesia: Combined spinal/ epidural.

Surgical approach: Posterolateral.

Main Steps and Reconstruction Techniques: A standard posterolateral incision was utilized. The gluteus maximus tendon was tenotomized to facilitate exposure while palpating and protecting the sciatic nerve. The tendon was repaired at the end of the case. The hip was dislocated, and a severely dysplastic femoral head was found. A large pseudoacetabulum was also noted.

Femoral registration: Using the Mako femoral protocol, a femoral array with reflective markers was set up. A 4.5 mm screw was placed on the lateral aspect of the greater trochanter and then touched by the femoral array to calibrate robot position. Using an array stylus, 32 points along the femoral head, neck and greater trochanter were registered and matched by the software to the three-dimensional representation of the patient's preoperative CT scan with a tolerated discrepancy of 0.5 mm. Once the model was built on the computer screen, the stylus was used to mark out the planned level of femoral neck resection. The femoral head was resected and retained for later use as an acetabular autograft (Fig. 5.81).

Acetabular exposure: The anterior capsule was then released off the proximal femur, and the femur was translated anteriorly. The reflected head of the rectus femoris was also released to permit visualization of the anterior border of the pseudoacetabulum. The location of the native acetabulum was confirmed through identification of the transverse acetabular ligament.

Acetabular registration: Three 1/8 inch threaded pins were placed in the iliac wing, and a pelvic array with reflective markers was secured. Within the surgical incision, a 4.5 mm screw was placed in the anterosuperior acetabular rim and touched with the array to help calibrate robot position. Then, using a stylus, 32 individual points along the pseudoacetabulum and acetabulum were registered which were matched by the software to the 3D representation of the patient's preoperative CT scan with a tolerance of less than 0.5 mm of registration error (Fig. 5.82).

Reaming: The Mako robot arm was then brought into the field with a 40 mm reamer attached. The reamer was directed to the desired trajectory of reaming in 40 degrees of abduction and 20 degrees of anteversion. Once this direction was confirmed, the arm was locked in this position and reaming commenced. The stereotactic interface of the Mako system displays the direction and depth of reaming of reaming on the computer screen in real time and does not permit any removal of bone greater than 0.5 mm outside of the predetermined hemisphere of resection. The acetabulum was progressively reamed until a 45 mm reamer removed the necessary bone to achieve a 1 mm press fit.

Grafting the pseudoacetabulum: The pseudoacetabulum was gently reamed with a 42 mm reamer until bleeding bone was encountered. On a back table, the femoral head was denuded of cartilage using a Midas burr, divided and then contoured to fill the pseudoacetabular deficiency. The graft was temporarily held with 2 K-wires, which were then replaced with three 4.5 mm titanium cancellous screws.

Cup placement: The Mako robot arm was again brought into the field, and the 45 mm reamer was used to re-establish a hemispherical cavity through an identical trajectory as before. A 46 mm Mako Restoris acetabular shell was then placed on the robotic arm, placed in a position of 40 degrees of abduction and 22 degrees of anteversion, and was impacted into place (Fig. 5.83). Seating to 0–1 mm of the acetabular surface was confirmed via the computer interface. Two posterosuperior 6.5 mm acetabular screws were then placed, followed by a trial liner.

Femoral preparation: The leg was then flexed, abducted and internally rotated. Evaluation of the femoral canal confirmed preoperative concerns for excessive anteversion. The femoral canal was accessed and reamed with the Smith & Nephew Emperion reamers. Proximal femur preparation followed to accommodate the proximal spout of the implant. After trialling with a standard offset neck and noting proximal impingement of the greater trochanter, an extended offset neck was then placed in 15 degrees of anteversion. Upon reducing the hip, it was found to be stable in all positions. The planned restoration was 20 mm, but the soft tissues were tight; thus 17 mm of leg length correction was accepted and confirmed with robotics. The trial components were then removed.

Final component placement: A 28 mm neutral Mako Restoris XLVE acetabular liner was placed. In the femur, a Smith & Nephew Emperion extended offset size 11 stem with a standard length small cone and #2 spout was then placed in the femur in 15 degrees of anteversion. A -3 mm Oxinium head was placed after cleaning the trunnion. The hip was reduced and found to be stable in all positions, with the same 17 mm restoration of leg length as before (Figs. 5.83 and 5.84).

5.24.8 Intraoperative Photos

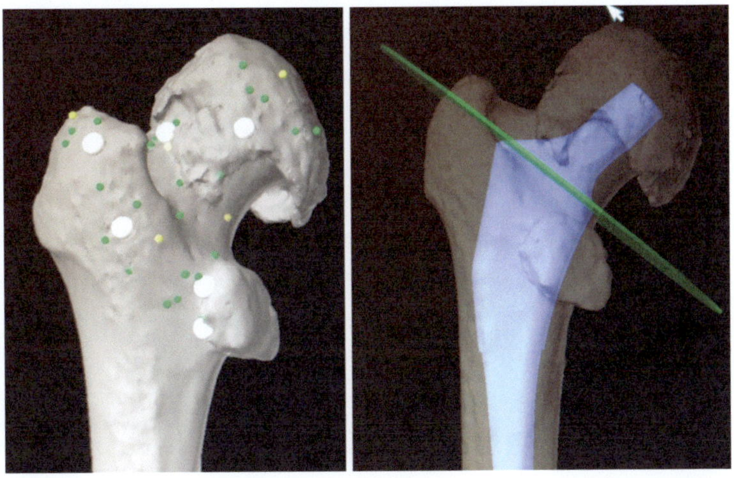

Fig. 5.81 *Left*: 3D reconstruction of proximal femur showing reference points (*green*, *yellow* and *white dots*). *Right*: 3D reconstruction with level of neck cut displayed with sample femoral implant (not the same design as final implant utilized)

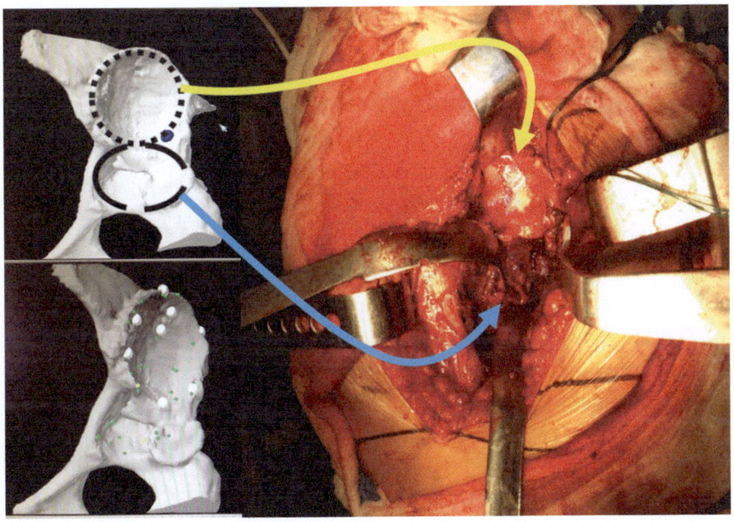

Fig. 5.82 Preoperative 3D reconstruction showing pseudoacetabulum (*dotted circle*) and true acetabulum (*lined circle*), with arrows pointing location of structures on the intraoperative photo. In the lower left, the intraoperative registration marks performed to confirm the preoperative image of the true bony surfaces

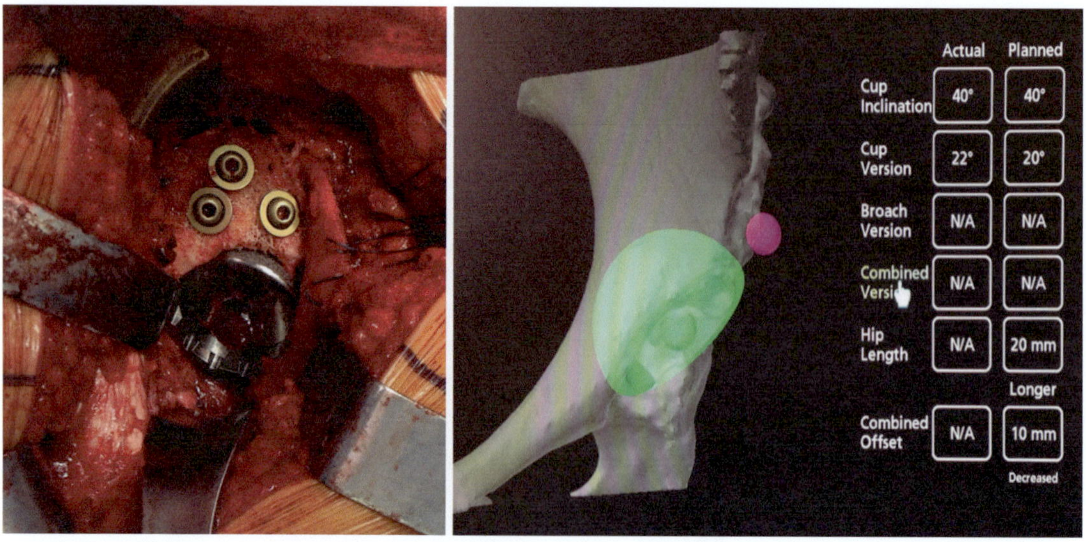

Fig. 5.83 Left: Intraoperative photo demonstrating femoral head autograft secured with three screws and successfully achieving lateral coverage for the final acetabular implant. Right: Corresponding 3D model showing, in real time, the position of the acetabular component. As indicated, the final component was placed in 40 degrees of inclination and 22 degrees of anteversion

5.24.9 Intraoperative Challenges

Challenges and solutions: The major challenges, in this case, were exposure, identification and restoration of the hip centre of rotation and addressing the superolateral acetabular bone loss. Exposure was achieved by releasing both the gluteus maximus and rectus femoris muscles as well as performing a circumferential capsular release. These steps which allowed the femur to translate anteriorly to expose both the pseudoacetabulum and native acetabulum properly. Robotic registration was then used to locate and prepare the acetabulum at the desired centre of rotation. The superolateral bone loss was address by placing a femoral head autograft.

Unanticipated problems and solution: None.

5.24.10 Postoperative Radiographs (Figs. 5.84 and 5.85)

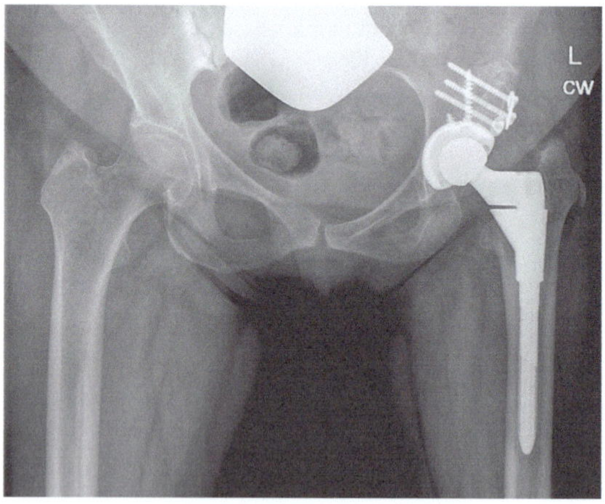

Fig. 5.84 Anteroposterior view of the pelvis showing the placement of the acetabular component at the level of the native acetabulum. The pseudoacetabulum has been supported with structural femoral autograft bone. Leg length discrepancy is significantly improved compared to the preoperative film. The femoral offset is similar to the contralateral side

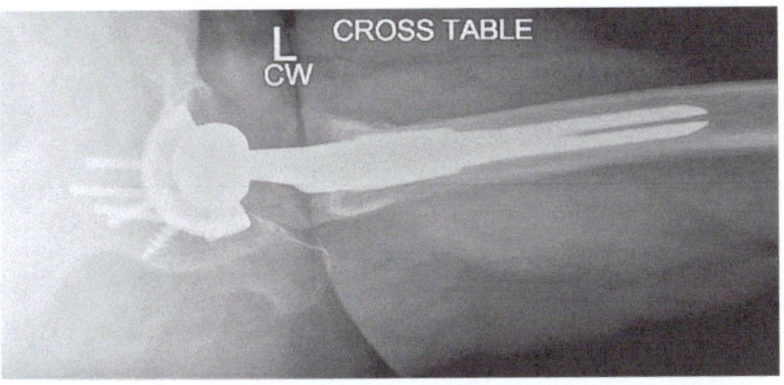

Fig. 5.85 Cross-table lateral view of the hip showing anteversion of the acetabular component, anteversion of the femoral prosthesis and both appropriate sizing and trajectory of the femoral prosthesis

5.24.11 Postoperative Management

Chemoprophylaxis and anticoagulant treatment period: The wound was closed in layers, and two subfascial drains were placed. These were removed on the second postoperative day. The patient was placed on aspirin for thromboprophylaxis.

Gait/limb loading until full loading: The patient was permitted to partially weight bear for six weeks and then progress to weight bearing as tolerated.

5.24.12 Follow-Up and Complications

No complications to date. We have 3-year follow-up with radiographs. She is currently able to ambulate an unlimited amount without an assistive device. She frequently walks 3–4 miles per day. She perceives her LLD as 0 and reports 0/10 pain.

5.24.13 Discussion

Advantages of the applied method:

1. Templating using robotic technology allows surgeons to scrutinize the preoperative CT scan carefully, anticipate intraoperative complexities and carefully plan their reconstruction strategy.
2. The haptic-guided arm greatly simplifies the reaming process and ensures that a hemispheric cavity is created in the direction and depth desired by the surgeon. The surgeon can reliably ream the acetabulum and place the acetabular component in the identical position to where they planned preoperatively.
3. The combined anteversion of both the acetabular and femoral components can be measured. This measurement is pertinent in this case due to the distorted anatomical relationships associated with hip dysplasia.
4. The femoral measurements permit reliable intraoperative assessment of leg length and offset, which were both critical variables in this case. Moreover, they may facilitate the preoperative or intraoperative decision for subtrochanteric femoral osteotomy for leg length equalization.
5. Intraoperative X-ray is not required to confirm optimal implant positioning and restoration of offset, centre of rotation and LLD.

Disadvantages of the method:

1. The preoperative CT scan exposes the patient to radiation.
2. While intraoperative time is reduced, the surgeon must dedicate time preoperatively to plan and three-dimensionally template the case.
3. Robotic systems are expensive up-front investments.
4. The Mako system can only be currently utilized with Mako and Stryker acetabular components.

Alternative evidence-based techniques for the case:

1. Reconstruction without the use of robot navigation is certainly possible. A caveat is that an intraoperative radiograph may be needed to confirm acetabular positioning.
2. Use of an 'ultraporous' acetabular component such as trabecular metal.
3. Alternatively restoring the superolateral acetabular bone defect with an 'ultraporous' metal augment such as trabecular metal.

4. Utilizing the 'cotyloplasty' technique [50] of performing a controlled perforation of the medial wall in the region of the cotyloid fossa to improve lateral coverage and avoid the need for a superolateral bone graft.

Why is the chosen technique better for this case?

1. Utilizing robot navigation simplified both femoral and acetabular preparation, permitted easy and reliable validation of acetabular positioning, and provided a reliable measurement of the restoration of both femoral offset and leg length discrepancy.
2. 'Ultraporous' acetabular components are appealing when reconstructing dysplastic hips due to usually small acetabular size and potential limits in implant-bone contact. Trabecular metal acetabular components have been utilized with success in the reconstruction of dysplastic hips, with long-term results demonstrating excellent survival and radiographic evidence of osseointegration [48]. Other implant manufacturers also offer 'ultraporous' acetabular components, although few have any medium to long-term follow-up.
3. The use of femoral head autografting to improve acetabular coverage in hip dysplasia has been extensively studied, with multiple publications demonstrating exceptional rates of the radiographic union in the presence of both cemented and cementless acetabular reconstruction [115–118]. Despite these positive results, the technique is still considered technically demanding and recent reviews have emphasized that achieving sufficient fixation of the graft with large fragment screws is critical [115]. Ultraporous metal augments have been well received in revision arthroplasty surgery for addressing acetabular wall and column defects and only short term results are available in the setting or primary reconstruction for hip dysplasia [119]. While these results are promising, the need for long-term follow-up and associated costs with using augments preclude them from being the preferred choice.
4. The 'cotyloplasty' technique [50] has been associated with excellent results and healing of the medial wall following controlled perforation [5, 41, 51]. The medial wall defect can then be filled with morcelized graft with or without the use of a wire mesh to control graft distribution. In the current case, this technique was not performed because (a) femoral head autografting is an excellent alternative that restores acetabular bone stock, and (b) restoring the patient's high femoral offset would have been more difficult (or perhaps not possible) by further medializing the hip centre of rotation. Further medialization of the hip centre of rotation combined with the concomitant inability to increase the femoral offset may increase the likelihood of trochanteric-pelvic and ischiofemoral impingement. It should also be stated that the 'cotyloplasty' is technically demanding, with concerns being raised of inducing a protrusion deformity or eventual component dissociation from the pelvis.

Indications and contraindications for your technique: We consider the use of robotic navigation for any complex primary hip arthroplasty where standard methods of acetabular positioning, restoration of offset, the centre of rotation, and leg length may not be reliably achieved using conventional techniques.

Learning curve and how to manage complications: As with any new technique, every step of robotic hip surgery does have a learning curve [120, 121]. The procedure can be broken down into several key steps: (1) preoperative templating in three dimensions, (2) intraoperative OR set-up, (3) array placement, (4) bone registration, (5) bone preparation and (6) intraoperative decision making with information provided by the robotic software. While all of above steps are manageable, they may initially appear foreign to surgeons who typically use traditional techniques. Domb [122] has published on the learning curve and surgical times when adopting robotic hip replacement. They reported decreased operative time and improved acetabular component position throughout their first 35 cases. To date, we have encountered two potential complications using robotic navigation. One potential complication is for software failure such that the intraoperative plan is not available or cannot be loaded. Although this is extremely rare, we templated using calibrated radiographs as a backup. The second potential complication involves a movement of the iliac screws needed to place the acetabular array. If the screws are too shallow or are accidentally manipulated during surgery, then the reference for position can be deleteriously affected, causing the surgeon to place the component in an inappropriate position if they follow the software only. Therefore, we take care to (1) achieve good fixation when placing the iliac screws, (2) make sure not to touch the array after it is calibrated, (3) use anatomic landmarks in addition to the computer software when preparing to ream and when placing the final implant.

Level of evidence concerning the superiority of this method against others: Early clinical and cadaveric data indicate that haptic-guided robotic systems can provide highly accurate and reliable acetabular cup positing. Pre- and postoperative comparative studies have shown that in the clinical setting, such robotic systems can produce postoperative implant positions that are identical to preoperative templating 80% of the time, with the remaining 20% being off-target by a maximum of 2 degrees [121]. While the optimal acetabular position to confirm hip stability remains a contentious topic, when aiming for contemporary, safe zones, robotic systems have been shown to provide more reliable results than conventional techniques [122]. With regard to reconstruction in the setting of hip dysplasia, no robot-specific published studies exist. Zhang and colleagues [123] examined 22 Crowe I patients who underwent computer-assisted (non-robotic) acetabular navigation. Within the 11 patients who underwent computer navigation, acetabular component measurements were significantly closer to their target abduction and anteversion compared to cups placed conventionally. The group also stated comment that navigation simplified the operating procedure and reduced the workload on the surgical team.

In conclusion, we report positive short terms results in this specific case of robot-assisted navigation for the reconstruction of Crowe III acetabular dysplasia. Our experience with this technology is concordant with the current literature in that it has provided reliable outcomes in achieving targeted implant positions and restoration of preoperative discrepancies in femoral offset and leg length discrepancies. We recognize that long-term studies are needed to determine if robotic THA leads to improved clinical outcomes and specifically if it decreases the incidence of complications. This latter requirement will be critical in justifying the increased costs associated with this exciting technology.

5.25 Case Title: Congenital Hip Disease: Hartofilakidis Type A

George Hartofilakidis and
Kalliopi Lampropoulou-Adamidou

5.25.1 Demographics

Age: Born in 1950 (51 years old at the index operation).
Sex: Female.
BMI: 23.5.

5.25.2 Relevant Past Medical History

Principal pathologies: Dysplasia of the left hip.
Previous surgical procedures: None.
Medication: None.
History of presenting complaint: Hip pain and limping was started around the age of 40.

5.25.3 Clinical Examination

Symptoms: Pain and limping.
Range of motion: Restricted painful motion up to 80° of flexion, 5° of abduction, 10° of adduction and rotational movements.

Main disability: Walking and daily activities.
Scoring if available: Pain: 2, Motion: 3, Walking: 3 (according to the Merle d'Aubigne and Postel scoring system as modified by Charnley).
Neurovascular evaluation: Intact.

5.25.4 Preoperative Radiological Assessment/Imaging (Figs. 5.86, 5.87 and 5.88)

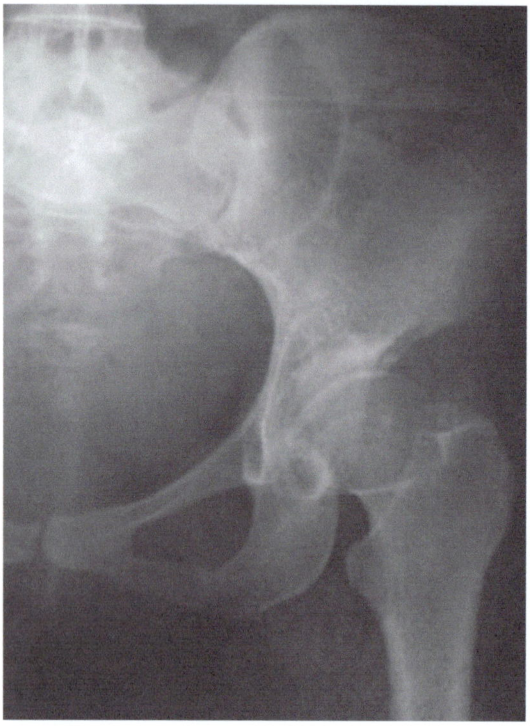

Fig. 5.86 Anteroposterior radiograph of the left hip at the age of 30, when dysplasia of the hip was diagnosed

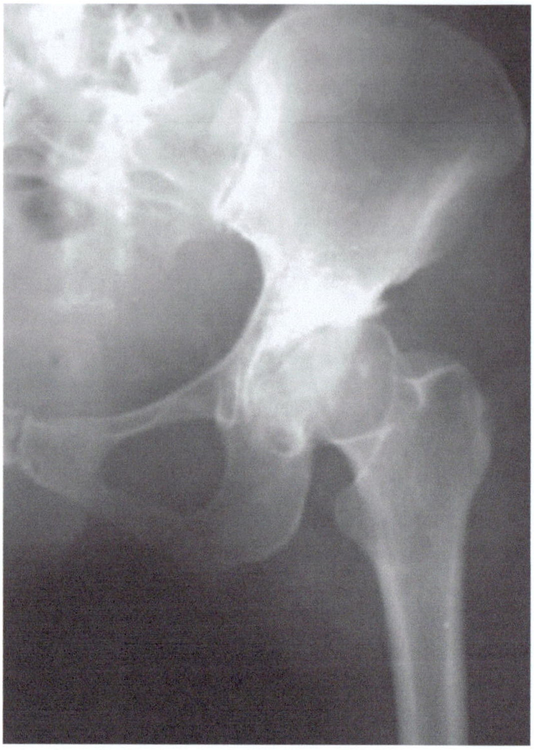

Fig. 5.87 Anteroposterior radiograph of the left hip at the age of 38. The patient remains without symptoms and has normal activity level

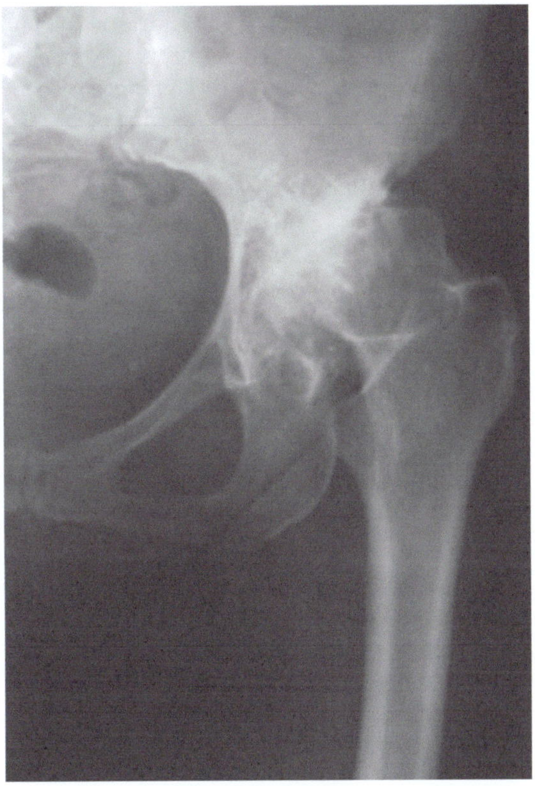

Fig. 5.88 Anteroposterior radiograph of the left hip at the age of 51, when total hip replacement was decided

5.25.4.1 Preoperative Planning (Figs. 5.86, 5.87 and 5.88)

Diagnosis: Dysplastic left hip.

Possible treatment options: Joint reconstruction.

Chosen treatment method: Joint reconstruction/ Total hip replacement.

Selection of implants if applicable and rational: Charnley low friction arthroplasty (LFA).

Templating: No.

5.25.5 Surgical Note

Patient's position: Supine.

Type of anaesthesia: General anaesthesia.

Surgical approach: Lateral transtrochanteric approach.

Main steps: Wide exposure with greater trochanter osteotomy, reconstruction of the acetabulum, reconstruction of the femur and osteosynthesis of greater trochanter with wires (Figs. 5.89 and 5.90).

5.25.5.1 Intraoperative Challenges

Challenges and solutions: Restoration of the normal centre of rotation.

5.25.6 Postoperative Radiographs (Figs. 5.89 and 5.90)

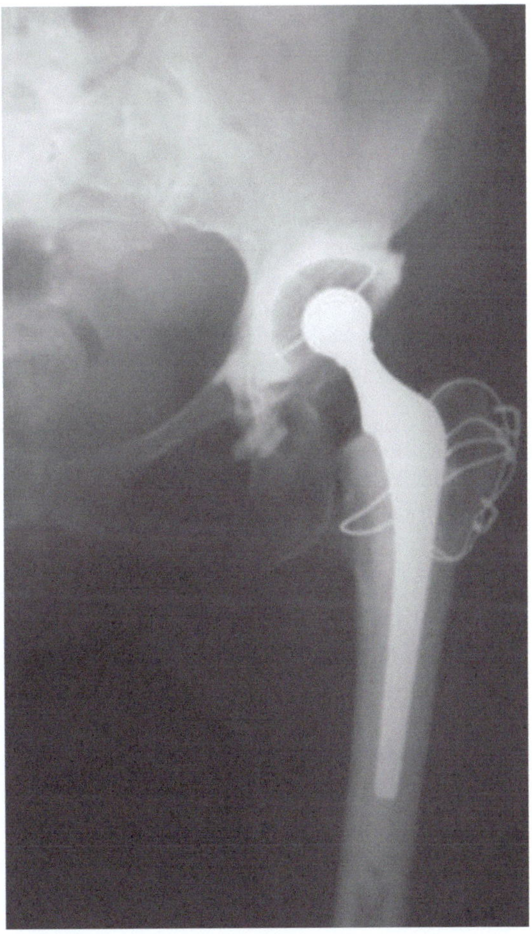

Fig. 5.89 Postoperative anteroposterior radiograph of the left hip

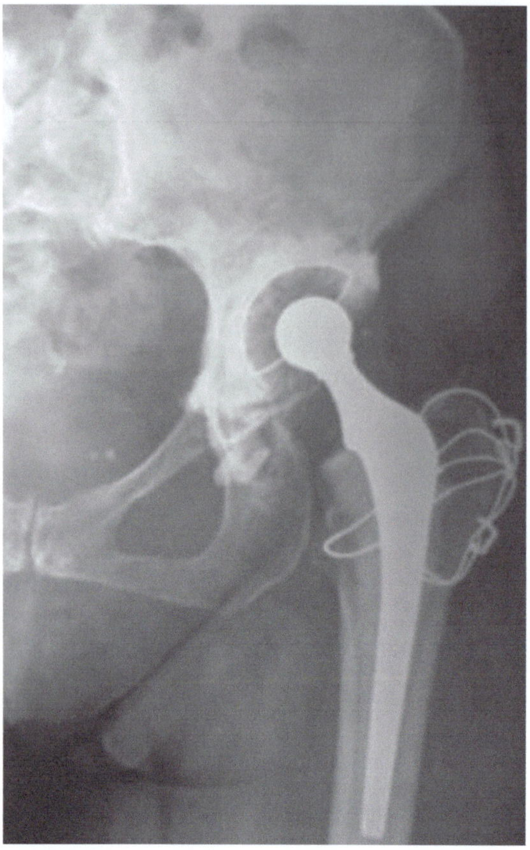

Fig. 5.90 Anteroposterior radiograph of the left 15 years postoperatively. Protheses are well fixed and there is no polyethylene wear. Greater trochanter is healed to its original bed. The patient is fully active and satisfied with the operation

5.25.6.1 Postoperative Management

Chemoprophylaxis and anticoagulant treatment period: Intraoperative cephalosporin administration and continuation for 2 days. Intravenous intraoperative heparin followed by postoperative administration of aspirin for 1 month.
Gait/limb loading until full loading: Bed rest for 2 weeks, progressive advancement of partial weight bearing to full weight bearing within the next 6 weeks.

5.25.7 Follow-up and Complications

There were no postoperative complications.

Scoring if available: Pain: 6, Motion: 4, Walking: 6 (according to the Merle d' Aubigne and Postel scoring system as modified by Charnley).

5.25.8 Discussion [124–128]

Advantages of the applied method: Joint replacement leading to pain relief and improvement of function and quality of life.
Disadvantages of the method: THR complications.
Indications and contraindications for your technique: Indications for joint replacement are the patient's pain, functional impairment with severe limping and psychological status. Contraindications are the poor surgeon's experience or absence of patient's consent to the possible complications and postoperative adaptations of daily life.

5.26 Case Title: Congenital Hip Disease: Hartofilakidis Type B

George Hartofilakidis and
Kalliopi Lampropoulou-Adamidou

5.26.1 Demographics

Age: Born in 1955 (38 years old at the index operation).
Sex: Female.
BMI: 27.

5.26.2 Relevant Past Medical History

Principal pathologies: Low dislocation of the left hip.
Previous surgical procedures: Subtrochanteric osteotomy of the subluxed left hip at the age of 12.
Medication: None.
Other: No.
History of presenting complaint: She was treated with closed reduction and immobilization in hip

spica for subluxation of the left hip at the age of 2, followed by a subtrochanteric osteotomy at the age of 12. Since then she had severe limping while pain started later around the age of 30.

5.26.3 Clinical Examination

Symptoms: Hip pain and severe limping.
Range of motion: Painful motion up to 100° of flexion, 20° of abduction, 20° of adduction, 20° of external rotation and 5° of internal rotation.
Specific tests: Positive Trendelenburg test.
Main disability: Walking and severe limping.
Scoring if available: Pain: 4, Motion: 5, Walking: 3 (according to the Merle d'Aubigne and Postel scoring system as modified by Charnley).
Neurovascular evaluation: Intact.

5.26.4 Preoperative Radiological Assessment/Imaging (Figs. 5.91, 5.92 and 5.93)

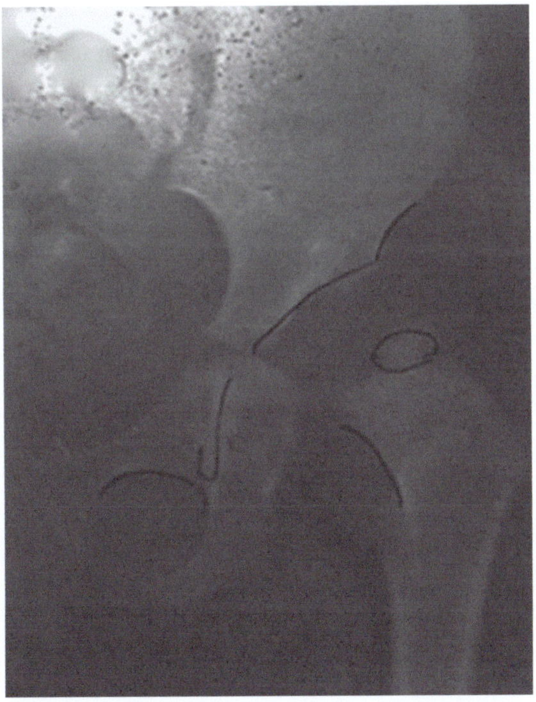

Fig. 5.91 Anteroposterior radiograph of the left hip with subluxation at the age of two

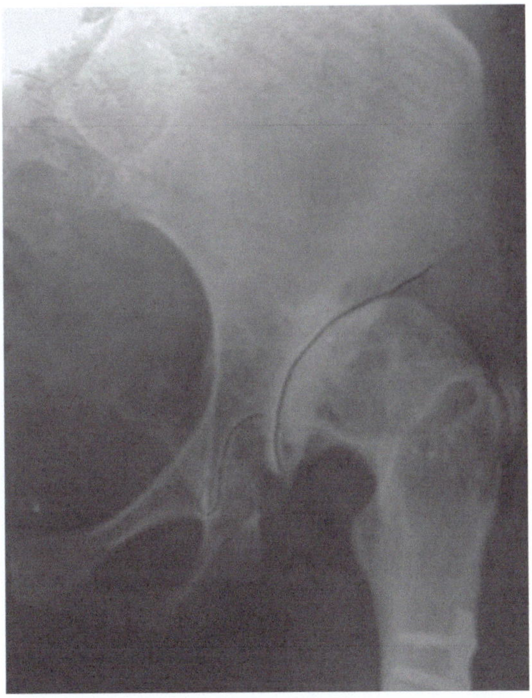

Fig. 5.92 Preoperative anteroposterior radiograph of the left hip at the age of 38

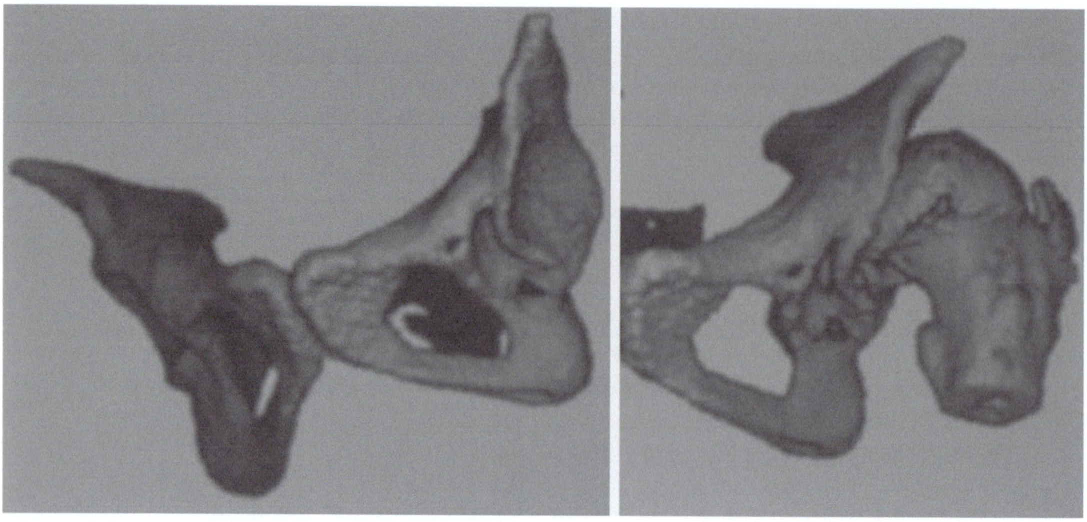

Fig. 5.93 Preoperative 3D-CT scan of the left hip

5.26.4.1 Preoperative Planning (Figs. 5.92 and 5.93)

Diagnosis: Low dislocation of the left hip.
Possible treatment options: Joint reconstruction.
Chosen treatment method: Joint reconstruction/ Total hip replacement.
Selection of implants if applicable and rational: Hybrid total hip arthroplasty.
Expected difficulties: Restoration of the normal centre of rotation and proper placement of the acetabular and femoral component.
Strategies to overcome difficulties: Wide exposure and identification and excision of the osteophyte that covers the superior rim of the true acetabulum.
Templating: No.

5.26.5 Surgical Note

Patient's position: Supine.
Type of anaesthesia: General anaesthesia.
Surgical approach: Lateral transtrochanteric approach.
Main steps: Wide exposure with greater trochanter osteotomy, reconstruction of the acetabulum at the level of the true acetabulum, reconstruction of the femur and osteosynthesis of greater trochanter with wires (Figs. 5.94 and 5.95).

5.26.6 Intra Operative Challenges

Challenges and solutions: Restoration of the normal centre of rotation.

5.26.7 Post-Operative Radiographs (Figs. 5.94 and 5.95)

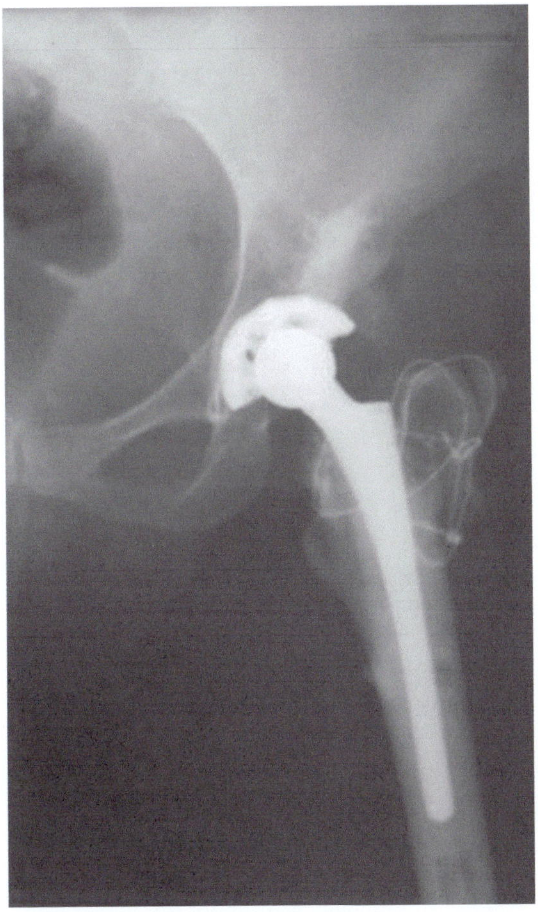

Fig. 5.94 Postoperative anteroposterior radiograph of the left hip

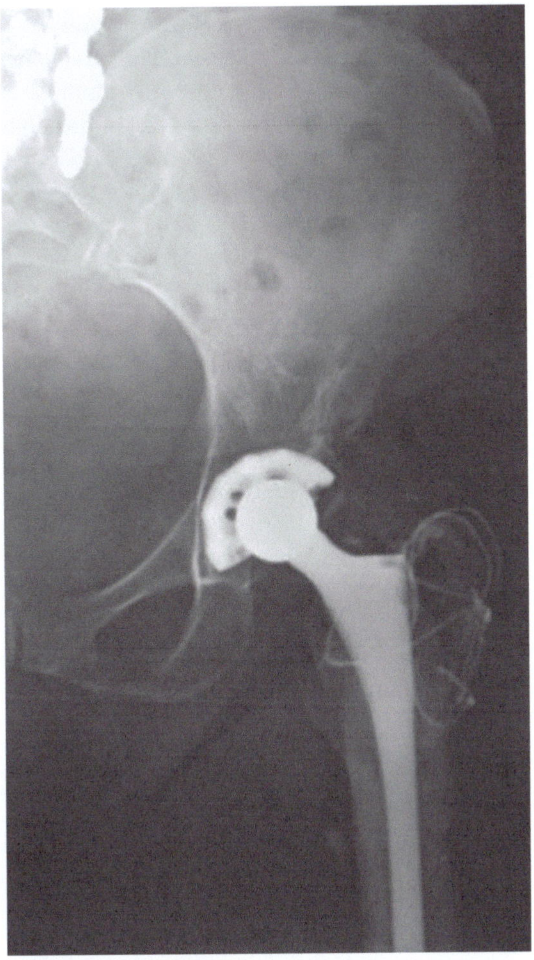

Fig. 5.95 Anteroposterior radiograph of the left hip 23 years postoperatively. Prostheses are well-fixed and there is no polyethylene wear. Greater trochanter is healed to its original bed. The patient is fully active and satisfied with the operation

5.26.7.1 Postoperative Management

Chemoprophylaxis and anticoagulant treatment period: Intraoperative cephalosporin administration and continuation for 2 days. Intravenous intraoperative heparin followed by postoperative administration of aspirin for 1 month.
Gait/limb loading until full loading: Bed rest for 2 weeks, progressive advancement of partial weight bearing to full weight bearing within the next 6 weeks.

5.26.8 Follow Up and Complications

There were no postoperative complications.
Scoring if available: Pain: 6, Motion: 5, Walking: 6 (according to the Merle d' Aubigne and Postel scoring system as modified by Charnley).

5.26.9 Discussion [124, 125, 127, 128, 129]

Advantages of the applied method: Joint replacement leading to pain relief and improvement of function and quality of life.
Disadvantages of the method: THR complications.
Indications and contraindications for your technique: Indications for joint reconstruction are the patient's pain, functional impairment with severe limping and psychological status. Contraindications are the poor surgeon's experience or absence of patient's consent to the possible complications and postoperative adaptations of daily life.

5.27 Case Title: Congenital Hip Disease: Hartofilakidis Type C

George Hartofilakidis and
Kalliopi Lampropoulou-Adamidou

5.27.1 Demographics

Age: Born in 1951 (42 years old at the index operation).
Sex: Female.
BMI: 22.

5.27.2 Relevant Past Medical History

Principal pathologies: High dislocation of the right hip.
Previous surgical procedures: None.
Medication: None.
Other: No.
History of presenting complaint: She had severe limping since infancy and pain started around the age of 35.

5.27.3 Clinical Examination

Symptoms: Pain and severe limping.
Range of motion: Fifteen degrees of flexion contracture, 15–110° of flexion, 10° of abduction, 10° of adduction, 10° of external rotation and 20° of internal rotation.
Specific tests: Positive Trendelenburg test.
Main disability: Walking and severe limping.

Scoring if available: Pain: 2, Motion: 4, Walking: 3 (according to the Merle d'Aubigne and Postel scoring system as modified by Charnley).
Neurovascular evaluation: Intact.

5.27.4 Preoperative Radiological Assessment/Imaging
(Figs. 5.96 and 5.97)

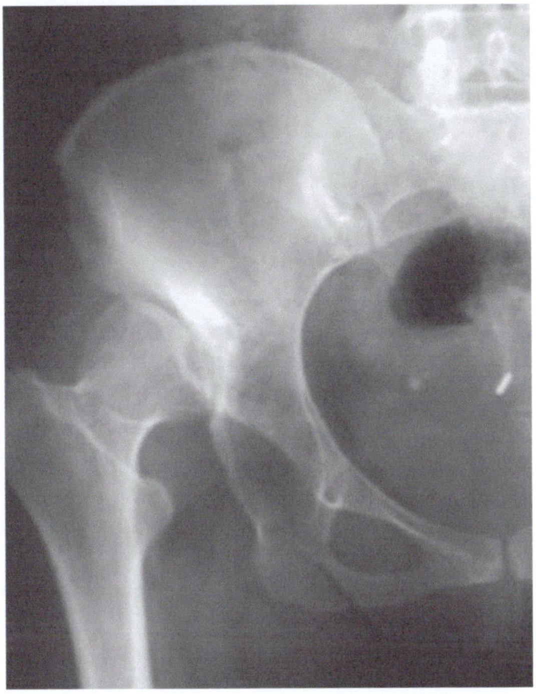

Fig. 5.96 Preoperative anteroposterior radiograph of the right hip at the age of 42

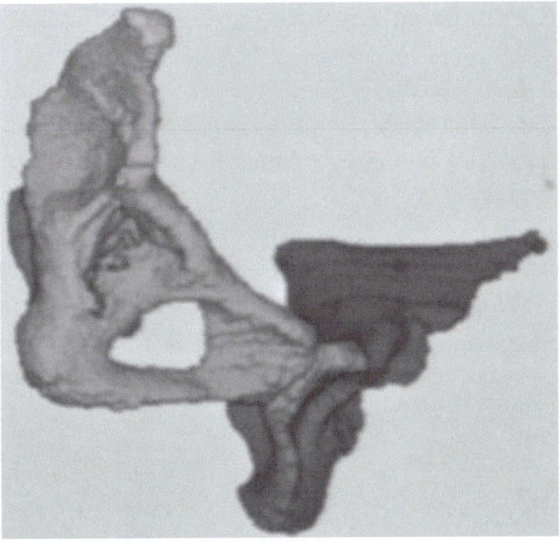

Fig. 5.97 Preoperative 3D-CT scan of the right hip

5.27.4.1 Preoperative Planning

Diagnosis: High dislocation of the right hip (Figs. 5.96 and 5.97).
Possible treatment options: Joint reconstruction.
Chosen treatment method: Joint reconstruction/ Total hip replacement.
Selection of implants if applicable and rational: Hybrid total hip arthroplasty.
Expected difficulties: Restoration of the normal centre of rotation, proper placement of the acetabular and femoral component and reduction of the hip.
Strategies to overcome difficulties: Wide exposure, identification of the true acetabulum and shortening of the femur.
Templating: No.

5.27.5 Surgical Note

Patient's position: Supine.
Type of anaesthesia: General anaesthesia.
Surgical approach: Lateral transtrochanteric approach.
Main steps: Wide exposure with greater trochanter osteotomy, reconstruction of the acetabulum at the level of the true acetabulum, reconstruction of the femur and shortening at the level of the femoral neck and osteosynthesis of greater trochanter with wires (Figs. 5.98 and 5.99).

5.27.6 Intraoperative Challenges

Challenges and solutions: Restoration of the normal centre of rotation.

5.27.7 Postoperative Radiographs (Figs. 5.98 and 5.99)

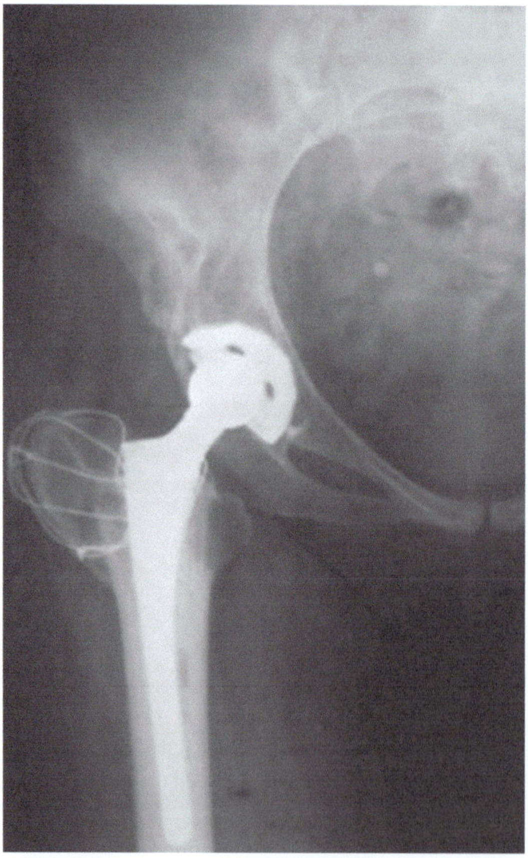

Fig. 5.98 Postoperative anteroposterior radiograph of the right hip after hybrid total hip arthroplasty

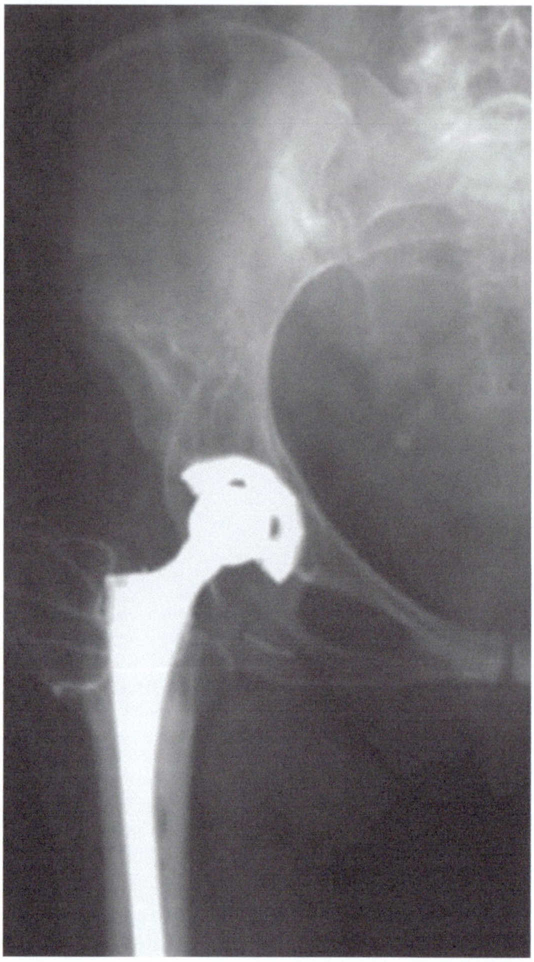

Fig. 5.99 Anteroposterior radiograph of the right hip 20 years postoperatively. Prostheses are well fixed and polyethylene wear is 2 mm. Greater trochanter are healed to its original bed. The patient is fully active and has a mild limping

5.27.7.1 Postoperative Management

Chemoprophylaxis and anticoagulant treatment period: Intraoperative cephalosporin administration and continuation for 2 days. Intravenous intraoperative heparin followed by postoperative administration of aspirin for 1 month.
Gait/limb loading until full loading: Bed rest for 2 weeks, progressive advancement of partial weight bearing to full weight bearing within the next 6 weeks.

5.27.8 Follow Up and Complications

There were no postoperative complications.
Scoring if available: Pain: 6, Motion: 5, Walking: 6 (according to the Merle d' Aubigne and Postel scoring system as modified by Charnley).

5.27.9 Discussion [18, 85, 125, 128, 130]

Advantages of the applied method: Joint replacement leading to pain relief and improvement of function and quality of life.
Disadvantages of the method: THR complications.
Indications and contraindications for your technique: Indications for joint reconstruction are the patient's pain, functional impairment with severe limping and psychological status. Contraindications are the poor surgeon's experience or absence of patient's consent to the possible complications and postoperative adaptations of daily life.

References

1. Gustke K. Hip pathologies that bedevil the dysplastic hip not for the shallow surgeon. Bone Joint J. 2013;95-B(Suppl A):31–6.
2. Kumar JN, Kumar JS, Wang VT, Das De S. Medium-term outcome of total hip replacement for dysplastic hips in Singapore. J Orthop Surg (Hong Kong). 2010;18:296–302.
3. Bicanic G, Barbaric K, Bohacek I, Aljinovic A, Delimar D. Current concept in dysplastic hip arthroplasty: techniques for acetabular and femoral reconstruction. World J Orthop. 2014;5(4):412–24.
4. Sakellariou VI, Christodoulou M, Sasalos G, Babis GC. Reconstruction of the acetabulum in developmental dysplasia of the hip in total hip replacement. Arch Bone Jt Surg. 2014;2(3):130–6.
5. Hartofilakidis G, Stamos K, Karachalios T, Ioannidis TT, Zacharakis N. Congenital hip disease in adults. Classification of acetabular deficiencies and operative treatmentwith acetabuloplasty combined with total hip arthroplasty. J Bone Joint Surg Am. 1996;78(5):683–92.
6. Argenson JN, Flecher X, Parratte S, Aubaniac JM. Anatomy of the dysplastic hip and consequences for total hip arthroplasty. Clin Orthop Relat Res. 2007;465:40–5.
7. Steppacher SD, Tannast M, Werlen S, Siebenrock KA. Femoral morphology differs between deficient and excessive acetabular coverage. Clin Orthop Relat Res. 2008;466:782–90.
8. Li PL, Ganz R. Morphologic features of congenital acetabular dysplasia: one in six is retroverted. Clin Orthop Relat Res. 2003;416:245–53.
9. Mast JW, Brunner RL, Zebrack J. Recognizing acetabular version in the radiographic presentation of hip dysplasia. Clin Orthop Relat Res. 2004;418:48–53.
10. Yasgur DJ, Stuchin SA, Adler EM, DiCesare PE. Subtrochanteric femoral shortening osteotomy in total hip arthroplasty for high-riding developmental dislocation of the hip. J Arthroplast. 1997;12:880–8.
11. Noble PC, Kamaric E, Sugano N, Matsubara M, Harada Y, Ohzono K, Paravic V. Three-dimensional shape of the dysplastic femur: implications for THR. Clin Orthop Relat Res. 2003;417:27–40.
12. Robertson DD, Essinger JR, Imura S, Kuroki Y, Sakamaki T, Shimizu T, Tanaka S. Femoral deformity in adults with developmental hip dysplasia. Clin Orthop Relat Res. 1996;327:196–206.
13. Iwase T, Hasegawa Y, Kawamoto K, Iwasada S, Yamada K, Iwata H. Twenty years' followup of intertrochanteric osteotomy for treatment of the dysplastic hip. Clin Orthop Relat Res. 1996;331:245–55.
14. Hartofilakidis G, Karachalios T. Total hip arthroplasty for congenital hip disease. J Bone Joint Surg Am. 2004;86(2):242–50.
15. Crowe JF, Mani VJ, Ranawat CS. Total hip replacement in congenital dislocation and dysplasia of the hip. J Bone Joint Surg Am. 1979;61:15–23.
16. Yiannakopoulos CK, Chougle A, Eskelinen A, Hodgkinson JP, Hartofilakidis G. Inter- and intraobserver variability of the Crowe and Hartofilakidis classification systems for congenital hip disease in adults. J Bone Joint Surg Br. 2008;90(5):579–83.
17. Yiannakopoulos CK, Xenakis T, Karachalios T, Babis GC, Hartofilakidis G. Reliability and validity of the Hartofilakidis classification system of congenital hip disease in adults. Int Orthop. 2009;33(2):353–8. Epub 2007 Nov 6
18. Hartofilakidis G, Babis GC, Lampropoulou-Adamidou K, Vlamis J. Results of Total hip Arthroplasty differ in subtypes of high dislocation. Clin Orthop Relat Res. 2013;471(9):2972–9.
19. Rogers BA, Garbedian S, Kuchinad RA, Backstein D, Safir O, Gross AE. Current concepts review total hip arthroplasty for adult hip dysplasia. J Bone Joint Surg Am. 2012;94:1809–21.
20. Bernasek TA, Haidukewych GJ, Gustke KA, Hill O, Levering M. Total hip arthroplasty requiring subtrochanteric osteotomy for developmental hip dysplasia: 5 to 14 year results. J Arthroplast. 2007;22(Suppl):145–50.
21. Boisgard S, Descampsa S, Bouillet B. Complex primary total hip arthroplasty. Orthopaed Traumatol. 2013;99S:S34–42.
22. Garvin KL, Bowen MK, Salvati EA, Ranawat CS. Longterm results of total hip arthroplasty in congenital dislocation and dysplasia of the hip. A follow-up note. J Bone Joint Surg Am. 1991;73(9):1348–54.

23. Shen B, Yang J, Wang L, Zhou ZK, Kang PD, Pei FX. Midterm results of hybrid total hip arthroplasty for treatment of osteoarthritis secondary to developmental dysplasia of the hip-Chinese experience. J Arthroplast. 2009;24:1157–63.
24. Lakstein D, Backstein D, Safir O, Kosashvili Y, Gross AE. Trabecular metal cup for acetabular defects with 50% or less host bone contact. Clin Orthop Relat Res. 2009;467(9):2318–24. Epub 2009 Mar 10
25. Georgiades G, Babis GC, Kourlaba G, Hartofilakidis G. Effect of Cementlessacetabular component orientation, position, and containment in total hip arthroplasty for congenital hip disease. J Arthroplast. 2010;25(7):1143–50.
26. Doehring TC, Rubash HE, Shelley FJ, Schwendeman LJ, Donaldson TK, Navalgund YA. Effect of superior and superolateral relocations of the hip center on hip joint forces. An experimental and analytical analysis. J Arthroplast. 1996;11(6):693–703.
27. Tanzer M. Role and results of the high hip center. Orthop Clin North Am. 1998;29(2):241–7.
28. Russotti GM, Harris WH. Proximal placement of the acetabular component in total hip arthroplasty. A long-term follow-up study. J Bone Joint Surg Am. 1991;73(4):587–92.
29. Kaneuji A, Sugimori T, Ichiseki T, Yamada K, Fukui K, Matsumoto T. Minimum Ten-year results of a porous acetabular component for Crowe I to III hip dysplasia using an elevated hip center. J Arthroplast. 2009;24:187–94.
30. Bicanic G, Delimar D, Delimar M, Pecina M. Influence of the acetabular cup position on hip load during arthroplasty in hip dysplasia. Int Orthop. 2009;33:397–402.
31. Cameron HU, Botsford DJ, Park YS. Influence of the Crowe rating on the outcome of total hip arthroplasty in congenital hip dysplasia. J Arthroplast. 1996;11(5):582–7.
32. Yoder SA, Brand RA, Pedersen DR, O'Gorman TW. Total hip acetabular component position affects component loosening rates. Clin Orthop Relat Res. 1988;228:79–87.
33. Hartofilakidis G, Stamos K, Karachalios T. Treatment of high dislocation of the hip in adults with total hip arthroplasty. Operative technique and long-term clinical results. J Bone Joint Surg Am. 1998;80:510–7.
34. Pagnano MW, Hanssen AD, Lewallen DG, Shaughnessy WJ. The effect of superior placement of the acetabular component on the rate of loosening after total hip arthroplasty. J Bone Joint Surg Am. 1996;78-A:1004–14.
35. Delimar D, Bićanić G, Pećina M, Korzinek K. Acetabular roof reconstruction with pedicled iliac graft: early clinical experience. Int Orthop. 2004;28:319–20.
36. Li H, Wang L, Dai K, Zhu Z. Autogenous impaction grafting in total hip arthroplasty with developmental dysplasia of the hip. J Arthroplast. 2013;28:637–43.
37. Morsi E, Garbuz D, Gross AE. Total hip arthroplasty with shelf grafts using uncemented cups. A long-term follow-up study. J Arthroplast. 1996;11(1):81–5.
38. Nousiainen MT, Maury AC, Alhoulei A, Backstein DJ, Gross AE. Long-term outcome of shelf grafts in total hip arthroplasty for developmental hip dysplasia. Orthopedics. 2009;32(9)
39. McQueary FG, Johnston RC. Coxarthrosis after congenital dysplasia. Treatment by total hip arthroplasty without acetabular bone-grafting. J Bone Joint Surg Am. 1988;70(8):1140–4.
40. Kobayashi S, Saito N, Nawata M, Horiuchi H, Iorio R, Takaoka K. Total hip arthroplasty with bulk femoral head autograft for acetabular reconstruction in developmental dysplasia of the hip. J Bone Joint Surg Am. 2003;85:615–21.
41. Inao S, Matsuno T. Cemented total hip arthroplasty with autogenousacetabular bone grafting for hips with developmental dysplasia in adults: the results at a minimum of ten years. J Bone Joint Surg Br. 2000;82:375–7.
42. Kim M, Kadowaki T. High long-term survival of bulk femoral head autograft for acetabular reconstruction in Cementless THA for developmental hip dysplasia. Clin Orthop Relat Res. 2010;468:1611–20.
43. Delimar D, Bohacek I, Pecina M, Bicanic G. Acetabular roof reconstruction with pedicled iliac graft: ten years later. Int Orthop. 2014;38:199–201.
44. Shinar AA, Harris WH. Bulk structural autogenous grafts and allografts for reconstruction of the acetabulum in total hip arthroplasty. Sixteen-year-average follow-up. J Bone Joint Surg Am. 1997;79:159–68.
45. Kwong LM, Jasty M, Harris WH. High failure rate femoral head allografts in total hip acetabula reconstructions at 10 years. J Arthroplast. 1993;8:341–6.
46. Mulroy RD, Harris WH. Failure of acetabularautogenous grafts in total hip arthroplasty. Increasing incidence: a follow- up note. J Bone Joint Surg Am. 1990;72:1536–40.
47. Siegmeth A, Duncan CP, Masri BA, Kim WY, Garbuz DS. Modular tantalum augments for acetabular defects in revision hip arthroplasty. Clin Orthop Relat Res. 2009;467:199–205.
48. Kamada T, Mashima N, Nakashima Y, Imai H, Takeba J, Miura H. Mid-term clinical and radiographic outcomes of porous tantalum modular acetabular components for hip dysplasia. J Arthroplasty. 2015;30(4):607–10.
49. Macheras GA, Kateros K, Koutsostathis SD, Tsakotos G, Galanakos S, Papadakis SA. The trabecular metal Monoblockacetabular component in patients with high congenital hip dislocation: a prospective study. J Bone Joint Surg Br. 2010;92(5):624–8.
50. Dunn HK, Hess WE. Total hip reconstruction in chronically dislocated hips. J Bone Joint Surg Am. 1976;58:838–45.
51. Dorr LD, Tawakkol S, Moorthy M, Long W, Wan Z. Medial protrusio technique for placement of a porous-coated, hemispherical acetabular component without cement in a total hip arthroplasty in patients who have acetabular dysplasia. J Bone Joint Surg Am. 1999;81:83–92.
52. Siebenrock KA, Tannast M, Kim S, Morgenstern W, Ganz R. Acetabular reconstruction using a roof rein-

forcement ring with hook for total hip arthroplasty in developmental dysplasia of the hip-osteoarthritis minimum 10-year followup results. J Arthroplast. 2005;20:492–8.
53. Gill TJ, Siebenrock K, Oberholzer R, Ganz R. Acetabular reconstruction in developmental dysplasia of the hip: results of the acetabular reinforcement ring with hook. J Arthroplast. 1999;14:131–7.
54. Pitto RP, Schikora N. Acetabular reconstruction in developmental hip dysplasia using reinforcement ring with a hook. Int Orthop. 2004;28:202–5.
55. Pignatti G, Stagni C, Fravisini M, Giunti A. Ceramic ceramic coupling. Total hip arthroplasty in young patients. Chir Organi Mov. 2003;88(4):369–75.
56. Numair J, Joshi AB, Murphy JC, Porter ML, Hardinge K. Total hip arthroplasty for congenital dysplasia or dislocation of the hip. Survivorship analysis and long-term results. J Bone Joint Surg Am. 1997;79(9):1352–60.
57. Sochart DH, Porter ML. Long-term results of cemented Charnley low-friction arthroplasty in patients aged less than 30 years. J Arthroplast. 1998;13(2):123–31.
58. Dorr LD, Jones RE, Padgett DE, Pagnano M, Ranawat AS, Trousdale RT. Robotic guidance in total hip arthroplasty: the shape of things to come. Orthopedics. 2011;34(9):652–5.
59. Dorr LD, Malik A, Dastane M, Wan Z. Combined anteversion technique for total hip arthroplasty. Clin Orthop Relat Res. 2009;467(1):119–27.
60. Sener N, Tözün IR, Asxik M. Femoral shortening and cementless arthroplasty in high congenital dislocation of the hip. J Arthroplast. 2002;17(1): 41–8.
61. Reikeraas O, Lereim P, Gabor I, Gunderson R, Bjerkreim I. Femoral shortening in total arthroplasty for completely dislocated hips: 3-7 year results in 25 cases. Acta Orthop Scand. 1996;67(1):33–6.
62. Paavilainen T. Total hip replacement for developmental dysplasia of the hip. Acta Orthop Scand. 1997;68(1):77–84.
63. Charity JA, Tsiridis E, Sheeraz A, Howell JR, Hubble MJ, Timperley AJ, Gie GA. Treatment of Crowe IV high hip dysplasia with total hip replacement using the Exeter stem and shortening derotational subtrochanteric osteotomy. J Bone Joint Surg Br. 2011;93(1):34–8.
64. Park MS, Kim KH, Jeong WC. Transverse subtrochanteric shortening osteotomy in primary total hip arthroplasty for patients with severe hip developmental dysplasia. J Arthroplast. 2007;22(7):1031–106.
65. Becker DA, Gustilo RB. Double-chevron subtrochanteric shortening derotational femoral osteotomy combined with total hip arthroplasty for the treatment of complete congenital dislocation of the hip in the adult. Preliminary report and description of a new surgical technique. J Arthroplast. 1995;10(3):313–8.
66. Cameron HU, Eren OT, Solomon M. Nerve injury in the prosthetic management of the dysplastic hip. Orthopedics. 1998;21(9):980–1.
67. Paavilainen T, Hoikka V, Solonen KA. Cementless total replacement for severely dysplastic or dislocated hips. J Bone Joint Surg Br. 1990;72(2):205–11.
68. Paavilainen T, Hoikka V, Paavolainen P. Cementless total hip arthroplasty for congenitally dislocated or dysplastic hips. Technique for replacement with a straight femoral component. Clin Orthop Relat Res. 1993;297:71–81.
69. Nercessian OA, Newton PM, Joshi RP, Sheikh B, Eftekhar NS. Trochanteric osteotomy and wire fixation: a comparison of 2 techniques. Clin Orthop Relat Res. 1996;333:208–16.
70. Menon PC, Griffiths WE, Hook WE, Higgins B. Trochanteric osteotomy in total hip arthroplasty: comparison of 2 techniques. J Arthroplast. 1998;13:92–6.
71. Thorup B, Mechlenburg I, Søballe K. Total hip replacement in the congenitally dislocated hip using the Paavilainen technique: 19 hips followed for 1.5–10 years. Acta Orthopaedica. 2009;80:259–62.
72. Bao N, Meng J, Zhou L, Guo T, Zeng X, Zhao J. Lesser trochanteric osteotomy in total hip arthroplasty for treating CROWE type IV developmental dysplasia of hip. Int Orthop. 2013;37:385–90.
73. Li X, Sun J, Lin X, Xu S, Tang T. Cementless total hip arthroplasty with a double chevron subtrochanteric shortening osteotomy in patients with Crowe type-IV hip dysplasia. Acta Orthop Belg. 2013;79: 287–92.
74. Masonis JL, Patel JV, Miu A, Bourne RB, McCalden R, Macdonald SJ, Rorabeck CH. Subtrochanteric shortening and derotational osteotomy in primary total hip arthroplasty for patients with severe hip dysplasia: 5-year follow-up. J Arthroplast. 2003;18:68–73.
75. Kawai T, Tanaka C, Ikenaga M, Kanoe H. Cemented total hip arthroplasty with transverse subtrochanteric shortening osteotomy for Crowe group IV dislocated hip. J Arthroplast. 2011;26:229–35.
76. Bruce WJ, Rizkallah SM, Kwon YM, Goldberg JA, Walsh WR. A new technique of subtrochanteric shortening in total hip arthroplasty: surgical technique and results of 9 cases. J Arthroplast. 2000;15:617–26.
77. Makita H, Inaba Y, Hirakawa K, Saito T. Results on total hip arthroplasties with femoral shortening for Crowe's group IV dislocated hips. J Arthroplast. 2007;22:32–8.
78. Neumann D, Thaler C, Dorn U. Femoral shortening and cementless arthroplasty in Crowe type 4 congenital dislocation of the hip. Int Orthop. 2012;36:499–503.
79. Koulouvaris P, Stafylas K, Sculco T, Xenakis T. Distal femoral shortening in total hip arthroplasty for complex primary hip reconstruction. A new surgical technique. J Arthroplast. 2008;23:992–8.
80. Lewallen DG. Neurovascular injury associated with hip arthroplasty. Instr Course Lect. 1998;47:275–83.
81. Eggli S, Hankemayer S, Muller ME. Nerve palsy after leg lengthening in total replacement arthroplasty for developmental dysplasia of the hip. J Bone Joint Surg (Br). 1999;81-B:843–5.

82. Edwards BN, Tullos HS, Noble PC. Contributory factors and etiology of sciatic nerve palsy in total hip arthroplasty. Clin Orthop Relat Res. 1987;218:136–41.
83. Prokopetz JJ, Losina E, Bliss RL, Wright J, Baron JA, Katz JN. Risk factors for revision of primary-total hip arthroplasty: a systematic review. BMC Musculoskelet Disord. 2012;13:251.
84. DiFazio F, Yong Shon W, Salvati EA, Wilson PD Jr. Long-term results of total hip arthroplasty with a cemented custom-designed swan-neck femoral component for congenital dislocation or severe dysplasia: a follow up note. J Bone Joint Surg Am. 2002;84-A:204–7.
85. Hartofilakidis G, Karachalios T, Georgiades G, Kourlaba G. Total hip arthroplasty in patients with high dislocation: a concise follow up, at a minimum of fifteen years, of previous reports. J Bone Joint Surg Am. 2011;93-A:1614–8.
86. Woolson ST, Harris WH. Complex total hip replacement for dysplastic or hypoplastic hips using miniature or microminiature components. J Bone Joint Surg Am. 1983;65-A:1099–108.
87. Dapuzzo MR, Sierra RJ. Acetabular considerations during total hip arthroplasty for hip dysplasia. Orthop Clin N Am. 2012;43:369–75.
88. Atilla B, Ali H, Aksoy MC, Cağlar O, Tokgözoğlu AM, Alpaslan AM. Position of acetabular component determines the fate of femoral head autographs in total hip replacement for acetabular dysplasia. J Bone Joint Surg Br. 2007;89(7):874–8.
89. Karachalios T, Hartofylakidis G. Congenital hip disease in adults: terminology, classification, pre-operative planning and treatment. J Bone Joint Surg Br. 2010;923:914–21.
90. Akiyama H, Kawanabe K, Yamamato K, Kuroda Y, So K, Goto K, Nakamura T. Cemented THA with subtrochanteric femoral shortening transverse osteotomy for severely dislocated hips: outcome with a 3 to 10 year follow-up period. J Orthop Sci. 2011;16(3): 270–7.
91. Togrul E, Ozkan C, Kalaci A, Gülsen M. A new technique of subtrochanteric shortening in total hip replacement for Crowe types III–IV dysplasia of the hip. J Arthroplasty. 2010;25(3):465–70.
92. Holinka J, Pfeiffer M, Hofstaetter JG, Lass R, Kotz RI, Giurea A. Total hip replacement in congenital high hip dislocation following iliofemoral monotube distraction. Int Orthop. 2011;35(5):639–45.
93. Filipenko VA, Tankut VA, Tankut AV, Zhigun AI, Bondarenko SE, Akramov VR. Hip arthroplasty at dysplastic coxarthrosis. "ARS Medica" Traumatol Orthop. 2011;17(53):352–7.
94. Park KS, Yoon TR, Song EK, Seon JK, Lee KB. Total hip arthroplasty in high dislocated and severely dysplastic septic hip sequelae. J Arthroplasty. 2012;27(7):1331–6.
95. Kiliçoğlu OI, Türker M, Akgül T, Yazıcıoğlu O. Cementless total hip arthroplasty with modified oblique femoral shortening osteotomy in Crowe type IV congenital hip dislocation. J Arthroplasty. 2013;28(1):117–25.
96. Traina F, De Fine M, Tassinari E, et al. Modular neck prostheses in DDH patients: 11-year results. J Orthop Sci. 2011;16(1):14–20.
97. Tamegai H, Otani T, Fujii H, et al. A modified S-ROM stem in primary total hip arthroplasty for developmental dysplasia of the hip. J Arthroplasty. 2013;28(10):1741–5.
98. Takao M, Ohzono K, Nishii T, et al. Cementless modular total hip arthroplasty with subtrochanteric shortening osteotomy for hips with developmental dysplasia. J Bone Joint Surg Am. 2011;93(6):548–55.
99. Oonishi H, Ohashi H, Oonishi H Jr, Kim SC. THA with hydroxyapatite granules at cement-bone interface: 15- to 20-year results. Clin Orthop Relat Res. 2008;466(2):373–9.
100. Fujita H, Katayama N, Iwase T, Otsuka H. Multicenter study of use of the Exeter stem in Japan: evaluation of 1000 primary THA. J Orthop Sci. 2012;17:370–6.
101. Fujita H, Okumura T, Hara H, Toda H, Harada H, Nishimura R, Tominaga T. Monitoring of blood pressure during total hip arthroplasty using the interface bioactive bone cement (IBBC) technique. J Orthop Sci. 2015;20(2):347–56.
102. Eskelinen A, Remes V, Ylinen P, Helenius I, Tallroth K, Paavilainen T. Cementless total hip arthroplasty in patients with severely dysplastic hips and a previous Schanz osteotomy of the femur. Acta Orthopedica. 2009;80:263–9.
103. Krych AJ, Howard JL, Trousdale RT, Cabanela ME, Berry DJ. Total hip arthroplasty with shortening subtrochanteric osteotomy in Crowe IV development dysplasia: surgical technique. J Bone Joint Surg. 2010;92:176–87.
104. Mahomed NN, Arndt DC, McGory BJ, Harris WH. The Harris hip score: comparison of patient self-report with surgeon assessment. J Arthroplasty. 2001;16(5):575–80.
105. Ng Vincent Y, Kean JR, Glassman AH. Limb-length discrepancy after hip arthroplasty: current concepts review. J Bone Joint Surg Am. 2013;95-A(15):1426.
106. Meermans G, Malik A, Witt J, Haddad F. Preoperative radiographic assessment of limb-length discrepancy in total hip arthroplasty. Clin Orthop Relat Res. 2011;469:1677–82.
107. Desai AS, Dramis A, Board TN. Leg length discrepancy after total hip arthroplasty: a review of literature. Curr Rev. Musculoskeletal Med. 2013;6:336–41.
108. Abdel MP, Stryker LS, Trousdale RT, et al. Uncemented acetabular components with femoral head autograft for acetabular reconstruction in developmental dysplasia of the hip: a concise follow-up report at a mean of twenty years. J Bone Joint Surg Am. 2014;96(22):1878–82.
109. Tsukada S, Wakui M. Bulk femoral head autograft without decortication in uncemented total hip arthroplasty: seven- to ten-year results. J Arthroplasty. 2012;27(3):437–44.
110. Abolghasemian M, Samiezadeh S, Jafari D, Bougherara H, Gross AE, Ghazavi MT. Dispalcement of the hip center of rotation after arthoplsty of Crowe

III and IV Dysplasia: a radiological and biomechanical study. J Arthoplasty. 2013;28:1031–5.
111. Nawabi DH, Meftah M, Nam D, Ranawat AS, Ranawat CS. Durable fixation achieved with medialized, high hip center cementless THAs for Crowe II and III Dysplasia. Clin Orthop Relat Res. 2014;472:630–6.
112. Hasegawa Y, Iwase T, Kanoh T, Seki T, Matsuoka A. Total hip arthroplasty for Crowe type IV developmental dysplasia. J Arthroplasty. 2012;27(9):1629–35.
113. Krych AJ, Howard JL, Trousdale RT, Cabanela ME, Berry DJ. Total hip arthroplasty with shortening subtrochanteric osteotomy in Crowe type-IV developmental dysplasia. J Bone Joint Surg Am. 2009;91(9):2213–21.
114. Sanchez-Sotelo J, Berry DJ, Trousdale RT, Cabanela ME. Surgical treatment of developmental dysplasia of the hip in adults: II. Arthroplasty options. J Am Acad Orthop Surg. 2002;10(5):334–44.
115. Hendrich C, Mehling I, Sauer U, et al. Cementless acetabular reconstruction and structural bone-grafting in dysplastic hips. J Bone Joint Surg Am. 2006;88:387–94.
116. Rodriguez JA, Huk OL, Pellicci PM, Wilson PD. Autogenous bone grafts from the femoral head for the treatment of acetabular deficiency in primary total hip arthroplasty with cement: long-term results. J Bone Joint Surg Am. 1995;77:1227–33.
117. Lee BP, Cabanela ME, Wallrichs SL, Ilstrup DM. Bone-graft augmentation for acetabular deficiencies in total hip arthroplasty: results of long-term follow-up evaluation. J Arthroplasty. 1997;12:503–10.
118. Spangehl MJ, Berry DJ, Trousdale RT, Cabanela ME. Uncemented acetabular components with bulk femoral head autograft for acetabular reconstruction in developmental dysplasia of the hip: results at five to twelve years. J Bone Joint Surg Am. 2001;83:1484–9.
119. Elganzoury I, Bassiony AA. Early results of trabecular metal augment for acetabular reconstruction in revision hip arthroplasty. Acta Orthop Belg. 2013;79(5):530–5.
120. Redmond JM, Gupta A, Hammarstedt JE, Petrakos AE, Finch NA, Domb BG. The learning curve associated with robotic-assisted total hip arthroplasty. J Arthroplasty. 2015;30(1):50–4.
121. Kanawade V, Dorr LD, Banks SA, Zhang Z, Wan Z. Precision of robotic guided instrumentation for acetabular component positioning. J Arthroplasty. 2015;30(3):392–7.
122. Domb BG, El Bitar YF, Sadik AY, Stake CE, Botser IB. Comparison of robotic-assisted and conventional acetabular cup placement in THA: a matched-pair controlled study. Clin Orthop Relat Res. 2014;72(1):329–36.
123. Zhang YZ, Chen B, Lu S, Yang Y, Zhao JM, Liu R, Li YB, Pei GX. Preliminary application of computer-assisted patient-specific acetabular navigational template for total hip arthroplasty in adult single development dysplasia of the hip. Int J Med Robot. 2011;7(4):469–74.
124. Hartofilakidis GC, Lampropoulou-Adamidou KI, Stathopoulos IP, Vlamis JA. The outcome of 241 Charnley total hip arthroplasties performed by one surgeon 30 to 40 years ago. J Arthroplast. 2015;30(10):1767–71.
125. Hartofilakidis G, Babis GC, Lampropoulou-Adamidou K. Congenital hip disease in adults. Italia: Springer-Verlag; 2014.
126. Roidis NT, Pollalis AP, Hartofilakidis GC. Total hip arthroplasty in young females with congenital dislocation of the hip, radically improves their long-term quality of life. J Arthroplast. 2013;28(7):1206–11.
127. Hartofilakidis G, Babis G, Georgiades G, Kourlada G. Trochanteric osteotomy in total hip replacement for congenital hip disease. J Bone Joint Surg (Br). 2011;93:601–17.
128. Karachalios T, Hartofilakidis G. Congenital hip disease in adults: terminology, classification, pre-operative planning and management. J Bone Joint Surg (Br). 2010;92(7):914–21.
129. Lampropoulou-Adamidou K, Georgiades G, Vlamis J, Hartofilakidis G. Charnley low-friction arthroplasty in patients 35 years of age or younger. Results at a minimum of 23 years. Bone Joint J. 2013;95-B:1052–6.
130. Karachalios T, Roidis N, Lampropoulou-Adamidou K, Hartofilakidis G. Acetabular reconstruction in patients with low and high dislocation: 20- to 32-year survival of an impaction grafting technique (named cotyloplasty). Bone Joint J. 2013;95-B:887–92.

6 Proximal Femoral Dysplasia

Eustathios Kenanidis, Panagiotis Kakoulidis,
Eleftherios Tsiridis, John Dundon,
Jonathan Vigdorchik, Antonia F. Chen,
and Richard H. Rothman

6.1 Current Concepts

E. Kenanidis, P. Kakoulidis, and E. Tsiridis

6.1.1 General

There is no consensus on the definition of the proximal femoral deformity (PFD) and also no validated scoring system for the severity of the disease [1, 2]. An unusual form of the upper part of the femur may be a deformity or an anatomic variation [2]. Berry considered that the need for special implants or techniques differentiates PFD from the typical spectrum of anatomic variability [2].

PFD can be recognized in different types of underlying diseases; these are classified into the following three categories [1, 3, 4]:

(a) Congenital: achondroplasia, dwarfism, and spondyloepiphyseal dysplasia
(b) Developmental: DDH that seems to be the most common reason
(c) Acquired: malunited proximal femoral fractures, prior femoral osteotomies, septic arthritis, metabolic bone diseases as osteoporosis, osteomalacia and rickets, Legg-Perthes-Calve and slipped femoral capitis, Paget disease, etc.

There is no universally accepted classification. Berry [2] proposed a classification that takes into account the anatomic site, the geometry of PFD, and the underlying disease. He supported that the anatomy and geometry of the PFD can affect the implant choice, size and positioning, and the need for osteotomy whether the underlying disease may influence the bone metabolism and the fixation method [2]. The anatomic site of the deformity may be the greater trochanter, the femoral neck, the metaphysis,

E. Kenanidis, M.D., Ph.D., M.Sc. (✉) · P. Kakoulidis, M.D.
Academic Orthopaedic Unit, Aristotle University Medical School, Thessaloniki, Greece

E. Tsiridis, M.D., Ph.D., F.A.C.S., F.R.C.S.
Academic Orthopaedic Unit, Papageorgiou General Hospital, Aristotle University Medical School, Thessaloniki, Greece
e-mail: etsiridis@doctors.org.uk

J. Dundon, M.D.
Orthopaedic Institute of New Jersey, Hackettstown, NJ, USA

J. Vigdorchik, M.D.
NYU Langone Health, NYU Langone Orthopaedic Hospital, New York, NY, USA
e-mail: Jonathan.Vigdorchik@nyumc.org

A.F. Chen, M.D., M.B.A.
Department of Orthopaedics, Harvard Medical School, Boston, MA, USA

Brigham and Women's Hospital, Boston, MA, USA
e-mail: Antonia.Chen@rothmaninstitute.com

R.H. Rothman, M.D., Ph.D.
Rothman Institute, Philadelphia, PA, USA

E. Tsiridis (ed.), *The Adult Hip - Master Case Series and Techniques*,
https://doi.org/10.1007/978-3-319-64177-5_6

or the diaphysis where torsional, angular, translational, and size deformities can be found [2].

The Dorr femoral bone classification assesses the morphology and the bone stock of the proximal femur radiographically [5]. The shape of the proximal femur is categorized based on the intramedullary canal to calcar isthmus ratio. The intramedullary canal isthmus is given by the distal endosteal contact points found 10 cm below the reference line through the mid-lesser trochanter. The intramedullary calcar isthmus is measured by the proximal endosteal contact points located 3 cm below the reference line through the mid-lesser trochanter. According to the Dorr classification, there are three different types of proximal femoral bone, namely:

1. Type A (CC ratio < 0.5): funnel-shaped with narrow canal and thick cortical walls.
2. Type B (CC ratio 0.5 < 0.75): has a moderate cortical wall. It is usually between A and C types.
3. Type C (CC ratio > 0.75): a wide cylindrical shape with seriously thin medial and posterior cortices.

Diseases as juvenile RA, achondroplasia, and spondyloepiphyseal dysplasia may be presented with very narrow proximal femoral canal whether RA, ankylosing spondylitis, or alcohol overuse consumption with too large canal. Dorr types I and II are usually managed with uncemented implants but type III with cemented [6]. Dorr types II and III are at greater risk for intraoperative fracture [6].

6.1.2 Technique Challenges

There are several technical difficulties that a surgeon could face intraoperatively. These usually concern the following:

1. A difficult exposure [2, 3].
2. The retained hardware from previous surgery. Channels, screw holes, bone remodelling, and broken hardware can be found following a former failed internal fixation [1].
3. A persisting infection [1].
4. The altered intraosseous relationship between the prosthesis and the proximal femur that can lead to:
   (a) Implant malposition [2, 3]
   (b) Abnormal fixation [2]
5. The increased risk of complications as femur perforations or fractures [1, 3].
6. A changed relationship between proximal femur and acetabulum and altered biomechanics (abductor lever arm) [2].
7. Hip instability caused by bony impingement [3].
8. Leg Length Discrepancy (LLD) [2].

6.1.3 Preoperative Evaluation

1. Perform careful preoperative planning.
2. Take full radiographic imaging of the femur (AP and profile X-rays views) and long leg standing AP X-ray to assess LLD [3, 4].
3. Perform CT scan with 3D reconstruction to thoroughly evaluate the deformity and to measure the width of the intramedullary cavity [3].
4. Exclude infection. Decide one- or two-stage procedure for the removal of existing implants, infection, or a very complex deformity [1, 3].
5. Evaluate the effect of the PFD on the decided exposure.
6. Individualize the treatment in each patient [3]; follow more straightforward operations in older patients with lower physical demands and complete anatomic reconstruction in younger more active patients.
7. Template on AP and lateral X-rays and choose one of the following treatment options [4]:
   (a) Correct the bone with osteotomy to fit the prosthesis [3, 7].
      - Find the apex of the angular deformity.
      - Find the dimensions of the wedge that need to be removed.
      - Decide for the length of the femoral component; usually a long revision implant at least two times the diameter beyond the site of the osteotomy [7].
   (b) Select a modular stem or custom implant to fit the femur [1].
   (c) Use implants to avoid an increased distal deformity. Possible options are short

stems, resurfacing prostheses [4], or undersized cemented prosthesis with reasonable alignment and continuous cement mantle [3].

8. Evaluate the need for bone grafting and intraoperative X-ray.
9. Evaluate possible effect on knee alignment, leg length, and hip biomechanics.

6.1.4 Specific Considerations Based on the Site of Deformity [2]

1. Greater trochanter (GT) deformity [2] poses difficulties to the exposure and alters biomechanics. There are usually two types of deformities:
   (a) GT that overhangs the femoral canal makes difficult the access to the canal and the reaming and increases the risk for fracture and varus position of the implant.
   (b) A high-riding GT abates the abduction power and raises the possibility of bony impingement to the pelvis at flexion and internal rotation. In marked deformity, evaluate the need for osteotomy or modular stems for fixation.
2. Femoral neck deformity [2] can affect implant alignment and rotation. Possible forms of deformities are:
   (a) Varus deformity: a unilateral deformity is usually associated with leg shortening. Elongate with stem and neck options and take care to avoid the risk of nerve palsy. In bilateral deformity, keep the length equal and use high offset stems to recreate anatomy and tension of the abductors.
   (b) Valgus deformity: in excessive valgus deformity, you may need modified implants with reduced metaphyseal flare.
   (c) Torsional deformities: these concern increased ante- or retroversion deformities of the neck. If the stem will be implanted in the same direction as the neck, then there is a danger of reduced movement or instability. Possible treatment options are:
      - Standard prosthesis implanted in a markedly different version than patient's neck. This is easier with cemented stems than uncemented stems and for extensively porous-coated distally fixed stems than metaphyseal-filling uncemented implants [2]. The use of small cemented stems increases the risk of suboptimal cement mantles and instability [3].
      - Modular cementless implants in a position that the proximal sleeve maximizes the contact with the proximal host bone and the stem obtains optimal joint stability. Modular stems (e.g., S-ROM) with distal flutes provide rotational stability and different offset stem solutions.
      - Subtrochanteric derotational osteotomy with a cylindrical extensively porous-coated femoral stem or modular tapered stem.
   (d) Metaphyseal deformity [2]: has noted diversity and usually results from trauma, prior surgery (e.g., osteotomy), and developmental reasons with large or small femoral canals.
      - Metaphyseal defects affect the choice of implant and the fixation method. Treatment options include standard implants, cemented stems of the appropriate size and geometry, and uncemented stems with a diaphyseal fixation that bypass the defect or modular implants. The fixation of uncemented proximally porous-coated monoblock metaphyseal-filling implants may be compromised with an inadequate fit and increased incidence of fracture.
      - Modular implants have advantages and often work well. The proximal sleeve maximizes contact with the deformity, and the stem offers joint stability and optimal diaphyseal contact. Modular implants are also ideal for a metaphyseal/diaphyseal mismatch, in very large (Dorr type C) and in very small femoral canals.
      - Osteotomy in this anatomical region has the disadvantage of small bony fragment produced that may be devascularized and compromise healing.
   (e) Diaphyseal defects [2] are usually traumatic complications and affect the implant alignment. Possible treatment options include:

- Shorter implant that ignores the deformity or small cemented stems.
- In the majority of patients, a transverse, oblique, or step-cut osteotomy is needed with cemented or uncemented implant. Uncemented implants are usually preferred because the cement at the site of osteotomy may compromise the healing. Long extensively porous-coated or modular prostheses are the implants of choice. The rotational stability that is obtained in the distal fragment with the S-ROM distal flutes allows rapid healing and weight bearing (in one stage).

6.1.5 Outcomes

There have been a modest number of studies that have examined the result of primary THA in patients with PFD using cemented or uncemented femoral components. Few studies are focused on the clinical outcomes of patients with PFD undergoing THA [1, 3, 7]. The majority of them demonstrate results from cohorts of patients suffering from pathologies that usually have PFD [8–14].

PFD can compromise implant fixation, whether cemented or uncemented implants are used [1]. Compromised fixation for cemented implants may be due to a weak implant alignment, a poor cement mantle or technique, or a poor bone-cement interface. Patients with PFD usually have a sclerotic bone that can lead to poorer cement interdigitation within the bone. PFD may also compromise fixation and initial fit of the prosthesis to the bone for uncemented stems [1]. Initial studies used cemented implants [7, 8, 10–12]. Later studies demonstrated that the use of uncemented implants is equally satisfactory [1, 13, 14].

Mortazavi et al. [1] reported on 58 THAs in 51 patients with PDF performed between 1998 and 2006 that were followed up prospectively. The cause of PFD in almost half of the group was hip dysplasia. Other reasons were previous femoral osteotomy for OA, proximal femoral fracture, Paget disease, coxa vara, Ollier's disease, and slipped capital femoral epiphysis. The vast majority of them were treated with uncemented prostheses. Revision stems were used in 25%, and in 23% of the hips, an osteotomy was required. The group was prospectively followed up for a mean of four years and showed significant improvement. There were two (3.5%) revisions in two patients for periprosthetic fracture and femoral loosening. The mechanical failure rate was 9% (5 hips).

Papaggelopoulos et al. [7] also showed the results of thirty one patients with PFD that were treated with cemented or uncemented THA and concurrent femoral osteotomy; twenty of them were primary and eleven revision THAs. There were nine cemented femoral THAs. There was a high rate of complications and reoperations (32%) demonstrating that THA with concurrent osteotomy is a very technically demanding technique. Complications included seven intraoperative femoral fractures, four osteotomy nonunions, four instabilities, four aseptic femoral loosening, one osteolysis and a deep infection.

6.1.6 Complications

Intraoperative or postoperative fractures and dislocations are the most frequent complications.

6.2 Case Title: Dysplasia Hartofilakidis Type 2 with an Excessive Valgus Neck-Shaft Angle of About 150° and Excessive Anteversion of the Neck

E. Kenanidis and E. Tsiridis

6.2.1 Demographics

Age: 75
Sex: Female

6.2.2 Relevant Past Medical History

Principal pathologies: Atrial fibrillation, arterial hypertension, dyslipidemia

Previous surgical procedures: Appendectomy, right THA nineteen years ago

Medication: Sotalol, aspirin, propafenone, irbesartan + hydrochlorothiazide, simvastatin, nitroglycerin

6.2.3 Preoperative Radiological Assessment/Imaging (Fig. 6.1)

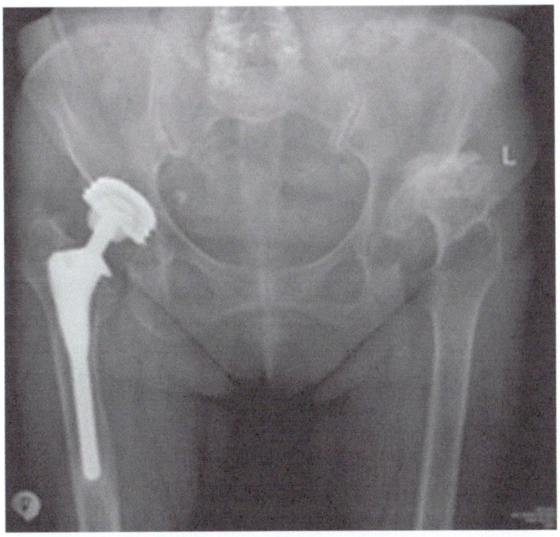

Fig. 6.1 AP x-ray of the left hip—congenital dysplasia of hip (Hartofilakidis type 2)

6.2.4 Preoperative Planning

Diagnosis: Osteoarthritis of left hip (Fig. 6.1)

Chosen treatment method: Uncemented acetabular shell Stryker Trident 50 mm, cancellous bone screw 6.5 mm (3×20 mm), polyethylene insert Stryker Trident X3 36 mm, cemented hip stem Stryker Exeter 37.5–2,150 mm, ceramic femoral head Stryker 36 mm, 0 mm

6.2.5 Surgical Note

A hybrid Exeter system was selected to compensate for the narrow femoral canal and the anteverted proximal femur and finally also for the small offset. The socket was elected to be inserted a few centimetres above the level of the teardrop to match the other side that has been replaced several years before. Deepening the acetabular reaming toward the inner plate provided us with significant coverage of the roof and the posterior wall of the component. Three screws were applied cranially for primary stability. The neck was cut short close to the lesser trochanter to maintain leg length equality. Early weight bearing was achieved following the surgery (Fig. 6.2).

Patient's position: Lateral decubitus

Type of anesthesia: General

Surgical approach: Mini-posterior

6.2.6 Postoperative Radiographs (Fig. 6.2)

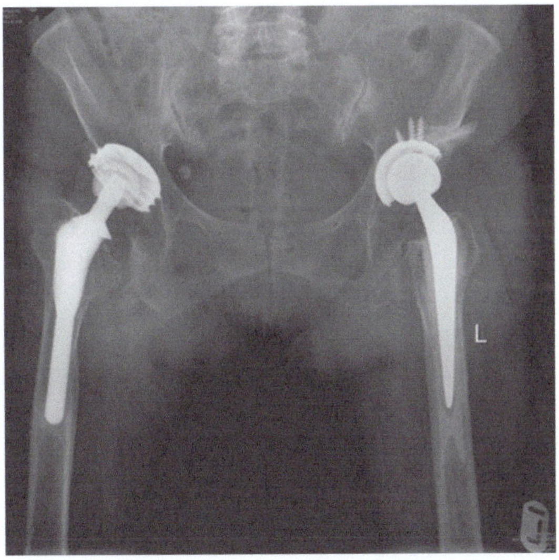

Fig. 6.2 AP of the left hip 1st day

6.2.7 Postoperative Management

Chemoprophylaxis and anticoagulant treatment period: Cefuroxime 750 mg (1 dose preoperatively, two doses postoperatively), vancomycin 500 mg (1 dose preoperatively, two doses postoperatively), enoxaparin 1 × 1 for thirty five days

Gait/limb loading until full loading: Partial weight bearing for 4 weeks and then full weight bearing as tolerated

6.2.8 Discussion

Hartofilakidis type 2 dysplasia is a challenge as the roof of the native acetabulum is usually missing or is too vertical to allow implant insertion safely. One of the methods to overcome this is to augment the roof with the femoral head autograft in a figure of 7 reconstruction or to mesh the defect and impact autografts underneath it or finally to insert a trabecular metal augment. Selecting a higher level to the native acetabulum to insert the socket was initially advocated by Ranawat; however the long-term results were disappowinting compared to the true site replacement. In our case, we lifted up the level of the join to match the other side; otherwise we would have ended up with a longer leg on the operated side. The latter option would have required possibly subtrochanteric shortening osteotomy to compensate for the leg length discrepancy, and the biomechanics of the left hip joint would have been different to the right hip joint regarding abductor leverage and strength, offset, and stability. For these reasons, it was elected to follow the strategy of the previous surgeon and implant a socket higher up. The result of the above -described process was a well-balanced pelvis, functioning abductors on both sides with a normal gait and walking pattern.

6.3 Case Title: Simultaneous Bilateral THA for Posttraumatic Arthritis Following Pelvic-Acetabular and Femoral Fractures

E. Kenanidis and E. Tsiridis

6.3.1 Demographics

Age: 36
Sex: Female
BMI: 30

6.3.2 Relevant Past Medical History

Principal pathologies: None

Previous surgical procedures: Car accident fifteen years back. Open-book pelvic fracture with pubic symphysis diastasis. Right side acetabular and femoral fracture and left side acetabular fracture dislocation

Medication: None

History of presenting complaint: Limping, leg length discrepancy, pain, complete reduction of the range of motion

6.3.3 Clinical Examination

Symptoms: Pain

Range of motion: Clinically minimal

Main disability: Pain

Scoring if available: HHS 60

Neurovascular evaluation: Intact

6.3.4 Preoperative Radiological Assessment/Imaging (Fig. 6.3)

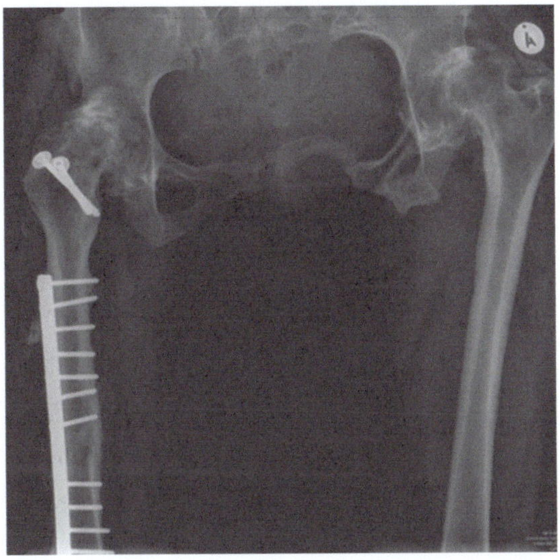

Fig. 6.3 Bilateral severe posttraumatic osteoarthritis. Right hip advanced osteonecrosis and left hip posterolateral subluxation. Evidence of open-book pelvic fracture posttraumatic fusion of the left sacroiliac joint complete dissociation of the pubis and a bone bridge developed to connect the two opposing end of the pubis. Left hemipelvis is externally rotated and abducted

6.3.5 Preoperative Planning

Diagnosis: Bilateral posttraumatic arthritis (Fig. 6.3)

Possible treatment options: One-stage reconstruction. Young and medically fit patient to withstand extensive surgery and blood loss. One-stage bilateral THA was elected to immediately balance the pelvis as both hips were severely affected and weight bearing was equally difficult on both sides.

Chosen treatment method: Left hip: uncemented acetabular shell DePuy Pinnacle 52 mm, cancellous bone screws 6.5 mm (2 × 25 mm, 1 × 20 mm), polyethylene DePuy 36 mm, uncemented femoral stem DePuy size 3 HI, 135 mm, ceramic femoral head DePuy 36 mm

Right Hip: Hybrid Exeter stem 37.5 mm offset and an uncemented acetabular component (Stryker) 52 mm × 36 mm and two stay screws through the shell, head ceramic 36 mm

Selection of implants if applicable and rational: Cemented stem to the right hip due to the proximal femoral deformity and the distal occlusion of the canal by the fracture

Expected difficulties: Acetabular reconstruction is expected to be challenging on both sides. It is also likely to find challenging the right femoral canal preparation due to the removal of proximal screws and screws through the proximal part of the plate.

Strategies to overcome difficulties: Special instruments for removal of screws, flexible reamers for femoral canal preparation

Templating: Necessary on both sides

6.3.6 Surgical Note

Left THA: Easy dislocation of the femoral head that was almost subluxated. Preparation of the acetabulum was found easier that though as the bone stock was sufficient front and back allowing for good inclination and fitting of the metal shell (52 mm with three supporting screws). The preparation of the canal was also easy and followed by the insertion of a straight non-anatomical proximally grid blasted tapered stem. Ceramic 36 mm head was used with an easy reduction and good stability (Fig. 6.4).

Right THA: Challenging dislocation as the femoral head was almost fussed with the socket. In times, we employed osteotomes to break bridges between head and socket; the head removed piecemeal with careful maneuvers. Preparation of the acetabulum was uneventful; however attention was made to remove the overhanging osteophytes and the very tight anterior capsule that was almost ossified. Attention was then turned to the femur. The osteotomy was easy as its height was not affecting the stem insertion planned to be cemented for easier fit through the expected proximal deformity. The proximal femur was then assessed. 2 × 6.5 mm partially threaded cancellous screws through the intertrochanteric line were found covered by bone around the distal flare of the greater trochanter. The washers helped us out to identify the screws and to remove them. A critical point during removal was the very tight perches of those screws to the medial cortex. The latter event made the removal challenging. It is often very difficult to start unscrewing those screws from the cortex as ossification around the screw threads is very robust. In our case, it was impossible to unscrew the screws with a screwdriver. The femur was turned externally until the inner tip of the screws was identified. Using screw removal cutting tubes over-drilling through the medial cortex helped us to mobilize this part of the screws and then remove them from the lateral cortex with less effort. The bone defects were filled immediately with corticocancellous grafts from the femoral head. Removing the proximal screws from the plate was easier as the pitch was cortical and the bonding to the medial wall was less robust. Another challenge was to open the femoral canal sufficient enough to enter the femoral rasps. Ossified diaphragms proximally in line with the screw track prohibited easy insertion of the rasps. Flexible reamers were used to break through them and open the canal for rasping. The procedure was completed using third-generation cementing technique. Easy reduction with a 36 mm ceramic head and an equal leg length and stable prosthesis were achieved (Fig. 6.5).

6.3.7 Postoperative Radiographs (Figs. 6.4 and 6.5)

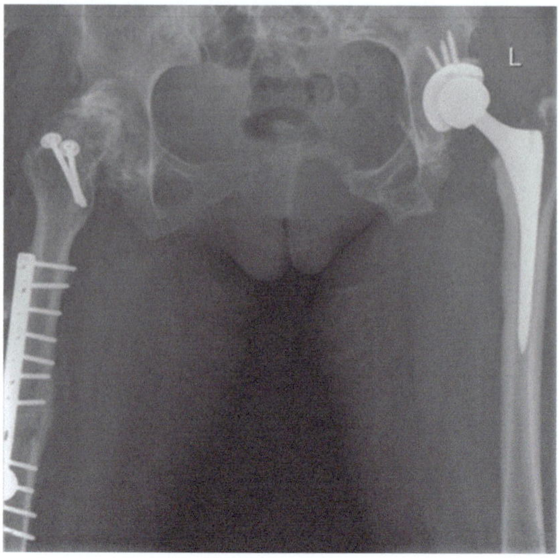

Fig. 6.4 Left THA well-positioned stem in line with the canal acetabulum well oriented

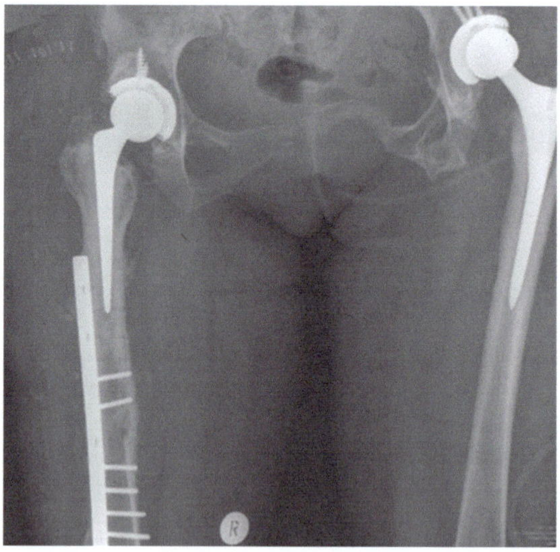

Fig. 6.5 Right hip, good acetabular orientation and stability. Stem well aligned with sufficient cement mantle stem proximal plate overlapping sufficient 1–2× ipsilateral femoral diameters at the level of insertion. Leg length equal. Pelvis well aligned and balanced

6.3.8 Postoperative Management

Chemoprophylaxis and anticoagulant treatment period: Teicoplanin one dose preoperatively and then two doses postoperatively for three days, enoxaparin 1 × 1 for the days of hospitalization then rivaroxaban 10 mg 1 × 1 for thirty days

Gait/limb loading until full loading: Partial weight bearing for six weeks and then weight bearing as tolerated

6.4 Case Title: DDH Hartofilakidis Type 1 Post-varus Proximal Femoral Osteotomy

E. Kenanidis and E. Tsiridis

6.4.1 Demographics

Age: 51
Sex: Female
BMI: 23

6.4.2 Relevant Past Medical History

Principal pathologies: Pain due to osteoarthritis, proximal femoral deformity iatrogenic, childhood varus osteotomy for DDH, shallow acetabulum, and altered biomechanics to the left hip lead to early osteoarthritis, arterial hypertension, dyslipidemia, and hypothyroidism

Previous surgical procedures: THA right hip

Medication: Simvastatin, ezetimibe, levothyroxine, atenolol

History of resenting complaint: Exacerbating pain gradually over the last four years, short limp and mild Trendelenburg

6.4.3 Clinical Examination

Symptoms: Pain, limitation in ROM

Range of motion: Flexion: 70^0, extension: -10^0, rotation impossible and add/abduction limited

Specific tests: Thomas positive 25°

Main disability: Pain, short limb

Scoring if available: HHS:70

Neurovascular evaluation: Intact, mild functional but not true Trendelenburg

6.4.4 Preoperative Radiological Assessment/Imaging (Fig. 6.6)

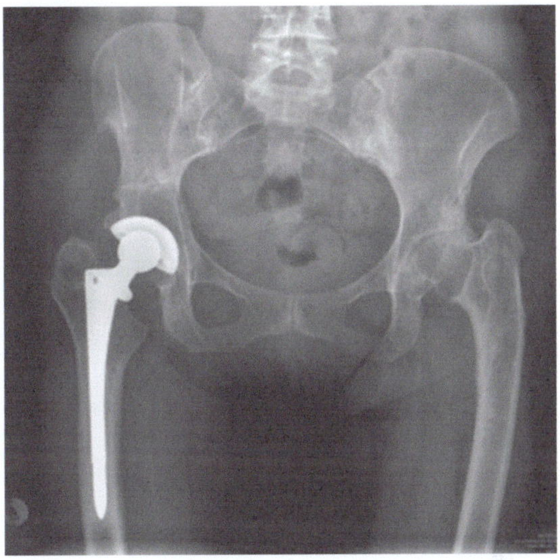

Fig. 6.6 Varus proximal femoral deformity from the previous osteotomy, capacious femoral canal with disuse osteoporosis, shallow acetabular fossa, and deficient anterior wall. Overriding greater trochanter obscuring the femoral canal to some extent increased anteversion and no obvious lesser trochanter

6.4.5 Preoperative Planning

Diagnosis: Osteoarthritis of left hip (Fig. 6.6)

Chosen treatment method: Uncemented acetabular shell Stryker Trident 50 mm, polyethylene Stryker Trident 32 mm, cemented hip stem Stryker Exeter 37.5, 150 mm, ceramic femoral head Stryker 32 mm, -4 mm

Selection of implants if applicable and rational: Cemented femoral component to compensate for the proximal femoral deformity. One should use an uncemented implant; a corrective valgus osteotomy should precede the implantation, and a long stem must be used.

Expected difficulties: Equal and adequate cement mantle in all Gruen zones

Strategies to overcome difficulties: Stem lateralization and acetabular medialization

6.4.6 Surgical Note

With the patient in lateral decubitus position using a mini-posterior approach, the hip was approached and easily dislocated. The osteotomy of the neck was low enough to prevent lengthening of the limb. The femur was displaced anteriorly behind the anterior wall retractor, and the acetabulum was cleared from osteophytes. The acetabular fossa was shallow, and the anterior wall was weak as expected. The reaming started as low as possible having identified the true floor using a curved osteotome. The anterior wall was protected, and the 50 mm reamer shaped the socket, and a 50 mm shell was inserted properly covered all around. Attention was then turned to the femur. Rasping started as lateral as possible to identify the canal from the piriformis fossa. The canal rasped to 37.5 mm number 0, and the lateral cortex was rasped additionally bringing the stem as lateral as possible thinning the lateral cortex. Only then the 37.5/0 rasp sat in the middle of the canal allowing us to continue without doing the corrective valgus osteotomy. The position of the rasp was checked with the C-arm taking an intraoperative radiograph which proved that the distance to the cortex was sufficient to allow a good cement mantle to be formed. Third-generation cementing technique and insertion of the stem allowed easy reduction and equal leg length on the contralateral side (Fig. 6.7).

6.4.7 Intraoperative Challenges

Challenges and solutions: Concentric rasping of the femur, lateralization of the femur, and medialization of the acetabular component

Thorough description of decision-making, including the reason for the final decision: Rasping the lateral cortex to the extent of reaching the cortex even rasping against the cortex is a valid solution for the stem to be inserted concentrically and to permit a proper two mm minimum cement mantle in all Gruen zones. The latter can be appreciated intraoperatively taking a radiograph to make sure that the expected mantle will be adequate.

6.4.8 Postoperative Radiographs (Fig. 6.7)

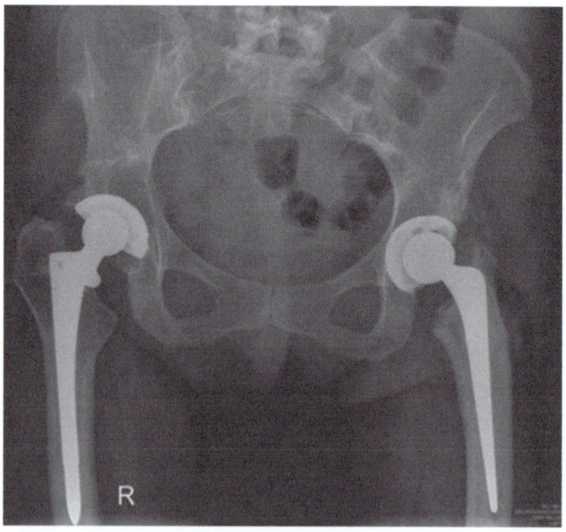

Fig. 6.7 Good cement mantle all around except possibly the top end of the zone 7 around the tip of the shoulder of the prosthesis. The stem is however in anteversion, and the true mantle is obscured to some extent. Intraoperatively the metaphyseal part of the cement mantle proximally was good and solid

6.4.9 Postoperative Management

Chemoprophylaxis and anticoagulant treatment period: Vancomycin 500 mg (one dose preoperatively and two doses postoperatively), cefuroxime 1.5 g (one dose preoperatively and two doses postoperatively), enoxaparin 1 × 1 for the days of hospitalization then rivaroxaban 10 mg 1 × 1 for thirty days

Gait/limb loading until full loading: Partial weight bearing for four weeks and then full weight bearing as tolerated

6.5 Case Title: Proximal Femoral Deformity

John Dundon and Jonathan Vigdorchik

6.5.1 Demographics

Age: 25
Sex: Female.
BMI: 33.0

6.5.2 Relevant Past Medical History

Principal pathologies: Proximal femoral deformity following surgery for developmental dysplasia of the hip

Previous surgical procedures: Periacetabular osteotomy, proximal femoral varus derotational osteotomy, removal of hardware, multiple previous hip arthroscopies with osteochondroplasty, and labral debridement and repair

Medication: None.

History of presenting complaint: The patient is a 25-year-old female with right hip pain since birth. The patient was born breech and has DDH originally treated with a Pavlik harness. This failed, and the patient ended up having multiple surgeries on her bilateral hips. The patient throughout her course has a right varus derotational osteotomy of the proximal femur, Ganz periacetaular osteotomy, and multiple hip arthroscopies with osteochondroplasty, none of which has provided durable relief. The patient now can only walk three blocks before pain limits her. She cannot put on her shoes and socks, has difficulty with stairs, and is unable to use public transport. The patient has failed nonoperative treatment with anti-inflammatories, injections, physical therapy, and assist devices and is now significantly limited by her pain. The patient denies any numbness or tingling, no previous neurovascular injury.

6.5.3 Clinical Examination

Symptoms: Coxalgic gait

Range of motion: Hip flexion 90^0, internal rotation 20^0, external rotation 40^0

Specific tests: Positive impingement testing, positive Stinchfield

Main disability: Limited and painful arc of motion

Scoring if available: Modified Harris Hip Score 31

Neurovascular evaluation: Motor 5/5, sensation normal, posterior tibial/dorsalis pedis pulses 2+

6.5.4 Preoperative Radiological Assessment/Imaging (Figs. 6.8, 6.9, and 6.10)

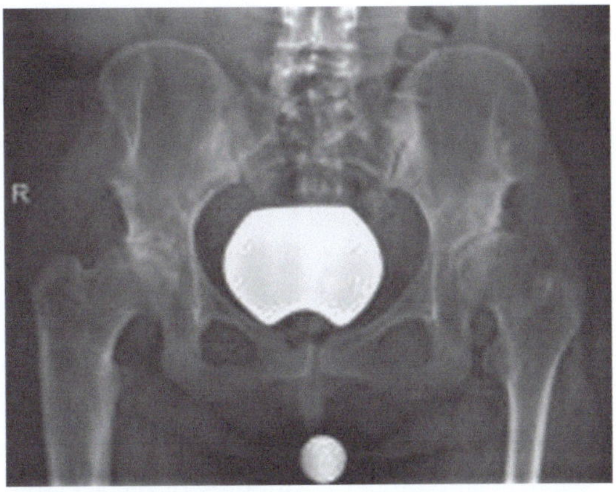

Fig. 6.8 Preoperative AP pelvis showing pelvic and proximal femoral deformities with degenerative changes

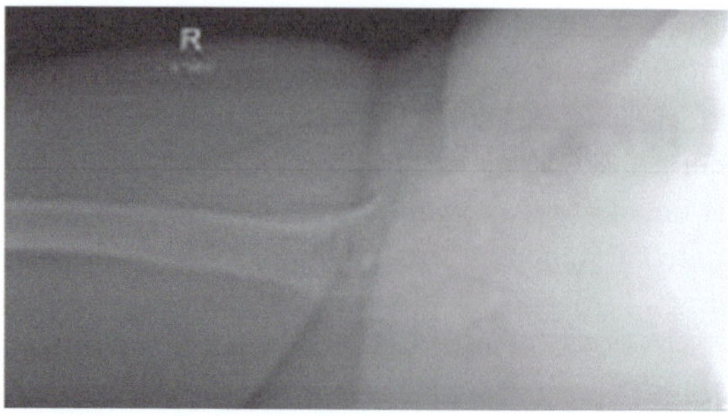

Fig. 6.9 Preoperative lateral of the right femur showing proximal femoral deformity

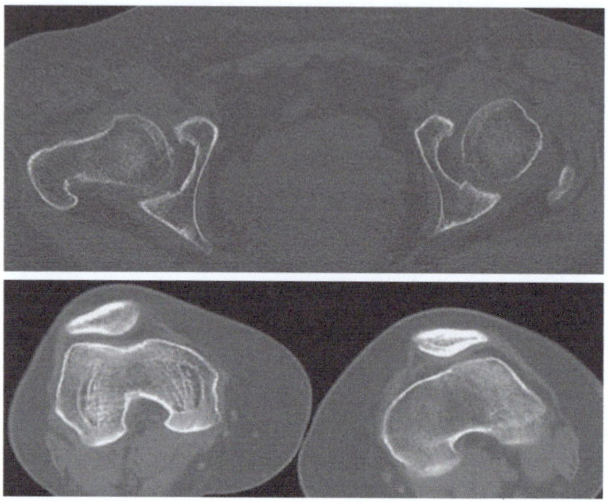

Fig. 6.10 Preoperative CT scan through the femoral neck and femoral condyles displaying neutral version of the femoral neck without any anteversion

6.5.5 Preoperative Planning

Diagnosis: Right proximal femoral deformity with associated degenerative changes following multiple previous operations for DDH. Left hip dysplasia with deficient bone laterally and superiorly (Figs. 6.8, 6.9 and 6.10)

Possible treatment options: Nonoperative management, total hip arthroplasty

Chosen treatment method: Total hip arthroplasty using MAKOplasty

Selection of implants if applicable and rational: For the acetabulum a MAKOplasty cup was used to ensure proper positioning of the acetabular component given the previous acetabular surgery and distortion of normal anatomy. The deformity of the ASIS from the previous operations negated the use of traditional computer navigation with ASIS registration. A DePuy S-ROM femoral stem was used in this case for multiple reasons. First, the modularity of proximal fit gave us the ability to obtain metaphyseal fit, to reduce the incidence of future stress shielding and bone loss associated with a distally fitting prosthesis. Secondly, this gave us the added advantage of adjusting the femoral anteversion as well given the previous surgical history of a derotational osteotomy and degree of femoral deformity.

Expected difficulties: We expected to deal with altered anatomy and reference points given previous proximal femoral and acetabular-sided surgery. The proximal femur was not only deformed and had altered version but was also vacuous, leading us to concerns as to whether a standard proximally fitting stem would give the fixation necessary for immediate weight bearing and ingrowth. There was also significant scar tissue from multiple previous surgeries making exposure more difficult.

Strategies to overcome difficulties: The plan was to use the MAKOplasty for the acetabular side to ensure proper cup placement and alignment, as well as for assessing leg length and offset. As for the femoral side, the modularity of the DePuy S-ROM would be instrumental in obtaining proper version and fit of the femoral component and helping to ensure the stability of the hip.

Templating: Preoperative templating was performed using the OrthoView software program for the S-ROM component and using the MAKOplasty software for the acetabulum.

6.5.6 Surgical Note

Patient's position: Left lateral decubitus

Type of anesthesia: Spinal

Surgical approach: Posterior approach

Main steps:

(1) Posterior approach to the hip was performed.

(2) The pelvic array was secured to the iliac wing using three pins.
(3) Release of the short external rotators and capsulotomy was performed.
(4) The greater trochanter and supra-acetabular marking pins were placed.
(5) The hip was dislocated, and our femoral neck cut was performed.
(6) The labral tissue and acetabular fossa were removed.
(7) We then registered our acetabulum with the computer program.
(8) Under the direction of the MAKOplasty program, our acetabulum was sized and reamed.
(9) Our acetabular component was impacted into correct position using the computer navigation and secured with screws.
(10) Our polyethylene liner was impacted into place.
(11) Our femur was prepared and reamed to size for the DePuy S-ROM.
(12) A trial reduction was performed. The hip was balanced from a soft tissue perspective ensuring appropriate tension and freedom from impingement.
(13) Final components were then impacted into place.

Reconstruction techniques: The S-ROM sleeve was placed in the proximal femur where the bone was located. In this patient, the sleeve was retroverted. Using the final stem, the femoral component was placed in ten degrees of anteversion (Figs. 6.11 and 6.12).

6.5.7 Intraoperative Challenges

Challenges and solutions: (1) Deficient acetabular bone—a small cup was used and placed appropriately medialized and 3 mm superior to ensure adequate bony coverage. (2) The femur was retroverted, and the canal was vacuous—we used an S-ROM component where we could appropriately size the sleeve to fit the proximal femur and then position the anteversion of the stem anatomically.

Unanticipated problems and solution: None

6.5.8 Postoperative Radiographs (Figs. 6.11 and 6.12)

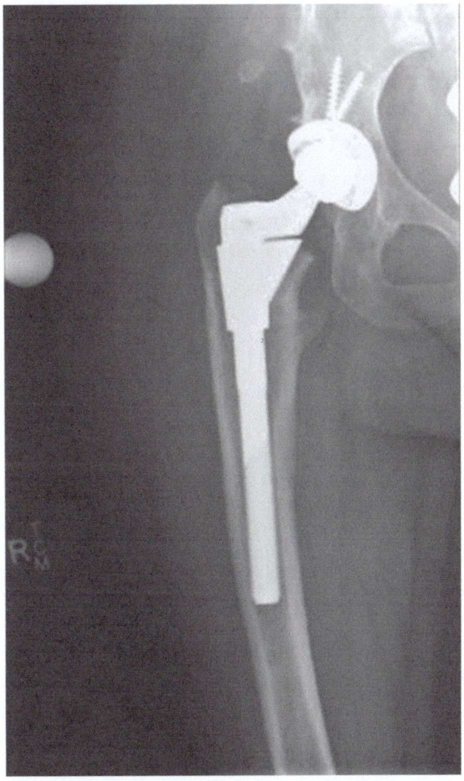

Fig. 6.11 Postoperative AP of the right hip

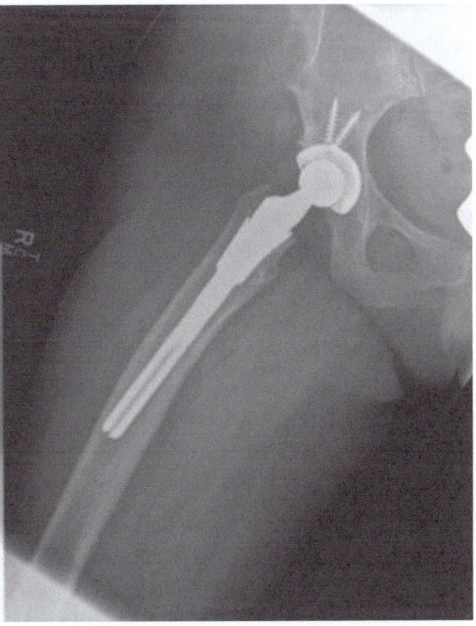

Fig. 6.12 Postoperative frog lateral of the right hip

6.5.9 Postoperative Management

Chemoprophylaxis and anticoagulant treatment period: Aspirin 325 mg orally twice daily along with sequential compression devices

Gait/limb loading until full loading: The patient was immediately made full weight bearing as tolerated.

6.5.10 Follow-Up and Complications

No complication

Scoring if available: Modified Harris Hip Score: 91

6.5.11 Discussion [1, 15, 16]

Advantages of the applied method: The advantage of using the MAKOplasty system is obtaining appropriate cup position (hip centre, abduction angle, anteversion) given the loss of normal anatomy and landmarks. Using this system we were able to obtain well-placed components in appropriate position and obtain hip stability even in a situation with highly altered anatomy. Using the S-ROM system gave us the flexibility to individualize her femoral implant reliably and obtain both metaphyseal and diaphyseal fixation. This method provides a reliable and reproducible method for dealing with complex problems associated with proximal femoral and acetabular deformity.

Disadvantages of the method: The disadvantages are the increased cost associated with the equipment necessary, the increased operative time associated with pin placement and acetabular mapping, and the learning curve associated with the use of this new technology.

Alternative evidence-based techniques for the case: Standard total hip arthroplasty could be performed as well without the assistance of the MAKOplasty technology.

Why is the chosen technique better for this case? Given the deformity of both the acetabulum and proximal femur, along with multiple previous surgeries creating deformity of the hip joint combined with the patient's obesity, we chose to proceed with robotic-assisted placement. There is good data showing the improved accuracy of the acetabular component with the restoration of leg length and offset using robotic-assisted surgery. With the given distortion of previous anatomic landmarks by prior surgery, we felt the best option for optimal component position in a young patient would be using MAKOplasty. A DePuy S-ROM femoral stem was used in this case for multiple reasons. Firstly the modularity of proximal fit gave us the ability to obtain metaphyseal fit, to reduce the incidence of future stress shielding and bone loss associated with a distally fitting prosthesis. Secondly this gave us the added advantage of adjusting the femoral anteversion as well given the previous surgical history and degree of femoral deformity. Studies have shown the modularity of the S-ROM is instrumental in compensating for proximal femoral deformity while achieving hip stability. In retrospective studies, this has shown the ability to compensate for deformity although the intraoperative and postoperative complications rates in these patients are high. This provides the ability to achieve cementless fixation in an otherwise difficult femur.

Indications and contraindications for your technique: Indications for the use of MAKOplasty would include any primary or revision hip arthroplasty. Indications for the use of S-ROM include metaphyseal/diaphyseal mismatch, proximal femoral deformity, and alterations in proximal femoral native version. Contraindications for this technique would be an active infection and the inability to comply with hip precautions, in line with standard total hip arthroplasty.

Learning curve and how to manage complications: There is a documented learning curve associated with the use of this technique, and familiarity with the equipment should be encouraged prior to use. Redmond et al. [15] described a learning curve during his experience, noting a shorter operative time, better acetabular component position, and fewer acetabular component outliers with increased experience with the technique.

Level of evidence concerning the superiority of this method against others: Level 3

6.6 Case Title: Primary Hip Arthroplasty—Proximal Femoral Deformity

Antonia F. Chen and Richard H. Rothman

6.6.1 Demographics

Age: 24
Sex: Female
BMI: 31.8 kg/m2

6.6.2 Relevant Past Medical History

Principal pathologies: Rheumatoid arthritis

Previous surgical procedures: Bilateral Charcot foot surgery, right hip surgery (unknown)

Medication: Tramadol, flaxseed oil

Other: Allergies—no known drug allergies

History of presenting complaint: This is a 24-year-old patient with significant right groin pain. The patient states that her pain has been present for years, as she underwent a previous surgery for her hip, and her pain is severe. This limits her activities of daily living, and her walking tolerance is reduced. Medication and activity modification have been minimally effective for greater than three months. Assistive walking devices did not improve her function. She had no complaints of numbness and tingling.

6.6.3 Clinical Examination

Symptoms: Pain with range of motion, antalgic gait

Range of motion: 0–90 degrees of flexion, 40 degrees abduction, 20 degrees adduction, 20 degrees external rotation, and 20 degrees internal rotation

Specific tests: The patient has negative Trendelenburg sign. She has a limb length discrepancy of 1.5 inches.

Main disability: Pain and limp

Neurovascular evaluation: Neurovascularly intact (5/5 quadriceps, 2+ dorsalis pedis pulses)

6.6.4 Preoperative Radiological Assessment/Imaging (Figs. 6.13, 6.14, and 6.15)

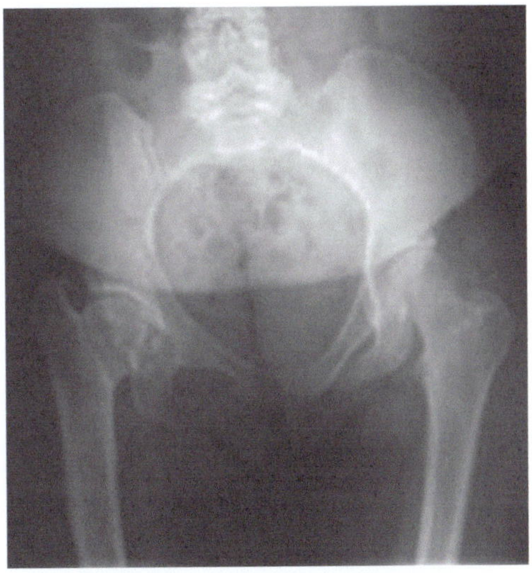

Fig. 6.13 Preoperative anteroposterior pelvis X-ray demonstrating degenerative joint disease

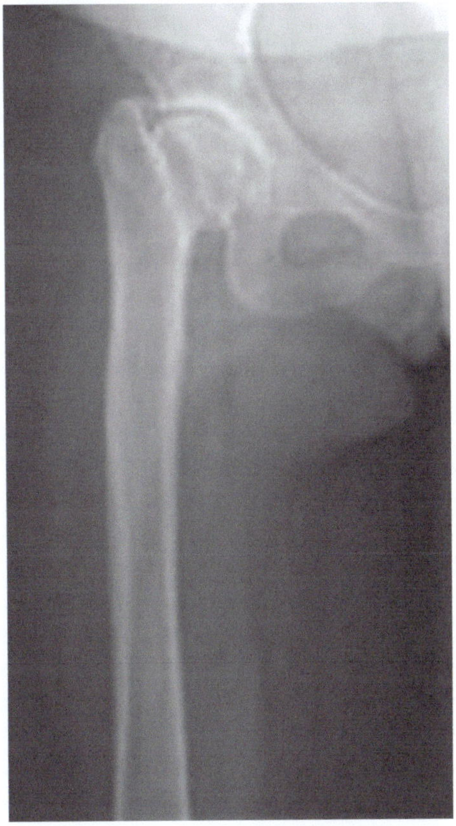

Fig. 6.14 Preoperative anteroposterior hip X-ray demonstrating degenerative joint disease and abnormal proximal femoral anatomy

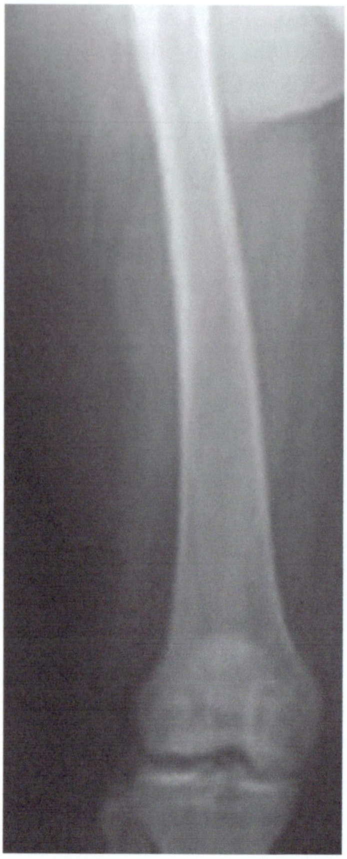

Fig. 6.15 Preoperative anteroposterior distal femur X-ray demonstrating a widened femoral canal

6.6.5 Preoperative Planning

Diagnosis: Degenerative joint disease with abnormal proximal femoral anatomy from congenital coxa vara (Figs. 6.13, 6.14 and 6.15)

Possible treatment options: Conservative therapy, valgus intertrochanteric osteotomy, total hip arthroplasty

Chosen treatment method: Total hip arthroplasty

Selection of implants if applicable and rational: Given the patient's abnormal femoral anatomy, a modular femoral implant was chosen so that version could be established to restore normal anatomy. A small acetabular cup was available given the patient's small stature. Various femoral head sizes were available, which were determined by the size of the acetabular cup.

Expected difficulties: The first expected difficulty was dislocation of the femoral head and resecting the femoral head, especially given the high-riding greater trochanter. Once the acetabulum was exposed, appropriate reaming has to be conducted to establish the appropriate hip centre. For the femur, appropriate femoral sizing was necessary to fill the canal of the widened femur, and femoral rotation has to be established appropriately to provide hip stability.

Strategies to overcome difficulties: Hip exposure was performed through the shortened abductors, taking care to preserve the abductors. To enable good exposure, the neck cut was made to fit the modular femoral component instead of the standard neck cut, which allowed for better acetabular exposure. Once the acetabulum was exposed, the hip centre was restored using the transverse acetabular ligament and delineation of the medial acetabular wall as anatomic landmarks. This provided adequate coverage of the acetabular component. Supplemental screw fixation was performed. For the femur, reaming was performed until there was a tight fit, and an appropriately sized body was used to fill the proximal femur. The femoral version was based on the distal femur, and a 32 head was used to provide additional stability.

Templating: Preoperative templating was performed for appropriate acetabular placement and femoral templating. It was noted that lower placement of the body of the femoral implant would be beneficial for restoring the hip centre.

6.6.6 Surgical Note

Patient's position: Supine

Type of anesthesia: Spinal

Surgical approach: Anterolateral

Main steps: Supine positioning, modified anterolateral gluteus medius splitting approach, acetabular cup (48 mm) placement with two screws, 32 neutral liner, and a modular femoral stem

Reconstruction techniques: A lateral incision was made to the hip, and a modified gluteus medius splitting approach was made. The high-riding greater trochanter was identified, and a femoral neck cut was made in a stepwise manner to fit the modular femoral component. The acetabulum was exposed, and the anatomic landmark of the transverse acetabular ligament was used to determine the height of the hip centre. The placement of the acetabular cup was determined by the medial wall, and anteversion and abduction were determined by anatomic landmarks. For the femur, reaming was performed to obtain a tight fit in the femoral canal, and the proximal body was placed against the proximal femoral cortex to allow for good ingrowth. The femoral version was selected on the distal femoral anatomy, and the hip was reduced and stable in all ranges of motion (Figs. 6.16 and 6.17).

6.6.7 Intraoperative Challenges

Challenges and solutions: Hip exposure—care was taken to preserve the abductors while obtaining adequate exposure given a high-riding greater trochanter. A generous femoral cut was performed to add to the exposure. Once the acetabulum was exposed, anatomical landmarks were crucial to creating an appropriate acetabular socket to place the acetabular cup. Deepening of the reamer was performed to medialize the cup and obtain adequate acetabular coverage. The femoral body and stem were chosen to fit the patient's anatomy and to ensure good bony ingrowth into the body. The version was determined not by the native femoral version but by the distal femur. The amount of limb lengthening should not exceed four cm to reduce the likelihood of nerve damage.

Unanticipated problems and solution: None

Thorough description of decision-making, including the reason for the final decision: Decision-making for acetabular component and femoral size was based on the intraoperative anatomy. A smaller acetabular cup was used to ensure that there was adequate coverage of the cup to allow for bony ingrowth. A large femoral stem was used given the patient's widened femoral canal. The body was chosen to provide proximal fixation, and the anteversion of the femoral stem was based on the distal femoral anatomy.

6.6.8 Postoperative Radiographs (Figs. 6.16 and 6.17)

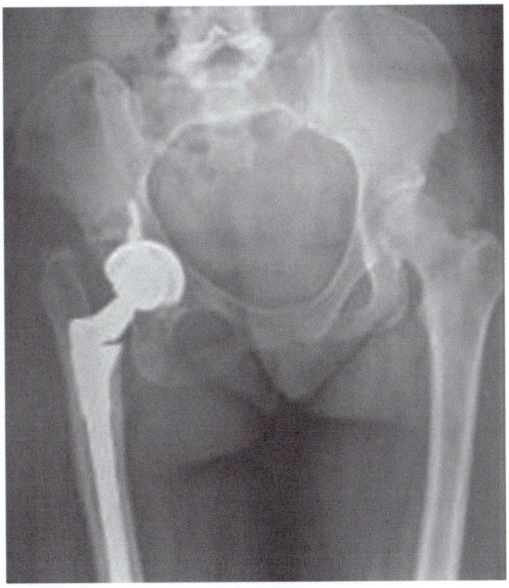

Fig. 6.16 Postoperative anteroposterior pelvis X-ray

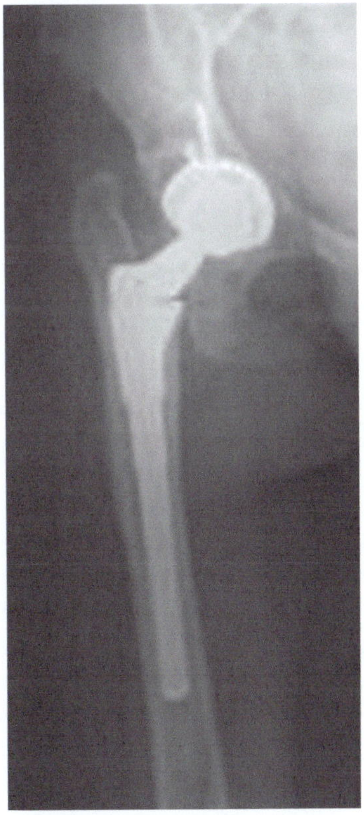

Fig. 6.17 Postoperative anteroposterior hip X-ray

6.6.9 Postoperative Management

Chemoprophylaxis and anticoagulant treatment period: The patient received two g of a first-generation cephalosporin 30 min prior to surgery and 24 h after surgery. Warfarin was given as anticoagulation for four weeks. The patient received compression mechanically during her hospital stay.

Gait/limb loading until full loading: Full weight bearing in the operative extremity.

6.6.10 Follow-Up and Complications

No postoperative complications were noted. There were no dislocations, infections, or wound problems.

6.6.11 Discussion

Advantages of the applied method: The advantage of performing a total hip arthroplasty is that this is definitive treatment where the patient can immediately weight bear after surgery. It is also a procedure that can be used to restore the hip centre and change the femoral anteversion to the anatomic location.

Disadvantages of the method: Performing a total hip arthroplasty in such a young patient will necessitate a revision or two within this patient's lifetime.

Alternative evidence-based techniques for the case: Previous studies have demonstrated that valgus intertrochanteric osteotomy can improve clinical outcomes [17].

Why is the chosen technique better for this case? In this case, there was evidence of cartilage destruction in the acetabulum. Thus, the best long-term solution in this patient was a total hip arthroplasty, as a valgus intertrochanteric osteotomy would not be appropriate with joint space narrowing.

Indications and contraindications for your technique: The indications for this procedure include joint space narrowing, evidence of cartilage destruction, and proximal femoral anatomy that cannot be surgically corrected by other means (e.g., femoral head sphericity). The contraindications for this procedure include inadequate bone stock for reconstruction and current septic arthritis.

Learning curve and how to manage complications: This procedure should be performed by experienced arthroplasty surgeons and not early in the learning curve for an orthopedic surgeon. Complications, such as sciatic nerve injury, should be initially treated conservatively by flexing the knee and extending the hip to relieve pressure on the nerve. Other complications such as limb length discrepancy should be discussed prior to surgery, as the patient must understand that their limb lengths may not be equal after surgery. This can be remedied with shoe lifts. Greater trochanteric fracture is more common in patients with high-riding greater trochanters, and this can be treated with claw fixation. Other complications, such as hematoma, periprosthetic joint infection, deep vein thrombosis, and pulmonary embolism, should be treated in the usual manner for patients undergoing total hip arthroplasty.

Level of evidence concerning the superiority of this method against others: Level IV studies demonstrated good implant survivorship with improvement in clinical outcome scores (Harris Hip Score) [4, 18].

References

1. Javad Mortazavi SM, Restrepo C, Kim PJW, Parvizi J, Hozack WJ. Cementless femoral reconstruction in patients with proximal femoral deformity. J Arthroplasty. 2011;26(3):354–9.
2. Berry DJ. Total hip arthroplasty in patients with proximal femoral deformity. Clin Orthopaed Relat Res. 1999;369:262–72.
3. Zaher NH. Total hip arthroplasty in patients with proximal femoral deformity. Pan Arab J Orth Trauma. 2004;8(2):167–73.
4. Boisgard S, Descamps S, Bouillet B. Complex primary total hip arthroplasty. Orthopaed Traumatol. 2013;99S:S34–42.
5. Dorr LD, Faugere MC, Mackel AM, Gruen TA, Bognar B, Malluche HH. Structural and cellular assessment of bone quality of proximal femur. Bone. 1993;14(3):231–42.

6. Nash W, Harris A. The Dorr type and cortical thickness index of the proximal femur for predicting peri-operative complications during hemiarthroplasty. J Orthop Surg (Hong Kong). 2014;22(1):92–5.
7. Papagelopoulos PJ, Trousdale RT, Lewallen DG. Total hip arthroplasty with femoral osteotomy for proximal femoral deformity. Clin Orthop Relat Res. 1996;332:151.
8. Shinar AA, Harris WH. Cemented total hip arthroplasty following previous femoral osteotomy: an average 16-year follow-up study. J Arthroplast. 1998;13:243.
9. Stuchin SA. Extra-articular deformities and the role of hip resurfacing - a proposed classification system. Bull NYU Hosp Jt Dis. 2009;67(2):135–7.
10. Ferguson GM, Cabanela ME, Ilstrup DM. Total hip arthroplasty after failed intertrochanteric osteotomy. J Bone Joint Surg Br. 1994;76:252.
11. Boos N, Krushell R, Ganz R, et al. Total hip arthroplasty after previous proximal femoral osteotomy. J Bone Joint Surg Br. 1997;79:247.
12. Iwase T, Hasegawa Y, Iwasada S, et al. Total hip arthroplasty after failed intertrochanteric valgus osteotomy for advanced osteoarthrosis. Clin Orthop Relat Res. 1999;364:175.
13. Parsch D, Jung AW, Thomsen M, et al. Good survival of uncemented tapered stems for failed intertrochanteric osteotomy: a mean 16 year follow-up study in 45 patients. Arch Orthop Trauma Surg. 2008;128:1081.
14. Suzuki K, Kawachi S, Matsubara M, et al. Cementless total hip replacement after previous intertrochanteric valgus osteotomy for advanced osteoarthritis. J Bone Joint Surg Br. 2007;89:1155.
15. Redmond JM, Gupta A, Hammarstedt JE, Petrakos AE, Finch NA, Domb BG. The learning curve associated with robotic assisted total hip arthroplasty. J Arthroplasty. 2015;30:50–4.
16. Kanawade V, Dorr LD, Banks SA, Zhang Z, Wan Z. Precision of robotic guided insrumentation for acetabular component positioning. J Arthroplasty. 2015;30:392–7.
17 Bartoníček J, Vávra J. Valgus intertrochanteric osteotomy for coxa vara of Bucholz-Ogden Types II and III in patients older than 30 years. Arch Orthop Trauma Surg. 2011;131(9):1211–7.
18 Murphy JM, Vanderhave KL, Urquhart AG. Total hip arthroplasty in adolescents with severe hip arthropathy and dysplasia associated with camptodactyly-arthropathy-coxa vara- pericarditis syndrome. J Arthroplasty. 2012;27(8):1581.e5–8. Clin Orthop Relat Res. 2013;471(9):2980–6

THA Following Previous Varus or Valgus Osteotomy

7

Eustathios Kenanidis, Panagiotis Kakoulidis, Eleftherios Tsiridis, Peter Mertens, Karl Brabants, William L. Griffin, Derek Ward, Javad Parvizi, Rajiv Merchant, and Eric Masterson

7.1 Current Concepts

E. Kenanidis, P. Kakoulidis, and E. Tsiridis

7.1.1 General

Proximal femoral osteotomy is a well-accepted joint-preserving treatment option in young patients with early symptomatic degenerative hip disease [1]. The primary goal of this procedure is to slow down the progression of osteoarthritic joint changes and to relieve pain, mainly through the realignment of the articular surfaces and redistribution of joint forces [2]. Additionally, it preserves the bone stock and delays THA and its possible harmful complications especially in young patients [1, 2].

There are various types of osteotomies, namely, the intertrochanteric varus or valgus osteotomy, the rotational osteotomy, the curved intertrochanteric osteotomies, etc. They are performed in selected patients with different underlying diseases as DDH, femoral head osteonecrosis, posttraumatic OA, rheumatoid arthritis, etc. [3–5].

Since the introduction of THA, the indication of hip osteotomies has been considerably altered and became relatively uncommon [2]. Furthermore, a substantial percentage of patients with a previous

E. Kenanidis, M.D., Ph.D., M.Sc. (✉) · P. Kakoulidis, M.D.
Academic Orthopaedic Unit, Aristotle University Medical School, Thessaloniki, Greece

E. Tsiridis, M.D., Ph.D., F.A.C.S., F.R.C.S.
Academic Orthopaedic Unit, Papageorgiou General Hospital, Aristotle University Medical School, Thessaloniki, Greece
e-mail: etsiridis@doctors.org.uk

P. Mertens, M.D. · K. Brabants, M.D.
ZNA Middelheim, Antwerp, Belgium
e-mail: peter.mertens@zna.be; carl.brabants@zna.be

W.L. Griffin, M.D.
OrthoCarolina Hip and Knee Center, Charlotte, NC, USA
e-mail: william.griffin@orthocarolina.com

D. Ward, M.D.
Division of Adult Reconstruction, University of California, San Francisco, CA, USA

J. Parvizi, M.D., F.R.C.S.
Sidney Kimmel School of Medicine, Philadelphia, PA, USA

Rothman Institute at Thomas Jefferson University, Philadelphia, PA, USA

R. Merchant, M.D., M.R.C.S., M.C.H.
Royal College of Surgeons in Ireland, Dublin, Ireland
e-mail: rajivmerchant@rcsi.ie

E. Masterson, B.Sc., M.Ch., F.R.C.S.I., F.R.C.S.
University of Limerick, Limerick, Ireland

Bon Secours Hospital Limerick, Limerick, Ireland

E. Tsiridis (ed.), *The Adult Hip - Master Case Series and Techniques*,
https://doi.org/10.1007/978-3-319-64177-5_7

osteotomy will be converted to THA in the mid- and long term [5]. The literature supports that over 50% of patients in the second decade from the osteotomy will need conversion to THA (60% at fifteen years, 18–30% at ten years) [2, 5].

7.1.2 Technical Challenges/ Difficulties

THA in patients with a previous proximal femoral osteotomy may be challenging chiefly due to the distorted anatomy of the femur. The possible technical difficulties that may be encountered in these surgical procedures are the following:

1. Residual proximal femoral deformity [6–8].
2. Occasionally need for a further corrective osteotomy before THA or trochanteric osteotomy [1, 8].
3. Sclerosis in the femoral metaphyseal region [6, 9].
4. Residual hardware [7, 9–11].
5. Challenging reaming of the femoral canal with higher intraoperative complication rate [1, 7, 11].
6. Risk for intraoperative cracks and fractures [1, 4].
7. Risk of instability due to malalignment, higher or lesser tension of abductors, impingement, and LLD.
8. Risk of varus or valgus malposition of the stem [12, 13].
9. Following the removal of the hardware, the cortical holes may compromise cement pressurization [7].
10. Difficult control of stem anteversion with a monoblock stem [6].
11. Longer operating time [3, 11, 12].
12. More extensive intraoperative blood loss [3, 11, 12].

7.1.3 Preoperative Planning

1. Perform a full clinical and radiological evaluation of the patient.
2. Take full-length AP and lateral X-rays.
3. CT is helpful to complete the evaluation of the deformity.
4. Template accurately.
5. Assess LLD.
6. Choose the implant to be used. Possible implant choices are the following:
   (a) A standard uncemented monoblock prosthesis.
   (b) A cemented prosthesis as it allows flexibility at insertion, however, it needs optimal positioning and optimal cement mantle for advantageous results.
   (c) Modular implants.
   (d) Custom-made prosthesis.

7.1.4 Published Results

Various studies have demonstrated the outcomes of conversion of the proximal femoral osteotomies to THA [1–19]. The majority of them are retrospective or prospective case series. There are also case control comparative studies with OA patients [3, 11, 12, 16]. There is a lack of high-quality studies. Except for the design and the other methodological concerns, the variety of underlying diseases and the different fixation techniques and implants that are used further render comparisons difficult [1–19].

These studies have sample sizes from 14 to 215 patients and a follow-up ranging from 4, 8 to 20 years [1–19]. The majority of them have mid-term follow-up. There is only one study reporting results on 20 years [4]. They demonstrated results for both cemented and uncemented implants. Concerning cementing techniques, they are usually referred to the outocomes of the first- [7, 8] and the second-generation [10] cementing technique. Many studies reported that the intraoperative time and the blood loss were increased compared to other groups of primary THAs [3, 11–13]. A recent systematic review [20] also demonstrated that THAs following previous osteotomies had a greater operative time and estimated blood loss. This is not however accepted as a reason for failure.

Inconsistent results have been reported about the complication rates, clinical outcomes, and implant survival [1–19]. Iwase et al. [9] published the results of 12 cemented and 18 uncemented THAs performed on patients with previous failed intertrochanteric valgus osteotomy. Survival at seven years was 100% for the cemented and 40% for the uncemented components [9]. First-generation cementing techniques reported inferior results in the long term compared to standard THA. Fergunson et al. [7] showed revision rate of 18% in 10 years using the first-generation cementing technique in 215 cemented THAs from previously failed intertrochanteric osteotomies. The second-generation cementing techniques significantly improved survivorship of stems [10]. Failures reported mainly due to an insufficient cement mantle supposedly caused by the irregular femoral anatomy [10].

Favorable results, however, have been reported for uncemented implants during the last years [4, 5, 14]. Merle et al. [4] evaluated 48 uncemented implants used for failed intertrochanteric osteotomies. The survival of stems due to aseptic loosening was 93% and for any reason 89% at 20 years. Parch et al. [14] also demonstrated survival of 91% for any reason and 93% for aseptic loosening at 15 years for 48 uncemented implants used for failed femoral osteotomies. It is questionable, however, if a conventional cementless stems may be used in a severe distortion of femoral anatomy. Custom-made or modular stems are reasonable in use in these cases.

A recent systematic review [20] reported no difference in survivorship between groups of THA following previous osteotomy and primary THA. The survival rate of THA following osteotomy ranged from 75 to 100%, and those of comparison group range from 94.1 to 100%, but no statistical significance existed. The majority of THA cohorts past osteotomy had a survivorship greater than 90% [1, 3, 12, 15, 16]. The reasons for revision involved the aseptic loosening, the recurrent dislocation, and the infection but there was no difference between groups.

7.2 Case Title: THA Following a Varus Osteotomy at Childhood for DDH. Flattened Head and Socket, Short Neck, and Neck Anteversion. Hartofilakidis 1 DDH

E. Kenanidis and E. Tsiridis

The alpha angle is <20%, and the socket is shallow. The patient has developed arthritis due to a chronic head deformity caused by osteonecrosis. The proximal femur appears to have some endosteal scalloping from the previous osteotomy (Fig. 7.1). Deepening the socket is always a safe way to cover the acetabular component. The shell was fitted snuggly, and no screws were necessary. The reason for using a cemented DDH Exeter stem was to compensate for the proximal femoral deformity. The best way to align the stem inside the femoral canal was to lateralize it as much as possible against the lateral wall. In addition to the latter, a short offset of 35.5 mm used in this case was necessary to accommodate the tight abductors. A low neck cut is necessary to avoid leg lengthening (Fig. 7.2).

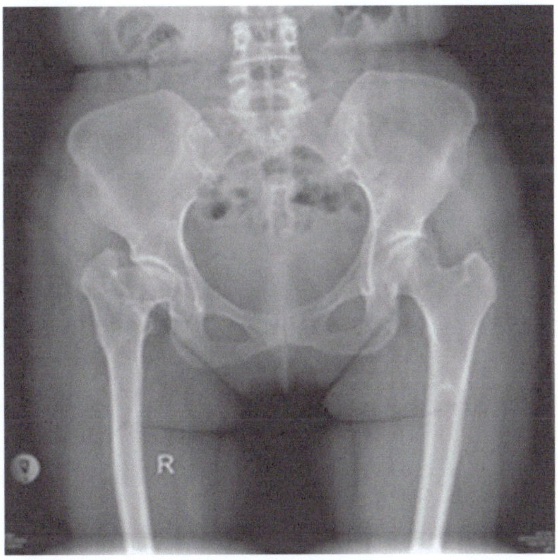

Fig. 7.1 AP x-ray of the right hip depicts the distorted proximal femoral anatomy following the previous osteotomy, the short anteverted neck and the shallow acetabulum

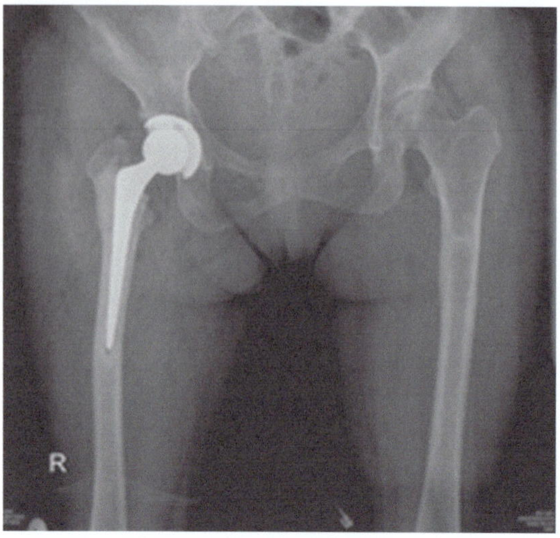

Fig. 7.2 Postoperative x-ray of the right hip depicts the hybrid THA with the cemented short offset Exeter stem

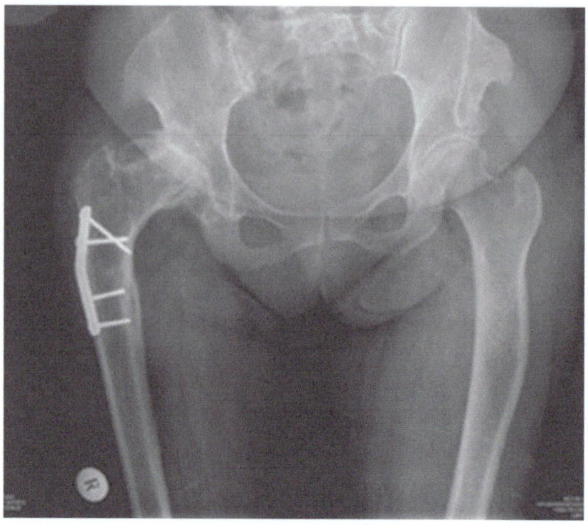

Fig. 7.3 AP pelvis x-ray demonstrating an end-stage rigth hip osteoarthritis following a previous varus osteotomy with retained hardware for DDH

7.3 Case Title: THA Primary Complex for DDH Hartofilakidis 2 and Subtrochanteric Varus Osteotomy

E. Kenanidis and E. Tsiridis

Right hip osteoarthritis. This pelvis is small and deformed. The anterior superior iliac spine on the right is disappeared as a Dunn osteotomy was possibly performed along with the varus subtrochanteric to bring the head to the socket (Fig. 7.3). The result was satisfactory for several years, however, predictably lead to osteonecrosis and arthritis. The head is flat, and the socket has an open alpha angle but enough depth to the medial wall to attempt reconstruction without grafting of the roof. There is also old metalwork in the place with cortical scalloping surrounding the screw end adjustment to the medial cortex. The canal is capacious Dorr type C but bowed proximally with a possibility of an endosteal bone bridge at the osteotomy healing site. The left hip appears better preserved. There is evidence of a varus subtrochanteric osteotomy that has been remodeled to a nearly normal-looking femur. There was no leg length discrepancy. A primary challenge for this THA was to remove the metalwork as the metal was soft and embedded into the bone. The first task was to perform the correct neck osteotomy to avoid leg lengthening. The acetabulum was flat, but digging down the teardrop let us ream concentrically to achieve good roof coverage without grafting it (medialization of the socket was necessary also to achieve better hip function). Attention was then turned to the femur. The rationale behind using a DDH short cemented Exeter stem with 35.5 mm offset is threefold: first to accommodate the existing short offset; second to fit the canal without reaching too low, thus avoiding varus placement of the stem; and third to easily adjust the leg length by deepening or leaving the stem proud as necessary. All the later are not easily achieved with an uncemented stem. The final result is satisfactory with equal leg length, good cement mantle around the stem, and a very limited lateralization of the stem (Fig. 7.4).

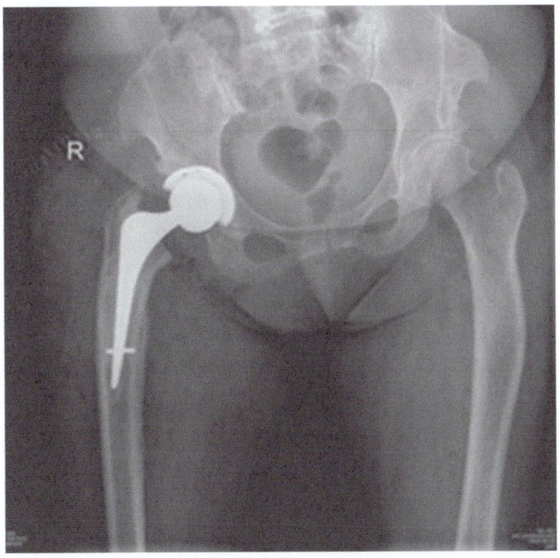

Fig. 7.4 AP x-ray of the first day showing the hybrid THA with a cemented, short offset Exeter stem

7.4 Case Title: Developmental Dysplasia of the Hip Hartofilakidis 1. Post Varus Proximal Femoral Osteotomy in Childhood

E. Kenanidis and E. Tsiridis

7.4.1 Demographics

Age: 41
Sex: Female
BMI: 25

7.4.2 Relevant Past Medical History

Principal pathologies: No clinical relevant medical history

Previous surgical procedures: DDH (1998) bilateral hip osteotomies varus right and valgus left

Medication: None

History of presenting complaint: Early right hip osteoarthritis with pain antalgic gait and short limp gate. Exacerbation of symptoms in the last two years

7.4.3 Clinical Examination

Symptoms: Pain

Range of motion: 0–90°, limited external and internal rotation

Specific tests: Thomas test positive at 30 degrees

Scoring if available: HSS: 70

Neurovascular evaluation: Intact

7.4.4 Preoperative Radiological Assessment/Imaging (Fig. 7.5)

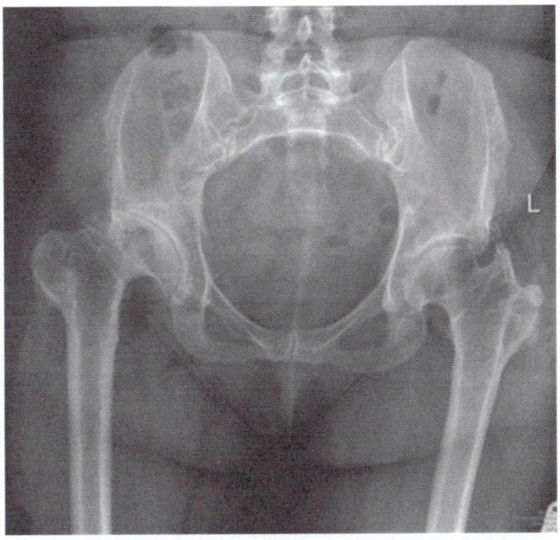

Fig. 7.5 AP X-ray of the right hip dysplasia of the proximal femur. It depicts a right hip varus osteotomy with metalwork removed, high-riding greater trochanter, flattened head, and elongated acetabulum. Significant lateralization of the acetabulum allowing potential roof coverage by deepening the acetabulum preparation while maintaining reasonable size of the socket implant

7.4.5 Preoperative Planning

Diagnosis: DDH Hartofilakidis 1 (Fig. 7.5)

Possible treatment options: A hybrid system is our choice due to the proximal femoral deformity. Equally an uncemented stem could be used; however, the junction of metaphysis/diaphysis is not predictably replaceable.

Chosen treatment method: Cemented hip stem Exeter 37.5–1,150 mm, ceramic femoral head 36 mm +2.5 mm, cancellous bone screw 6.5 mm (2 × 20 mm), uncemented acetabular shell 52 mm, acetabular liner 36 mm / 52 mm

Selection of implants if applicable and rational: the cemented stem is better situated in the proximal femoral dysplasia. Alternatively, a custom-made stem or a carefully templated uncemented nonanatomical tapered stem could fit this femur.

Expected difficulties: Acetabular reconstruction may need roof augmentation.

Strategies to overcome difficulties: Cemented stem to overcome the proximal femoral deformity and adjust leg length and offset

Templating: Current templating using the Exeter system in AP and lateral views 100% magnification

7.4.6 Surgical Note

With the patient in lateral decubitus position and using mini-posterior approach, the hip was exposed. The primary finding was the short relation of the soft tissues to the head and neck including the sciatic nerve that was identified and released proximally and distally to control its tension for the subsequent lengthening of the hip. The sort rotators and the posterior capsule were tagged using Ethibond suture number 5. The dislocation was difficult due to the significant capsular adhesions and shortening of the neck. The head was trimmed using an osteotome to facilitate dislocation and to approach the anterior part of the capsule, and the shrank rectus femoris tendon. The dislocation was done gradually and an extensive anterior capsular release performed that was redundant and thickened. The fibrotic tissue around the tensor fascia lata proximally and around the greater trochanter was released. The hip was eventually dislocated, and the neck was divided low to allow for leg length equalization avoiding the need for shortening osteotomy. Division of the rectus femoris tendon to help anterior displacement of the proximal femur.

Acetabular Preparation

The socket was found shallow and elongated. The anterior wall was identified as well as the posterior wall that was significantly strong and solid. The transverse ligament was recognised at the bottom of the socket, and the true floor was found after digging down the medial wall just above the transverse ligament. A small-diameter reamer 44 mm was then used to initiate the reaming and to establish the medial wall. The orientation of the reamer was vertical down to the teardrop and backward against the posterior wall. The subsequent reaming enlarged the diameter without changing the orientation of the socket. That brought us up to 51 mm diameter reamer with good roof coverage; a 52 mm uncemented shell was then inserted tightly and two 30 mm screws put against the roof. Throughout the process of acetabular reaming, attention was pointed toward the anterior wall to avoid thinning and fracture; thus, power was directed backward as the posterior wall was robust and stable. Another point of reference was the transverse ligament against which the reaming was directed and then upward against the roof where the acetabulum contains the largest amount of cancellous bone. Employing the above maneuver, the roof was shaped to cover the periphery of the shell.

Stem Preparation

The stem was easily inserted binding the canal through the piriformis fossa. Limited to zero degrees of anteversion to compensate for the already anteverted neck and proximal femur was used. Protection of the greater trochanter was of great importance to maintain the abductors. Third-generation cementing technique as described in previous sections of the book was employed using the Exeter system and a 37.5 mm offset stem and a 36 mm ceramic head +2.5 mm. Easy reduction and equal leg length were established (Fig. 7.6).

7.4.7 Postoperative Radiographs (Figs. 7.6 and 7.7)

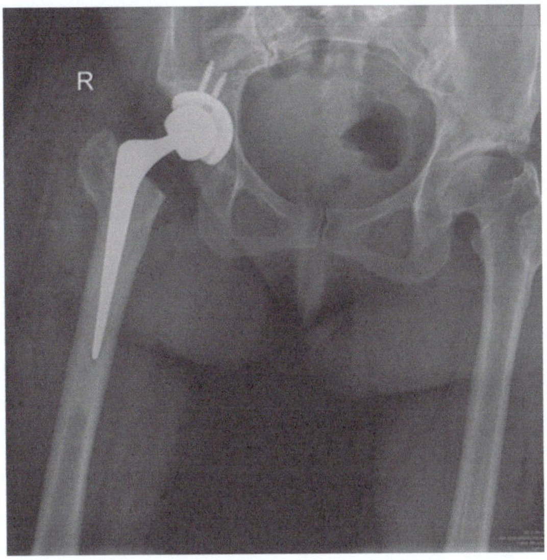

Fig. 7.6 Proper cementation and alignment of the stem. AP x-ray of the right hip at the first postoperative day

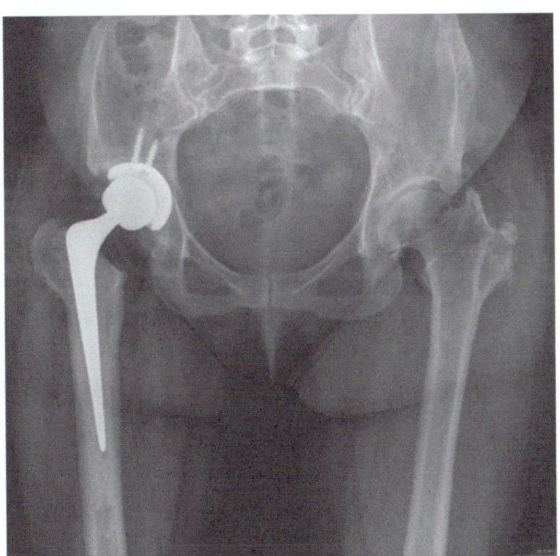

Fig. 7.7 AP X-ray of the right hip at the first postoperative month. The acetabular component is a few mm above the teardrop deep inside the cancellous bone of the socket roof with good coverage and screw purchase unchanged at 12-month follow-up

7.4.8 Postoperative Management

Chemoprophylaxis and anticoagulant treatment period: Vancomycin 500 mg (one dose preoperatively and two doses postoperatively), cefuroxime 1.5 g (one dose preoperatively and two doses postoperatively), enoxaparin 1x1 for 35 days

Gait/limb loading until full loading: Partial weight bearing for 4 weeks and then full-weight bearing as tolerated

7.5 Case Title: THA Following a Previous Proximal Femoral Osteotomy

Peter Mertens and Karl Brabants

7.5.1 Demographics

Age: 40
Sex: F
BMI: 24

7.5.2 Relevant Past Medical History

Principal pathologies: Coxarthrosis following a previous proximal femoral osteotomy

Previous surgical procedures: Proximal femoral osteotomy

Medication: Paracetamol

History of presenting complaint: After a corrective osteotomy at 8 years, the patient complained of progressive pain, limping, and limitation of mobility. A limb shortening of 3 cm is noted. Endorotation of the leg

7.5.3 Clinical Examination

Symptoms: Pain, limping, internal rotation of the leg

Range of motion: Flexion 40°, impossible rotation, extension 0°

Main disability: Limping, pain, leg - shortening

Neurovascular evaluation: Intact

7.5.4 Preoperative Radiological Assessment/Imaging (Figs. 7.8, 7.9, and 7.10)

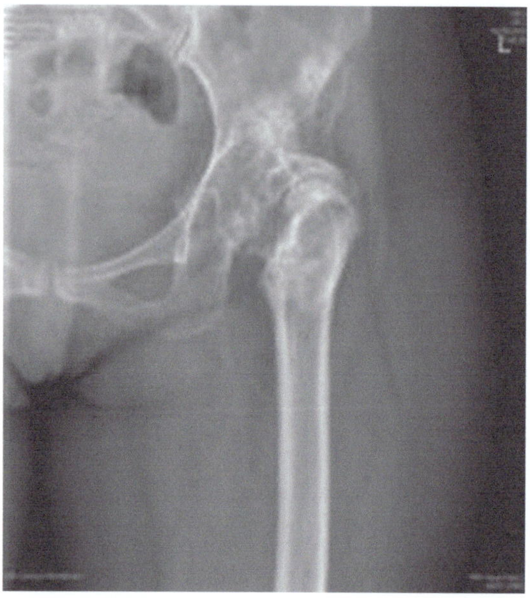

Fig. 7.8 AP x-ray of the left hip

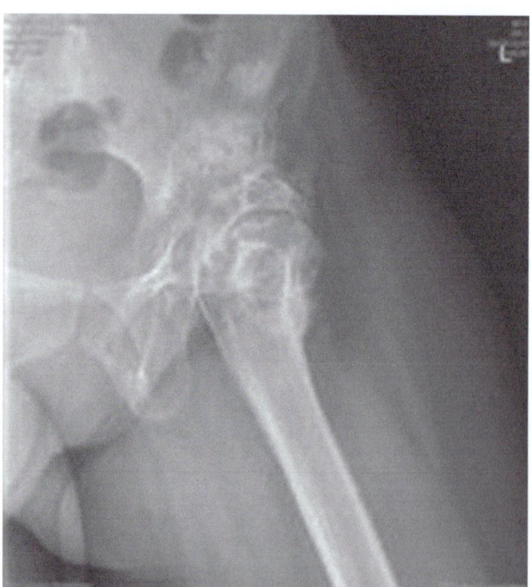

Fig. 7.9 Lateral x-ray of the left hip

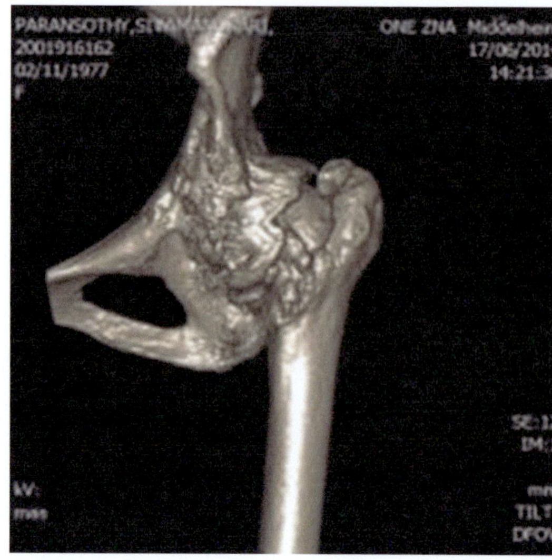

Fig. 7.10 Preoperative CT to evaluate the acetabulum

7.5.5 Preoperative Planning

Diagnosis: Secondary coxarthrosis (Figs. 7.8, 7.9, and 7.10)

Possible treatment options: Osteotomy + THR

Chosen treatment method: THR

Selection of implants if applicable and rational: R3 cup and Spectron cemented hip prosthesis (Smith & Nephew)

Expected difficulties: The instability and the abnormal anatomy due to the previous trochanteric osteotomy, the size of the stem (small patient), the plate at the distal femur (problems with the length of long stems) and the correction of the endorotation

Strategies to overcome difficulties: A cemented and an uncemented stem were available.

7.5.6 Surgical Note

Patient's position: Lateral decubitus

Type of anesthesia: General

Surgical approach: Anterolateral approach

Main steps: Osteotomy of the femoral neck. Visualization of the acetabulum, reaming to achieve an adequate coverage of the cup. Fixation with three screws. Reaming for the femoral stem (Figs. 7.11 and 7.12)

7.5.7 Intraoperative Challenges

Challenges and solutions: Due to the previous trochanteric osteotomy, the trochanter was rotated and caused impingement and instability perioperatively.

Unanticipated problems and solution: A decision was made to use a cemented stem in the most stable position, not taking the trochanter into account.

Thorough description of decision-making, including the reason for the final decision: The rotated trochanter was not anticipated. Possible solutions were derotation osteotomy, fixation with plate or long stem, or usage of a short cemented stem with sufficient offset to avoid impingement. A short tapered cementless stem was tested, but no fixation was achieved preoperatively, and the posterior impingement problem was not solved. Then a cemented stem was used and rotated to avoid impingement and correct the malrotation

7.5.8 Postoperative Radiographs (Figs. 7.11 and 7.12)

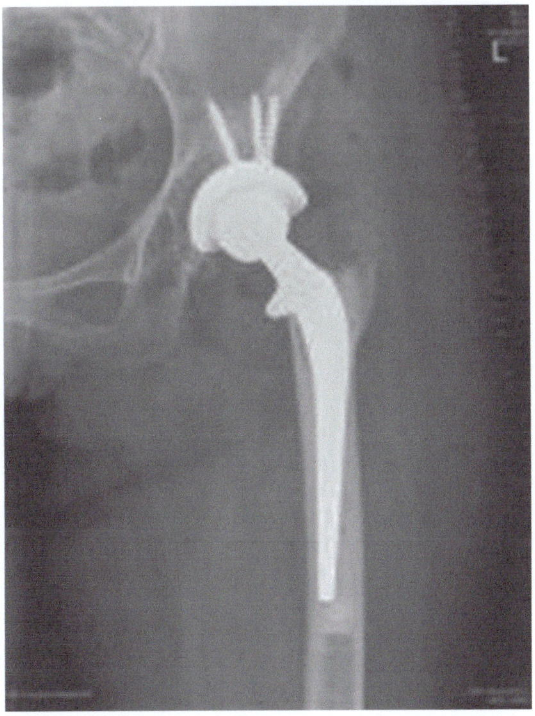

Fig. 7.11 AP x-ray of the left THA

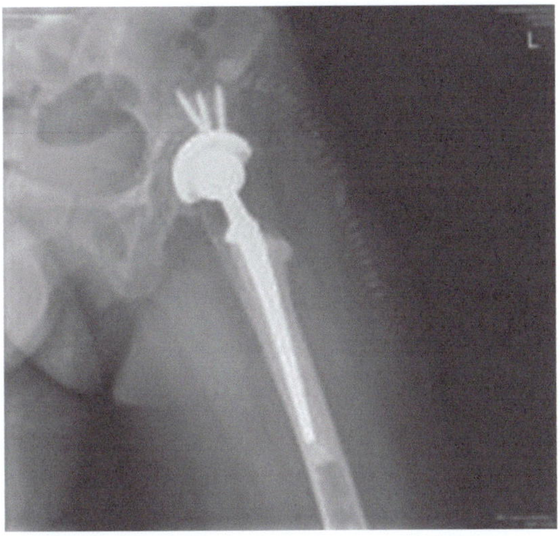

Fig. 7.12 Lateral x-ray of the left THA

7.5.9 Postoperative Management

Chemoprophylaxis and anticoagulant treatment period: Rivaroxaban 10 mg for 30 days

Gait/limb loading until full loading: Partial weight bearing for six weeks

7.5.10 Discussion [21–23]

Advantages of the applied method: Straightforward procedure, no healing of osteotomy necessary, lengthening possible

Disadvantages of the method: Abductor insufficiency, prolonged physiotherapy necessary

Alternative evidence-based techniques for the case: A high-cost custom-made implant

Why is the chosen technique better for this case? Less invasive, immediate weight bearing is tolerated. Low cost

Learning curve and how to manage complications: Planning is needed; evaluation of the acetabulum and trochanteric area is necessary. All options (cemented cup, cemented and cementless stem, revision stem) should be available. The patient should even have consented to a Girdlestone procedure.

7.6 Case Title: Conversion (Childhood Proximal Femoral Osteotomy to Total Hip)

William L. Griffin

7.6.1 Demographics

Age: 50
Sex: Female
BMI: 32

7.6.2 Relevant Past Medical History

Principal pathologies: DDH right hip

Previous surgical procedures: Proximal femoral osteotomy as a child. Contralateral left total hip 2 years prior

History of presenting complaint: Increased pain, decreased ROM, sense of instability, and LLD over the past year unresponsive to NSAIDs

7.6.3 Clinical Examination

Symptoms: Pain with weight bearing and ROM of the right hip

Range of motion: 30° flexion contracture. Flexes to 80°. No rotation

Specific tests: Infection workup—Negative (ESR and CRP—normal)

Main disability: Pain and difficulty walking

Neurovascular evaluation: Neurovascular exam—normal

7.6.4 Preoperative Radiological Assessment/Imaging (Figs. 7.13 and 7.14)

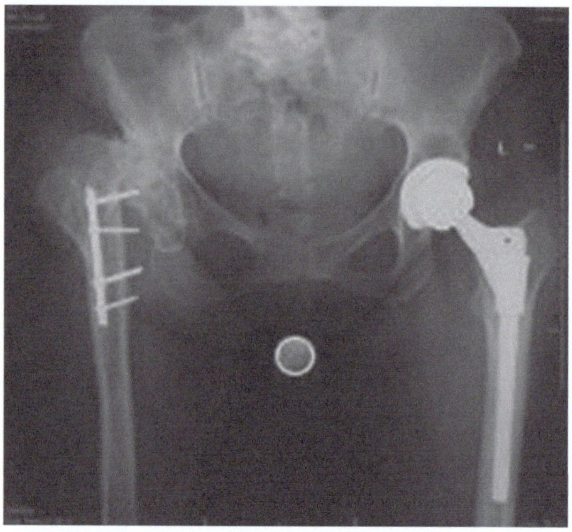

Fig. 7.13 AP pelvis: left, THA; right, Crowe III dysplasia with end-stage degenerative changes. Retained proximal femoral plate from prior proximal femoral osteotomy, now intramedullary due to bone overgrowth

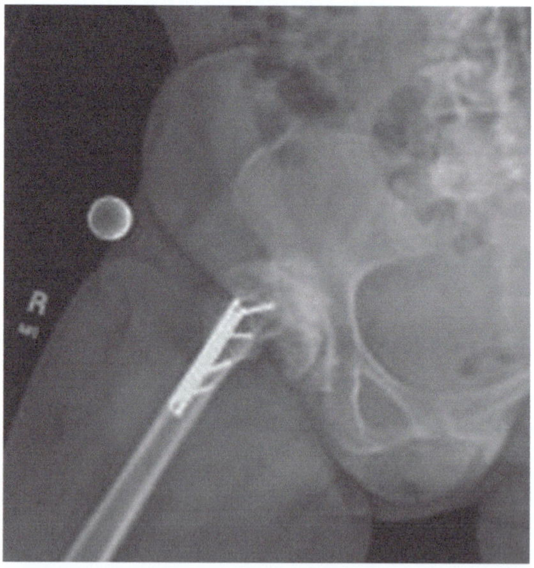

Fig. 7.14 Lateral X-ray right hip: demonstrating minimal femoral bow and a small canal diameter

7.6.5 Preoperative Planning

Diagnosis: Severe degenerative changes in the right hip due to DDH, with intramedullary retained hardware from the previous osteotomy (Figs. 7.13 and 7.14)

Possible treatment options: Right THA with removal of the hardware using either a trapdoor osteotomy or an extended trochanteric osteotomy

Chosen treatment method: Same

Selection of implants if applicable and rational: Cementless small acetabular component with medialization to obtain coverage support and press-fit fixation. A stem that will fit in this very small canal, allow anteversion adjustments, and bypass the cortical defect laterally. High-speed burr for lateral trapdoor osteotomy. Screw removal set for anticipated difficulty removing the old hardware

Expected difficulties: The hardware has been in place for 48 years. Removal will be difficult due to bone overgrowth. Cup fixation will be difficult in this dysplastic acetabulum. Regain as much length as possible without too much tension on the sciatic nerve.

Strategies to overcome difficulties: Open through of the bone to expose the retained plate using a pencil tip high-speed burr. Screw removal set. Use a small-diameter stem that will fit the narrow canal and allow for intraoperative adjustments to anteversion, offset, and ability to bypass lateral defect.

7.6.6 Surgical Note

Patient's position: Lateral

Type of anesthesia: General

Surgical approach: Posterior, to allow for more extensile approach if needed

Main steps: (1) Careful dislocation in this stiff hip to avoid fracture. (2) Femoral neck cut. (3) Release of gluteus maximus tendon and partial anterior capsulectomy to allow for adequate acetabular exposure and release of flexion contracture. Iliopsoas remained quite tight and also required a release. (4) Acetabular reaming to the true floor, medialization provides better superior support. Supplemental screw fixation. (5) Lateral trap door osteotomy to expose the retained plate. Removal of the plate and screws. (6) Flexible reamer to enlarge femoral canal. (7) Assess the soft tissue tension to determine the anticipated femoral head position relative to the trochanter.

Reconstruction techniques: Plate removal required removal of the screw heads with a carbide bit, then plate removal, followed by screw removal with the screw removal equipment. Center of rotation was made nearly anatomic with medialization of the acetabular reaming to the medial wall to allow for press-fit fixation and then the use of a + 4 mm lateralized polyethylene insert to restore offset. Femoral fixation was obtained using a monoblock small stature Wagner stem to allow for adjustments in anteversion and leg length while bypassing the lateral stress riser (Fig. 7.15).

7.6.7 Intraoperative Challenges

Challenges and solutions: (1) Cup fixation and position—Medialization for improved coverage and a lateralized poly to restore offset. (2) Hardware removal—Femoral osteotomy using a trapdoor technique and high-speed burr. Screw removal set for this 48-year-old plate and screws

Unanticipated problems and solution: Screw heads cold welded to plate. High-speed carbide bit to remove screw heads and then plate removal, followed by reverse threaded screw removal equipment

Thorough description of decision-making, including the reason for the final decision: Femoral reconstruction could have been achieved with a modular SROM-type implant to allow for anteversion and offset adjustments; however, the proximal femoral integrity was not strong enough for support of proximal sleeve fixation, and we elected to use a monoblock Wagner-style stem with more distal fixation.

7.6.8 Postoperative Radiographs (Fig. 7.15)

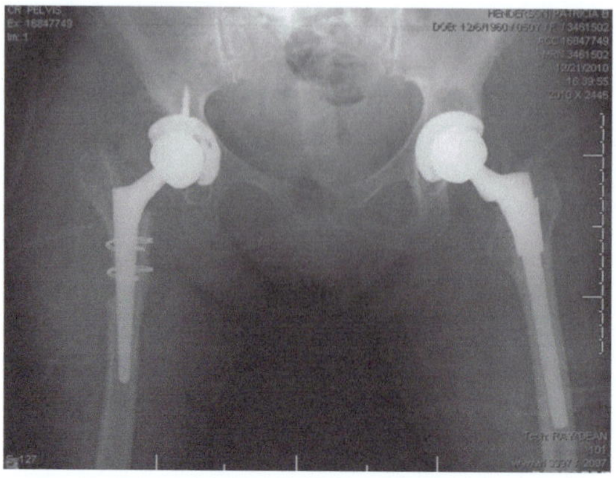

Fig. 7.15 Postoperative AP pelvis X-ray: Acetabulum medialized to the medial wall. Larger than anticipated acetabular size due the wider than expected AP dimension of the native acetabulum. Trapdoor osteotomy secured with cerclage wires. Monoblock Wagner stem with distal fixation to protect weakened proximal femur

7.6.9 Postoperative Management

Chemoprophylaxis and anticoagulant treatment period: Standard DVT prophylaxis for high-risk patients was used in this case (Coumadin × 4 weeks).

Gait/limb loading until full loading: Due to the weakened nature of the femur, the patient was limited to touchdown weight bearing for six weeks.

7.6.10 Follow Up and Discussion [24–26]

Alternative evidence-based techniques for the case: This particular case provided a number of unusual challenges including (1) acetabular fixation, (2) hardware removal, (3) femoral fixation, and (4) leg length discrepancy along with soft tissue balancing. There may have been a number of different ways to handle these challenges, and there is no entirely correct answer. Ideally I prefer to remove the least amount of retained hardware that I can get away with, but in this case, I don't think this was an option. Both acetabular and femoral fixation could have been achieved with the use of cement. However, the damaged femur is not suited for adequate cement technique.

Learning curve and how to manage complications: Preoperative planning is crucial in these complex cases. The severe dysplasia alone requires planning to accommodate small acetabular and femoral sizes, acetabular fixation, and soft tissue contractures. The retained hardware adds another level of complexity to the case. Hardware removal requires planning for osteotomies, screw and plate removal difficulties, and the equipment needed to overcome these difficulties. Finally, femoral fixation in a damaged femur can be difficult, and backup options may be required.

7.7 Case Title: Total Hip Arthroplasty After Proximal Femoral Osteotomy

Derek Ward and Javad Parvizi

7.7.1 Demographics

Age: 48
Sex: Female
BMI: 27 kg/m^2

7.7.2 Relevant Past Medical History

Principal pathologies: Developmental dysplasia of the hip

Previous surgical procedures: Proximal femoral osteotomy (subtrochanteric, valgus producing)

Medication: Tramadol

History of presenting complaint: The patient presented with worsening left hip discomfort and a severe limp. The patient had a history of dysplasia with corrective proximal femoral surgery at a young age but had developed pain in her groin as a young adult. Conservative measures were employed, and the patient was able to function with varying degrees of pain until the prior six months when the pain became unbearable.

7.7.3 Clinical Examination

Symptoms: Pain with ambulation and hip range of motion. Pain with prolonged sitting

Range of motion: Left hip extension to 10°, flexion to 85°, external rotation to 15°, internal rotation to -5°, abduction to 10°, and adduction to 15°

Specific tests: Positive Trendelenburg gait, positive Trendelenburg sign, 1.5 cm limb length discrepancy with the left limb shorter, significant pain with straight leg raise, and the Stinchfield maneuver

Main disability: Pain with walking, difficulty with activities of daily living secondary to hip pain

Scoring if available: SF-36 outcome value 54. WOMAC outcome value 14. Harris Hip Score 48 points

Neurovascular evaluation: 2+ dorsalis pedis pulse, feet are warm and well perfused, motor function intact

7.7.4 Preoperative Radiological Assessment/Imaging (Figs. 7.16 and 7.17)

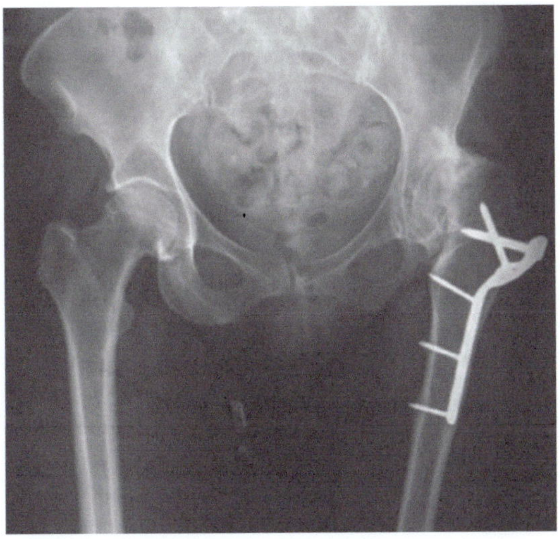

Fig. 7.16 Preoperative low AP pelvis showing left hip coxarthrosis with prior osteotomy hardware

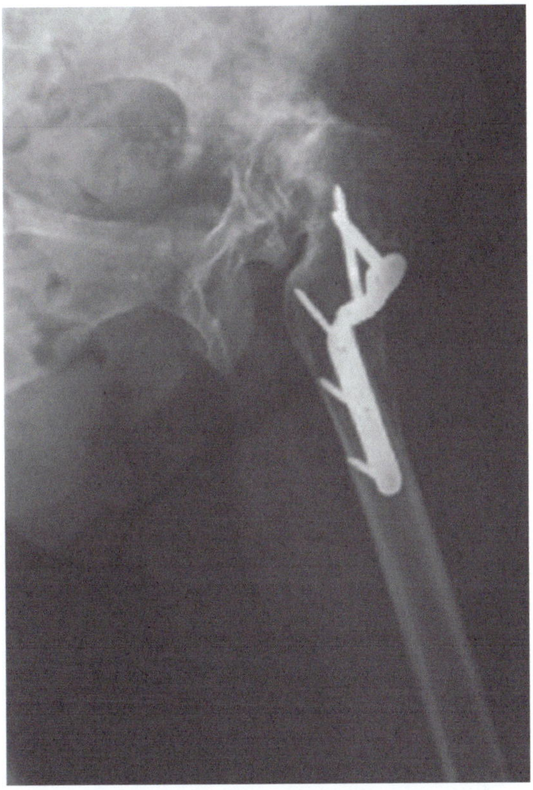

Fig. 7.17 Preoperative lateral x-ray of the left hip

7.7.5 Preoperative Planning

Diagnosis: Left hip coxarthrosis secondary to hip dysplasia in the setting of prior proximal femoral osteotomy and retained hardware (Figs. 7.16 and 7.17)

Possible treatment options: (1) Single-stage hardware removal, proximal femoral osteotomy, and uncemented total hip arthroplasty. (2) Single-stage hardware removal, proximal femoral osteotomy, and hybrid total hip arthroplasty with cemented femoral component. (3) Single-stage partial hardware removal and short-stem uncemented total hip arthroplasty. (4) Staged hardware removal with secondary uncemented or hybrid total hip arthroplasty with proximal femoral osteotomy. (5) Hip resurfacing

Chosen treatment method: Single-stage removal of hardware, proximal femoral osteotomy, and uncemented total hip arthroplasty

Selection of implants if applicable and rational: A modular femoral stem was utilized. The choice of this implant was based on the need for a proximal femoral osteotomy to correct the underlying deformity and the need to bypass the osteotomy for appropriate distal fixation combined with the ability of the implant to control the femoral version independent of distal fixation.

Expected difficulties: (1) Removal of hardware. (2) Need for a biplanar osteotomy. (3) Poor femoral and acetabular bone quality. (4) Shallow, anteverted, lateralized acetabulum with poor bone stock. (5) Risk of intraoperative fracture with hardware removal. (6) Possible presence of infection

Strategies to overcome difficulties: Appropriate hardware removal equipment and fixation options were made available. Equipment to allow for intraoperative flexibility and complications was made available including periprosthetic fracture fixation options and proximal femoral replacement. The removal of hardware was complicated by osseous overgrowth of the lateral plate as well as difficulty removing the screws. A metal-cutting burr was necessary for partial plate removal, while the main motion of the plate is retained as removal would have significantly compromised osseous integrity. A broken screw removal set was also used including trephines. The osteotomy was performed with the plate in place. Multiple cables were used, both as prophylaxis for fracture given poor bone quality and for stability of the osteotomy.

Templating: Osteotomy templating was done based on preoperative imaging.

7.7.6 Surgical Note

Patient's position: The patient was placed in a supine position with a 5 cm bump under the pelvis. This allowed for excellent intraoperative assessment of limb length.

Type of anesthesia: The patient received a spinal anesthesia.

Surgical approach: A direct lateral approach was utilized.

Main steps: Antibiotics and tranexamic acid were given. The patient's prior incision was incorporated and extended proximally and distally. Once the fascia was incised, the greater trochanter and vastus lateralis ridge were identified. The proximal aspect of the hardware was identified, and osseous overgrowth was removed over the proximal screw holes. The proximal screws were removed with some difficulty, and the proximal aspect of the plate was removed using a metal-cutting burr. A split was made in the abductors, and the anterior 40% of the abductors were incorporated into the capsulotomy and exposure. The hip was dislocated, the neck cut made, and the femoral head removed. Retractors were placed, and the acetabulum was reamed and a press-fit cup impacted into place. The proximal lateral aspect of the femur was then exposed to approach the planned osteotomy site. The remaining screws were removed with varying difficulty and screw breakage. The appropriate osteotomy site was at the level of the lateral plate; however, due to significant bone overgrowth, the choice was made to perform the osteotomy around the plate. The osteotomy was performed using a Gigli saw. The femoral canal distally was then reamed to an appropriate size implant for distal fixation. The proximal portion of the femur was then reamed to the appropriate size. The deformity was then corrected and trials placed. Trial reductions were performed, and the version was adjusted appropriately for stability. The final femoral component was placed, and a standard, layered closure was performed (Figs. 7.18 and 7.19).

Reconstruction techniques: Uncemented revision modular stem with primary press-fit acetabular component. Osteotomy fixed around the revision femoral stem using cables

7.7.7 Intraoperative Challenges

Challenges and solutions: A few major challenges were highlighted by this case. First, it is important to anticipate that any prior hardware, particularly those that have been in place for decades, are at times difficult to remove. Thus, all necessary equipment to remove the hardware including a broken screw set, high-speed burr, and any specialized removal equipment need to be available. Second, the presence of severe deformity necessitates an osteotomy. The type, location, and extent of the osteotomy need to be determined preoperatively based on detailed templating. The latter will determine what type of femoral component may be needed. The bone stock encountered in these patients is also unpredictable, and hence various modes of fixation for the stem need to be considered and made available during surgery.

Unanticipated problems and solution: We did not fully anticipate needing to retain the distal portion of the plate, and performing the osteotomy around this hardware was technically challenging. The solution to this was to recognize that removing the plate would have compromised the structural integrity of the proximal femur and increased the risk of nonunion. Performing the osteotomy with the plate in place required the use of a Gigli saw.

Thorough description of decision-making, including the reason for the final decision: The key of solution in our case was the estimation that given the retained hardware, the anticipated difficulty of removal, and the need for an osteotomy, a distal fixation would be important. With the need for an osteotomy choosing an uncemented implant where stability is independent of the osteotomy healing is also ideal. Given the proximal deformity and underlying dysplasia, an implant that allows for intraoperative adjustment of femoral version is also very helpful. The osteotomy was necessary in order to realign the patient's proximal femur to obtain fixation and restore the appropriate anatomy and biomechanics.

7.7.8 Postoperative Radiographs (Figs. 7.18 and 7.19)

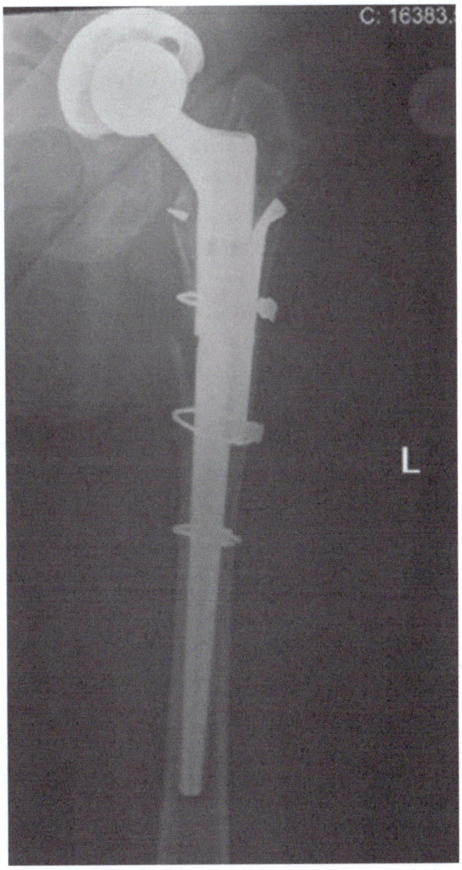

Fig. 7.18 Postoperative AP demonstrating appropriate fit of the modular revision stem as well as retained hardware and cable fixation

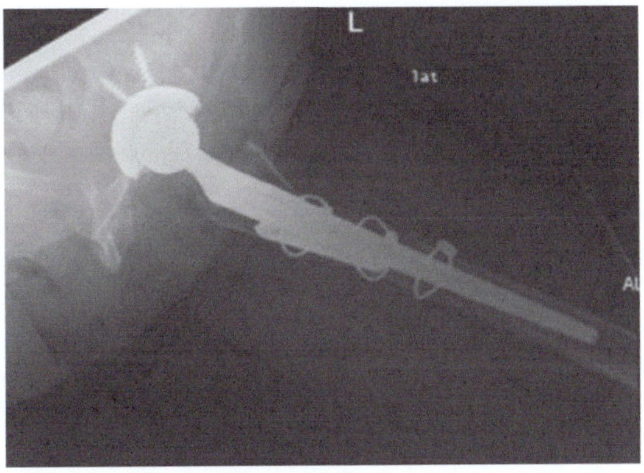

Fig. 7.19 Postoperative lateral

7.7.9 Postoperative Management

Chemoprophylaxis and anticoagulant treatment period: The patient was placed on standard postoperative antibiotics for 24 h. Aspirin 81 mg PO BID was utilized for DVT prophylaxis for four weeks.

Gait/limb loading until full loading: The patient was made touchdown weight bearing for six weeks.

7.7.10 Follow-Up and Complications

No complications at the last follow-up 4 years status post-procedure.

Scoring if available: SF-36 outcome value improved from 54 to 90. WOMAC outcome value improved from 14 to 6. HHS also improved from 48 points to 87 points.

7.7.11 Discussion

Advantages of the applied method: The advantages using a modular, distal-engaging femoral component include improved flexibility when dealing with a proximal osteotomy as well as intraoperative adjustment of femoral version.

Disadvantages of the method: Disadvantages of this method include the need for removal of all screws and prolonged recovery time associated with healing an osteotomy as well as the risks of nonunion.

Alternative evidence-based techniques for the case: Alternative techniques include partial removal of screws and use of a short femoral stem, a cemented implant with or without an osteotomy, or a hip resurfacing.

Why is the chosen technique better for this case? The use of distal fixation bypasses the issues of proximal poor bone stock, and the osteotomy allows for improved hip biomechanics.

Indications and contraindications for your technique: Indications include patients with appropriately healthy distal bone stock to employ cementless fixation. Contraindications include very poor bone stock in the osteopenia or osteoporotic patient or prior hardware that precludes removal.

Learning curve and how to manage complications: The surgeon should have multiple plans in place as well as all necessary equipment for primary, secondary, and tertiary options. An appropriately extensile approach should be chosen. Complications of particular import include nonunion of the osteotomy which may necessitate revision surgery and bone grafting. Optimization of the patient to prevent this complication is warranted including appropriate nutrition and smoking cessation. Stable fixation is paramount.

Level of evidence concerning the superiority of this method against others: Proximal femoral deformities encountered during primary total hip arthroplasty stem from a variety of disorders and encompass a spectrum of challenges. Deformity may result from prior femoral neck or proximal femur fracture, dysplasia, prior osteotomy, Paget's disease, fibrous dysplasia, and congenital bowing to name a few. Management of deformity includes considerations for prior hardware and surgical approach, risk of dislocation, canal stenosis, engagement of the chosen prosthesis and subsequent risk for loosening, as well as the possible need for osteotomy (for shortening or realignment). The majority of evidence for treatment of proximal femoral deformity lies in small case series with the most common use of osteotomy in primary total hip from series of patients with hip dysplasia and high hip dislocations. A series published from our institution of 56 hips with proximal femoral deformities treated with uncemented prosthesis showed that non-primary components were utilized in 25% of cases and 23% of cases required an osteotomy. In this series, patients had significant functional improvement. The revision rate was 3.5%, and the mechanical failure (radiographic failure plus revision) rate was 9% (5 hips) at an average follow-up of 4 years [25]. Charity et al. reported on 15 hips with Crowe IV dysplasia undergoing THA with a subtrochanteric osteotomy and a cemented prosthesis with a mean follow-up of 114 months. All of the patients had significant improvement in functional scores and range of motion. One femur had to be revised for nonunion [27]. A similar retrospective study by Krych et al. of uncemented prostheses in 24 patients with Crowe IV hip dysplasia also showed significant improvements in function and hip scores. In this series, there were two nonunions and one loosening of the femoral stem [28]. These series demonstrated that both cemented and non-cemented components may be used with success. All the case series demonstrate a relatively higher complication rate than standard primary total hip replacement but with overall good outcomes.

7.8 Case Title: Total Hip Replacement in the Setting of a Previous Proximal Femoral Valgus Osteotomy

Rajiv Merchant and Eric Masterson

7.8.1 Demographics

Age: 51 years
Sex: Female

7.8.2 Relevant Past Medical History

Principle Pathologies: Long-standing bilateral dislocated hips

Previous Surgical Procedures: Bilateral Schanz (valgus) osteotomies some years ago. The plate had been removed from the left side, and broken screws were left in situ. The plate on the right side remained in situ. The screws were of the old flat-head design.

Medication: Not on significant medication

7.8.3 History of Presenting Complaint/Clinical Examination

Pain in both hips: Difficulty in range of movement with reduced walking distance. Considerable reduction in the ability to perform daily activities. Extremely poor walking with a marked bilateral Trendelenburg gait using two crutches.

7.8.4 Preoperative Radiological Assessment/Imaging (Figs. 7.20 and 7.21)

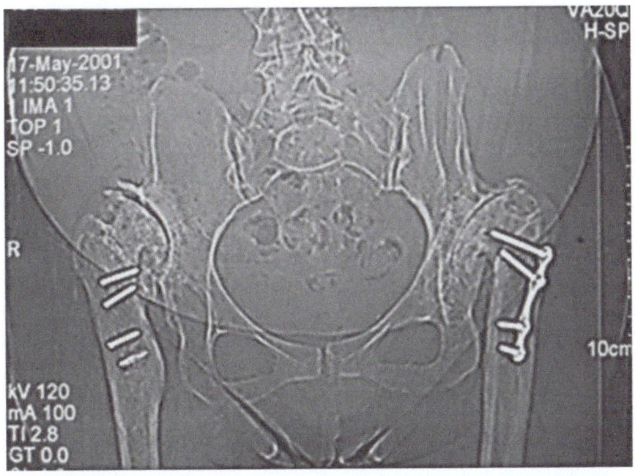

Fig. 7.20 CT scanogram showing the preoperative deformity

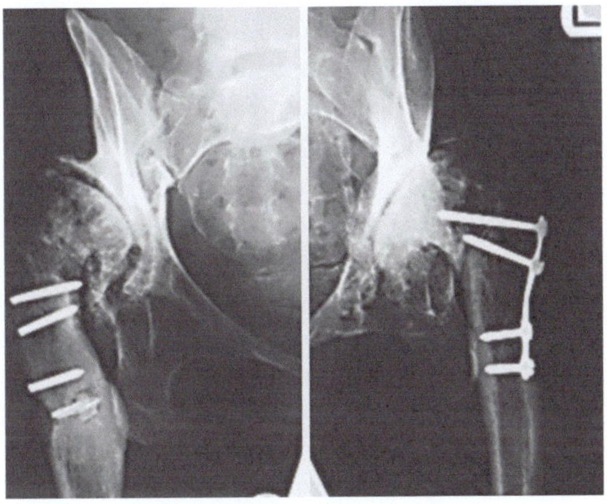

Fig. 7.21 Plain AP radiographs

7.8.5 Preoperative Planning (Figs. 7.20 and 7.21)

Diagnosis: Bilateral developmental dysplasia of the hip with chronic dislocation and false acetabuli. Previous varus osteotomies both sides (Figs. 7.20 and 7.21)

Possible treatment options: (1) Nonoperative management with walking aids and analgesia. (2) Bilateral total hip replacements

Chosen treatment method: Removal of metal, trochanteric slide osteotomy, uncemented cup in anatomical position, and CDH stem implantation

7.8.6 Selection of Implants and Rationale

Acetabular components: Porous-coated Mallory-Head shell (Biomet, Zimmer Biomet, Warsaw, Indiana) and RingLoc ArCom Acetabular Liner with a high wall (Biomet, Zimmer Biomet, Warsaw, Indiana)

Femoral Components: CDH total hip system porous and HA-coated femoral stem (Biomet, Zimmer Biomet, Warsaw, Indiana), a modular head 22.2 mm with -5 neck (Biomet, Zimmer Biomet, Warsaw, Indiana)

Rationale: Uncemented components were chosen due to the relatively young age of the patient and good-quality bone. A high posterior lipped polyethylene insert was used to minimize the risk of dislocation. Specialized CDH system was used due to the complex nature of the femoral reconstruction.

Expected Difficulties: (1) Removing the existing metalwork. (2) The extent of soft tissue contracture. (3) Appropriate cup orientation and combined version in the absence of a normal femoral anatomy

Strategies to overcome difficulty: Extent of femoral resection required, size of the trochanteric fragment, the diameter of the femoral canal, and acetabular size using the AP diameter must be assessed.

7.8.7 Surgical Note

Patient's position: On the side with an anterior support at the abdomen and posterior sacral support. A cushion was used under bony prominences and torso. Arms were positioned on arm boards.

Type of anesthesia: Spinal anesthesia

Surgical approach: A trochanteric slide osteotomy

Main steps: A broken screw removal set was used to extract the old metalwork. A trochanteric slide osteotomy was performed to keep the attached musculature. The remaining proximal femur was resected. The true acetabulum was identified and cleared. It was reamed up to 42 mm. No further reaming was possible due to the thinning of the anterior column. A same size Mallory-Head shell was inserted and fixation augmented with one self-tapping low-profile screw. The femoral canal was prepared to size 11 mm. An 11 femoral CDH stem was trialled with a –5 mm neck 22.5 mm head. The reduction was stable in all range of movement. The sciatic nerve was found to be under mild tension. After implantation, the trochanter was reduced and fixed with a cable grip and two cables. The soft tissue was closed with 2 Vicryl, 0 Vicryl, and 2-0 Nylon (Fig. 7.22). One month later, a similar procedure was performed for the left hip except for an 8 mm CDH femoral stem used (Fig. 7.23).

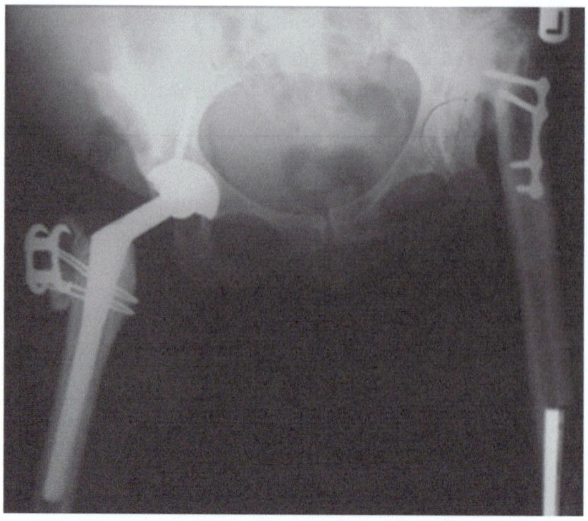

Fig. 7.22 Left THR with the head in anatomical location, comparison with the deformity on the right

Reconstruction techniques: The angulated dislocated femur was resected. A trochanteric slide osteotomy facilitated keeping the muscular attachment which was then reduced to the remaining femur.

7.8.8 Intraoperative Challenges

Challenges and solutions: **(1)** Visualizing and identifying the acetabulum. The acetabulum was identified by removing a large volume of the redundant capsule. A bone lever was then introduced into the obturator foramen inferiorly to obtain an adequate view. **(2)** Protection of the sciatic nerve. The hip was reduced with the knee in a flexed position and then gradually extended along with continually assessing the tension on the nerve. **(3)** Reattaching the osteotomy. The receiving surfaces were made even using a burr.

7.8.9 Postoperative Radiographs (Figs. 7.23 and 7.24)

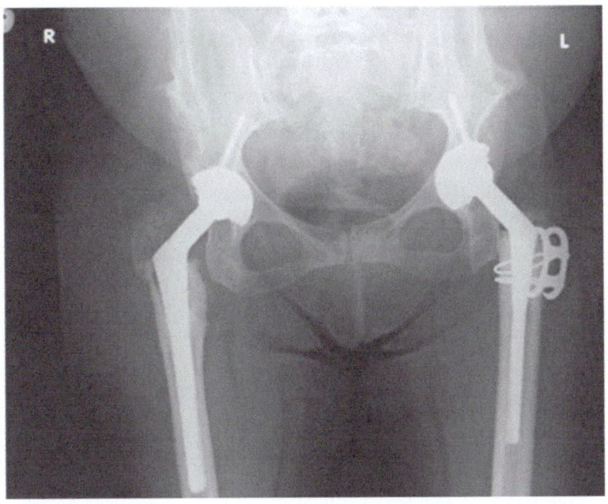

Fig. 7.23 Postoperative X-ray 3 years after surgery

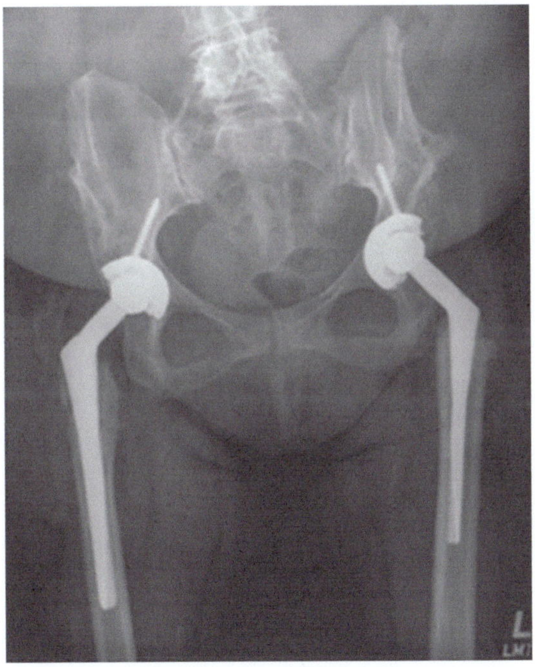

Fig. 7.24 X-ray 10 years after surgery

7.8.10 Postoperative Management

Chemoprophylaxis and anticoagulant treatment: Two doses of IV cefuroxime 750 mg. Three days of subcutaneous enoxaparin 40 mg and then switched to rivaroxaban 10 mg oral for 32 days. Mechanical thromboprophylaxis in the form of TED stockings was applied for six weeks.

Gait/limb loading until full loading: The patient was nursed in an abduction and hip flexion for 48 hours postsurgery due to stretching of the sciatic nerve. Non-weight bearing for six weeks

7.8.11 Follow-Up and Complications

The right total hip replacement required removal of Dall-Miles cable grip due to soft tissue irritation 1 year after surgery. She was left with a persistent trochanteric nonunion.

The left total hip replacement dislocated two days postsurgery. The patient underwent closed reduction of the hip. On screening, the instability manifested in full extension and force external rotation. This was managed in a hip spica applied to the patient standing and hip in mild abduction and flexion for six weeks. Two months later, the patient underwent revision surgery on the left hip due to recurrent instability. The acetabular liner was removed, and the high lip was oriented anteriorly as opposed to posterior. The head was changed from -5 neck to 0 mm neck. A small piece of the ischium which was impinging on the hip was removed. The patient was then placed in a hip spica cast for six weeks as treated previously.

7.8.12 Discussion

Advantage of the applied method: Adequate exposure. Due to the number of previous surgeries, it is anticipated that finding the true acetabulum and appropriate reaming would be challenging. Exposure is key. A traditional anterolateral of posterior approach is not sufficient. Also due to the chronic shortening, a proximal femoral resection would be essential to prevent stretching of the sciatic nerve. Therefore, a trochanteric slide osteotomy can allow for both resection and exposure.

Disadvantages of the method: Problems of the bone union can occur after osteotomy as was the case in our patient.

Alternative evidence-based techniques: The above case is a Crowe IV-type dysplastic hip with previous non-arthroplasty surgeries. Any arthroplasty procedure needs to be tailored to the patient due to high variability. While a one-size-fits-all approach may not be adequate, in the literature, two general types of procedures have been described. The first is a sequential resection of the femur along with a greater trochanter osteotomy. This allows for the abductors to remain attached, albeit with an increased risk of nonunion and possible difficulty in seating the final implant. It is also not possible to use cemented stems as there is no medial support in the remaining femur [29]. The other type of femoral reconstruction described is a subtrochanteric osteotomy, which has the advantages of preserving the metaphysical bone, derotating the femur, and allowing shortening osteotomies as required [28].

Why the chosen technique is better: It is the senior authors' experience that acetabular exposure and femoral implantation and assessment of version are easier with the technique described above.

Indications and contraindications of your technique: This technique is useful in Crowe IV-type DDH. It must not be used if the trochanteric bone stock is poor from the outset and if a large segment of femur needs to be excised. This technique must also be used with caution as serial trialing can cause injury to the sciatic nerve.

Learning curve and how to manage complications: In our experience, the above patient experiences significant morbidity due to her left hip dislocations. In hindsight it was noted that her femoral stem may have been slightly anteverted. Achieving appropriate version can be challenging, especially in the absence of normal bone anatomy. This case was performed at a time when appropriate abduction braces were not available. It is the authors' routine practice to apply an abduction brace after complex reconstruction/revision hip arthroplasty.

References

1. Haverkamp D, de Jong PT, Marti RK. Intertrochanteric osteotomies do not impair long-term outcome of subsequent cemented total hip arthroplasties. Clin Orthop Relat Res. 2006;444:154.
2. Zweifel J, Hönle W, Schuh A. Long-term results of intertrochanteric varus osteotomy for dysplastic osteoarthritis of the hip. Int Orthop (SICOT). 2011;35:1–12.
3. Kawasaki M, Hasegawa Y, Sakano S, et al. Total hip arthroplasty after failed transtrochanteric rotational osteotomy for avascular necrosis of the femoral head. J Arthroplast. 2005;20(5):574.
4. Merle C, Marcus R. Streit & Moritz Innmann & Tobias Gotterbarm & Peter R. Aldinger Long-term results of cementless femoral reconstruction following intertrochanteric osteotomy International Orthopaedics (SICOT). 2012;36:1123–8.
5. Breusch SJ, Lukoschek M, Thomsen M, Mau H, Ewerbeck V, Aldinger PR. Ten-year results of uncemented hip stems for failed intertrochanteric osteotomy. Arch Orthop Trauma Surg. 2005;125:304–9.
6. Suzuki K, Kawachi S, Matsubara M, Morita S, Jinno T, Shinomiya K. Cementless total hip replacement after previous intertrochanteric valgus osteotomy for advanced osteoarthritis. J Bone Joint Surg (Br). 2007;89-B:1155–7.
7. Ferguson GM, Cabanela ME, Ilstrup DM. Total hip arthroplasty after failed intertrochanteric osteotomy. J Bone Joint Surg Br. 1994;76-B:252.
8. Boos N, Krushell R, Ganz R, et al. Total hip arthroplasty after previous proximal femoral osteotomy. J Bone Joint Surg Br. 1997;79(2):247.
9. Iwase T, Hasegawa Y, Iwasada S, et al. Total hip arthroplasty after failed intertrochanteric valgus osteotomy for advanced osteoarthrosis. Clin Orthop Relat Res. 1999;364:175.
10. Shinar AA, Harris WH. Cemented total hip arthroplasty following previous femoral osteotomy: an average 16-year follow-up study. J Arthroplast. 1998;13(3):243–53.
11. Park K-S, Tumin M, Peni I, Yoon T-R. Conversion total hip arthroplasty after previous transtrochanteric rotational osteotomy for osteonecrosis of the femoral head. J Arthroplast. 2014;29:813–6.
12. Lee YK, Ha YC, Kim KC, et al. Total hip arthroplasty after previous transtrochanteric anterior rotational osteotomy for femoral head osteonecrosis. J Arthroplast. 2009;24(8):1205.
13. Takegami Y, Komatsu D, Seki T, Ishiguro N, Hasegawa Y. Total hip arthroplasty after failed curved intertrochanteric varus osteotomy for avascular necrosis of the femoral head Nagoya. J Med Sci. 2016;78(1):89–97.
14. Parsch D, Jung AW, Thomsen M, Ewerbeck V, Aldinger PR. Good survival of uncemented tapered stems for failed intertrochanteric osteotomy: a mean 16 year follow-up study in 45 patients. Arch Orthop Trauma Surg. 2008;128:1081–5.
15. Rijnen WH, Lameijn N, Schreurs BW, et al. Total hip arthroplasty after failed treatment for osteonecrosis of the femoral head. Orthop Clin North Am. 2009;40(2):291.
16. Soballe K, Boll KL, Kofod S, et al. Total hip replacement after medial-displacement osteotomy of the proximal part of the femur. J Bone Joint Surg Am. 1989;71(5):692.

17. Benke GJ, Baker AS, Dounis E. Total hip arthroplasty after upper femoral osteotomy: a clinical review. J Bone Joint Surg Br. 1982;64-B:570.
18. Echeverri A, Shelley P, Wroblewski BM. Long-term results of hip arthroplasty for failure of previous surgery. J Bone Joint Surg. 1988;70b:49–51.
19. Suominen S, Antti-Poika I, Santavirta S, et al. Total hip replacement after intertrochanteric osteotomy. Orthopedics. 1991;14:253.
20. Duncan S. ScottWingerter, Angela Keith, Susan a. Fowler, John Clohisy. Does previous osteotomy compromise Total hip Arthroplasty? A systematic review. J Arthroplast. 2015;30:79–85.
21. Takao M, et al. Cementless modular total hip arthroplasty with subtrochanteric shortening osteotomy for hips with developmental dysplasia. J Bone Joint Surg Am. 2011;93:548–55.
22. Bali K, et al. Subcapital osteotomy of the femoral neck for patients with healed slipped capital femoral epiphysis. Bone Joint J. 2014;96-B:1441–8.
23. Imbuldeniya AM, et al. Cementless total hip replacement without femoral osteotomy in patients with severe developmental dysplasia of the hip. Bone Joint J. 2014;96-B:1449–54.
24. Woodcock J, Larson AN, Mabry TM, Stans AA. Do retained pediatric implants impact later total hip arthroplasty? J Pediatr Orthop. 2013;33(3):339–44.
25. Mortazavi SM, Restrepo C, Kim PJ, Parvizi J, Hozack WJ. Cementless femoral reconstruction in patients with proximal femoral deformity. J Arthroplasty. 2011;26(3):354–9.
26. Faldini C, Miscione MT, Chehrassan M, Acri F, Pungetti C, d'Amato M, Luciani D, Giannini S. Congenital hip dysplasia treated by total hip arthroplasty using cementless tapered stem in patients younger than 50 years old: results after 12-years follow-up. J Orthop Traumatol. 2011;12(4):213–8.
27. Charity JA, Tsiridis E, Sheeraz A, Howell JR, Hubble MJ, Timperley AJ, et al. Treatment of Crowe IV high hip dysplasia with total hip replacement using the Exeter stem and shortening derotational subtrochanteric osteotomy. J Bone Joint Surg Br. 2011;93:34–8. https://doi.org/10.1302/0301-620X.93B1.24689.
28. Krych AJ, Howard JL, Trousdale RT, Cabanela ME, Berry DJ. Total hip arthroplasty with shortening subtrochanteric osteotomy in Crowe type-IV developmental dysplasia: surgical technique. J Bone Joint Surg Am. 2010;92(Suppl 1 Pt 2):176–87. https://doi.org/10.2106/JBJS.J.00061.
29. Perry KI, Berry DJ. Femoral considerations for total hip replacement in hip dysplasia. Orthop Clin North Am United States. 2012;43(3):377–86.

8 Posttraumatic Hip Osteoarthritis

Eustathios Kenanidis, Vasileios Lampridis, Iakovos Vlastos, Eleftherios Tsiridis, Goran Bicanic, Zoran Sulje, Domagoj Delimar, Bogdan Deleanu, John B. Meding, E. Michael Keating, and Tatsuya Sueyoshi

8.1 Current Concepts

E. Kenanidis, V. Lampridis, I. Vlastos, and E. Tsiridis

8.1.1 General

Posttraumatic hip osteoarthritis is usually the result of complex injuries of the acetabulum or intraarticular hip fractures. Acetabular fractures are severe injuries with increased morbidity [1]. The prevalence of acetabular fractures has a bimodal distribution: a young group following a high-energy trauma and an older group with frequent falls and osteoporosis [2, 3]. The gold standard of treatment for displaced fractures is the open reduction and internal fixation that aims to restore the joint congruency and to avoid the development of posttraumatic osteoarthritis. Nonoperative treatment is indicative for minimally displaced (<2 mm) acetabular fractures [4]. Posttraumatic arthritis can be also the result of failed internal fixation of hip fractures [5].

Posttraumatic OA results from imperfect reduction or failed fracture fixation, missed or untreated osteochondral defects or chondrolysis due to trauma and avascular necrosis of the head [6]. Sufficient anatomic reduction of acetabular fractures is usually achieved; however, in some

E. Kenanidis, M.D., Ph.D., M.Sc. (✉)
V. Lampridis, M.D., M.Sc. (H.C.M.), F.E.B.O.T. · I. Vlastos, M.D.
Academic Orthopaedic Unit, Aristotle University Medical School, Thessaloniki, Greece

E. Tsiridis, M.D., Ph.D., F.A.C.S., F.R.C.S. (✉)
Academic Orthopaedic Unit, Papageorgiou General Hospital, Aristotle University Medical School, Thessaloniki, Greece
e-mail: etsiridis@doctors.org.uk

G. Bicanic, M.D., Ph.D.
Al Zahra Hospital Dubai, Dubai, UAE
e-mail: goran@bicanic.eu

Z. Sulje, M.D.
Department of Orthopaedic Surgery and Traumatology, University Hospital Centre Zagreb, Zagreb, Croatia

D. Delimar, M.D., Ph.D.
University of Zagreb, School of Medicine, Zagreb, Croatia

Department of Orthopaedic Surgery, University Hospital Centre Zagreb, Zagreb, Croatia
e-mail: domagoj.delimar@kbc-zagreb.hr

B. Deleanu, M.D., Ph.D.
Pius Branzeu Emergency Clinical County Hospital, Timisoara, Romania

Victor Babes University of Medicine and Pharmacy, Timisoara, Romania

J.B. Meding, M.D. · E. Michael Keating, M.D.
The Center for Hip and Knee Surgery, St. Francis Hospital, Mooresville, IN, USA

T. Sueyoshi, M.D., Ph.D.
Kobe City Medical Center General Hospital, Kobe, Japan

E. Tsiridis (ed.), *The Adult Hip - Master Case Series and Techniques*,
https://doi.org/10.1007/978-3-319-64177-5_8

series secondary hip arthritis has been reported at a range of 17–67% [1, 2, 7, 8]. Immediate total hip arthroplasty is an option in older patients with a fracture pattern that either has significant involvement of the posterior wall and comminution or associated significant impaction of the femoral head articular surface. This, however, represents a small subset of patients [9].

Posttraumatic hip arthritis has a diverse clinical picture. The possible patterns of deformity are the following:

(a) Hip arthritis with residual incongruency of the fracture after ORIF.
(b) Displaced acetabular or femoral head fractures following conservative treatment.
(c) Hip arthritis due to failed internal fixation of the acetabulum or femoral head. Loose hardware, columnar fracture nonunion or malunion, subluxation and avascular bone fragments are other possible findings.
(d) Complex fractures with persistent dislocation.

The potential technical challenges or difficulties that a surgeon could face during THA for posttraumatic hip OA are the following [8–10]:

1. Residual pelvic deformity
2. Acetabular bone loss
3. Possible non-united fractures or necrotic fracture fragment/osteonecrosis
4. Retained hardware
5. Undetected infection
6. Heterotopic ossification
7. Extensive scarring
8. Risk of sciatic nerve injury
9. Longer operating time and higher transfusion need

8.1.2 Indications for Delayed THA Following Acetabular Fractures

1. Posttraumatic hip arthritis [6]
2. Avascular necrosis of the femoral head [11]
3. A salvage procedure following failed ORIF
4. Pain and stiffness interfering with daily motions, followed by radiological signs compatible with advanced arthritis, articular incongruity or osteonecrosis [9]

8.1.3 Preoperative Planning [6, 9]

- Exclude infection. Blood tests (CRP, ESR) and joint aspiration for aerobic and anaerobic cultures will be needed. In case of infection, follow a two-stage procedure: remove the hardware, debride and implant a joint spacer. Following a period of antibiotic administration, proceed with THA. This has been correlated with good long-term results [6].
- Take full AP and lateral X-rays, inlet and outlet view and CT to evaluate the acetabular deformity.
- In case of severely affected acetabulum, you may need intraoperative X-rays to identify the true acetabulum for cup placement.
- Understand the principal pathology and alterations that have happened to the acetabulum. Template preoperatively and decide implants to use. In case of severe deformities, revision reconstruction techniques are employed.
- Large heads, dual mobility cups or constrained liners must be present to deal with the instability that is frequent in posttraumatic OA.
- Evaluate the integrity and function of sciatic nerve, and consider intraoperative electromyography monitoring.
- Assess LLD and make a plan to restore it.

8.1.4 Surgical Considerations

- Individualize each patient.
- Choose the appropriate approach. The approach must be able to expand to the posterior columns if necessary and to remove the hardware [10]. The standard posterior approach seems to be reasonable due to better visualization of columns and sciatic nerve. Other approaches, however, may occasionally be used.
- Find the sciatic nerve and protect it [9].
- In the presence of heterotopic ossification, remove all the bone that cause symptoms, impede the approach or lead to impingement. To prevent reoccurrence, think of prophylactic radiation therapy [9].
- With the exception of infection, remove only the screws or hardware that compromises the placement of the cup [9].

- Confirm the continuity of the anterior and posterior columns. In case of residual mobility, reconstruct the columns and the acetabulum.
- Find the true floor and reconstruct the cup. Restore the hip centre of rotation to reach better results [6].
- Achieve stable fixation and cup coverage of at least 70–75%. Cemented or uncemented cups may be used.
- Although in the majority of patients, an uncemented hemispherical acetabular component is all that is needed, in the presence of acetabular bone loss, necrosis or nonunion be prepared to apply principles of revision THR [9].
- Check the possible bony impingement between the trochanter and the pelvis, leading to a high risk of postoperative dislocation [9].

8.1.5 Published Results

THA following acetabular fractures is reported to have inferior results than the primary non-traumatic THA [3, 6, 12, 13]. This is mainly attributed to the younger age of patients and the complexity of the traumatic THA procedure. Recent however studies reported better results [10]. There is limited information in the literature concerning the postoperative course of posttraumatic THA following acetabular fractures [7]. These are usually retrospective and comparative case -control studies, with sample size ranging from 21 to 75 patients and a mean follow-up from 2.5 to 20 years [2, 3, 6, 8, 10, 11, 14–20]. The vast majority of studies reported results till ten years of follow-up except a recent research from Von Roth et al. [8] that reached twenty years post-op results. Survival for any reason was reported to range from 57 [8] to 100% [10].

Their minimal level of evidence, the lack of long-term results for new implants [8], the non-reported severity of acetabular fractures and the lack of high-quality prospective comparative studies between cemented and uncemented implants for different fracture patterns do not give us reasonable answers for their course of these arthroplasties.

Von Roth et al. [8] recently reported twenty years results of a small cohort of sixty six patients with posttraumatic OA treated with previous implant designs THA. The 20-year survivorship of the acetabular component free from revision for aseptic loosening was 71%, and free from revision for any reason was 57%. The type of the acetabular fixation (cemented or uncemented) was not associated with a difference in survivorship. Although survival for aseptic loosening was 69% for cemented acetabular components and 75% for uncemented acetabular components, this difference was not significant ($p = 0.6$).

Ranawat et al. [6] reported 79% survival for any reason and 97% for aseptic loosening in his series of thirty two patients with posttraumatic OA treated with THA. Revision surgery was significantly correlated with nonanatomic restoration of the hip centre and a history of infection.

In a recent systematic meta-analysis, Makridis et al. [4] analysed the outcome of early and delayed THA following acetabular fracture in 645 patients. He reported that the mean 10-year survival of late THAs implanted in cases of posttraumatic hip OA was 76% for the cup and 85% for the stems. The 10-year survival for uncemented cups was better but non-significant than cemented (86.7% vs. 81%, $p = 0.163$). The same was also true for uncemented vs. cemented stems (91% vs. 89%, $p = 0.652$).

Previous reports raised the problem of cemented acetabular fixation to be as high as 50% [3]. Recent however results are better and even better for the uncemented cups. The increased failure rate of cemented acetabular components was attributed to factors such as the relatively younger population, the abnormal anatomy after trauma, the sclerotic bone bed, the loss of acetabular bone stock and complications involving the previous hardware [3]. Schreurs et al. [19], however, evaluated twenty hips that were reconstructed with acetabular bone impaction grafting and a cemented THA after acetabular fracture and then were monitored for an average of 9.5 years. Survival rate was 100% at ten years and 80% at fifteen years.

In a recent retrospective comparative study [2], the inferior outcomes of posttraumatic THA were reported. The 10-year survivorship after THA was lower in patients with a previous acetabular fracture than in the matched cohort

(70% vs. 90%, $p < 0.001$). There was no difference in the 10-year survival rate for those patients treated conservatively or with internal fixation. Patients with previous acetabular fracture had significant greater risk of infection (7% vs. 0% OR, 11.79; $p = 0.028$), dislocation (11% vs. 3; OR, 4.36; $p = 0.048$) or heterotopic ossification (43% vs. 16%; OR, 3.93; $p = 0.001$).

8.1.6 Complications

The rate of complications of posttraumatic OA treated with THA was reported to be higher than of primary THA [2, 6]. The possible reported complications are:

1. Instability/dislocation

   Ranawat et al. [6] reported 9% of dislocation in his series of thirty two patients and Morison et al. [2] 11%. Bellabarba et al. [18], however, reported no dislocations.
2. Infection

   The increased risk for infection is mainly attributed to multiple prior surgeries and retained hardware from previous acetabular reconstruction [2]. In a recent review, Makridis et al. [4] reported 5.6% incidence of infection for posttraumatic THA as a whole that was higher than this of conventional hip arthroplasty. Ranawat et al. [6] reported 16% rate of infection and Morison et al. [2] 7%. Weber [16] and Bellabarba et al. [18], however, demonstrated no infections in their series.
3. Iatrogenic nerve injuries [10, 11].
4. Aseptic loosening probably greater due to the younger patients.
5. Intraoperative periprosthetic femoral fractures.
6. Heterotopic ossification

   It is consistently reported. Makridis et al. [4] reported 30% incidence of heterotopic ossification; however, only one further processed to revision surgery for Brooker IV. Morison et al. [2] published 43% of heterotopic ossification in his series.
7. Other less reported complications are DVT, bilateral paraesthesia, femoral artery injury and nonunion of the trochanteric osteotomy site [4].

8.2 Case Title: Revision THA for a Failed Gamma Nail in An Octogenarian

E. Kenanidis and E. Tsiridis

Misplacement of the nail and cut out of the hip screw. There is a significant subtrochanteric extension, and no abductors left. Revision to a long cemented Exeter stem, calcar reconstruction with metal mesh and an attempt to reattach the greater trochanter and the abductors. Constrained cemented liner (Stryker) to secure hip against dislocation (Fig. 8.1).

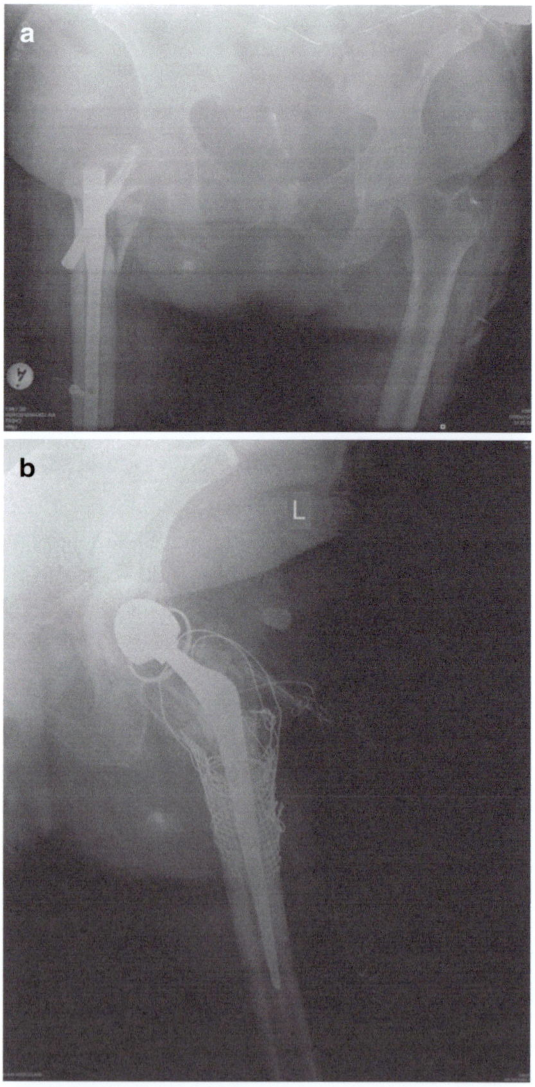

Fig. 8.1 (**a**) Preoperative pelvic x-ray. (**b**) Postoperative x-ray of the left hip

8.3 Case Title: Primary THA Impaction Acetabular Autografting for Posttraumatic Osteoarthritis Following Acetabular Fracture Fixation Complicated by Heterotopic Ossification Brooker IV of Gluteus Medius and Minimus

E. Kenanidis and E. Tsiridis

8.3.1 Demographics

Age: 45
Sex: Male
BMI: 30

8.3.2 Relevant Past Medical History

Principal pathologies: Acetabular fracture following a road traffic accident treated with ORIF complicated by HO Brooker 4

Previous surgical procedures: Acetabular ORIF 24 months back

Medication: None

History of presenting complaint: Pain, hip ankylosis, shortening and external rotation of the limb and palpable ossification of the hip abductors

8.3.3 Clinical Examination

Symptoms: Pain, inability to walk due to fixed flexion deformity and ankyloses

Specific tests: Thomas test positive at 40°

Main disability: Limited function of the right hip

Scoring if available: HHS < 70

Neurovascular evaluation: Intact

8.3.4 Preoperative Radiological Assessment/Imaging (Figs. 8.2 and 8.3)

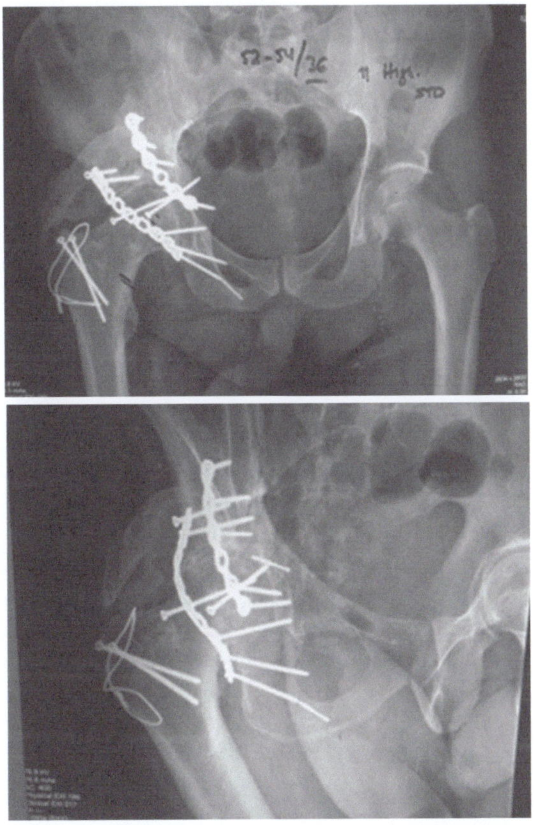

Figs. 8.2 and 8.3 Anterior and posterior wall Matta plates for the ORIF. Screws and wires around the greater trochanter applied for the trochanteric osteotomy to approach the hip during fixation. HO Brooker 4 bridging GT and superior acetabular fossa with complete ankylosis of the hip and damage of the gluteus medius and minimus

8.3.5 Preoperative Planning

Diagnosis: Posttraumatic osteoarthritis and Brooker 4 HO right hip (Figs. 8.2 and 8.3)

Possible treatment options: Primary THA, in the case of abductor insufficiency constrained liner

Chosen treatment method: Acetabulum cemented constrained liner 46 mm, head 22 mm and Exeter stem 44 mm offset, size 2

Selection of implants if applicable and rational: Cemented impaction autografting of the acetabulum due to the incongruity of the acetabular fossa and the lack of the bone stock

Expected difficulties: Safe removal of the HO, bleeding and acetabular reconstruction

Strategies to overcome difficulties: Single-dose local radiation 800 cGy on day one postoperatively

Templating: Done

8.3.6 Surgical Note

With the patient in lateral decubitus position and a posterior approach excising the previous scar, the hip was approached. The sciatic nerve was identified with some difficulty starting from the insertion of the gluteus maximus to the linea aspera that was partially detached to facilitate hip dislocation. The sciatic nerve was tracked and fried from adhesions all the way up to the piriformis muscle and tagged using artery rubber bands. The joint was then assessed. Significant muscle ossification was evident with complete ossification of gluteus medius and minimus. The bony bridge was strong and palpable underneath a very thin layer of gluteus maximus that was overlaying it. A blunt straight retractor was placed between the GM and the HO, and a sharp broad osteotome was used to start removing the HO from the back. Aggressive bone removal leads to bleeding that was easily controlled by tamponade. The anterior part of the HO was more challenging to remove as it was reaching the lesser trochanter medially. Eventually, the hip was mobilized enough to see the neck all around, but the head was not possible to dislocate, and the decision was made to osteotomize the neck in situ and remove a salami slice to dislocate the proximal femur anteriorly. That was done successfully, and further removal of HO was then possible especially from the anterior acetabular wall. Wide excision of the capsule was also done to facilitate the mobilization of the femur. Eventually the proximal femur was retracted anteriorly behind the anterior wall, and the acetabulum was exposed. The head was still in and not possible to be extracted using the corkscrew. It was then decided to remove it piecemeal and that was possible using sharp osteotomes. Care was taken to divide it into large fragments to use it later for the acetabular reconstruction. The head was eventually removed leaving behind an uneven cavity deep to the inner plate classifying the acetabulum as Paprosky 2B. In addition, the posterior wall was heavily compromised by the fracture relying entirely on the reconstruction plate. The decision was then made to proceed to impaction autografting using the femoral head to reconstruct the acetabular cavity for cemented implant insertion. The femoral head was then manually divided in chips 2–3 cm large for impaction grafting. The grafting started using the proper impactors until a new endo-acetabular cancellous substrate was created looking like cobblestone. The cavity was measured with a 46 mm reamer and found concentric, and then a third-generation cementing technique leads to the insertion of a cemented constrained liner 46 mm (Stryker). The decision was based on the complete lack of abductors following the removal of HO. Attention was then turned to the femur; the metalwork from the greater trochanter was easily removed, and the canal was approached without any difficulty. The cancellous bone was very weak from disuse, and decision was made to proceed to a cemented Exeter stem 44 mm, size 2. The reduction was easy with a 22 mm head, and the hip was stable. Leg length was equal to the contralateral and the external rotation recovered to the neutral position. Postoperatively day one, the patient received 800 cGy single-dose radiation locally to reduce HO recurrence (Fig. 8.4).

8.3.7 Intraoperative Challenges

Challenges and solutions: Removing the HO from the anterior acetabular wall and impaction autografting of the Paprosky 2B socket

Unanticipated problems and solution: Bleeding that was tamponated successfully and complete damage to the hip abductors that was compensated with the constrained liner. Uncemented shell was not considered as the acetabulum was uneven and further reaming would have led to further thinning of the anterior and posterior wall that were already compromised. Especially the posterior wall was relying largely upon the posterior plate fixation.

Thorough description of decision-making, including the reason for the final decision: Impaction autografting was necessary to reconstruct the socket, and uncemented implant deemed unsuitable as the bone stock was insufficient to support the metal shell all around especially posteriorly.

8.3.8 Postoperative Radiographs (Fig. 8.4)

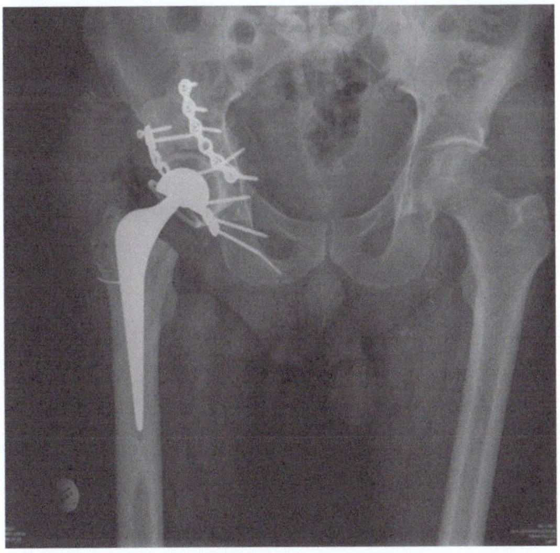

Fig. 8.4 Impaction autografting lateralizing the socket to the appropriate acetabular/pelvic profile. Extensive removal of HO with success especially anteriorly down to the ischial tuberosity. A standard well-executed cemented Exeter stem with equal leg length

8.3.9 Postoperative Management

Chemoprophylaxis and anticoagulant treatment period: Vancomycin 500 mg (one dose preoperatively and two doses postoperatively), cefuroxime 1,5 gr (one dose preoperatively and two doses postoperatively) and tinzaparin 1 × 1 for 35 days

Gait/limb loading until full loading: Partial weight bearing for four weeks and then full weight bearing as tolerated

8.3.10 Follow-Up and Complications

No complication

Scoring: HHS 90

8.4 Case Title: THA Hybrid for Hip Fracture

E. Kenanidis and E. Tsiridis

A 65-year-old with a displaced left hip fracture and shortening and valgus displacement. Whilst ORIF is not indicated at this age group to a high risk of osteonecrosis, the patient is too young for hemiarthroplasty. A hybrid THA was elected to address the matter with a 36 mm head for stability.

Easy adjustment of the leg length and a 36 mm head to address potential early instability reported in the literature for the THA following hip fractures (Fig. 8.5).

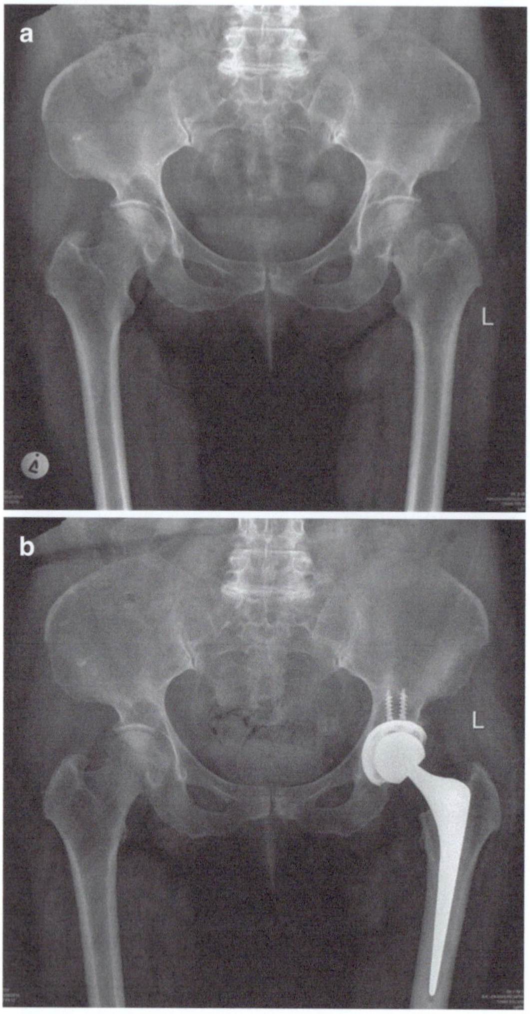

Fig. 8.5 (**a**) Preoperative pelvic x-ray. (**b**) Postoperative pelvic x- ray showing the hybrid left THA

8.5 Case Title: Open Book Pelvis and Acetabular Fracture with Roof Contained Defect

E. Kenanidis and E. Tsiridis

Open book fracture with diastasis of the symphysis pubis and acetabular destruction with a contained roof defect. The acetabulum was reconstructed using impaction autografting of the roof (femoral head) and a full tantalum revision socket to bridge the defects. An HXLP liner coupled with a ceramic 36 mm head and an uncemented stem for the reconstruction (Fig. 8.6).

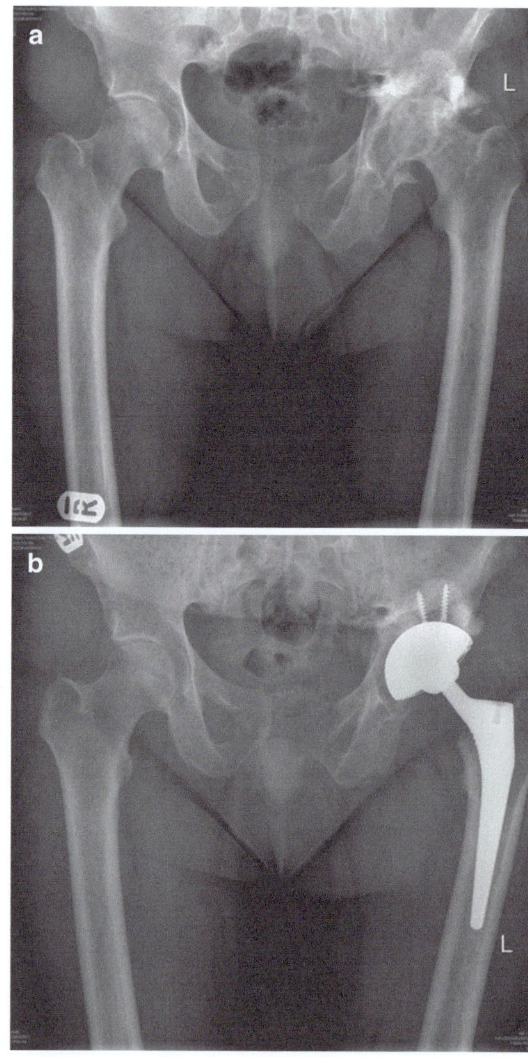

Fig. 8.6 (**a**) Preopartive pelvic x-ray demonstrating the open book fracture with diastasis of the symphysis pubis and a left acetabular contained defect. (**b**) Postoperative pelvic x-ray of the THA showing the acetabular reconstruction with impaction autografting and a full tantalum cup and an uncemented femoral stem

8.6 Case Title: Total Hip Arthroplasty After Pertrochanteric Fracture and Osteosynthesis with DHS

Goran Bicanic, Zoran Sulje, and Domagoj Delimar

8.6.1 Demographics

Age: 73
Sex: Female
BMI: 33.1

8.6.2 Relevant Past Medical History

Principal pathologies: Arterial hypertension and diabetes mellitus type 2

Previous surgical procedures: In 2013 after a fall on the left hip, the patient sustained a pertrochanteric fracture, treated with osteosynthesis with DHS.

Medication: Glimepirid, metformin, lisinopril, nebivolol, alprazolam, escitalopram and ketoprofen

History of presenting complaint: One year after the pertrochanteric fracture and the osteosynthesis with DHS, the patient started to complain because of the pain especially in flexion of the hip, the decreased range of motion (ROM) and the leg length discrepancy (progressive shortening of the operated leg).

8.6.3 Clinical Examination

Symptoms: Pain during walking, decreased range of motion and two cm abbreviation of the left (operated) leg

Range of motion: Completely blocked internal rotation

Main disability: Pain and decreased range of motion

Neurovascular evaluation: Without pathology

8.6.4 Preoperative Radiological Assessment/Imaging (Figs. 8.7 and 8.8)

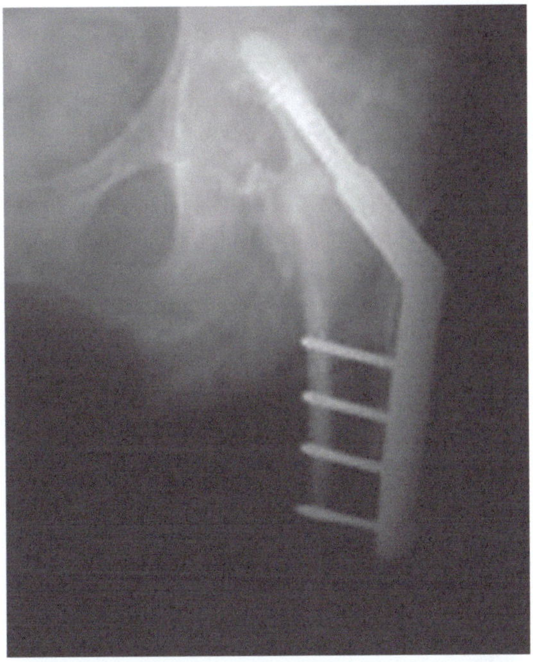

Fig. 8.7 Preoperative X-ray (AP)

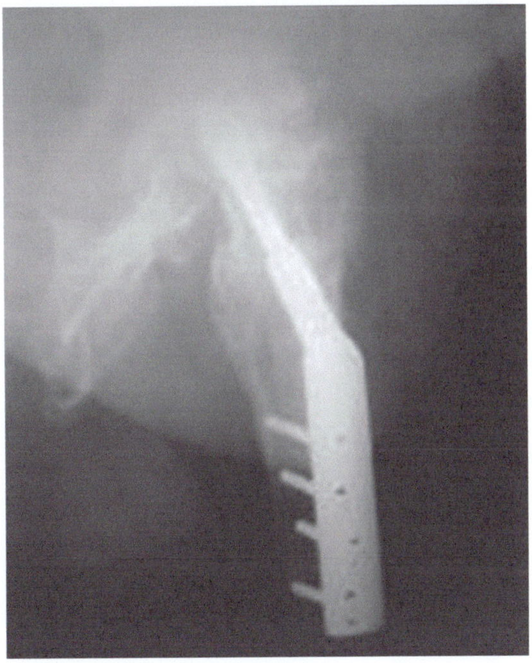

Fig. 8.8 Preoperative X-ray (Lowenstein)

8.6.5 Preoperative Planning

Diagnosis: Posttraumatic hip arthritis (Figs. 8.7 and 8.8)

Possible treatment options: Physical therapy, hardware removal or hip arthroplasty

Chosen treatment method: Hip arthroplasty

Selection of implants if applicable and rational: Cemented or cementless hip arthroplasty. For the acetabular side, trabecular metal is an option. Whenever possible, we aim to implant a cementless hip endoprosthesis. Only in case of severe osteoporosis, the femoral stem would be cemented, if one cannot achieve excellent primary stability. With the severe destruction of the acetabulum for better primary stability, we would choose trabecular metal acetabulum as it gives better primary stability and better possibility for bone ingrowth.

Expected difficulties: Hardware removal is sometimes challenging with the need to extend the approach (in this case distally). Increased probability of infection because of the previous operation. Possible difficulties with endoprosthesis implantation because of sclerosis of the femoral canal and lack of spongious bone.

Strategies to overcome difficulties: Detailed preoperative planning and ensuring availability of all the necessary equipment (for hardware removal)

Templating: A standard templating was performed but with the option for downsizing of the femoral component, since with the sclerosis of the femoral canal (at the level of the screws) sometimes does not allow to implant the planned size.

8.6.6 Surgical Note

Patient's position: Supine position

Type of anaesthesia: Spinal anaesthesia

Surgical approach: Direct lateral (extended distally for hardware removal)

Main steps: Hardware removal followed by standard implantation of the endoprosthesis (Fig. 8.9)

8.6.7 Intraoperative Challenges

Challenges and solutions: Complete removal of the plate and screws. Sometimes there can be breakage of the screws. An option is to make first the femoral neck resection and to remove DHS from inside.

Unanticipated problems and solution: If the DHS is in the acetabulum, it can destroy the posterior wall of the acetabulum. For this case, a trabecular metal acetabulum is an excellent option for achieving primary stability.

Thorough description of decision-making, including the reason for the final decision: For the straightforward case with hardware removal, no significant adjustment of the standard technique is necessary. Removal of the hardware and standard hip arthroplasty are usually possible, but additional options for hardware removal should be available (broken screw removal and options for acetabular and femoral reconstruction).

8.6.8 Postoperative Radiographs (Figs. 8.9)

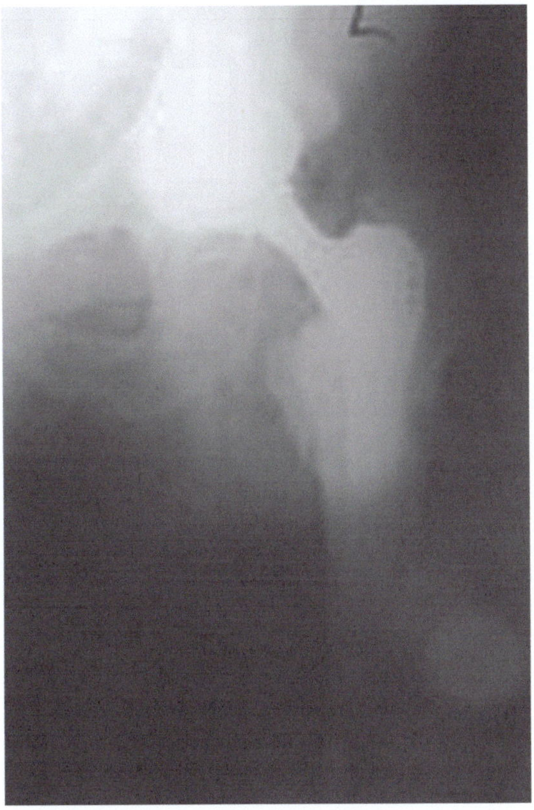

Fig. 8.9 Postoperative x-ray of the THA

8.6.9 Postoperative Management

Chemoprophylaxis and anticoagulant treatment period: Chemoprophylaxis 7–10 days with cephalosporins until intraoperative cultures are received (until negative) and anticoagulant treatment for six weeks

Gait/limb loading until full loading: Weight bearing as tolerated (with crutches)

8.6.10 Follow-Up and Complications

No complication

8.6.11 Discussion [2, 21, 22]

Advantages of the applied method: For this case, the hardware removal and the standard hip arthroplasty is easy for the orthopaedic surgeon and a good option for the patient.

Disadvantages of the method: Need for an extended approach and increased possibility of periprosthetic infection

Alternative evidence-based techniques for the case: Two-stage arthroplasty: first hardware removal and after healing standard hip arthroplasty

Why is the chosen technique better for this case? One-stage operation with reduced recovery time

Indications and contraindications for your technique: Indications: any posttraumatic arthritis with the need for hardware removal. Contraindications: suspicion of infection

Learning curve and how to manage complications: The learning curve is short.

Level of evidence concerning the superiority of this method against others: Level 5, expert opinion

8.7 Case Title: Total Hip Arthroplasty After Acetabular and Femoral Fracture and Osteosynthesis with Plate and Screws

Goran Bicanic, Zoran Sulje, and Domagoj Delimar

8.7.1 Demographics

Age: 58
Sex: Male
BMI: 32.4

8.7.2 Relevant Past Medical History

Principal pathologies: Mb Gilbert

Previous surgical procedures: Fractured left acetabulum and osteosynthesis with screws, fractured left humerus and osteosynthesis with humeral nail and fractured left femur and osteosynthesis with plate and screws

Medication: Desloratadine

History of presenting complaint: Very shortly after the osteosynthesis of the left hip, he started to complain about the tenderness of the hip, the crepitus and the decreased range of motion. He underwent physical therapy but without any improvement.

8.7.3 Clinical Examination

Symptoms: Pain on walking and on any movement of the hip, limping and decreased range of motion

Range of motion: Flexion 110°, extension 0°, external and internal rotation blocked

Main disability: Pain and limited range of motion

Neurovascular evaluation: Without pathology

8.7.4 Preoperative Radiological Assessment/Imaging (Figs. 8.10 and 8.11)

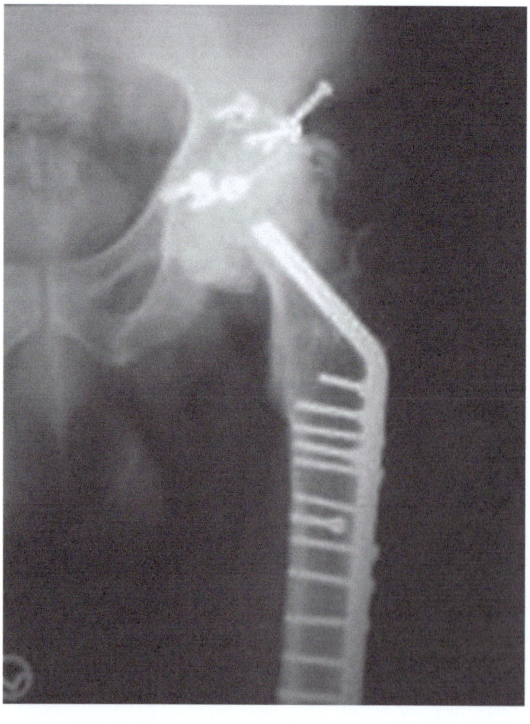

Fig. 8.10 Preoperative X-ray (AP)

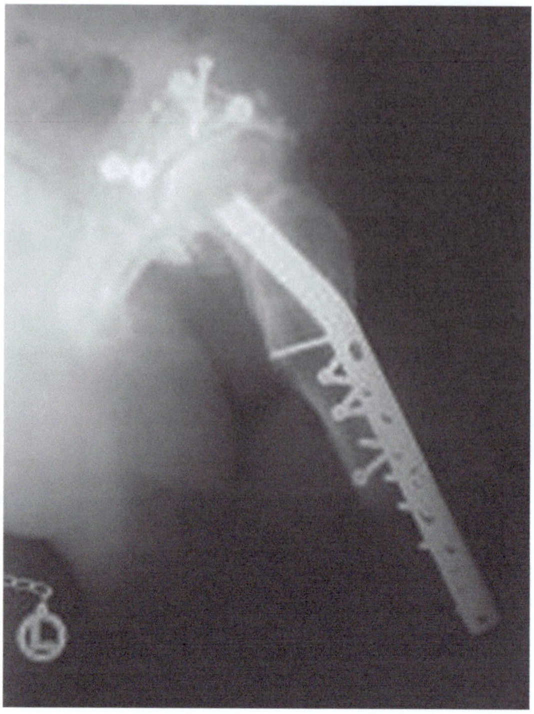

Fig. 8.11 Preoperative X-ray (Lowenstein)

8.7.5 Preoperative Planning

Diagnosis: Posttraumatic hip arthritis (Figs. 8.10 and 8.11)

Possible treatment options: Physical therapy, hardware removal or hip arthroplasty

Chosen treatment method: Total hip arthroplasty

Selection of implants if applicable and rational: Cemented or cementless hip arthroplasty. For the acetabular side, trabecular metal is an option. Whenever possible, we aim to implant cementless hip endoprosthesis. Only in case of severe osteoporosis, the femoral stem would be cemented, if one cannot achieve excellent primary stability. With the severe destruction of the acetabulum for better primary stability, we would choose trabecular metal acetabulum as it gives better primary stability and better possibility for bone ingrowth.

Expected difficulties: Hardware removal is sometimes challenging with the need to extend the approach. There is an increased probability of infection because of the previous operation. Possible difficulties with the endoprosthesis implantation because of the sclerosis of the femoral canal and the lack of spongious bone. Also, it is *not* necessary to remove all the hardware the from the acetabular side, since it can produce unnecessary tissue damage. Removal of the screws is only essential if the screws are protruding in the acetabulum.

Strategies to overcome difficulties: Detailed preoperative planning and ensuring the availability of all the necessary equipment (for hardware removal). The proper preoperative planning is required for the selection of the approach since some approaches cannot be extended proximally. In some cases, bone grafting could be necessary, and therefore availability of bone grafts should be provided.

Templating: A standard templating was performed but with the option for downsizing of the femoral component since with the sclerosis of the femoral canal (at the level of the screws) sometimes does not allow to implant the planned size.

8.7.6 Surgical Note

Patient's position: Supine

Type of anaesthesia: Spinal anaesthesia

Surgical approach: Direct lateral (extended distally for hardware removal)

Main steps: Hardware removal followed by standard implantation of the endoprosthesis (Fig. 8.12)

Reconstruction techniques: Not needed for this case

8.7.7 Intraoperative Challenges

Challenges and solutions: Complete removal of the plate and screws on the femoral side and implantation of the acetabular component without removal of the acetabular hardware.

Unanticipated problems and solution: If the screws of the previous acetabular osteosynthesis are protruding in the acetabulum, then an extension of the approach is needed for screw removal, bone grafting at the place of the screws and the acetabular reconstruction with trabecular metal. For this case, a trabecular metal acetabulum is an excellent option for achieving primary stability.

Thorough description of decision-making, including the reason for the final decision: For the straightforward case with hardware removal, no significant adjustment of the standard technique is necessary. Care must be taken with the preoperative planning to ensure that no screws are protruding in the acetabulum. Removal of the hardware and standard hip arthroplasty are usually possible, but additional options for hardware removal should be available (broken screw removal and options for acetabular and femoral reconstruction).

8.7.8 Postoperative Radiographs (Fig. 8.12)

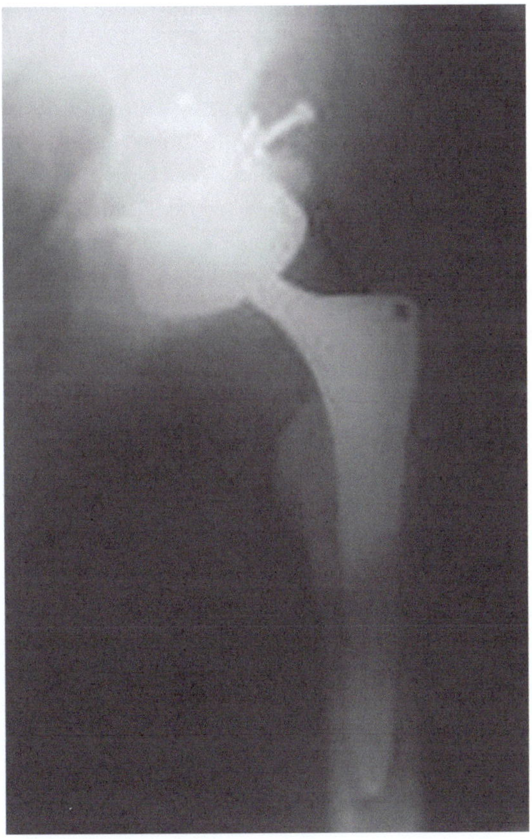

Fig. 8.12 Postoperative x-ray of the THA

8.7.9 Postoperative Management

Chemoprophylaxis and anticoagulant treatment period: Chemoprophylaxis 7–10 days with cephalosporins until intraoperative cultures are received (until negative) and anticoagulant treatment for six weeks

Gait/limb loading until full loading: Weight bearing as tolerated (with crutches)

8.7.10 Follow-Up and Complications

No complication

8.7.11 Discussion [8, 21, 22]

Advantages of the applied method: For this case, the hardware removal and the standard hip arthroplasty is easy for the orthopaedic surgeon and a good option for patient.

Disadvantages of the method: Need for an extended approach and increased possibility of periprosthetic infection. Sometimes removal of the hardware can be challenging.

Alternative evidence-based techniques for the case: Two-stage arthroplasty: first hardware removal and after healing standard hip arthroplasty

Why is the chosen technique better for this case? One-stage operation with reduced recovery time

Indications and contraindications for your technique: Indications: any posttraumatic arthritis with the need for hardware removal. Contraindications: suspicion of infection

Learning curve and how to manage complications: The learning curve is short.

Level of evidence concerning the superiority of this method against others: Level 5, expert's opinion

8.8 Case Title: Total Hip Arthroplasty After Fractured Acetabulum

Goran Bicanic, Zoran Sulje, and Domagoj Delimar

8.8.1 Demographics

Age: 56
Sex: Male
BMI: 29.2

8.8.2 Relevant Past Medical History

Principal pathologies: Ulcerative colitis

Previous surgical procedures: Following a bilateral pubic ramus fracture, the patient was treated with osteosynthesis with two screws. The acetabular fracture was treated conservative. The initial operation was performed in a regional general hospital.

Medication: Pantoprazole, mesalazine, promazine and warfarin

History of presenting complaint: Recovery of the fractured pelvis was not successful. He walked with crutches, but soon because of an increased pain and decreased range of motion in the right hip, he could only move by a wheelchair.

8.8.3 Clinical Examination

Symptoms: Pain during walking, decreased the range of motion and shortening of the right leg

Range of motion: Completely blocked rotations in the right hip. Decreased hip flexion

Main disability: Pain and decreased range of motion

Neurovascular evaluation: Without pathology

8.8.4 Preoperative Radiological Assessment/Imaging (Fig. 8.13)

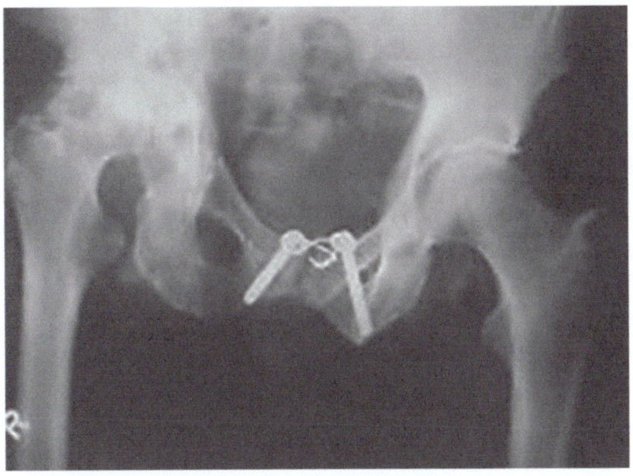

Fig. 8.13 Preoperative X-ray (AP)

8.8.5 Preoperative Planning

Diagnosis: Posttraumatic hip arthritis (Fig. 8.13)

Possible treatment options: Physical therapy and hip arthroplasty

Chosen treatment method: Hip arthroplasty

Selection of implants if applicable and rational: Cemented or cementless hip arthroplasty. For the acetabular side, trabecular metal is an option. Whenever possible, we aim to implant cementless hip endoprosthesis. With the severe destruction of the acetabulum for better primary stability, we would choose trabecular metal acetabulum as it gives better primary stability and better possibility for bone ingrowth.

Expected difficulties: Because of the severe destruction of acetabulum and the lack of bone stock, there is a difficulty in the implantation of the acetabular component and an increased probability of infection because of the previous operation. Restoring the centre of rotation is also challenging.

Strategies to overcome difficulties: The detailed preoperative planning and ensuring availability of all the necessary equipment. Providing there is bone graft available for a possible acetabular reconstruction

Templating: Standard templating for THA

8.8.6 Surgical Note

Patient's position: Supine position

Type of anaesthesia: Spinal anaesthesia

Surgical approach: Direct lateral

Main steps: Standard implantation of the endoprosthesis (Fig. 8.14)

Reconstruction techniques: Not needed for this case

8.8.7 Intraoperative Challenges

Challenges and solutions: Implantation of the acetabular component can be challenging when the fracture of the acetabulum is treated conservatively because of the possible significant destructions, acetabular and femoral head irregularities. Depending on the preoperative planning, one should aim to restore the true centre of rotation or should opt to put the acetabulum in a more proximal position (maximum up to 3 cm above the ideal centre of rotation but usually acceptable up to 1 cm). The latter is technically easier and, so far, the published literature accepts three cm as maximum that can be tolerated as acceptable. In some cases, bone grafting is necessary to provide sufficient bone stock and bone ingrowth over the acetabulum.

Unanticipated problems and solution: If there is lack of the bone stock in the acetabulum, as in this case, trabecular metal acetabulum is an option for achieving primary stability (together with bone grafting). Trabecular metal augments can also be used.

Thorough description of decision-making, including the reason for the final decision: The acetabulum was placed in a more proximal position which provided good primary fixation and then secondary stability. Offset and leg length was reconstructed with a larger neck (head). Therefore, the abductor muscle strength was not compromised.

8.8.8 Postoperative Radiographs (Fig. 8.14)

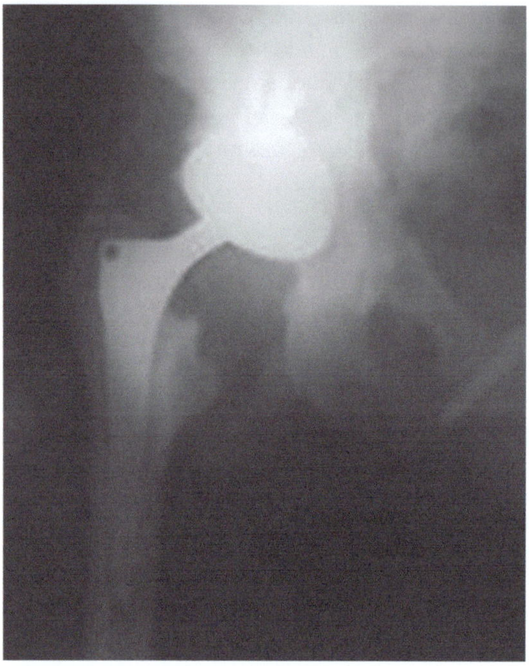

Fig. 8.14 Postoperative x-ray of the THA

8.8.9 Postoperative Management

Chemoprophylaxis and anticoagulant treatment period: Chemoprophylaxis 7–10 days with cephalosporins until intraoperative cultures are received (until negative) and anticoagulant treatment for six weeks

Gait/limb loading until full loading: Weight bearing as tolerated (with crutches)

8.8.10 Follow-Up and Complications

Periprosthetic infection. Two months after implantation of the endoprosthesis, the patient started to complain because of redness around the wound and fever. We cleaned the wound; the intraoperative cultures showed that it was infection with *Pseudomonas aeruginosa*, so we started antibiotic treatment with cephalosporins. After two years, he again noticed redness around the postoperative scar. We have done a revision surgery where we changed the head and acetabular liner together with the long course of i.v. antibiotics; the infection is still present.

8.8.11 Discussion [21–23]

Advantages of the applied method: This method is easy, and there is no need for additional bone grafting, augments or any acetabular reconstruction. Standard techniques and approaches can be utilized just bearing in mind that additional care must be taken to reconstruct the leg length and offset.

Disadvantages of the method: If the ideal centre of rotation is not achieved, then the long-term results could be less than expected.

Why is the chosen technique better for this case? There is an increased possibility of infection for all cases of previous surgery, especially when done in emergency departments. Therefore, minimizing operative time and making arthroplasty as simple as possible is an advantage.

Indications and contraindications for your technique: Indications: any posttraumatic arthritis with the destruction of the acetabulum in the proximal direction. Contraindications: suspicion of infection. If there is a large destruction of the acetabulum in the proximal direction, sometimes it is necessary to reconstruct the ideal centre of rotation with either bone grafting or specific acetabular implants (oblong or metal augments for acetabulum).

Learning curve and how to manage complications: The learning curve is short.

Level of evidence concerning the superiority of this method against others: Level 5, expert opinion

8.9 Case Title: Avascular Necrosis of the Femoral Head at 2 Years After Pertrochanteric Fracture Surgery

Deleanu Bogdan

8.9.1 Demographics

Age: 67 years
Sex: Male
BMI: 24

8.9.2 Relevant Past Medical History

Principal pathologies: Hypertension

Previous surgical procedures: Dynamic interlocking trochanteric gamma nail on the right hip

Medication: None

Other: Smoking history

History of presenting complaint: At six months postoperatively, following the dynamic interlocking trochanteric gamma nail on the right hip, the patient presented moderate pain on the right hip and limited joint mobility with no history of recent trauma. The anteroposterior radiograph revealed incipient avascular necrosis of the femoral head, Ficat stage 2. Despite that the gamma nail was in a good position, we considered that the source of the pain was the intolerance to the implant. At two years postoperatively, the gamma nail on the right hip was removed. Then the course of the patient was satisfactory, with a small limitation of the hip mobility and a decrease in the level of local pain. After the implant removal, the patient was kept under observation and conservative treatment, to prevent further damage to the right hip and allow the healing to occur. In time, the symptoms increased progressively, including a limping and stiffness in the hip joint and pain without effort.

8.9.3 Clinical Examination

Symptoms: Moderate pain in the right hip that increased progressively and does not respond to anti-inflammatory medication

Range of motion: Limited flexion-extension and adduction-abduction on the right hip

Main disability: Walked with a cane

Neurovascular evaluation: Good

8.9.4 Preoperative Radiological Assessment/Imaging (Figs. 8.15, 8.16, and 8.17)

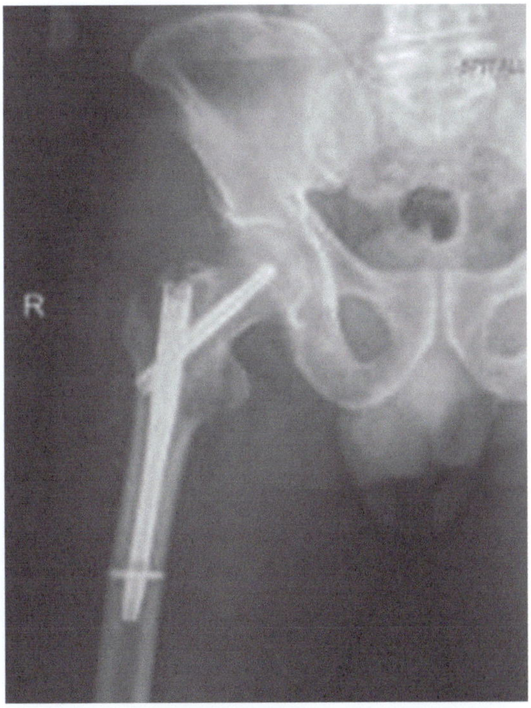

Fig. 8.15 Anteroposterior X-ray of the hip with gamma nail

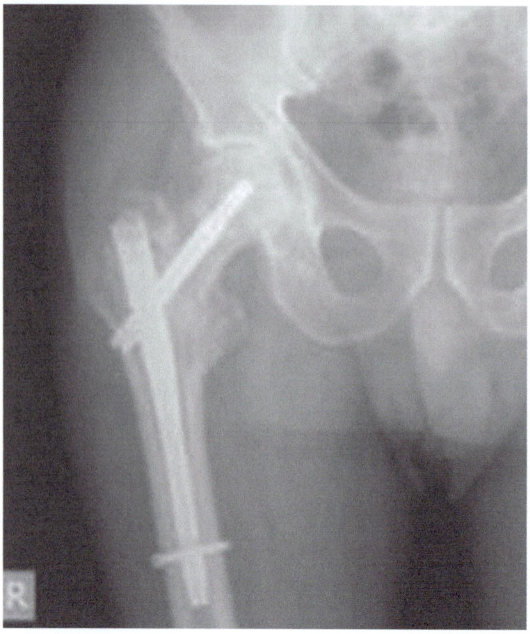

Fig. 8.16 Anteroposterior X-ray of the hip at 6 months postoperatively

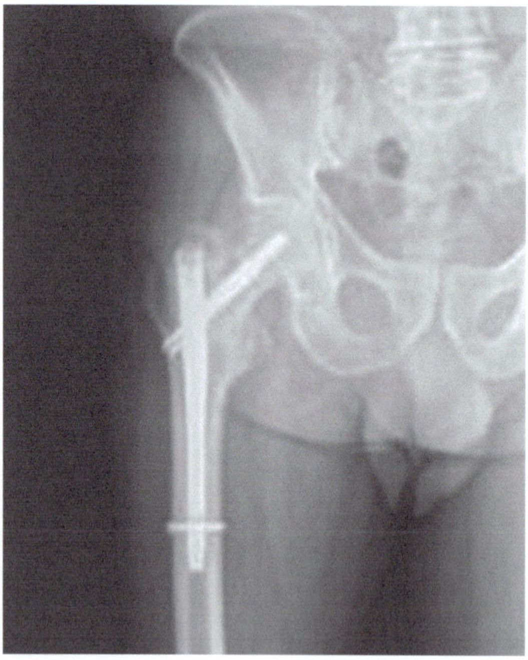

Fig. 8.17 Anteroposterior X-ray of the hip at 2 years postoperatively

8.9.5 Preoperative Planning

Diagnosis: Avascular necrosis of the femoral head Ficat stage 4 and secondary osteoarthritis of the right hip (Figs. 8.15, 8.16, 8.17 and 8.18)

Possible treatment options: Core decompression of the femoral head and total hip arthroplasty

Chosen treatment method: The gamma nail on the right hip was removed, and after six months, uncemented total hip arthroplasty was performed.

Selection of implants if applicable and rational: Total hip arthroplasty using uncemented porous-coated femoral stems

Expected difficulties: Because the patient had a pertrochanteric fracture, we expected challenges in introducing the femoral stem.

Templating: Template acetabular component (number 48) and template femoral component (number 10)

8.9.6 Surgical Note

Patient's position: Supine position

Type of anaesthesia: Spinal anaesthesia

Surgical approach: Lateral approach Hardinge

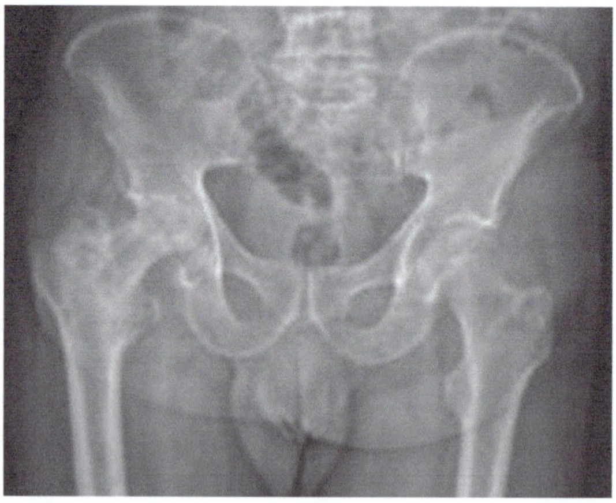

Fig. 8.18 Anteroposterior X-ray of the hip after gamma nail was removed

Main steps: Incision, superficial dissection, deep dissection (do not extend more than 3–5 cm above greater trochanter to prevent injury to superior gluteal nerve), expose anterior joint capsule and remove it, dislocate the hip by flexing and adducting and gently internally rotating the hip

Reconstruction techniques: Perform the osteotomy of the femoral head with an oscillating saw, complete the excision of the labrum, begin the bony preparation of the acetabulum, ream the acetabulum with a bone-conserving cheese grater, insert the acetabular component and then expose and prepare the femur (Fig. 8.19).

8.9.7 Intraoperative Challenges

Challenges and solutions: The difficulty to introducing the femoral stem because the bone tissue was rough, and we introduced a femoral component number 7.5 (number 10 was at preoperative planning) uncemented prosthesis type Taperloc Biomet.

Unanticipated problems and solution: Having regard that the opening of the femoral canal was difficult, we started with osteosynthesis reamers, first the small ones, progressively increasing, and then we used prosthesis broaches.

Thorough description of decision-making, including the reason for the final decision: We introduced a smaller femoral component because we did not want to force and produce a femoral shaft fracture.

8.9.8 Postoperative Radiographs (Fig. 8.19)

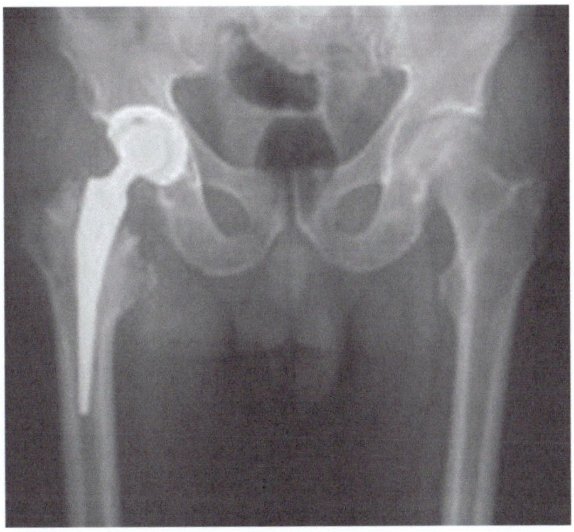

Fig. 8.19 Anteroposterior X-ray of the hip with total hip arthroplasty

8.9.9 Postoperative Management

Chemoprophylaxis and anticoagulant treatment period: Anticoagulant for thirty days postoperative

Gait/limb loading until full loading: Partial weight bearing on the right lower limb for six weeks

8.9.10 Follow-Up and Complications

No postoperative complication

Scoring: Before arthroplasty, the Harris Hip Score (HHS) was 58 and then 74 at 45 days postoperatively, 82 at four months and 90 at the first postoperative year.

8.9.11 Discussion [24–26]

Advantages of the applied method: Reduce hip pain, restore lost mobility and improve the overall quality of life.

Disadvantages of the method: None

Alternative evidence-based techniques for the case: Core decompression of the femoral head

Why is the chosen technique better for this case? Because of the secondary osteoarthritis of the right hip

Indications and contraindications for your technique: Arthritis of the hip

Learning curve and how to manage complications: Minor infections of the wound are treated with antibiotics. Major or deep infections may require more surgery and removal of the prosthesis. Sometimes after a hip replacement, one leg may feel longer or shorter than the other. Your orthopaedic surgeon will make every effort to make your leg lengths even but may lengthen or shorten your leg slightly to maximize the stability and biomechanics of the hip. Some patients may feel more comfortable with a shoe lift after surgery. This occurs when the ball comes out of the socket. If the ball does come out of the socket, a closed reduction usually can put it back into place without the need for more surgery. In situations in which the hip continues to dislocate, further surgery may be necessary.

Level of evidence concerning the superiority of this method against others: There are a few advantages in using bone cement in joint replacement surgeries: bone cement allows a surgeon to affix prosthetic joint components to a bone that is slightly porous from osteoporosis; a small amount of antibiotic material can be added to the bone cement, helping to decrease the risk of postsurgical infection.

8.10 Case Title: Total Hip Arthroplasty After Femoral Fracture Surgery

John B. Meding, E. Michael Keating, and Tatsuya Sueyoshi

8.10.1 Demographics

Age: 48 years
Sex: Male
BMI: 26 kg/Sqm

8.10.2 Relevant Past Medical History

Principal pathologies: Malunion of femur fracture with retained hardware

Previous surgical procedures: ORIF of femur fracture

Medication: Oxycodone/acetaminophen

Other: Active hunter and outdoorsman

History of presenting complaint: Sustained femur fracture twenty years prior and now with three years history of progressive right hip pain and use of a cane

8.10.3 Clinical Examination

Symptoms: Right groin pain with walking and at night

Range of motion: 90 degrees of flexion, 30 degrees abduction, 10 degrees adduction, −20 degrees of IR and 30 degrees of ER. SLR to 70 degrees

Specific tests: Severe pain with flexion and IR

Main disability: Pain and activity restrictions

Scoring if available: Harris Hip Score 43 points

Neurovascular evaluation: No focal loss

8.10.4 Preoperative Radiological Assessment/Imaging (Figs. 8.20, 8.21, and 8.22)

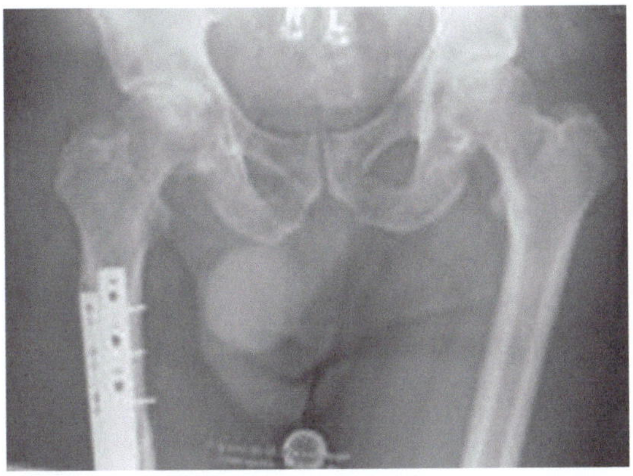

Fig. 8.20 Preoperative pelvic AP view

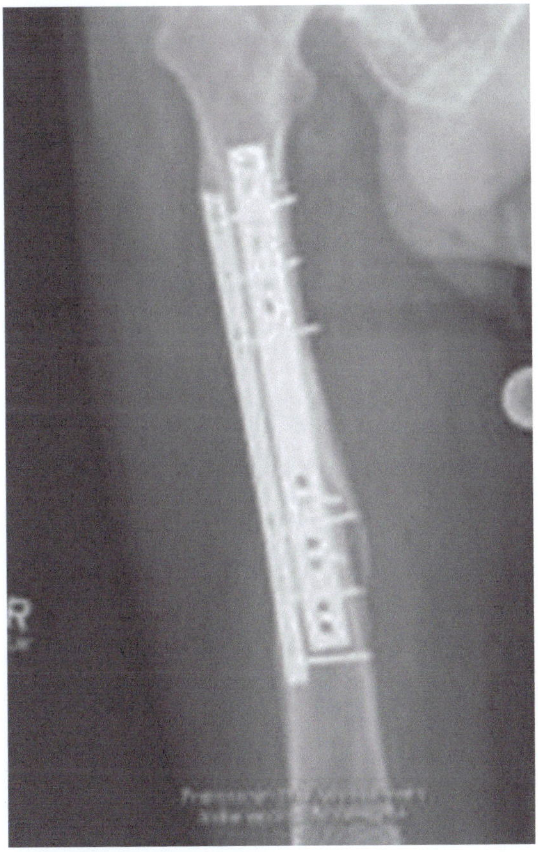

Fig. 8.21 Preoperative femoral AP view

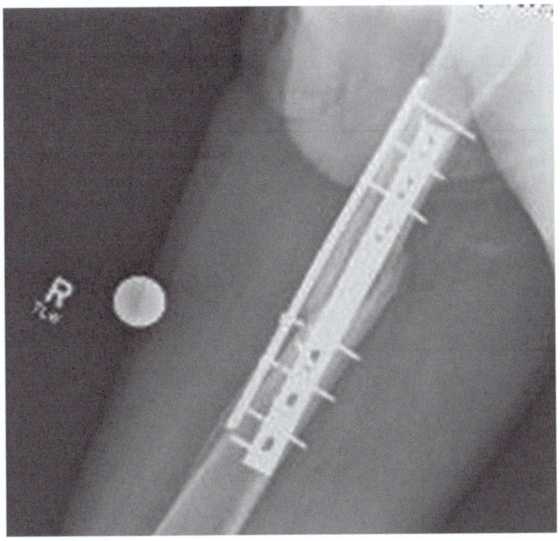

Fig. 8.22 Preoperative femoral lateral view

Other: Note retained screws that would interfere with placement of standard length stem.

8.10.5 Preoperative Planning

Diagnosis: Hip osteoarthritis after femoral fracture with retained hardware (Figs. 8.20, 8.21 and 8.22)

Possible treatment options: Total hip arthroplasty, resurfacing of the hip joint, hemiarthroplasty of the hip joint and short-stem THA

Chosen treatment method: Total hip arthroplasty

Selection of implants if applicable and rational: Cementless implants are preferred for both acetabular and femoral sides. Cemented implants take a risk of extravasation of cement from the fracture site, screw holes and defects after previous hardware removal. Some surgeons prefer modular versatile and distally fixed prosthesis [27, 28]. Consider where the femoral stem is fixed as the loading stress may induce a postoperative fracture. For the example suggested, we used Taperloc Microplasty stem (Biomet, Inc., IN, USA).

Expected difficulties: There may be altered anatomical structures. Ectopic ossifications are sometimes observed even if they don't appear on X-rays. Vastus lateralis muscle or other muscles often have stiffness and scar tissues due to the previous surgery.

Strategies to overcome difficulties: An extensible approach should be performed to get a better view of the surgical field via anterolateral approach. Blood transfusion or intraoperative blood recollection system (such as a cell saver) may be needed.

Templating: The importance of preoperative planning cannot be never overemphasized. X-ray evaluation should include not only typical AP and lateral views of the hip but also standing full leg AP and lateral views to check out a limb length discrepancy, an inclination of the pelvis and a posture. Computed tomography (CT) images are more accurate in evaluating the bony deformity of the femur. Template the planned implant for femoral and acetabular sides. Plan the removal of screws or plates to implant a new prosthesis. Previously implanted hardware would be minimally removed to avoid a postoperative fracture.

8.10.6 Surgical Note

Patient's position: Lateral decubitus position

Type of anaesthesia: General anaesthesia without epidural anaesthesia

Surgical approach: Posterior and anterior approach is not recommended because it is sometimes difficult to extend a surgical field or an implant removal on a supine position.

Main steps: After posterior approach, the femoral head is dislocated before the previous hardware removal notice that the fracture is well healed. Tissue specimens were taken for bacteriologic testing, and frozen sections were used to confirm absence of active infection. After an exposure of the hip joint, the socket was prepared in a usual fashion to a planned size and implant. After reaming and rasping at the proximal femur, it was evident that the medial plate and screws as well as the proximal screws of lateral plate required removal.

Reconstruction techniques: Uncemented THA (Figs. 8.23 and 8.24)

8.10.7 Intraoperative Challenges

Challenges and solutions: Retained hardware. Hardware removed through a separate incision

Unanticipated problems and solution: Utilization of the previous medial incision was required.

Thorough description of decision-making, including the reason for the final decision: Because medial plate required removal, the leg was prepped for a medial incision facilitating plate removal.

8.10.8 Postoperative Radiographs (Figs. 8.23 and 8.24)

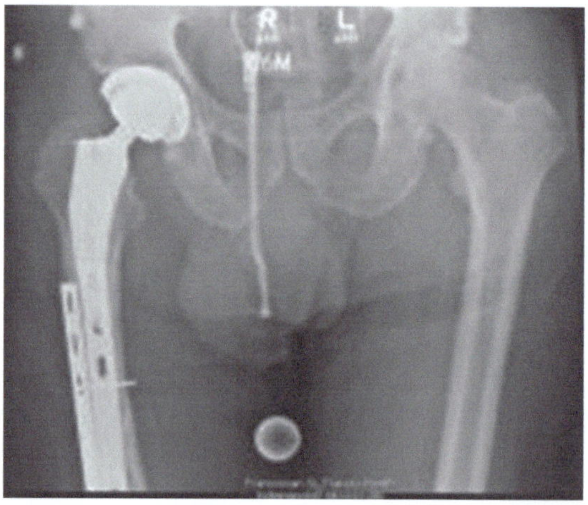

Fig. 8.23 Postoperative six months. AP view

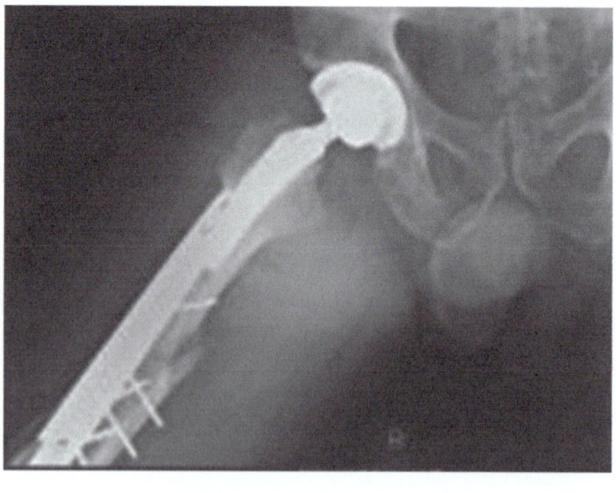

Fig. 8.24 Postoperative six months. Lauenstein view

Other: Note hardware removed.

8.10.9 Postoperative Management

Chemoprophylaxis and anticoagulant treatment period: Vancomycin 1000 mg perioperative. Heparin sodium 1500 units IV intraoperative. ECASA 325 mg Q day for six weeks

Gait/limb loading until full loading: WBAT POD#1

8.10.10 Follow-Up and Complications

Scoring if available: At 10 years post-op: Harris Hip Score 98, no pain. Ambulates without support

8.10.11 Discussion [5]

Advantages of the applied method: After hardware removal relatively straightforward THA

Disadvantages of the method: Two incisions required.

Why is the chosen technique better for this case? Immediate WBAT

Indications and contraindications for your technique: Perhaps one may consider hardware removal as a separate procedure, but this is not needed.

Learning curve and how to manage complications: Need to be familiar with the medial approach to the femur

References

1. Giannoudis PV, Grotz MR, Papakostidis C, Dinopoulos H. Operative treatment of displaced fractures of the acetabulum. A meta-analysis. J Bone Joint Surg Br. 2005;87:2–9.
2. Morison Z, Moojen DJF, Nauth A, Hall J, McKee MD, Waddell JP, Schemitsch EH. Total hip arthroplasty after acetabular fracture is associated with lower survivorship and more complications. Clin Orthop Relat Res. 2016;474:392–8.
3. Romness DW, Lewallen DG. Total hip arthroplasty after fracture of the acetabulum. Long-term results. J Bone Joint Surg Br. 1990;72(5):761–4.
4. Makridis KG, Obakponovwe O, Bobak P, Giannoudis PV. Total hip arthroplasty after acetabular fracture: incidence of complications, reoperation rates and functional outcomes: evidence today. J Arthroplast. 2014;29:1983–90.
5. Archibeck MJ, Carothers JT, Tripuraneni KR, White RE Jr. Total hip arthroplasty after failed internal fixation of proximal femoral fractures. J Arthroplast. 2013;28(1):168–71.
6. Ranawat A, Zelken J, Helfet D, Buly R. Total hip arthroplasty for posttraumatic arthritis after acetabular fracture. J Arthroplast. 2009;24(5):759–67.
7. Mont MA, Elmallah RK. CORR insights: total hip arthroplasty after acetabular fracture is associated with lower survivorship and more complications. Clin Orthop Relat Res. 2016;474:399–401.
8. von Roth P, Abdel MP, Scott Harmsen W, Berry DJ. Total hip arthroplasty after operatively treated acetabular fracture. A concise follow-up, at a mean of twenty years, of a previous report investigation performed at the Mayo Clinic, Rochester, Minnesota. J Bone Joint Surg Am. 2015;97:288–91.
9. Sierra RJ, Mabry TM, Sems SA, Berry DJ. Acetabular fractures: the role of total hip replacement. Bone Joint J. 2013;95-b(suppl a):11–6.
10. Zhang L, Zhou Y, Li Y, Xu H, Guo X, Zhou Y. Acetabular fractures: a 5-year follow-up study. J Arthroplast. 2011;26(8):1189–93.
11. Sermon A, Broos P, Vanderschot P. Total hip replacement for acetabular fractures. Results in 121 patients operated between 1983 and 2003 injury. Int J Care Injured. 2008;39:914–21.
12. Malkin C, Tauber C. Total hip arthroplasty and acetabular bone grafting for unreduced fracture dislocation of the hip. Clin Orthop Relat Res. 1985;201:57.
13. Rogan I, Weber F, Solomon L. Total hip replacement following fracture dislocation of the acetabulum. J Bone Joint Surg Br. 1979;61-B:252.
14. Khurana S, Nobel TB, Merkow JS, Walsh M, Egol KA. Total hip arthroplasty for posttraumatic osteoarthritis of the hip fares worse than THA for primary osteoarthritis. Am J Orthop. 2015;44(7):321–5.
15. Lai O, Yang J, Shen B, Zhou Z, Kang P, Pei F. Midterm results of uncemented acetabular reconstruction for posttraumatic arthritis secondary to acetabular fracture. J Arthroplast. 2011;26(7):1008–13.
16. Weber M, Berry DJ, Harmsen WS. Total hip arthroplasty after operative treatment of an acetabular fracture. J Bone Joint Surg Am. 1998;80(9):1295–305.
17. Berry DJ, Halasy M. Uncemented acetabular components for arthritis after acetabular fracture. Clin Orthop Relat Res. 2002;405:164–7.
18. Bellabarba C, Berger RA, Bentley CD, Quigley LR, Jacobs JJ, Rosenberg AG, Sheinkop MB, Galante JO. Cementless acetabular reconstruction after acetabular fracture. J Bone Joint Surg Am. 2001;83-A(6):868–76.
19. Schreurs BW, Zengerink M, Welten ML, van Kampen A, Slooff TJ. Bone impaction grafting and a cemented cup after acetabular fracture at 3–18 years. Clin Orthop Relat Res. 2005;437:145–51.
20. Lizaur-Utrilla A, Sanz-Reig J, Serna-Berna R. Cementless acetabular reconstruction after acetabular

fracture: a prospective, matched-cohort study. J Trauma Acute Care Surg. 2012;73(1):232–8.
21. Rodriguez-Merchan E. Coxarthrosis after traumatic hip dislocation in the adult. Clin Orthop Relat Res. 2000;377:92–8.
22. Kraus P, Braud J, Whatley J. Total hip arthroplasty after previous fracture surgery. Clin North Am. 2015;46(2):193–213.
23. Guerado E, Cano JR, Cruz E. Fractures of the acetabulum in elderly patients. An update. Injury. 2012;43(Suppl 2):33–41.
24. Kamal D, Traistaru R, Alexandru DO, Grecu DC, Mogoanta L. Epidemiologic study of avascular necrosis of femoral head. Curr Health Sci J. 2013;39(3):169–74.
25. Barquet A, Mayora G, Guimaraes JM, Suárez R. Avascular necrosis of the femoral head following trochanteric fractures in adults: a systematic review. Injury. 2014;45(12):1848–58.
26. Mallina R, Dinah F. Avascular necrosis of femoral head a rare complication of a common fracture in an octogenarian. Geriatr Orthop Surg Rehabil. 2013;4(3):74–7.
27. Thakur RR, Deshmukh AJ, Goyal A, et al. Management of failed trochanteric fracture fixation with cementless modular hip arthroplasty using a distally fixing stem. J Arthroplasty. 2011;26:398–403.
28. Abouelela AA. Salvage of failed trochanteric fracture fixation using the revitan curved cementless modular hip arthroplasty. J Arthroplasty. 2012;27:1382–8.

THA Following Pediatric Hip Diseases (Legg-Calvé-Perthes/ Slipped Capital Femoral Epiphysis)

9

Eustathios Kenanidis, Panagiotis Kakoulidis, Vasileios Lampridis, Michail E. Klontzas, Eleftherios Tsiridis, Jan F.A. Somers, Ran Schwarzkopf, Andrew Brian Old, Jens Vanbiervliet, and Jean-Pierre Simon

E. Kenanidis, M.D., Ph.D., M.Sc. (✉) ·
P. Kakoulidis, M.D. ·
V. Lampridis, M.D., M.Sc. (H.C.M.), F.E.B.O.T.
Academic Orthopaedic Unit, Aristotle University Medical School, Thessaloniki, Greece

M.E. Klontzas, M.D.
Imperial College London, Biological Systems Engineering Lab, London, UK

E. Tsiridis, M.D., Ph.D., F.A.C.S., F.R.C.S.
Academic Orthopaedic Unit, Papageorgiou General Hospital, Aristotle University Medical School, Thessaloniki, Greece
e-mail: etsiridis@doctors.org.uk

J.F.A. Somers, M.D.
Department of Surgery, Yan Yperman Hospital, Ypres, Belgium
e-mail: orthosomers@telenet.be

R. Schwarzkopf, M.D., M.Sc.
Department of Orthopaedic Surgery, NYU Langone Health Orthopaedic Hospital, Hospital for Joint Diseases, New York, NY, USA
e-mail: schwarzk@gmail.com

A.B. Old, M.D.
Premier Orthopaedics, Penn Medicine Chester County Hospital, West Chester, PA, USA

J. Vanbiervliet, M.D.
Yan Yperman Hospital, Ypres, Belgium

J.-P. Simon, M.D., Ph.D.
University Hospitals Leuven, Leuven, Belgium

9.1 Current Concepts

E. Kenanidis, P. Kakoulidis, V. Lampridis, M.E. Klontzas, and E. Tsiridis

Legg-Calvé-Perthes disease (LCPD) represents a type of idiopathic avascular necrosis of the femoral head which typically develops during childhood [1, 2]. Its etiology is considered to be multifactorial but is unknown; genetic, constitutional, and environmental factors have been implicated [3]. Despite receiving treatment, some patients initially develop morphological changes in the femoral head and secondarily an acetabular deformity, femoroacetabular in congruency, and an abnormal hip movement that could lead to early-onset secondary osteoarthritis [1, 4]. In a current prospective cohort, 5% of LCPD patients underwent THA at twenty years after non-operative treatment [5]. Stulberg classification is used as a prognostic tool of hip osteoarthritis at skeletal maturity [2]; Stulberg types III–V are more susceptible to the development of early secondary hip osteoarthritis [1].

Slipped capital femoral epiphysis (SCFE) is the most common hip disorder in adolescence [5, 6]. It is a Salter-Harris type I fracture through the proximal femoral physis, leading to slippage of the upper femoral epiphysis in a backward direction through the hypertrophic zone

E. Tsiridis (ed.), *The Adult Hip - Master Case Series and Techniques*, https://doi.org/10.1007/978-3-319-64177-5_9

[5, 6]. As a result, the femoral head remains in the acetabulum, and the neck is displaced anteriorly and externally rotated [6]. Its etiology is controversial; genetic, constitutional, and endocrine factors have been implicated. Delayed or missed diagnosis often leads to anatomic and biomechanical hip changes and unusual kinematics resulting in secondary hip osteoarthritis in the fourth to fifth decade of life [5].

Patients with SCFE and LCPD represent a minority group among patients treated with primary THA [7]. SCFE and LCPD disease were reported to be responsible for 0.6% of primary THAs in the Nordic Arthroplasty Registry Association [7], varying from 1.3% in Norway and 1.0% in Denmark to 0.1% in Sweden. In Denmark, Perthes disease was responsible for 0.6% of primary THAs and SCFE 0.4%, while in Sweden the percentages were 0.1% and 0.02%, respectively [7].

9.1.1 THA Indications

Advanced symptomatic degenerative joint disease.

9.1.2 Anatomic Alterations and Technical Difficulties

The altered anatomy in SCFE and LCDP patients makes the THA surgery technically demanding. The most usual anatomic changes and technical challenges found in these patients are the following:

LCDP:

1. Multi-planar deformities of the femoral head (typically flattening and widening) [1]
2. Incongruency between the acetabulum and the femoral head [1]
3. Shallow, enlarged, and retroverted acetabulum [2]
4. Elongated greater trochanter [1]
5. Short femoral neck (due to growth disturbance)
6. Multi-planar deformities are usually complicated by previous surgical procedures undertaken during childhood (pelvic and proximal femoral osteotomies and soft tissue procedures) [1]
7. Alterations in the normally expected proximal femoral anatomy [2]
8. Soft tissue contractures [2]
9. The relatively young age of patients [4]

SCFE:

1. Loss of the neck-head offset [5]
2. Femoroacetabular impingement [5]
3. Loss of the peripheral articular cartilage in the superior quadrant of the femoral head [5]
4. Previous surgical procedures that were undertaken during childhood [8]
5. Coxa vara [5]
6. Relatively young patient age [8]
7. Soft tissue contractures [8]

9.1.3 Preoperative Planning

1. Biplanar radiographs, anteroposterior and lateral radiographs
2. Computed tomography with 3D reconstruction to evaluate the upper femoral part shape and the need for special custom-made implants

9.1.4 Published Results

Limited number of cohorts and registry data give us information about the natural course of THA in SCFE and LCP patients [1, 2, 5–14]. These are usually retrospective small case series of more than ten to less than one hundred patients [1, 2, 5, 6, 8, 9, 12–14]. The mean age of patients at the time of THA ranges from thirty two to fifty six years old. They report midterm results with a mean follow-up period between 4,5 and 11 years [1, 2, 5–8, 10–14] with only one small study reaching fifteen years of follow-up [9]. Uncemented or hybrid implants are usually used. Modular neck [5] and custom-made prostheses [1] were also be used to restore the proximal femoral anatomy, optimizing the metaphyseal bone contact and the leg length. Hesham Al-Khateeb [1] et al. reported 100% and 79% survival rates, respectively, for femoral and acetabular components of fifteen primary THAs for LCPD patients, using custom-made cementless femoral components at a mean of 10.1 years.

Pediatric hip diseases often have been reported to have inferior results following THA compared to primary osteoarthritis of the hip [7]. The mean survival rate in the previously mentioned studies ranged from 81 to 98% [1, 2, 5–14]. The old implant designs and inconsistent surgical techniques might play an important role in determining the initial poor results. In one of the largest case series, Baghdadi et al. [2] evaluated the results of ninety THAs retrospectively, in patients suffering from LCDP at a mean of eight years postoperatively; cementless and hybrid implants were used. The survival rate for the whole cohort was 89%, for cementless arthroplasties 90%, and hybrid 86%. Traina et al. [5] demonstrated 92.8% overall survival for thirty two THAs performed in patients with SCFE.

Recent reports, however, from the Danish, the Norwegian, and the Swedish Hip Arthroplasty Registries [7, 10, 11, 14] gave different information. Based on a follow-up of 540 patients reported to the Norwegian Arthroplasty Register during 1987–2007, Lehmann et al. [10] reported the quality of life of patients with pediatric hip disease treated with THA below forty years old compared to healthy age-matched controls. Although the reasons were unclear, SCFE patients who had been operated had a better quality of life than the other groups.

Using combined data from the Danish, the Norwegian, and the Swedish Hip Arthroplasty Registries, Engesaeter et al. [7] reported a comparable risk ratio for revision for any reason, between the combined group LCPD/SCFE (2335 THAs) and the OA group (288,435 THAs) at 7 years; the relative risk was 0.85 (CI, 0.72–1.0). Similar results were obtained with the aseptic loosening (RR 0.81; CI, 0.63–1.0), with the dislocation (RR 0.72; CI, 0.44–1.2), and with the infection as endpoint (RR 1.0; CI, 0.56–1.6). There was a lower risk of revision for any reason for the combined group of LCDP/SCFE (n = 2335) compared to the DDH (n = 12,068) (RR 0.82; CI, 0.67–0.99) and for the dislocation as endpoint (RR 0.56; CI, 0.33–0.95), but not for the aseptic loosening (RR 0.84; CI, 0.63–0.1.1) and infection as endpoint. There was no difference comparing the SCFE and the LCPD groups.

Thillemann et al. [11] using data from the Danish National Registry also found no statistically significant differences in the risk of revision between Morbus LCPD, epiphysiolysis, and primary osteoarthritis during the early postoperative phase and later follow-up. Data from the New Zealand Registry [14] also demonstrated comparable results of revision rate and Oxford Hip Score for THA between a group of primary osteoarthritis and secondary osteoarthritis due to SCFE.

9.1.5 Complications

Aseptic loosening, wound infection, heterotopic ossification, intraoperative fracture, sciatic nerve palsy, and leg length discrepancy are the most common described complications in the literature [1, 2, 5–14]. Traina et al. [5] reported fifteen out of thirty two cases of heterotopic ossification in patients with SCFE treated with THA. Baghdadi et al. [2] showed 16% of complications in his series of ninety LCDP patients undergoing THA. There were nine intraoperative fractures, three nerve palsies, and a sepsis. The increased rate of nerve palsies in some studies [2, 5] was attributed to the limb lengthening and the inadequate soft tissue release.

9.2 Case Title: Perthes with Avascular Necrosis and Arthritis

E. Kenanidis and E. Tsiridis

Typical Perthes with a short neck, a high-riding greater trochanter, and a flattened socket. In this particular case, the neck was varus anyway, thus leading to a high-riding GT after shortening. One of the main difficulties of such case was to approach the socket as well as to tension properly the abductors.

The hip was in varus, so the neck cut was low to prevent lengthening and also to simulate varus anatomy. The resultant high-riding GT is not compromising the range of motion except for the abduction. Recovering the offset was difficult due to the persistent shrinkage of the abductors. An uncemented socket snuggly fitted into a deepened acetabulum and was fully covered by bone. A straight stem fitted well the Dorr type A femur (Fig. 9.1).

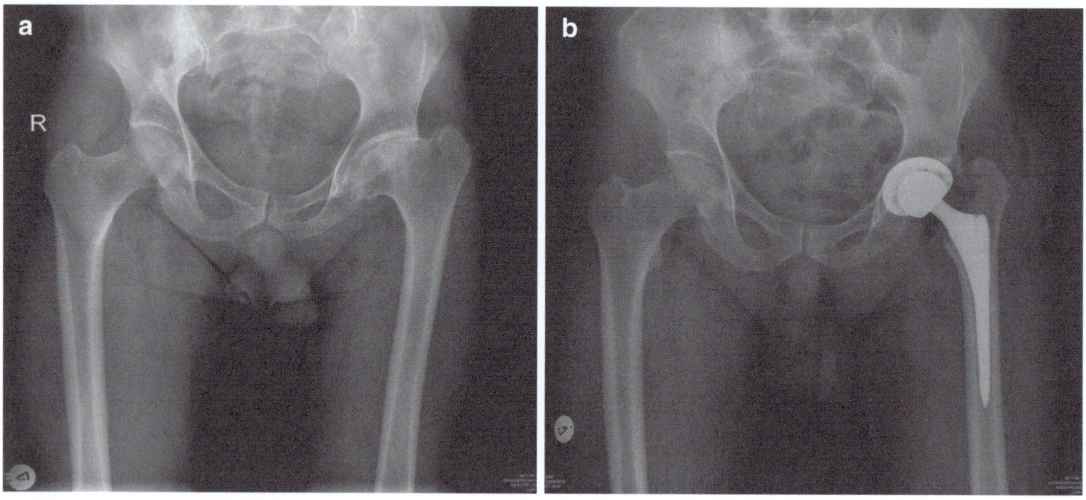

Fig. 9.1 (**a**) Preoperative x-ray of the pelvis (**b**) Postoperative x-ray of the first day

9.3 Case Title: THA for Perthes with Short Neck, Flattened Head, and Shallow Socket

E. Kenanidis and E. Tsiridis

The typical Perthes development with a short neck and a flattened head; the socket is shallow and flat corresponding to the head. The anterior and posterior walls are weak. The offset is minimal and the abductors short and shrunken (Fig. 9.2a).

During shell insertion, the posterior wall sustained a crack fracture adjacent to the roof heading to the iliac wing. The shell was reinforced with three long screws and the fracture fixed using a 3.5 mm one-third tubular plate (Fig. 9.2b and c). The femur was treated with a 35.5 mm offset cemented DDH Exeter stem to compensate for the short offset and the shrunk abductors. Low neck cut maintained the leg length equal. Attention must be taken to release the sciatic nerve due to its proximity to the neck. An intraoperative photo of the reconstruction demonstrates the plate position around the roof and the posterior wall of the socket (Fig. 9.2c). The approach was mini-posterior with the short rotators, and the capsule tagged with Ethibond 5/0 suture to protect the sciatic nerve (see next the retractor).

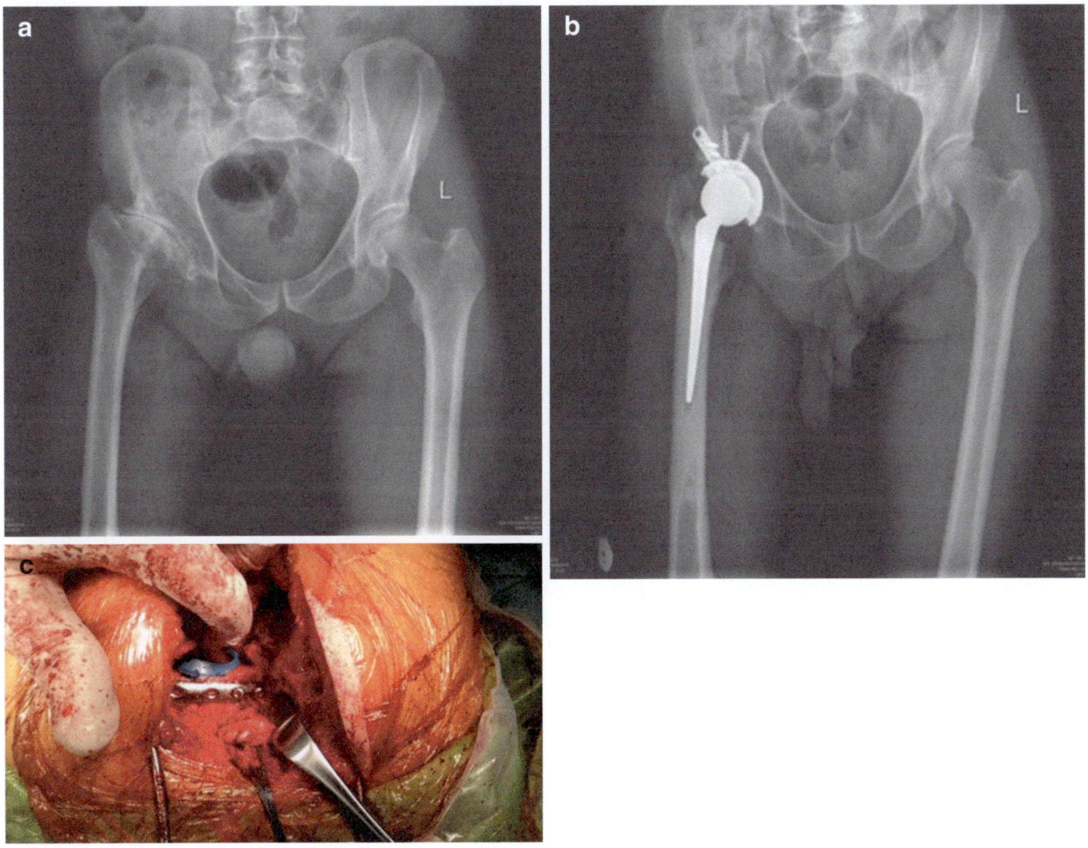

Fig. 9.2 (**a**) Preoperative pelvic x-ray (**b**) Postoperative pelvic x-ray (**c**) Intraoperative photo depicting the plate reconstruction of the posterior wall

9.4 Case Title: THA for Perthes and Proximal Femoral Deformity Post-Varus Osteotomy at Childhood Complicated by an Acute Periprosthetic Acetabular Fracture

E. Kenanidis and E. Tsiridis

9.4.1 Demographics

Age: 66
Sex: Female
BMI: 20

9.4.2 Relevant Past Medical History

Principal pathologies: Perthes operated when the patient was five years of age with valgus osteotomy, ovarian cancer under surveillance in remission, osteoporosis, and pain.

Previous surgical procedures: Ovariectomy for cancer but no metastatic disease at present.

Medication: Alendronate and calcium.

History of presenting complaint: Pain and reduced ROM

9.4.3 Clinical Examination

Symptoms: Pain and short limp gait (approximately 2.5 cm)

Range of motion: Flexion 60°, extension 10°, rotation, abduction and adduction limited

Specific tests: Thomas positive 25 degrees

Main disability: Pain and short limp gait

Scoring if available: HHS:80

Neurovascular evaluation: Intact

9.4.4 Preoperative Radiological Assessment/Imaging (Fig. 9.3)

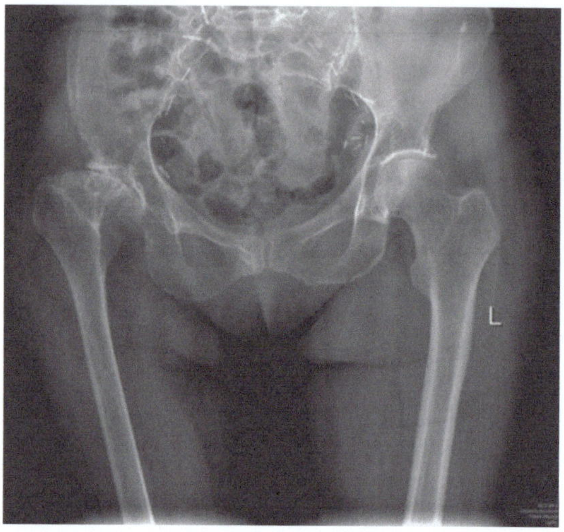

Fig. 9.3 Preoperative pelvic x-ray demonstrating a typical Perthes deformity with a flattened head and short neck. The acetabulum is swallowed and dysplastic. There is anteversion of the proximal femur, and the femoral canal is narrow and osteoporotic. Ill developed acetabulum

9.4.5 Preoperative Planning

Diagnosis: Osteoarthritis of the right hip, dysplasia from Perthes, and postsurgical valgus osteotomy at young age (Fig. 9.3).

Possible treatment options: Cemented Exeter hybrid appropriate for the narrow femoral canal and the short offset.

Chosen treatment method: Uncemented acetabular shell Stryker Trident 46 mm, cancellous bone screws (2 × 25 mm), cemented hip stem Stryker Exeter 35.5, 125 mm, polyethylene 32 mm, and ceramic femoral head Stryker 32 mm.

Selection of implants if applicable and rational: Exeter hybrid for the availability of offsets and sizes.

Expected difficulties: Acetabular reaming

Strategies to overcome difficulties: A variety of offsets available and available treatment options for acetabular complications, i.e., fractures, etc.

9.4.6 Surgical Note

With the patient in lateral decubitus position and using a mini-posterior approach, the hip was exposed. Dislocation was easy; however, relations were too close to the bone due to shortening of the neck and the head flattening over the years. Easy osteotomy exposed the acetabulum that was flattened out and shallow. Reaming of the socket was aiming toward the inner wall to create roof and walls for the shell. During shell insertion (46 mm shell with 32 mm inner diameter liner), however, a minor hairline fracture occurred in the superior posterior aspect of the acetabulum due to cortical thinning. An immediate action was taken to stabilize the fracture regardless of the limited extension of it. A pelvic plate (Matta System Stryker), with six holes, cortical bone screws (1 × 36 mm, 1 × 26 mm), and cancellous bone screws (1 × 45mm, 1 × 40mm), was contoured to accommodate the superior roof and the posterior wall safely and was applied with the shell in situ. In addition, screws were put through the shell to secure fixation. The result was satisfactory regarding the acetabular implant stability, and attention then turned to the femur. Third-generation cementing technique and an implant with short offset 35.5 mm fitted the canal and the short offset of the hip. A 32 mm ceramic head used and the hip was easily reduced; the hip was stable and the leg length equal to the contralateral side (Fig. 9.4).

9.4.7 Intraoperative Challenges

Challenges and solutions: Acute periprosthetic acetabular fracture.

Thorough description of decision-making, including the reason for the final decision: Exeter cemented stem to address the small offset and the narrow femoral canal.

9.4.8 Postoperative Radiographs (Fig. 9.4)

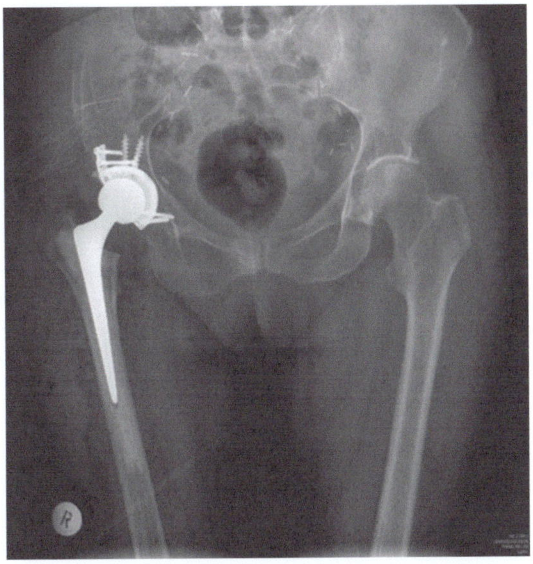

Fig. 9.4 Equal leg length and good femoral cement mantle. The acetabular component is well oriented, and the plate is clearly positioned on the roof and the posterior wall. Well-placed stay screws through the acetabular shell for extra stability

9.4.9 Postoperative Management

Chemoprophylaxis and anticoagulant treatment period: Vancomycin 500 mg (one dose preoperatively, two doses postoperatively), cefuroxime 1,5 gr (one dose preoperatively, two doses postoperatively), enoxaparin 1 × 1 for the days of hospitalization, and the rivaroxaban 10 mg 1 × 1 for thirty days

Gait/limb loading until full loading: Partial weight bearing for eight weeks and then full weight bearing as tolerated

9.5 Case Title: Primary Complex Hip Arthroplasty for Previous Legg-Calvé-Perthes Disease

Somers J.F.A.

9.5.1 Demographics

Age: 41
Sex: Male
BMI: 24

9.5.2 Relevant Past Medical History

Principal pathologies: Bilateral LCP (Legg-Calvé-Perthes) disease at the age of 5

Previous surgical procedures: Bilateral subtrochanteric osteotomy at the age of 6 (painful hips due to insufficient acetabular coverage); hip arthroscopy at the age of 40

Medication: NSAID

Other: No other medical morbidities

History of presenting complaint: At the age of 5, diagnosis of LCP with painful hips and limping. The patient was treated with rest and bracing. At the age of 6 bilateral subtrochanteric osteotomies and bracing for one year. Postoperatively there was no pain in the hips, but developed shortening of the left leg. The patient used shoe lift for more than thirty years. He started work at eighteen (manual labor) and experienced no pain until the age of thirty five. Then a growing pain at the left hip arrived that was treated with oral analgesics. Due to increasing pain, he was advised for THR, but the patient declined, thinking that he was too young for hip replacement surgery. He asked for other treatment option and hip arthroscopy was then offered. Hip arthroscopy revealed torn labrum and extensive cartilage damage. He experienced less pain for six months but then returned to the clinic with increasing pain and disability in the left hip/groin and growing limping.

9.5.3 Clinical Examination

Symptoms: Pain upon loading, pain at rest and at night, limp

Range of motion: Decreased ROM with flexion 75°, abduction 10°, adduction 15°, internal rotation 0°, and external rotation 25°; extension deficit 5°

Specific tests: Painful hip impingement test, Trendelenburg +

Main disability: Functional

Scoring if available: UCLA 3/10, modified Charnley score 9/18

Neurovascular evaluation: Normal

9.5.4 Preoperative Radiological Assessment/Imaging (Figs. 9.5 and 9.6)

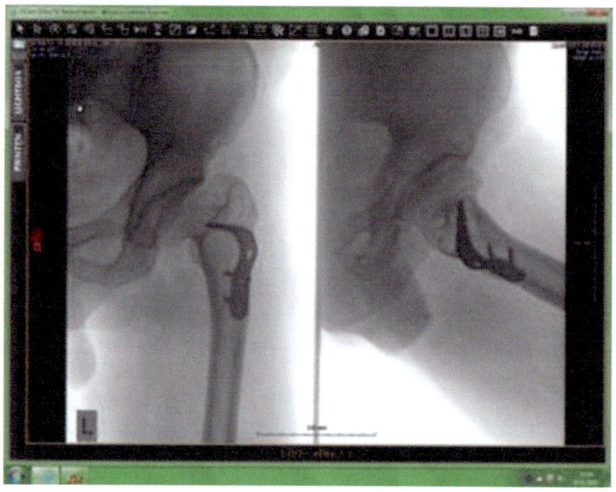

Fig. 9.5 Preoperative X-ray of the left hip showing deformed mushroom-shaped femoral head, shortening, overgrowth of the greater trochanter, and decreased abductor lever arm. Hook plate in situ for thirty five years after subtrochanteric osteotomy at the age of 6. Bowing of proximal femur. Narrow femoral canal

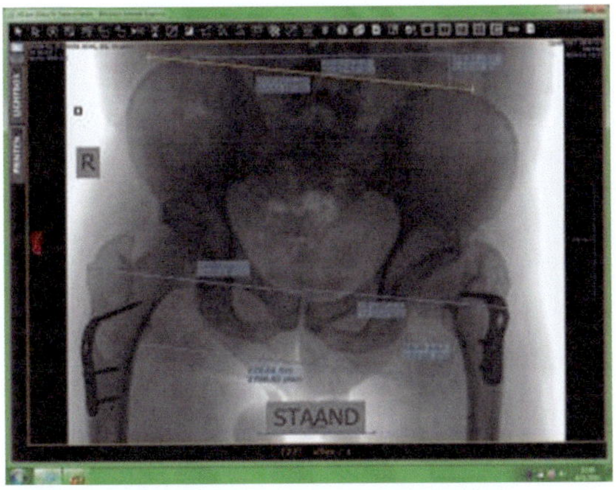

Fig. 9.6 Preoperative measurements showing pelvic tilt due to shortening of the left leg, LLD of 26 mm measured on the pelvis, and 35 mm on the femur, reduced abductor lever arm of 15 mm

9.5.5 Preoperative Planning

Diagnosis: Secondary osteoarthritis due to LCP with coxa brevis and coxa plana, weakness of abductors and important leg length discrepancy (Fig. 9.5)

Possible treatment options: THR, hip arthrodesis

Chosen treatment method: THR with restoration of leg length and abductor lever arm

Selection of implants if applicable and rational: Hard-on-hard bearing if possible; thin femoral implant with sufficient offset; proven track record for implants; therefore choice was made for Trident cup with ceramic liner and Exeter stem with alumina ceramic head

Expected difficulties: Mismatch between the femoral offset and the small femoral implant; LLD; recreation of the abductor lever arm; if a cemented stem is used, then a possible cement leak; stress riser of the femur after removal of the previous implant and a risk of femoral fracture; very narrow femoral canal with previous surgery; difficult entry in the femoral canal; insufficient stability for press-fit cup, screws in acetabular shell; difficult implant removal; overgrowth of the greater trochanter with shortened abductor lever arm

Strategies to overcome difficulties: Preoperative planning; use of extra small implants (Asiatic Exeter); recreate the abductor lever arm partially from the acetabular side; use of high-speed burr femur; plug cortical holes to prevent cement leak; use of intraoperative X-rays if possible; recreate proper tension on the abductors and recreate the abductor lever arm – sometimes use of distalization/osteotomy of the greater trochanter.

Templating: Plan under -correction of the LLD of 5 mm, planning of 20 mm gain; plan to implant the acetabular component slightly lateralized to gain offset if the femoral offset cannot be gained from the stem; plan to increase the abductor lever arm by 10–15 mm. Gain in femoral offset and LLD allows distalization and lateralization of trochanter by femoral implant (Fig. 9.6).

9.5.6 Surgical Note

Patient's position: Lateral

Type of anesthesia: General

Surgical approach: Posterolateral

Main steps: Standard posterolateral approach. Identification and protection of the sciatic nerve. Attention to the lateral femur and exposure of the hook plate. Removal of the plate that was fully ingrown. Attention to hip joint. Release of the piriformis, the conjoined tendon and the quadratus femoris muscle. Psoas tenotomy. Full capsular release 360° and dislocation. Femoral neck osteotomy and removal of the deformed head. Attention was then turned to the acetabulum that is shallow. The standard preparation of the acetabulum for a cementless socket, hereby deliberately not medializing to the medial floor. Trident cup 56 mm with three screws. Ceramic insert Trident. Attention to the femur. Challenging entry due to the absence of normal intramedullary canal and corticalization. Use of high-speed burr and preparation for cemented Exeter stem. Although we were prepared for the use of Asiatic small stems, these have their tip at the level of the distal holes of the plate and there was a risk to act as stress risers. Therefore, we further proceed to open the canal with the burr until a trial stem CDH large—37.5 mm offset number 0—could be introduced. The broach was too large for entry. The trial reduction showed good restoration of the leg length and the offset by lengthening ±20 mm. Stability was satisfactory with no impingement. Exeter cement plug in the femoral canal and plugging of the lateral femoral holes with spongious bone and bone wax and thorough cleaning of the femoral canal. Excellent dry bone bed after drying with peroxide. Third-generation cementing technique according to the Exeter technique with three units of simplex and tobramycin bone cement. Pressurization from 2′ to 6′ and introduction of preheated Exeter CDH large stem 37.5 mm offset number 0 with 15° anteversion. Application of a "horse collar" and further pressurizing the cement until full curing at 10′. Alumina ceramic head 32 mm +0 mm. No closure of capsule and no reinsertion of short external rotators. Hemostatic matrix solution and closure in layers. Pressure bandage 24 h; no drain (Figs. 9.7 and 9.8).

9.5.7 Intraoperative Challenges

Challenges and solutions: (1) LLD—beware of overcorrection aiming for 5 mm less than the ideal (overcorrection is not well tolerated). (2) Recreation of the abductor lever arm—ideally when the cup is seating in the anatomical position this would require femoral offset stem of 44 mm; this would not be possible to enter in the femoral canal (narrow and bowed after osteotomy)—a choice is to lateralize the acetabulum and gain the abductor lever arm length. (3) Difficult entry to the femoral canal—use of high-speed burr. (4) Cement leak—plug the canal and removal of cement extrusion after curing. (5) Cup stability—use sufficient number of screws.

Unanticipated problems and solution: Breakage of the previous screw in femur—use of hollow drill over screw for removal

9.5.8 Postoperative Radiographs (Figs. 9.7 and 9.8)

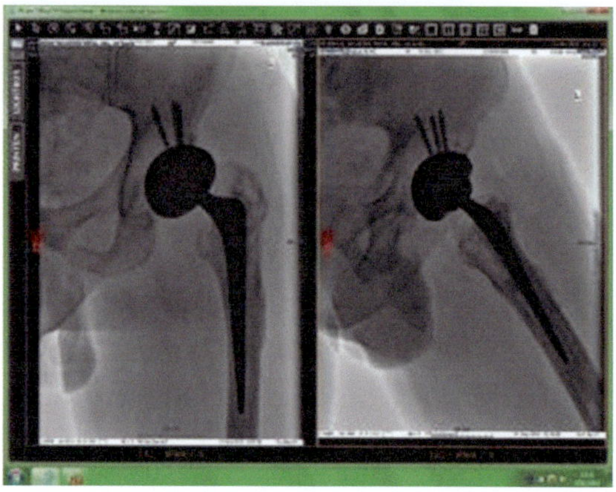

Fig. 9.7 AP and lateral post-op X-rays, showing proper cementing technique and fixation of the acetabular component

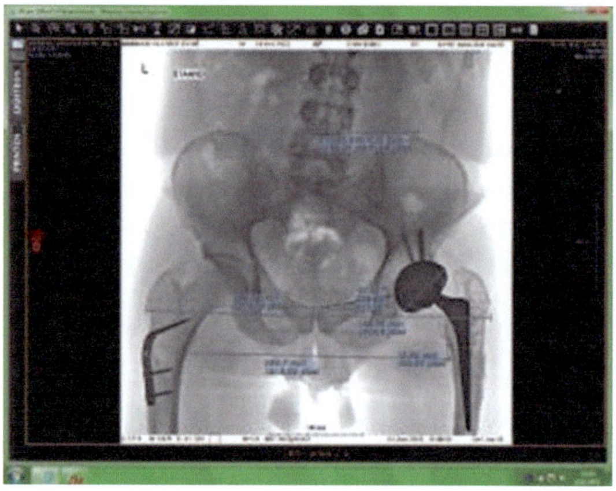

Fig. 9.8 Post-op measurements with good restoration of abductor lever arm; reasonable balance of the pelvis (6 mm difference) with deliberate slight undercorrection of leg length and cup angle of 47°. Contralateral hip without apparent osteoarthritis

9.5.9 Postoperative Management

Chemoprophylaxis and anticoagulant treatment period: Foot pumps and aspirin

Gait/limb loading until full loading: Full weight bearing permitted from the first postop day

9.5.10 Follow-Up and Complications

No complication

Scoring: UCLA 7/10, regained full employment manual labor, Trendelenburg negative, clinically minimal pelvic tilt but feels no LLD, good mobility, modified Charnley score 18/18

9.5.11 Discussion [1, 15, 16]

Advantages of the applied method: Proven design, hard-on-hard bearing in young patient, recreation of the proper pelvic balance and leg length restoration, recreation of the abductor lever arm

Disadvantages of the method: Small Exeter stem, lateralized acetabular shell

Alternative evidence-based techniques for the case: use of a cementless short stem, a modular neck femoral implant and a highly cross-linked polyethylene

Why is the chosen technique better for this case? Long follow-up for taper slip design principle; absence of modularity; ceramic on ceramic has the lowest wear rate.

Indications and contraindications for your technique: No contraindications

Learning curve and how to manage complications: Beware of overlengthening

Level of evidence concerning the superiority of this method against others: There is overwhelming evidence that the taper slip principle with the Exeter stem gives excellent long-term results. The bone will be loaded physiologically, and the aseptic loosening rate is almost 0 at 20 years if a proper cementing technique is used. Ceramic-on-ceramic bearings have the lowest wear rate, and we are unaware of cases of squeaking with the Trident cup if it is used against an Exeter stem. All cases of squeaking described are with cementless stems. Although we cannot rule the possibility of squeaking out, the incidence with the use of a cemented stem is extremely low. The only alternative method to recreate the anatomy properly (with restoration of the abductor lever arm and to avoid post-op abductor insufficiency and possible limping) is by using modular implants. These are more prone to fretting corrosion at the modular interfaces and do not have a similar long-term follow-up, nor do they achieve as high survival percentages in the medium and long-term as the used implants. Sometimes distalization of the greater trochanter is mandatory. If the recreation of the abductor lever arm can be recreated with the implants only, possible complications of distalization of the greater trochanter can be avoided (nonunion, hardware problems).

9.6 Case Title: Complex Total Hip Arthroplasty After Slipped Capital Femoral Epiphysis

R. Schwarzkopf and A.B. Old

9.6.1 Demographics

Age: 50 years old
Sex: Male
BMI: 28

9.6.2 Relevant Past Medical History

Principal pathologies: Slipped capital femoral epiphysis

Previous surgical procedures: Percutaneous in situ screw fixation of bilateral slipped femoral capital epiphysis in bilateral hips in 1979

Medication: Blood pressure control, NSAIDs for pain control

Other: Patient has hypertension treated with beta blockers

History of presenting complaint: A patient is a 50-year-old man with a 3-year history of severe debilitating bilateral hip pain and loss of range of motion. The patient complained of pain, instability, and reported restricted motion in both hips.

9.6.3 Clinical Examination

Symptoms: Bilateral hip pain, severely restricted range of motion

Range of motion: Bilateral hip exam showed obligatory external rotation. The patient had no internal rotation and fixed the external rotation.

Main disability: Restricted ambulation secondary to pain

Neurovascular evaluation: +2 dorsalis pedis bilaterally, neurologically intact

9.6.4 Preoperative Radiological Assessment/Imaging (Fig. 9.9)

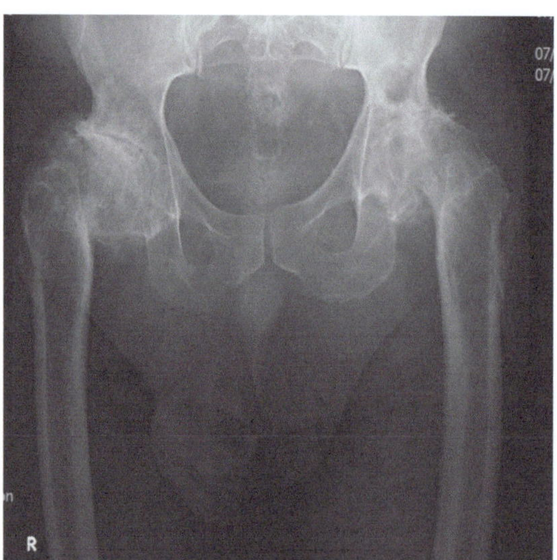

Fig. 9.9 Anteroposterior radiograph of the pelvis. Severe secondary osteoarthritis from dysplasia secondary to slipped capital femoral epiphysis (SCFE). Classic SCFE deformity with posterior and inferior subluxation of the femoral epiphysis

Preoperative Planning

Diagnosis: Bilateral hip arthritis (Fig. 9.9)

Possible treatment options: Conservative nonsurgical management

Chosen treatment method: Bilateral total hip arthroplasty

Selection of implants if applicable and rational: Smith and Nephew Emperion modular hip system. The femoral component is made up of two separate parts, the stem and the sleeve. This allows the surgeon to maximize both metaphyseal and diaphyseal fixation by sizing the two components independently. The second added advantage with this modular system is the ability to dial in the desired version of the femoral stem and allows the surgeon intraoperative flexibility to accommodate for the dysplasia that comes with a displaced femoral epiphysis.

Strategies to overcome difficulties: Preoperative planning should be the foundation that all surgeries are built upon. Never is this more true in total hip arthroplasty following any dysplasia. Successful replacement requires preemptive planning on the surgeon's behalf. This helps maximize efficiency in the OR but also provides a guide to help the surgical team achieve their goals. It is important to reestablish leg length but also stability. This requires accurate restoration of version, neck length, and offset.

Templating: Templating should be considered an important aspect of the preoperative plan. This allows the surgeon to begin to visualize the necessary boney cuts and implant positioning. It is also important to establish any special instruments or implant sizes that may be required to ensure things go as smoothly as possible in the operating room and the necessary equipment is available.

9.6.5 Surgical Note

Patient's position: Lateral decubitus

Type of anesthesia: Spinal regional

Surgical approach: Modified lateral Hardinge approach

Main steps: A standard incision was made in the midline of the femur, centered over the greater trochanter. Sharp dissection was performed through the skin and subcutaneous tissue down to the level of the tensor fascia lata (TFL). Strict hemostasis was obtained with electrocautery bovie. Centering over the greater trochanter and in line with the skin incision, the TFL was incised allowing access to the gluteus medius (GM) and vastus lateralis (VL) below. The anterior one-third of the GM and VL were separated and brought anteriorly in standard fashion. The anterior capsule was then incised in an inverted T along the anterior femoral neck. Given the version of the neck and head and the fixed external rotation hip contracture, an in situ femoral neck cut was performed. The femoral head was then removed using a corkscrew inserted with power. Following sequential reaming, a Smith and Nephew, 56 mm outer diameter (three-hole hemispherical Stiktite-coated shell) cup was impacted into position. This allowed for a 36-mm-sized head to be used. A neutral (zero degree) highly cross-linked polyethylene (XLPE) liner was then impacted into the cup after two screws were placed into the superior posterior safe zone.

Attention was then turned to the femur. Standard access to the femoral canal was obtained using a boxed osteotome and canal find. An opening reamer was then used followed by a metaphyseal rasp. Once the proximal femur has been prepared, the canal was sequentially reamed until cortical chatter was felt. The distal femur was sized to a 15 stem, 150 mm length. Next, a proximal reamer was used for the metaphysis. A size small sleeve was then trialled and found to be a good fit. The neck was then attached, and the appropriate version was dialed into the trial component. The trial was reduced with a 36 mm, +4 mm 12/14 taper head. The hip was taken through a range of motion and found to be stable. The final component was impacted, and the final head put on before the hip was reduced. The hip was taken through range of motion and found to be stable. A standard multilayer closure was performed (Figs. 9.10 and 9.11).

9.6.6 Intraoperative Challenges

Challenges and solutions: It's important to establish equal leg lengths and ultimately to achieve a stable hip. With fixed external rotation contractures, it is best not to destabilize the posterior structures including the short external rotators and the capsule. Therefore, the decision was made to use a modified Hardinge approach leaving the posterior stabilizers intact. If it is not possible to dislocate the femoral head, an in situ neck cut can be used to remove the femoral head safely.

Unanticipated problems and solution: None, proper planning and implant selection will help avoid unexpected problems.

9.6.7 Postoperative Radiographs (Figs. 9.10 and 9.11)

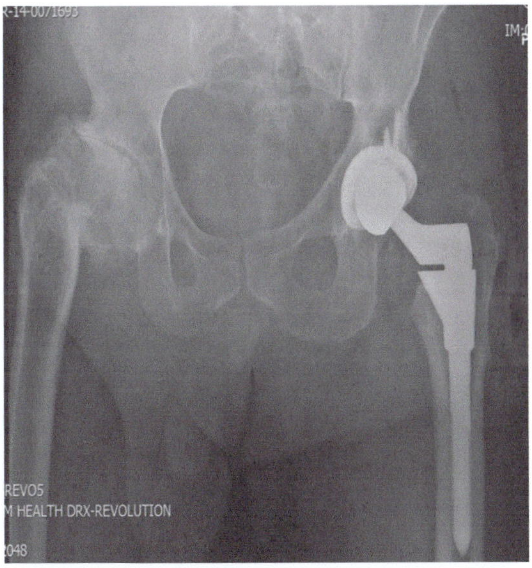

Fig. 9.10 An AP pelvis following the left hip replacement. The patient has been lengthened knowing that the right hip can be matched at a later date

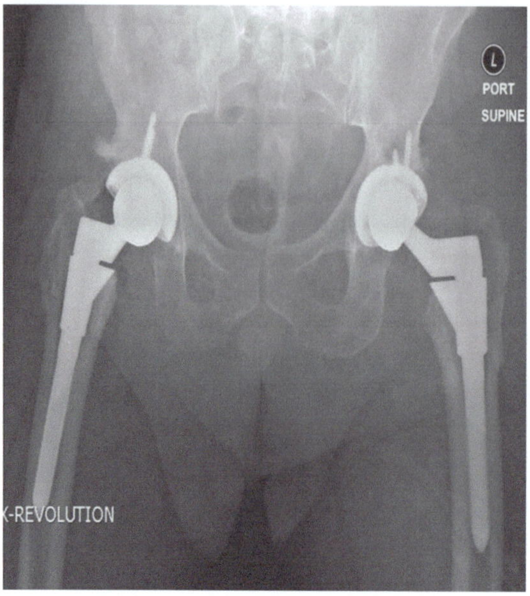

Fig. 9.11 AP pelvis following the right hip replacement. The image shows restoration of equal leg lengths and appropriate offset

9.6.8 Postoperative Management

Chemoprophylaxis and anticoagulant treatment period: The patient was placed on four weeks of aspirin 325 mg PO BID.

Gait/limb loading until full loading: Postoperatively the patient was made weight bearing as tolerated. At final follow-up, the patient was ambulating without a cane.

9.6.9 Discussion [17–22]

Advantages of the applied method: The advantages include retained inherent stability by leaving the posterior structures intact with the lateral approach. Use of the modular stem allowed for multiple points, metaphysis and diaphysis, of fixation for the stem but also intraoperative flexibility regarding the metaphyseal sleeve position and ability to dial in the appropriately needed neck anteversion.

Alternative evidence-based techniques for the case: Total hip resurfacing is a controversial topic secondary to concerns regarding metal-on-metal bearings and the high complication rate. However, there is literature to support the use of hip resurfacing in younger male patients with good bone stock in the hands of experienced surgeons. Amstutz et al. [18] reported on 21 patients (24 hips) that were treated with resurfacing following childhood dysplasias (this included both SCFE and Legg-Calvé-Perthes). Of the ten patients who had SCFE, none required reoperation in the reported follow-up period.

A second alternative could be the use of a cemented implant to allow for secure stem fixation and the intraoperative ability to dial in the desired implant version of the neck. The Exeter Group described a 10–17-year follow-up of cemented THA for 107 patients with 130 hips [19]. This cohort included three patients with an underlying diagnosis of SCFE. One of these patients required a revision surgery secondary to acetabular loosening although the cemented stems had 100% survivorship in their study.

Why is the chosen technique better for this case? Although hip resurfacing is a potential option for young males with good bone stock, the current standard of care would suggest a THA should be performed. Hip resurfacing is incredibly technically demanding and is limited to the femoral neck length and offset options. Large femoral heads require large cups that can lead to impingement. Metal-on-metal bearing is currently controversial given the system exposure to increased metal ions and the possible risk of pseudotumor. There is also the added risk of femoral neck fracture secondary to technical error or advancement of AVN secondary to the compromised blood supply following SCFE. With the advent of tantalum cups and the demonstrated failure rate of cemented acetabular components in young patients, a press-fit cup is likely all that is required. Cemented stems have documented longevity in the young; however, cement adds time to the case in the operating room along with possible complications such as hypotensive episodes (although rare). Modular press-fit stems have shown good survivorship and allow for intraoperative and patient-specific neck length, offset, and version options.

Indications and contraindications for your technique: Indications – just as in any patient with arthritis, post-SCFE patients must have debilitating pain and loss of function before being considered for operative intervention. Contraindications include infection and poorly controlled modifiable risk factors such as diabetes, poor nutrition, smoking, and substance abuse or dependency.

Level of evidence concerning the superiority of this method against others: Modular press-fit stems were introduced in the 2000s to address femoral anteversion, offset, bone loss, and metaphyseal/diaphyseal mismatch. In a level 3 evidence study, Le and colleagues prospectively assessed thirty one hips after primary total hip arthroplasty treated with a modular femoral component [22]. Thc patients were evaluated for both clinical and radiographic outcomes at a minimum of 15-year follow-up. There were no femoral revisions for aseptic loosening; all hips had radiographic evidence of bone ingrowth. They reported two infections. Stress shielding was seen in 74% (23 hips) and osteolysis in 58% (18 hips). They had no stem junction breakage.

9.7 Case Title: THR for Old SCFE

J.F.A. Somers, J. Vanbiervliet, and J.P. Simon

9.7.1 Demographics

Age: 37
Sex: Male
BMI: 27

9.7.2 Relevant Past Medical History

Principal pathologies: SCFE

Previous surgical procedures: Bilateral pinning in situ

Medication: Painkillers

History of presenting complaint: Independent farmer, painful left hip, and long-standing shortening of the left leg

9.7.3 Clinical Examination

Symptoms: Stiffness and pain +++ of the left hip

Range of motion: Extremely limited at the left hip

Main disability: Pain during activity and at night

Neurovascular evaluation: normal

9.7.4 Preoperative Radiological Assessment/Imaging (Figs. 9.12, 9.13, and 9.14)

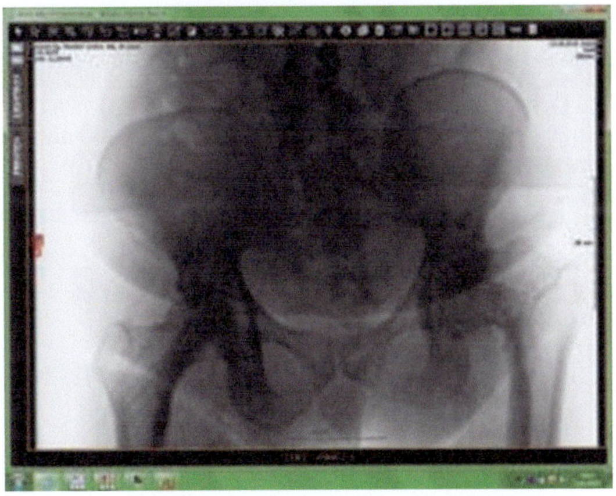

Fig. 9.12 AP pelvis showing leg length discrepancy of 30 mm

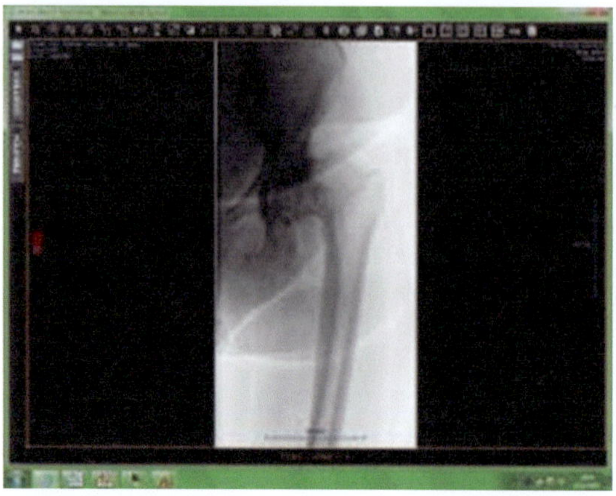

Fig. 9.13 AP hip showing narrow femoral canal

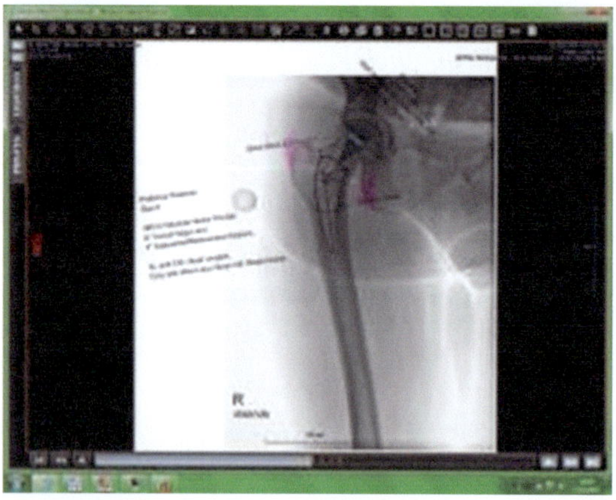

Fig. 9.14 Preop templating of the other hip for normal kinematics

9.7.5 Preoperative Planning

Diagnosis: SCFE (Figs. 9.12 and 9.13)

Possible treatment options: THR

Chosen treatment method: THR

Selection of implants if applicable and rational: Cementless cup, ceramic on ceramic, short cementless stem, modular neck

Expected difficulties: Insufficient acetabular wall posterior, narrow femoral canal, stiffness

Strategies to overcome difficulties: Screw in the cup, short stem, full capsular release

Templating: use other hip (Fig. 9.14)

9.7.6 Surgical Note

Patient's position: Lateral decubitus

Type of anesthesia: General

Surgical approach: Posterolateral

Main steps: Standard posterolateral approach. Identification and protection of the sciatic nerve. Release of the piriformis, the conjoined tendon and the quadratus femoris muscle. Capsular release and dislocation. Femoral neck osteotomy. Psoas release. The standard preparation of the acetabulum for a cementless socket. Use of the transverse ligament for the correct alignment. Cup cementless 56 mm. Intraoperative testing of cup stability and use of an extra screw for initial stability. Ceramic liner insert. Then attention was turned to the femur and broaching. Preserve short stem nr 6 to 15° anteversion. Trial reduction with modular neck straight short shows a good restoration of leg length and offset with head 36 mm + 4 mm. Stability was satisfactory in full ROM. No impingement. Placement of definitive modular neck and a ceramic head. Reduction. Reinsertion of conjoined tendon/piriformis with nonabsorbable suture. Hemostatic matrix solution and closure in layers. Pressure bandage 24 h; no drain (Figs. 9.15 and 9.16).

9.7.7 Intraoperative Challenges

Challenges and solutions: Leg length discrepancy and stability after full release; use modular neck and template on the opposite side

9.7.8 Postoperative Radiographs (Figs. 9.15 and 9.16)

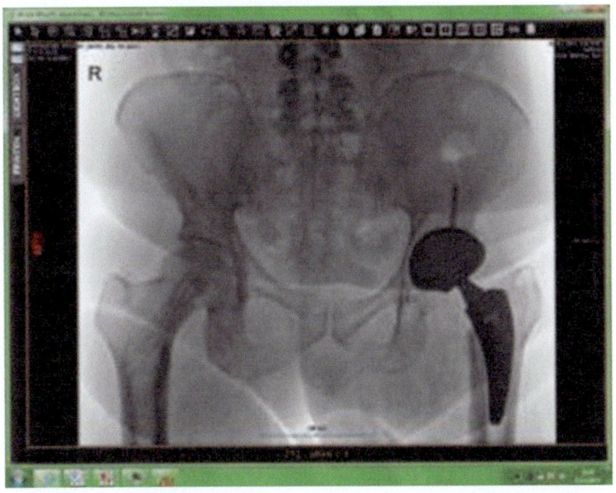

Fig. 9.15 AP pelvis showing correction of the leg length and the abductor lever arm

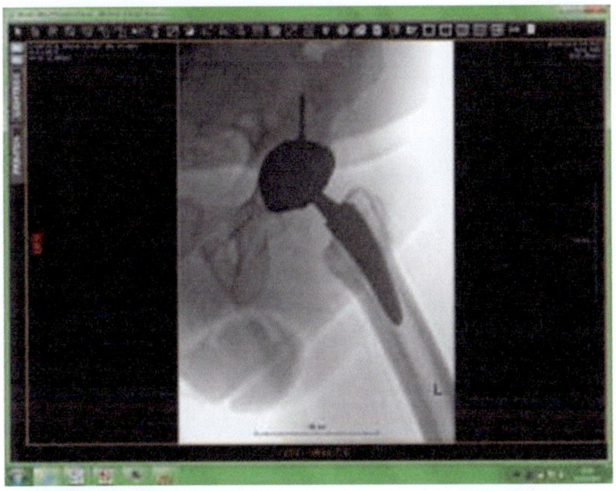

Fig. 9.16 Profile post-op

9.7.9 Postoperative Management

Chemoprophylaxis and anticoagulant treatment period: Foot pumps and aspirin for four weeks

Gait/limb loading until full loading: Full weight bearing

9.7.10 Follow-Up and Complications

No complication

Scoring: At work after six months, having no pain and good mobility

9.7.11 Discussion

Advantages of the applied method: Full restoration of the normal anatomy and kinematics, hard-on-hard bearing in young patient

Disadvantages of the method: Short follow-up of used implants, modular neck

Alternative evidence-based techniques for the case: Cemented stem-type Exeter

Why is the chosen technique better for this case? Modularity allows perfect restoration of anatomy; used necks have proven track record [5, 23]. Ceramic on ceramic has the lowest wear rate.

Indications and contraindications for your technique: Can be used for most cases with SCFE. Avoid long varus modular necks if high BME.

9.8 Case Title: Primary Complex Hip Arthroplasty for Previous Slipped Capital Epiphysis

J.F.A. Somers, Jens Vanbiervliet, and Jean-Pierre Simon

9.8.1 Demographics

Age: 18
Sex: Female
BMI: 26

9.8.2 Relevant Past Medical History

Principal pathologies: Slipped capital epiphysis of the left hip during childhood at the age of 10

Previous surgical procedures: Reduction and fixation of the femoral head with a cannulated screw at the age of 10. Arthroscopic rinsing at the age of 17

Medication: None

Other: Generalized joint hyperlaxity

History of presenting complaint: After the initial treatment for SCFE with in situ pinning, this teenager developed secondary osteoarthritis in a very early stage. At the age of fifteen, she was suffering from pain and was on daily pain medication. At the age of 17, an arthroscopic debridement was attempted, but extensive cartilage damage was found, and she did not improve after surgery. At the age of 18, she was experiencing pain day and night and was using a crutch. She was limping, and her walking perimeter was limited to a hundred of m. She was taking simple analgesia orally on a daily basis.

9.8.3 Clinical Examination

Symptoms: Pain

Range of motion: Flexion 80°, abduction 25°, adduction 15°, external rotation 25°, internal rotation 10°; all painful

Specific tests: Trendelenburg test +, impingement test +

Main disability: Pain during activity and at rest; night pain

Neurovascular evaluation: Normal

9.8.4 Preoperative Radiological Assessment/Imaging (Figs. 9.17, 9.18, and 9.19)

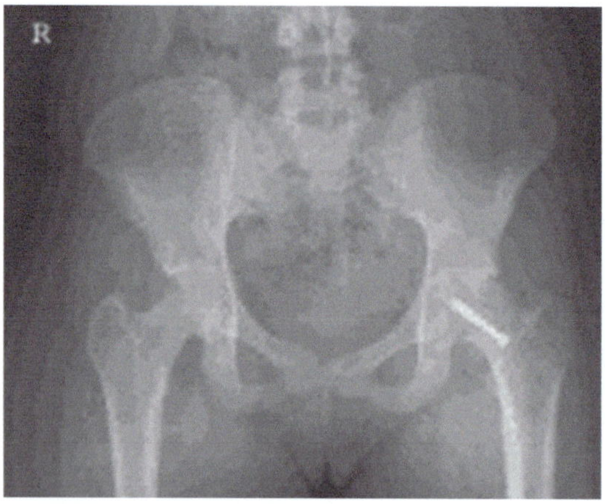

Fig. 9.17 AP pelvis

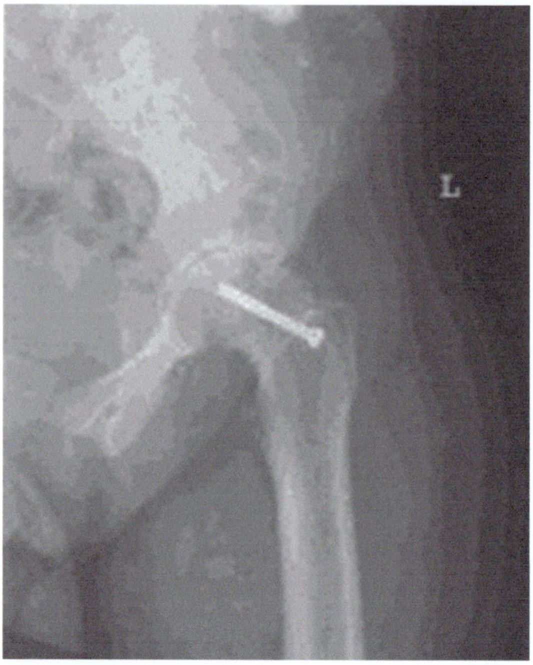

Fig. 9.18 Lateral view

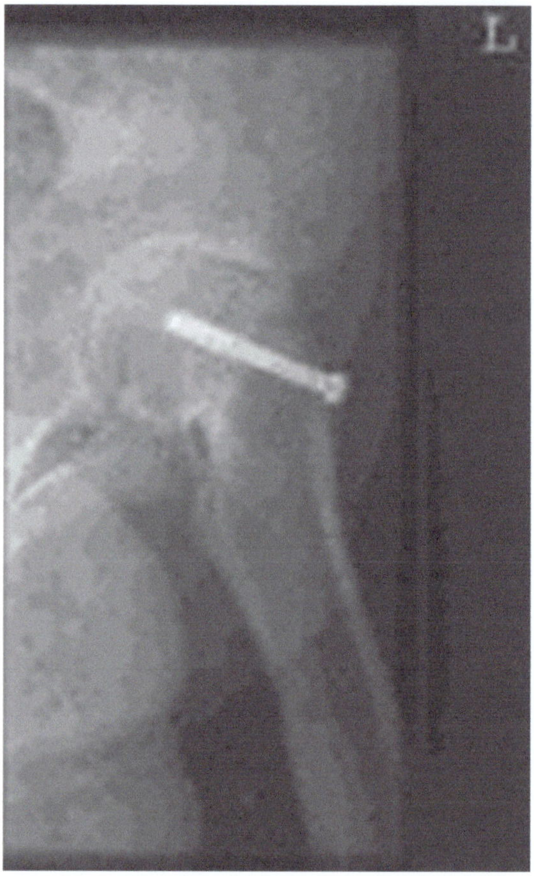

Fig. 9.19 Lateral view

9.8.5 Preoperative Planning

Diagnosis: Osteoarthritis of the left hip (Figs. 9.17, 9.18, and 9.19)

Possible treatment options: Total hip arthroplasty or hip arthrodesis but no hip resurfacing because of the femoral neck distortion

Chosen treatment method: THA

Selection of implants if applicable and rational: Stryker Exeter V40 stem size 0 (offset 44), Stryker 32 mm femoral head (offset 0 mm), 52 mm Zimmer Trilogy acetabular cup with highly cross-linked polyethylene liner (+ 10-degree elevated rim), one 6.5 mm diameter screw (50 mm)

Expected difficulties: Narrow femoral canal; screw at the level of femoral cut; higher risk of dislocation; extremely young age; two previous surgeries, beware of the possibility of low-grade infection; retroversion of the acetabulum (ischial spine sign) and coxa profunda—difficulty with cup stability and positioning

Strategies to overcome difficulties: Conventional surgical approach with appropriate intraoperative view; use of proven implants; extremely careful to recreate anatomy and correct leg length; intraoperative frozen section (Feldman criteria)

9.8.6 Surgical Note

Patient's position: Lateral decubitus

Type of anesthesia: General anesthesia

Surgical approach: Posterolateral approach

Main steps: Standard posterolateral approach. Identification and protection of the sciatic nerve. Release of the piriformis, the conjoined tendon and the quadratus femoris muscle. Capsular release and dislocation. Femoral neck osteotomy and careful dislodging of the head of the screw from the lateral proximal femur. Prelevation of three soft tissue specimens for pathology: frozen section and use of Feldman criteria (<5 polymorphonuclear cells per high power field in 3 × 3 fields means no infection), negative. The standard preparation of the acetabulum for a cementless socket. Use of the transverse ligament for the correct alignment. Intraoperative testing of cup stability and use of an extra screw for initial stability. Trial insert. Attention was then turned to the femur and standard preparation for cemented Exeter stem. Trial reduction showed good restoration of leg length and offset with 44 mm offset stem. Satisfactory stability but at the limit of deep flexion with adduction and internal rotation and no impingement. Decision for elevated rim liner. Placement of highly cross-linked elevated rim liner and attention back to the femur. Exeter cement plug and thorough cleaning of the femoral canal. Excellent dry bone bed after drying with peroxide. Third-generation cementing technique according to the Exeter technique with three units of simplex and tobramycin bone cement. Pressurization from 2′ to 6′ and the introduction of preheated Exeter universal stem 44 mm offset nr 0 to 15° anteversion. Application of "horse collar" and further pressurizing the cement until full curing at 10′. Alumina ceramic head 32 mm + 0 mm. Reduction. Closure of posterior capsule and reinsertion of conjoined tendon/piriformis with nonabsorbable suture. Hemostatic matrix solution and closure in layers. Pressure bandage 24 h; no drain (Figs. 9.20 and 9.21).

9.8.7 Intraoperative Challenges

Challenges and solutions: retroversion of the acetabulum, cup stability, screw fixation; narrow femoral canal with relatively high femoral offset; use the Exeter slimmest stem with appropriate offset; stability of hip in a patient with generalized hyperlaxity, 32 mm ceramic head and elevated rim liner.

9.8.8 Postoperative Radiographs (Figs. 9.20 and 9.21)

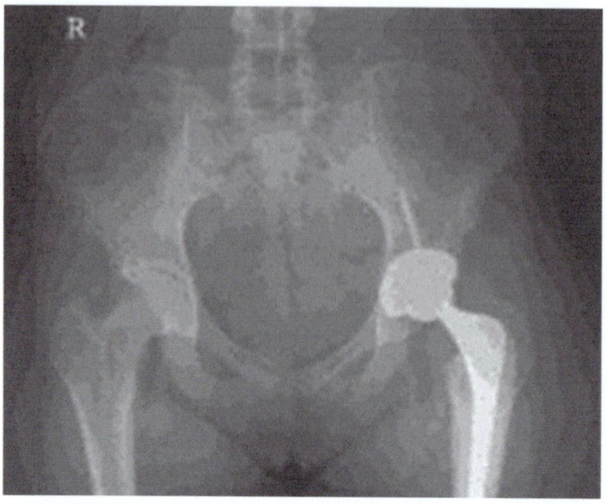

Fig. 9.20 AP pelvis

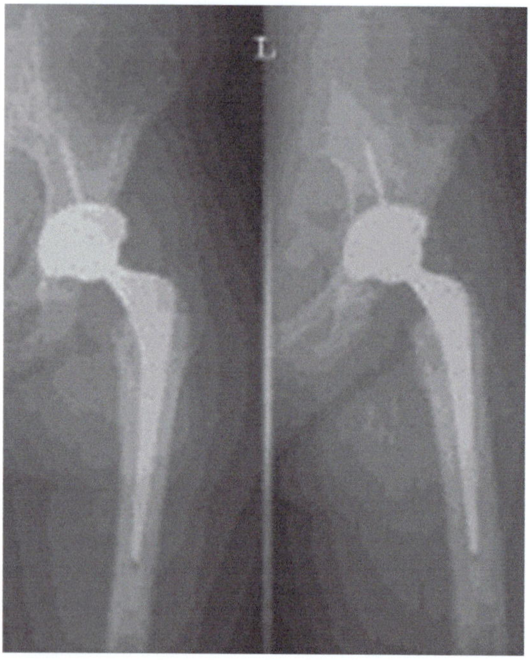

Fig. 9.21 Lateral view

9.8.9 Postoperative Management

Chemoprophylaxis and anticoagulant treatment period: Mechanical prophylaxis with foot pumps; LMWH for three weeks

Gait/limb loading until full loading: Full weight bearing allowed as from day one postoperatively

9.8.10 Follow-Up and Complications

No complications

Scoring: HHS 100 /WOMAC 100/UCLA 8 at 1- and 5-year FU

9.8.11 Discussion [6, 15, 24]

Advantages of the applied method: Perfect restoration of anatomy with low risk of intraoperative femoral fracture, very long-term success of taper slip principle/Exeter stem, long-term success of Trilogy cup, low wear characteristics of highly cross-linked polyethylene, very low risk of implant-related problems in the first 10–20 years, no risk of thigh pain

Disadvantages of the method: No hard-on-hard bearing used

Alternative evidence-based techniques for the case: Ceramic-on-ceramic bearing has better wear characteristics but higher risk of dislocation—squeaking—ceramic liner fracture; cementless stems

Why is the chosen technique better for this case? Highest success rate for femoral Exeter stem compared to any other stem type, with proven preservation of femoral bone stock; literature shows 80% success at ten years only for cementless THA due to short-term complications.

Learning curve and how to manage complications: Recreation of leg length and offset with Exeter philosophy; cementing technique

References

1. Al-Khateeb H, Kwok IH, Hanna SA, Sewell MD, Hashemi-Nejad A. Custom cementless THA in patients with Legg-Calvé-Perthes disease. J Arthroplast. 2014; 29(4):792–6.
2. Baghdadi YM, Larson AN, Stans AA, Mabry TM. Total hip arthroplasty for the sequelae of Legg-Calvé-Perthes disease. Clin Orthop Relat Res. 2013;471(9):2980–6.

3. Mazloumi SM, Ebrahimzadeh MH, Kachooei AR. Evolution in diagnosis and treatment of Legg-Calvé-Perthes disease. Arch Bone Joint Surg. 2014;2(2):86–92.
4. Larson AN, Sucato DJ, Herring JA, Adolfsen SE, Kelly DM, Martus JE, Lovejoy JF, Browne R, Delarocha A. A prospective multicenter study of Legg-Calvé-Perthes disease: functional and radiographic outcomes of nonoperative treatment at a mean follow-up of twenty years. J Bone Joint Surg Am. 2012;94:584–92.
5. Traina F, De Fine M, Abati CN, Bordini B, Toni A. Outcomes of total hip replacement in patients with slipped capital femoral epiphysis. Arch Orthop Trauma Surg. 2012;132(8):1133–9.
6. Schoof B, Citak M, O'Loughlin PF, Kendoff D, Haasper C, Gehrke T, Gebauer M. Eleven year results of total hip arthroplasty in patients with secondary osteoarthritis due to slipped capital femoral epiphysis. Open Orthop J. 2013;7:158–62.
7. Engesæter LB, Engesæter IØ, Fenstad AM, Havelin LI, Kärrholm J, Garellick G, Pedersen AB, Overgaard S. Low revision rate after total hip arthroplasty in patients with pediatric hip diseases. Acta Orthop. 2012;83(5):436–41.
8. Traina F, De Fine M, Sudanese A, Calderoni PP, Tassinari E, Toni A. Long-term results of total hip replacement in patients with Legg-Calvé-Perthes disease. J Bone Joint Surg Am. 2011;93(7):e25.
9. Pietrzak K, Strzyzewski W, Pucher A, Kaczmarek W. Total hip replacement after Legg-Calvé-Perthes disease. Chir Narzadow Ruchu Ortop Pol. 2011;76(3):129–33.
10. Lehmann TG, Engesaeter IØ, Laborie LB, Lie SA, Rosendahl K, Engesaeter LB. Total hip arthroplasty in young adults, with focus on Perthes' disease and slipped capital femoral epiphysis: follow-up of 540 subjects reported to the Norwegian Arthroplasty register during 1987–2007. Acta Orthop. 2012;83(2):159–64.
11. Thillemann TM, Pedersen AB, Johnsen SP, Søballe K. Danish hip Arthroplasty registry. Implant survival after primary total hip arthroplasty due to childhood hip disorders: results from the Danish hip Arthroplasty registry. Acta Orthop. 2008;79(6):769–76.
12. Lim YW, Kim MJ, Lee YS, Kim YS. Total hip arthroplasty in patient with the sequelae of Legg-Calvé -Perthes disease. Hip Pelvis. 2014;26(4):214–9.
13. Larson AN, McIntosh AL, Trousdale RT, Lewallen DG. Avascular necrosis most common indication for hip arthroplasty in patients with slipped capital femoral epiphysis. J Pediatr Orthop. 2010;30(8):767–73.
14. Boyle MJ, Frampton CM, Crawford HA. Early results of total hip arthroplasty in patients with slipped upper femoral epiphysis compared with patients with osteoarthritis. J Arthroplast. 2012;27(6):1003–7.
15. Bedard NA, Callaghan JJ, Stefl MD, Liu SS. Systematic review of literature of cemented femoral components: what is the durability at minimum 20 years followup? Clin Orthop Relat Res. 2015;473(2):563–71.
16. Costa CR, Johnson AJ, Naziri Q, Mont MA. Review of total hip resurfacing and total hip arthroplasty in young patients who had Legg-Calvé-Perthes disease. Orthop Clin North Am. 2011;42(3):419–22.
17. Helms NJ, Lewallen LW, McIntosh AL, Sierra RJ. Total hip arthroplasty in the young: special emphasis on post-SCFE patients. J Pediatr Orthop. 2013;33(Suppl 1):S137–42.
18. Amstutz HC, Su EP, Le Duff MJ. Surface arthroplasty in young patients with hip arthritis secondary to childhood disorders. Orthop Clin North Am. 2005;36(2):223–30.
19. Lewthwaite SC, Squires B, Gie GA, Timperley AJ, Ling RS. The Exeter Universal hip in patients 50 years or younger at 10-17 years' followup. Clin Orthop Relat Res. 2008;466(2):324–31.
20. Sandiford NA, Duncan CP, Garbuz DS, Masri BA. Tapered, fluted titanium stems in revision total hip arthroplasty: role and results in contemporary practice. Instr Course Lect. 2015;64:359–66.
21. Hoberg M, Konrads C, Engelien J, Oschmann D, Holder M, Walcher M, Rudert M. Outcome of a modular tapered uncemented titanium femoral stem in revision hip arthroplasty. Int Orthop. 2015;39(9):1709–13.
22. Le D, Smith K, Tanzer D, Tanzer M. Modular femoral sleeve and stem implant provides long-term total hip survivorship. Clin Orthop Relat Res. 2011;469(2):508–13.
23. Somers JFA. Metal ion levels in ceramic-on-ceramic THR with modular necks. Hip Int. 2015;25(5):484–7.
24. Ling RS, Charity J, Lee AJ, et al. The long-term results of the original Exeter polished cemented femoral component: a follow-up report. J Arthroplasty. 2009;24(4):511–7.

Osteonecrosis

10

Eustathios Kenanidis, Anastasios Nektarios Tzavellas, Andreas Leonidou, Eleftherios Tsiridis, Arkan S. Sayed-Noor, Bakir Kadum, Karl Brabants, Peter Mertens, and Bogdan Nikolae Deleanu

10.1 Current Concepts

E. Kenanidis, A.N. Tzavellas, A. Leonidou, and E. Tsiridis

Osteonecrosis of the femoral head (ONFH) is a multifactorial debilitating condition that may lead to progressive destruction of the hip joint (Fig. 10.1). The incidence of the disease increases among the third and fifth decade of life [1]. ONFH is the diagnosis of 5–12% of annually performed THAs in the USA [1, 2]. The pathogenesis of the disease has not been fully delineated; it is probably a multifactorial process where the genetic predisposition plays a crucial role [3, 4]. The main risk factors that have been associated with the pathogenetic mechanism of ONFH are hip fracture and dislocation, corticosteroids or excessive alcohol consumption, coagulation disorders and haemoglobinopathies [4]. Fat and air embolization, autoimmune and storage diseases, smoking and hyperlipidaemia have also been implicated [1, 5].

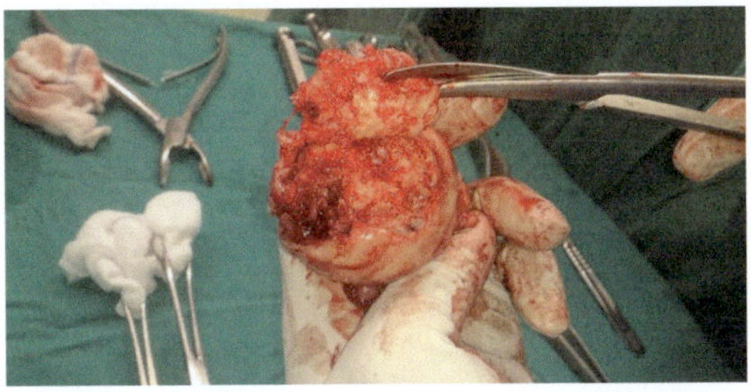

Fig. 10.1 Ficat IV osteonecrosis of the femoral head. Complete collapse and fragmentation of the head cartilage with subchondral necrosis and sclerosis

There is no consensus on the optimal treatment algorithm of the disease [6]; this results from the lack of high-level studies in the literature [3, 4]. Sixteen major classification systems have been developed that help in the prognosis, the treatment decision and the outcome

E. Kenanidis, M.D., Ph.D., M.Sc. (✉)
A.N. Tzavellas, M.D., M.Sc.
Academic Orthopaedic Unit, Aristotle University Medical School, Thessaloniki, Greece

A. Leonidou, P.G.Dip., M.Sc., F.R.C.S.
Reading Shoulder Unit, Reading, UK
e-mail: leonidou@doctors.org.uk

E. Tsiridis, M.D., Ph.D., F.A.C.S., F.R.C.S.
Academic Orthopaedic Unit, Papageorgiou General Hospital, Aristotle University Medical School, Thessaloniki, Greece
e-mail: etsiridis@doctors.org.uk

A.S. Sayed-Noor, M.D., Ph.D., F.R.C.S. · B. Kadum, M.D., Ph.D.
Department of Surgical & Perioperative Sciences, Umeå University, Umeå, Sweden

K. Brabants, M.D. · P. Mertens, M.D.
ZNA Middelheim, Antwerp, Belgium
e-mail: carl.brabants@zna.be; peter.mertens@zna.be

B.N. Deleanu, M.D., Ph.D.
Pius Branzeu Emergency Clinical County Hospital, Timisoara, Romania

Victor Babes University of Medicine and Pharmacy, Timisoara, Romania

E. Tsiridis (ed.), *The Adult Hip - Master Case Series and Techniques*,
https://doi.org/10.1007/978-3-319-64177-5_10

comparison. The Ficat classification is the more commonly used [7].

Different conservative and surgical options based on the stage of the disease have been proposed. The extent and the location of the necrotic lesion, the presence of bone marrow edema and the underlying disease are the main prognostic factors [4, 8]. Weight-bearing portion lesions and non-idiopathic diseases compared to idiopathic have the worse prognosis.

The few clinical studies have not yet established the usefulness of the pharmacological agents as the anticoagulants, the lipid-lowering agents, the bisphosphonates, the antioxidants and the vasoactive substances in the treatment of ONFH [9, 10]. Limited evidence also exists for other used nonoperative procedures as the extracorporeal shock wave treatment and the pulsed electromagnetic therapy [11].

Surgical treatment is divided into head-preserving procedures (percutaneous drilling, core decompression with or without non-vascularized grafts, stem cells, or biologic adjuncts, vascularized bone grafting, rotational osteotomies, tantalum rod insertion) (Fig. 10.2 a, b) for the early stages of the disease [12, 13] and arthroplasty including both resurfacing and THA for the advanced stages [4].

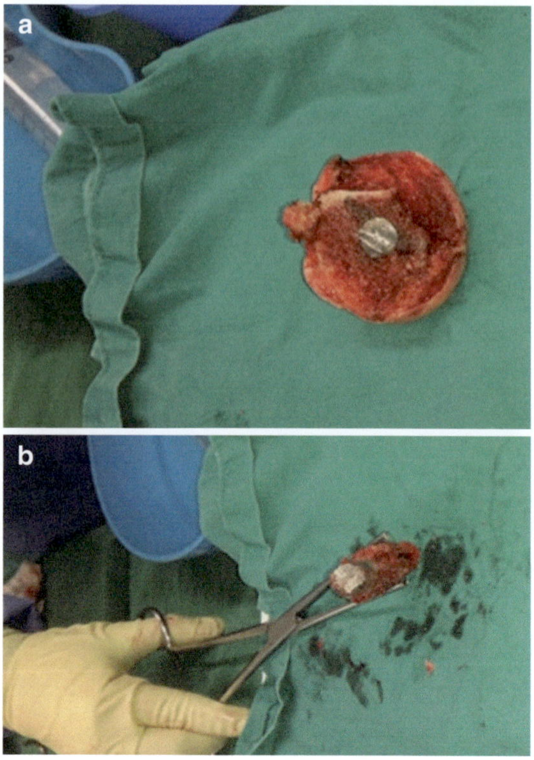

Fig. 10.2 (**a**, **b**). Tantalum rode removal from a femoral neck and head during THA for osteonecrosis. The rode has TA cover, and the core is solid titanium. It is necessary to have a powerful cutting *s*aw to divide it. Removing it from the neck may be challenging and may cause fracture of the greater trochanter.

10.1.1 THA Indication

THA seems to be the most effective treatment modality in the pain management and the functional recovery based on the severity of the disease but also on the patient-specific factors (age, symptoms, prognostic factors) [1]. The primary indications of THA are considered the following [1, 4]:

- The collapse of the femoral head or the presence of large osteonecrotic lesion in the pre-collapse stages
- The advanced painful degenerative changes of the femoral head with acetabular involvement and joint destruction
- Failure of the head-preserving methods

10.1.2 Preoperative Planning

- There is great variability of the patients suffering from ONFH. The underlying disease and the stage of ONFH seriously affect the severity of surgery. They are usually younger patients with increased preoperative ROM compared to long-standing OA patients [14].
- Manage carefully perioperatively and optimize the patient's medical conditions to improve outcomes [1].
- Remember that the bone quality of the acetabulum or the proximal femur may be compromised by the underlying disease, the use of

pharamacological agents as corticosteroids or the luck of weight bearing [1].

- Ream gently the acetabulum and impact the implant as the usual associated subchondral sclerosis may not be present [1].
- The previous femoral head-preserving surgical methods could alter the proximal femur anatomy (previous osteotomy, core decompression or bone graft).
- In specific patients, especially those exposed to high dose of corticosteroids, the necrotic lesion may extend into the calcar providing inadequate support to the femoral component.

10.1.3 Published Results

There is a lack of consensus in the literature about the most appropriate arthroplasty type and fixation for ONFH patients, mainly due to the lack of high level of evidence studies [4, 15, 16].

Historically, the reported results of previous cemented THA cohorts for ONFH were devastating. The high reported failure rates of 37–53% [14, 17–19] were attributed to the first generation of cement, the older implants, the relative young age of patients and the inferior bone quality.

During the last years, the results of THA for ONFH patients have improved considerably [1]. ONFH patients are now considered to have similar failure rates after THA than the general population [20–26]. In a recent systematic review, Johansson et al. [16] evaluated 2593 patients who received THA for ONFH. The overall survival rate of the primary THAs was 87%. This was more or less attributed to the first-generation cement and the worse technique used. THAs performed after 1990 had better results than THAs performed before 1990. The mean survival rate of the THAs before 1990 was 83% at a mean follow-up of 9 years whether those following 1990 was 97% at a mean follow-up of 6 years (odds ratio = 3.8). Following 1990, the results were comparable with the reported survival rate for primary THA for OA in different national registries (Swedish, New Zealand, Danish, Australian) [16]. The group of patients that undergone THA after 1990 had a significantly greater percentage of cementless implants (89% vs. 28%) ($p < 0.001$) and a higher proportion of men ($p < 0.001$). The underlying disease had a predictive value of the survival. Patients suffering from sickle cell disease, renal failure and/or transplant and Gaucher disease had significant higher than the overall risk. Patients suffering from systemic lupus erythematosus ($p < 0.001$), idiopathic disease ($p = 0.005$) and heart transplant ($p = 0.027$) had significantly lower risk than the overall. The corticosteroid use was not an independent risk factor for revision compared to the total risk ($p = 0.097$) [16].

However, even in these high-risk groups, the results of THR have improved over time, so that the underlying disease is not considered as a predictor of poor outcomes by many authors [27–29]. This is attributed to the improved medical and surgical management and the modern prosthetic designs, including cementless acetabular and femoral fixation [27–29]. Ilyas et al. [27] reported no femoral stem revision on eighteen consecutive sickle cell patients with a mean age of twenty eight years that had undergone simultaneous bilateral cementless bipolar hip replacements at a mean follow-up of 5.7 years. Chang et al. [29] evaluated seventy four cementless THRs in fifty two patients suffering from osteonecrosis of the femoral head after kidney transplantation; there was 96.6% cumulative implant survivorship at a mean follow-up of 10.2 years.

Recent tribological advances as ultrahigh cross-linked polyethylene and ceramic bearings showed promising results for THA in patients suffering from osteonecrosis in midterm results [30, 31]. Min et al. [30] reported 100% survival, with the exception of infection, in 162 THRs with highly cross-linked polyethylene bearings at a mean of 7.2 years of follow-up. Kim et al. [31] also showed 100% survivorship (excluding infection) for seventy three THRs for osteonecrosis using alumina ceramic heads on highly cross-linked polyethylene at a mean follow-up of 8.5 years. To address cup osteolysis [32], the use of titanium or tantalum highly porous acetabular cups has been proposed.

Studies reporting on primary THR following previous hip joint-preserving procedures at midterm follow-up supported no affection of the outcomes [33–35]. Kawasaki et al. [33] reported on fifteen failed trans-trochanteric rotational osteotomies for ONFH converted to THR at a mean follow-up of five years; there were no significant differences in the implant survivorship, the stability or the Harris Hip Score compared with a matched group of sixteen hips that underwent primary THR. Helbig et al. [35] demonstrated no complications or component loosening on fifteen THAs previously treated with core decompression at a mean follow-up of fifty four months.

The proper type of fixation of THAs for ONFH is also conflicting in the literature [16]. Two papers comparing uncemented and cemented THA in osteonecrotic hips provide better short- and long-term outcomes for the cementless group. Bedard et al. [36] found that the revision rates due to loosening were significantly lower in the uncemented group after ten years of follow-up of sixty six patients that had undergone either cementless or cemented THA. Yu et al. [37] reported that the incidence of postoperative complications and revision rate of the cemented group were significantly higher than those of the uncemented group 30.7% vs 12,5% and 23.1% vs 0, respectively, at approximately four years of follow-up.

Resurfacing arthroplasty is an option in a young ONFH patient. Current indications for resurfacing are patients with high functional demand, good bone quality especially of the neck, no anatomical deformities and avascular osteonecrosis in Ficat III or IV stage osteonecrosis involving less than 50% of the femoral head [38, 39]. It is not indicated in men older than sixty five and women older than fifty years old [4]. The female fertility, a femoral head size smaller than 46 mm, renal insufficiency and a known metal allergy are further contraindications. Patient selection is critical for the survivorship of resurfacing THA [38, 39]. The results after resurfacing in osteonecrosis are comparable to the patients treated for coxarthrosis [4, 40]. Hemiresurfacing arthroplasty (HRA) of the femoral head has reemerged as a viable option in the young patient subgroup. In a systematic review [41] of published studies that evaluated the outcomes of hemiresurfacing arthroplasty (HRA) in patients with osteonecrosis from 1950 to 2014, a total of 430 patients from fourteen published studies were identified. The mean follow-up was 69 months. The overall success rate was 74%. One hundred two (21%) revision surgeries were required; the main reasons were the acetabular cartilage wear (43%), the acetabular protrusion and the continuing groin pain.

Short stems are another potential solution for the arthroplasty treatment of ONFH. A recent review [42] of the existing literature regarding the outcome of short-stem arthroplasty in ONFH, included few studies usually with short-term results in patients with progressive ONFH [43–46]. The short- to medium-term results showed predominantly good outcomes; however, longer follow-up studies are needed.

10.2 Case Title: Bilateral Staged THA and Revision. Primary THA on the Right for Osteonecrosis Following Fibular Vascularized Autograft and Revision to a Cemented Liner into the In Situ Metal Shell on the Left THA

E. Kenanidis and E. Tsiridis

10.2.1 Demographics

Age: 45
Sex: Male
BMI: 28

10.2.2 Relevant Past Medical History

Principal pathologies: Pain and inability to walk on the left; short limp gate and pain on the right.

Previous surgical procedures: Vascularized fibular graft fifteen years back for corticosteroid-induced osteonecrosis following treatment for lymphoma.

Medication: None.

History of presenting complaint: Pain and inability to walk on the left; short limp gate and pain on the right.

10.2.3 Clinical Examination

Symptoms: Left THA, instability, sense of dislocating the hip, pain on weight bearing; right hip, short limb four cm and pain in all directions.

Range of motion: Left THA, instability apprehension to dislocate in extreme ranges unable to test properly due to latter symptoms; right hip, flexion 60, extension −10, unable to perform internal and external rotation, abduction and adduction.

Specific tests: Shot limp gate, Thomas positive at 25 degrees for the right hip.

Main disability: Pain and instability short limp gate.

Scoring if available: HHS right: 60; HHS left: 80.

Neurovascular evaluation: Intact.

10.2.4 Preoperative Radiological Assessment/Imaging (Fig. 10.3)

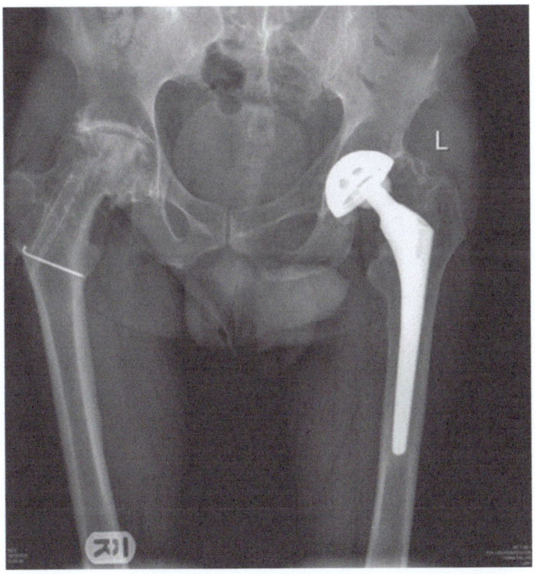

Fig. 10.3 The preoperative radiograph right hip: femoral head osteonecrosis stage IV with advanced collapse and deformity. Arthritis and deformity of the socket. Obvious vascularized fibular autograft with sclerotic margins through the neck; K-wire holding the graft and the vascular anastomosis in place. Left THA: dorsal migration of the ceramic femoral head into the XLPoly liner indicating wear and instability with no evidence of polyethylene debris osteolysis around the joint

10.2.5 Preoperative Planning

Diagnosis: Osteonecrosis of the femoral head right hip and osteoarthritis of the right hip. The left THA has liner wear that needs revision (Fig. 10.3).

Possible treatment options: Left THA: remove the acetabular implant and revise to uncemented or retain the metal shell if stable drill through the screw holes to allow cement interdigitation and cement an HXLP into it. Right: uncemented THA; the quality of the bone is excellent, and the patient is young.

Chosen treatment method: Right THA: Corail fully coated anatomical double-tapered stem (DePuy) size 12; acetabulum, 54 mm shell and 36 mm HXLP (DePuy).

Left hip revision: 46 mm HXLP (Stryker) cemented inside the metal shell in situ

Selection of implants if applicable and rational: Stable implants can be retained during revision, and cementing a liner into a cell is a well-established technique especially when the shell was multihole thus allowing the creation of several peg holes for the cement interdigitating.

Expected difficulties: Right hip, removing the K-wire may be a challenge. Also rasping the femoral canal may be difficult as the proximal canal is occluded by the graft.

Strategies to overcome difficulties: Implant availability if necessary to remove the shell with an "explant device" (Zimmer) in the left THA.

Templating: Yes on the right for adjusting the leg length and the femoral neck cut and hip offset.

10.2.6 Surgical Note

Left THA revision first procedure: With the patient in lateral decubitus and a posterior approach, the hip was exposed easily. The dislocation revealed a worn liner and an intact femoral head with no signs of metallosis or poly debris. The bone segments were found intact both around the femur and the acetabulum. The femoral head was easily removed to allow better access to the acetabulum and then was retracted anteriorly behind an anterior retractor taking care not to scratch (wrapped up with a gauge) the taper that was 12/14 standard. The acetabular liner was removed easily using a lip elevator and a sharp blow at the periphery approximately near the 13–14.00 hours. The shell was exposed and vigorously checked for stability. There was no interface space between the implant and the bone, and curved chisels were unable to enter the interface. The decision was then made to retain the shell and cement a liner into it. Another reason for doing so was the availability of several screw holes in the periphery (multihole shell) to allow cement peg creation for better cement stability. Trail liner was selected and was found that 46 mm HXLP would enable enough cement to a min of 2 mm around it for fixation to the inner shell. Drilling through the screw holes with a 6.5 mm drill gave many good and deep enough holes for cement insertion and pressurization against the bone. One mix (40 mg) of Palacos cement was prepared and inserted and pressurized as per third-generation cementing technique, especially into the predrilled holes. At 6 min the liner was inserted tightly and pressurized strongly against the shell. The orientation was fine-tuned easily as space was existing between the liner and the shell to adjust according to the correct direction. The result was satisfactory, and a ceramic head was elected according to the stability and the offset to provide a good function to the hip (Fig. 10.4).

Right hip THA second procedure (*3 months later*): With the patient in lateral decubitus position and a mini-posterior approach the hip was exposed. There were adhesions around the joint that made the approach rather challenging and necessitated the identification tagging and freeing the sciatic nerve to a significant length to avoid injury to it. The hip was not easy to dislocate due to arthritis causing protrusion and fusions in several places. The neck was divided with the hip located into the socket, and effort was then made to move around the proximal femur. The dislocation then was even more challenging due to adhesion; thus, another slice of the bone was taken down from the remaining head to allow space for the dislocation. After significant capsulotomy to the front of the joint, the proximal femur was more free, and the femur was displaced anteriorly with a retractor. The head was then extracted from the socket using a corkscrew with some difficulty. The ream of the acetabulum was cleared from the osteophytes, and the preparation of the acetabulum started. The shape of the socket was "rocket" looking with a sharp medialization to the inner plate and rough surfaces all around. Care was taken to protect the medial wall and sharp, curved osteotomes used to create the flor prior to using reamers. Then reamers used to smoothen down the periphery up to 52 mm providing an excellent bleeding bone bed for shell insertion. Autograft chips 1–2 cm long impacted snuggly against the cortical inner plate for the cancelization of the surface prior to implant insertion (we call this "primary impaction autografting"). An acetabular, 54 mm shell and 36 mm HXLP (DePuy), was inserted so tightly that screws were deemed not necessary for primary stability. Attention then turned to the femur. Removing the K-wire was a challenge as it cannot be taken out from the top. The entry site was identified buried under the bone, at the beginning of the greater trochanter's flare. The pin was only possible to be removed from there by pulling off the bone. The proximal femoral canal was also a minor challenge as it was occluded by the fibular autograft. The most striking finding was apparent sclerosis, i.e. the non-union between the fibular cortex and the neck cancellous bone. An interface was evident with sclerosis all around. The fibular graft was taken down using a speed burr, and the canal was freed from occlusion allowing the operation to continue in a standard way. A "Corail" fully coated anatomical double tapered stem (DePuy) size 12 was inserted and tested for offset stability and range of movement; a 36 mm ceramic head used for the reduction. Stability was excellent and the leg length recovered fully (Fig. 10.5).

10.2.7 Intraoperative Challenges

Challenges and solutions: Right THA, removing the K-wire and the opening of the proximal femoral canal as described above.

Unanticipated problems and solution: None.

10.2.8 Postoperative radiographs (Figs. 10.4 and 10.5)

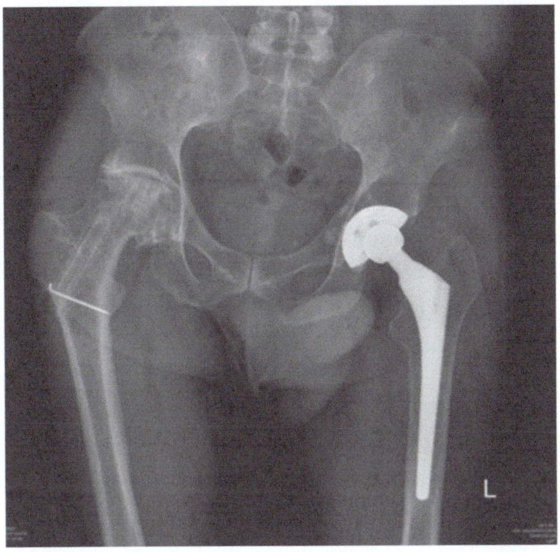

Fig. 10.4 Left hip revision: the most interesting point is the cement extrusion through the newly created peg holes which are apparent all around through the shell and the nice fitting of the HXLP liner into the in situ shell

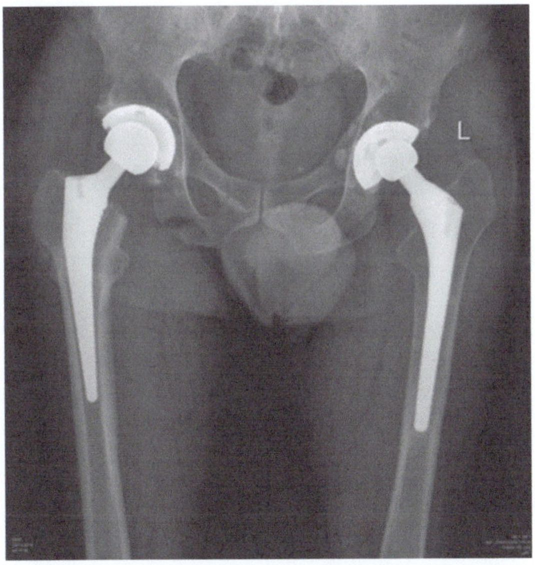

Fig. 10.5 Right THA: standard THA, observe the tip end of the fibular graft at the flare of the greater trochanter and the narrowing of the canal medial and lateral. It is also interesting to appreciate the equalization of the leg length due to extensive capsular releases at front and back and the final good balancing of the pelvis

10.2.9 Postoperative Management

Chemoprophylaxis and anticoagulant treatment period: Vancomycin 500 mg (one dose preoperatively and two doses postoperatively) and cefuroxime 750 mg (one dose preoperatively and two doses postoperatively). Enoxaparin 1x1 for the days of hospitalization then rivaroxaban 10 mg 1 × 1 for thirty days.

Gait/limb loading until full loading: Partial weight bearing for four weeks and then full weight bearing as tolerated.

10.2.10 Follow-Up and Complications

No complication.
Scoring: Left HHS: 95; right HHS: 100.

10.3 Case Title: Primary THA for Paprosky 2A Due to Idiopathic Osteonecrosis and Chronic Osteoarthritis. TM Acetabular Shell and Solid Cancellous Autografting of the Medial Wall

E. Kenanidis and E. Tsiridis

10.3.1 Demographics

Age: 71
Sex: Male
BMI: 25

10.3.2 Relevant Past Medical History

Principal pathologies: Neglected chronic osteoarthritis following idiopathic osteonecrosis. The complete distortion of the head and the acetabulum with a severe bone loss on both sites.

Previous surgical procedures: None.

Medication: Antihypertensives.

History of presenting complaint: Pain, short limb, limited external rotation and fixed flexion deformity.

10.3.3 Clinical Examination

Symptoms: Pain and LLD.

Range of motion: Flexion: 70⁰; extension: -20⁰; internal and external rotation: 10⁰; abduction/adduction: limited.

Specific tests: Thomas test: +35.

Main disability: Inability to walk.

Scoring if available: HHS < 70.

Neurovascular evaluation: Intact.

10.3.4 Preoperative Radiological Assessment/Imaging (Fig. 10.6)

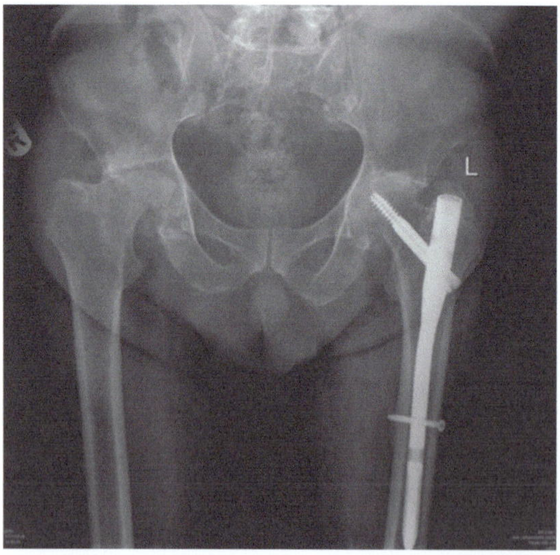

Fig. 10.6 The half femoral head is missing on the right. This is a chronic osteonecrosis with advanced bone loss and sclerotic deformation. The acetabulum has been compromised as well following the shape of the femoral head, leading to significant bone loss and pathological protrusion deformity of the socket. Overall diffuse osteopenia or osteoporosis. Evidence of "pathological" fracture due to osteoporosis on the left (intertrochanteric fracture treated with gamma-nail two years back)

10.3.5 Preoperative Planning

Diagnosis: Osteonecrosis and severe arthritis, bone loss and acetabular protrusion (Fig. 10.6).

Possible treatment options: Acetabular site, needs medial grafting and lateralization of the implanted shell. Should one use an uncemented implant, TM choice may have a better grip on the periphery of the sclerotic acetabulum and allow for better osseointegration of the graft.

Chosen treatment method: Uncemented acetabular cup 56 mm/36 mm. Trabecular socket (Zimmer) and Exeter cemented stem, 44 mm offset, size 3.

Selection of implants if applicable and rational: Hybrid to address the bone reconstruction of the socket with autografting and cemented femoral stem for better fixation due to age and osteoporosis.

Expected difficulties: Reconstructing the acetabulum and dealing with the sclerotic ream of the socket.

Strategies to overcome difficulties: Solid autografting of the medial wall to lateralize the acetabular implant.

Templating: Done.

10.3.6 Surgical Note

With the patient in lateral decubitus position and under general anaesthesia, the hip was approached using a mini-posterior approach. Hip dislocation was challenging as the head was deeply situated into the acetabular fossa and surrounded by inflammatory scar tissue. Dislocation revealed a well-deformed and sclerotic acetabulum with severe bone loss classified as Paprosky 2A. After neck osteotomy, the femur was displaced anteriorly, and attention turned to the acetabular reconstruction. Reaming started with a large reamer as the inner plate was compromised and the periphery enlarged. Reaming up to 54 mm exposed bleeding cancellous bone, and a trial socket was placed successfully. The bottom of the acetabular fossa though was "empty". A large segment of the femoral head that was sclerotic and dead was removed, and the remaining was cleared from cartilage and cortical bone and was shaped to fit

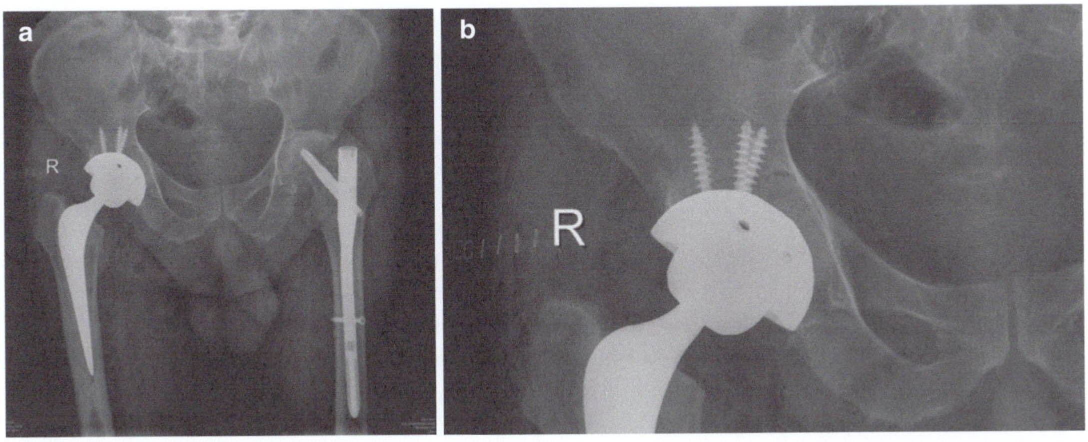

Fig. 10.7 **a** and **b** Good lateralization of the socket. Cancellous autograft against the deformed and deficient medial wall allowed a well-shaped acetabulum to be formed. Reconstruction using a TA shell for better peripheral grip and better osteo-integration to the autograft

the medial defect (see enlarged photo postoperatively). The autograft was impacted solidly into the medial wall, and on the top of it, a TA shell 56 mm (Zimmer) was placed with three vertical stability screws. The shell was solidly engaged by the periphery of the acetabulum. Attention then turned to the femoral side and a routine third-generation cemented Exeter stem 44/3 inserted with success. Stable reduction and good leg length were established with a 36 mm head (Fig. 10.7a, b).

10.3.7 Intraoperative Challenges

Challenges and solutions: Reaming the socket without compromising the walls until bleeding cancellous bone was exposed. Grafting the medial wall.

Unanticipated problems and solution: Sclerotic acetabular periphery.

Thorough description of decision-making, including the reason for the final decision: Uncemented TA shell for the socket and autografting the medial wall to lateralize the acetabular component successfully and recover the centre of rotation. Only a TM shell could grip snuggly with a sclerotic acetabular fossa. A cemented liner would have faced with the problem of sclerosis with no easy solution. In addition, the large uncemented shell allowed a 36 mm head to be used for better overall stability.

10.3.8 Postoperative Radiographs (Fig. 10.7a, b)

10.3.9 Postoperative Management

Chemoprophylaxis and anticoagulant treatment period: Vancomycin 500 mg (one dose preoperatively and two doses postoperatively), cefuroxime 750 mg (one dose preoperatively and two doses postoperatively) and tinzaparin 1 × 1 for 35 days.

Gait/limb loading until full loading: Partial weight bearing for 4 weeks. Then full weight bearing as tolerated.

10.3.10 Follow-Up and Complications

No complication.

Scoring: HHS: 95.

10.4 Case Title: Osteonecrosis of the Femoral Head

Arkan S. Sayed-Noor and Bakir Kadum

10.4.1 Demographics

Age: 49 years
Sex: Female
BMI: 30.8

10.4.2 Relevant Past Medical History

Principle pathologies: Hypertension for seven years and mild depression for three years.

Previous surgical procedures: None.

Medication: Metoprolol tablet 100 mg/day and citalopram tablet 20 mg/day.

Other: None.

10.4.3 History of Present Complaint

In March 2013, the patient was referred to our orthopaedic department by her general practitioner (GP). She had complained of pain in the left buttock for five months. The pain was mainly on exertion although she had aches at rest in the evening, especially when she had overloaded her legs during the day. No traumatic events or previous problems in the spine, pelvis or lower limbs were reported in the history. According to the referral letter, the physical examination had shown diffuse tenderness in the gluteal and trochanteric regions with slight limitation of the internal rotation of the left hip compared to the right. The range of motion (ROM) of the left hip, including the femoroacetabular impingement tests, was otherwise comparable to the right side and within normal limits. Possibly, a very mild wasting of the left thigh muscles was also noted. The distal neurovascular status was normal regarding ROM, reflexes, sensation and circulation. The Trendelenburg sign was bilaterally negative. A plain X-ray was ordered by the GP and showed no abnormalities apart from small osteophytes on the lateral aspects of femoral head bilaterally (Fig. 10.8). The pain was considered as muscular and was suspected to be related to the gluteal muscle/tendons with or without the involvement of the trochanteric bursae. The patient was treated with nonsteroidal anti-inflammatory tablets (naproxen tablet 500 mg twice daily) plus paracetamol 1 g two to four times daily. A basic exercise programme for the spine and hips was also given. This treatment did not help alleviate the pain. The patient noted a reduction in her walking distance due to pain.

According to our regional protocol, a GP cannot refer patients for magnetic resonance imaging (MRI) for the pelvis and hip; only an orthopaedic surgeon can do this. The GP, therefore, chose to refer the patient to our department for further evaluation.

In her visit to our department, the patient showed antalgic gait with limping, reduced internal rotation and thigh muscle wasting on the left compared to the right side. At that time, the patient underwent an MRI of the pelvis and hips. This showed an area of low intensity (oedema) at the upper part of the femoral head on the T1-weighted images and of high intensity on the T2-weighted images. The pathological area was estimated to involve approximately 20% of the femoral head (Fig. 10.9). Mild bilateral tendinosis of the gluteus medius tendons was also noted. No other abnormalities were found. The MRI findings were therefore suggestive of early-stage osteonecrosis of the femoral head (ONFH) (Ficat stage I, Steinberg stage IB). A computed tomography (CT) was also done to rule out a subchondral fracture, and CT showed no pathological changes. This was followed by a haematological workup. This included a complete blood profile, C-reactive protein, erythrocyte sedimentation rate (ESR) and lipid profile. Apart from a cholesterol level of 240 mg/dL (6.2 mmol/L), all other parameters were within normal ranges.

After discussing the findings with the patient and giving her information about the existing evidence for the management of early-stage ONFH, conservative treatment was started with observation, protected weight bearing, ROM exercise, statins (simvastatin 20 mg once a day) and alendronate (70 mg once a week). A follow-up visit was planned for four weeks later. Unfortunately, the patient could not attend this visit because of a cold-like illness that was diagnosed by the GP to be a side effect of the statin treatment. The statin was therefore stopped. The patient attended another follow-up visit three months later, complaining at that time of severe pain in the groin and buttock with walking difficulty. A new X-ray examination showed the segmental collapse of the upper lateral part of the femoral head (Fig. 10.10) (Ficat stage III, Steinberg stage IVB). The patient was admitted the same day to the orthopaedic ward for pain relief and mobilization. The patient was scheduled for total hip arthroplasty (THA) to be done in July to August 2013.

10.4.4 Clinical Examination

Symptom: Left buttock pain with some radiation to the groin, limping with walking difficulty.

Range of motion: Reduced internal rotation (10 degrees compared to 25 degree on the right side) and thigh muscle wasting of 1–2 cm in diameter in mid-thigh point compared to the right side. Otherwise, ROM was within normal range.

Specific tests: Femoroacetabular impingement tests and Trendelenburg sign were normal. Tenderness over the gluteal and trochanteric regions.

Scores: WOMAC functional score was 70 (0 best and 100 worst), and EQ-5D for the quality of life was 0.37 (0 worst and 1.0 best).

Neurovascular evaluation: Normal distal motor and sensory status. Normal circulation.

10.4.5 Preoperative Radiological Assessment/Imaging (Figs. 10.8, 10.9, and 10.10)

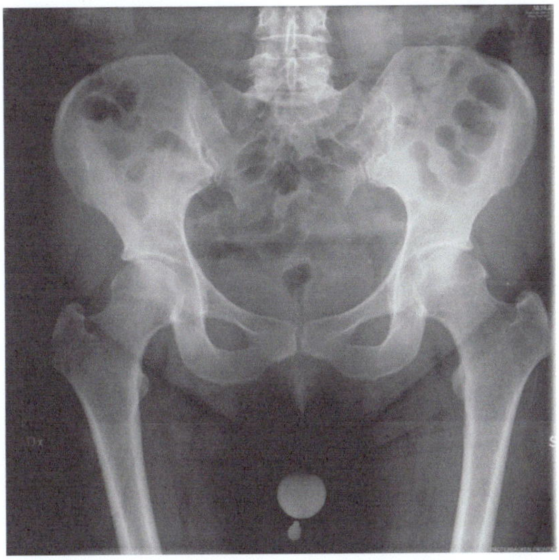

Fig. 10.8 Apart from small osteophytes on the lateral aspect of the femoral head, no other abnormalities were seen on the plain X-ray taken by the GP

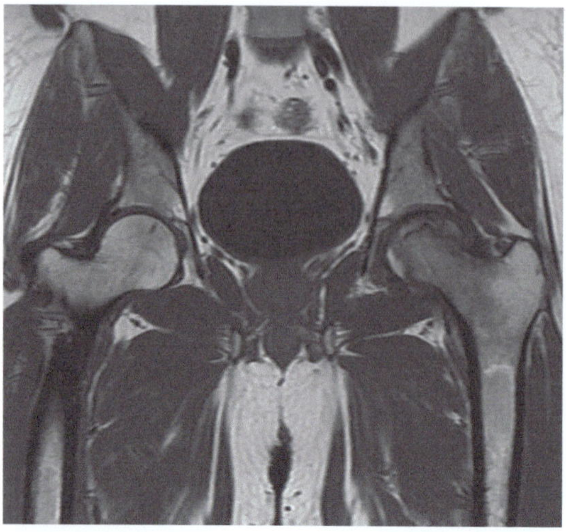

Fig. 10.9 MRI of the pelvis and hips. This showed an area of low intensity (oedema) at the upper part of the left femoral head, suggestive of an early stage of ONFH (Ficat stage I, Steinberg stage IB). The pathological area was estimated to involve approximately 20% of the femoral head

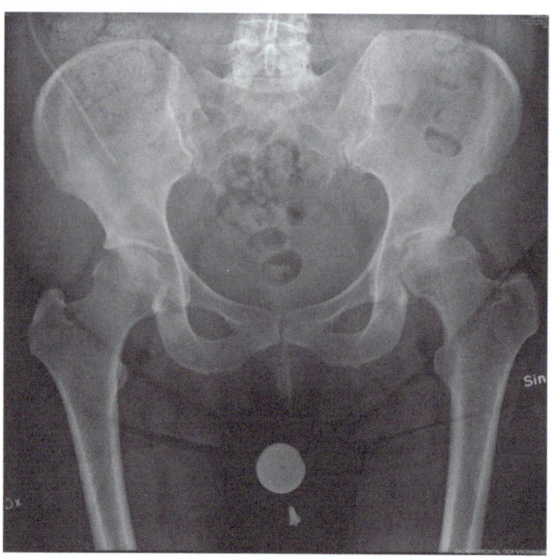

Fig. 10.10 A new X-ray examination showed the segmental collapse of the upper lateral part of the femoral head (Ficat stage III, Steinberg stage IVB)

10.4.6 Preoperative Planning

Diagnosis: ONFH with the segmental collapse of the upper lateral part of the femoral head (Ficat stage III, Steinberg stage IVB) (Fig. 10.10).

Possible treatment options: In symptomatic patients with a segmental collapse of the femoral head, THA is the option of choice.

Chosen treatment method: THA.

Selection of implants: We chose a non-cemented cup and a cemented stem with metal on highly crossed-linked polyethylene bearings.

Expected difficulties: The degree of the segmental collapse was no more than 20% of the femoral head, with no bony loss on the acetabular side. However, we expected the bone quality of the acetabular floor to be poor, and we were prepared to put a cemented cup in this case. The BMI was not high enough to give technical difficulties.

Templating: We used the Mdesk™ (RSA BioMedical, Umeå, Sweden) system to choose the size of the cup and stem as well as the neck length and caput-collum-diaphyseal (CCD) angle. Our routine was to use a 32 mm head size.

10.4.7 Surgical Notes

Patient's position: Lateral decubitus with pelvic immobilizer. The surgeon checked for the proper positioning of the patient on the operating table.

Type of anaesthesia: Spinal with sedation.

Surgical approach: Posterior (posterolateral) approach according to Moore.

Main steps: Sharp dissection of the fascia lata and fascia over gluteus maximus and blunt dissection along the fibres of this muscle. Identification of the short external rotators that are cut from their trochanteric attachment with a cautery. Preservation of the piriformis muscle attachment. Meticulous haemostasis. Capsulotomy and posterior dislocation of the hip. Femoral neck osteotomy 1–1.5 cm proximal to the lesser trochanter. Use curved retractors to allow adequate exposure of the acetabulum. Removal of the labrum and osteophytes. Check for the bone quality of the acetabular floor with a curette. Careful successive reaming of the acetabular floor and repeated irrigation. When the subchondral bone is adequately exposed, the suitable acetabular cup size is measured. As we planned to use the Trilogy non-cemented cup

(Zimmer, USA), we chose one size bigger than the last reamer. The cup was fixed by press-fit techniques aiming for a 45 degrees inclination and 25 degrees anteversion. Despite good fixation, we chose to insert three screws to ensure rotational stability. The liner is then fixed to the cup using the locking ring. The femoral canal is then exposed using suitable retractors for the proximal femur. As we planned to use the cemented Lubinus stem (Link, Germany), successive rasping and repeated irrigation were done until adequate contact with cortical bone was achieved and the stem size was measured, one size less than the last rasp. The stem is then cemented using a third-generation cementing technique. The suitable neck length was measured to ensure good prosthetic stability, ROM and minimal leg length discrepancy. The short external rotators were refixed to the trochanter using osteo-suturing. The fascia lata and fascia over gluteus maximus are sutured with polydioxanone (PDS), the subcutaneous tissue is sutured with Vicryl, and the skin is closed with Monocryl, Ethilon or staples (Fig. 10.11).

Reconstruction techniques: In this patient, no reconstruction was needed since there were no bony defects or loss.

10.4.8 Intraoperative Challenges

Challenges and solutions: The bone quality of the acetabular floor was considered poor as the surgeon noted wide trabecular spaces and soft spots when using the curette. However, no bone graft was needed, and the non-cemented cup achieved an adequate fixation using the press fit techniques together with the additional screw fixation.

Unanticipated problems and solutions: Routinely, we use a 32 mm head size. When the cemented stem was fixed, and the suitable neck length was tested, the surgeon noted that the prosthetic stability was not optimal as the jumping distance was not long enough. This was managed by changing the head size to 36 mm. The cup liner was changed accordingly. With this head size, prosthetic stability improved.

Thorough description of decision-making, including the reason for the final decision: The choice of THA as the final treatment option was inevitable since non-surgical treatment was unsuccessful with the progression of clinical and radiological manifestations. The segmental collapse could not be managed by a joint-preserving modality like core decompression or grafting. We had different options regarding the choice of prosthetic type and bearings. We chose the hybrid model (non-cemented cup and cemented stem) because of our previous favourable experience, as well as the good reports of this combination in the arthroplasty registries. The bearing using metal on polyethylene was suitable for the age and level of activity of the patient. The preoperative templating, as well as the intraoperative evaluation, were the cornerstones in choosing the size of the components as well as the prosthetic neck length and head size.

10.4.9 Postoperative Radiographs (Fig. 10.11)

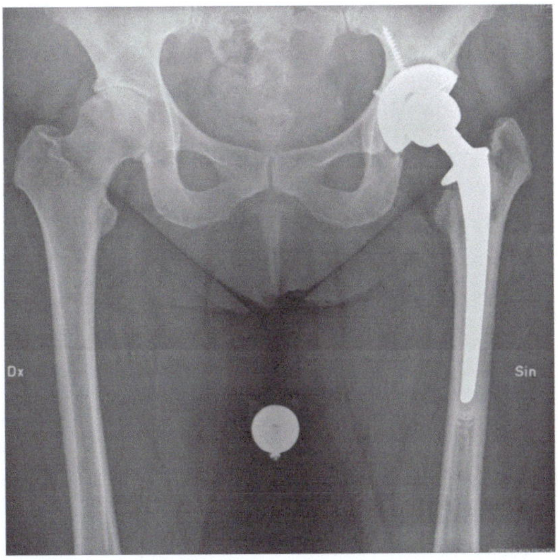

Fig. 10.11 Postoperative X-ray. Note the ongoing segmental collapse of the contralateral femoral head. Bilaterality is common in ONFH. Also, note the minute space between the acetabular bed and the metal backing of the acetabular cup. These tiny spaces are usually filled with the bone when the osseointegration between the cup and the bone is completed. It is recommended to have 75% direct bone contact between the cup and the bone

10.4.10 Postoperative Management

Chemoprophylaxis and anticoagulant treatment period: Intravenous anti-staphylococcus antibiotics (cloxacillin 2 g, four doses) were given perioperatively according to our routine. The first dose was given thirty min before the operation, the second two h after the first, the third eight hours after the second and the fourth eight hours after the third dose. Regarding anticoagulant treatment, dalteparin (low-molecular weight heparin), 5000 IE was given subcutaneously once a day for ten days.

Gait/limb loading until full loading: Immediate weight bearing with full loading was allowed postoperatively. However, crutches were recommended as assistance during the first six weeks after the operation.

10.4.11 Follow-Up and Complications

Report of postoperative complications and their management: Redness of the wound edge was noted during stitch removal. This redness was treated with observation and wound toilet. Wound swab showed no bacterial growth. No antibiotics were needed. The patient also reported a feeling of leg length discrepancy (operated limb felt longer). Clinical and radiological leg length measurement showed a leg length discrepancy of less than ten mm. Explanation and reassurance were enough to manage this point. No other postoperative problems were encountered.

Scores: The WOMAC functional score was 35 at three months and 25 at twelve months follow-up. The EQ-5D for the quality of life was 0.67 at three months and 0.73 at twelve months follow-up.

10.4.12 Discussion

ONFH is a progressive condition that typically affects active people in the 20 to 40 years age range. About 10% of primary THAs in the USA and 3.5% in Sweden are annually done for ONFH. The prevalence has increased during the last two to three decades, possibly due to increasing prevalence of predisposing factors. Bilateral disease is common. The pathophysiology is not fully understood. However, the disease is thought to result from a common pathway involving ischaemic changes of the femoral head secondary to intravascular occlusion or extravascular pressure. In their *current concept review*, Mont et al. [47] discussed the potential biomarkers and genes that may play a role in the aetiology of ONFH. Direct trauma (with or without fracture or dislocation) can obliterate the blood circulation to the femoral head, while elevated circulating lipid levels in patients with chronic corticosteroid use, alcohol intake or hyperlipidaemia can give rise to microembolism with intravascular damage. Other predisposing factors include pregnancy, smoking, haemoglobinopathies/coagulation disorders, radiation, caisson disease and autoimmune disease. In 40% of cases, no obvious cause is found, i.e. it is idiopathic. In our patient, no apparent predisposing factor was found apart from hyperlipidaemia.

The clinical picture can be misleading, especially in early stages where symptoms are too mild and plain radiographs are normal. Therefore, a high index of suspicion is required if early diagnosis is to be made. Plain radiographs should include AP and lateral and frog-leg projections. The latter can show changes like sclerosis, cystic changes or the crescent sign in a better way than the AP and lateral views. Patients with predisposing factors presenting with groin or buttock pain and normal radiographs should be considered for MRI to rule out the possibility of ONFH. The changes in MRI are typical in most cases, and a CT scan is only required if it is unclear whether there is a subchondral fracture or not. Other modalities like bone scan, positron emission tomography, X-ray absorptiometry or histological studies are rarely used. The radiological changes of ONFH should be differentiated from other conditions like metastasis, subchondral insufficiency fractures and idiopathic transient osteoporosis of the hip.

There are different classification systems for ONFH. The Ficat and ARCO/Steinberg systems are commonly used in clinical practice despite limited reliability. The main parameter in these classification systems is the presence or absence of bony collapse, as patients with pre-collapse changes can be considered for non-surgical treatment, while patients with collapse often require THA. However, it is still unknown which factors affect the progression of the pre-collapse to collapse stage. Some think that the size and site of the lesions can play a role. Subchondral lesions involving more than 15% of the femoral head are thought to progress to collapse more than smaller lesions located in a more caudal site. In our patient, the lesion involved nearly 25% of the femoral head and was located in the subchondral upper part of the femoral head.

The treatment of ONFH depends on several factors, e.g. site and size of the lesion and the presence or absence of collapse [2, 47]. Patients with pre-collapse lesions involving less than 15% of the femoral head can be considered for non-surgical treatment, e.g. observation, protected weight bearing, analgesia and bisphosphonate. Statins can be added in patients with hyperlipidaemia, such as in our patient. However, there is a paucity of evidence about the efficacy of this treatment in preventing lesion collapse. Some authors recommend joint-preserving surgical intervention such as core decompression with or without bone grafting or multiple drilling for pre-collapse lesions especially those located subchondrally and involving more than 15% of the femoral head. Other treatment options at this stage include angular and rotational proximal femoral trans-trochanteric osteotomies to shift the lesion away from the joint-loaded surface. These treatment modalities have shown good outcome in symptom relief and preventing lesion collapse in more than 60% of cases. When collapse takes place or in young patients with a crescent sign on plain radiographs, joint replacement is often required. In this regard, some authors recommend hemi-surfacing arthroplasty in patients with no acetabular cartilage changes. This option requires, however, meticulous patient selection and is technically demanding. Moreover, studies have shown that hemi-surfacing arthroplasty is less predictable in symptom relief compared with THA. We have no personal experience with this type of arthroplasty.

The other option in patients with femoral head collapse is THA. The choice of prostheses type and bearings in THA depends on the age of the patient, the bone quality and the degree of osteoarthritis. In young (<50 year) active patients, we recommend non-cemented cup and stem with ceramic or metal head and a highly cross-linked polyethylene liner. Studies have shown an increased risk of wear and aseptic loosening in this patient category compared to older patients. However, the overall satisfaction and functional outcome were comparable in both groups.

In our patient, we chose a non-cemented cup and a cemented stem with metal on highly crossed-linked polyethylene bearings because of the patient's activity level and our good experience in using this combination. There was no technical difficulty in implanting the prosthesis. During the operation, we noted that the prosthetic stability was not optimal as the jumping distance was not long enough. This was managed by changing the head size from 32 mm to 36 mm. With this head size, the prosthetic stability improved, and no dislocation occurred during the follow-up period.

In summary, ONFH is a challenging entity with unclear pathophysiological changes and unpredictable natural history. Early diagnosis and intervention seem to improve outcome. Patients are often young and active, demanding durable treatment solutions, and there is an urgent need for more high-level evidence in the literature regarding the efficacy of the available treatment options in different disease stages.

10.5 Case Title: Femoral Head Osteonecrosis

Karl Brabants and Peter Mertens

10.5.1 Demographics

Age: 23
Sex: Female
BMI: < 20

10.5.2 Relevant Past Medical History

Principal pathologies: Septic arthritis of the left hip at the age of three years.

Previous surgical procedures: Trauma at the age of 3 years.

Medication: None.

History of presenting complaint: After a septic arthritis of the left hip at three years, the patient developed a dysplastic hip and a global hypotrophy of the left hemipelvis and leg. Pain, limping and limitation of mobility: limited flexion, adduction contracture. Shortening of six cm, partially in the hip, partially in the dystrophic limb.

10.5.3 Clinical Examination

Symptoms: Pain, limping, limb shortening of six cm.

Range of motion: Flexion 70°, endorotation contracture of 10°, full extension possible.

Specific tests: No muscular weakness in the left leg.

Main disability: Limping, pain, leg shortening, limitation of mobility, no Trendelenburg sign (!).

Neurovascular evaluation: EMG, normal conductions—due to the hypotrophy of the left leg, a Doppler was performed to exclude vascular origin of this hypotrophy or hypovascularization of the leg. Pulsations were normal at the groin and knee (triphasic signals) and decreased in a. tibialis anterior + posterior (monophasic signals).

10.5.4 Preoperative Radiological Assessment/Imaging (Figs. 10.12, 10.13, and 10.14)

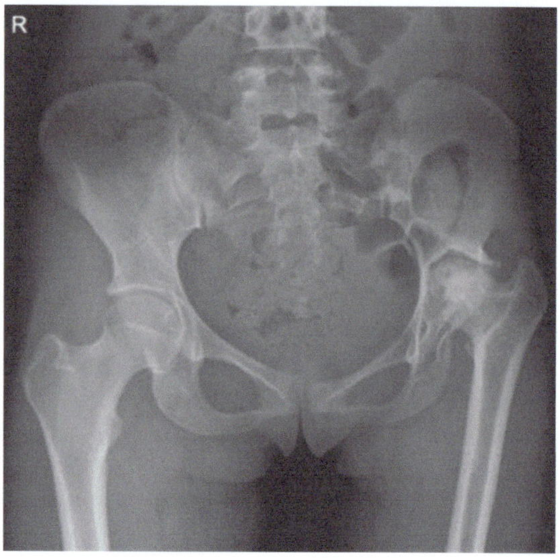

Fig. 10.12 AP pelvis X-ray

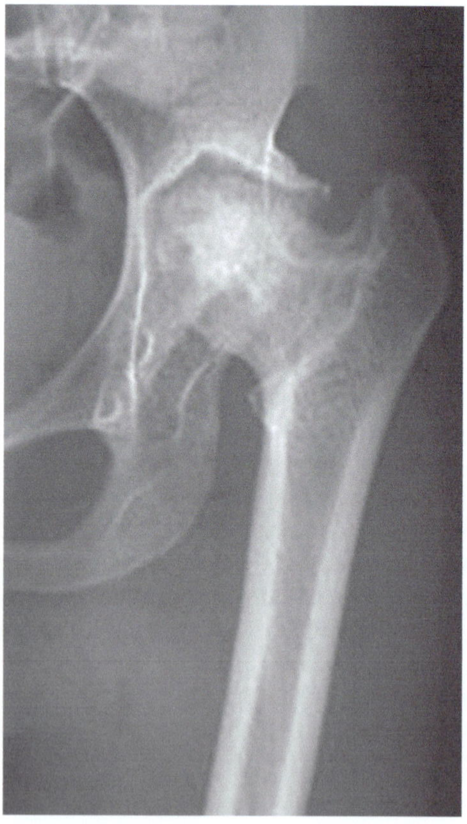

Fig. 10.13 AP hip X-ray

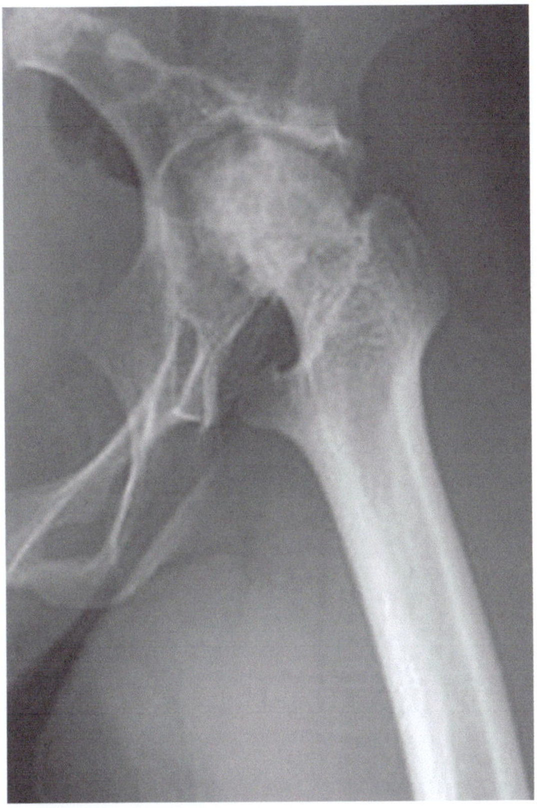

Fig. 10.14 Lateral hip X-ray

10.5.5 Preoperative Planning

Diagnosis: Secondary coxarthrosis after septic arthritis/dysplasia (Figs. 10.12, 10.13 and 10.14).

Possible treatment options: Primary THA with or without trochanter or extended femoral osteotomy.

Chosen treatment method: Primary THA.

Selection of implants if applicable and rational: Trilogy cup (uncemented, Zimmer)—Anthology stem size 1, standard offset (uncemented S&N), Oxinium head 32–3 (S&N). Preference for uncemented cup due to the high reported failure of acetabular reconstruction with cemented cups (16–50% at more than ten years' follow-up), probably caused by younger patient age and non-anatomic placement (1).

Expected difficulties: Stiffness of the hip with fibrosis and shortening of periarticular capsule and muscles. High centre of rotation and expected difficulties to keep it distal. Shallow acetabulum (dystrophy). Overhang of trochanter major. Anteversion of the femoral head. Small size of the femur due to hypotrophy. Lean patient; increased offset non-desirable (aesthetic and to avoid trochanter pain). Intension to avoid a trochanteric osteotomy (expecting difficulties of reattachment, intension to avoid a Trendelenburg gait).

Strategies to overcome difficulties: A cemented and uncemented stem was available; multihole cup available, options for trochanter osteotomy or extended femoral osteotomy; trochanteric plate (Accord S&N) and cable wires available; homologous bone grafts available.

10.5.6 Surgical Note

Patient's position: Lateral decubitus.

Type of anaesthesia: General.

Surgical approach: Anterolateral approach (Hardinge).

Main steps: Approach. Osteotomy of the femoral neck. Visualization of the acetabulum, reaming to achieve good coverage of the cup. Fixation with two screws. Entering the femoral canal, femoral reaming, enlargement of the proximal femur.

10.5.7 Intraoperative Challenges

Challenges and solutions: It was hard to reach the acetabulum due to the extreme periarticular fibrosis. After the neck osteotomy, it was impossible to keep the centre of rotation distally. On the other hand, we would like to avoid a trochanteric or extended osteotomy due to our fear of having difficulties to reattach the greater trochanter after lengthening of the legand to avoid Trendelenburg gait. We accepted the high acetabular position. Using a bigger acetabular component, we corrected somewhat the acetabular offset and the centre of rotation. No problems with acetabular containment.

Unanticipated problems and solution: There were difficulties to enter the proximal femur due to the deformation of the calcar and extreme sclerosis at the proximal metaphysis. There was a need of drill to enter the femoral canal. We expected a very small canal, but it was even too small for the smallest stem size. We had to reshape calcar and proximal metaphysis with spherical cutters and enlarge the proximal canal by reaming up to eleven mm over a drill guide. Nevertheless, a small longitudinal fissuration occurred during the introduction of the final stem (Anthology 1, standard offset). This was treated by removal of the stem, subtrochanteric cerclage (Dall Miles cable wiring) followed by the reintroduction of the same stem (Figs. 10.15 and 10.16).

10.5.8 Postoperative Radiographs (Figs. 10.15 and 10.16)

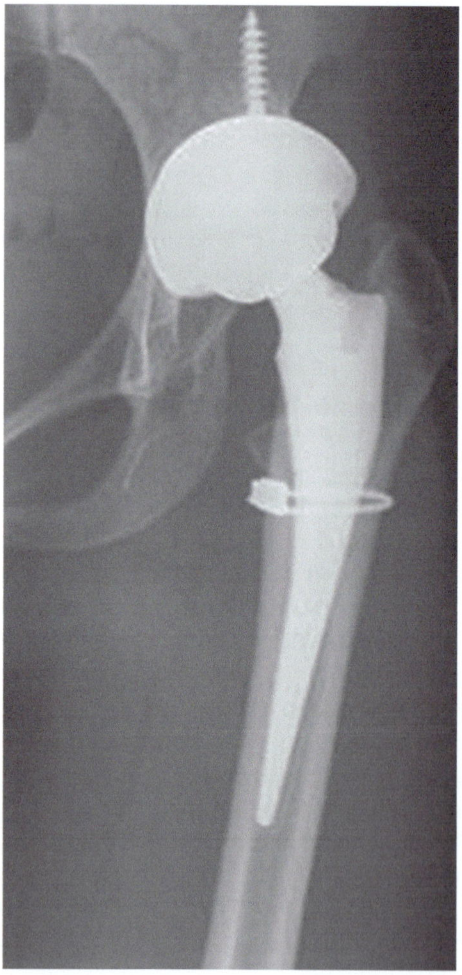

Fig. 10.15 AP X-ray of the first postoperative year

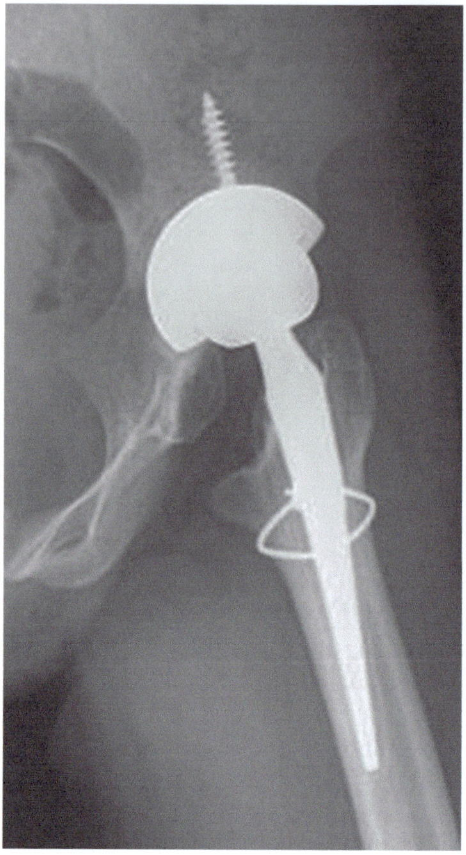

Fig. 10.16 Lateral hip X-ray of the first postoperative year

10.5.9 Postoperative Management

Chemoprophylaxis and anticoagulant treatment period: Rivaroxaban 10 mg for thirty five days.

Gait/limb loading until full loading: Partial weight bearing for six weeks (20 kg, two crutches).

10.5.10 Follow-Up and Complications

No complications, no subsidence, fast recovery, very happy patient, negative Trendelenburg sign and walking with a heel elevation of 1.5 cm.

10.5.11 Discussion [48–50]

Advantages of the applied method: The most straightforward procedure technically, avoiding possible complications of a shelf graft and femoral osteotomy.

Disadvantages of the method: The shortening was decreased to three cm. It is uncertain if we will gain the full length with extended femoral osteotomy.

Alternative evidence-based techniques for the case: A custom-made implant but very it is a very expensive technique.

Why is the chosen technique better for this case? The easiest solution, less invasive, low cost, good conditions for later revision (probably given the young age of this patient).

Indications and contraindications for your technique: Preoperative check of vascular condition is mandatory; hypertrophy can be associated with lack of a main vessel; surgery can be catastrophic in such a situation.

10.6 Case Title: Combined Bilateral Femoral Head Necrosis and Pertrochanteric Fracture

Bogdan Nikolae Deleanu

10.6.1 Demographics

Age: 66
Sex: Female
BMI: 26 kg/m^2

10.6.2 Relevant Past Medical History

Principal pathologies: None.

Medication: None.

History of presenting complaint: The patient sustained a left pertrochanteric fracture caused by a fall from the same height, associated with primary hip OA treated with a long-stem THA. At her 1-year follow-up visit, she had no pain in the left hip, with excellent ROM (flexion of 105°, abduction 32°). Then the patient presented intense pain of her right hip associated with a progressing limp for five months. The X-ray revealed stage VI femoral head avascular necrosis (AVN), with the proximal migration of the femoral head with a secondary acetabular rim destruction. She was scheduled for a primary right THA. A few days after the visit, she sustained a fall from the same height that resulted in extreme pain over the already painful right hip and pain and deformation of the normal anatomy of the right arm. She was diagnosed with a right pertrochanteric fracture (Figs. 10.17 and 10.18).

10.6.3 Clinical Examination

Symptoms: Non-weight bearing, the hip was extremely painful on palpation and mobilization.

Range of motion: Right lower limb was externally rotated by approximately 30° and shortened by approximately seven cm.

Specific tests: Pelvic AP emergency X-ray. Hip AP X-ray, thoracic and shoulder AP X-ray.

Main disability: Non-weight bearing, painful hip and arm.

Scoring if available: Harris Hip Score was 68, and the WOMAC score 64,8. At 1 year postoperatively, the patient was ambulant with a Harris Hip Score of 84 and a WOMAC score of 81.1.

Neurovascular evaluation: Distal pulses present, distal sensibility and motor control present.

10.6.4 Preoperative Radiological Assessment/Imaging (Figs. 10.17 and 10.18)

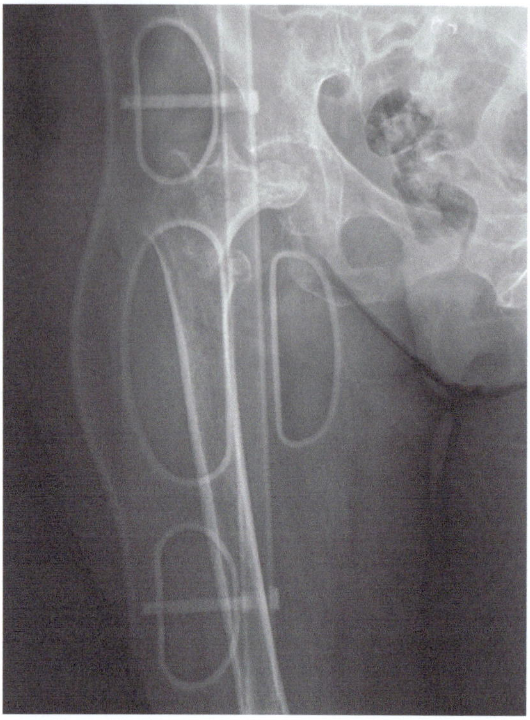

Fig. 10.17 Emergency X-ray of the right hip showing a simple intertrochanteric fracture associated with femoral head stage IV AVN, with the femoral head impacted in the acetabular rim. No bone or soft tissue malignancies detected

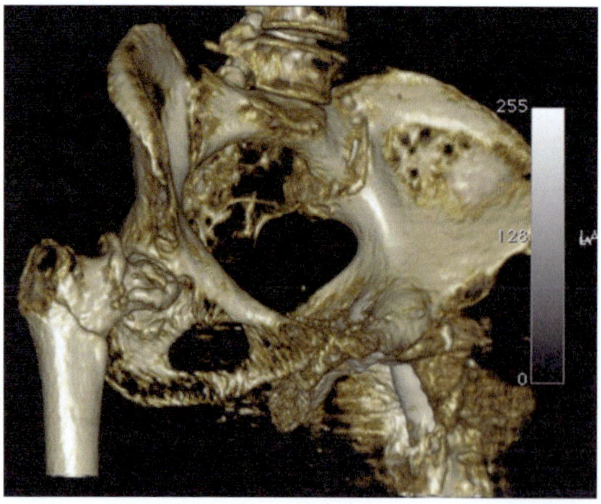

Fig. 10.18 Pelvic 3D CT scan showing a simple intertrochanteric fracture associated with femoral head stage IV AVN, with the femoral head impacted in the acetabular rim

10.6.5 Preoperative Planning

Diagnosis: Left hip pertrochanteric fracture Evans II. Femoral head AVN stage VI. Secondary left hip OA (Figs. 10.17 and 10.18).

Possible treatment options: IM nailing (short nail) with a CMD; nail extraction and total hip arthroplasty after fracture consolidation. SHS fixation of the trochanteric fracture. SHS extraction and THA after fracture consolidation. THA with a long stem with diaphyseal support.

Chosen treatment method: THA with a long stem with diaphyseal support. (Revitan Straight, Zimmer, Warsaw, IN, USA).

Selection of implants if applicable and rational: Although it is a more difficult and more invasive surgery, this option allows for only one surgical intervention and also addresses both the traumatic and the degenerative pathologies of the same hip. While IM nailing is a relatively fast and uncomplicated surgery, based on the preoperative imaging, we expected to have difficulty to abduct the leg for nail insertion, and the acetabular impaction could lead difficulties in reducing the fracture in both AP and lateral views. Similar problems would be encountered for SHS with the added larger incision. Both implants would only address the traumatic pathology and would not allow for early postoperative mobilization. Furthermore, the second surgery would need to remove the first implant causing significant bleeding, as proven by various studies. The femoral component would need to be implanted on a consolidated fracture making reaming difficult and prolonged with further bleeding and infection risk.

Expected difficulties: Reaming of the femoral canal for a straight femoral component should consider the anatomical curvature of the femur. It also should be done in such a way that it would not create a three-point support of the stem.

Strategies to overcome difficulties: Plan the reaming, and check with intraoperative X-rays if in doubt.

Templating: No digital templating was performed. We used printed templates on printed digital X-rays.

10.6.6 Surgical Note

Patient's position: Supine on OR table.

Type of anaesthesia: Spinal.

Surgical approach: Lateral approach to the hip (Hardinge).

Main steps: Skin incision, lateral approach. Expose the capsule; remove the femoral head with the fractured part of the trochanter, without the muscular insertions. Ream the acetabulum with primary reamers, implant the uncemented primary acetabular component, and insert the poly liner. Open the femoral canal (endosteal approach), and ream the femur with progressive reamers until the taper-like shape of the femoral canal is obtained for a 5 cm distance. Determine the size of the proximal and the distal component, and assemble them on the instrument table. Implant the resulting femoral component using the press-fit technique. Attach trochanteric fragments with thick sutures. Perform trial reduction and select the femoral head. Apply the femoral head and reduce the prosthesis. Routine closure.

Reconstruction techniques: Total hip arthroplasty with a long femoral stem (Fig. 10.19).

10.6.7 Intraoperative Challenges

Challenges and solutions: The femoral neck osteotomy cannot be performed because of the fracture pattern. So retaining the trochanteric fragments with the muscle insertions must be preserved and attached to the prosthesis with thick sutures or wires, reaming the femoral canal as described above.

10.6.8 Postoperative Radiographs (Fig. 10.19)

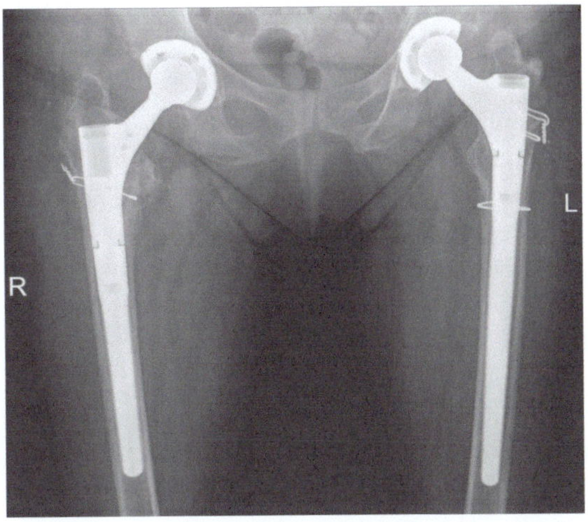

Fig. 10.19 Postoperative X-ray of the first year, showing bilateral primary THA with uncemented acetabular shell and modular femoral components with radiographic union for both pertrochanteric fractures

10.6.9 Postoperative Management

Regular THA postoperative rehabilitation protocol with partial progressive weight bearing two days postoperatively and full weight bearing at six weeks postoperatively.

10.6.10 Discussion [51–55]

Advantages of the applied method: While other surgeries might be faster or minimally invasive, they would also require a second surgery with increased OR times and intraoperative bleeding. So, this technique solves both the traumatic and the degenerative problem in the same surgery and allows for early postoperative mobilization. This is the maximum benefit-to-risk ratio to the patient.

Disadvantages of the method: The selected implant is more costly in the first stage than a CMD or an SHS. The combined cost is almost equivalent. Also, the first surgery is more time consuming and more laborious with longer OR time and increased blood loss, so a better preoperative assessment of the patient should be done.

Alternative evidence-based techniques for the case: None other than those discussed.

Why is the chosen technique better for this case? One surgery, better postoperative mobilization, less potential for complications.

Indications and contraindications for your technique: It is a long, unreamed, femoral stem with diaphyseal support option, so it can be used in all THA situations where the trochanteric region is compromised.

Learning curve and how to manage complications: Relatively similar to a primary THA regarding the approach and the concept. More difficult to insert due to its modular design and the press fit nature of a straight implant in a curved bone.

Level of evidence concerning the superiority of this method against others: 2b.

References

1. Zalavras CG, Lieberman JR. Osteonecrosis of the femoral head: evaluation and treatment. J Am Acad Orthop Surg. 2014;22(7):455–64.
2. Moya-Angeler J, Gianakos AL, Villa JC, Ni A, Lane JM. Current concepts on osteonecrosis of the femoral head. World J Orthop. 2015;6(8):590–601.
3. Zalavras CG, Vartholomatos G, Dokou E, Malizos KN. Genetic background of osteonecrosis: associated with thrombophilic mutations? Clin Orthop Relat Res. 2004;422:251–5.
4. Scaglione M, Fabbri L, Celli F, Casella F, Guido G. Hip replacement in femoral head osteonecrosis: current concepts. Clin Cases Miner Bone Metabol. 2015;12(Suppl. 1):51–4. Supplement to n.3 2015
5. Lieberman JR, Roth KM, Elsissy P, Dorey FJ, Kobashigawa JA. Symptomatic osteonecrosis of the hip and knee after cardiac transplantation. J Arthroplast. 2008;23(1):90–6.
6. Issa K, Pivec R, Kapadia BH, Banerjee S, Mont MA. Osteonecrosis of the femoral head: the total hip replacement solution. Bone Joint J. 2013;95-B(11 Suppl A):46–50.
7. Mont MA, Marulanda GA, Jones LC, Saleh KJ, Gordon N, Hungerfor DS, et al. Systematic analysis of classification systems for osteonecrosis of the femoral head. J Bone Joint Surg Am. 2006;88(Suppl 3):16–26.
8. Mont MA, Zywiel MG, Marker DR, McGrath MS, Delanois RE. The natural history of untreated asymptomatic osteonecrosis of the femoral head: a systematic literature review. J Bone Joint Surg Am. 2010;92(12):2165–70.
9. Glueck CJ, Freiberg RA, Sieve L, Wang P. Enoxaparin prevents progression of stages I and II osteonecrosis of the hip. Clin Orthop Relat Res. 2005;435:164–70.
10. Chen CH, Chang JK, Lai KA, Hou SM, Chang CH, Wang GJ. Alendronate in the prevention of collapse of the femoral head in nontraumatic osteonecrosis: a two-year multicenter, prospective, randomized, double-blind, placebo-controlled study. Arthritis Rheum. 2012;64(5):1572–8.
11. Wang CJ, Wang FS, Huang CC, Yang KD, Weng LH, Huang HY. Treatment for osteonecrosis of the femoral head: comparison of extracorporeal shock waves with core decompression and bone grafting. J Bone Joint Surg Am. 2005;87(11):2380–7.
12. Gangji V, De Maertelaer V, Hauzeur JP. Autologous bone marrow cell implantation in the treatment of non-traumatic osteonecrosis of the femoral head: five year follow-up of a prospective controlled study. Bone. 2011;49(5):1005–9.
13. Eward WC, Rineer CA, Urbaniak JR, Richard MJ, Ruch DS. The vascularized fibular graft in precollapse osteonecrosis: is long-term hip preservation possible? Clin Orthop Relat Res. 2012;470(10):2819–26.
14. Ortiguera CJ, Pulliam IT, Cabanela ME. Total hip arthroplasty for osteonecrosis: matched-pair analysis of 188 hips with long-term follow-up. J Arthroplast. 1999;14(1):21–8.
15. Lavernia CJ, Villa JM. Total hip arthroplasty in the treatment of osteonecrosis of the femoral head: then and now. Curr Rev Musculoskelet Med. 2015;8(3):260–4.
16. Johannson HR, Zywiel MG, Marker DR, Jones LC, McGrath MS, Mont MA. Osteonecrosis is not a predictor of poor outcomes in primary total hip arthroplasty: a systematic literature review. Int Orthop. 2011;35(4):465–73.
17. Cornell CN, Salvati EA, Pellicci PM. Long-term follow-up of total hip replacement in patients with osteonecrosis. Orthop Clin North Am. 1985;16:757–69.
18. Stauffer RN. Ten-year follow-up study of total hip replacement. J Bone Joint Surg Am. 1982;64-A:983–90.
19. Chandler HP, Reineck FT, Wixson RL, McCarthy JC. Total hip replacement in patients younger than thirty years old: a five-year follow-up study. J Bone Joint Surg Am. 1981;63-A:1426–34.

20. Issa K, Naziri Q, Rasquinha VJ, et al. Outcomes of primary total hip arthroplasty in systemic lupus erythematosus with a proximally-coated cementless stem. J Arthroplasty. 2013;28(9):1663–6.
21. Baek SH, Kim SY. Cementless total hip arthroplasty with alumina bearings in patients younger than fifty with femoral head osteonecrosis. J Bone Joint Surg Am. 2008;90-A:1314–20.
22. Issa K, Johnson AJ, Naziri Q, et al. Hip osteonecrosis: does prior hip surgery alter outcomes compared to an initial primary total hip arthroplasty? J Arthroplasty. 2014;29(1):162–6.
23. Mont MA, Seyler TM, Plate JF, Delanois RE, Parvizi J. Uncemented total hip arthroplasty in young adults with osteonecrosis of the femoral head: a comparative study. J Bone Joint Surg Am. 2006;88-A(Suppl):104–9.
24. Seyler TM, Bonutti PM, Shen J, Naughton M, Kester M. Use of an alumina-on alumina bearing system in total hip arthroplasty for osteonecrosis of the hip. J Bone Joint Surg Am. 2006;88-A(Suppl):116–25.
25. Wang TI, Hung SH, Su YP, et al. Noncemented total hip arthroplasty for osteonecrosis of the femoral head in elderly patients. Orthopedics. 2013;36:271–5.
26. Issa K, Naziri Q, Maheshwari AV, et al. Excellent results and minimal complications of total hip arthroplasty in sickle cell hemoglobinopathy at mid-term follow-up using cementless prosthetic components. J Arthroplasty. 2013;28(9):1693–8.
27. Ilyas I, Moreau P. Simultaneous bilateral total hip arthroplasty in sickle cell disease. J Arthroplast. 2002;17:441–5.
28. Marulanda GA, Minniti CP, Ulrich SD, Seyler TM, Mont MA. Perioperative management for orthopaedic patients with sickle cell anaemia. J Orthop Surg. 2009;17:346–50.
29. Chang JS, Han DJ, Park SK, Sung JH, Ha YC. Cementless total hip arthroplasty in patients with osteonecrosis after kidney transplantation. J Arthroplast. 2013;28:824–7.
30. Min BW, Lee KJ, Song KS, Bae KC, Cho CH. Highly cross-linked polyethylene in total hip arthroplasty for osteonecrosis of the femoral head: a minimum 5-year follow-up study. J Arthroplast. 2013;28:526–30.
31. Kim YH, Choi Y, Kim JS. Cementless total hip arthroplasty with alumina-on-highly cross-linked polyethylene bearing in young patients with femoral head osteonecrosis. J Arthroplast. 2011;26:218–23.
32. Kim YH, Kim JS, Park JW, Joo JH. Contemporary total hip arthroplasty with and without cement in patients with osteonecrosis of the femoral head: a concise followup, at an average of seventeen years, of a previous report. J Bone Joint Surg [Am]. 2011;93-A:1806–10.
33. Kawasaki M, Hasegawa Y, Sakano S, Masui T, Ishiguro N. Total hip arthroplasty after failed transtrochanteric rotational osteotomy for avascular necrosis of the femoral head. J Arthroplast. 2005;20:574–9.
34. Ball ST, Le Duff MJ, Amstutz HC. Early results of conversion of a failed femoral component in hip resurfacing arthroplasty. J Bone Joint Surg Am. 2007;89-A:735–41.
35. Helbig L, Simank HG, Kroeber M, et al. Core decompression combined with implantation of a demineralised bone matrix for non-traumatic osteonecrosis of the femoral head. Arch Orthop Trauma Surg. 2012;132:1095–110.
36. Bedard NA, Callaghan JJ, Liu SS, Greiner JJ, Klaassen AL, Johnston RC. Cementless THA for the treatment of osteonecrosis at 10-year follow-up: have we improved compared to cemented THA? J Arthroplast. 2013;28(7):1192–1199. Epub 2013 Feb 12. doi:10.1016/j.arth.2012.09.008.
37. Yu L, Qi C, Yu T, Meng Q, Zhao X, Liu K, Cai Y. A comparative study on short-termeffectiveness between cemented and uncementedtotal hip arthroplasty for osteonecrosis of femoral headafterrenal transplantation. ZhongguoXiu Fu Chong JianWaiKeZaZhi. 2013 Dec;27(12):1409–13.
38. Quesada MJ, Marker DR, Mont MA. Metal-on-metal hip resurfacing: advantages and disadvantages. J Arthroplast. 2008;23(7 suppl):69–73.
39. Nunley RM, Della Valle CJ, Barrack RL. Is patient selection important for hip resurfacing? Clin Orthop Relat Res. 2009;467(1):56–65.
40. Maus U, Roth A, Tingart M, Rader C, Jager M, Noth U, Reppenhagen S, Heiss C, Beckmann J. S3 guideline. Part 3: non-traumatic avascular necrosis in adults - surgical treatment of Atraumatic avascular femoral head necrosis in adults. Z Orthop Unfall. 2015;153(5):498–507.
41. Seung-Ju K, Dong-Geun K, Sung Bae P, Jong Hun K. Is hemiresurfacing arthroplasty for osteonecrosis of the hip a viable solution? J Arthroplast. 2015;30:987–92.
42. Floerkemeier T, Budde S, Gronewold J, Radtke K, Ettinger M, Windhagen H, von Lewinski G. Short-stem hip arthroplasty in osteonecrosis of the femoral head. Arch Orthop Trauma Surg. 2015;135:715–22.
43. Zeh A, Weise A, Vasarhelyi A, Bach AG, Wohlrab D. Medium-term results of the Mayo short-stem hip prosthesis after avascular necrosis of the femoral head. Z Orthop Unfall. 2011;149(2):200.
44. Floerkemeier T, Tscheuschner N, Calliess T, Ezechieli M, Floerkemeier S, Budde S, Windhagen H, von Lewinski G. Cementless short stem hip arthroplasty METHA as an encouraging option in adults with osteonecrosis of the femoral head. Arch Orthop Trauma Surg. 2012;132(8):1125.
45. Fink B, Ruther W. Partial and total joint replacement in femur head necrosis. Orthopade. 2000;29(5):449.
46. Karatosun V, Gunal I, Unver B, Gultekin A. Thrust plate prosthesis for osteonecrosis of the femoral head: short-term results of 15 patients followed 2–6 years. J Orthop Sci. 2006;11(5):450.
47. Mont MA, Cherian JJ, Sierra RJ, Jones LC, Lieberman JR. Nontraumatic osteonecrosis of the

femoral head: where do we stand today? A ten-year update. J Bone Joint Surg Am. 2015;97(19):1604–27.
48. Takao M, et al. Cementless modular total hip arthroplasty with subtrochanteric shortening osteotomy for hips with developmental dysplasia. J Bone Joint Surg Am. 2011;93:548–55.
49. Liebermann JR, Berry DJ. Advanced reconstruction hip. Hip Society, AAOS 2006, chapter 16, pp. 115–20.
50. Goel SC. Management of sequelae of septic arthritis of hip in infancy, JK-practitioner. Rev Article. 2003;10(3):169–75.
51. Haentjens P, Lamraski G. Endoprosthetic replacement of unstable, comminuted intertrochanteric fracture of the femur in the elderly, osteoporotic patient: a review. Disabil Rehabil. 2005;27:1167–80.
52. Liu X-Z, Yang W, Yang S-H, Xu W-H, Ye S-N. Total hip arthroplasty for treatment of elderly patients with comminuted intertrochanteric fracture accompanied by femoral head necrosis. Chinese J Traumatol (English Ed). 2008;11:359–63.
53. Weiss RJ, Kärrholm J, Hailer NP, Beckman MO, Stark A. Salvage of failed trochanteric and subtrochanteric fractures using a distally fixed, modular, uncemented hip revision stem. Acta Orthop. 2012;83:488–92.
54. Dean BJF, Matthews JJ, Price A, Stubbs D, Whitwell D, Gibbons CMLH. Modular endoprosthetic replacement for failed internal fixation of the proximal femur following trauma. Int Orthopaed (SICOT). 2011;36:731–4.
55. Pui CM, Bostrom MP, Westrich GH, Valle CJD, Macaulay W, Mont MA, Padgett DE. Increased complication rate following conversion total hip arthroplasty after cephalomedullary fixation for intertrochanteric hip fractures: a multi-center study. J Arthroplasty. 2013;28:45–7.

11 Neurologic Diseases: Parkinson's Disease

Eustathios Kenanidis, Andreas Leonidou, Michael Potoupnis, Eleftherios Tsiridis, Aristotelis Kourtis, and Richard P. Baker

11.1 Current Concepts

E. Kenanidis, A. Leonidou, M. Potoupnis, and E. Tsiridis

Parkinson's disease (PD) is a neurodegenerative disease that is caused by the loss of function of dopaminergic neurons in the substantia nigra [1]. Typical clinical manifestations are the tremor, bradykinesia, rigidity, contractures, dystonia, postural instability and impaired mobility [1, 2]. This relatively rare pathologic condition (1–2% of >60 years population) [2] also includes non-motor symptoms as cognitive decline, depression and impairment of the autonomic nervous system. Gait abnormalities and loss of bone mass often predispose to falls and fracture [1]. Musculoskeletal problems and degenerative joint disease are usual sources of pain in these patients.

PD patients treated with hemiarthroplasty for hip fractures revealed increased postoperative mortality and risk of complications [2–5]. Previous hip fracture studies reported rate of hip dislocation up to 37% and a high rate of mortality in the early, within 6 months, postoperative period, up to 47% [5].

11.1.1 Indications for THA

- Painful degenerative joint disease
- Medically fit patients
- Early stages of the disease
- PD patients that are under close medical supervision

11.1.2 Contraindications

- Late disease stages
- Not closely monitored patients
- Patients omitting their medication [6]

E. Kenanidis, M.D., Ph.D., M.Sc. (✉)
Academic Orthopaedic Unit, Aristotle University Medical School, Thessaloniki, Greece

A. Leonidou, Pg.Dip., M.Sc., F.R.C.S.
Reading Shoulder Unit, Reading, UK
e-mail: leonidou@doctors.org.uk

M. Potoupnis, M.D., Ph.D. ·
E. Tsiridis, M.D., Ph.D., F.A.C.S., F.R.C.S.
Academic Orthopaedic Unit, Papageorgiou General Hospital, Aristotle University Medical School, Thessaloniki, Greece
e-mail: mikepot@otenet.gr; etsiridis@doctors.org.uk

A. Kourtis, M.D.
Athens Medical Centre, Athens, Greece

Southmead Hospital, Bristol, UK

University of Bristol, Bristol, UK

R.P. Baker, M.D., M.Sc., M.B.Ch.B., F.R.C.S.
Avon Orthopaedic Centre, Southmead Hospital, North Bristol NHS Trust, Bristol, UK

E. Tsiridis (ed.), *The Adult Hip - Master Case Series and Techniques*,
https://doi.org/10.1007/978-3-319-64177-5_11

11.1.3 Preoperative Planning

PD patients require careful pre-, peri- and post-operative medical management to minimize complications [4, 7].

11.1.3.1 Non-surgical Considerations

- PD patient should take his medication; a neurologist must fully monitor and optimize the pharmacological management of the patient [6].
- Customize the muscle relaxants before surgery [2] to minimize interaction with anaesthetic agents.
- Assess the bone mineral density to prevent possible fracture and further loss of bone mass [1, 7].
- To avoid complications use aggressive medical management concerning extended antibiotic prophylaxis, respiratory physiotherapy, early mobilization and prevention of pressure sores [2].

11.1.3.2 Surgical Considerations

- Reduce the risk of instability and abductor dysfunction. Regardless the muscle tone that is occasionally satisfactory or even faulty giving the impression that is adequate due to stiffness, the risk of instability is high [2, 8]. Adiadochokinesia and rigidity may increase the forces around the joint leading to dislocation [2, 8]. Options to prevent the risk of dislocation are larger heads, dual mobility implants or constrained liners [9–11].
- Use of cemented fixation in case of diffuse osteoporosis.

11.1.4 Published results

There is lack of information in the literature for PD patients undergoing THA. There are few reports [1, 8, 12, 13], usually small series of PD patients treated with THA; these include operations performed between the 1970s and the mid-1990s, limiting generalization of their results in the current clinical setting. Few recent cohorts [1, 12] and reports from national registries [8, 13] have been added for the postoperative course of these patients.

Cohorts' sample size extends up to 107 THAs [12]. Jämsen et al. reported on 857 PD patients undergoing TKA or THA [8]. Mean age ranged from over 60 to 76 years old with a mean follow-up period from 17.2 to 85.2 months. Both cemented and uncemented implants were used.

Good short-term results were reported for survivorship and pain relief. Weber et al. reported survivorship free of reoperation to be 93% at 5 years [2]. Jämsen demonstrated survival at 1 and 3 years 98.0% and 96.8%, respectively [8].

Most series supported the improvement of the functional outcome in the early post-op period but deteriorated as the underlying neurological condition worsened. The primary satisfactory outcome in patients with PD is followed at the later stages of the disease with a dramatical lessening of functional ability; however, pain relief is probably maintained [12]. The long-term outcomes are not well recorded as only about one-third of patients survived to 10 years [8].

11.1.5 Complications

11.1.5.1 Longer Hospitalization

Data from Finnish Registry demonstrated that PD patients had longer mean perioperative hospitalization compared to matched controls (9 vs. 7 days, $p < 0.001$) [8].

11.1.5.2 Increased Perioperative Mortality

Previous hip fracture studies reported increased perioperative mortality in PD patients [2–4]; this was not proved for elective THA treatment. Weber et al. reported that 6 out of 98 died within 6 postoperative months following THA [12]. Jämsen, however, reported that 1-year mortality was similar but higher in longer follow-up for the Parkinson group compared to matched controls (HR 1.94, 95% CI 1.68–2.25) [8]. Increased mortality was associated with higher age (HR per increment of 1 year 1.07, 95% CI 1.05–1.09), male gender (HR 1.14, 95% CI 1.01–1.28), cardiovascular disease (HR 1.43, 95% CI 1.10–1.86) and diabetes (HR 1.50, 95% CI 1.03–2.16) [8]. Prolonged hospitalization and mortality were associated with psychiatric conditions and accumulating comorbidity, particularly with cardiovascular disease [8].

11.1.5.3 Hip Instability/Dislocation

Dislocations and infection seem to be the most frequent postoperative complications and the main reasons for revision [2, 3, 8, 11–13]. Results concerning dislocation, however, are controversial. Weber et al. reported no dislocation at the group of primary THA and 12% at revision THA, results similar to matched controls [12]. Meek et al. [13] reported results from patients with Parkinson treated with THA between 1996 and 2004 as reported in the Scottish National Arthroplasty Registry. They found that dislocation rate after THA was not significantly different (even lower) in patients with PD (annually 0–0.46) than in control group [13]. They suggested that this unexpectedly low rate may have been due to successful pharmacological treatment that maintained muscle tone. On the contrary Jämsen et al. reported that 6.1% of PD patients from the Finnish Registry experienced hip dislocation, the majority of whom during the first postoperative year [8]. PD was associated with a higher rate almost two-fold of hip dislocations compared with controls, till the end of the first postoperative year throughout the follow-up (HR 2.33, 95% CI 1.02–5.32). There was no difference after 1 year (HR 1.29, 95% CI 0.58–2.93) [8]. Adductor contracture is commonly found and tenotomies considered necessary to prevent dislocation in small percentage of patients.

11.1.5.4 Bacterial Infections

PD seems to predispose the patient to bacterial infections during the postoperative period. Weber et al. [12] reported that the most common complication was urinary tract infection in postoperative period [12] and that infection was the most common postoperative complication (5,6%) in their series [12]. Jämsen, however, reported similar 1-year surgical site infection rate than matched controls [8].

11.1.5.5 Increased Rate of Postoperative Complications

The majority of the studies reported considerable postoperative comorbidity and complications in PD patients [1–3, 8, 12, 13]. Except for dislocation and infection, cognitive impairment, sacral decubitus, DVT, trochanteric nonunion, transient peroneal nerve palsy, pulmonary embolism and haematoma were also reported.

11.2 Case Title: THA and Primary Impaction Autografting for a Malunited Acetabular Fracture with Central Head Dislocation and Neurological Deficit

E. Kenanidis and E. Tsiridis

Apparent malunited acetabular fracture with central hip dislocation (Fig.11.1). The inner

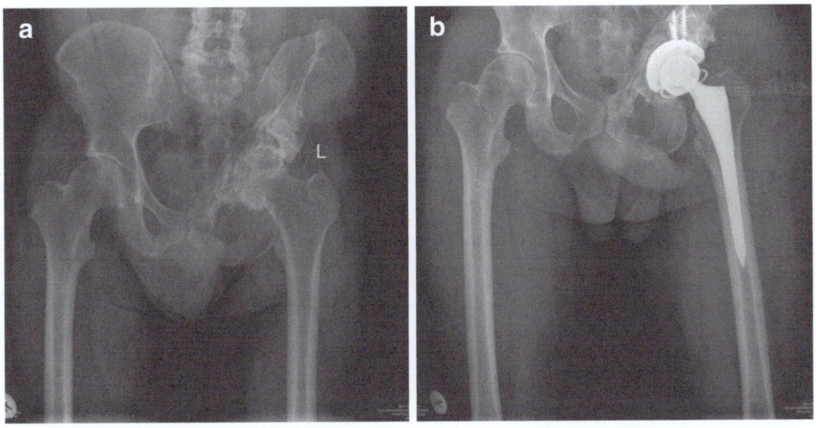

Fig. 11.1 (**a**) Preoperative x-ray (*left*) (**b**) Postoperative x-ray of the first day (*right*)

plate has moved inwards, and the roof is osteoporotic and deficient. The patient suffers from a neurological deficit on this site with reduced power 3/5 to normal and defective abductors due to trauma.

An important issue was to recover the centre of rotation and to lateralize the socket enough to get the limb out to length. Impaction autografting was important both for the latter and to also recover the bone defects that are apparent in the preoperative radiograph. Building up the socket leading to the condensed opaque postoperative radiograph demonstrating the reconstruction of the acetabular cavity. The shell was easily then inserted into a well-shaped bed and stabilized with three long screws. An uncemented shell and constrained liner (Stryker) used to compensate for the neurological deficiency and the abductor damage. The femur was easily addressed with a double-tapered straight proximally coated uncemented stem (DePuy) (Fig.11.1).

11.3 Case Title: THA Cemented with Constrained Liner for Multiple Sclerosis, Instability and Osteoporosis

E. Kenanidis and E. Tsiridis

Multiple sclerosis is a devastating neurological condition that debilitates relatively young individuals. This is the case of a 60-year-old Caucasian female who suffered from MS since the age of 35. Her mobility was fair with a pair of walking aids. She sustained an osteoporotic femoral neck fracture and was treated with a cemented THA (Fig.11.2).

Cemented constrained liner and cemented stem compensated for the osteoporotic bone on both sides and the instability due to MS (Fig.11.2).

11.4 Case Title: Primary Cemented THA+ PLAD + Primary Acetabular Impaction Autografting in an Octogenarian with Dementia and Pseudoparkinsonism

E. Kenanidis and E. Tsiridis

11.4.1 Demographics

Age: 81
Sex: Female

11.4.2 Relevant Past Medical History

Principal pathologies: Dyslipidaemia, diabetes type II, arterial hypertension

Previous surgical procedures: Resected polyps of colon in 2005

Medication: Rabeprazole, losartan, aspirin, nebivolol, inj. insulin aspart

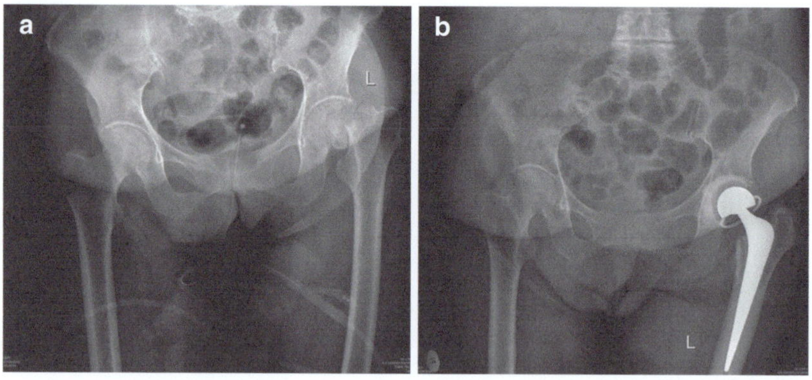

Fig. 11.2 (**a**) Preoperative x-ray of the left femoral neck fracture (*left*) (**b**) Postoperative x-ray (*right*)

11.4.3 Clinical Examination

Painful right hip. Limited ROM and inability to walk due to pain and instability. History of falls and high risk of hip fracture. The patient was advised to consider elective surgery to prevent free fall and fracture. Evidence was provided to support the THA option versus risk of fracture and morbidity and mortality data explained prior obtaining consent form.

Scoring if available: HHS: 70

Neurovascular evaluation: Generalized muscle weakness, abductor wasting, pseudoparkinsonism from anti-depressant consumption

11.4.4 Preoperative Radiological Assessment/Imaging (Fig.11.3)

Severe osteoarthritis; complete and global distortion of the cartilage both in the head and the acetabular site; subchondral cysts on either side of the joint. Generalized osteoporosis with significant bone loss in the proximal femur. Femur type IV Dorr. Acetabular erosion to the bottom end adjacent to the inner plate of the acetabulum. Sclerotic margins around the inner periphery of the acetabulum with limited cancellous bone medially. Challenging reaming expected with limited cancellous bone available and need for primary impaction autografting may be considered to compensate for the bone loss.

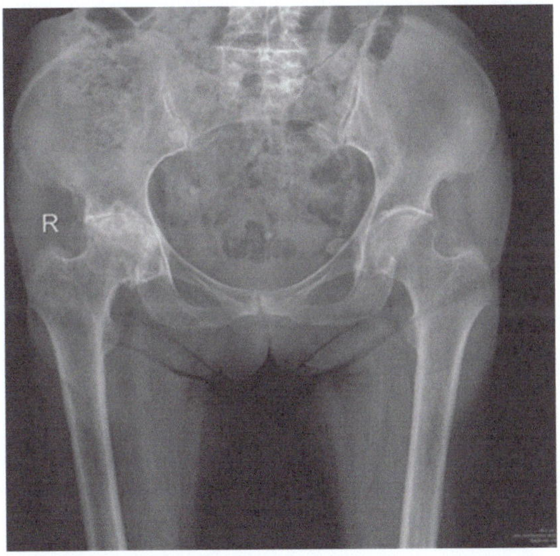

Fig. 11.3 Severe osteoarthritis; complete and global distortion of the cartilage both in the head and the acetabular site; subchondral cysts on either side of the joint. Generalized osteoporosis with significant bone loss in the proximal femur. Femur type IV Dorr. Acetabular erosion to the bottom end adjacent to the inner plate of the acetabulum. Sclerotic margins around the inner periphery of the acetabulum with limited cancellous bone medially. Challenging reaming expected with limited cancellous bone available and need for primary impaction autografting may be considered to compensate for the bone loss

11.4.5 Preoperative Planning

Diagnosis: Osteoarthritis of right hip

Chosen treatment method: Cemented RimFit Stryker Exeter 46 mm/28 mm, posterior lip augmentation device (PLAD) DePuy 28 mm, cemented hip stem Stryker Exeter 37.5–1/150 mm, femoral head Stryker 28 mm/0 mm

11.4.6 Surgical Note

With the patient in a standard table and lateral decubitus position, a mini-posterior approach was performed using standard equipment. Easy approach due to muscle relaxation and wasting. Evident of abductor deficiency with fatty degeneration in places was noticed. Easy exposure of the acetabulum and retractor placement at the front of the anterior wall of the acetabulum and below the transverse ligament inferiorly. Careful dislocation to avoid intraoperative fracture of the femur. Following the head removal, the femur was retracted anteriorly behind the anterior retractor. Clearance of the redundant anterior capsule and partial release of the rectus femoris tendon to achieve better anterior retraction. Reaming started with small reamers to explore the inner plate and actual depth of the acetabulum. Sclerotic acetabulum inner surface was difficult to ream. A curved osteotome was used to scratch the sclerotic bone in places before using larger reamers. The latter helped us to expose cancellous bone; however, the inner plate and part of the socket periphery remained sclerotic as expected. Primary impaction grafting was then employed.

Primary impaction autografting and cementation technique: The femoral head was denuded from the cartilage and the osteophytes using the saw. Then it was divided into segments perpendicular to its axis leading to several bony discs available for grafting. A powerful bone cutter (Rowngner or Louwer) was used to prepare large chips of at least 1–2 cm each from cancellous bone. The chips were introduced into the reamed acetabular bed and were impacted one next to the other tightly with special impactors until a neo-cancellization of the acetabulum was made. The strength of the construct was tested manually with a curette, and only when the grafted bed was robust enough to resist scratching off the inner plate of the acetabulum, the impaction was stopped. Third-generation cementation technique was then used to insert the implant. Proper drying of the acetabulum and suction drain placed on the roof of the acetabulum used to dry the bed. Keyholes using a 6mm drill established at the rim of the roof and near the pubic and ischial acetabular extensions. Palacos cement with gentamicin was used for cementation. The cement was pressurized against the wall using the appropriate device from the Exeter system up until 5 min. To premeasure all-polyethylene cup was then introduced using the special inserter to adjust the abduction, anteversion and inclination of the component. Steady pressurization of the implant against the cement up until 13 min. Socket size was 46 mm with inner 28mm diameter for a 28mm head.

Attention then was turned to the femoral preparation: The lower limb was turned around to expose the upper end of the osteotomized femur. The entry near to the popliteal fossa was made using the box chisel, and the canal was identified. It was evident that the bone was severely osteoporotic. Reaming was then started until a 37.5mm offset size 1 Exeter rasp stem was inserted tight. Trial reduction with a 28mm standard head was then found appropriate for abductor tension and offset. The leg length was assessed, and the stem position in depth was marked on the bone using the dotted system on the rasp stem.

Third-generation cementing technique was employed for the femur: Washing thoroughly and drying the canal using suction drain and impacting a swab inside the canal to reduce blood rebound before cementation. A cement plug was measured and inserted in the appropriate depth size 12. Palacos cement with gentamicin was inserted retrograde at 4 min using the suction aspiration in the canal to reduce blood rebound. The canal was occluded with the special cement pressurizer used with the cement gun to maintain pressure and inject more cement during the process until fat globules were extruded from the proximal femoral cortex indicating appropriate pressurization. Approximately at 8 min, the stem was inserted using the cement centralizer to the predetermined length. The proximal cement mantle was then pressurized using the horseshoe collar pressurizer and the unique device on top of it to maintain position and pressure up until the end of the cement setting at 13 min. Trial reduction and final head 28 mm standard were inserted (Figs. 11.4 and 11.5).

PLAD insertion: To prevent dislocations a PLAD was elected to be inserted. The position of the PLAD is 6–12.00. PLAD is double-faced: a metal face on the top for the screw insertion and a polyethylene face for the interface with the socket. PLAD has an extended inner lip that goes over the neck-head junction limiting the risk of dislocation; in addition by raising the posterior edge of the acetabular component, it also reduces the risk of dislocation when the hip is in flexion and internal rotation. Attention must be taken to place the screws well into the polyethylene rim of the socket without compromising the thickness of the liner. The screws, therefore, go through the polysocket and then through the cement mantle to the surrounding bone. Care must be taken to remove all the polyethylene debris from the drilled holes. It is advisable to do all screws available usually six. Positioning the PLAD too far in will compromise the ROM of the hip and too far out won't protect the hip ROM from dislocation; thus, appropriate placement and previous experience are essential for the correct placement of the PLAD. In our case, a 28 mm PLAD was used. The 22–28 mm PLADs are available in the market by DePuy Johnson and Johnson (Figs. 11.4 and 11.5).

Patient's position: Lateral decubitus

Type of anaesthesia: General

Surgical approach: Mini posterior

11.4.7 Postoperative Radiographs (Figs. 11.4 and 11.5)

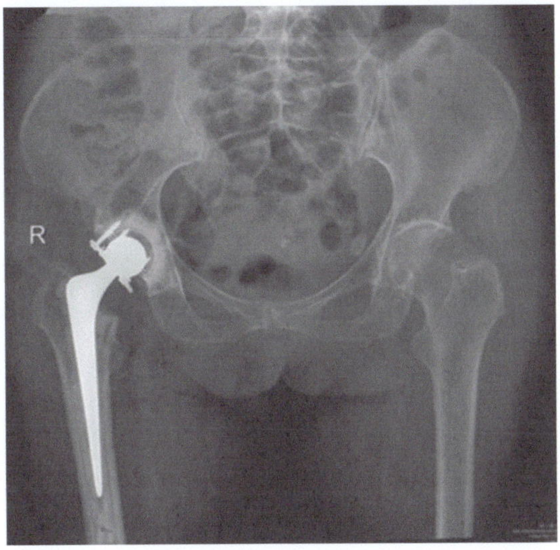

Fig. 11.4 AP of the right hip first day

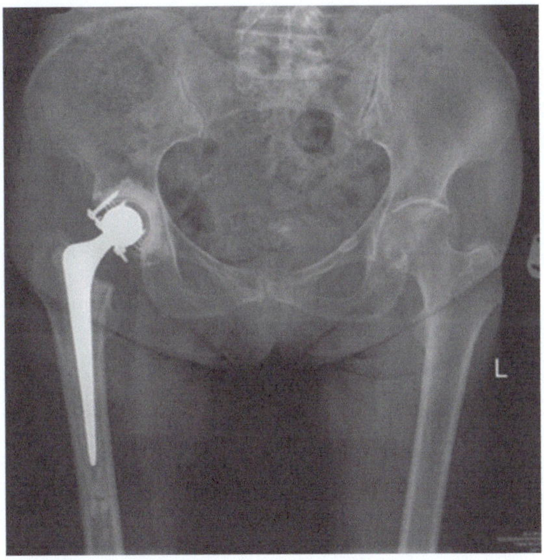

Fig. 11.5 AP of the right hip first month

Good cement mantle on both sites of the femur and acetabulum with at least 2 mm width impaction grafting of the acetabulum brought the polyethylene laterally recovering the centre of rotation and the appropriate offset of the hip joint (Figs. 11.4 and 11.5).

11.4.7.1 Postoperative Management

Chemoprophylaxis and anticoagulant treatment period: Cefuroxime 750 mg (one dose preoperatively and two doses postoperatively), vancomycin 500 mg (one dose preoperatively and two doses postoperatively), enoxaparin 1 × 1 for 35 days

Gait/limb loading until full loading: Partial weight bearing for four weeks and then as tolerated

11.5 Case Title: Primary Arthroplasty for Parkinson's Disease

A. Kourtis and R. Baker

11.5.1 Demographics

Age: 74
Sex: Female
BMI: 24

11.5.2 Relevant Past Medical History

Principal pathologies: Osteoarthritis left hip, Parkinson's disease

Previous surgical procedures: Nil

Medication: Sinemet CR, Sinemet Plus, Madopar, Stalevo, Requip XL, amantadine, oxycodone, paracetamol, temazepam, citalopram, Laxido

Others: Nil

History of Presenting Complaint: A 74-year-old female had a year of left groin and buttock pain which rapidly deteriorated over three months. The pain kept the patient awake at night, and all activities of daily living were affected. Due to the rapid deterioration and increase in pain, the patient requested total hip replacement.

11.5.3 Clinical Examination

Symptoms: Pain not controlled with opioid medication. The patient was wheelchair bound outside of her house and could only mobilize holding furniture. Stable Parkinson's disease.

Range of motion: Flexion, 60°; obligatory internal rotation when hip flexed; internal rotation, -10°; external rotation, 5°; abduction, 10°; adduction, 10°. The pain was reproduced during all movements.

Specific tests: Fixed flexion deformity 30°

Main disability: Pain during all movements with associated rest pain and night pain. Stiffness in the hip. Husband has to help with foot social care and dressing.

Neurovascular evaluation: Sciatic and femoral nerves intact. Shuffling gait, generalized hypertonia, uncontrolled rhythmic tremor

11.5.4 Preoperative Radiological Assessment/Imaging

11.5.4.1 Preoperative Planning

Diagnosis: Osteoarthritis of the left hip (Figs. 11.6, 11.7, and 11.8)

Possible treatment options: Cemented left total hip replacement (THR). Hybrid THR with a

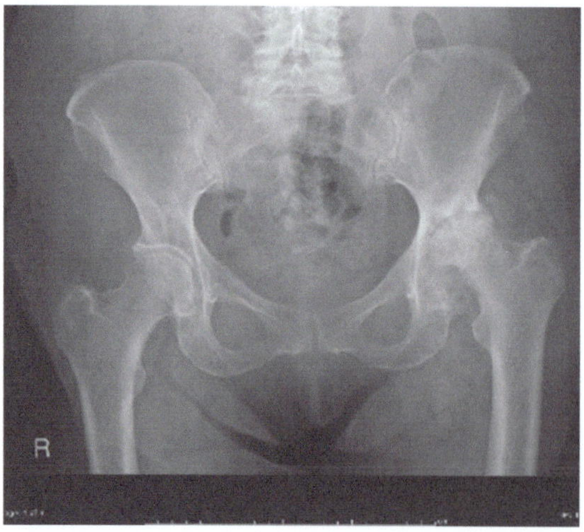

Fig. 11.6 AP view of both hip joints. Osteoarthritis of the left hip with a migration of femoral head superiorly and laterally

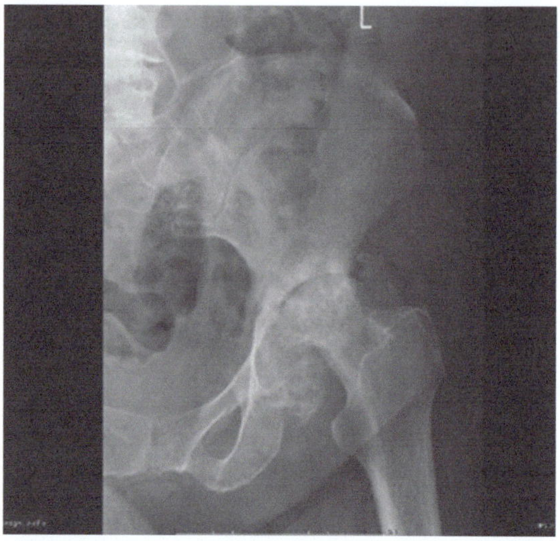

Fig. 11.7 Iliac Judet views of the left hip

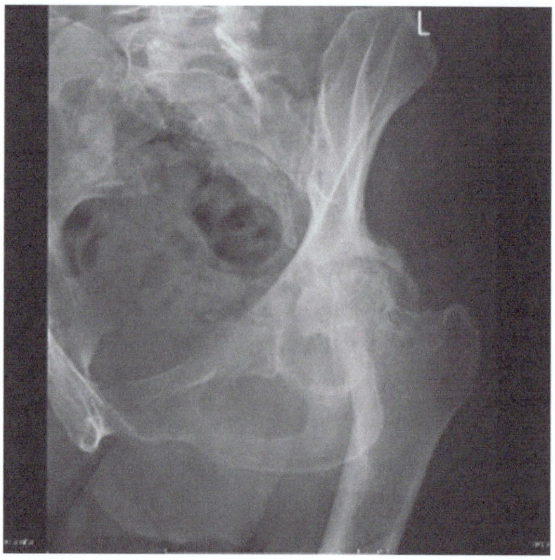

Fig. 11.8 Obturator Judet view of left hip

large femoral head +/− a lipped liner. Hybrid THR with a dual mobility or constrained liner

Chosen treatment method: Hybrid left total hip replacement with a constrained liner

Selection of implants if applicable and rational: Cemented stem due to osteoporotic "stove type" femur and risk of fracture and poor press fit with an uncemented stem

Expected difficulties: Patient at risk of involuntary movements and high risk of falls with a progressive neurological condition. Risk of dislocation greater than a patient without neurological condition

Strategies to overcome difficulties: High hip center with superior and lateral acetabular erosion secondary to the osteoarthritic process. The operation performed for pain relief with little improvement in mobility expected, high hip center accepted and planned for preoperatively. Albeit unlikely, we had acetabular augments on standby increase socket more complicated than anticipated.

Templating: Digital

11.5.5 Surgical Note

Patient's position: Lateral position

Type of anesthesia: Spinal injection and general anesthesia

Surgical approach: Posterior approach with repair of short external rotators

Main steps: Neck cut as per preoperative templating. Acetabular reaming to fit socket shape without attempting to ream down to true floor

Reconstruction techniques: Uncemented hemispherical acetabular cup with a minimum of three screws, a constrained polyethylene liner and a cemented femoral stem. An abductor tenotomy (release) was required at the end due to contracture formation of the left hip.

11.5.6 Intraoperative Challenges

Challenges and solutions: Correct positioning of the acetabular and the femoral components. Optimal press fit and excellent fixation with screws are crucial. Careful positioning of the implants with thorough preparation.

Unanticipated problems and solution: Nil

Thorough description of decision making, including the reason for the final decision: Low-demand patient needed one operation for pain relief and minimization of complications. The patient would be at increased risk of dislocation with her progressive neurological condition and frequent falls. Capturing the femoral head decreases this risk.

11.5.7 Postoperative Radiographs (Figs. 11.9 and 11.10)

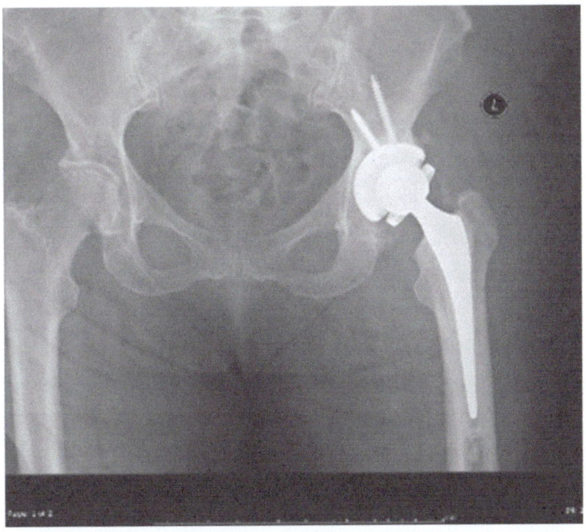

Fig. 11.9 AP view of a left hybrid total hip replacement with a constrained liner and screw fixation

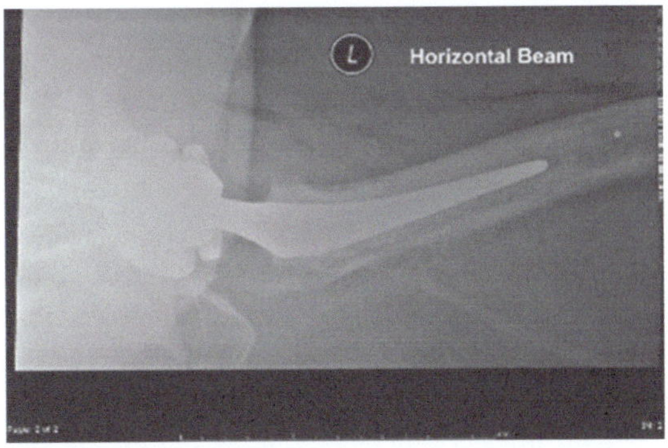

Fig. 11.10 Lateral view of a left hybrid total hip replacement

11.5.7.1 Postoperative Management

Chemoprophylaxis and anticoagulant treatment period: Dabigatran 150 mg once daily for 28 days. Day 4 large hematoma appeared and wound remained dry. Patient switched to per os aspirin 150 mg once daily.

Gait/limb loading until full loading: Full weight bearing immediately

11.5.8 Follow-Up and Complications

No postoperative complications, other than haematoma.

11.5.9 Discussion

Advantages of the applied method: A total hip replacement with a constrained liner reduces the risk of dislocation significantly. A patient with a progressive neurological condition who has a late complication following surgery may be unable to tolerate any future procedures. Dislocation following THA in patients with Parkinson's disease has been shown to have lower rates of dislocation [13] and higher rates [8] compared to standard cases. There were lower rates of dislocation in data from the Scottish National Joint Registry—but no implant details were available—and presumably cases with a capture cup may have been included in this analysis.

Disadvantages of the method: Dissociation of the components and increased interfacial stresses resulting in acetabular loosening and early failure. If they dislocate, they need an open reduction.

Alternative evidence-based techniques for the case: Cemented or hybrid total hip replacement with a large femoral head—both have increased risk of dislocation [14]. Hybrid THR with a dual mobility system.

Why the chosen technique is better for this case? One operation, low-demand patient unlikely to loosen implant and high-risk dislocation avoided

Indications and contraindications for this technique:

Indications: The constrained liner is a robust solution for patients with advanced neuromuscular disorders such as Parkinson's disease.

Contraindications: Patients diagnosed with Parkinson's disease at early stages with proper neuromuscular function and low risks for recurrent falls and dislocations. Poor acetabular bone stock

Level of evidence concerning the superiority of this method against others: Level 3

References

1. Mathew PG, Sponer P, Kucera T, Grinac M, Knízek J. Total hip arthroplasty in patients with Parkinson's disease. Acta Med (Hradec Kralove). 2013;56(3):110–6.
2. Qucally JM, Abdulkarim A, Mulhall KJ. Total hip replacement in patients with neurological conditions. J Bone Joint Surg Br. 2009;91(10):1267–73.
3. Clubb VJ, Clubb SE, Buckley S. Parkinson's disease patients who fracture their neck of femur: a review of outcome data. Injury. 2006;37:929–3.
4. Kraay MJ, Bigach SD. The neuromuscularly challenged patient: total hip replacement is now an option. Bone Joint J. 2014;96-B(11 Suppl A):27–31.
5. Coughlin L, Templeton J. Hip fractures in patients with Parkinson's disease. Clin Orthop. 1980;148:192–5.
6. Brennan KA, Genever RW. Managing Parkinson's disease during surgery. BMJ. 2010;341:c5718.
7. Zuckerman LM. Parkinson's disease and the orthopaedic patient. J Am Acad Orthop Surg. 2009;17:48–55.
8. Jämsen E, Puolakka T, Peltola M, Eskelinen A, Lehto MU. Surgical outcomes of primary hip and knee replacements in patients with Parkinson's disease: a nationwide registry-based case-controlled study. Bone Joint J. 2014;96-B(4):486–91.
9. Li J, Zheng W, Zhao J, Liu D, Xu W. Large diameter metal on metal total hip replacement for femoral neck fractures with neurological conditions: a retrospective assessment. Indian J Orthop. 2014;48(6):605–11.
10. Park KS, Seon JK, Lee KB, Yoon TR. Total hip arthroplasty using large-diameter metal-on-metal articulation in patients with neuromuscular weakness. J Arthroplast. 2014;29(4):797–801. Epub 2013 Sep 17

11. Hayward RMK, Bindi SMF, Wallace M. Outcomes of dual-mobility acetabular cup for instability in primary and revision total hip arthroplasty. J Orthop Traumatol. 2015;16:9–13.
12. Weber M, Cabanela ME, Sim FH, Frassica FJ, Harmsen WS. Total hip replacement in patients with Parkinson's disease. Int Orthop. 2002;26(2):66–8.
13. Meek RM, Allan DB, McPhillips G, Kerr L, Howie CR. Epidemiology of dislocation after total hip arthroplasty. Clin Orthop. 2006;447:9–18.
14. Berry DJ, von Knoch M, Schleck CD, Harmsen WS. Effect of femoral head diameter and operative approach on risk of dislocation after primary total hip arthroplasty. J Bone Joint Surg Am. 2005;87:2456–63.

12 Sickle Cell Disease

Eustathios Kenanidis, Panagiotis Kakoulidis, Panagiotis Lepetsos, Michael Potoupnis, Eleftherios Tsiridis, Emre Toğrul, Bülent Atilla, Duy L. Phan, and Ran Schwarzkopf

12.1 Current Concepts

E. Kenanidis, P. Kakoulidis, P. Lepetsos, M. Potoupnis, and E. Tsiridis

Sickle cell disease (SCD) is an autosomal recessive disorder caused by a point mutation in the β-globin chain of haemoglobin that forms haemoglobin S [1, 2]. Under low oxygen tension, the abnormal erythrocytes are susceptible to sickling. The abnormal haemoglobin and erythrocytes produce hemolytic anaemia and reduced hemopoiesis, recurrent pain episodes, as well as chronic end-organ damage and infarction [2]. The most usual orthopedic manifestations of the disease are the following [3]:

1. Osteonecrosis

The sickling of the red blood cells causes vascular congestion and microvasculature thrombosis in the bone. The resulting ischemia, enhanced by the increased intraosseous pressure, produces bone infarction and necrosis [3]. The incidence of osteonecrosis of the femoral head ranges from 3 to 50% based on the sickle cell genotype [3] of the haemoglobinopathy. Bilateral hip involvement is also possible [4].

2. Pyogenic infection

The SCD patients are vulnerable to bacteremia and hematogenous seeding in their bones and joints [5]. The latter is mainly attributed to the immunodeficiency secondary to a splenic auto-infarction [3]. *Staphylococcus aureus* is the most usual cause of osteomyelitis in SCD [6];

E. Kenanidis, M.D., Ph.D., M.Sc. (✉) · P. Kakoulidis, M.D
Academic Orthopaedic Unit, Aristotle University Medical School, Thessaloniki, Greece

P. Lepetsos, M.D., Ph.D., M.Sc.
Fourth Orthopaedic Department, KAT Hospital, Athens, Greece
e-mail: plepetsos@med.uoa.gr

E. Tsiridis, M.D., Ph.D., F.A.C.S., F.R.C.S. · M. Potoupnis, M.D., Ph.D
Academic Orthopaedic Unit, Papageorgiou General Hospital, Aristotle University Medical School, Thessaloniki, Greece
e-mail: etsiridis@doctors.org.uk; mikepot@otenet.gr

E. Toğrul, M.D.
Ortopedia Hospital, Adana, Turkey

B. Atilla, M.D.
Faculty of Medicine, Hacettepe University, Ankara, Turkey

D.L. Phan, M.D.
Kaiser Permanente, Oakland, CA, USA

R. Schwarzkopf, M.D., M.Sc.
Department of Orthopaedic Surgery, NYU Langone Health Orthopaedic Hospital, Hospital for Joint Diseases, New York, NY, USA

E. Tsiridis (ed.), *The Adult Hip - Master Case Series and Techniques*, https://doi.org/10.1007/978-3-319-64177-5_12

Salmonella typhi, however, is the most characteristic organism [3].

3. Bone marrow hyperplasia [3]

The chronic anaemia of the SCD patients causes increased bone marrow erythropoiesis and hyperplasia. It results in widening of the medullary canal and thinning of the trabeculae and cortices especially in the metaphyses of long bones. It causes substantial intraoperative technical difficulties during a THA (intramedullary reaming, prosthesis fitting, insertion, and fixation) [3, 6].

12.1.1 Indications for THA

Advances in medical therapy resulted in a longer life of SCD patients [2, 3]. Subsequently, THA has increased popularity in this group of patients. The primary indications for THA in SCD patients are the following [2, 3]:

1. Medical fitness to undergo elective surgery
2. Continuous, disabling hip pain that is uncontrolled to nonsurgical management

12.1.2 Preoperative Planning [2, 3]

The surgeon cooperating with a haematologist familiar to SCD patients must have in mind to:

1. Prevent a sickle cell crisis: avoid acidosis, manage fluids, and oxygenate adequately [1].
2. Evaluate the cardiac status and fluid balance. There is high incidence of congestive heart failure in SCD patients [2].
3. Find a remote infection that puts in danger the prosthetic implant. Chronic ulcers are the primary sources of infection [3, 4, 7].
4. Consider a preoperative transfusion or plasmapheresis to improve oxygen carrying capacity [2]. It is supported that an SCD patient should have a postoperative Hb >10 g/dL and Hct > 30% [2]. In a randomized study [8], however, an aggressive preoperative transfusion was not helpful to prevent overall and sickle cell-related complications.
5. Use autologous donation, phenotypically matched blood, and leukocyte-depleted blood to decrease alloimmunization rate that occurs in 20–30% of SCD patients [6].
6. Consider pain management techniques for patients.
7. Although unproven, the epidural anaesthesia in this population may decrease the rate of sickling and subsequent crisis via a temporary sympathectomy, peripheral vasodilatation and decreased peripheral vascular resistance in the lower extremities [9].

12.1.3 Intraoperative Considerations [3]

We can expect technical difficulties during the operation due to the well-established changes in the bones and the excessive blood loss [8]. Recurrent bone changes include [3]:

1. Broadening of the medullary canal
2. Trabecular and cortical thinning due to marrow hyperplasia
3. Small isolated areas of sclerosis
4. Canal elimination from repeated episodes of marrow infarction

The technical difficulties during bony preparation and implantation usually involve:

1. Bone quality:
   - The poor bone quality increases acetabular fracture risk during cementless implantation.
   - An intraoperative femoral perforation and fracture of the thin metaphyseal cortices during the reaming or component insertion are reported to be high (4.9–18.2%) [3]. Therefore, a stepwise preparation of the femur is required to avoid penetration and fracture.
   - Occasionally use narrow femoral stems, and prepare difficult femurs under an image intensifier using speed burrs.
2. Acetabular protrusion:
   - High incidence.
   - It limits the extent of the medial reaming and may require a medial bone grafting or structural acetabular support.

- Hip dislocation may be difficult [2, 3]. Better divide the femoral neck in situ before removing the head rather than taking the risk of a femoral shaft fracture while forcibly dislocating the hip.

12.1.4 Published Results

Several [4, 6–18] studies provide outcomes for the effectiveness of cemented or uncemented THA in patients with sickle cell disease. These are various case series and cohort studies of 7–244 patients reporting 7–312 THAs. The patients' age ranges from 10 to 58 years. The mean follow-up period was between 3.3 and 13 years. The failure and revision rates range from 0% in small series to as high as 63% at a mean follow-up of 6.5 years [13]. Recent studies, however, reported more favourable results concerning aseptic loosening, independently of the fixation method [16–18].

Despite the high complication and revision rate, several studies [6, 7, 10–15] have shown that THA provides pain relief and increased function to SCD patient [4, 9, 11, 14, 18]. Hernigou et al. [18] in a series of 312 fully cemented THA in sickle cell patients with mean age of 32 years and mean follow-up of 13 years, reported 91% and 86% survivorship of both components after 10–15 years, respectively. Despite the high percentage of complications in this cohort, 64% of patients were free of pain. Recently Gulati et al. [16] reported improved Harris Hip Score from 42 preoperatively to 92 postoperatively in a mean follow-up of 3.8 years.

The reported survivorship is strictly endangered compared with age-matched THA controls [3]. Comparing, however, the seven years follow-up results of cementless hip replacement between sicklers and other osteonecrotic patients, Issa et al. [17] found that implant survivorship (95% vs. 97%), HHS (87 vs. 88), and radiographic findings were similar among the groups [17].

Cemented vs. cementless fixation. No high-quality prospective comparative studies are comparing cemented vs. cementless fixation for THA in SCD [3]. Cementless cup fixation seems to be favourable based on the reported results of implant loosening. The selection of the type of fixation of the femoral prosthesis in patients with SCD is controversial. Hickman et al. [14] reported no loosening of thirteen uncemented cups at six years, and Ilyas et al. [4] aseptic loosening of 1 out of 18 uncemented cups at a mean follow-up of 5.7 years. Cemented cup fixation has a poorer prognosis with revision rate for aseptic loosening up to 33% [6]. Acurio and Friedman [10] showed a statistically significant lower rate of aseptic loosening for uncemented (22%) compared with cemented (59%) ($p < 0.05$) in 25 sickle cell patients. This information, however, cannot be considered as definite. In a recent cohort study, Hernigou et al. [18] reported only 8% cup and 5% stem aseptic loosening in 312 full cemented THAs at a mean of fourteen years follow-up.

A possible disadvantage of cementless fixation is the difficulty to achieve a biologic fixation in avascular and necrotic SCD bone [3]. A cementless acetabular fixation is usually enhanced with screws. The use of cement may cause thermal necrosis of the already infarcted bone, a greater incidence of infection, and septic or aseptic loosening [4, 10]. Advantages of a cemented fixation are considered the additional hemostasis through tamponade effect on intramedullary bleeding, the decreased risk of femoral perforation, and the avoidance of biologic fixation in avascular/necrotic bone [3, 8, 9, 14].

The cemented fixation is expected to fail due to an acetabular protrusion and the lack of viable cancellous bone. The primary impaction grafting using the femoral head could be an option when the cemented fixation is elected to overcome acetabular sclerosis and other deformities or defects. However, the quality of such a bone is not ideal, and the uncontained defects should never be reconstructed using this technique. Finally, a proximal femoral deformity and lack of homogenous endosteal canal dimensions can be managed better with a cemented implant.

Overall the femoral fixation is dependent on multiple factors including the shape of the femoral canal and the bone quality. Cemented femoral fixation has the advantage of an easier fitting, bleeding control, and initial implant stability compared to the uncemented fixation; long-term comparative results, however, are not available.

12.1.5 Complications

The medical and surgical complications are increased in patients with SCD undergoing THA. The reported complication rates vary from 18% to 80% [6, 7, 10–15]. In the greater reported cohort, Hernigou et al. demonstrated 27% medical and 13% orthopedic complications [18]. Perfetti et al. [19] supported that SCD patients had 152% higher risk of complications ($p < 0.001$), 42% longer length of stay ($p < 0.001$), and 19% higher hospital charges ($p < 0.001$) for THA than matched controls.

12.1.5.1 Immediate

- Greater blood loss and tranfusion rate during THA in SCD compared to unaffected THA patients [8].
- Increased cardiopulmonary, neurological and mental status complications.
- Greater frequency of major transfusion reactions due to alloimmunization [6]. The reported incidence of reactions in studies ranged from 1 to 12% [6, 10, 18].
- A sickle cell crisis and acute chest syndrome (ACS) is reported up to 17% [8]. ACS is a form of acute lung injury that is mainly clinically diagnosed, and it is a major cause of morbidity and mortality.

12.1.5.2 Short Term

- Greater reported postoperative rate of wound infections 16–25% in some series [7, 10–13].

12.1.5.3 Late

- The late periprosthetic infection due recurrent bacteremia is higher compared to the general population [10–13]. Hernigou et al. [18] reported a late infection rate of 3% as the main late postoperative complication.
- A hip dislocation is reported up to 26% [14], possibly due to an earlier septic or aseptic loosening of the implant.

12.2 Case Title: Cementless Hip Arthoplasty and Adductor Tenotomy for Femoral Head Necrosis in a Patient Suffering from Sickle Cell Anaemia

Emre Toğrul and Bülent Atilla

12.2.1 Demographics

Age: 19
Sex: Female
BMI: 16.2

12.2.2 Relevant Past Medical History

Principal pathologies: Femoral head avascular necrosis related to sickle cell disease.

Previous surgical procedures: None.

Medication: None.

Other: Sickle cell anemia.

History of presenting complaint: Patient was complaining of left hip pain.

12.2.3 Clinical Examination

Symptoms: Leg length discrepancy, pain and limitation on movement, and restriction of abduction due to contracture.

Range of motion: Restricted internal rotation on the left hip.

Specific tests: X-rays taken in a neutral standing (weight bearing) position and measurements taken on the X-ray picture.

Main disability: Pain on the left side and restricted movement, leg length discrepancy (1 cm), abduction restriction (10°), and abduction contracture.

Scoring if available: Harris Hip Score is 77.5.

Neurovascular evaluation: There isn't any sign of neurovascular dysfunction.

12.2.4 Preoperative Radiological Assessment/Imaging (Figs. 12.1 and 12.2)

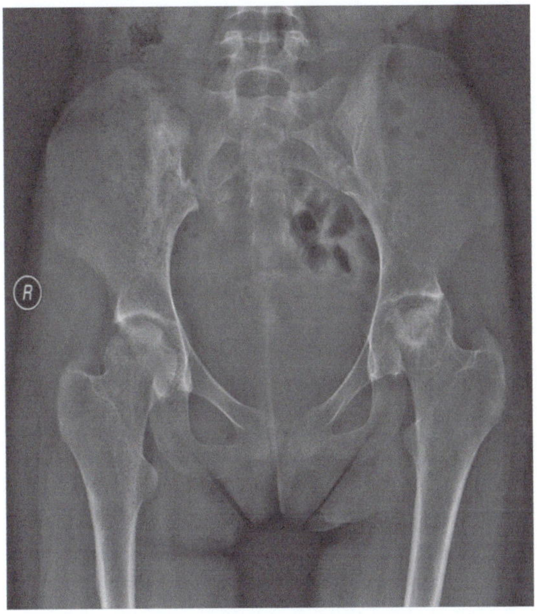

Fig. 12.1 Osteonecrosis of the left femoral head

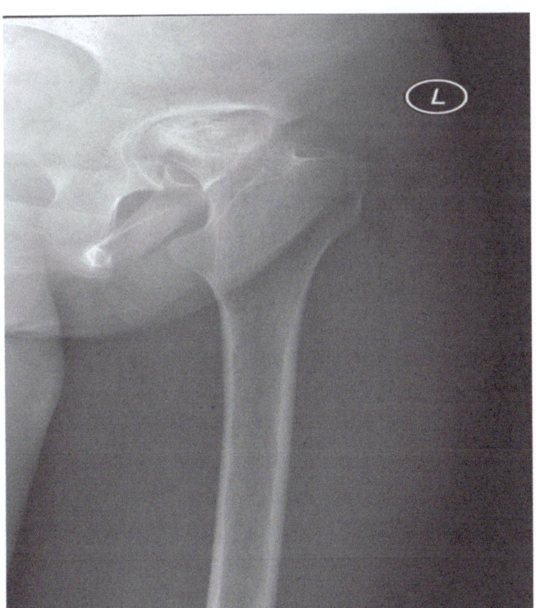

Fig. 12.2 Sickle cell anaemia may present with a diffuse patch sclerosis and ingrowth of new bone formation around the femoral shaft. There may be a periosteal hypertrophy as in the osteomyelitis. The bony changes tend to obliterate the femoral canal leading to a complicated femoral reaming process

12.2.5 Preoperative Planning

Diagnosis: Avascular necrosis of the femoral head due to sickle cell anemia (Figs. 12.1 and 12.2).

Possible treatment options: There is no other possible treatment option than arthroplasty surgery regarding the late stage of avascular necrosis and the collapsed femoral head.

Chosen treatment method: Cementless total hip arthroplasty and adductor tenotomy.

Selection of implants if applicable and rational: Titanium M/L Taper Hip Prosthesis Femoral Stem (Zimmer), ceramic insert, Trilogy IT Acetabular System, Biolox delta Ceramic Femoral Head.

Expected difficulties: Technical problems in the operation because of the long-standing deformities, the poor bone quality, and the presence of sclerosis due to intramedullary necrosis obliterating the medullary canal. They include a risk of intraoperative fracture of the femur, excessive bleeding, coexisting infections (e.g., urinary), unanticipated pain, inability to equalise the leg length, increased infection risk etc.

12.2.6 Strategies to Overcome Difficulties

Bleeding: Using hypotensive anesthesia, tissue-preserving surgical dissection, and preparing blood products.

Intraoperative fracture of the femur: Using the correct surgical technique to reduce the possibility of femur fracture.

Pain: Using distal venting hole in the femur, supporting fluid intake, giving oxygen therapy, and using PCA to minimise the pain.

Infection control: Preoperative patient screening (e.g., FBC, urine culture). In case of a detected preoperative infection, treat before surgery (e.g., urinary tract infection). Skin preparation. Care for asepsis.

Inability to equalize the leg length: Preoperative control/measurement.

12.2.7 Surgical Note

Patient's position: Lateral decubitus position. Secure fixation is mandatory to avoid pelvic rotation intraoperatively.

Type of anesthesia: Spinal epidural anesthesia.

Surgical approach: Minimally invasive surgery via a posterior approach.

Main steps: a. Exposure and joint dislocation, b. Femoral head cut, C. Acetabular reaming, d. Reaming of the femoral canal, e. Implantation of trial components, f. Hip reduction and evaluation of the hip stability, g. Implantation of the permanent acetabular cup and the femoral component, h. Trial reduction, i. Implantation of the femoral head and evaluation of the hip stability, k. Evaluation of the abduction and adductor tenotomy.

Reconstruction techniques: Posterior capsule repair.

12.2.8 Intraoperative Challenges

Challenges and solutions: The sickle cell disease is a life-threatening condition; the endarteritis due to a vascular occlusion by the sickled red blood cells leads to a multisystem disorder. Patients with sickle cell disease may present hepatosplenomegaly, pulmonary problems related to pneumonia and infarct, leg ulcers, cardiomegaly, and psychiatric disorders including drug abuse and suicide attempt.

Bleeding: Anemia is a common preop finding that we can manage with a preoperative blood transfusion, careful surgical technique, and supporting of the patient with blood products (erythrocyte suspension). Crystalloid replacement is needed throughout the operation to maintain the hydration and to keep the hematocrit at the desired level.

Intraoperative bone fracture due to low bone quality/hard canal preparation: The periosteal cortex is often very thin that increases the risk of femoral fracture and perforation.

Breaking the chain of infection control: Care for asepsis.

Inability to equalise the leg length: After implantation of the prosthesis, check the equality of leg length with the patient at the supine position.

Unanticipated problems and solution: None.

12.2.9 Postoperative Radiographs (Fig. 12.3)

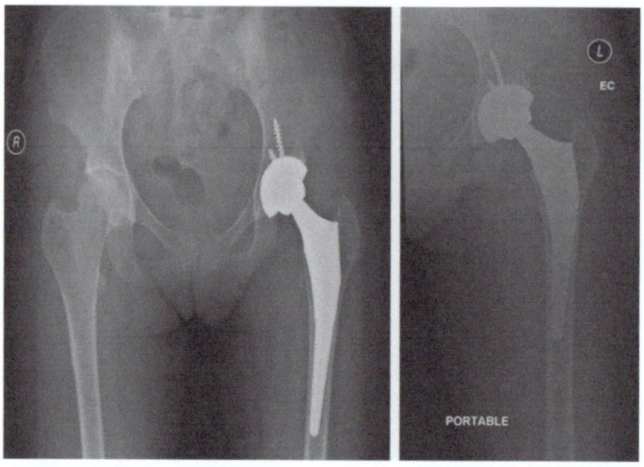

Fig. 12.3 Postoperative AP pelvis X-ray of the patient. Cementless fixation with a proximal metaphyseal canal filling stem

12.2.10 Postoperative Management

Chemoprophylaxis and anticoagulant treatment period: The anticoagulant treatment (low-molecular-weight heparin (LMWH) was started 12 h after surgery. The patient received injection OD for 4 days during hospital stay and LMWH for 10 days after discharge home. On the 8th day, the patient was started oral antiplatelet (aspirin 300 mg) OD for 6 weeks.

Gait/limb loading until full loading: The patient was able for full loading at the first postoperative day. An epidural catheter was left in situ for 2–3 days to enhance lower limb perfusion. Vigilance should be maintained postoperatively, till there is no risk of respiratory depression.

12.2.11 Follow-Up and Complication

There were no complications postoperatively.

Scoring: Harris Hip Score is 95.65.

12.2.12 Discussion

Sickle cell disease (SCD) is a genetically transmitted multisystem disease caused by the substitution of valine for glutamic acid at the sixth position in the beta chain of hemoglobin. Osteonecrosis of the femoral head is one of the common skeletal problems in sickle cell disease, more frequently seen in young adults; when progressed to fragmentation and collapse of the femoral head, the head-preserving treatment is no longer beneficial, and total hip arthroplasty is the only alternative.

The management of patients suffering from sickle cell disease is a considerable challenge. A multidisciplinary approach is needed with an experienced hematologist, anesthetist, and surgeon. Careful hematologic management is mandatory; the hematocrit level should not rise above 40% at any time; optimally, it should be kept between 28 and 34%. Throughout the operative procedure, a proper oxygenation, hydration, and peripheral perfusion should be maintained. The oxygenation should be kept above 97% at all times to prevent sickling crisis. Historically total hip replacement has reported with a poor prognosis in these patients however arthroplasty remains the only option to treat the severe disability caused by the disease.

Advantages of the applied method: Reduced bleeding and infection risk and patient compliance

Disadvantages of the method: Hard learning curve.

Alternative evidence-based techniques for the case: Femoral head preserving techniques, such as core decompression with or without biological enhancement techniques, may be used for patients at earlier stages of osteonecrosis. Based on the natural history of the avascular necrosis in sickle cell anemia that tends to progress, a procedure like femoral osteotomy, that makes hip arthroplasty more difficult, is not recommended. Related advantages of cemented THA are to overcome bone integration into the prosthesis and to reduce the associated risk of infection by adding antibiotic to the cement [18].

Why is the chosen technique better for this case? Cementless prosthesis has long survival, reduced risk of bleeding.

Indications and contraindications for your technique: Indications: degenerative coxarthrosis. Contraindications: life-threatening illness.

Learning curve and how to manage complications: Using the correct surgical technique and being careful to minimize risk of femur fracture. Giving right anteversion position to minimize the dislocation risk. Inability to equalize the leg length, after placing the prosthesis to check the equality of leg length during surgery by giving the supine position.

12.3 Case Title: Conversion THA in Sickle Cell Patient

Duy Phan and Ran Schwarzkopf

12.3.1 Demographics

Age: 39
Sex: Male
BMI: 24.7 kg/m^2

12.3.2 Relevant Past Medical History

Principal pathologies: Sickle cell anemia, hip avascular necrosis, cerebrovascular accidents, and deep vein thrombosis.

Previous surgical procedures: Bilateral total hip arthroplasty, right hip prosthesis explant with irrigation and debridement and antibiotic spacer placement, splenectomy, and cholecystectomy.

Medication: Benadryl, Dilaudid, fentanyl patches, Coumadin, docusate sodium, senna, calcium, and vitamin D.

Other: No tobacco, alcohol, or drug abuse.

History of presenting complaint: The patient is a 39-year-old male with a history of sickle cell anemia and bilateral hip avascular necrosis. He underwent right total hip arthroplasty in November 2004 and left total hip arthroplasty in November 2005. He was doing well with ambulation in the interval period, however, started to have pain in the right hip and was diagnosed with a periprosthetic joint infection with subsequent hip explantation, debridement, and antibiotic spacer placement in September 2013. Patient completed a course of intravenous antibiotics. These surgeries were all performed at an outside hospital. Due to the complexity of the case, he was unable to follow up with his original surgeon for the second-stage revision surgery and was referred to our specialty institution for evaluation in December 2014. He was ambulating as tolerated but with pain at the right hip with weight bearing and range of motion of the hip. This pain initially started after placement of the antibiotic spacer and had not subsided. He otherwise denied fevers, chills, or any other systemic symptoms.

12.3.3 Clinical Examination

Symptoms: Pain with weight bearing and ambulation.

Range of motion: At the right lower extremity, surgical incisions about the hip are healed without erythema, swelling, or drainage. Limited hip range of motion with forward flexion of 60°, abduction of 30°, and internal and external rotation of 15°, with slight crepitus felt in all planes. 5/5 strength with hip flexors and extensors. Full knee range of motion with 5/5 strength with quadriceps and hamstrings. Full ankle range of motion with 5/5 strength gastrocnemius-soleus complex and tibialis anterior. Limb length discrepancy was 2.7 cm.

Specific tests: CRP and ESR were within normal range.

Main disability: Pain.

Neurovascular evaluation: Neurologically intact at the right lower extremity from L2 to S1. Palpable the dorsalis pedis and posterior tibialis pulses.

12.3.4 Preoperative Radiological Assessment/Imaging (Figs. 12.4, 12.5, and 12.6)

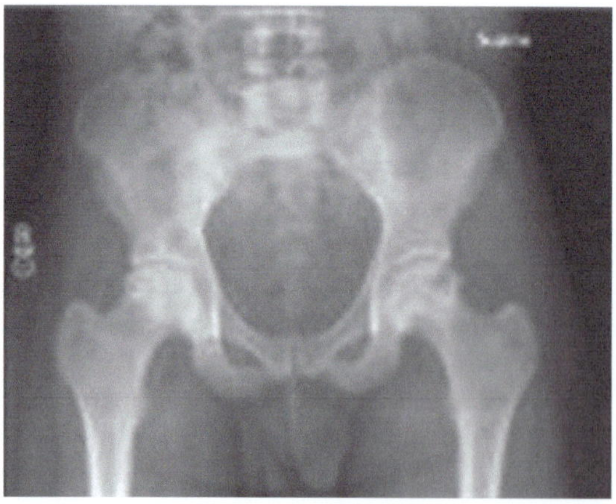

Fig. 12.4 AP pelvis showing right hip avascular necrosis with subchondral sclerosis and flattening of the femoral head

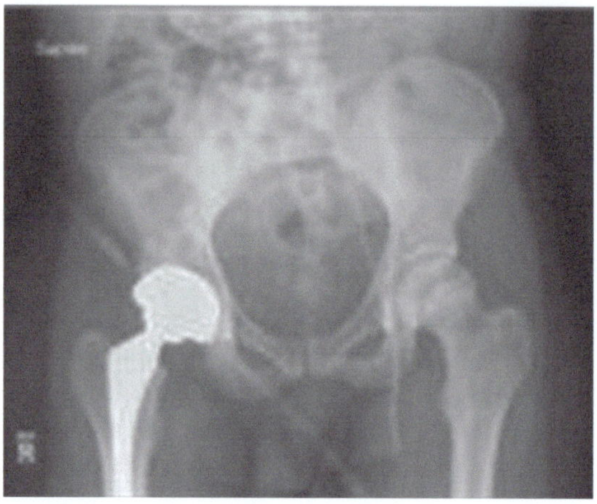

Fig. 12.5 AP pelvis showing postsurgical changes with right total hip arthroplasty

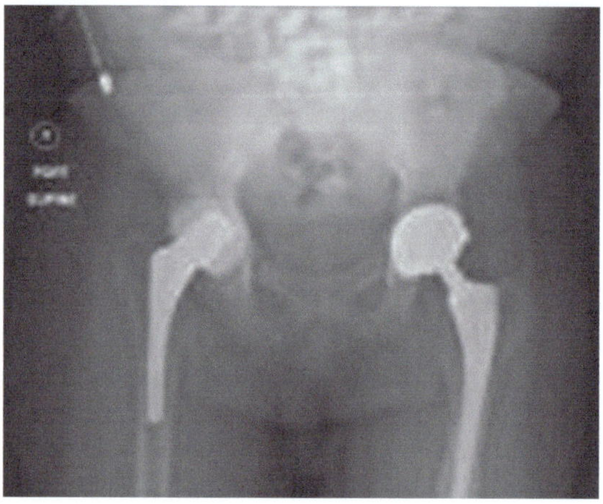

Fig. 12.6 AP pelvis, ten years after primary THA, showing postsurgical changes due to first-stage revision THA for a chronic periprosthetic joint infection with right hip antibiotic spacer placement. The original press-fit stem was kept and matched with a unipolar cement spacer; there has also been interval left total hip arthroplasty

12.3.5 Preoperative Planning

Diagnosis: Right hip periprosthetic joint infection at post resection status and placement of antibiotic spacer.

Possible treatment options: Revision right total hip arthroplasty, right hip fusion, and resection arthroplasty.

Chosen treatment method: Revision right total hip arthroplasty.

Selection of implants if applicable and rational: (1) Fluted tapered titanium stem with a modular sleeve to allow for bypassing the previous spacer, or another possible stress riser area into the femoral diaphysis and adjusting femoral neck version. (2) Trabecular metal revision shell with screws to have both initial fixation and bone ingrowth. (3) Oxinium femoral head to decrease wear rates due to the patient's young age. (4) Dual mobility cup to prevent impingement and dislocation due to increased dislocation risk in complex revision surgery.

Expected difficulties: (1) Removal of the antibiotic spacer as well as of a well-ingrown extendedly coated stem. (2) Avoiding an excessive protrusion of the acetabulum during the acetabular reaming and preparation. (3) Exposing and maintaining sufficient bone stock in the femur and acetabulum to allow for press-fit implants but avoiding an iatrogenic fracture. (4) Patient's sickle cell condition and his tendency for severe sickling events. (5) High risk of recurrent periprosthetic joint infection due to his history of the previous infection and sickle cell disease [19].

Strategies to overcome difficulties: (1) The hardware extraction set was called for, which included burrs, micro-saws, and flexible osteotomes to allow for hardware removal without significant bone loss. (2) Extended trochanteric osteotomy was planned to facilitate a controlled explantation of the well-ingrown stem if removal from the top is not possible (3) Gently reaming in the acetabulum and femur, with intraoperative X-ray to ensure adequate implant position and to rule out an intraoperative fracture. (4) Preoperative hospital admission for preoperative fluid and blood transfusion and close monitoring of hydration and hemoglobin status. Closely followed by treating hematologist.

Templating: Preoperative digital templating was performed to ensure restoration of leg length and offset lost by the extended use of the antibiotic spacer and protrusio acetabuli.

12.3.6 Surgical Note

Patient's position: Left lateral decubitus.

Type of anesthesia: Regional/spinal with sedation.

Surgical approach: Modified Kocher-Langenbeck utilising and resecting the previous scars.

Main steps: After the patient was positioned on the table, a posterolateral incision was made through the skin down to the underlying fascia. The fascia was incised longitudinally distally and the gluteus maximus muscle splint bluntly proximally. The sciatic nerve was identified and carefully retracted. A pseudocapsule was observed overlying the femoral greater trochanter and femoral neck and sharply dissected. Synovial fluid samples were obtained and sent for immediate analysis of WBC count and differential as well as tissue for frozen section analysis. Both results returned negative for an acute infection. A thorough synovectomy was completed, and the hip was then dislocated. The femoral head was able to be manually removed, whereas the femoral stem required more work. Flexible osteotomes were used to break the bone-prosthesis interface, and the stem was extracted. A small amount of bone loss was observed anteriorly, but the femur did not have any evidence of fracture. To avoid any periprosthetic fractures during the femoral preparation prophylactic, wires were placed around the femur. The acetabulum was debrided of scar tissue to expose the rim. The anterior and posterior columns did not have evidence of fracture.

Reconstruction techniques: Sequential reaming was performed in the acetabulum until endosteal contact and bleeding bone were observed. Care was taken to not excessively medialize due to the preexisting protrusion. Cancellous bone chips were placed to fill in the medial acetabular wall defect. A trabecular metal revision acetabular cup was then impacted into place, and multiple screws were placed for stability. The dual mobility cup was then cemented into place in the desired anteversion and abduction angles. Cerclage wires were placed around the proximal femur for prophylaxis to prevent fracture. The femur was then sequentially reamed, and a trial stem, collar, neck, and head were placed in the desired anteversion restoring the planned leg length and offset. The hip was reduced and found to be stable in all planes. Intraoperative imaging was obtained which showed an acceptable position of the components. The hip was dislocated; the final stem, collar and head were then impacted into place; the hip reduced and again was taken through a range of motion and found to be stable. The wound was soaked for 3 min in dilute betadine solution (0.35%) followed by irrigation with 1 L of normal saline. The sciatic nerve was again identified and found to be without any great tension. The wound was closed in multiple layers and covered with a sterile dressing. The patient was then extubated and transferred to the postoperative care unit in a stable condition.

12.3.7 Intraoperative Challenges

Challenges and solutions: The main challenges of the presented case included the removal of a fully coated well-ingrown stem, avoiding a further acetabular protrusion and achieving acetabular component fixation, and the increased risk of dislocation.

12.3.8 Postoperative Radiographs (Figs. 12.7 and 12.8)

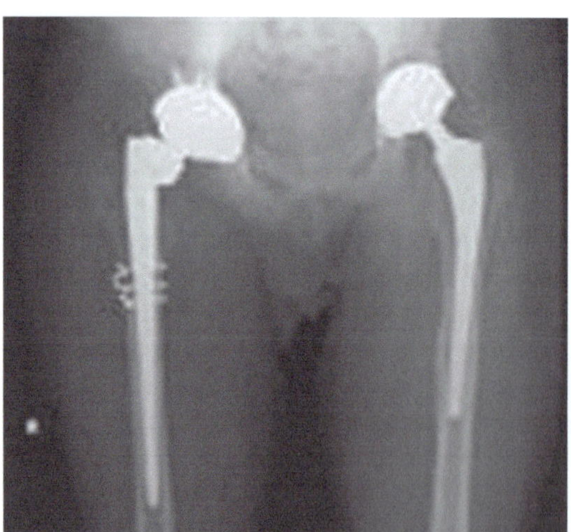

Fig. 12.7 AP pelvis January 2015 showing revision right total hip arthroplasty. Note the multiple screws in the acetabular cup as well as cerclage wires around the femur to ensure stability

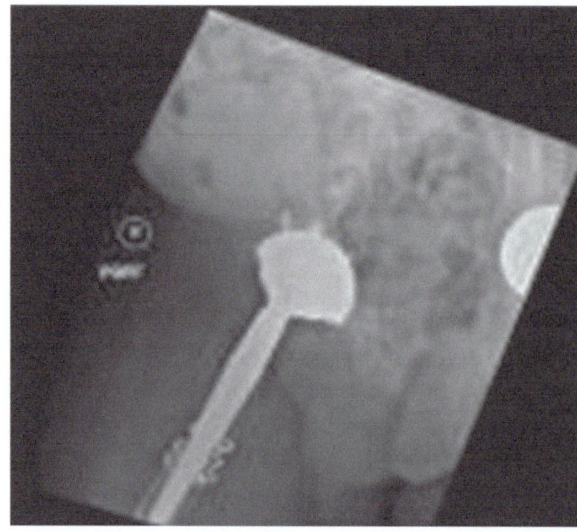

Fig. 12.8 Cross-table lateral of the right hip again showing revision right total hip arthroplasty

12.3.8.1 Postoperative Management

Chemoprophylaxis and anticoagulant treatment period: Sequential compression devices; Coumadin with the desired INR from 1.8 to 2.3 for 3 weeks to avoid an excessive postoperative bleeding, increasing after 3 weeks to an INR from 2.0 to 2.5 for chronic DVT prophylaxis due to a long history of thrombotic events.

Gait/limb loading until full loading: Weight bearing as tolerated with upper extremity support.

12.3.9 Follow-Up and Complications

No notable postoperative complications; the patient has healed his incision, she has no evidence of infection, and she has not had a dislocation event or reoccurrence of DVT. In the final follow-up, signs of bony ingrowth into the stem and cup are observed with no evidence of implant subsidence or motion.

12.3.10 Discussion

Advantages of the applied method: The used technique facilitated a safe removal of the current antibiotic spacer and reimplantation of a total hip arthroplasty. The use of dual mobility articulation in complex revision surgery has been shown to decrease the risk of dislocation.

Disadvantages of the method: Increased risk of femoral fracture both during the extraction of the retained femoral stem as well as during the preparation and implantation of the revision femoral stem. Femoral preparation is particularly challenging in patients with sickle cell disease due to the focal medullary sclerosis that develops as a consequence of the repeated intraosseous vascular events and bone infarcts.

Alternative evidence-based techniques for the case: Other surgical techniques would include the use of a cemented femoral component, which would decrease the risk of an intraoperative femoral fracture. For the acetabular reconstruction, a technique utilizing more allograft bone placement could be considered due to the patient's relatively young age and may lead to an increased bone stock that may be beneficial if future revision surgeries are needed.

Why the chosen technique is better for this case? The technique utilised in this case was chosen both due to its advantages in long-term survival due to bony ingrowth and implant stability, as well as the surgeons' familiarity and level of comfort with both the implants and the technique.

Indications and contraindications for your technique: There are no absolute contraindications for the chosen acetabular reconstruction technique. Regarding to the femoral reconstruction, in cases where the bone stock of the femoral isthmus is not enough to secure implantation of a tapered press-fit stem then a different technique such as impaction grafting and cementation should be considered.

Learning curve and how to manage complications: The learning curve for complex revision surgery is acceptable; the most important stepping stone for mastering revision hip surgery is a solid training foundation in arthroplasty surgery as well as a subspecialty training (fellowship) in adult hip reconstruction surgery. Most common intraoperative complications would be femoral and acetabular fractures; the surgeon has to be comfortable with complex femoral reconstruction techniques including osteosynthesis. For the acetabulum, the surgeon should feel comfortable with treating a situation of pelvic disassociation.

Level of evidence concerning the superiority of this method against others: There are no randomized studies evaluating the different treatment options for such complex revision hip cases. We do have enough literature evidence to support press-fit implants for both the acetabulum and femur in such complex reconstruction cases [17, 20, 21].

References

1. Hammer M, Geier KA, Aksoy S. Perioperative care for patients with sickle cell who are undergoing total hip replacement as treatment for osteonecrosis. Orthop Nurs. 2003;22(6):384–97.
2. Kamath AF, Mcgraw MH, Israelite CL, Kamath AF, Mcgraw MH, Israelite CL. Surgical management of osteonecrosis of the femoral head in patients with sickle cell disease. World J Orthop. 2015;6(10):776–82.
3. Jeong GK, Ruchelsman DE. Total hip arthroplasty in sickle cell hemoglobinopathies. J Am Acad Orthop Surg. 2005;13:208–17.
4. Ilyas I, Moreau P. Simultaneous bilateral total hip arthroplasty in sickle celldisease. J Arthroplast. 2002;17:441–5.
5. Poignard A, Bouhou M, Homma Y, Hernigou P. Septic arthritis of the hip in adults with sickle cell anemia. Orthop Rev. 2011;3:e1.
6. Moran MC, Huo MH, Garvin KL, Pel-licci PM, Salvati EA. Total hip arthroplasty in sickle cell hemoglobinopathy. Clin Orthop. 1993;294:140–8.
7. Gunderson C, D'Ambrosia RD, Shoji H. Total hip replacement in patients with sickle-cell disease. J Bone Joint Surg Am. 1977;59:760–2.
8. Vichinsky EP, Neumayr LD, Haberkern C, Earles AN, Eckman J, Koshy M, Black DM. The perioperative complication rate oforthopedic surgery in sickle cell disease: report of the National sickle cell surgery study group. Am J Hematol. 1999;62:129–38.
9. Clarke HJ, Jinnah RH, Brooker AF, Michaelson JD. Total replacement of the hip for avascular necrosis in sickle cell disease. J Bone Joint Surg Br. 1989;71:465–70.
10. Acurio MT, Friedman RJ. Hip arthroplasty in patients with sickle-cell haemoglobinopathy. J Bone Joint Surg Br. 1992;74:367–71.
11. Bishop AR, Roberson JR, Eckman JR, Fleming LL. Total hip arthroplasty inpatients who have sickle-cell hemoglo-binopathy. J Bone Joint Surg Am. 1988;70:853–5.
12. Epps C, Castro O. Complications of total hip replacement in sickle cell disease. Orthop Transactions. 1978;2:236–7.
13. Hanker GJ, Amstutz HC. Osteonecrosis of the hip in the sickle cell diseases: treatment and complications. J Bone Joint Surg Am. 1988;70:499–506.
14. Hickman JM, Lachiewicz PF. Results and complications of total hip arthroplastiesin patients with sickle-cell hemoglobin-opathies: role of cementless components. J Arthroplast. 1997;12:420–5.

15. Al-Mousawi F, Malki A, Al-Aradi A, Al-Bagali M, Al-Sadadi A, Booz MM. Total hip replacement in sickle cell disease. Int Orthop. 2002;26:157–61.
16. Gulati Y, Sharma M, Bharti B, Bahl V, Bohra I. Short term results of cementless total hip arthroplasty in sicklers. Indian J Orthop. 2015;49(4):447–51.
17. Issa K, Naziri Q, Maheshwari AV, Rasquinha VJ, Delanois RE, Mont MA. Excellent results and minimal complications of total hip arthroplasty in sickle cell hemoglobinopathy at mid-term follow-up using cementless prosthetic components. J Arthroplast. 2013;28:1693–8.
18. Hernigou P, Zilber S, Filippini P, Mathieu G, Poignard A, Galacteros F. Total THA in adult osteonecrosis related to sickle cell disease. Clin Orthop Relat Res. 2008;466:300–8.
19. Perfetti DC, Boylan MR, Naziri Q, Khanuja HS, Urban WP. Does sickle cell disease increase risk of adverse outcomes following total hip and knee Arthroplasty? A Nationwide database study. J Arthroplast. 2015;30:547–51.
20. Hug KT, Gupta AK, Wellman SS, Bolognesi MP, Attarian DE. Creation of a femoral cortical window to facilitate total hip arthroplasty in patients with sickle cell hemoglobinopathies. J Arthroplasty. 2013;28(2):323–5. doi:10.1016/j.arth.2012.06.021. Epub 2012 Aug 3. PMID: 22,868,077
21. Patel YD, Szczech BW, Patel S, Issa K, Kapadia BH, Mont MA. Management strategies for total hip arthroplasty in sickle cell patients. J Long Term Eff Med Implants. 2014;24(2–3):219–24.

Arthrodesis: Ankylosis 13

Eustathios Kenanidis, Panagiotis Kakoulidis, Panagiotis Lepetsos, Eleftherios Tsiridis, Merrill A. Ritter, Tatsuya Sueyoshi, Lazaros A. Poultsides, Georgios K. Triantafyllopoulos, and Michael M. Alexiades

13.1 Current Concepts

E. Kenanidis, P. Kakoulidis, P. Lepetsos, and E. Tsiridis

There are two types of hip ankylosis [1]:

1. **Spontaneous**: as a result of trauma, infection, hemophilia, or ankylosing spondylitis
2. **Surgical**: a rare technically challenging salvage procedure that is a viable option in young selected patients who are not ideal candidates for Total Hip Arthroplasty (THA) [2]

The optimal position for hip arthrodesis ranged between 20° and 30° of flexion, 5° and 10° of external rotation, 5° of adduction, and optimal Leg Length Discrepancy (LLD) < 2 cm [1, 3, 4]. Hip arthrodesis allows most patients to live a pain-free life for many years. It, however, affects gait and alters the biomechanics of the adjacent joints, mainly the lumbosacral spine and the ipsilateral knee [5] leading to increased incidence of degenerative diseases and pain in the next decades [1, 6, 7].

Beaulé et al. [6] supported that surgical ankylosis is indicated in active young adults with a

E. Kenanidis, M.D., Ph.D., M.Sc. (✉) · P. Kakoulidis, M.D.
Academic Orthopaedic Unit, Aristotle University Medical School, Thessaloniki, Greece

P. Lepetsos, M.D., Ph.D., M.Sc.
Fourth Orthopaedic Department, KAT Hospital, Athens, Greece
e-mail: plepetsos@med.uoa.gr

E. Tsiridis, M.D., Ph.D., F.A.C.S., F.R.C.S.
Academic Orthopaedic Unit, Papageorgiou General Hospital, Aristotle University Medical School, Thessaloniki, Greece
e-mail: etsiridis@doctors.org.uk

M.A. Ritter, M.D.
Center for Hip and Knee Surgery, Mooresville, IN, USA

T. Sueyoshi, M.D., Ph.D.
Kobe City Medical Center General Hospital, Kobe, Japan

L.A. Poultsides, M.D., M.Sc., Ph.D.
New York University School of Medicine, New York, NY, USA

Department of Orthopaedic Surgery, Division of Adult Reconstruction, New York Langone Orthopaedic Hospital, New York Langone Medical Center, New York, NY, USA
e-mail: PoultsidesL@hss.edu

G.K. Triantafyllopoulos, M.D., M.Sc.
Hospital for Special Surgery, New York, NY, USA

M.M. Alexiades, M.D.
Department of Rehabilitation and Associate Orthopaedic, Hospital for Special Surgery, New York, NY, USA

Weill Cornell Medical College, New York, NY, USA
e-mail: AlexiadesM@hss.edu

E. Tsiridis (ed.), *The Adult Hip - Master Case Series and Techniques*,
https://doi.org/10.1007/978-3-319-64177-5_13

severe monoarticular disease, greater physical demands and minimal preexisting arthritis, or traumatic malalignment or instability of the lumbar spine, ipsilateral knee, and contralateral hip [6]. Conversion of hip arthrodesis to THA is used to halt the degenerative process of adjacent joints and improve the function [8]. Due to the consistent long-term results of hip arthrodesis [7, 9], only 1/5 of patients with hip ankylosis proceed to conversion to THA [7, 9, 10] at early middle age. It is supported that the time of conversion to THA was affected by the age of the patient at the index arthrodesis [11]. Patients that underwent ankylosis at >15 years old converted to THA at a mean of 24 years compared with patients aged ≤15 years old at the time of arthrodesis that turned at an average of 41 years ($p < 0.0001$) [11].

13.1.1 Indications for Conversion of Hip Arthrodesis to THA [1, 5, 12, 13]

1. Progressive, disabling pain or instability from the lumbosacral spine, ipsilateral knee, and contralateral hip
2. Limited function resulting from hip fusion or malpositioning
3. Painful nonunion of the hip
4. Planned ipsilateral knee replacement (especially when arthrodesis is malpositioned)
5. Fractures around the arthrodesis
6. Significant limb-length discrepancy (>3 cm)

It is crucial to define the origin of pain indeed and understand the functional demands and expectations of the patient to explore the necessity of the procedure.

13.1.2 Contraindications [1, 5, 12, 13]

1. Active infection of the hip (absolute contraindication)
2. Uncooperative or unrealistic patient for this procedure that has significant expected complication rate
3. Aesthetic reasons or expectations to recover the LLD fully.

13.1.3 Preoperative Evaluation [1, 2]

1. Take a complete patient history concerning hip ankylosis. Determine:
   - The index etiology of the procedure
   - The type (spontaneous or surgical)
   - The time since the procedure
   - Possible complications (e.g., infection, venous thromboembolism, nerve palsy, nonunion, repeat operations)
2. Perform a thorough physical examination. Assess:
   (a) Leg-length discrepancy
      - This may be difficult, particularly in a malpositioned arthrodesis.
      - Ask for long-leg films or CT scanogram.
      - Keep in mind that >3 cm correction of LLD increases the risk of neurovascular damage.
   (b) Neurovascular status
   (c) Pelvic obliquity, kyphoscoliosis of the lumbosacral spine
   (d) Range of motion and stability of adjacent joints
   (e) The functional integrity of the hip abductors
      - It is a prognostic factor of ambulation and risk of dislocation following conversion to THA.
      - Manual examination may be non useful due to atrophy and lack of motion.
      - EMG and MRI can be helpful (muscle integrity, fatty infiltration, and size).
   (f) The previous incision/s
3. Perform a thorough radiographic evaluation.
   - Routine pelvic and hip x-rays, Judet views, and CT.
   - Assess the location of retained hardware, and delineate the acetabular columns.
4. Particularly for patients with a history of infection:
   - Obtain microbiology records to find the previous infectious microorganism.
   - Perform preoperative laboratory studies (WBC count, ESR, and CRP), hip aspiration, and MRI to identify persistent foci of osteomyelitis.

- Take 5–6 samples of tissue and bone for microbiology and histopathology tests intraoperatively.
- In persistent sepsis, perform two-stage THA (resection and antibiotic spacers).

13.1.4 Surgical Technique

Several surgical approaches have been reported, including lateral approach with transtrochanteric osteotomy, a lateral approach with tenotomy of the anterior aspect of the gluteus medius, an anterolateral approach, and posterior, posterolateral, and anterior approach [4, 8, 14–16].

Regardless of the surgical approach used, the surgeon must [1, 4]:

1. Expose adequately to remove retained hardware.
2. Identify and preserve the hip abductor muscles.
3. Identify the acetabular columns using certain landmarks as the inferior border of the acetabulum, the transverse acetabular ligament, the sciatic notch, and the anterior superior iliac spine.
4. Determine the level of the femoral neck osteotomy. This is usually at the junction of the femoral neck with the ilium.
5. Use the radiolucent table and intraoperative fluoroscopy to identify the level of neck osteotomy and orient the reaming.
6. Take care not to place the cup in an excessively cephalic position. Medialize the hip rotation center.
7. Identify, protect, and avoid tension to the sciatic nerve intraoperatively and following reduction of the implants.
8. Select implant and fixation method depending on the quantity and quality of available bone stock. Cemented cup fixation remains an option in select cases as in extreme sclerosis associated with radiation necrosis. In uncemented cups, use screws to optimize cup stability. A large head, dual mobility, or a constrained liner may be useful to compensate for instability.
9. Optimize LLD and restore femoral offset to avoid impingement and instability.
10. In patients with bilateral ankylosed hips, there is an increased risk of suboptimal cup position due to permanent pelvic obliquity [17–19].

13.1.5 Published Results

Several studies [8, 10–15, 17–34] have reported outcomes of surgical or spontaneous ankylosed hips converted to THA. Information however for this infrequently performed procedure remains limited as many of them referred to previous decades, with small sample size (usually <50 patients) and relatively short periods of follow-up. They consist of case series of 12–187 patients corresponding to 13–208 hips. Only one series has more than 100 patients [11]. The mean duration since hip fusion ranges from 11 to 36 years. Mean age at the time of THA was 29 to 60 years with mean follow-up ranging from 1 to 17 years. Six cohorts have a minimum of 9 years follow-up [11–14, 17, 20]. In these six studies, survivorship ranges from 74% (55% to 93%) to 96% (92% to 98%).

Conversion of hip arthrodesis to THR requires special considerations:

1. It has diminishing frequency as arthrodesis is a relatively rare procedure replaced by arthroplasty in young ages [4].
2. Functional improvement was noticed in all series; however, the majority of them reported lower scores than routine primary THA [5, 13, 21, 29]. Villanueva [5] and Richards et al. [13] reported inferior outcomes in conversion of hip arthrodesis to THA than primary and revision THA. Fernandez-Fairen et al. [14] however, reported comparable results with primary THA at long-term follow-up.
3. Improvement in walking ability and gait pattern and the need for walking aid were unpredictable [10, 12, 15, 22, 24, 25, 28]. The main reasons of remaining Trendelenburg gait were the incomplete recovery of the abductor function and extensor muscles and insufficient restoration of femoral offset.

Improvement in persistent limping was noticed till two years [22, 23].
4. The amount and extent of pain relief in the surrounding joints and lumbosacral spine vary in different series. Several authors [16, 25, 26] reported relief of pain in the majority of patients whether other [10] less favorable results (pain improvement in 50%). In a recent systematic review [4], back pain or ipsilateral knee pain relief was reported at 49–86% and 22–86%, respectively, with patients reporting neither back nor knee pain reaching up to 31 and 66%, respectively.
5. Decreased Range of Motion (ROM) is expected due to scarring, contraction, and devascularization of soft tissue around the hip, repeated operations, and a long-standing hip arthrodesis resulting in muscle atrophy before conversion [21–23, 26].
6. Better results were reported for conversion following previous spontaneous than surgical fusion [4, 12]. Peterson et al. [12] reported 5% failure in previous spontaneous vs. 33% in surgical fusion. Reikerås [29] et al. reported a negative correlation between older patient's age at the index arthrodesis as well as between duration of arthrodesis and outcome. Joshi et al. [11] reported higher functional scores following conversion THA in patients aged >15 years at the time of hip ankylosis.
7. The recovery period is usually longer than that following primary or revision THA reaching completion at 1 year. Functional improvement may be extended up to 3 years [10, 21].
8. The patient needs to have realistic expectations. The mean reported patient satisfaction following conversion THA was 63–100% [4]. Several authors, however, indicated that patients would undergo the operation again though they had suboptimal pain relief [31, 32].

13.1.6 Complications

1. It is a technically demanding procedure with a high risk of complications ranging from 11 to 54% [4, 10, 13]. Complication rate seems to be comparable to revision than primary THA [4].
2. Local complications were more frequent than systematic including mainly infection, mechanical failure, loosening, persistent pain, dislocation, fracture, nerve palsy, heterotopic ossification, and persistent restriction in ROM [10, 16, 29, 32]. The risk for infection was greater in cases of previous septic arthritis [2, 11, 29].
3. Although frequently controversial, the reported risk factors for failure are young age at fusion [11] (patients <15 years at fusion worse results), age <50 years at the time of conversion [12, 20], multiple previous surgical procedures (altered proximal femoral geometry leading to suboptimal component positioning and fixation) [22], surgical (worse) vs. spontaneous arthrodesis [12, 20], and duration of arthrodesis >30 years [1, 3, 5, 11, 12] and the condition of muscle status [5].

13.2 Hip Fusion Takedown to Total Hip Arthroplasty

Merrill A. Ritter and Tatsuya Sueyoshi

Converting a well-fixed hip fusion to a total hip replacement carries with it not only the complications of a major surgery but those associated with this particular condition. The hip fusion may have solved the particular problem back then but carries with it the new issues of no hip motion and added difficulties thru the spine. The conversion, therefore, has the fundamental challenge of the unknown concerning mainly the etiology of the fusion, the progressive destruction and the vialbility of the muscles, the presence of hardware and its destruction.

Previous surgery: Familiarize yourself with the nuances of the previous type of surgery, such as muscle transfer, osteotomies, and hardware application.

Approach: The surgeon should be comfortable with all approaches to the hip in that the previous surgeon may have used many. Every muscle despite its condition has to be maintained. Retraction, therefore, has to be all but avoided in that the muscles will probably pull apart or off their attachment to the bone. Retractor like

Cobras will do more damage than good. Increase the exposure to avoid retraction.

Hardware: Plates, screws, and wires of all makes and metals have been used. One needs to be aware of the types of screws and screw heads, whether the implants are covered with bone and muscle, what happens if part of the implant is broken now or while trying to remove it and the exposure to remove it. Have all types of equipment to remove any plate or screw and trephines to get the ones that break. Remember to make the approach too large rather than too small.

Operation: Following the approach and hardware removal, amputate the femoral neck up as close to the femoral head-neck junction as possible. Try to avoid a trochanteric osteotomy. Once again be careful as to retraction and now manipulation as it may damage to whatever muscles remain. Ream right into the remaining femoral head or whatever is in that area. Ream carefully in that the bone may be very osteoporotic. If the fusion was extra-articular, you have to find the original hip area. Do not put the hip in a new region. Because of the high probability of dislocation, put the largest acetabular component in so that a large femoral head can be used. At this point, a well-fixed cementless socket should be positioned in a little more anteversion once again because of dislocation. Be prepared to cement the socket. Have them in the room or rough up the back of polyethylene insert. If you have never cemented a socket, then maybe you should not do this operation. It is not unusual to have a very osteoporotic acetabulum that will not hold a cementless socket. These are easy to cement in that the trabecular bone is so prominent. Dry it well and keep it dry by supra-acetabular suction.

The femoral procedure should be standard utilizing a cementless component. The biggest concern is the previous holes for screws and if any were not removed with the other hardware. Once again because of the osteoporosis, make sure the femoral component is longer than the last hole by plenty of room. Have long stem prostheses available. Before inserting the final prosthesis, check the hip thru the extremes of motion to see if it will dislocate and what you might need to do to avoid it. Dislocation is your biggest acute problem.

Before closure, you now have to decide as to whether or not you are going to apply a single hip spica. If you have any concern about dislocation, consider on the need for a single hip spica. Hopefully, you informed the patient that this is a possibility. If you use a hip spica, I will leave it on for 4–6 weeks.

Postoperatively: Heterotopic ossification is a concern, and most likely you should use Indocin for two weeks. Everything else would be as you like. Rehab will be long and the patient may need a cane forever. Every patient we have done has been elated with the operation despite the cast in a few occasions and the extended rehab. We have been involved with 19 cases (Figs. 13.1, 13.2, 13.3 and 13.4). Two have been revised for acetabular loosening. These were poorly cemented sockets.

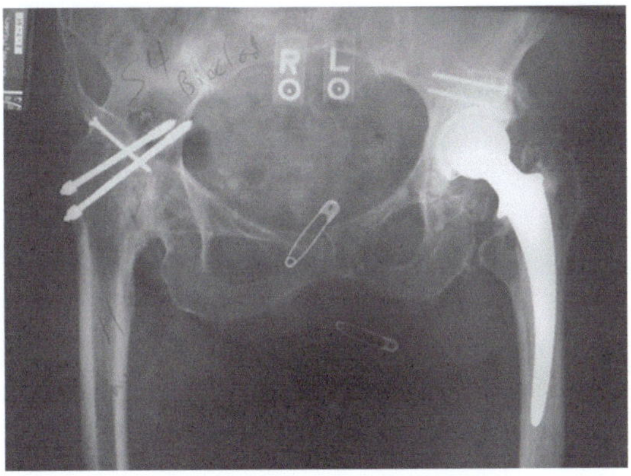

Fig. 13.1 56-year-old female had a right hip fusion in 1960 for an unknown reason. She had a left hip replacement in 1991, elsewhere

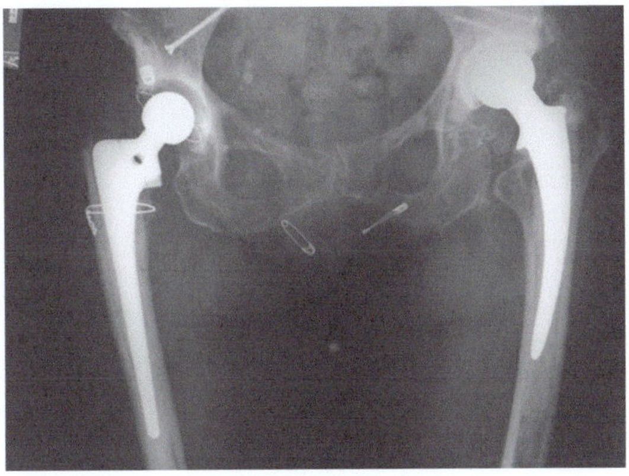

Fig. 13.2 At age 86, 1991, we took down the fusion and inserted a cemented calcar stem and an all poly cup. The patient died in 2009, 105 years old, 19 years postoperative

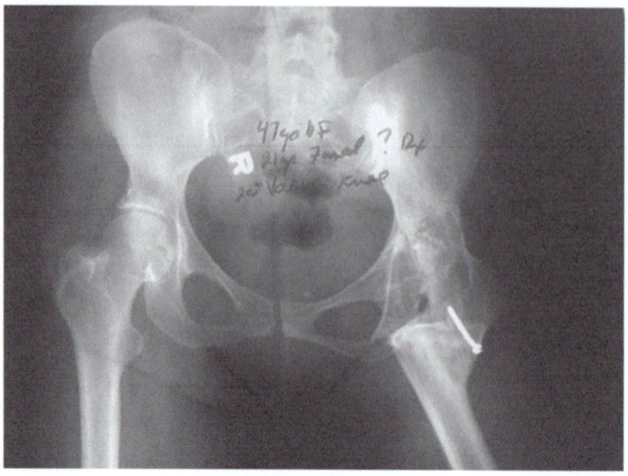

Fig. 13.3 18-year-old female had a left hip fusion for questionable tuberculosis in 1950

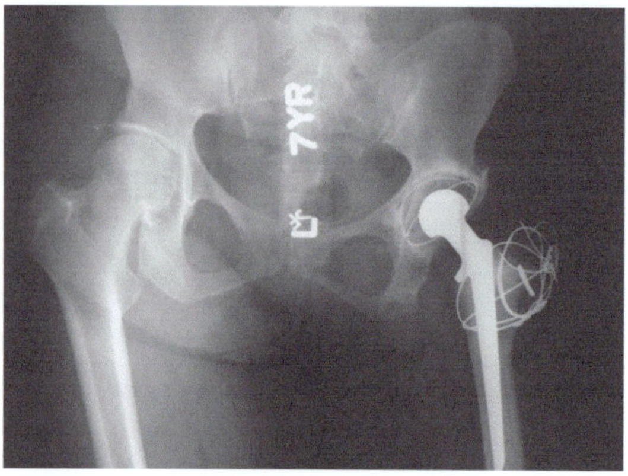

Fig. 13.4 We took down the fusion in 1981 and inserted a cemented T-28 stem and a cemented all poly cup. She was 47 years old. She died 21 years postoperative

Fortunately, we had no dislocations, but we were very aggressive as to avoid this possibility.

13.3 Case Title: Conversion of Arthrodesis to Total Hip Arthroplasty Via Direct Anterior Approach

Lazaros A. Poultsides, Georgios K. Triantafyllopoulos, and Michael M. Alexiades

13.3.1 Demographics

Age: 55 years old
Sex: Female
BMI: 32.9

13.3.2 Relevant Past Medical History

Principal pathologies: Obesity, hyperlipidemia.

Previous surgical procedures: Right hip arthrodesis, left total hip arthroplasty.

Medication: Ezetimibe 20 mg p.o. every other day, simvastatin 40 mg p.o. every other day, aspirin 81 mg p.o. once a day.

History of presenting complaint: The patient had a history of multiple right hip injuries as a child in Russia beginning at the age of 4. She was dislocated several times and was treated with a right hip fusion at the age of 10 in Russia.

13.3.3 Clinical Examination

Symptoms: Limp, low back pain.

Range of motion: (Right hip) 20 degrees fixed flexion deformity, external/internal rotation = 0/0, abduction/adduction = 0/0.

Main disability: Limb-length discrepancy, patient unable to reciprocate stairs, compensating lumbar spine scoliosis.

Neurovascular evaluation: Within normal limits.

13.3.4 Preoperative Radiological Assessment/Imaging (Figs. 13.5 and 13.6)

Others: Preoperatively, the patient had an MRI to evaluate the status of the abductors which revealed them intact but atrophied.

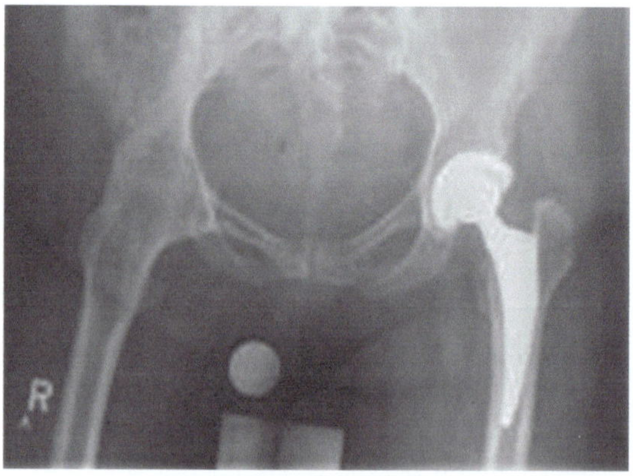

Fig. 13.5 Anteroposterior (AP) view of the pelvis. The right hip is fused without the presence of any hardware

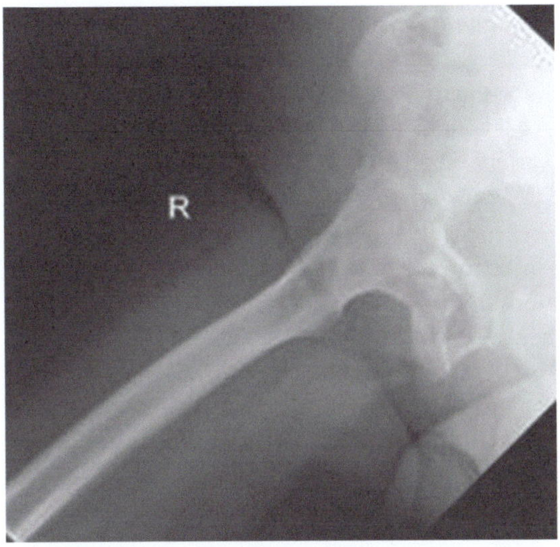

Fig. 13.6 Lateral view of the right hip

13.3.5 Preoperative Planning

Diagnosis: Fused right hip.

Possible treatment options: Conversion to total hip arthroplasty via posterior, direct lateral, anterolateral, or direct anterior approach.

Chosen treatment method: Conversion of right hip fusion to total hip arthroplasty via direct anterior approach.

Selection of implants if applicable and rational: We selected a press-fit hemispherical cup and a flat-tapered wedge stem, along with a ceramic-on-plastic bearing with highly cross-linked UHMWPE. The use of press-fit components was feasible since preoperative imaging revealed adequate bone stock at both the iliac bone and the femur. Considering patient's age, a ceramic head was selected in order to achieve a minimum polyethylene wear rate. We also opted for a large-diameter head and a high-wall acetabular liner, taking into account the anticipated hip abductor weakness to reduce dislocation risk.

Expected difficulties: Absent anatomical landmarks for cup positioning.

Strategies to overcome difficulties: Reaming of the iliac bone for insertion of the acetabular component under fluoroscopic imaging.

Templating: We templated for a 50 mm G7 cup (Biomet Inc., Warsaw, IN) and a size 8, standard offset Taperloc Microplasty stem (Biomet Inc., Warsaw, IN). The neck cut was determined at 10 mm from the lesser trochanter based on preoperative templating.

13.3.6 Surgical Note

Patient's position: The patient was placed in the supine position with both lower extremities prepped and draped.

Type of anesthesia: Regional anesthesia (combined spinal and epidural).

Surgical approach: The Direct anterior approach of the right hip.

Main steps: An approximate 8 cm longitudinal incision was made starting superolateral and distal to the anterior superior iliac spine, which was carried down to the level of the tensor fascia lata. The tensor fascia lata was divided, and blunt dissection was done to identify the interval between the tensor fascia lata and the sartorius. The ascending branch of the lateral femoral circumflex artery was identified and cauterized. The fat pad between the gluteus medius and the rectus femoris was identified and dissected to the deep interval. A triangular region of the capsule, which showed signs of significant atrophy, was then excised. The site of hip arthrodesis was identified. Under fluoroscopy, the appropriate femoral neck osteotomy level was identified, the neck cut was performed, and a second, more proximal cut was made removing a ring of bone. The proximal femur was freed from the acetabulum, allowing thus appropriate leg moving and position. Afterward, under direct fluoroscopic visualization, the proximal part of the femoral neck and head was removed using an oscillating saw paying attention to be coplanar with the native acetabular opening mouth and anteverted to the sagittal plane.

Reconstruction techniques: The desired position of the cup was determined with fluoroscopy, and, with sequential reaming under fluoroscopic imaging and up to a 48 mm reamer, an adequately medialized concavity was created on the iliac bone for cup insertion. Then, a 50 mm press-fit acetabular component was impacted into place. Supplemental fixation

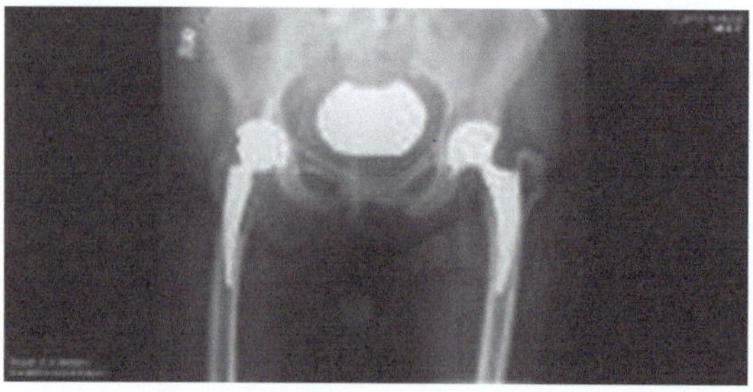

Fig. 13.7 Postoperative AP pelvis radiographic view demonstrating well-positioned implants and restoration of leg-length equality

of the cup was achieved with two screws, and the final polyethylene liner was inserted. Next, an Omni-Tract hook was placed around the proximal femur at the level of the gluteus maximus insertion and the lesser trochanter, and the right lower extremity was placed in hyperextension, adduction, and external rotation. After soft-tissue releases of the superior capsule, the femoral canal was sequentially broached up to the appropriate size. A standard offset trial neck and a 36 mm +0 trial femoral head were inserted, and a trial reduction was made. The hip was found to be stable in all range of motion. Of note, a high-wall polyethylene insert was inserted to provide additional coverage posterosuperiorly due to the relative abductor deficiency. The final implants were then inserted, and the hip was reduced. Due to the preexisting fixed flexion deformity and in order to bring the hip joint in neutral position, additional release of the anteriosuperior capsule and pie-crusting of iliopsoas tendon were performed. This surgical step facilitated limb-length equalization. The wound was closed in a standard fashion (Fig. 13.7).

13.3.7 Intraoperative Challenges

Challenges and solutions: As already stated, it was not possible to safely determine any clear anatomic landmarks for cup positioning, due to the previous arthrodesis. In order to overcome this obstacle, the acetabulum was prepared by reaming under direct fluoroscopic visualization.

Unanticipated problems and solution: During preparation of the acetabulum, we noted that the bone quality of the iliac bone was very poor. Again, fluoroscopy assisted with avoiding inadvertent breaching of the medial wall.

Thorough description of decision making, including the reason for the final decision: In order to reestablish the acetabulum, we identified the most proximal margin of the obturator foramen with fluoroscopy, where we positioned one Aufranc retractor; this location provided us the most inferior part of the acetabular fossa. Two additional Hohmann retractors were placed at the anterior and the posterior wall, respectively. This gave us an approximate localization of the "native" acetabulum and determined the "safe spot." Then, under fluoroscopic guidance, we performed sequential reaming, paying close attention to be concentric, not to migrate proximally and thus elevate the new center of rotation. We also preserve sufficient bone stock of the anterior and posterior acetabular wall to adequately medialize the cup providing a better functional level arm for the abductors.

13.3.8 Postoperative Radiographs (Fig. 13.8)

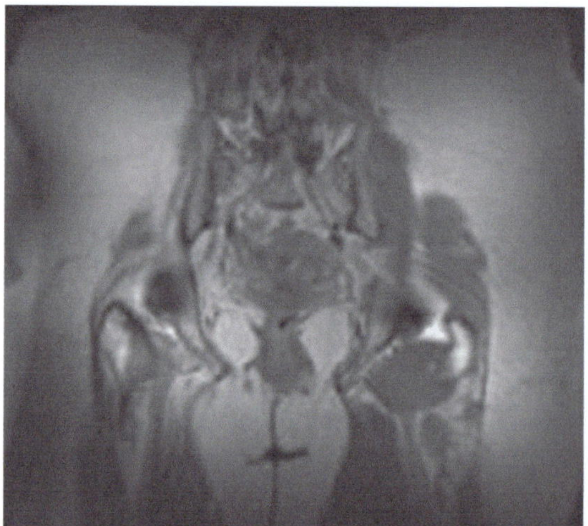

Fig. 13.8 Coronal T1-weighted MRI of the pelvis. The MRI was performed for investigating right hip pain and a Trendelenburg gait which were developed after a fall; note the significant atrophy of the right gluteus medius and the detachment of its insertion on the greater trochanter

13.3.9 Postoperative Management

Chemoprophylaxis and anticoagulant treatment period: Cefazolin 2 g i.v. × 2 doses; aspirin 325 mg twice a day for 4 weeks.

Gait/limb loading until full loading: Weight bearing as tolerated.

13.3.10 Follow-up and Complications

The patient developed cellulitis at the right buttock area postoperatively, which was treated with amoxicillin p.o. 16 months post-conversion; the patient sustained a fall on her right buttock, after which she developed right hip pain and Trendelenburg gait, while previously asymptomatic. The diagnostic workup (MRI) revealed partial tearing of the right gluteus medius (Fig. 13.8). The patient underwent open surgical repair of the hip abductors which resulted in resolution of pain and Trendelenburg gait at four months postop.

13.3.11 Discussion

Advantages of the applied method: The use of the direct anterior approach for converting a hip arthrodesis to total hip arthroplasty offers the benefit of sparing muscles that have undergone atrophy and are already weakened due to the long-standing disuse. Therefore, a more rapid rehabilitation can be expected. Moreover, the use of intraoperative fluoroscopy with this approach facilitates appropriate positioning of the acetabular component, as well as restoration of the desired leg length. Determining leg-length equality is also more straightforward with this approach, as both lower extremities are prepped and draped making side-to-side comparisons very easy intraoperatively. Finally, considering the abductor weakness generally seen in these patients, the direct anterior approach may be associated with a reduced risk for posterior dislocation postoperatively, along with less damage to the abductors compared to direct lateral and anterolateral approaches.

Disadvantages of the method: Perhaps the main disadvantage of the technique is the potentially less extensile exposure compared to traditional approaches (including trochanteric osteotomy). Some surgeons may not feel very comfortable with the limited access to the hip joint for such a complex case and in obese patients. However, we feel that familiarization with the technique and ample use of fluoroscopy can help the surgeon overcome this limitation. Moreover, recent reports have demonstrated that the anterior approach can be safely extended both proximally and distally, providing thus excellent visualization. Finally, there may be some wound-healing concerns with the direct anterior approach, especially in obese patients.

Alternative evidence-based techniques for the case: Conversion of a fused hip to total hip arthroplasty has been previously reported with the use of different approaches, including direct lateral, posterior, and use of trochanteric osteotomy [4]. The selection of the technique depends on surgeon preference, the presence of hardware and previous incisions, as well as the surgical plan. In general, the complication rate with the conversion of hip arthrodesis to total hip arthroplasty is high [4].

Why the chosen technique is better for this case? As stated earlier, with the direct anterior approach, we avoided further impairment of the already atrophied hip musculature. Besides, the ancillary use of fluoroscopy facilitated restoration of the normal hip biomechanics. Finally, the straightforward in situ osteotomy of the femoral neck under fluoroscopic visualization was assisted with hip dislocation and exposure.

Indications and contraindications for your technique: Even though the direct anterior approach to the hip is indicated for total hip arthroplasty in patients with a straightforward anatomy, we believe that the surgeon that routinely uses the technique for primary cases can also apply it for conversion of hip arthrodesis to arthroplasty. In general, a contraindication for this approach is the presence of severe deformity at the proximal femur. As demonstrated by the present case, obesity is not an insurmountable impediment to the technique.

Learning curve and how to manage complications: When transitioning practice to direct anterior approach, it is accepted that a minimum number of 50 cases are necessary for mastering the technique. Therefore, we believe that a surgeon accustomed to the direct anterior approach can apply it to perform a conversion of a fused hip to total hip arthroplasty relatively easy, paying attention to the critical steps.

Level of evidence concerning the superiority of this method against others: In the literature, there are two retrospective series of 37 and 9 patients, respectively, with fused hips converted to total hip arthroplasty using the direct anterior approach (level IV studies) [35, 36]. Even though these reports suggest similar outcomes with previous studies incorporating different techniques, there are no comparative studies among the various approaches to this date.

References

1. Swanson MA, Huo MH. Total hip arthroplasty in the ankylosed hip. J Am Acad Orthop Surg. 2011;19(12):737–45.
2. Whitehouse MR, Duncan CP. Conversion of hip fusion to total hip replacement technique and results. Bone Joint J. 2013;95-B(Supple A):114–9.
3. Sponseller PD, McBeath AA, Perpich M. Hip arthrodesis in young patients: a long-term follow-up study. J Bone Joint Surg Am. 1984;66(6):853–9.
4. Jain S, Giannoudis PV. Arthrodesis of the hip and conversion to total hip arthroplasty a systematic review. J Arthroplasty. 2013;28(9):1596–602.
5. Villanueva M, Sobrón FB, Parra J, Rojo JM. Conversion of arthrodesis to total hip arthroplasty: clinical outcome, complications, and prognostic factors of 21 consecutive cases. HSS J. 2013;21:138–44.
6. Beaulé PE, Matta JM, Mast JW. Hip arthrodesis: current indications and techniques. J Am Acad Orthop Surg. 2002;10(4):249–58.
7. Callaghan JJ, Brand RA, Pedersen DR. Hip arthrodesis: a long-term follow-up. J Bone Joint Surg Am. 1985;67(9):1328–35.
8. Scemama C, Lestrat V, Combourieu B, Judet T. Anterior approach for total hip arthroplasty conversion of hip fusion. Int Orthop. 2015;28:1821–5.
9. Sofue M, Kono S, Kawaji W, Homma M. Long term results of arthrodesis for severe osteoarthritis of the hip in young adults. Int Orthop. 1989;13:129–33.
10. Hamadouche M, Kerboull L, Meunier A, Courpied JP, Kerboull M. Total hip arthroplasty for the treatment of ankylosed hips: a five to twenty-one-year follow-up study. J Bone Joint Surg Am. 2001;83-A:992–8.
11. Joshi AB, Markovic L, Hardinge K, Murphy JCM. Conversion of a fused hip to total hip arthroplasty. J Bone Joint Surg Am. 2002;84-A:1335–41.
12. Peterson ED, Nemanich JP, Altenburg A, Cabanela ME. Hip arthroplasty after previous arthrodesis. Clin Orthop Relat Res. 2009;467:2880–5.
13. Richards CJ, Duncan CP. Conversion of hip arthrodesis to total hip arthroplasty: survivorship and clinical outcome. J Arthroplast. 2011;26:409–13.
14. Fernandez-Fairen M, Murcia-Mazón A, Torres A, Querales V, Murcia A. Is total hip arthroplasty after hip arthrodesis as good as primary arthroplasty? Clin Orthop Relat Res. 2011;469:1971–83.
15. Aderinto J, Lulu OB, Backstein DJ, Safir O, Gross AE. Functional results and complications following conversion of hip fusion to total hip replacement. J Bone Joint Surg (Br). 2012;94-B(Suppl):36–41.
16. Kim YH, Oh SH, Kim JS, Lee SH. Total hip arthroplasty for the treatment of osseous ankylosed hips. Clin Orthop Relat Res. 2003;414:136–48.
17. Kim YL, Shin SI, Nam KW, et al. Total hip arthroplasty for bilaterally ankylosed hips. J Arthroplast. 2007;22:1037–41.
18. Wang W, Huang G, Huang T, Wu R. Bilaterally primary cementless total hip arthroplasty in patients with ankylosing spondylitis. BMC Musculoskelet Disord. 2014;15:344.
19. Ye C, Liu R, Sun C, Lin J, Li H, Re H, Sun B, Sun Q, Yang L. Cementless bilateral synchronous total hip arthroplasty in ankylosing spondylitis with hip ankylosis. Int Orthop (SICOT). 2014;38:2473–247.
20. Strathy GM, Fitzgerald RHJ. Total hip arthroplasty in the ankylosed hip. A ten-year follow-up. J Bone Joint Surg Am. 1988;70-A:963–6.
21. Morsi E. Total hip arthroplasty for fused hips; planning and techniques. J Arthroplast. 2007;22: 871–5.
22. Kilgus DJ, Amstutz HC, Wolgin MA, Dorey FJ. Joint replacement for ankylosed hips. J Bone Joint Surg Am. 1990;72-A:45–54.
23. Abdel-Aal A, Bakr H, Mahran M. Total hip arthroplasty for fused hips. Orthopedics. 2010;33:400–4.
24. Lubahn JD, Evarts CM, Feltner JB. Conversion of ankylosed hips to total hip arthroplasty. Clin Orthop Relat Res. 1980;153:146–52.
25. Brewster RC, Coventry MB, Johnson EW. Conversion of the arthrodesed hip to a total hip arthroplasty. J Bone Joint Surg Am. 1975;57-A:27–30.
26. Amstutz HC, Sakai DN. Total joint replacement for ankylosed hips. Indications, technique, and preliminary results. J Bone Joint Surg Am. 1975;57-A:619–25.
27. Kempf I, Jenny JY. Total prosthesis after ankylosis of the hip joint. Report of 22 cases. Int Orthop. 1991;15:239–43.

28. Rittmeister M, Starker M, Zichner L. Hip and Knee Replacement After Longstanding Hip Arthrodesis. Clin Orthop Relat Res. 2000;371:136–45.
29. Reikerås O, Bjerkreim I, Gundersson R. Total hip arthroplasty for arthrodesed hips. 5- to 13-year results. J Arthroplast. 1995;10:529–31.
30. Hardinge K, Williams D, Etienne A, MacKenzie D, Charnley J. Conversion of fused hips to low friction arthroplasty. J Bone Joint Surg (Br). 1977;59-B: 385–92.
31. Rutz E, Schäfer D, Valderrabano V. Total hip arthroplasty after hip joint ankylosis. J Orthop Sci. 2009;14(6):727.
32. Schäfer D, Dick W, Morscher E. Total hip arthroplasty after arthrodesis of the hip joint. Arch Orthop Trauma Surg. 2000;120:176–8.
33. Siavashi B, Mohseni N, Zehtab MJ, Ramim T. Clinical outcomes of total hip arthroplasty in patients with ankylosed hip. Arch Bone Jt Surg. 2014;2(1):25–30. Epub 2014 Mar 15
34. Ye C, Liu R, Sun C, Lin J, Li H, Re H, Sun B, Sun Q, Yang L. Cementless bilateral synchronous total hip arthroplasty in ankylosing spondylitis with hip ankylosis. Int Orthop. 2014;38(12):2473–6.
35. Scemama C, Lestrat V, Combourieu B, Judet T. Anterior approach for total hip arthroplasty conversion of hip fusion. Int Orthop. 2016;40(9): 1821–5.
36. Tamaki T, Oinuma K, Miura Y, Shiratsuchi H. Total hip arthroplasty through a direct anterior approach for fused hips. Hip Int. 2015;25(6):549–52.

Paget's Disease

14

Eustathios Kenanidis, Andreas Leonidou, Grigorios T. Sakellariou, Michael Potoupnis, and Eleftherios Tsiridis

14.1 Current Concepts

E. Kenanidis, A. Leonidou, G.T. Sakellariou, M. Potoupnis, and E. Tsiridis

14.1.1 General

Paget's disease is a chronic non-metabolic disease characterized by loss of the local rhythm of bone turnover [1]. This pathologic entity also known as osteitis deformans has increased incidence following 50 years old and shows great geographic variation [1, 2].

The primary abnormality is an osteoclastic dysfunction leading to an excessive bone resorption that is followed by rapid but non-woven new bone formation with an anarchic microstructure [2–5]. The newly formed bone is prone to deformity and fracture, especially in the weight-bearing extremities. The disease is usually asymptomatic [1]. This localized chronic osteopathy may have monostotic (25%) or polyostotic (75%) skeletal and nonskeletal manifestations [1, 2, 4].

Skeletal manifestations usually involve pelvis, femur, tibia, spine, and skull [2]. Bone deformities as coxa vara, femoral bowing, acetabular protrusion, bone size expansion, and fragility fractures [1] are usually encountered. There is also bone hypervascularity and altered joint biomechanics leading to OA development [3]. Hip OA is frequent in Paget's disease patients demonstrating commonly medial or concentric narrowing of joint space [6]. The nonskeletal manifestations include skin temperature changes, neurologic complications, deafness, and heart failure [1].

14.1.2 Indications for THA

Severe degenerative joint disease [3].

14.1.3 Preoperative Planning

- Be sure that the source of pain is from arthritic joint [3]. Other potential sources of hip pain include bone pain caused by disease activity,

E. Kenanidis, M.D., Ph.D., M.Sc. (✉)
G.T. Sakellariou, M.D.
Academic Orthopaedic Unit, Aristotle University Medical School, Thessaloniki, Greece

A. Leonidou, Pg.Dip., M.Sc., F.R.C.S.
Reading Shoulder Unit, Reading, UK
e-mail: leonidou@doctors.org.uk

E. Tsiridis, M.D., Ph.D., F.A.C.S., F.R.C.S. ·
M. Potoupnis, M.D., Ph.D
Academic Orthopaedic Unit, Papageorgiou General Hospital, Aristotle University Medical School, Thessaloniki, Greece
e-mail: etsiridis@doctors.org.uk; mikepot@otenet.gr

E. Tsiridis (ed.), *The Adult Hip - Master Case Series and Techniques*,
https://doi.org/10.1007/978-3-319-64177-5_14

stress fracture, radiculopathy, and Paget's sarcoma [3].

- Evaluate the patient thoroughly to detect and treat extraskeletal manifestations of the disease. A cardiac evaluation is valuable; patients suffering from the polyostotic disease also have heart enlargement and altered the left ventricular function [3].
- Assess the activity of Paget's disease measuring sALP and hydroxyproline [3]. Suppression therapies with bisphosphonates are indicated to improve the symptoms and reduce the complications as intraoperative and postoperative blood loss and the rapid postoperative osteolytic bone resorption due to hypervascularity [5]. Perform hip arthroplasty when ALP is in its lowest level [1, 4].
- Use preoperative autologous blood donation.
- Take full-length radiographs for templating to assess the degree of deformity and the extent of bone involvement [3]. Go through the x-rays to explore the presence of a stress fracture on the tension side of the bone or soft tissue mass that could raise the suspicion of sarcomatous change; in this case, CT or MRI may be used [3].
- Select the arthroplasty implants correctly [3]. An antiprotrusio cage for acetabular protrusion, femoral osteotomy for femoral bowing, and custom prosthesis may be needed.

14.1.4 Intraoperative Planning [3]

- Use extensile approach when necessary.
- Reduce the intraoperative blood loss using preoperatively bisphosphonates and intraoperative blood salvage to facilitate cement fixation of implants and fasten the surgery [4, 5].
- Release soft tissue broadly in patients with severe contractures.
- Extremely sclerotic acetabular bone may make reaming involved and endanger the appropriate placement of the acetabulum [3].
- Before you implant an uncemented acetabular cup, ream sufficiently in periphery and then fix with additional screws [3].
- In acetabular protrusion, possible treatment options include a medial acetabular bone grafting, an oversized hemispherical cup, an antiprotrusio cage, and lateral offset acetabular liners [3].
- Use concurrent osteotomy when component alignment is difficult [7]. Avoid diaphyseal osteotomies if possible [3]. Adjust bone cuts to avoid excessive resection of bone.
- Use sharp rasps and reamers, burr, or drill to allow ease of access into the intramedullary canal.
- Coxa vara increases the possibility of placing the femoral stem in varus positioning [6].
- Trochanteric or realignment osteotomies may be necessary for adequate exposure and prevention of varus alignment [6].
- Use uncemented components especially when the bone is very sclerotic, or a concurrent osteotomy is done; in a sclerotic bone, the interdigidation of cement is compromised, and cement extravasation into the fracture is prevented.
- Be aware that in elderly, there is increased rate of intraoperative fracture using anatomic stems.

14.1.5 Postoperative Planning

- Continue medical treatment if the disease activity is high. Increased disease activity has been related with an increased rate of implant loosening [3].
- Administer prophylaxis against heterotopic ossification.
- Monitor closely for cardiac complications [3].

14.1.6 Published results

There is lack of high-level studies in the literature. They are usually small cohorts giving medium- to long-term results [2, 4, 8–14]. There is debate concerning the use of cemented or uncemented implants [4, 8, 15].

Cemented THA for Paget's disease patients is moderately documented. Several cohort studies [2, 9–12] of previous decades reported excellent to good results in 70–86% of the cases. They consisted of 21–80 patients, aged 67.4–72.4 years with a mean follow-up from 2.1 to 10.4 years. Merkow et al. [12] reported 9.5% revision rate within 5 postoperative years on 21 cemented THAs for Paget's disease. McDonald et al. [11] demonstrated significantly increased revision rate (15%) for aseptic loosening of 52 cemented THAs in patients with Paget's disease compared to an unselected total hip population. Cemented THA in Paget's disease patients is considered a viable option; however, concern has been raised for an overall increased incidence of symptomatic and asymptomatic radiographic loosening [2, 9–12] at long-term (up to 40% around the cup in some series) [11]. Pagetic bone is sclerotic and prone to bleeding, so cement penetration, and interdigitation may be compromised limiting long-term fixation [4, 8].

Cementless fixation has been reported lately with quite promising results. There are several case reports and case series studies [4–8, 13–15] with a sample size of 1–39 patients and mean age ranging from 68 to 78 years old. The follow-up period ranged from an average of 5.5 to 12.5 years. Imbuldeniya et al. [8] showed 86% survival for both stem and cup with revision and 95.5% with aseptic loosening as the end point, at 10 years follow-up of 33 uncemented THAs for Paget's disease. The mean Harris hip score increased from 56 to 83 at the latest follow-up. A cementless fixation is a viable option (Fig. 14.1); however, its advantages over cemented are questionable [8]. There has been concern about the possible effect of the active disease on the implant fixation and that altered quality, and morphological features of pagetic bone may influence bone ingrowth of cementless implants [4, 8].

14.1.7 Complications

Heterotopic ossification occurs at a range of 23–52% of patients with Paget's disease undergoing THA [2, 9–12, 14]. The risk is comparable to that in patients with a previous history of heterotopic ossification, hypertrophic OA, or post-traumatic arthritis [3]. The precise etiology is unknown; however, it is not related to disease activity and patients function; the majority of HO cases, however, are of minor severity. Preoperative and postoperative radiation are needed. Other complications include increased blood loss (due to hypervascularity of bone, the technical difficulty of the procedure, and the need for concomitant procedures, such as osteotomy, which prolong the length of surgery), periprosthetic

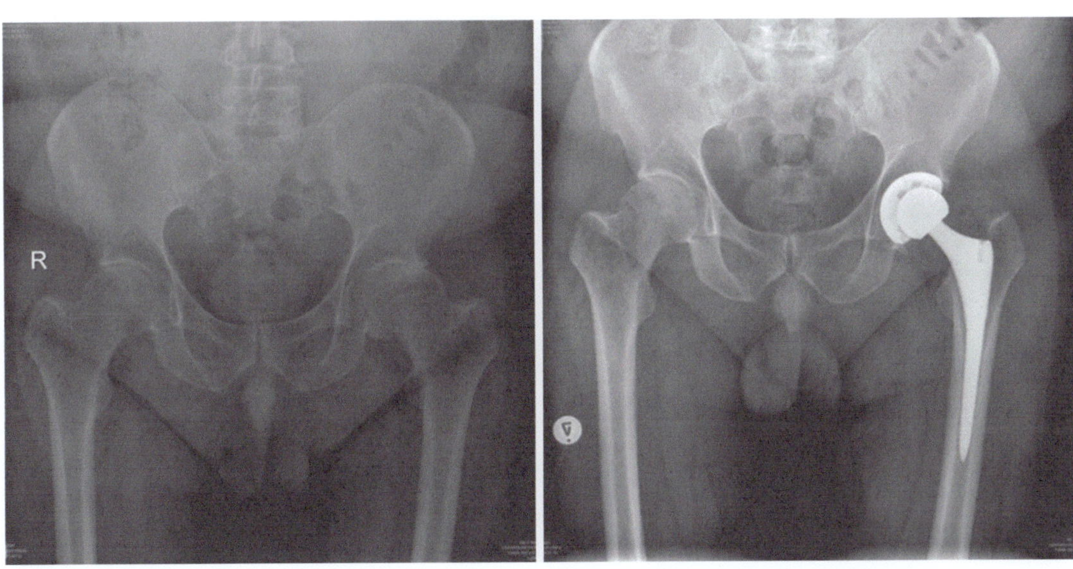

Fig. 14.1 Paget disease in a relatively young individual with a typical early bowing of the femurs and sclerosis of the iliac wings. Preoperative (*left*) and postoperative THA radiograph

fracture, nonunion of trochanteric osteotomy, malignant transformation, and deep venous thrombosis [3].

Paget in a relatively young individual with a typical early bowing of the femurs and sclerosis of the iliac wings.

References

1. Lewallen DG. Total hip arthroplasty in special cases hip arthroplasty in patients with paget's disease. Clin Orthop Relat Res. 1999;369:243–50.
2. Sochart DH, Porter ML. Charnley low-friction arthroplasty for Paget's disease of the hip. J Arthroplast. 2000;15(2):210–9.
3. Parvizi J, Klein GR, Sim FH. Surgical management of Paget's disease of bone. J Bone Miner Res. 2006;21(Suppl 2):P75–82.
4. Lusty PJ, Walter WL, Walter WK, Zicat B. Cementless hip arthroplasty in Paget's disease at medium-term follow-up (average of 6.7 years). J Arthroplast. 2007;22(5):692–6.
5. Wegrzyn J, Pibarot V, Chapurlat R, Carret JP, Béjui-Hugues J, Guyen O. Cementless total hip arthroplasty in Paget's disease of bone: a retrospective review. Int Orthop. 2010;34(8):1103–9.
6. Dunlop DJ, Donnachie NJ, Treacy RBC, Treacy RBC. Failure after customized curved femoral stems in Total hip Arthroplasty for Paget's disease. J Arthroplast. 2000;15(3):398–401.
7. Alexakis PG, Brown BA, Hohl WM. Porous hip replacement in Paget's disease. An 8-2/3-year follow up. Clin Orthop Relat Res. 1998;350:138–42.
8. Imbuldeniya AM, Tai SM, Aboelmagd T, Walter WL, Walter WK, Zicat BA. Cementless hip arthroplasty in Paget's disease at long-term follow-up (average of 12.3 years). J Arthroplast. 2014;29(5):1063–6.
9. Ludkowski P, Wilson-MacDonald J. Total arthroplasty in Paget's disease of the hip. A clinical review and review of the literature. Clin Orthop Relat Res. 1990;255:160–7.
10. Stauffer RN, Sim FH. Total hip arthroplasty in Paget's disease of the hip. J Bone Joint Surg Am. 1976;58(4):476–8.
11. McDonald DJ, Sim FH. Total hip arthroplasty in Paget's disease. A follow-up note. J Bone Joint Surg Am. 1987;69(5):766–72.
12. Merkow RL, Pellicci PM, Hely DP, Salvati EA. Total hip replacement for Paget's disease of the hip. J Bone Joint Surg Am. 1984;66(5):752–8.
13. Kirsh G, Kligman M, Roffman M. Hydroxyapatite-coated total hip replacement in Paget's disease: 20 patients followed for 4-8 years. Acta Orthop Scand. 2001;72(2):127–32.
14. Parvizi J, Schall DM, Lewallen DG, Sim FH. Outcome of uncemented hip arthroplasty components in patients with Paget's disease. Clin Orthop Relat Res. 2002;403:127–34.
15. Hozack WJ, Rushton SA, Carey C, Sakalkale D, Rothman RH. Uncemented total hip arthroplasty in Paget's disease of the hip: a report of 5 cases with 5-year follow-up. J Arthroplast. 1999;14(7):872–6.

15 Autoimmune and Inflammatory Diseases: Rheumatoid Arthritis

Eustathios Kenanidis, Panagiotis Kakoulidis, Grigorios T. Sakellariou, Michael Potoupnis, and Eleftherios Tsiridis

15.1 Current Concepts

E. Kenanidis, P. Kakoulidis, G.T. Sakellariou, M. Potoupnis, and E. Tsiridis

Rheumatoid arthritis (RA) is an autoimmune disease that is characterised by peripheral and systematic inflammatory polyarthritis, resulting in joint deformity and destruction [1]. RA affects 1% of the white and 5.3% of Native Americans as well as 2% of women and 0.5% of men in the UK [2].

Almost one-fourth of them will need total joint arthroplasty (elbow, knee, hip, shoulder) throughout their life [2, 3]. The prevalence however of THA and TKA in RA patients has been reduced almost 40% from 1990 to nowadays due to the optimization of therapy [3, 4]. It remains, however, the third most common indication for lower limb joint replacement in Northern Europe and North America [5].

RA patients undergoing THA are considered a unique group, different than OA patients; there is a decreased likelihood of a favourable outcome and higher complication rates [6–8]. The RA patients have the following characteristics:

1. Younger age
2. A chronic systemic inflammation
3. Polyarticular joint involvement
4. Use of immune suppressive and disease-modifying drugs that influence bone and soft tissue properties
5. Compromised biomechanical properties of both soft tissue and bone

Indications: Total hip arthroplasty is a surgical intervention carried out on the end-stage arthritis patients [1].

15.1.1 Preoperative Evaluation

- Take a full history and a thorough clinical, laboratory, and radiological examination [2].
- Assess the atlantoaxial instability with neutral, lateral, flexion and extension radiographs [2]. RA patients have increased the risk of cervical spine instability, reported high up to 44% in some series of patients referred for THA [9]. Go

E. Kenanidis, M.D., Ph.D., M.Sc. (✉) ·
P. Kakoulidis, M.D. · G.T. Sakellariou, M.D
Academic Orthopaedic Unit, Aristotle University Medical School, Thessaloniki, Greece

E. Tsiridis, M.D., Ph.D., F.A.C.S., F.R.C.S. ·
M. Potoupnis, M.D., Ph.D
Academic Orthopaedic Unit, Papageorgiou General Hospital, Aristotle University Medical School, Thessaloniki, Greece
e-mail: etsiridis@doctors.org.uk; mikepot@otenet.gr

E. Tsiridis (ed.), *The Adult Hip - Master Case Series and Techniques*,
https://doi.org/10.1007/978-3-319-64177-5_15

for further evaluation with MRI at abnormal radiographic findings [10]. Symptoms as occipital headache, weakness of limbs, bladder and bowel dysfunction, and long track should be considered as alerts for cervical spine evaluation [10, 11]. Cervical instability may cause sudden death or paraplegia and other neurological complications at surgery. Findings on MRI as basilar invagination, C1–2 or subaxial instability, with ≤13 mm space available for the spinal cord, or myelopathy usually question the time of intervention; cervical stabilisation before THA is then a reasonable option [2, 10, 11].

- Employ regional anaesthesia to avoid neck hyperextension or airway obstruction due to an inflammation of cricoarytenoid joints. When the regional anesthesia is impossible, a general anesthesia should be mediated through a fiber-optic-guided nasotracheal intubation [2].
- Evaluate the cardiopulmonary system sufficiently. RA patients have increased cardiovascular and pulmonary morbidity and mortality rate than the general population; this risk, however, has been controlled and lessened with DMARD therapy [5].
- Choose the appropriate joint to perform surgery in case of a polyarticular involvement. Consider first the most painful joint; when however the upper extremity involvement affects the ability to manage canes and walkers, then first consider upper extremity joint. In case of multiple impaired lower extremity joints, evaluate whether the knee and foot deformities (fixed equinus deformity of the foot, excessive varus- valgus) will compromise rehabilitation and begin from them [2, 12].
- Adjust the antirheumatic therapy preoperatively that has anti-inflammatory and immunosuppressive action [2]. The continuation of drugs increases the risk of wound healing and infection; however, the stoppage increases the likelihood of flare, thereby compromising the rehabilitation [2]. There are recommendations for the preoperative management of these drugs; their validity and applicability, however, are questioned as there are limited statistical evidence and clinical data [13, 14].

15.1.1.1 Synthetic DMARDs

1. Methotrexate: the international task force [15] recommends continuation through the perioperative period. Discontinuation of MTX seems to increase the risk of infection. In an RCT study of 388 rheumatoid patients, Grennan et al. [16] compared RA patients that continued or discontinued MTX with a control group of RA patients never treated with MTX. The RA patients that stopped MTX before the elective surgery had increased the infection rate compared to patients continuing MTX (15% vs 2% infection rate) [16].
2. Hydroxychloroquine: as it is not an immunosuppressive drug, continuation throughout the perioperative period is recommended [2].
3. Leflunomide: the reported results are conflicting [15, 17, 18]. It is considered safer to stop the medication until there is evidence of a satisfactory wound healing, normal bowel, and kidney function postoperatively.

15.1.1.2 Corticosteroids

They are potent anti-inflammatory and immunosuppressive agents widely prescribed in RA patients; they have a minor, however, disease-modifying role [2, 5]. The perioperative management of these drugs is not clarified. There are limited reported data [5]. Corticosteroids impair wound healing, increase the risk of infection in a dose-dependent manner [19] and possibly suppress the adrenal axis intra- or postoperatively [20]. The EULAR recommendations propose that an RA patient undergoing THA must receive a single, intraoperative supplemental dose of 100 mg hydrocortisone [13, 14].

15.1.1.3 Biologic Agents

The anti-TNF factors increase the infection risk during the first six months postoperatively [21]. There are, however, limited data and no randomised controlled trials in RA patients undergoing arthroplasty [2, 22]. It is recommended to stop biological agents preoperatively and start them two weeks postoperatively when the sutures are out [2]. Different preoperative and postoperative period recommendations exist for individual drugs (from 1 preoperative week stop for etanercept to 4 months for rituximab) [2].

15.1.2 Intraoperative Challenges

- The technical challenges of performing THR in patients with RA are mainly due to bone loss, osteopenia, and protrusio acetabuli [5].
- Protrusio acetabuli: This is a technical difficulty due to medial wall deficiency. Hirst et al. [23] described three categories of protrusion acetabuli. Bone grafting in the first two types and possibly an extra cage will be needed in the third type.

15.1.3 Published Results

There are several cohort and case series, comparative studies with OA patients or data from registries for RA patients treated with THA [24–65]. They reported data from cemented [24–39], uncemented [40–56], or hybrid [57] THAs for RA patients. Case series and cohort studies demonstrated mid- to long-term results of cemented and uncemented THAs, ranging from 2 to 25 years [24–56]. The sample size usually ranges from 20 to 200 patients; however, there are studies with up to 1000 patients [28] and also data from registries [58–65]. The survival of the implants ranged from 75 to 98%. The reported results, however, are not homogenous making difficult the extraction of conclusions. There was a trend toward uncemented THA for RA patients during the last years [7]. There is not, however, enough high-level evidence to support cemented or uncemented implants for THA in RA. The nature of the disease and the continuous change in the treatment also play a role.

Several cohort and case series studies [24–39] with sample size up to 1553 patients and follow-up from 2 to 25 years have reported outcomes of cemented THA in RA. Wroblewski et al. [27] demonstrated the results of 292 Charnley low-friction cemented arthroplasties in 195 young patients with an established diagnosis of RA. The mean age of patients at the time of surgery was 38 years, and the mean follow-up 15 years. The survival for any reason was 74% at 25 years. There were 41 hip revisions mainly of the cup. In one of the greatest studies, Lehtimaki et al. [28] followed up a cohort of 1153 consecutive Charnley low-friction arthroplasties in 1086 RA patients. The overall survival was 90.5% at ten years and 83% at fifteen years. Survival of the stem was 90.5% at ten years and 89.9% at fifteen years and for the cup 93.6 and 87.1%, respectively. In a recent systematic review of the literature on clinical and radiological results of cemented THA in RA, Zwartele et al. [6] reported that an increased risk of cemented THA for aseptic loosening of the cup and stem for RA patients was found in older but not in recent studies and none of the registries supported this finding.

Although the compromised rheumatic bone is a risk of mechanical complications in THA, the uncemented arthroplasty gain ground during the last years [7]. Several case series [40–56] are consisting of 20–190 patients with a mean follow-up period from 3.3 to 12.5 years. In a recent study, Haraguchi et al. [40] evaluated 191 uncemented THAs performed in 149 rheumatoid patients between 1998 and 2005. The implant survival at 17 years were 99.5% for the stems, 93.9% for the cups, and 90.8% for the liners. The highly cross-linked polyethylene has better survival compared with conventional polyethylene and alumina-bearing surface. Jana et al. [50] also reported 98.1% survival at ten years for porous-coated stems in rheumatoid patients. A recent systematic review supported the use of uncemented THA in rheumatoid patients [7]. The authors advocated that uncemented THA for RA did not have inferior results, and despite the more frequent mechanical complications of the stem, it is an equivalent solution for RA THAs. There was an increased reported rate of mechanical complications, as acetabular fractures and migration of the cup in 9 out of 22 studies and proximal femoral fractures and subsidence of the stem in 14 out of 20 studies of the review [7]. Reevaluating six studies comparing uncemented to cemented THA, the overall failure rate ratio (uncemented/cemented) for the cup was 0.6 (95% CI, 0.14–2.60) and for the stem 0.71 (95% CI, 0.06–8.55), both favoring uncemented fixation.

There are also conflicting data from the national registries [58–65]. The Finnish registry showed better results for cementless stems both in young and in older patients with RA [60, 62]. Eskelinen et al. [60] evaluated 2557 THAs performed between 1980 and 2003 in patients aged less than 55 years old from the Finnish arthroplasty registry. The proximally circumferentially porous-coated uncemented stems had 89% survival for aseptic loosening at 15 years. The risk of stem revision due to aseptic loosening was higher with cemented stems than with proximally porous-coated uncemented stems implanted during the same period (RR: 2.4, $p < 0.001$). The risk of the cup revision was significantly higher for all the uncemented than for all-polyethylene cemented cups for any reason. The 55 years or older patients from the same registry, [62] had comparable results for cemented and uncemented THAs with survival about 80% at 15 years. Hailer et al. [61], however, reported inferior results for uncemented arthroplasties. They evaluated 170.413 cemented or fully uncemented THA for rheumatoid patients between 1992 and 2007. There were 1.5 times increased the risk for revision of uncemented compared to cemented THA for any reason and aseptic loosening. The risk of aseptic loosening for uncemented cups was higher (RR: 1.8; CI: 1.6–2.0) but lesser for uncemented stems compared to cemented (RR: 0.4; CI: 0.3–0.5). There was also an elevated risk for revision of uncemented stems for periprosthetic fracture during the first 2 years.

15.1.4 Complications

The most frequently reported complications for THA in RA are the infection, dislocation, periprosthetic fractures, aseptic loosening, and venous thromboembolism. Results, however, from different studies are inconclusive and non-consistent.

1. Periprosthetic infection: The increased risk of infection for RA patients undergoing THA has not been fully estimated. There is also non- consistent evidence of the effect in infection risk of concomitant treatment in RA patients and non-consistent definition of infection and RA in the majority of studies [66]. Ravi et al. [66] recognized no increased risk of infection for rheumatoid patients undergoing THA compared to OA. In a recent systematic review of the literature on clinical and radiological results of cemented THA in RA, the authors recognised that the reported results so far are inconclusive to support an elevated infection risk in cemented THA of RA patients [6]. However, due to the under -registration of infection, the authors recognised that RA patients have a mild increased risk of infection in cemented THA. Schrama et al. [67] tried to compare the risk of revision for infection following THA for RA and OA patients using data from the Norwegian registry. The rheumatoid patients had 1.3 higher risk for revision than OA patients; this risk, however, was more evident since 2001. Singh et al. [59] demonstrated that RA is a risk factor for readmission during the first 90 days following THA and that this risk is increased during the last years. The two most common readmission reasons were joint prosthesis infection (10.2%) and septicemia (10.2%) in RA.
2. Hip dislocation: Zwartele et al. recognised mildly increased the risk for instability following THA for RA patients [6]; there was estimated, however, the under- registration of this complication in different series. In a recent meta-analysis, Ravi et al. [66] evaluated 40 studies reporting >200 TKAs or THAs between 1990 and 2011. There were 2.16 times increased the risk for dislocation following THA in RA patients compared to OA. This was attributed to the lower soft tissue quality in RA and possible differences in surgical approach, head size, anatomic differences as protrusion acetabuli, the upward migration and destruction of the acetabular roof, collapse of the femoral head, soft tissue

laxity, less hip abductor strength, or the use of bone cement between groups [66].

3. Venous thromboembolism: An increased risk for venous thromboembolism has not been proved [66, 68]. In a recent systematic review [68], RA patients were not found to have increased risk for DVT or bleeding following joint arthroplasty.
4. Periprosthetic fractures: Sidler et al. [69] demonstrated that RA was recognized as a general but an independent risk factor for intra- and postoperative periprosthetic femoral fractures following THA.

15.2 Case Title: Primary THA Rheumatoid Arthritis and Corticosteroid-Induced Osteonecrosis

E. Kenanidis and E. Tsiridis

15.2.1 Demographics

Age: 52
Sex: male
BMI: 28

15.2.2 Relevant Past Medical History

Principal pathologies: rheumatoid arthritis and chronic use of corticosteroids

Previous surgical procedures: uncemented THA contralateral side 15 years back (Fig. 15.1)

Medication: steroids, antibodies, methotrexate

Others: steroid -induced osteoporosis

History of presenting complaint: pain and short limp gate

15.2.3 Clinical Examination

Symptoms: pain, short limp

Range of motion: flexion: 60; extension: -10; int/external rotation: 0–10; abd/adduction: 10

Specific tests: Thomas test positive

Main disability: pain inability to walk

Scoring if available: HHS < 70

Neurovascular evaluation: intact

15.2.4 Preoperative Radiological Assessment/Imaging (Fig. 15.1)

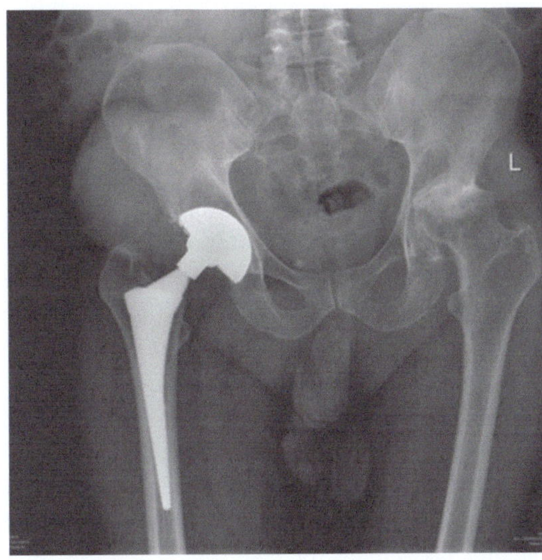

Fig. 15.1 Right hip uncemented modular THA. Left hip typical V- shaped head osteonecrosis, Ficat-Arlet classification 4 with collapse and reduction of the joint space

15.2.5 Preoperative Planning

Diagnosis: femoral head osteonecrosis Ficat-Arlet classification 4, arthritis, shortening, external rotation (Fig. 15.1)

Possible treatment options: THA

Chosen treatment method: hybrid THA: uncemented acetabular cup 52mm/36mm (Stryker), ceramic head 36mm, cemented stem 44mm offset size 2

Selection of implants if applicable and rational: hybrid with cemented stem to address the corticosteroid-induced osteoporosis

Expected difficulties: the capsular adhesions and contracture from chronic inflammation; a potential bone loss

Strategies to overcome difficulties: on the day of surgery, hydrocortisone 50–75 mg or methylprednisolone 10–15 mg intravenously can be used with the dose tapered to the routine corticosteroid dose in 1–2 days to avoid Addison's crisis.

Templating: done

15.2.6 Surgical Note

With the patient in lateral decubitus position and a mini - posterior approach, the hip was approached. Adhesions and contractures were evident, and the hip was dislocated with some difficulty but without a problem. Extensive anterior and posterior capsulectomy was performed to allow lengthening of the limp. The head was deformed and collapsed, and the cartilage over it was wiped off the subchondral bone and plicate like the "accordion bellows." The subchondral bone was in places sclerotic and nonviable. The femoral head osteotomy revealed adequate bleeding bone in the remaining neck, and the femur was displaced anteriorly for the preparation of the acetabulum. The reaming of the socket was uneventful, and a 52 mm shell was tightly inserted needing no screws for stability. Attention then was turned to the femur. A third-generation cementing technique was employed to insert a 44/2 Exeter stem successfully (Fig. 15.2). Leg length was trialled, and equal LL was achieved to the contralateral side. The THA was stable, and the sciatic nerve was intact.

15.2.7 Intraoperative Challenges

Challenges and solutions: extensive releases of adhesions due to chronic inflammation and joint disease.

Thorough description of decision making, including the reason for the final decision: removing part of the anterior capsule was deemed necessary to allow correction of the length and the fixed flexion deformity.

15.2.8 Postoperative Radiographs (Fig. 15.2)

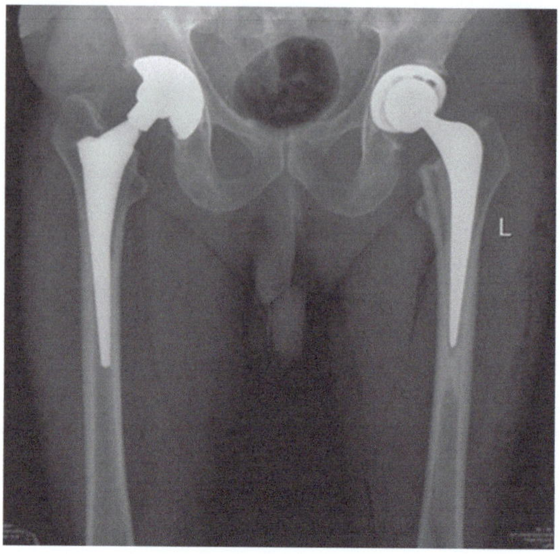

Fig. 15.2 Straightforward Exeter hybrid THA with equal leg length. A self-criticism point was the thin mantle in Gruen zones 6 and 7 and around the shoulder of the prosthesis. The latter could be a projection but never the less if existing may reduce the strength of the cement mantle in this region

15.2.9 Postoperative Management

Chemoprophylaxis and anticoagulant treatment period: vancomycin 500 mg (one dose preoperatively and two doses postoperatively), cefuroxime 750 mg (one dose preoperatively and two doses postoperatively), and tinzaparin once daily for 35 days

Gait/limb loading until full loading: partial weight bearing for four weeks; then weight bearing as tolerated

15.2.10 Follow-Up and Complications

No complication

Scoring if available: HHS: 95

15.3 Case Title: Primary Bilateral Hybrid Exeter THA for Psoriatic Arthritis

E. Kenanidis and E. Tsiridis

The selection of hybrid implants was based on the existing knowledge that people who have inflammatory arthritis and receive corticosteroids also suffer from advanced osteoporosis; thus, the cemented implant is indicated, especially on the femoral side. On the acetabular side, there is evidence that cemented and uncemented implants may perform equally well, though for the case of rheumatoid arthritis in our opinion, as the addition of two to three roof screws is of paramount importance to maintain the stability of the socket until osseointegration appears onto the cell surface. An uncemented femoral stem in our opinion is not a good choice because there is not enough cancellous bone to support the metaphyseal part of the prosthesis.

Acetabular side: advanced erosion with subchondral cysts and osteoporosis of the socket along with mild protrusion appearance on both sides (Fig. 15.3). The reaming of the socket should be done with great care to avoid bridging the inner plate of the socket or damaging the anterior or posterior wall. Graft reinforcement using autograph from the femoral head was necessary to reconstruct the inner plate using primary impaction grafting technique. Socket introduction should be done with great care to avoid fracturing the posterior wall or roof of the socket. Long reinforcement screws of significant length, i.e., more than 25–30 mm, should be added to maintain the initial stability of the socket. It is advisable to under ream by 1 mm the socket, as the bone is expected to be too soft during the shell introduction.

Femoral side: osteoporosis around the greater trochanter may increase the risk of fracture during stem insertion. This is particularly important when someone is using uncemented implants with shoulders; thus, our decision to use cemented Exeter stem would overcome the latter problem (Fig. 15.4). One should take care not to remove too much of the cancellous bone of the metaphysis during the reaming process, as the latter may lead to cement on cortex cementation, which is not biomechanically sound. Care must also be taken to plug the canal adequately to pressurise the cement using third-generation cementing technique and stop the profound bleeding during cement insertion—that is not uncommon in inflammatory arthritis patients. Gentle insertion of the actual stem is usually guaranteed using cemented implants.

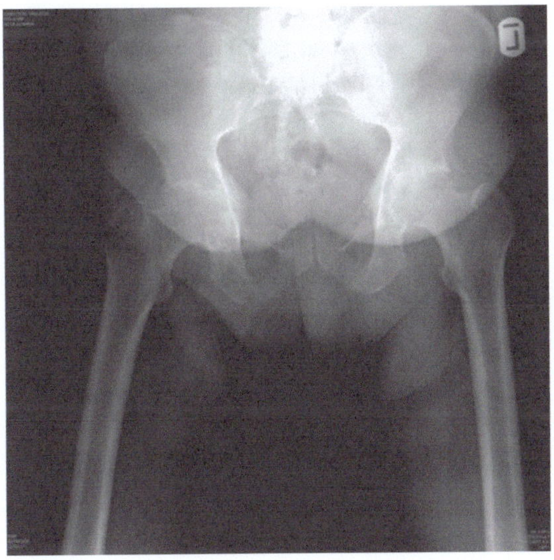

Fig. 15.3 Preoperative x-ray

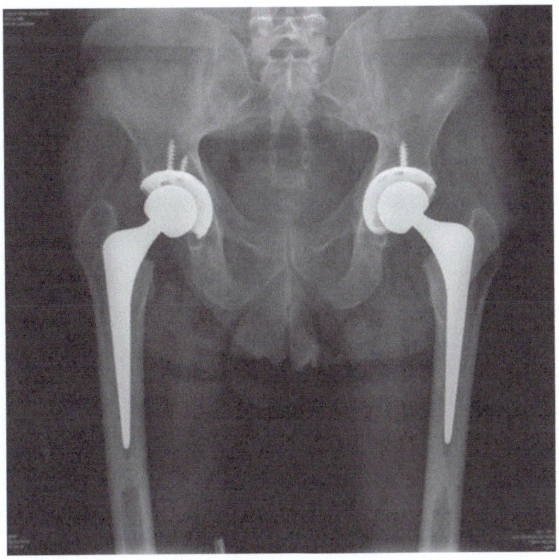

Fig. 15.4 Postoperative x-ray

15.4 Case Title: Bilateral Simultaneous THAs-Lupus Erythematosus

E. Kenanidis and E. Tsiridis

15.4.1 Demographics

Age: 40
Sex: female
BMI: 25

15.4.2 Relevant Past Medical History

Principal pathologies: lupus erythematosus, global bilateral hip arthritis, bilateral femoral head osteonecrosis from chronic use of corticosteroids (Fig. 15.5)

Previous surgical procedures: none

Medication: azathioprine, hydroxychloroquine, prednisolone

History of presenting complaint: pain, reduced ROM

15.4.3 Clinical Examination

Symptoms: pain

Range of motion: limited

Main disability: pain

Scoring if available: HHS: 80

Neurovascular evaluation: intact

15.4.4 Preoperative Radiological Assessment/Imaging (Fig. 15.5)

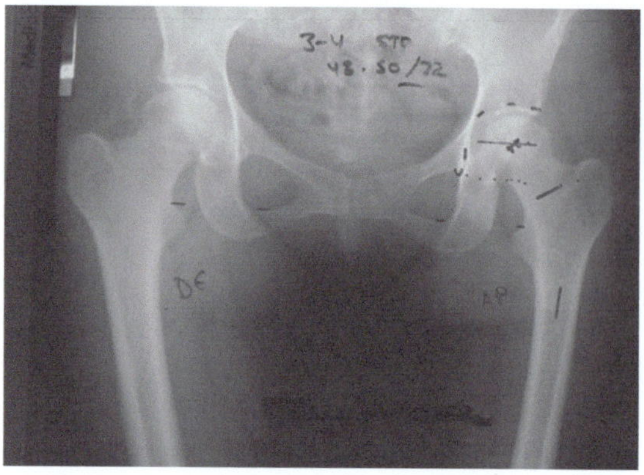

Fig. 15.5 Bilateral global arthritis. The typical distraction of the articular cartilage without significant architectural deformity as in osteoarthritis and lack of osteophytes. Central areas of osteonecrosis as demarcated V - shaped radiopaque signals in both hips. Templating outlines potential sizes and alignment of the implants

15.4.5 Preoperative Planning

Diagnosis: bilateral osteonecrosis of femoral head and arthritis.

Possible treatment options: cemented or uncemented THAs. Our algorithm of treatment indicates uncemented approach only for the young patients with good bone quality.

Chosen treatment method: bilateral: uncemented acetabular shell PINNACLE DePuy 48mm, polyethylene acetabular liner DePuy 32mm, uncemented femoral hip stem size 3 standard DePuy, ceramic femoral head DePuy 32mm.

Selection of implants if applicable and rational: intraoperative decision making for the implant choice. In this case, we selected uncemented option and simultaneous bilateral procedure due to young age and good general health status.

Templating: done preoperatively as per radiograph above.

15.4.6 Surgical Note

Azathioprine was stopped one week preoperatively, hydroxychloroquine was not, and prednisolone was continued perioperatively. The anesthetist maintained the continuous corticosteroid infusion to prevent Addison's crisis during surgery. The patient was draped for the right hip THA first. In lateral decubitus position and using a mini posterior approach, the hip was exposed and replaced using uncemented components. The quality of the bone was judged intraoperatively efficient, and the cemented option was abandoned. A straightforward approach to both acetabulum and femur and good fitting of the implants. Acetabular component shell was 48 mm with a 32 mm HXLP, and a size 3 uncemented proximally coated and double tapered femoral implants with standard offset (DePuy) were used (Fig. 15.6). The patient was then turned to the other side and was redraped. The surgical personnel repeated the preparation face as per primary THA from the beginning. Uneventful left THA using the same implants and sizes.

15.4.7 Postoperative Radiographs (Fig. 15.6)

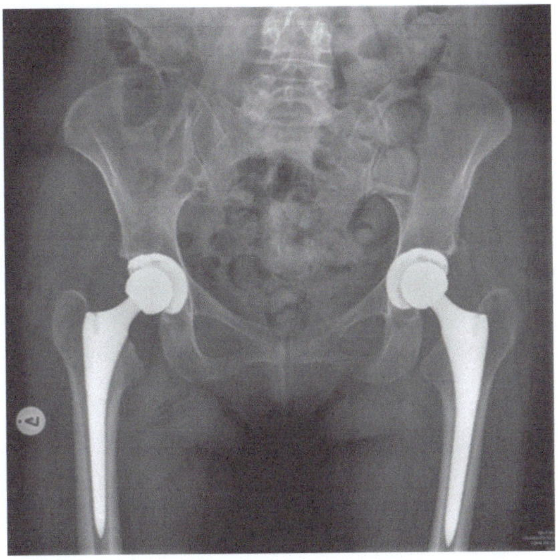

Fig. 15.6 Bilateral simultaneous THAs significant similarities in terms of implantation and implant sizes. Good alignment and orientation of implants

15.4.8 Postoperative Management

Chemoprophylaxis and anticoagulant treatment period: cefuroxime 1,5 gr (one dose preoperatively and two doses postoperatively), vancomycin 500 mg (one dose preoperatively and two doses postoperatively), enoxaparin 1x1 for the days of hospitalisation, and then rivaroxaban for 30 days

Gait/limb loading until full loading: partial weight bearing for four weeks; then as tolerated

References

1. Mosleh-Shirazi MS, Ibrahim M, Pastides P, Khan W, Rahman H. An insight into methods and practices in hip Arthroplasty in patients with rheumatoid arthritis. Int J Rheumatol. 2015;2015:140–3.
2. Goodman SM, Figgie M. Lower extremity Arthroplasty in patients with inflammatory arthritis: preoperative and perioperative management. J Am Acad Orthop Surg. 2013;21:355–63.
3. Louie GH, Ward MM. Changes in the rates of joint surgery among patients with rheumatoid arthritis in California, 1983–2007. Ann Rheum Dis. 2010;69(5):868–71.
4. Hekmat K, Jacobsson L, Nilsson JA, et al. Decrease in the incidence of total hip arthroplasties in patients with rheumatoid arthritis: results from a well defined population in South Sweden. Arthritis Res Ther. 2011;13(2):R67.
5. Clement ND, Breusch SJ, Biant LC. Lower limb joint replacement in rheumatoid arthritis. J Orthop Surg Res. 2012;7:27.
6. Zwartelé R, Pφll RG. Cemented total hip arthroplasty in rheumatoid arthritis. A systematic review of the literature. Hip Int. 2013;23(2):111–22.
7. Zwartelé RE, Witjes S, Cornelis Doets H, Stijnen T, Po¨ll RG. Cementless total hip arthroplasty in rheumatoid arthritis:a systematic review of the literature. Arch Orthop Trauma Surg. 2012;132:535–46.
8. Bongartz T, Halligan CS, Osmon DR, et al. Incidence and risk factors of prosthetic joint infection after total hip or knee replacement in patients with rheumatoid arthritis. Arthritis Rheum. 2008;59(12):1713–20.
9. Neva MH, Häkkinen A, Mäkinen H, Hannonen P, Kauppi M, Sokka T. High prevalence of asymptomatic cervical spine subluxation in patients with rheumatoid arthritis waiting for orthopaedic surgery. Ann Rheum Dis. 2006;65(7):884–8.
10. Takatori R, Tokunaga D, Hase H, Mikami Y, Ikeda T, Harada T, Imai K, Nishimura T, An HS, Inoue N, Kudo T. Three-dimensional morphology and kinematics of the craniovertebral junction in rheumatoid arthritis. Spine. 2010;35:1278–84.
11. Roche CJ, Eyes BE, Whitehouse GH. The rheumatoid cervical spine: signs of instability on plain cervical radiographs. Clin Radiol. 2002;57:241–9.
12. Wilkinson JM, Stanley D, Getty CJM. Surgical management of the rheumatoid patient. Curr Orthop. 2004;18:357–70.
13. Hoes JN, Jacobs JW, Boers M, et al. EULAR evidence-based recommendations on the management of systemic glucocorticoid therapy in rheumatic diseases. Ann Rheum Dis. 2007;66(12):1560–7.
14. van der Goes MC, Jacobs JW, Boers M, et al. Patient and rheumatologist perspectives on glucocorticoids: an exercise to improve the implementation of the European League Against Rheumatism (EULAR) recommendations on the management of systemic glucocorticoid therapy in rheumatic diseases. Ann Rheum Dis. 2010;69(6):1015–21.
15. Visser K, Katchamart W, Loza E, et al. Multinational evidence-based recommendations for the use of methotrexate in rheumatic disorders with a focus on rheumatoid arthritis: integrating systematic literature research and expert opinion of a broad international panel of rheumatologists in the 3E initiative. Ann Rheum Dis. 2009;68(7):1086–93.
16. Grennan DM, Gray J, Loudon J, Fear S. Methotrexate and early postoperative complications in patients with rheumatoid arthritis undergoing elective orthopaedic surgery. Ann Rheum Dis. 2001;60(3):214–7.
17. Fuerst M, Möhl H, Baumgärtel K, Rüther W. Leflunomide increases the risk of early healing complications in patients with rheumatoid arthritis undergoing elective orthopedic surgery. Rheumatol Int. 2006;26(12):1138–42.
18. Tanaka N, Sakahashi H, Sato E, Hirose K, Ishima T, Ishii S. Examination of the risk of continuous leflunomide treatment on the incidence of infectious complications after joint arthroplasty in patients with rheumatoid arthritis. J Clin Rheumatol. 2003;9(2):115–8.
19. Grijalva CG, Chen L, Delzell E. Initiation of tumor necrosis factor-α antagonists and the risk of hospitalization for infection in patients with autoimmune diseases. JAMA. 2011;306(21):2331–9.
20. Marik PE, Varon J. Requirement of perioperative stress doses of corticosteroids: a systematic review of the literature. Arch Surg. 2008;143(12):1222–6.
21. Galloway JB, Hyrich KL, Mercer LK, et al. Anti-TNF therapy is associated with an increased risk of serious infections in patients with rheumatoid arthritis especially in the first 6 months of treatment: updated results from the British Society for Rheumatology biologics register with special emphasis on risks in the elderly. Rheumatology (Oxford). 2011;50(1):124.
22. Galloway JB, Hyrich KL, Mercer LK, et al. Risk of septic arthritis in patients with rheumatoid arthritis and the effect of anti-TNF therapy: results from the British Society for Rheumatology biologics register. Ann Rheum Dis. 2011;70(10):1810–4.
23. Hirst P, Esser M, Murphy JC, Hardinge K. Bone grafting for protrusion acetabuli during total hip replacement. A review of the Wrightington method in 61 hips. J Bone Joint Surg Br. 1987;69:229–33.
24. Dutka J, Sosin P, Skowronek P, Sorysz T. Total hip arthroplasty in rheumatoid arthritis: results of 12-years follow-up. Chir Narzadow Ruchu Ortop Pol. 2009;74(4):202–6.
25. Kirk PG, Rorabeck CH, Bourne RB, Burkart B. Total hip arthroplasty in rheumatoid arthritis: comparison of cemented and uncemented implants. Can J Surg. 1993;36(3):229–32.
26. Poss R, Maloney JP, Ewald FC, Thomas WH, Batte NJ, Hartness C, Sledge CB. Six- to 11-year results of total hip arthroplasty in rheumatoid arthritis. Clin Orthop. 1984;182:109–16.
27. Wroblewski BM, Siney PD, Fleming PA. Charnley low-frictional torque arthroplasty in young rheumatoid and juvenile rheumatoid arthritis: 292 hips followed for an average of 15 years. Acta Orthop. 2007;78(2):206–10.

28. Lehtimaki MY, Kautiainen H, Lehto MU, Hamalainen MM. Charnley low-friction arthroplasty in rheumatoid arthritis. A survival study up to 20 years. J Arthroplast. 1999;14:651–61.
29. Onsten I, Besjakov J, Carlsson AS. Improved radiographic survival of the Charnley prosthesis in rheumatoid arthritis and osteoarthritis. Results of new versus old operative techniques in 402 hips. J Arthroplast. 1994;9(1):3–8.
30. Rosenberg WW, Schreurs BW, de Waal Malefijt MC, Veth RP, Slooff TJ. Impacted morsellized bone grafting and cemented primary total hip arthroplasty for acetabular protrusion in patients with rheumatoid arthritis: an 8- to 18-year follow-up study of 36 hips. Acta Orthop Scand. 2000;71(2):143–6.
31. Creighton MG, Callaghan JJ, Olejniczak JP, Johnston RC. Total hip arthroplasty with cement in patients who have rheumatoid arthritis. A minimum ten-year follow-up study. J Bone Joint Surg Am. 1998;80:1439–46.
32. Ranawat CS, Dorr LD, Inglis AE. Total hip arthroplasty in protrusion acetabuli of rheumatoid arthritis. J Bone Joint Surg Am. 1980;62(7):1059–65.
33. Johnsson R, Ekelund L, Zygmunt S, et al. Total hip replacement with spongious bone graft for acetabular protrusion in patients with rheumatoid arthritis. Acta Orthop Scand. 1984;55(5):510–3.
34. Severt R, Wood R, Cracchiolo A 3rd, Amstutz HC. Long-term follow-up of cemented total hip arthroplasty in rheumatoid arthritis. Clin Orthop. 1991;265:137–45.
35. Wessinghage D, Kisslinger E. [Long-term results after cemented total hip arthroplasty in chronic polyarthritis]. [article in German]. Orthopade. 1998;27(6):381–91.
36. Unger AS, Inglis AE, Ranawat CS, Johanson NA. Total hip arthroplasty in rheumatoid arthritis. A long-term follow-up study. J Arthroplast. 1987;2:191–7.
37. Chmell MJ, Scott RD, Thomas WH, Sledge CB. Total hip arthroplasty with cement for juvenile rheumatoid arthritis. Results at a minimum of ten years in patients less than thirty years old. J Bone Joint Surg Am. 1997;79:44–5.
38. Tang WM, Chiu KY. Primary total hip arthroplasty in patients with rheumatoid arthritis. Int Orthop. 2001;25(1):13–6.
39. Matewski D, Szymkowiak E, Gumanski R, Puchała J, Sniegowski M. Outcome of total hip replacement in rheumatic arthritis. Ortop Traumatol Rehabil. 2005;7(6):633–8.
40. Haraguchi A, Nakashima Y, Miyahara H, Esaki Y, Okazaki K, Fukushi JI, Hirata G, Ikemura S, Kamura S, Sakuraba K, Fujimura K, Akasaki Y, Yamada H. Minimum 10-year results of cementless total hip arthroplasty in patients with rheumatoid arthritis. Mod Rheumatol. 2016;15:1–7.
41. Yuasa T, Maezawa K, Nozawa M, Kaneko K. Cementless total hip arthroplasty for patients with rheumatoid arthritis: a more than 10-year follow-up. Eur J Orthop Surg Traumatol. 2016;26(6):599–603.
42. Lu N, Yang Y, Chen H, Li W, Pu B, Liu L. Cementless total hip arthroplasty and impacted bone grafting for protrusio acetabuli in patients with rheumatoid arthritis. Zhongguo Xiu Fu Chong Jian Wai Ke Za Zhi. 2015;29(2):160–2.
43. Bause L. Short stem total hip arthroplasty in patients with rheumatoid arthritis. Orthopedics. 2015;38(3 Suppl):S46–50. https://doi.org/10.3928/01477447-20150215-56.
44. Matsushita I, Morita Y, Ito Y, Motomura H, Kimura T. Long-term clinical and radiographic results of cementless total hip arthroplasty for patients with rheumatoid arthritis: minimal 10-year follow-up. Mod Rheumatol. 2014;24(2):281–4.
45. Carl HD, Ploetzner J, Swoboda B, Weseloh G, Mueller LA. Cementless total hip arthroplasty in patients with rheumatoid arthritis using a tapered designed titanium hip stem minimum: 10-year results. Rheumatol Int. 2011;31(3):353–9.
46. Zwartele R, Peters A, Brouwers J, Olsthoorn P, Brand R, Doets C. Long-term results of cementless primary total hip arthroplasty with a threaded cup and a tapered, rectangular titanium stem in rheumatoid arthritis and osteoarthritis. Int Orthop. 2008;32(5):581–7. Epub 2007 Jul 3
47. Arnold P, Schüle B, Schroeder-Boersch H, Jani L. Review of the results of the ARO multicenter study. Orthopade. 1998;27(6):324–32.
48. Effenberger H, Lassmann S, Hilzensauer G. Cementless hip prosthesis in patients with rheumatoid arthritis. Orthopade. 1998;27(6):354–65.
49. Loehr JF, Munzinger U, Tibesku C. Uncemented total hip arthroplasty in patients with rheumatoid arthritis. Clin Orthop. 1999;366:31–8.
50. Jana AK, Engh CA Jr, Lewandowski PJ, et al. Total hip arthroplasty using porous-coated femoral components in patients with rheumatoid arthritis. J Bone Joint Surg Br. 2001;83:686.
51. Keisu KS, Orozco F, McCallum JD 3rd, Bissett G, Hozack WJ, Sharkey PF, Rothman RH. Cementless femoral fixation in the rheumatoid patient undergoing total hip arthroplasty: minimum 5-year results. J Arthroplast. 2001;16(4):415–21.
52. Walker KR, Kyle RF, Gustilo RB. Noncemented femoral components in total hip arthroplasty for patients with rheumatoid arthritis. Minn Med. 1996;79(7):27–31.
53. Thomason HC 3rd, Lachiewicz PF. The influence of technique on fixation of primary total hip arthroplasty in patients with rheumatoid arthritis. J Arthroplast. 2001;16(5):628–34.
54. Cracchiolo A 3rd, Severt R, Moreland J. Uncemented total hip arthroplasty in rheumatoid arthritis diseases. A two- to six-year follow-up study. Clin Orthop Relat Res. 1992;277:166–74.
55. Lachiewicz PF. Porous-coated total hip arthroplasty in rheumatoid arthritis. J Arthroplast. 1994;9:9–15.
56. Katsimihas M, Taylor AH, Lee MB, Sarangi PP, Learmonth ID. Cementless acetabular replacement in patients with rheumatoid arthritis: a 6- to 14-year prospective study. J Arthroplast. 2003; 18(1):16–22.
57. Ito H, Tanino H, Yamanaka Y, Minami A, Matsuno T. Intermediate- to long-term results after hybrid total

hip arthroplasty in patients with rheumatoid arthritis. J Arthroplast. 2013;28(2):309–14.
58. Schrama JC, Espehaug B, Hallan G, et al. Risk of revision for infection in primary total hip and knee arthroplasty in patients with rheumatoid arthritis compared with osteoarthritis: a prospective, population-based study on 108,786 hip and knee joint arthroplasties from the Norwegian Arthroplasty register. Arthritis Care Res (Hoboken). 2010;62(4):473–9.
59. Singh JA, Inacio MC, Namba RS, Paxton EW. Rheumatoid arthritis is associated with higher ninety-day hospital readmission rates compared to osteoarthritis after hip or knee arthroplasty: a cohort study. Arthritis Care Res (Hoboken). 2015;67(5):718–24.
60. Eskelinen A, Paavolainen P, Helenius I, Pulkkinen P, Remes V. Total hip arthroplasty for rheumatoid arthritis in younger patients: 2,557 replacements in the Finnish Arthroplasty register followed for 0-24 years. Acta Orthop. 2006;77(6):853–65.
61. Hailer N, Garellick G, Karrholm J. Uncemented and cemented primary total hip arthroplasty in the Swedish hip Arthroplasty register. Acta Orthop. 2010;81:34–41.
62. Mäkelä KT, Eskelinen A, Pulkkinen P, Virolainen P, Paavolainen P, Remes V. Cemented versus cementless total hip replacements in patients fifty-five years of age or older with rheumatoid arthritis. J Bone Joint Surg Am. 2011;93(2):178–86.
63. Hallan G, Lie S, Furnes O, et al. Medium- and long-term performance of 11, 516 uncemented primary femoral stems from the Norwegian arthroplasty register. J Bone Joint Surg Br. 2007;89(12):1574–80.
64. Furnes O, Lie SA, Espehaug B, Vollset SE, Engesaeter LB, Havelin LI. Hip disease and the prognosis of total hip replacements. A review of 53,698 primary total hip replacements reported to the Norwegian Arthroplasty register 1987-99. J Bone Joint Surg Br. 2001;83(4):579–86.
65. Rud-Sorensen C, Pedersen AB, Johnsen SP, Riis AH, Overgaard S. Survival of primary total hip arthroplasty in rheumatoid arthritis patients. Acta Orthop. 2010;81(1):60–5.
66. Ravi B, Escott B, Shah PS, Jenkinson R, Chahal J, Bogoch E, Kreder H, Hawker G. A systematic review and meta-analysis comparing complications following Total joint Arthroplasty for rheumatoid arthritis versus for osteoarthritis. Arthritis Rheum. 2012;64(12):3839–49.
67. Schrama JC, Fenstad AM, Dale H, Havelin L, Hallan G, Overgaard S, Pedersen AB, Kärrholm J, Garellick G, Pulkkinen P, Eskelinen A, Mäkelä K, Engesæter LB, Fevang BT. Increased risk of revision for infection in rheumatoid arthritis patients with total hip replacements. Acta Orthop. 2015;86(4): 469–76.
68. Mameli A, Marongiu F. Thromboembolic disease in patients with rheumatoid arthritis undergoing joint arthroplasty: update on prophylaxes. World J Orthop. 2014;5(5):645–52.
69. Sidler-Maier CC, Waddell JP. Incidence and predisposing factors of periprosthetic proximal femoral fractures: a literature review. International Orthopaedics (SICOT). 2015;39:1673–82.

16 Ceramic on Ceramic

Eustathios Kenanidis, Panagiotis Kakoulidis, and Eleftherios Tsiridis

16.1 Current Concepts

E. Kenanidis, P. Kakoulidis, and E. Tsiridis

Alumina ceramic is a highly oxidized ceramic that is formed by the fusion of microscopic grains of alumina (Al_2O_3) and/or zirconia (ZrO_2) ceramic powder into a solid phase. During the process of sintering known as "hot isostatic pressing," the agents are pressed above 1000 bars and sintered at 1600 °C [1]. Then, the components are polished to get the finest surface possible. This hard material is also hydrophilic and highly polished and has better biocompatibility than metal ions. These unique characteristics were used in THA to decrease wear rate and osteolysis [1].

The originally introduced ceramic heads in the 1970s were alumina oxide, which has better wear characteristics than zirconia oxide. However, the increased rate of fracture of the first-generation ceramics, squeaking and edge wear metal debris put under question its general use [2]. Since then ceramics have been continuously improved. Through evolvement of generations, the increased purity and strength, the reduced grain size, the increased smoothness of the material, and the addition of hot isostatic pressure thus improved tribological characteristics [2]. The fourth generation of CoC articulation is composed of an alumina matrix material consisting of 75% alumina, 24% zirconia, and 1% mixed oxides (BIOLOX delta) [3]. Delta ceramics have eliminated the risk of fragility and currently are in use as hard on hard or hard on poly couples [3].

Its use increased to one fourth of all THAs as reported in Wales and Great Britain Registry; however, still the ceramic on poly remains the prime choice as HXLP has improved the tribology of the couple.

16.1.1 Advantages

(a) High hardness [1, 4]

Ceramics are harder than metals and can be better polished to a much lower surface roughness. These characteristics provide high resistance to abrasion and major scratches and minimal wear rate [1, 4].

E. Kenanidis, M.D., Ph.D., M.Sc. (✉)
P. Kakoulidis, M.D.
Academic Orthopaedic Unit, Aristotle University Medical School, Thessaloniki, Greece

E. Tsiridis, M.D., Ph.D., F.A.C.S., F.R.C.S (✉)
Academic Orthopaedic Unit, Papageorgiou General Hospital, Aristotle University Medical School, Thessaloniki, Greece
e-mail: etsiridis@doctors.org.uk

E. Tsiridis (ed.), *The Adult Hip - Master Case Series and Techniques*,
https://doi.org/10.1007/978-3-319-64177-5_16

(b) Great wettability [1, 4]

The excellent wettability ensures uniform distribution of synovial fluid between implant surfaces. This feature guarantee fluid film lubrication and very low friction between the articulating surfaces [1, 4].

(c) High elastic modulus [2]
(d) Low wear rate

In vitro studies demonstrated wear rate of <0.1 mm^3 per million cycles [5]. In vivo studies, however, showed higher rate mainly due to edge loading and impingement to the neck [6]; it is however certainly lower than the wear of MoP (1.8 mm^3 per million cycles) [4]. Sphericity and clearance between ceramic head and cup affect wear production. The optimal deviation from sphericity is usually ±1 μm and clearance between the two components 20–50 μm [1].

(e) Wear particle size

CoC articulations produce smaller particles than MoP. There is usually a bimodal particle size range (smaller particles 5–90 nm and greater 0.05–3.2 μm) [7].

(f) Decreased biologic activity of ceramic particles

Ceramic particles have reduced biologic and specific activity compared to polyethylene particles [8, 9]. The usual reaction to alumina wear debris is fibrocystic with very few macrophages and no giant cells [1, 10]. They are considered to be biologically inert, but if released in sufficient numbers, ceramic particles can produce osteolysis similar but less intense to that induced by polyethylene particles [4, 11].

(g) Minimal rate of osteolysis

Several reports have confirmed the low rate of osteolysis in CoC THAs [11–16]. It is mainly attributed to the low wear rate and inert material. Hamadouche et al. [17] reported undetectable wear on plain radiographs for 51 patients who have undergone cemented CoC THA at 20 years at cup and femur. Hernigou et al. [18] identified better the osteolysis on CT than plain radiographs at 20 years postoperatively. Ceramic wear particles can induce osteolytic cytokine production by human macrophages, but the necessary volumetric concentration of the particles to generate this response was extremely high. True osteolysis can only be observed in abnormal situations such as poor implant positioning, irregular contact, or following an instability of the components [19].

(h) Technically easier revision

Revision THA in case of CoC is considered easier to perform due to the lack of foreign body reaction and osteolysis. Removal of the acetabular component, however, especially the denucleation of the ceramic liner from the metal shell is somehow challenging especially in the presence of screws.

(i) Possibility to use greater head size and increase stability
(j) Excellent biocompatibility
(k) Advantaging solution in younger patients

16.1.2 Disadvantages

1. Fractures of ceramic implants/head or liner

Ceramics are brittle materials with no ductility and limited bending strength or ability to deform; thus, they fracture without warning [1]. This complication is unique to this bearing couple [2]. Following cyclic loads applied to a ceramic component, tiny flaws created during material manufacturing or implantation can act as stress risers leading to crack propagation throughout the material and finally to catastrophic failure through fracture [2, 20]. There are several proposed reasons for head fracture including increased body weight, high activity level, the hammering of the femoral head, and imprisonment of a foreign body between the morse taper and the ball, but the principal cause is certainly material quality.

Hannouche et al. [1] speculated that fractures initiate at implantation acting as a stress riser that propagates and leads subsequently to a fracture. Francesco Traina et al. [21] in a retrospective case-control study found that the malposition of the acetabular component out of the optimal range of anteversion of 15+/−10 was the reason of fracture. It produced neck-cup impingement marginal head subluxation and edge loading of the liner's rim or the metal back rim, i.e., in cases of high-profile locking mechanisms of the shell leading subsequently to liner failure.

The reported risk of ceramic head fracture was 0.26–13.14 for the earlier generations, but newer generations (BIOLOX delta) showed a minimal risk of fracture (0.004–0.015%) due to a general improvement of materials [22]. The reported risk of ceramic liner fracture was reported to be greater for "sandwich type" than monoblock metal ceramic implant [23]. In a multicenter study, there was no fracture of new a monoblock liner (BIOLOX delta) at three years [24].

2. Squeaking and Clicking

The definition of squeaking is obscure. Noise generating from CoC and MoM is not a universally accepted term. Swanson et al. [24] defined squeaking as an audible sound emanating from the hip with movement. Some other definitions include grinding, clicking, or grating that is reproducible or which can be heard by other people. The squeaking affects the quality of patients' life and implant survival.

The reason is more or less unknown. There are many theories, but probably the reason is multifactorial. Two main hypotheses are supporting that the sound is generated by the extra-articular impingement of the femoral neck on the acetabular component [25, 26] or by the increased friction of the bearing couple [27].Acetabular mal-orientation and extra-articular impingement of the femoral neck on the acetabular component have been proposed [24]. The neck rim impingement produces edge loading and localized wear called strip wear [28, 29]. The microseperation theory of the femoral head supported that micro-subluxation during gait is the causing factor of eccentrical loading and strip wear [30, 31]. Parvizi et al. proposed that the noise is femoral implant design dependent permitting impingement of the neck to the metallic cup [32]. Restrepo et al. [33] demonstrated that the prevalence of squeaking was seven times higher for patients who had received a titanium molybdenum-zirconium-iron-alloy stem as compared to those who received a titanium-aluminum-vanadium-alloy stem. Individual stem types have been implicated [34].

There are studies [35, 36] where the incidence of squeaking was almost 0% and other with 5–10% [37, 38]. In a recent meta-analysis from the Australian Registry, Owen et al. [34] studied 16,828 CoC THAs with a mean follow-up ranging from 22 to 249 months. The average incidence of squeaking was 4.2%, but the rate for revision for squeaking was 0.2%. There was the significantly lower incidence (1.2%) in self-reporting studies than in that where there was a specific questionnaire (4.5%) ($p = 0.002$). There was lower but nonsignificant incidence between studies lasting less than 100 months compared to other with duration >100 months. In another meta-analysis by Stanat and Capozzi, the mean rate was estimated at 2.4% [39].

3. Ceramic Liner Rim Damage

It is a direct harm of the liner rim by the neck of the stem. The ceramic fragments produced accelerate the wear production, impingement, and dislocation [40].

4. Revision Concerns of CoC THAs

The lack of precise data available on the revision of CoC THAs creates a lot of concerns. Firstly, identification of impeding catastrophic failure is difficult as there are no radiological signs [4]. A high degree of clinical suspicion is needed.

Removal also of a ceramic liner from a metal shell that is stable may be challenging [4]. In the absence of screws, a well-fixed metal shell can be removed with ream cutters swiveling around the bone-metal interface. In the case of screws, removing the ceramic liner is a change;

direct perpendicular sharp impact in the liner/shell interface especially if the ceramic liner is proud or overhanging may lead to the liner dissociation [4].

During the revision of the ceramic head, a question arises as to whether we have to revise a stable stem. The removal of a ceramic head could damage the cone and initiate stress risers and propagate cracks to the newly implanted ceramic head [41]. Using metallic sleeves to overlap the cone may provide a "fresh" cone/ceramic interface. It is strongly recommended to exclude the possibility that the retained stem taper is damaged by close gross visual evaluation [41].

5. Increased cost of the prosthesis
6. Demanding surgical technique
7. Concern about instability due to less availability of neck length and liners
8. Stress shielding of the pelvis bone

It applies for all hard on hard THAs, but no studies at the moment have identified loss of bone stock at revision THA.

16.1.3 Reported Results

Previous studies reported less favorable results. Cemented cup fixation was related with disadvantageous results. Iwakiri et al. reported an 8-year survival rate of 90.7% with revision for any reason and 94.4% with revision for alumina failure as the end point for 77 cemented CoC THAs [42]. Hamadouche et al. [17] also evaluated retrospectively 118 CoC THAs at 20 years. Cementless cup survival for any reason was 85.6%, while for cemented cup survival was 61.2%.

Results, however, have been improved during the last years (Fig. 16.1). Survival seems to depend on the implant generation, type, and design of the implant and with fixation and surgical technique (cementless or cemented); thus, the interpretation of studies depends on them [4].

Systematic reviews showed the variable longevity of implants ranging from 73 to 100% at a mean follow-up of 31–240 months [43]. Recently, excellent results with uncemented CoC THAs have been reported [44–46]. In a study from HSS, Molloy et al. [45] reported 98% survival rate for 301 uncemented CoC THAs at ten years. Seo et al. [46] demonstrated 96.5% at 6.5 years for any reason for 301 uncemented third-generation CoC THAs. New-generation ceramic implants showed a survival rate of 92–99% at ten years [44, 47–49]; these are more promising results however not better than reported so far results for MoP.

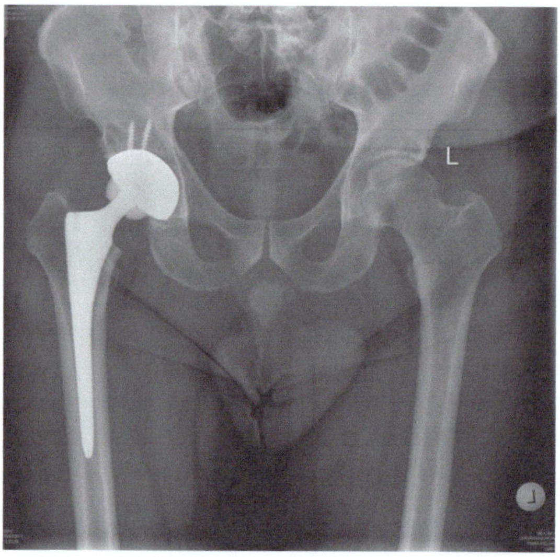

Fig. 16.1 Postoperative radiograph of an uncemented C-C couple in a young physician operated on for osteonecrosis of the femoral head

In a recent meta-analysis, Si et al. [50] evaluated the results of 13 RCTs to compare the outcomes between CoC and CoP; they evaluated a total of 2.488 patients. The wear rate was lower in CoC than CoP THA; however, only 2 out of 13 RCTs gave wear rate results. The incidence of component-related noise and overall ceramic fracture in CoC group were 14.73 times and 6.02 times higher than CoP THA, respectively. There were no significant differences in rates of radiolucent line formation (>1 mm), osteolysis, loosening, revision with follow-up ≥five years, intraoperative femoral fracture, dislocation, deep infection, deep venous thrombosis, and leg length discrepancy between groups. The authors supported that there is no clear evidence of the superiority of CoC to CoP and more high-level studies are needed.

References

1. Hannouche D, Zaoui A, Zadegan F, Sedel L, Nizard R. Thirty years of experience with alumina-on-alumina bearings in total hip arthroplasty. Int Orthop. 2011;35:207–13.
2. Su EP. Ceramic-ceramic bearing: too unpredictable to use it regularly. HSS J. 2012;8:287–90.
3. Massina P, Lopesb R, Massonc B, Mainard D, The French Hip & Knee Society (SFHG). Does Biolox® Delta ceramic reduce the rate of component fractures in total hip replacement? Orthop Traumatol Surg Res. 2014;100:S317–21.
4. Gallo J, Goodmanb SB, Lostaka J, Janouta M. Advantages and disadvantages of ceramic on ceramic total hip arthroplasty: a review. Biomed Pap Med Fac Univ Palacky Olomouc Czech Repub. 2012;156(3):204–12.
5. Williams S, Schepers A, Isaac G, Hardaker C, Ingham E, van der Jagt D, Breckon A, Fisher J. The 2007 Otto Aufranc award. Ceramic-on- metal hip arthroplasties: a comparative in vitro and in vivo study. Clin Orthop Relat Res. 2007;465:23–32.
6. Lusty PJ, Watson A, Tuke MA, Walter WL, Walter WK, Zicat B. Wear and acetabular component orientation in third generation alumina-on- alumina ceramic bearings: an analysis of 33 retrievals. J Bone Joint Surg Br. 2007;89(9):1158–64.
7. Fisher J, Jin Z, Tipper J, Stone M, Ingham E. Tribology of alternative bearings. Clin Orthop Relat Res. 2006;453:25–34.
8. Catelas I, Huk OL, Petit A, Zukor DJ, Marchand R, Yahia L. Flow cytometric analysis of macrophage response to ceramic and poly- ethylene particles: effects of size, concentration, and composition. J Biomed Mater Res. 1998;41(4):600–7.
9. Kubo T, Sawada K, Hirakawa K, Shimizu C, Takamatsu T, Hirasawa Y. Histiocyte reaction in rabbit femurs to UHMWPE, metal, and ceramic particles in different sizes. J Biomed Mater Res. 1999;45(4):363–9.
10. Petit A, Catelas I, Antoniou J, Zukor DJ, Huk OL. Differential apoptotic response of J774 macrophages to alumina and ultra-high-molecular-weight polyethylene particles. J Orthop Res. 2002;20: 9–15.
11. Catelas I, Petit A, Zukor DJ, Marchand R, Yahia L, Huk OL. Induction of macrophage apoptosis by ceramic and polyethylene particles in vitro. Biomaterials. 1999;20(7):625–30.
12. Bohler M, Mochida Y, Bauer TW, Plenk H Jr, Salzer M. Wear debris from two different alumina-on-alumina total hip arthroplasties. J Bone Joint Surg Br. 2000;82:901–9.
13. Brown C, Williams S, Tipper JL, Fisher J, Ingham E. Characterisation of wear particles produced by metal on metal and ceramic on metal hip prostheses under standard and microseparation simulation. J Mater Sci Mater Med. 2007;18:819–82.
14. Fye MA, Huo MH, Zatorski LE, Keggi KJ. Total hip arthroplasty performed without cement in patients with femoral head osteonecrosis who are less than 50 years old. J Arthroplast. 1998;13:876–81.
15. Gualtieri G, Nigrisoli M, Dallari D, Catamo L, Gualtieri I. A study of the mechanical and biological behavior of bioceramic hip arthroplasty followed-up after more than 10 years. Chir Organi Mov. 1993;78:213–22.
16. Huo MH, Martin RP, Zatorski LE, Keggi KJ. Ceramic total hip replacement done without cement. Long term follow-up study. Orthop Trans. 1995;19:400–1.
17. Hamadouche M, Boutin P, Daussange J, Bolander ME, Sedel L. Alumina-on-alumina total hip arthroplasty: a minimum 18.5-year follow-up study. J Bone Joint Surg Am. 2002;84-A:69–7.
18. Hernigou P, Zilber S, Filippini P, Poignard A. Ceramic ceramic bearing decreases osteolysis: a 20-year study versus ceramic-polyethylene on the contralateral hip. Clin Orthop Relat Res. 2009;467:2274–80.
19. Hatton A, Nevelos JE, Matthews JB, Fisher J, Ingham E. Effects of clinically relevant alumina ceramic wear particles on TNF-alpha production by human peripheral blood mononuclear phagocytes. Biomaterials. 2003;24:1193–204.
20. Willmann G. Ceramic femoral head retrieval data. Clin Orthop Relat Res. 2000;379:22–8.
21. Traina F, De Fine M, Bordini B, Toni A. Risk factors for ceramic liner fracture after total hip arthroplasty. Hip Int. 2012;22(06):607–14.
22. Huet R, Sakona A, Kurtz SM. Strength and reliability of alumina ce- ramic femoral heads: review of design, testing, and retrieval analysis. J Mech Behav Biomed Mater. 2011;4(3):476–83.
23. Szymanski C, Gueriot S, Boniface O, Deladerriere JY, Luneau S, Maynou C. Sandwich type ceramic liner fracture rate with the atlas III socket: a study of 144 primary total hip replacements at a mean 74 months' follow-up. Orthop Traumatol Surg Res. 2011;97(5):494–500.
24. Swanson TV, Peterson DJ, Seethala R, Bliss RL, Spellmon CA. Influence of prosthetic design on squeaking after ceramic-on-ceramic total hip arthroplasty. J Arthroplast. 2010;25(Suppl):36–42.
25. Eichmann TH, Clarke IC, Gustafson GA. Squeaking in a ceramic on ceramic total hip. In: Lazannec JY, Dietrich M, editors. Bioceramics in joint arthroplasty. Germany: Steinkopff Verlag; 2004. p. 187–92.
26. Ecker TM, Robbins C, van Flandern G, et al. Squeaking in total hip replacement: no cause for concern. Orthopedics. 2008;31:875–6. 84
27. Walter WL, Lusty PJ, Watson A, et al. Stripe wear and squeaking in ceramic Total hip bearings. Semin Arthroplast. 2006;17:190–5.
28. Taylor S, Manley MT, Sutton K. The role of stripe wear in causing acoustic emissions from alumina ceramic-on-ceramic bearings. J Arthroplast. 2007;22(7 Suppl 3):47–51.
29. Glaser D, Komistek RD, Cates HE, Mahfouz MR. Clicking and squeak- ing: in vivo correlation of

sound and separation for different bearing surfaces. J Bone Joint Surg Am. 2008;90(Suppl 4):112–20.
30. Chevillotte C, Trousdale RT, Chen Q, Guyen O, An KN. The 2009 frank Stinchfield award: "hip squeaking": a biome- chanical study of ceramic-on-ceramic bearing surfaces. Clin Orthop Relat Res. 2010;468:345–50.
31. Nevelos J, Ingham E, Doyle C, Streicher R, Nevelos A, Walter W, Fisher J. Microseparation of the centers of alumina-alumina artificial hip joints during simulator testing produces clinically relevant wear rates and patterns. J Arthroplast. 2000;15:793–5.
32. Parvizi J, Adeli B, Wong JC, Restrepo C, Rothman RH. A squeaky reputation: the problem may be design-dependent. Clin Orthop Relat Res. 2011;469(6):1598–605.
33. Restrepo C, Post ZD, Kai B, Hozack WJ. The effect of stem design on the prevalence of squeaking following ceramic-on-ceramic bearing total hip arthroplasty. J Bone Joint Surg Am. 2010;92(3):550–7.
34. Owen H. An estimation of the incidence of squeaking and revision surgery for squeaking in ceramic-on-ceramic total hip replacement a meta-analysis and report from the Australian d., orthopaedic association national joint registry. Bone Joint J. 2014;96-B:181–7.
35. Park YS, Park SJ, Lim SJ. Ten-year results after cementless THA with a sandwich-type alumina ceramic bearing. Orthopedics. 2010;33(11):796.
36. Sugano N, Takao M, Sakai T, Nishii T, Miki H, Ohzono K. Eleven- to 14-year follow-up results of cementless total hip arthroplasty using a third-generation alumina ceramic-on-ceramic bearing. J Arthroplast. 2012;27(5):736–41.
37. Chevillotte C, Pibarot V, Carret JP, Bejui-Hugues J, Guyen O. Nine years follow-up of 100 ceramic-on-ceramic total hip arthroplasty. Int Orthop. 2011;35(11):1599–604.
38. Jarrett CA, Ranawat AS, Bruzzone M, Blum YC, Rodriguez JA, Ranawat CS. The squeaking hip: a phenomenon of ceramic-on-ceramic total hip arthroplasty. J Bone Joint Surg Am. 2009;91(6):1344–9.
39. Stanat SJ, Capozzi JD. Squeaking in third- and fourth-generation ceramic-onceramic total hip arthroplasty: meta-analysis and systematic review. J Arthroplast. 2012;27:445–53.
40. Stafford GH, Islam SU, Witt JD. Early to mid-term results of ceramic- on-ceramic total hip replacement: analysis of bearing-surface-related complications. J Bone Joint Surg Br. 2011;93(8):1017–20.
41. Hannouche D, Delambre J, Zadegan F, Sedel L, Nizard R. Is there a risk in placing a ceramic head on a previously implanted trunion? Clin Orthop Relat Res. 2010;468(12):3322–7.
42. Iwakiri K, Iwaki H, Minoda Y, Ohashi H, Takaoka K. Alumina inlay failure in cemented polyethylene-backed total hip arthroplasty. Clin Orthop Relat Res. 2008;466(5):1186–92.
43. Zywiel MG, Sayeed SA, Johnson AJ, Schmalzried TP, Mont MA. Survival of hard-on-hard bearings in total hip arthroplasty: a sys- tematic review. Clin Orthop Relat Res. 2011;469(6):1536–46.
44. Kress AM, Schmidt R, Holzwarth U, Forst R, Mueller LA. Excellent results with cementless total hip arthroplasty and alumina-on-alumina pairing: minimum ten-year follow-up. Int Orthop. 2011;35(2):195–200.
45. Molloy D, Jack C, Esposito C, Walter WL. A mid-term analysis suggests ceramic on ceramic hip Arthroplasty is durable with minimal wear and low risk of squeak. HSS J. 2012;8:291–4.
46. Seo BH, Ryu DJ, Kang JS, Kyoung H. Primary total hip arthroplasty using 3rd generation ceramic-on-ceramic articulation moon. Hip Int. 2016;26(5):468–73.
47. D'Antonio JA, Capello WN, Naughton M. Ceramic bearings for total hip arthroplasty have high survivorship at 10 years. Clin Orthop Relat Res. 2012;470(2):373–81.
48. Boyer P, Huten D, Loriaut P, Lestrat V, Jeanrot C, Massin P. Is aluminaon-alumina ceramic bearings total hip replacement the right choice in patients younger than 50 years of age? A 7- to 15-year follow-up study. Orthop Traumatol Surg Res. 2010;96(6):616–22.
49. Lee YK, Ha YC, Yoo JJ, Koo KH, Yoon KS, Kim HJ. Alumina-on-alumina total hip arthroplasty: a concise follow-up, at a minimum of ten years, of a previous report. J Bone Joint Surg Am. 2010;92(8):1715–9.
50. Si H-b, Zeng Y, Cao F, Pei F-x, Shen B. Is a ceramic-on-ceramic bearing really superior to ceramic-on-polyethylene for primary total hip arthroplasty? A systematic review and meta-analysis of randomised controlled trials. Hip Int. 2015;25(3):191–8.

17 Tumor Resection

Eustathios Kenanidis, Panagiotis Kakoulidis, Eleftherios Tsiridis, Anthony Viste, Michael J. Taunton, Mathew P. Abdel, Simon Cowie, and Richard P. Baker

17.1 Current Concepts

E. Kenanidis, P. Kakoulidis, and E. Tsiridis

The proximal femur is a typical anatomic location for primary malignant or benign tumors and metastatic disease [1, 2]. The improvement of the surgical management of tumors of the proximal femur amalgamated with advances in the field of neoadjuvant chemotherapy, and radiotherapy further improved the patients' function and quality of life during the last yearsHindquarter amputation remains an option especially for aggressive sarcomas of the proximal femur; however, limb salvage is now more than ever a feasible option [2]. Reconstructive surgery is the method of choice to achieve limb salvage and retention of function [3].

Proximal femoral reconstruction (PFR) has definitive benefits in the treatment of patients with low-grade pathology who have undergone curative resection margin surgery, offering a good to an excellent functional outcome and survival rates over 90%. The main reconstructive options for PFR are allograft–prosthesis composites [4–8] and custom [9–11] or modular megaprostheses [1, 6, 12–16].

Several tertiary orthopaedic oncology units provided level III or IV evidence studies of proximal femoral reconstruction for primary

E. Kenanidis, M.D., Ph.D., M.Sc. (✉) · P. Kakoulidis, M.D.
Academic Orthopaedic Unit, Aristotle University Medical School, Thessaloniki, Greece

E. Tsiridis, M.D., Ph.D., F.A.C.S., F.R.C.S. (✉)
Academic Orthopaedic Unit, Papageorgiou General Hospital, Aristotle University Medical School, Thessaloniki, Greece
e-mail: etsiridis@doctors.org.uk

A. Viste, M.D., Ph.D.
Hospices Civils de Lyon, CHU Lyon Sud, Lyon, France

Service de Chirurgie Orthopédique et Traumatologique, Lyon, France

M.J. Taunton, M.D. · M.P. Abdel, M.D.
Department of Orthopaedic Surgery, Mayo Clinic College of Medicine, Mayo Clinic, Rochester, MN, USA
e-mail: Taunton.Michael@mayo.edu; Abdel.Matthew@mayo.edu

S. Cowie, M.R.C.S., B.M.B.S., B.Med.Sci.
Southmead Hospital, North Bristol Trust, Bristol, UK

R.P. Baker, M.D., M.Sc., M.B.ChB., F.R.C.S
Avon Orthopaedic Centre, Southmead Hospital, North Bristol NHS Trust, Bristol, UK

E. Tsiridis (ed.), *The Adult Hip - Master Case Series and Techniques*, https://doi.org/10.1007/978-3-319-64177-5_17

malignant or benign bone tumors [1, 2, 12, 14, 17–24]. The sample size range from 20 to 150 patients with a mean follow-up from 2 to 12 years and patient's age from 2 to 88 years. The origin of metastatic lesions is either the lung or breast, and the main primary malignant bone tumor is osteosarcoma [1, 2, 12, 14, 17, 18–26].

The survival of the prostheses depends on many parameters including the age of patients, the type of tumor, benign or malignant, the presence or absence of metastases, etc. Following clearance of a tumor at the margin and adjuvant therapy, the reported survival ranged from 47 to 97% [1, 2, 14, 17–21, 26]. Effective adjuvant treatments have improved the survival and the limb salvage rates in patients with malignancies. Although the majority of studies mentioned the use of adjuvant chemotherapy and radiotherapy in patients, they don't, however, give details of the protocol followed, the inclusion criteria and length of follow-up, making comparison difficult [3].

The types of implants used in each study also vary depending on the patient's age, the implant and allograft availability and cost, as well as the surgeon expertise [3]. There is ongoing debate concerning the most appropriate type of implant for young patients who have a disease-free acetabulum. The unipolar endoprosthesis is considered the treatment of choice in these patients to permit further acetabular development [17, 26]. Instability is the main reason for concern and failure [17, 26]. Van Kampen et al. [26] reported results of 40 hip replacements in children between 2 and 15 years old for malignant disease. Unipolar proximal femoral arthroplasty failed in all children at ten years mainly due to pain or subluxation. The total PFR in older children was considered an appropriate alternative to offer additional stability [17, 26].

Allograft–prosthetic composites, compared to mega-prostheses, restore the bone stock and offer a tendon reattachment and presumably superior function [2, 3]. The high complication rate however due to infections, nonunions, and fractures usually overcome the advantages. The modular prostheses are the implant of choice for PFA. They offer long-term survival; they are more cost-effective and steadily available and thus reduce the time of surgery and the risk of complications from bed rest compared to custom-made prostheses [1, 2, 14, 17, 19, 22, 24–26]. A hemiarthroplasty offers additional stability compared to total PFA [1, 14, 19, 26]. It is considered beneficial in elderly patients or patients with metastasis with a life expectancy fewer than five years [3]. Appropriate abductor repair or direct repair on the allograft–prosthesis composite, constrained liners, or dual mobility cups may further reduce the risk of dislocation.

The results of patients with a primary malignant disease are much better than those with metastatic pathology [2, 19]. Chandrasekar et al. [19] reported the results of 131 cemented unipolar PFR in patients with primary malignant or metastatic disease. The survival rate was 82.3% for one year and 44.2% at five years for patients with primary malignant process compared to 55.3% and 12%, respectively, in patients with metastases.

The overall revision rate following PFA is usually higher compared with primary total hip arthroplasty [2, 3]. Deep infection, fracture, dislocation, and aseptic loosening are the main complications of endoprosthesis [27]. Other reasons for reoperation include the need for conversion from bipolar/unipolar to total PFR in a young patient to decrease the risk of instability and improve functional results [17, 26]. In older adults with bipolar PFR and pain from an acetabular protrusion, a revision to either a cemented or uncemented acetabular component is usually needed. Local tumor recurrences [1, 14, 19, 24, 26] require revision surgery, limb amputation, or no further surgery due to advanced disease and poor prognosis.

Dislocations were more common in patients with total PFR compared to a bipolar or unipolar prosthesis and usually treated with closed reduction [1, 18, 21]. Malnutrition, long duration of surgery, chemotherapy, multiple previous operations, irradiated soft tissue, and local soft tissue condition are all well-known risk factors for infection in these patients [1, 14, 18, 19, 21, 24]. Infection is managed with a two-stage-procedure with a good outcome. Prolonged suppressive antibiotic treatment or excisional arthroplasty or amputation are options in more burdened patients [1, 14, 19, 24, 28]. Jacofsky et al. [28] reported four infections out of 42 THA made for the salvage of failed treatment of pathological proximal femoral fractures. Three patients underwent resection arthroplasty, and one experienced debridement as well as one stage reimplantation. Sokolovski et al. [18] also reported six cases of late infection in a series of 44 patients. Four of these cases were treated conservatively with antibiotics, while in the other two a revision endoprosthesis hip replacement was performed.

Symptomatic leg length discrepancy (>2 cm), venous thromboembolic events, and sciatic nerve palsy are other reported complications [2, 14, 17, 19, 26]. The use of extendable proximal femoral arthroplasties diminishes the risk in the pediatric population [26].

17.2 Case Title: Primary Total Hip Arthroplasty Following Oncologic Resection

A. Viste, M.J. Taunton, and
M.P. Abdel

17.2.1 Demographics

Age: 51 years
Sex: Female
BMI: 27 kg/m2

17.2.2 Relevant Past Medical History

Principal pathologies: Metastatic adenoid cystic carcinoma with multiple bony, lung, and soft tissue metastases.

Previous surgical procedures: Tumor debulkings, cryoablation, and cementoplasty of the right acetabulum.

Medication: Methadone, hydromorphone, intrathecal infusion device.

History of Presenting Complaint: Metastasis to the right hip (femur and acetabulum) with pathologic femoral neck and posterior column fractures.

17.2.3 Clinical Examination

Symptoms: Significant pain in the right groin and thigh for the past year with inability to ambulate.

Range of motion: 0–90 degrees of flexion, −20 degrees of internal rotation, 5 degrees of external rotation, 10 degrees of abduction, no adduction.

Specific tests: Log rolling test positive; Stinchfield's test positive.

Main disability: Unable to bear weight; wheelchair bound.

Neurovascular evaluation: Quadriceps and iliopsoas are weak with 2/5 strength. Otherwise, neurovascularly intact.

17.2.4 Preoperative Radiological Assessment/Imaging (Figs. 17.1, 17.2, and 17.3)

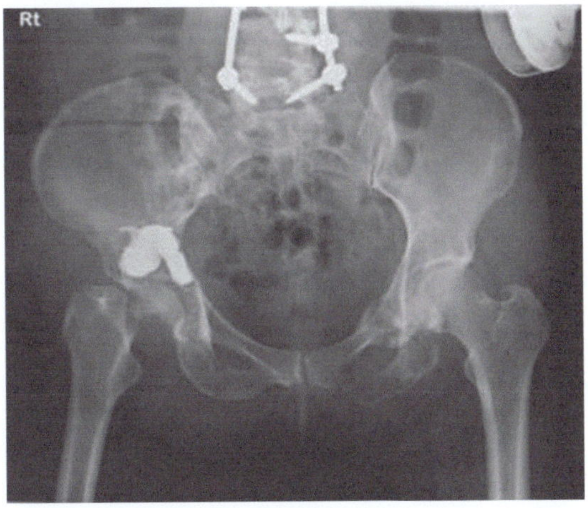

Fig. 17.1 AP pelvis radiograph: reveals lytic lesions of the right femoral head and neck with pathologic fracture, cementoplasty in the acetabulum, and large supra-acetabular lytic lesion

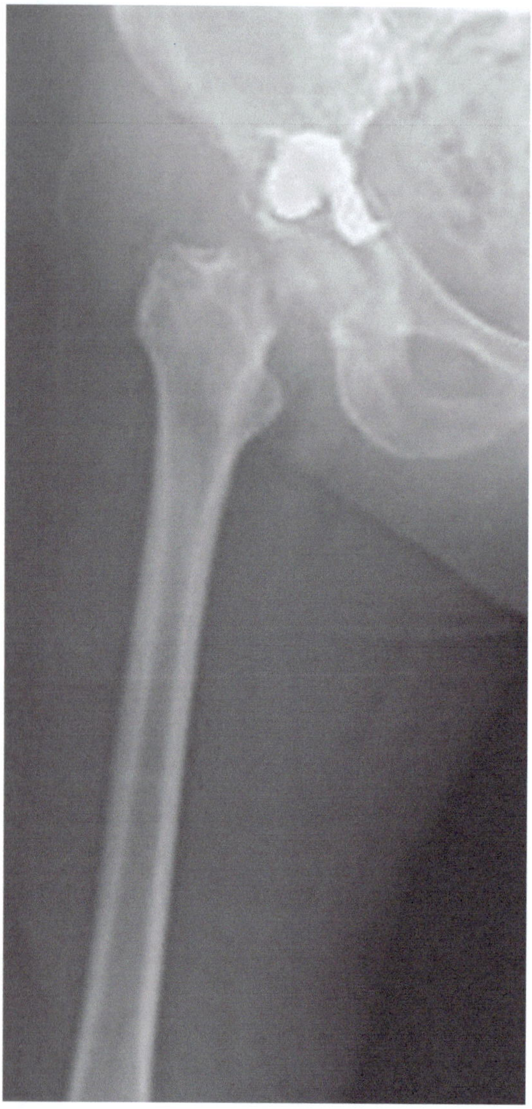

Fig. 17.2 AP right hip: radiograph reveals no additional metastatic lesions in the femur

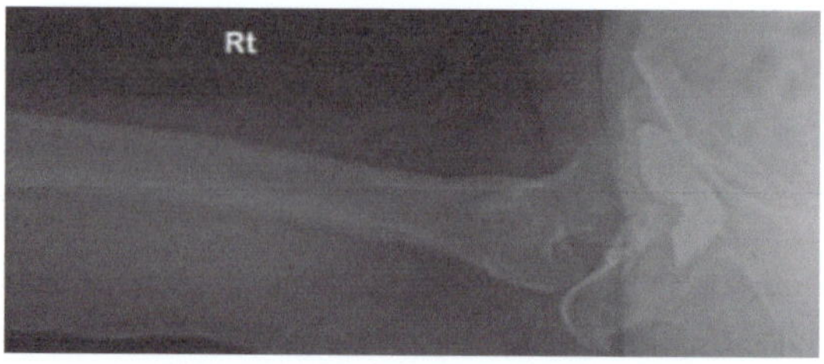

Fig. 17.3 Cross-table lateral of right hip: radiograph completed prior to pathologic femoral neck fracture reveals cementoplasty in the acetabulum and a pathologic fracture through the posterior column

17.2.5 Preoperative Planning

Diagnosis: Pathologic fracture of the posterior column and femoral neck secondary to metastatic disease (Figs. 17.1, 17.2 and 17.3).

Possible treatment options: Hemiarthroplasty, Girdlestone procedure, complex acetabular reconstruction with cup–cage construct and total hip arthroplasty (THA).

Chosen treatment method: Complex acetabular reconstruction with cup–cage construct and THA.

Selection of implants if applicable and rational: Highly porous tantalum acetabular component with multiple superior and inferior screws, tantalum augments, reinforcement cage, considering larger femoral head vs dual-mobility construct (high risk of dislocation), considering uncemented femoral stem if acceptable bone quality.

Expected difficulties: Massive acetabular bone loss, posterior column pathologic fracture, previous cementoplasty, prior pelvic radiation inhibiting bone ingrowth and soft tissue quality, pathologic femoral neck fracture increasing risk of instability.

Strategies to overcome difficulties: Highly porous tantalum acetabular component, multiple supplemental screws both superiorly and inferiorly, tantalum augments, reinforcement cage, larger femoral head.

Templating: Template size of the acetabular component in the anatomic location to determine if tantalum augments are required. Templating also assists with limb lengths

17.2.6 Surgical Note

Patient's position: Lateral decubitus.

Type of anesthesia: General endotracheal anesthesia and psoas block.

Surgical approach: Posterolateral.

Main steps: Complete pathologic femoral neck fracture; removal of femoral head; superb acetabular exposure; removal of previous cement in acetabulum; debulk tumor; assess the presence of pelvic discontinuity by moving superior and inferior halves of acetabulum; evaluate the bone loss; touch ream to the bleeding bone; determine the need for superior and posterior tantalum augments; place augments with screws; place acetabular component in optimal orientation; cement must be placed between augments and acetabular component to unitize; place multiple screws (6–10) in acetabular component superiorly and inferiorly; attempt to place screws through cup, augment, and into the host bone; optimize stability with large femoral head or dual-mobility construct; long cemented stem if multiple metastatic lesions in femur or if radiated femur (otherwise, uncemented is acceptable).

Reconstruction techniques: Tantalum revision acetabular component; multiple superior and inferior screws; tantalum augments; reinforcement cage with screws through cage, cup, and into the host bone; 36 mm polyethylene liner cemented in place; uncemented stem (Figs. 17.4 and 17.5).

17.2.7 Intraoperative Challenges

Challenges and solutions: Posterior wall defect treated with tantalum augment combined with pathologic pelvic discontinuity treated with superior and inferior screws through acetabular component and reinforcement cage.

Unanticipated problems and solution: See above.

Thorough description of decision-making, including the reason for the final decision: See above.

17.2.8 Postoperative Radiographs (Figs. 17.4 and 17.5)

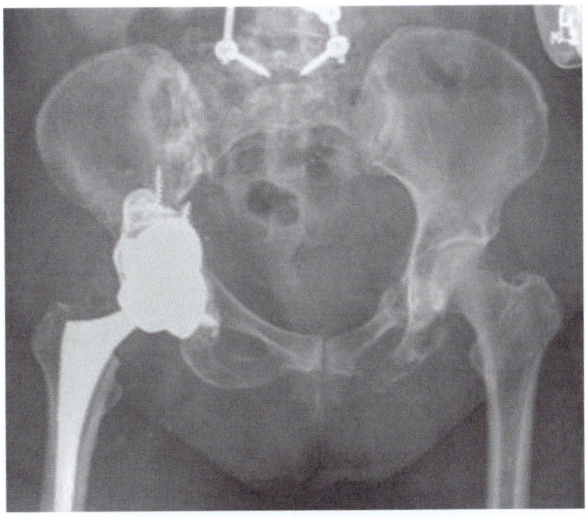

Fig. 17.4 AP pelvis radiograph: postoperative radiograph depicting massive acetabular reconstruction with tantalum acetabular component and augments, supplemental screws, reinforcement cage, and uncemented stem

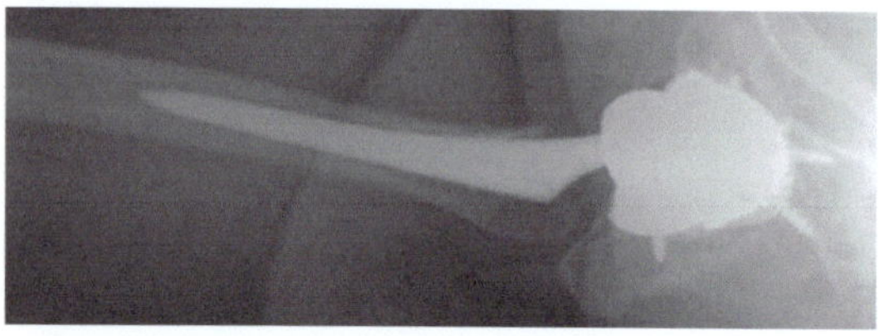

Fig. 17.5 Cross-table lateral of right hip: this radiograph is particularly helpful to reveal the position of the acetabular component and placement of multiple supplemental screws

17.2.9 Postoperative Management

Chemoprophylaxis and anticoagulant treatment period: Warfarin for 12 weeks, sequential compression devices, and encouraged ambulation.

Gait/limb loading until full loading: Partial weight bearing for three months.

17.2.10 Follow-Up and Complications

No complications.

17.2.11 Discussion

Advantages of the applied method: A solid initial mechanical construct that allows for biologic fixation even in cases of radiation, pathologic lesions, and pelvic discontinuities.

Disadvantages of the method: Risk of postoperative instability and deep periprosthetic infection.

Alternative evidence-based techniques for the case: Girdlestone arthroplasty, Harrington technique, use of a cemented stem.

Why the chosen technique is better for this case? See above.

Indications and contraindications for your technique: Metastatic or primary oncologic processes of the acetabulum and pelvic discontinuities.

Learning curve and how to manage complications: Requires a surgeon who completes a large volume of revision procedures, as well as availability of all revision implants.

Level of evidence concerning the superiority of this method against others: See references [29–31].

17.3 Case Title: A Surgical Technique for Salvage of a Failed Femoral Intercalary Spacer

Simon Cowie and Richard Baker

17.3.1 Demographics

Age: 48 years old
Sex: Female
BMI: 24

17.3.2 Relevant Past Medical History

Principal pathologies: High-grade pleomorphic liposarcoma.

Previous surgical procedures: Primary surgical procedure—mid-diaphyseal resection of the femur and subsequent intercalary diaphyseal endoprosthesis (OsteoBridge IDSF, Merete®20, USA). Excision of a 12.3 cm mid-diaphyseal femoral segment. Proximally a 12 × 110 mm and distally 12 × 130 mm stems had been fixed in situ using Palacos R-G PMMA cement (Heraeus Medical GmbH, Germany) and two locking screws proximally and distally. The intercalary body had been built to 130 mm (using a 70mm and 60mm body) and assembled with accurate rotational alignment and leg length under image intensifier control. A gracilis transfer flap was utilized to fill the soft tissue defect. Confirmed on histological examination, clear margins, and 100% necrosis of the lesion.

Medication: Simple analgesia.

Other: Preoperative radiotherapy before the primary procedure. Before the revision surgery, the patient was restaged showing no local or distant recurrence of malignancy.

History of presenting complaint: Initial presentation—3-month history of growing, focal, mid-thigh pain, and swelling with worsening tolerance of ambulation and knee bend after the primary intercalary spacer. No systemic symptoms identified. Subsequent presentation—11 months postoperatively the patient was referred to our orthopedic unit with “knee instability.”

17.3.3 Clinical Examination

Symptoms: Mid-thigh pain with radiation to the knee, "knee instability."

Range of motion: Full passive range of movement hip and knee joints; however, clear evidence of uncontrollable rotational instability between the proximal and distal femur.

Specific tests: Nil required.

Main disability: Pain (ambulatory). "Knee instability" during gait. Uncontrollable rotational instability between the proximal and distal femur.

Neurovascular evaluation: Complete neurological examination grossly intact lower limb. Except L3 power MRC 4/5 to affected limb presumed secondary to pain.

17.3.4 Preoperative Radiological Assessment/Imaging (Figs. 17.6 and 17.7)

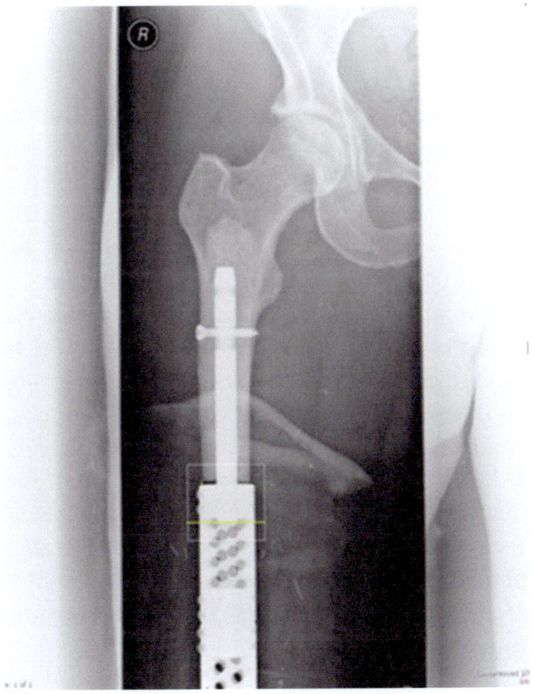

Fig. 17.6 Postprimary surgery indicating gap between proximal femur and intercalary device with distal part proximal stem at level of first holes

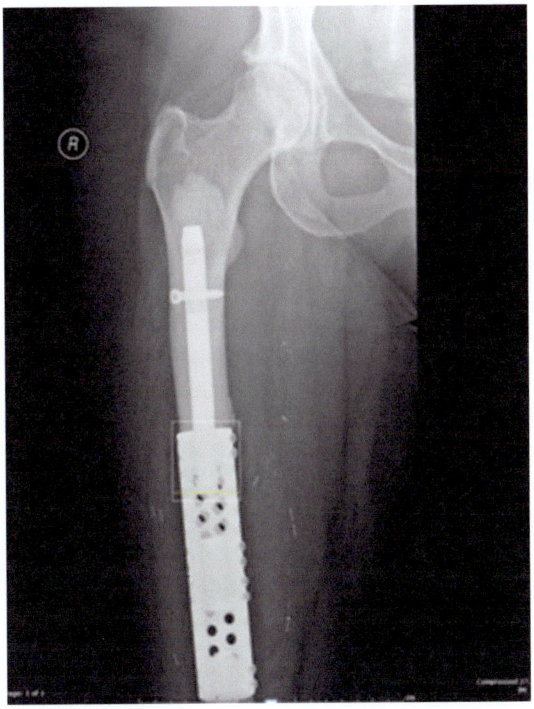

Fig. 17.7 Failed intercalary space with loss of gap and telescoping of the proximal stem to the level of third holes. Radiographic evidence of failed intercalary device

17.3.5 Preoperative Planning

Diagnosis: Failed femoral intercalary spacer at the junction of its body and proximal stem. Likely attributable to the implant appearing not seated against the bone proximally on the immediate postoperative radiographs and therefore led to subsidence of the stem in the proximal body (Figs. 17.6 and 17.7).

Possible treatment options: (1) Revision diaphyseal endoprosthesis. (2) Revision diaphyseal endoprosthesis with orthogonal plating. (3) Vascularized autografting. (4) Allograft.

Chosen treatment method: Revision diaphyseal endoprosthesis with orthogonal plating.

Selection of implants if applicable and rational: Intercalary diaphyseal endoprosthesis (OsteoBridge IDSF, Merete®20, USA). Primary surgery used this system. Two orthogonal plates (AXSOS, Stryker, USA) were chosen for rotational stability.

Expected difficulties: (1) Removal of matt cemented intercalary spacer stems if required. A significant challenge could be encountered in trying to remove the stemmed components with risk of fracture, the need to bivalve the femur leading to a risk of secondary fracture, and potential nonunion and increased morbidity associated with prolonged surgical time. (2) Possible further femoral resection. (3) Rotational control. (4) Development of construct to tolerate load, strain, and reproduction of similar characteristics as pre-existing bony tissue to withstand forces and full weight bearing postoperatively for accelerated rehabilitation. (5) Consideration of failure secondary to infection (no preoperative suspicion). (6) Recurrence of high-grade pleomorphic liposarcoma.

Strategies to overcome difficulties: (1) If well fixed, leave the original stems in situ. (2) Total femoral replacement would be the preferred option. (3) Orthogonal plating to control rotational instability. (4) Replace intercalary spacer bodies; tighten all screws as per manufacturer guidelines and orthogonal plate. (5) Multiple intraoperative microbiology sampling for enrichment and extended cultures. (6) Histological specimens for recurrence.

Templating: Nil required as known sizes of the intercalary system from previous surgery (stem and intercalary body). Preoperative planning identified no apparent tumor recurrence (MRI—proviso artifact in tissues near implant) or fracture, and an X-ray revealed good bone stock; therefore total femoral replacement not indicated.

17.3.6 Surgical Note

Patient's position: Supine. Radiolucent table.

Type of anesthesia: General anesthesia with spinal.

Surgical approach: Direct lateral through the old incision with a lifting of local gracilis flap.

Main steps: (1) Intraoperative assessment for reconstruction planning. Identified; (a) a significant fluid-filled cavity heavily stained with titanium debris encasing the implant. Multiple microbiology samples sent (nb subsequent microbiology tests all negative at extended culture). Histology negative for tumor recurrence but confirmed metal debris. (b) Failure of the mid-diaphyseal intercalary spacer at the level of the proximal body and proximal cemented stem interface causing rotation around its axis and telescoping of up to 15 mm.

The intercalary spacer stems are matt coated and were found to be well fixed at revision surgery. We opted to leave the stems in situ due to the significant potential difficulties in removing them. (2) Reconstruction and stabilization.

Reconstruction techniques: The loose intercalary spacer body was removed and replaced with a repeat 70mm and 60mm bodies with its 16 screws tightened as per manufacturer guidelines. Two orthogonal plates were sited anteriorly and laterally under image intensifier guidance to control rotation, reinforce construct stability and to prevent a repeated implant failure (Fig. 17.8).

17.3.7 Intraoperative Challenges

Challenges and solutions: (1) Rotational control and construct stability—orthogonal anterior and lateral plating supporting reconstructed intercalary body. The majority of intraoperative challenges had been identified as part of the preoperative planning. See comments below.

Unanticipated problems and solution: Nil specific to this case. We would strongly highlight the need for preoperative planning and consideration of surgical technique for loose stem removal if evident intraoperatively. Differing surgical procedure in the form of further femoral resection and total femoral replacement should be considered if preoperative planning CT/MRI identified potential tumor recurrence and further bony involvement requiring resection.

Thorough description of decision-making, including the reason for the final decision: Thorough surgical preoperative planning and assessment (outlined above) meant likely surgical plan for stem stability evaluation and, if well integrated, change of intercalary bodies only if well fixed, and orthogonal plating for rotational stability and construct strength. Plating was considered essential as the body stem junction had already failed previously in a short time, and we didn't wish to rely on the same construct. Given the well-fixed stems and no clinical evidence of further sarcoma involvement (including preoperative radiographic evidence), additional femoral resection was not required. Allograft treatment would have increased surgical morbidity with no expected long-term gain and a higher chance of construct failure before its incorporation. Stability and construct strength/durability was the main aim for accelerated rehabilitation, full ambulation, and early discharge from the hospital.

17.3.8 Postoperative Radiographs (Fig. 17.8)

17.3.9 Postoperative Management

Chemoprophylaxis and anticoagulant treatment period: Enoxaparin 40 mg until discharged from hospital (28 days total)

Gait/limb loading until full loading: Full weight bearing with no restrictions to physiotherapy from day 1 postoperatively.

17.3.10 Follow-Up and Complications

No immediate, short-term, or medium-term follow-up complications were identified during admission or formal clinic reviews.

17.3.11 Discussion

Advantages of the applied method: (1) Reduced surgical morbidity. (2) Reduced chance of construct

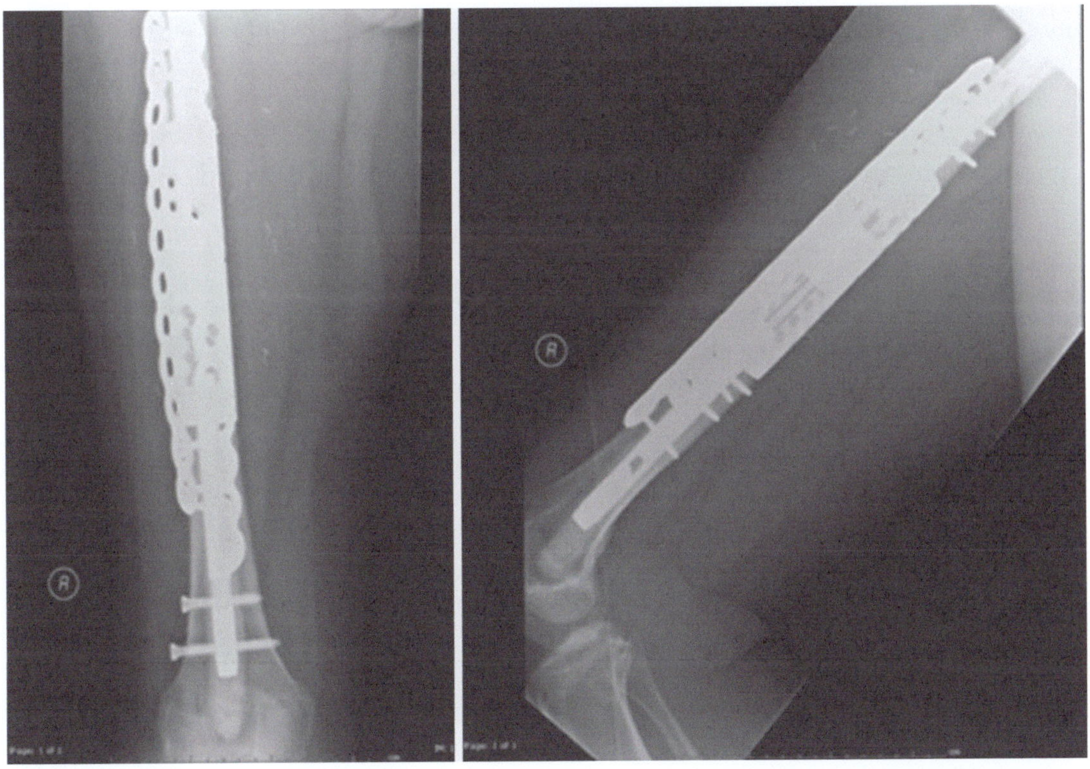

Fig. 17.8 Postrevision AP/LAT radiographs with revised intercalary spacer and orthogonal plate fixation. Radiographic evidence of revision technique

failure as a multi-planar control. (3) Eliminated concerns are nonunion through bivalving femur or autografting. (4) Accelerated full weight-bearing rehabilitation postoperatively.

Disadvantages of the method: (1) Increased risk of periprosthetic fracture and possible infection compared to revision intercalary spacer only.

Alternative evidence-based techniques for the case: Multiple options for segmental reconstruction exist. Examples include diaphyseal endoprosthesis [32, 33] vascularized autografts [34], allografts [35, 36], and total femoral replacement. One must be aware at primary surgery that endoprosthesis failure is also widely documented in the literature [32, 33, 35].

Why is the chosen technique better for this case? Failure can often be attributed to either mechanical (fixation stability) or biological (graft integration) failures. Mechanical and biological failures often arise from the insufficient stability of the initial fixation. For prevention of repeated construct failure and increased rotational control, we would recommend additional orthogonal plating in revision for a failure of the primary surgical fixation in this way.

Indications and contraindications for your technique: Indications—(1) revision surgery for failed intercalary space with well-fixed stems. Contraindications—(1) no contraindications identified.

Learning curve and how to manage complications: We describe a simple yet effective technique to achieve anatomic and functional reconstruction with minimal additional morbidity associated with the revision of a failed intercalary spacer. If a recurrent failure of intercalary spacers is apparent in the literature, then the question remains whether the addition of orthogonal plates should be considered as part of the primary surgery.

Level of evidence concerning the superiority of this method against others: None available.

References

1. Menendez LR, Ahlmann ER, Kermani C, Gotha H. Endoprosthetic reconstruction for neoplasms of the proximal femur. Clin Orthop Relat Res. 2006;450:46–51.
2. Potter B, Chow V, Adams S, Letson GD, Temple HT. Endoprosthetic proximal femur replacement: metastatic versus primary tumours. Surg Oncol. 2009;18(4):343.
3. Thambapillary S, Dimitriou R, Makridis KG, Fragkakis EM, Bobak P, Giannoudis PV. Implant longevity, complications and functional outcome following proximal femoral Arthroplasty for musculoskeletal tumors: a systematic review. J Arthroplast. 2013;28(8):1381–5.
4. Fox EJ, Hau MA, Gebhardt MC, Hornicek FJ, Tomford WW, Mankin HJ. Long-term follow-up of proximal femoral allografts. Clin Orthop Relat Res. 2002;397:106–13.
5. Donati D, Giacomini S, Gozzi E, Mercuri M. Proximal femur reconstruction by an allograft prosthesis composite. Clin Orthop Relat Res. 2002;394:192–200.
6. Farid Y, Lin PP, Lewis VO, Yasko AW. Endoprosthetic and allograft–prosthetic composite reconstruction of the proximal femur for bone neoplasms. Clin Orthop Relat Res. 2006;442:223–9.
7. McGoveran BM, Davis AM, Gross AE, Bell RS. Evaluation of the allograft–prosthesis composite technique for proximal femoral reconstruction after resection of a primary bone tumour. Can J Surg. 1999;42(1):37–45.
8. Zehr RJ, Enneking WF, Scarborough MT. Allograft–prosthesis composite versus megaprosthesis in proximal femoral reconstruction. Clin Orthop Relat Res. 1996;322:207–23.
9. Kabukcuoglu Y, Grimer RJ, Tillman RM, Carter SR. Endoprosthetic replacement for primary malignant tumors of the proximal femur. Clin Orthop Relat Res. 1999;358:8–14.
10. Unwin PS, Cannon SR, Grimer RJ, Kemp HBS, Sneath RS, Walker PS. Aseptic loosening in cemented custom-made prosthetic replacements for bone tumours of the lower limb. J Bone Joint Surg Br. 1996;78(1):5–13.
11. Bickels J, Meller I, Henshaw RM, Malawer MM. Reconstruction of hip stability after proximal and total femur resections. Clin Orthop Relat Res. 2000;375:218–30.
12. Donati D, Zavatta M, Gozzi E, Giacomini S, Campanacci L, Mercuri M. Modular prosthetic replacement of the proximal femur after resection of

a bone tumour: a long-term follow-up. J Bone Joint Surg Br. 2001;83(8):1156–60.
13. Finstein JL, King JJ, Fox EJ, Ogilvie CM, Lackman RD. Bipolar proximal femoral replacement prostheses for musculoskeletal neoplasms. Clin Orthop Relat Res. 2007;459:66–75.
14. Ogilvie CM, Wunder JS, Ferguson PC, Griffin AM, Bell RS. Functional outcome of endoprosthetic proximal femur replacement. Clin Orthop Relat Res. 2004;426:44–8.
15. Sharma S, Turcotte RE, Isler MH, Wong C. Experience with cemented large segment endoprostheses for tumors. Clin Orthop Relat Res. 2007;459:54–9.
16. Zeegin EN, Aponte-Tinao LA, Hornicek FJ, Gebhardt MC, Mankin HJ. Survivorship analysis of 141 modular metallic endoprostheses at early follow-up. Clin Orthop Relat Res. 2004;420:239–50.
17. Chandrasekar C, Grimer R, Carter S, Tillmann RM, Abudu A, Jeys LM. Unipolar proximal femoral endoprosthetic replacement for tumour. The risk of revision in young patients. J Bone Joint Surg Br. 2009;91:401–4.
18. Sokolovski V, Voloshin V, Aliev M, Zubikov VS, Saravanan SA, Martynenko DV, Nisichenko DV, Strelnikov KN. Total hip replacement for proximal femoral tumours: our midterm results. Int Orthop. 2006;30(5):399–402.
19. Chandrasekar C, Grimer R, Carter S, et al. Modular endoprosthetic replacement for tumours of the proximal femur. J Bone Joint Surg Br. 2009;91(1):108.
20. Langlais F, Lambotte J, Colin P, et al. Long-term results of allograft composite total hip prostheses for tumours. Clin Orthop Relat Res. 2003;414:197.
21. Gosheger G, Hillmann A, Lindner N, et al. Soft tissue reconstruction of megaprosthesis using a trevira tube. Clin Orthop Relat Res. 2001;393:264.
22. Bruns J, Delling G, Gruber H, et al. Cementless fixation of megaprosthesis using a conical fluted stem in the treatment of bone tumours. J Bone Joint Surg Br. 2007;89(8):1084.
23. Holt G, Christie M, Schwartz H. Trabecular metal endoprosthetic limb salvage reconstruction of the lower limb. J Arthroplasty. 2009;24(7):1079.
24. Orlic D, Smerdelj M, Kolundzic R, et al. Lower limb salvage surgery: modular endoprosthesis in bone tumour treatment. Int Orthop. 2006;30(6):458.
25. Hattori H, Mibe J, Matsuoka H, et al. Surgical management of metastatic disease of the proximal femur. J Orthop Surg. 2007;15(3):295.
26. van Kampen M, Grimer R, Carter S, et al. Replacement of the hip in children with a tumour in the proximal part of the femur. J Bone Joint Surg Am. 2008;90(4):785.
27. Graci C, Maccauro G, Mura Torp F, Spinelli MS, Rosa MA, Fabbriciani C. Infection following bone tumor resection and reconstruction with tumoral prostheses: a literature review. Int J Immunopathol Pharmacol. 2010;23(4):1005–13.
28. Jacofsky OJ, Haidukewych GJ, Zhang H, Sim FH. Complication and results of arthroplasty for savage of failed treatment of malignant pathologic fractures of the hip. Clin Orthop Relat Res. 2004;427:52–6.
29. Joglekar SB, Rose PS, Lewallen DG, Sim FH. Tantalum acetabular cups provide secure fixation in THA after pelvic irradiation at minimum 5-year followup. Clin Orthop Relat Res. 2012;470(11):3041–7.
30. Khan FA, Rose PS, Yanagisawa M, Lewallen DG, Sim FH. Surgical technique: Porous tantalum reconstruction for destructive nonprimary periacetabular tumors. Clin Orthop Relat Res. 2012;470(2):594–601.
31. Rose PS, Halasy M, Trousdale RT, Hanssen AD, Sim FH, Berry DJ, Lewallen DG. Preliminary results of tantalum acetabular components for THA after pelvic radiation. Clin Orthop Relat Res. 2006;453:195–8.
32. Abudu A, Carter SR, Grimer RJ. The outcome and functional results of diaphyseal endoprostheses after tumour excision. J Bone Joint Surg Br. 1996;78:652–7.
33. Aldlyami E, Abudu A, Grimer RJ, Carter SR, Tillman RM. Endoprosthetic replacement of diaphyseal bone defects: long-term results. Int Orthop. 2005;29:25–9.
34. Ozger H, Akgul T, Yildiz F, Topalan M. Biological reconstruction of the femur using double free vascularized fibular autografts in a vertical array because of a large defect following wide resection of an osteosarcoma: a case report with 7 years of follow-up. J Pediatr Orthop B. 2013;22(1):52–8.
35. Alman BA, De Bari A, Krajbich JI. Massive allografts in the treatment of osteosarcoma and Ewing sarcoma in children and adolescents. J Bone Joint Surg Am. 1995;77:54–64.
36. Ozaki T, Hillmann A, Bettin D, Wuisman P, Winkelmann W. Intramedullary, 86 antibiotic-loaded cemented, massive allografts for skeletal reconstruction: 26 cases compared with 19 uncemented allografts. Acta Orthop Scand. 1997;68:387–91.

Part IV

Revision Hip Arthroplasty Acetabulum

18 Acetabular Impaction Grafting (AIG)

Eustathios Kenanidis, Eleftherios Tsiridis, Martin Buttaro, Eduardo García-Cimbrelo, and Eduardo García-Rey

18.1 Current Concepts

E. Kenanidis and E. Tsiridis

AIG was first described as a primary hip arthroplasty technique by Hastings and Parker in 1975 for rheumatoid patients with acetabular protrusion [1]. It was subsequently used for revision THR by Slooff [2, 3]. Initially, AIG was described as a cemented implantation technique. Now it can be used with a cementless acetabular component as well [4–6].

E. Kenanidis, M.D., Ph.D., M.Sc. (✉)
Academic Orthopaedic Unit, Aristotle University Medical School, Thessaloniki, Greece

E. Tsiridis, M.D., Ph.D., F.A.C.S., F.R.C.S.
Academic Orthopaedic Unit, Papageorgiou General Hospital, Aristotle University Medical School, Thessaloniki, Greece
e-mail: etsiridis@doctors.org.uk

M. Buttaro, M.D.
Hospital Italiano de Buenos Aires, Buenos Aires, Argentina
e-mail: martin.buttaro@hospitalitaliano.org.ar

E. García-Cimbrelo, M.D., Ph.D.
E. García-Rey, M.D., Ph.D.
Hospital Universitario La Paz-Idi Paz, Madrid, Spain

18.1.1 Objectives

- AIG involves robust impaction of bone chips into a contained acetabular defect. A segmental defect must be converted to a contained using metal mesh or porous tantalum augments [7].
- The impacted bone provides a steady, cancellous host bed that restores bone stock and enables proper cementation of the acetabular component at the true centre of rotation, recreating the acetabular anatomy and biomechanics [7, 8].

18.1.2 Indications [7, 8]

1. Bone loss due to:
   (a) The osteolysis that follows an aseptic implant loosening
   (b) A treated infection
   (c) An implant removal at revision surgery (iatrogenic)
2. Protrusio acetabuli
3. Dysplasia
4. Trauma as a previous healed acetabular fracture
5. Contained acetabular defects or segmental that are converted to contained

E. Tsiridis (ed.), *The Adult Hip - Master Case Series and Techniques*,
https://doi.org/10.1007/978-3-319-64177-5_18

18.1.3 Contraindications

1. Non-contained large peripheral or central segmental defects (type 3 and type 4 Paprosky defects/pelvic discontinuity) [8]. This technique, however, was employed efficiently in several patients in different cohorts [9, 10].
2. Unhealed acetabular fracture [8].
3. Untreated infection [8].
4. When bony in-growth and initial press-fit stability on the rim is impossible for the uncemented AIG (severe osteoporosis, osteonecrosis, irradiation, metabolic bone disorders, tumours) [7].

18.1.4 Cemented Technique [6–8]

(a) Adequately expose the anterior and posterior columns of the acetabulum and identify the teardrop.
(b) Remove the failed implant and all the cement and fibrous tissue to identify the margins of the defect.
(c) Promote the bleeding of the host bone surface to assist the incorporation of the bone graft. If the bone is sclerotic, careful surface reaming and or multiple drill holes may encourage neovascularisation.
(d) A contained defect must be exposed. Use an appropriately sized acetabular impactor placed in the correct orientation within the cavity to delineate the presence of any peripheral segmental defect.
(e) Reconstruct an uncontained to contained defect with the use of mesh. Trim a rim mesh appropriately to fit using an impactor as a guide to its final location. Secure the rim mesh with small screws placed at 1 cm intervals around the margin. Bicortical screws are ideal (Fig. 18.1).
(f) Use porous tantalum metal wedges alternatively in case of an extensive segmental defect reconstruction [11, 12].
(g) Section the head into two or four segments and produce chips of 0.8–1 cm [3] using large rongeurs. Washed fresh frozen allograft is the ideal bone graft as it reduces graft recoil and enhances chip impaction.

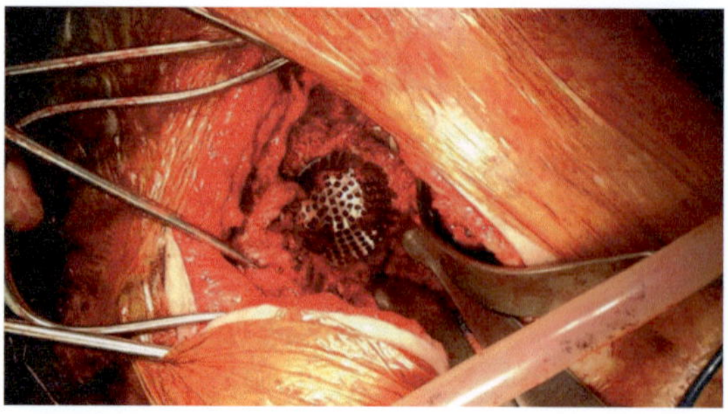

Fig. 18.1 Paprosky 3A medial wall acetabular mesh before impaction grafting to support the graft

Impaction grafting is a dynamic process, and impaction forces should provide a 'cobblestone looking' bed after the impaction. Following IG, the grafted bed is impossible to scratch off the host bone.

(h) Initially pack the chips in the apex of the cavity, into cysts and around screws using small impactors. Then impact layers of the graft into the cavity. Never use reverse reaming as it thins out the graft and reduces the strength of the construct. Avoid excessive graft thickness on the medial floor.
(i) Wash gingerly the grafted bed through a specially designed mesh and dry as preparing for proper third-generation cementing technique.
(j) Form a solid circumferential bed similar to the cortical bone at least 5 mm thick for cementing of the socket.
(k) Third-generation cementing technique is then performed including drying of the bed, creation of peg holes, retrograde cement insertion, pressurisation for 3–5 min against the bed, insertion of poly and continuous pressurisation into the adjusted position until cement setting.

18.1.5 Uncemented Technique

- The technique is based on different principles. It involves the use of a cementless hemispherical cup with screws for initial socket stability. The uncemented component must have a good ream fit. It must achieve press-fit fixation on the rim, whilst AIG restores the bone loss in segmental defects [7]. Graft loading is not possible directly via the uncemented socket immediately after surgery.

(a) Ream the acetabulum using hemispherical reamers to allow press-fit fixation.
(b) Use the trial prosthesis to identify defects.
(c) Impact the morselized bone graft into the defect with tamps.
(d) Use routinely a press-fit porous-coated titanium cup 1 to 2 mm larger than the last trial [7].
(e) Use a minimum of two screws regardless the apparent stability of the prosthesis [7].

18.1.6 Advantages

1. Correction of cavitary and segmental defects [8]
2. Restoration of the acetabular anatomy, biomechanics and recreation of the correct hip rotation centre [6, 7]
3. Replacement of the acetabular bone stock, a particular advantage in the younger patient [6–8]
4. Established technique with good published results [8]
5. Technically demanding, but reproducible technique
6. Treatment option in cemented and uncemented revision, for aseptic loosening and treated infection
7. Used in the primary settings of protrusio acetabuli, dysplasia and trauma [8]
8. Effective in technically challenging patients as rheumatoid [13] and younger than 55 years patients [14–17]

18.1.7 Disadvantages

1. Technically demanding and time consuming [6]
2. Expensive and resource-intensive technique. It requires fresh frozen allograft ideally from a femoral head [7]
3. Not reproducible in less experienced hands [18]
4. Not suitable or secure for large segmental defects [19]
5. Full weight bearing may delay up to 3 months postoperatively [19]

18.1.8 Cemented Acetabular Reconstruction

Published results: Several cohort studies are presently available [1, 2, 3, 9, 10, 13–18, 20–32]. These case series are comprised up of 334 patients. They range in follow-up from some months to 25 years [20]. The majority of them reported satisfactory mid- to long-term results. Schreurs BW et al. [24] reported survivorship for any reason of 79% at 15 years. He also showed 87% survival rate with aseptic loosening as the endpoint and 75% survival for any reason at a follow-up of 20–25 years (the longest follow-up) [20]. The results of the largest series [25] concerning more than 300 patients treated with AIG and a cemented cup for revision THA, demonstrated overall survivorship 91.6% with revision for aseptic loosening and 89.1% with revision for any reason at a mean follow-up of 5.8 years. In another large study, Gilbody et al. [31] reported 85.9% survival with aseptic loosening as the endpoint at 13.5 years for 304 revision THAs treated with cemented component and AIG and metal mesh.

In the majority of studies, the survival with aseptic loosening as the endpoint ranged from 83 to 96% at midterm. There were also reports of similar procedures that reported much higher failure rates [18]. Risk factors associated with failures included combined segmental and cavitary defects, malpositioned components and the use of allograft rather than autograft. Van Haaren et al. [18] reported a survivorship for aseptic loosening of only 72% at a mean follow-up of 7.2 years in 71 cemented AIG revisions. The majority of failures concerned type III and type IV defects which were considered as AIG contraindications.

For large segmental defects, there are also good short-term results in a combination of the IBG with trabecular metal augments [10]. In 98 type IIIA and 83 type IIIB defects re-revised for a major acetabular loss with a cemented cup and AIG, the survival rate was 84% and 82% at eight years, respectively [10].

Cemented AIG has also been used successfully for the management of bone loss in younger patients [14–17]. Schreurs et al. [14] reported 80% survivorship for any reason and 91% for aseptic loosening at 25 years, for 42 hips in 37 patients younger than 50 years. Busch et al. [15] demonstrated survival rate 73% at 20 years and 52% at 25 years for any reason as well as 85% at 20 and 77% at 25 years for aseptic loosening in a small group of young patients less than 50 years treated with AIG and cemented cup. In another small cohort study comprised of 86 THAs in patients with mean age 46.4, Te Stroet showed 87% survival for any reason and 97% for aseptic loosening at 10 years' follow-up [17].

Schreurs et al. [13] showed that this technique might be efficient for the management of bone loss in the revision of patients suffering from Rheumatoid Arthritis (RA). In a cohort of twenty eight RA patients receiving revision hip arthroplasty with AIG and cemented cup, the survival was 80% for any reason and 85% for aseptic loosening at a mean of twelve years.

Several studies demonstrated the significance of the amount of bone loss and the type of the defect with the survival using this technique [10, 28, 32]. Iwase et al. [28] demonstrated that the extent of the bone defect affected the outcome of an acetabular revision when a cemented cup and AIG were used. The maximum acetabular defect distance (MADD), that is radiographically indicating the greatest depth of the grafted layer, affected cup survival. The group of patients with 'MADD ≤20 mm' showed higher survivorship as far as the aseptic loosening was concerned, compared with the group with 'MADD ≥ 20 mm' (95% vs 74%, $p = 0.034$). The group where none or one mesh was used showed greater survival compared with the group where two meshes were used (96% vs 73%, $p = 0.044$) [28].

Garcia Rey [30] also demonstrated the importance of the extent of bone loss as well as its topography with the survival of the technique. He followed up 204 revision THAs treated with AIG and cemented cup for a mean of 10 years. One hundred hips were Paprosky type 3A and 104 type 3B. The survival rate for loosening at 15 years was 83% for Group 3A and 73% for Group 3B ($p = 0.04$). The survivorship for loosening at 15 years was greater in the cases where no mesh was used 89%, followed by medial mesh 85%, lateral mesh 80% and medial and lateral meshes 54% ($p = 0.008$). Lateral segmental defects and subsequent lateral mesh use were found the most important factors associated with loosening ($p = 0.008$; hazard ratio: 2.942; 95% CI: 1.328–6.516) indicating other reconstruction options.

To our knowledge, there are no prospective trials comparing IBG revision to other forms of acetabular reconstruction.

18.1.9 Cementless AIG Revision

Published results: AIG and cementless porous-coated component with screws is now a well-established method for primary THA and acetabular revision.

Studies provide encouraging short- and mid-term results of cup reconstruction with AIG and porous-coated cup [4, 5, 33–38]. These are small cohort studies comprised of 19 to 127 patients with a mean follow-up of 32–144 months. The mean overall reported survival rate ranges from 89.5 to 95.85 and the survival for aseptic loosening, not less than 94% [4, 5, 33–38].

An uncemented hemispherical cup reconstruction with AIG alone is mainly recommended for Paprosky type 1, and some type 2 defects, where a press-fit fixation at the ream for the cup can be achieved [7]. The more host bone contact that can be achieved, the better the likelihood of long-term success. Implant surface contact with <40–50% of native bone has been associated with a higher rate of failure [37]. Although this is a robust long-time belief, other studies did not support it [38].

18.1.10 Complications [8]

1. The host cavity must be contained (a) primarily by the host walls in the case of a cavitary defect or (b) if segmental defect is present then make it contained using mesh or porous tantalum augments.
2. Fill the superior defect initially for loading stability.
3. Avoid placing excessive graft medially, which can lateralize the acetabular component.
4. Peripheral impaction after packing of the main cavity is a vital step in producing a densely packed bone bed to cement successfully.
5. Early migration of the cup if graft gets absorbed early. The rate of migration decreases as graft incorporates.

6. Significant cup migration in large uncontained defects reconstructed using large meshes may result in fatigue failure of the mesh and overall failure.

18.2 Case Title: Revision THA Using Impaction Bone Grafting for the Socket and Stem for Aseptic Loosening

E. Kenanidis and E. Tsiridis

Polyethylene-induced osteolysis with severe socket bone loss Paprosky type 2B and femoral bone loss Paprosky 3A. There is also proximal femoral dilatation and ballooning thinning the cortex and risking fracture. The acetabular site was reconstructed using a marginal roof mesh to contain the small defect followed by impaction grafting of the acetabular bed and accepting a cemented HXLP (Stryker). The femur was prophylactically wired to prevent a fracture from hoop stresses, and a long 205 mm and 44 mm offset cemented Exeter stem (Stryker) was inserted using the third-generation cementing technique. The reason for selecting impaction allografting for reconstructing the femur was based on patient's young age. Biological reconstruction is occasionally preferable for young individuals pending on contained and reconstructable defects (Fig. 18.2).

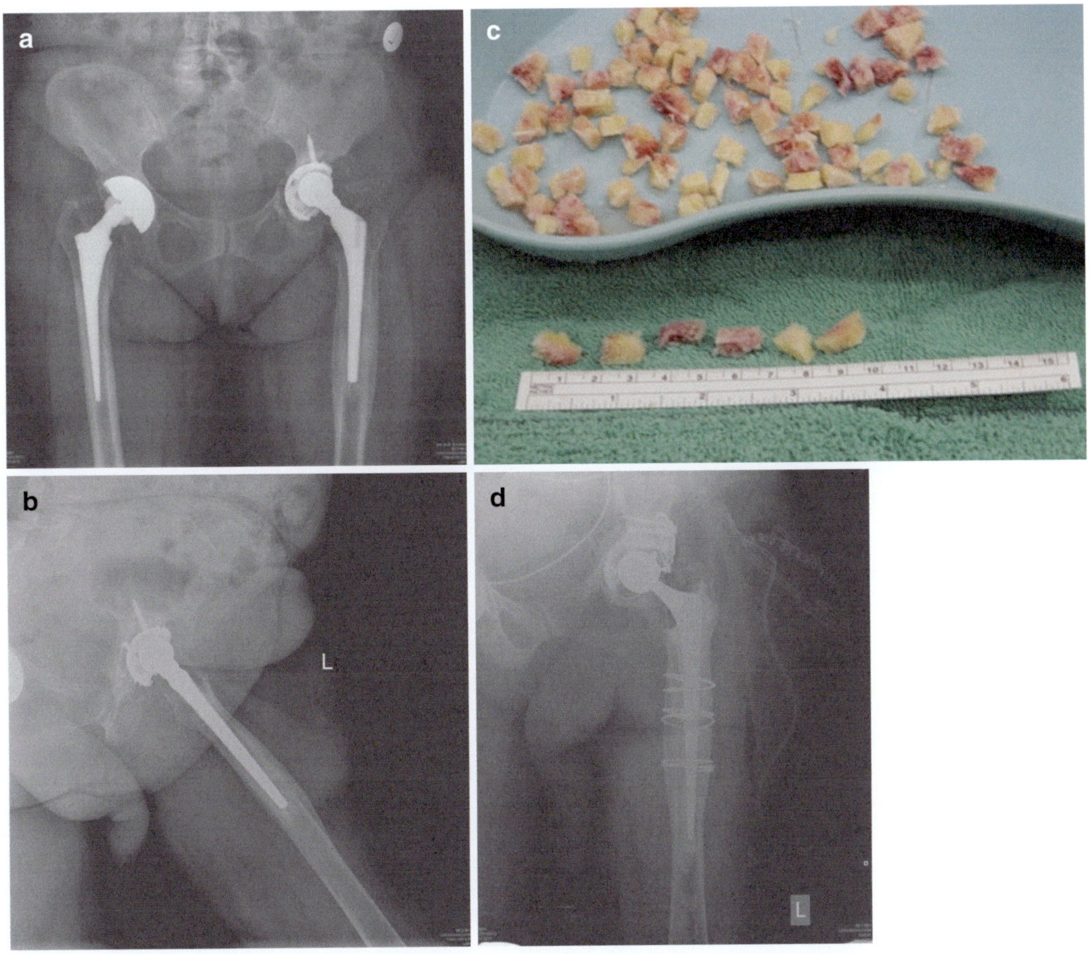

Fig. 18.2 (**a**, **b**) Preoperative AP and Lateral x-rays of the left hip (**c**) bone chips used for the acetabular impaction grafting and (**d**) postoperative x-ray of the left hip

18.3 Case Title: Re-revision THA Acetabulum Paprosky 2A Defect Using Impaction Grafting and Constrained Liner

E. Kenanidis and E. Tsiridis

18.3.1 Demographics

Age: 79
Sex: Male
BMI: 30

18.3.2 Relevant Past Medical History

Principal pathologies: arterial hypertension, dyslipidaemia, prostate hyperplasia.

Previous surgical procedures: AMIS primary two years back, acetabular component loosening six months postoperatively, the first revision to a larger uncemented socket and head to increase stability. Injury to abductors and positive Trendelenburg.

Medication: b-blockers and statins.

History of presenting complaint: pain and limping following revision procedure.

18.3.3 Clinical Examination

Symptoms: pain and instability due to positive Trendelenburg.

Range of motion: full ROM but painful, unable to abduct further to 20°.

Specific tests: unable to stand on the left leg.

Scoring: HHS 70.

Neurovascular evaluation: left hip abductor wasting injury to the superior gluteal nerve during the first revision procedure.

18.3.4 Preoperative Radiological Assessment/Imaging

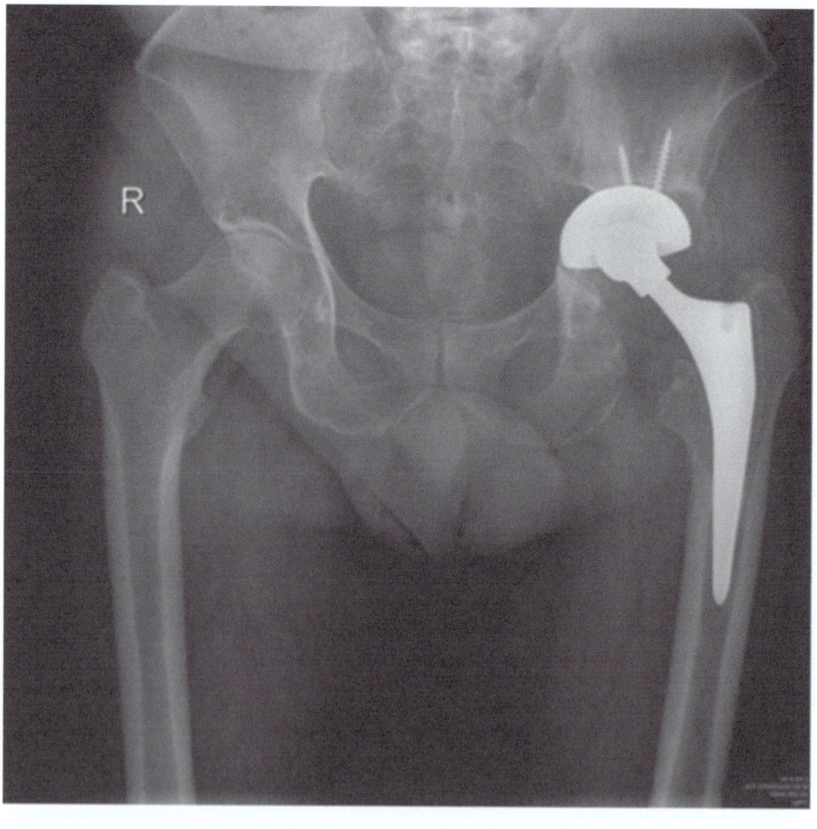

Fig. 18.3 Contained defect but medial wall compromise that could be classified as Paprosky 2B (medial wall absent but periphery intact)

18.3.5 Preoperative Planning

Diagnosis: loose left acetabular component Paprosky type 2A defect contained but medial wall absent (Fig. 18.3).

Possible treatment options: revision acetabulum using impaction grafting.

Chosen treatment method: medial wall mesh Stryker X-change SM, screws for mesh (4 × 35 mm,1 × 25 mm), impaction allografting and constrained cemented acetabular insert Stryker Trident 50 mm and femoral head 28 mm metal.

Selection of implants if applicable and rational: re-revision with instability and positive Trendelenburg. A constrained liner was available to use.

Strategies to overcome difficulties: joint aspiration performed prior to surgery and microbiology testing send ten days before the revision. No microorganisms were grown over a 10-day enhanced culture. A bone scan Tc-99 m was performed that reviled loosening of the acetabular component and a subsequent Indium-111 WBC scintigraphy confirmed aseptic loosening alone.

18.3.6 Surgical Note

With the patient in lateral decubitus position and a posterior approach, the hip was exposed. Six samples were sent for microbiology testing including soft and bone tissues. The stem was found solidly fixed. The femoral head was easily removed, and then the composite stem femur was retracted anteriorly behind the anterior retractor. The greater trochanter was denuded entirely from the abductors solidifying our original decision for the use of a constrained liner. The exposure and the removal of the loose acetabular component was easy. The acetabulum was then accessed for its congruency. The ream was intact though deformed in places, and the medial wall was compromised significantly. Reaming with subsequent reamers was performed until the cancellous bone was exposed up to size 54 mm. Impaction allografting was elected to be performed. An octopus-shaped medial wall mesh of medium size (Stryker) was placed on top of the medial wall defect and stabilized with two peripheral screws. The roof was reinforced with a small marginal roof mesh (Stryker) and screws. Impaction acetabular grafting using morselized large 1 cm washed out cheeps was performed with the special impactors until the cavity on top and medial was filled with new cancellous and stable allograft. Stability was manually tested. Then a trial reduction using a trial constrained liner was performed to adjust for the leg length and stability. Then a cemented constrained component size 50 mm (Stryker) was cemented into the grafted socket using third-generation cementing technique (Fig. 18.4 a, b).

18.3.7 Postoperative Radiographs (Fig. 18.4)

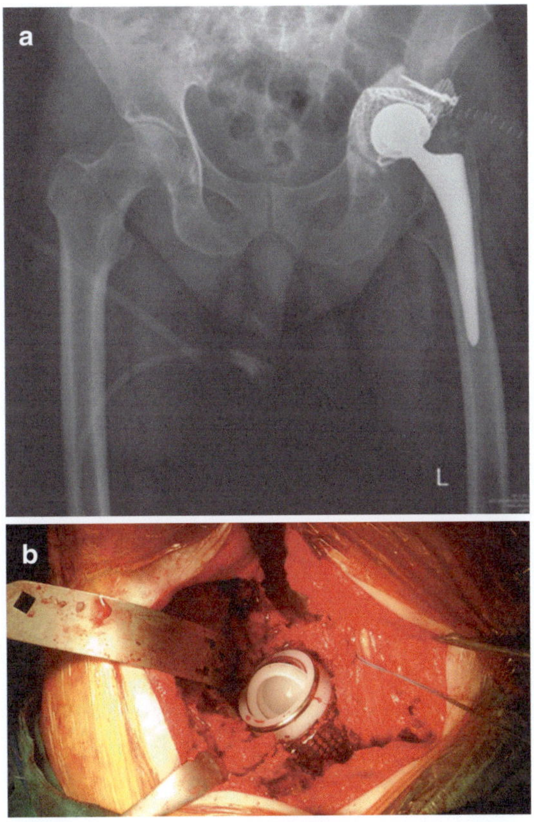

Fig. 18.4 (**a**) Medial wall mesh and marginal mesh on the roof. Impaction grafting and constrained liner. Leg length equal after reduction. (**b**) Intraoperative picture

18.3.8 Postoperative Management

Chemoprophylaxis and anticoagulant treatment period: vancomycin 500 mg (one dose preoperatively and two doses postoperatively), cefuroxime 750 mg (one dose preoperatively and two doses postoperatively), enoxaparin 1 × 1 for the days of hospitalization then rivaroxaban 10 mg 1 × 1 for thirty days

Gait/limb loading until full loading: partial weight bearing for six weeks and then weight bearing as tolerated.

18.4 Case Title: Acetabular Impaction Grafting

Martin Buttaro

18.4.1 Demographics

Age: 79
Sex: female
BMI: 22

18.4.2 Relevant Past Medical History

Principal pathologies: hip ankylosis in 1954 due to DDH (Fig. 18.5).

Previous surgical procedures: primary and acetabular revision right THA in 1974 (Fig. 18.6).

History of Presenting Complaint: right hip pain.

18.4.3 Clinical Examination

Symptoms: pain

Range of motion: severely altered

Main disability: unable to walk more than one hundred metres

Scoring if available: Merle DÁubigne 6 out of 18 points

Neurovascular evaluation: normal

18.4.4 Preoperative Radiological Assessment/Imaging (Figs. 18.5, 18.6, and 18.7)

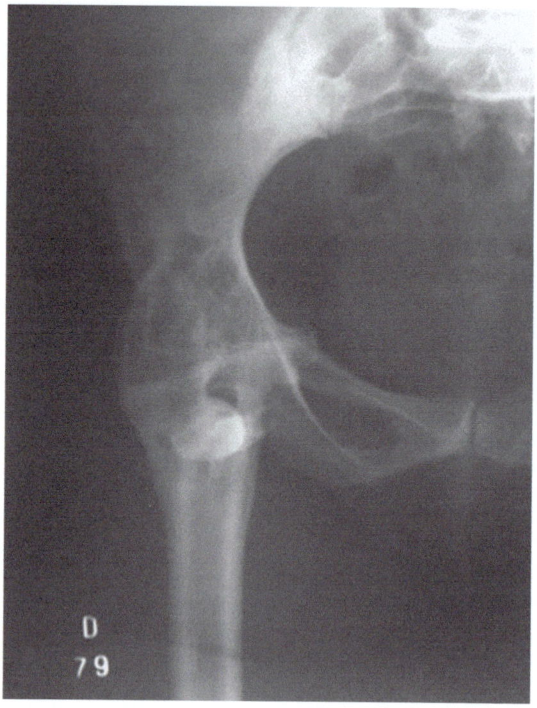

Fig. 18.5 Anteroposterior right hip radiograph of the patient in 1974, when a right Charnley total hip arthroplasty was indicated

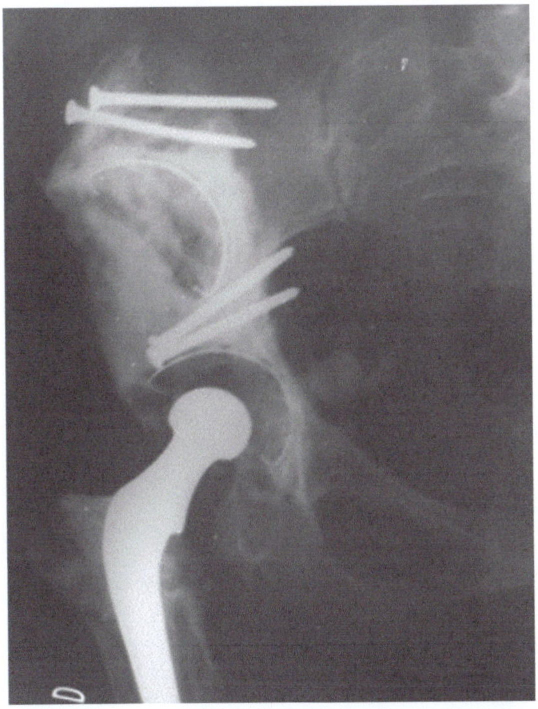

Fig. 18.6 Anteroposterior right hip radiograph showing a Charnley total hip arthroplasty with two cemented cups, the upper one was first cemented, forty eight hours later the patient was sent to the operating room again, and a new cemented cup in the proper position was implanted

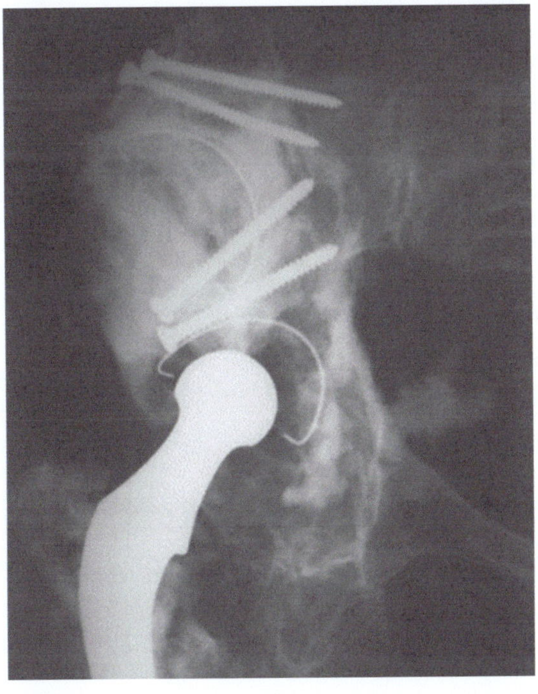

Fig. 18.7 Anteroposterior right hip radiograph depicting acetabular loosening and massive bone loss thirty four years postoperatively. We indicated revision hip surgery with a trabecular metal cup and augment

18.4.5 Preoperative Planning

Diagnosis: acetabular loosening of a right THA (Fig. 18.7).

Possible treatment options: revision THA.

Chosen treatment method: bone reconstruction with strut and cancellous impaction grafting.

Selection of implants if applicable and rational: we planned to use a jumbo tantalum cup, but due to the amount of bone loss, that cup was not possible to be implanted (Figs. 18.8 and 18.9).

Strategies to overcome difficulties: we tailored an allograft belonging to a proximal femur and impacted it between the anterior and posterior columns; then we fixed it with two screws to the iliac bone and two screws to the ischium, and then we cemented a cup (Figs. 18.9, 18.10, 18.11, 18.12, 18.13 and 18.14).

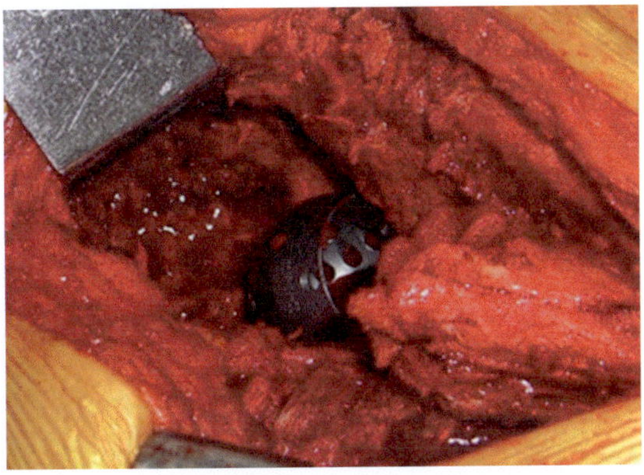

Fig. 18.8 Intraoperative view showing the massive bone loss as determined by the number 52 reamer

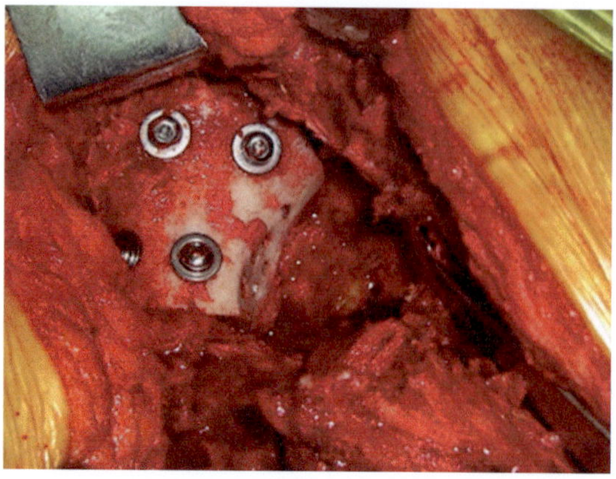

Fig. 18.9 A proximal femur was tailored to be impacted between the anterior and posterior column of the acetabulum and then fixed with four screws, two directed to the iliac bone and two to the ischium. After achieving stability of the strut, the morselized bone graft was impacted in the medial wall. The strut allograft was reamed, and some holes were performed for cement penetration

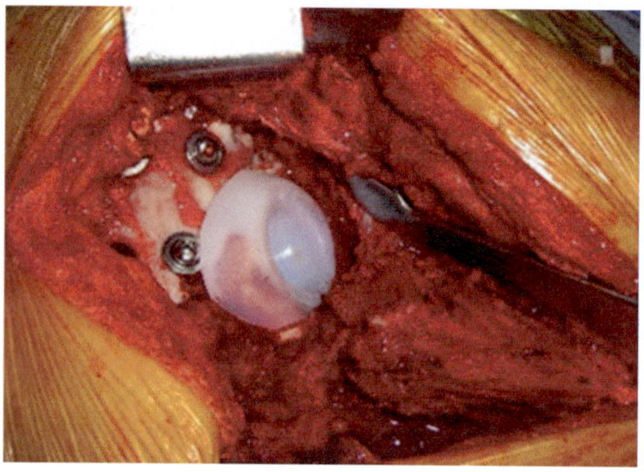

Fig. 18.10 An Ogee cemented cup was cemented, and femoral reconstruction was performed with impaction grafting and a long cemented stem

18.4.6 Surgical Note

Patient's position: lateral decubitus.
Type of anaesthesia: hypotensive epidural.
Surgical approach: posterolateral.
Main steps: see above.
Reconstruction techniques: see above.

18.4.7 Intraoperative Challenges

Challenges and solutions: massive bone defect, unable to be reconstructed with trabecular metal technology (Fig. 18.8).

18.4.8 Postoperative Radiographs (Figs. 18.11, 18.12, 18.13, and 18.14)

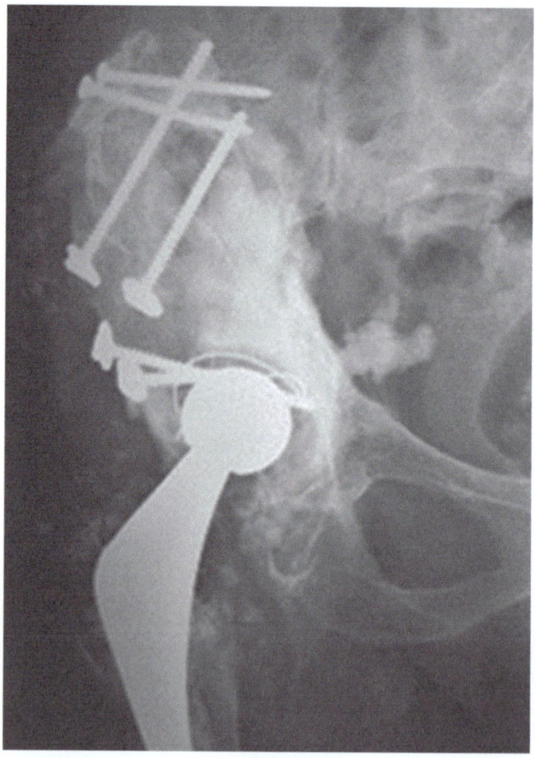

Fig. 18.11 Immediate postoperative radiographs showing the anatomical centre of rotation

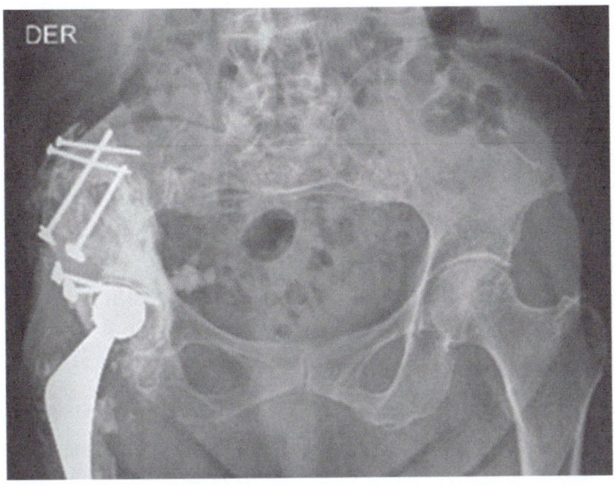

Fig. 18.12 Anteroposterior both hips radiograph at seven years' follow-up

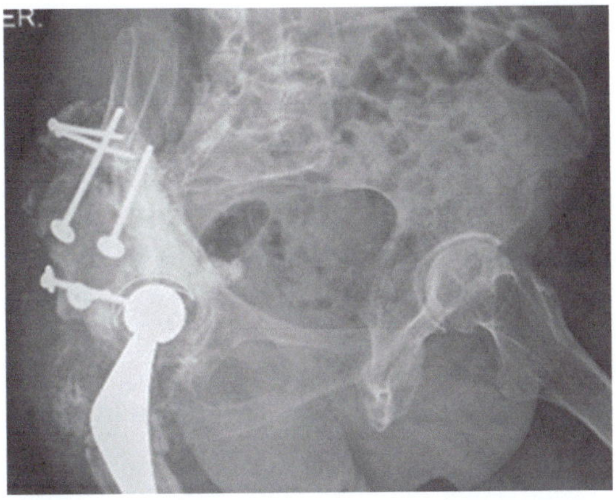

Fig. 18.13 Oblique obturator view at seven years' follow-up

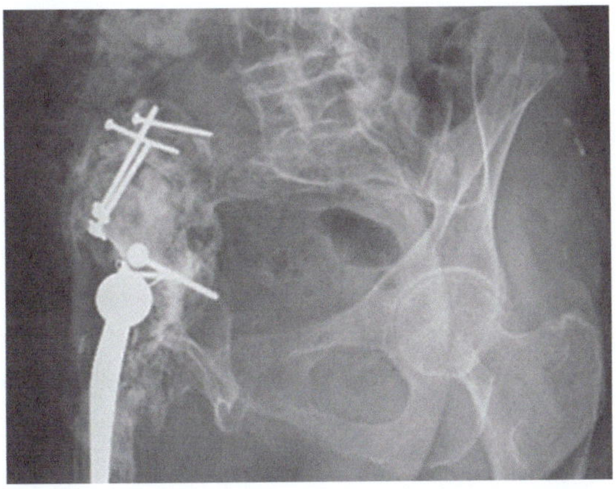

Fig. 18.14 Oblique iliac view at seven years' follow-up

18.4.9 Postoperative Management

Chemoprophylaxis and anticoagulant treatment period: enoxaparin for four weeks.

Gait/limb loading until full loading: three months of non-weight bearing and three months of partial weight bearing, then full weight bearing.

18.4.10 Follow-Up and Complications

Scoring: 14 points Merle DÁubigne score.

18.4.11 Discussion [26, 39, 40]

Advantages of the applied method: bone reconstruction.

Disadvantages of the method: old patient.

Alternative evidence-based techniques for the case: no alternatives.

Why is the chosen technique better for this case: the only one we found.

Indications and contraindications for your technique: indication is the bone loss and contraindication is the active infection.

Learning curve and how to manage complications: prolonged learning curve.

Level of evidence concerning the superiority of this method against others: low level.

18.5 Case Title: Acetabular Impaction Grafting

Eduardo García-Cimbrelo and Eduardo García-Rey

18.5.1 Demographics

Age: 78
Sex: female
BMI: 28

18.5.2 Relevant Past Medical History

Principal pathologies: high blood pressure.

Previous surgical procedures: cemented total hip replacement right side 1986 due to primary osteoarthritis.

Medication: enalapril.

History of presenting complaint: groin pain which requires daily oral analgesics and the use of a cane for walking outdoors during the last six months.

18.5.3 Clinical Examination

Symptoms: groin pain during everyday activities. Evident limp which requires the use of a cane. Difficulty putting on her shoe.

Range of motion: flexion of the right hip is limited to 70°, internal rotation is abolished, and the abduction of the hip is only 10–15°.

Specific tests: positive straight leg raising.

Main disability: walking restriction.

Scoring: 2-3-3 Merle-D'Aubigne and Postel scale.

Neurovascular evaluation: normal.

18.5.4 Preoperative Radiological Assessment/Imaging (Fig. 18.15)

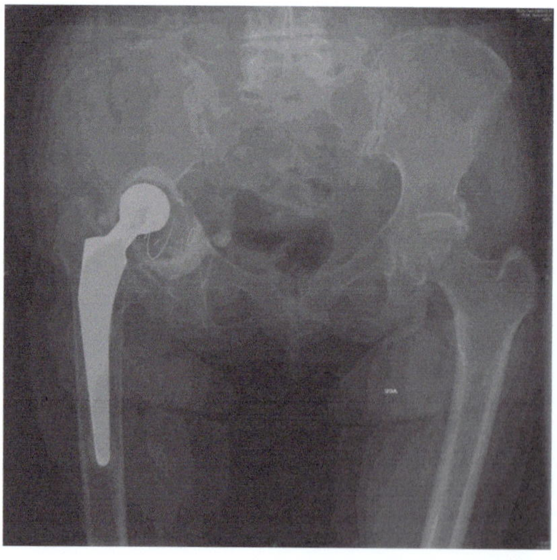

Fig. 18.15 Loosened cemented right hip with an acetabular bone defect larger than 30%

18.5.5 Preoperative Planning

Diagnosis: loosened cemented cup with a large acetabular bone defect Paprosky type 3A (Fig. 18.15).

Possible treatment options: extra-large uncemented cup, cage reconstruction, acetabular impaction bone grafting.

Chosen treatment method: acetabular impaction bone grafting.

Selection of implants if applicable and rational: rim and medial metallic mesh fixed with screw for uncontained defect and morselized bone allograft and a cemented cup.

Expected difficulties: large segmental bone defects after removal of the previous implant.

Strategies to overcome difficulties: use of metallic meshes.

18.5.6 Surgical Note

Patient's position: Lateral decubitus.

Type of anaesthesia: spinal.

Surgical approach: posterolateral.

Main steps: previous approach, removal of the debris, the fibrous tissue and the loosened implant. The stem is fixed.

Reconstruction techniques: fixation of both metallic meshes to the rim and medial wall, morselized bone allograft chips from two frozen femoral heads with size range 0.7–1 cm made by rongeur, impaction using appropriate instrumentation X-change (Stryker) and cementation of a contemporary cup 50 mm using antibiotic-loaded gentamicin cement (Palacos) (Figs. 18.16 and 18.17).

18.5.7 Intraoperative Challenges

Challenges and solutions: convert an uncontained defect to a contained acetabular bone defect.

Unanticipated problems and solution: large segmental defects, use of metallic meshes.

Thorough description of decision making, including the reason for the final decision: the planned surgery was finally done after removal of the previous implant and fibrous tissue.

18.5.8 Postoperative Radiographs (Figs. 18.16 and 18.17)

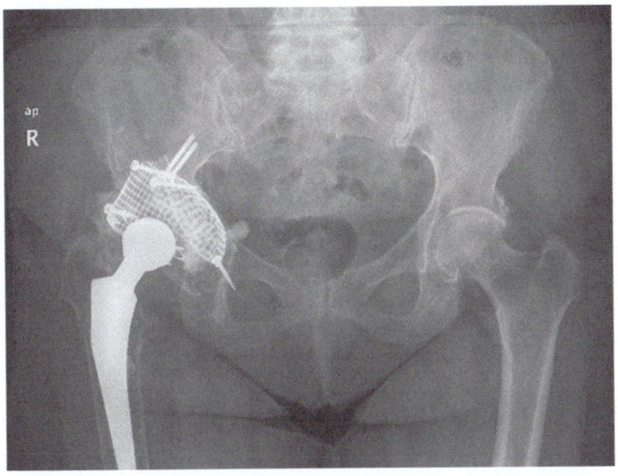

Fig. 18.16 Restoration of the hip rotation centre after acetabular impaction bone grafting and a cemented cup with the use of two metallic meshes

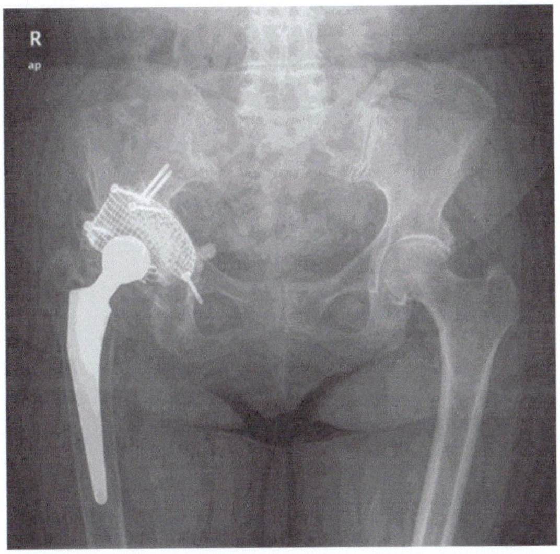

Fig. 18.17 No signs of loosening four years after surgery. Trabecular remodelling changes can be observed

18.5.9 Postoperative Management

Chemoprophylaxis and anticoagulant treatment period: subcutaneous low-weight molecular heparin during six weeks.

Gait/limb loading until full loading: partial toe-touch weight bearing during eight weeks and use of a cane thereafter. The patient still use the cane outdoors for long walking distances.

18.5.10 Follow-Up and Complications

Scoring: 6-5-5 Merle-D'Aubigne and Postel scale

18.5.11 Discussion [10, 20, 25]

Advantages of the applied method: restoration of the hip rotation centre and bone stock after converting and uncontained defect to a contained cavitary defect.

Disadvantages of the method: large segmental rim acetabular defects.

Alternative evidence-based techniques for the case: trabecular augments combined with acetabular impaction bone grafting.

Why is the chosen technique better for this case: after stabilization of segmental defect with the use of meshes, bone allograft form femoral heads allows to restore bone stock.

Indications and contraindications for your technique: moderate and severe acetabular bone defects without pelvic discontinuity.

Learning curve and how to manage complications: stabilization of segmental defects before doing impaction, especially on the rim. According to Nijmegen recommendations, the use of meshes can convert an uncontained defect to a cavitary bone defect. The principles of using large bone chips of around 1 cm and firm impaction are critical to the success of the technique. Larger segmental bone defects of the roof of the acetabulum remain challenging even with the use of a lateral mesh, so the newer lateral trabecular augmentations in combination with impaction bone grafting may help to solve this problem.

Level of evidence concerning the superiority of this method against others: long-term results from the original group and other independent series around the world.

References

1. Hastings DE, Parker SM. Protrusio acetabuli in rheumatoid arthritis. Clin Orthop Relat Res. 1975;108:76–83.
2. Slooff TJ, Huiskes R, van Horn J, Lemmens AJ. Bone grafting in total hip replacement for acetabular protrusion. Acta Orthop Scand. 1984;55:593–6.

3. Slooff TJ, Buma P, Schreurs BW, et al. Acetabular and femoral reconstruction with impacted graft and cement. Clin Orthop Relat Res. 1996;324:108–15.
4. Lee JM, Nam HT. Acetabular revision total hip arthroplasty using an impacted morselized allograft and a cementless cup: minimum 10-year follow-up. J Arthroplast. 2011;26:1057–60.
5. Palm L, Jacobsson SA, Kvist J, et al. Acetabular revision with extensive allograft impaction and uncemented hydroxyapatite-coated implants:results after 9 (7-11) years follow-up. J Arthroplast. 2007;22: 1083–91.
6. Deirmengian GK, Zmistowski B, O'Neil JT, Hozack WJ. Management of acetabular bone loss in revision total hip arthroplasty. J Bone Joint Surg Am. 2011;93A:1842–52.
7. Ibrahim MS, Raja S, Haddad FS. Acetabular impaction bone grafting in total hip replacement. Bone Joint J. 2013;95-B(Supple A):98–102.
8. Petheram TG, Howell JR. The Exeter method-acetabular impaction grafting with cemented reimplantation. Oper Orthop Traumatol. 2014;26(2):114–25.
9. Buckup J, Salinas EA, Valle AG, Boettner F. Treatment of large acetabular defects: a surgical technique utilizing impaction grafting into a metallic mesh. HSS J. 2013;9(3):242–6.
10. Garcia-Cimbrelo E, Cruz-Pardos A, Garcia-Rey E, Ortega-Chamarro J. The survival and fate of acetabular reconstruction with impaction grafting for large defects. Clin Orthop Relat Res. 2010;468:3304–13.
11. Gill K, Wilson MJ, Whitehouse SL, Timperley AJ. Results using trabecular metal™ augments in combination with acetabular impaction bone grafting in deficient acetabula. Hip Int. 2013;23:522–8.
12. Borland WS, Bhattacharya R, Holland JP, Brewster NT. Use of porous trabecular metal augments with impaction bone grafting in management of acetabular bone loss. Acta Orthop. 2012;83:347–52.
13. Schreurs BW, Luttjeboer J, Thien TM, de Waal Malefijt MC, Buma P, Veth RP, Slooff TJ. Acetabular revision with impacted morselized cancellous bone graft and a cemented cup in patients with rheumatoid arthritis. A concise follow-up, at eight to nineteen years, of a previous report. J Bone Joint Surg Am. 2009;91(3):646–51.
14. Schreurs BW, et al. Acetabular reconstruction with impaction bone-grafting and a cemented cup in patients younger than fifty years old. J Bone Joint Surg Am. 2004;86:2385–92.
15. Busch VJ, Gardeniers JW, Verdonschot N, et al. Acetabular reconstruction with impaction bone-grafting and a cemented cup in patients younger than fifty years old: a concise follow-up at twenty to twenty-eight years, of a previous report. J Bone Joint Surg Am. 2011;93:367–71.
16. Comba F, Buttaro M, Pusso R, Piccaluga F. Acetabular revision surgery with impacted bone allografts and cemented cups in patients younger than 55 years. Int Orthop. 2009;33:611–6.
17. Te Stroet MA, Rijnen WH, Gardeniers JW, van Kampen A, Schreurs BW. Satisfying outcomes scores and survivorship achieved with impaction graftingfor revision THA in young patients. Clin Orthop Relat Res. 2015;473(12):3867–75.
18. van Haaren EH, Heyligers IC, Alexander FGM, Wuisman PIJM. High rate of failure of impaction grafting in large acetabular defects. J Bone Joint Surg (Br). 2007;89-B:296–300.
19. Colo E, Rijnen WH, Schreurs BW. The biological approach in acetabular revision surgery: impaction bone grafting and a cemented cup. Bone Joint J. 2014;96-B(2):188–94.
20. Schreurs BW, Keurentjes JC, Gardeniers JW, et al. Acetabular revision with impacted morsellised cancellous bone grafting and a cemented acetabular component: a 20 to 25year follow-up. J Bone Joint Surg (Br). 2009;91-B:1148–53.
21. Comba F, Buttaro M, Pusso R, Piccaluga F. Acetabular reconstruction with impacted bone allografts and cemented acetabular components: a 2 to 13 year follow- up study of 142 aseptic revisions. J Bone Joint Surg (Br). 2006;88-B:865–9.
22. Garcia-Cimbrelo E, Cordero J. Impacted morsellised allograft and cemented cup in acetabular revision surgery. A five to nine year follow-up study. Hip Int. 2002;12:281–8.
23. Schreurs BW, et al. Acetabular reconstruction with impacted morsellised cancellous bone graft and cement: a 10- to 15-year follow-up of 60 revision arthroplasties. J Bone Joint Surg Br. 1998;80:391–5.
24. Schreurs BW, et al. Acetabular revision with impacted morsellised cancellous bone grafting and a cemented cup: a 15- to 20- year follow-up. J Bone Joint Surg Br. 2004;86:492–297.
25. Rigby M, Kenny PJ, Sharp R, et al. Acetabular impaction grafting in total hip replacement. Hip Int. 2011;21:399–408.
26. Buttaro MA, Comba F, Pusso R, Piccaluga F. Acetabular revision with metal mesh, impaction bone grafting, and a cemented cup. Clin Orthop Relat Res. 2008;466:2482–90.
27. Azuma T, Yasuda H, et al. Compressed allograft chips for acetabular reconstruction in revision hip arthroplasty. J Bone Joint Surg Br. 1994;76(5):740–4.
28. Iwase T, Ito T, Morita D. Massive bone defect compromises postoperative cup survivorship of acetabularrevision hip arthroplasty with impaction bone grafting. J Arthroplast. 2014;29(12):2424–9.
29. Arumugam G, Nanjayan SK, Quah C, Wraighte P, Howard P. Revision hip arthroplasty using impacted cancellous bone and cement: a long-term follow-up study. Eur J Orthop Surg Traumatol. 2015;25(8):1279–84.
30. García-Rey E, Madero R, García-Cimbrelo E. THA revisions using impaction allografting with mesh is durable for medial but not lateral acetabular defects. Clin Orthop Relat Res. 2015;473(12):3882–91.
31. Gilbody J, Taylor C, Bartlett GE, Whitehouse SL, Hubble MJ, Timperley AJ, Howell JR, Wilson MJ.

Clinical and radiographic outcomes of acetabular impaction grafting without cage reinforcement for revision hip replacement: a minimum ten-year follow-up study. Bone Joint J. 2014;96-B(2):188–94.

32. van Egmond N, De Kam DC, Gardeniers JW, Schreurs BW. Revisions of extensive acetabular defects with impaction grafting and a cement cup. Clin Orthop Relat Res. 2011;469(2):562–73. https://doi.org/10.1007/s11999-010-1618-8. Epub 2010 Oct 8.
33. Dorairajan A, Reddy RM, Krikler S. Outcome of acetabular revision using an uncemented hydroxyapatite-coated component: two to five year results and review. J Arthroplast. 2005;20:209–18.
34. Lachiewicz PF, Poon ED. Revision of a total hip arthroplasty with a Harris-Galante porous-coated acetabular component inserted without cement: a follow-up note on the results at five to twelve years. J Bone Joint Surg Am. 1998;80:980–4.
35. Tanzer M, Drucker D, Jasty M, McDonald M, Harris WH. Revision of the acetabular component with an uncemented Harris-Galante porous-coated prosthesis. JBone Joint Surg [Am]. 1992;74-A:987–94.
36. Jasty M. Jumbo cups and morsalized graft. Orthop Clin North Am. 1998;29:249–54.
37. Garcia-Cimbrelo E. Porous-coated cementless acetabular cups in revision surgery:a 6 to 11 year follow-up study. J Arthroplast. 1999;14:397–406.
38. Patel S, Sukeik M, Haddad FS. Initial implant stability predicts migration but not failure in cementless acetabular revision with bone grafting. J Arthroplast. 2013;28:832–7.
39. Te Stroet MA, Keurentjes JC, Rijnen WH, Gardeniers JW, Verdonschot N, Slooff TJ, Schreurs BW. Acetabular revision with impaction bone grafting and a cemented polyethylene acetabular component: comparison of the Kaplan-Meier analysis to the competing risk analysis in 62 revisions with 25 to 30 years follow-up. Bone Joint J. 2015;97-B(10):1338–44. https://doi.org/10.1302/0301-620X.97B10.34984. PMID: 26430007
40. Colo E, Rijnen WH, Schreurs BW. The biological approach in acetabular revision surgery: impaction bone grafting and a cemented cup. Hip Int. 2015;25(4):361–7. doi:10.5301/hipint.5000267. Epub 2015 May 20. PubMed PMID: 26044533

19 Trabecular Metal Augments

Eustathios Kenanidis, Ioannis Nakopoulos, Eleftherios Tsiridis, Pedro Dantas, Vasco V. Mascarenhas, Sérgio Gonçalves, Michael J. Feldstein, Matthew S. Austin, William J. Hozack, William L. Griffin, Savyasachi C. Thakkar, James D. Slover, Julie Shaner, and Javad Parvizi

19.1 Current Concepts

E. Kenanidis, I. Nakopoulos, and E. Tsiridis

Porous trabecular metal augments are uncemented hemispheric or elliptical components used for the management of severe acetabular bone loss [1]. Based on the unique characteristics of trabecular metal, they can be used instead of structural allograft to reconstruct major acetabular bone defects [1]. They are made of porous metal tantalum or titanium alloys, and they are available in different shapes and sizes [2]. The basic forms include the half-moon augments appropriate for minor column defects and the buttress augments with anterior of posterior

E. Kenanidis, M.D., Ph.D., M.Sc. (✉) ·
I. Nakopoulos, M.D.
Academic Orthopaedic Unit, Aristotle University Medical School, Thessaloniki, Greece

E. Tsiridis, M.D., Ph.D., F.A.C.S., F.R.C.S. (✉)
Academic Orthopaedic Unit, Papageorgiou General Hospital, Aristotle University Medical School, Thessaloniki, Greece
e-mail: etsiridis@doctors.org.uk

P. Dantas, M.D. · S. Gonçalves, M.D., M.Sc.
Hospital Curry Cabral, Lisbon, Portugal

V.V. Mascarenhas, M.D., M.Sc., M.B.A.
UIME (MSK Imaging Unit), Hospital da Luz, Lisbon, Portugal

M.J. Feldstein, M.D., S.M
Kaiser Permanante, Oakland, CA, USA
e-mail: Michael.Feldstein@rothmaninstitute.com

M.S. Austin, M.D.
Rothman Institute Orthopaedics, Philadelphia, PA, USA
e-mail: Matt.Austin@rothmaninstitute.com

W.J. Hozack, M.D.
Sidney Kimmel Medical School at Thomas Jefferson University, Rothman Institute Orthopaedics, Philadelphia, PA, USA
e-mail: william.hozack@rothmaninstitute.com

W.L. Griffin, MD (✉)
OrthoCarolina Research Institute, Charlotte, NC, USA

OrthoCarolina Hip and Knee Center, Charlotte, NC, USA
e-mail: William.Griffin@orthocarolina.com

S.C. Thakkar, MD
Department of Adult Hip & Knee Reconstruction Surgery, MedStar Georgetown University Hospital and MedStar Washington Hospital Center, Washington, DC, USA

J.D. Slover, MD
Department of Adult Hip & Knee Reconstruction Surgery, New York University Hospital for Joint Diseases, New York, NY, USA

J. Shaner, MD
Temple University Hospital, Philadelphia, PA, USA

J. Parvizi, M.D., F.R.C.S
Sidney Kimmel School of Medicine, Philadelphia, PA, USA

Rothman Institute at Thomas Jefferson University, Philadelphia, PA, USA

E. Tsiridis (ed.), *The Adult Hip - Master Case Series and Techniques*,
https://doi.org/10.1007/978-3-319-64177-5_19

columnar extensions to compensate for anterosuperior or posterosuperior acetabular defects [1, 3]. For superior segmental defects, more than 30 mm above the acetabulum, a figure of seven augments may also be used [1].

19.1.1 Objective

They are employed to reconstruct major acetabular defects contributing to the acetabular component stability [4]. The augments fill the defects, united with the acetabular cup, and provide structural support to the acetabular component until bone ingrowth occurs [1]. Also, they are used to restore the COR and hip biomechanics [1].

They are applied:

(a) With TM sockets [1]
(b) In the distraction technique for pelvic discontinuity [5–7]
(c) In the cup-cage technique [8]
(d) With the impaction grafting technique [9]

19.1.2 Indications

There are no absolute indications for their usage. They have been used however based on the following indications:

- An acetabular component uncovering higher than 40%. A contact of the component with the remaining host bone <60% in type III defects renders bone ingrowth uncertain [1, 10].
- Combined defects of the columns and the roof [11].
- An excessive bone loss from the anterior or posterior column and loss of stability resulting from intraoperative preparation to implant a jumbo cup [11].
- Restoration of the hip centre of rotation [12].

19.1.3 Contraindications

- The young age (<35 years) is considered as a relative contraindication. In this group of patients, multiple coming revision procedures are expected [11].

19.1.4 Surgical Technique [1, 11, 13]

The augments are fixed first to the host bone with screws, then to the acetabular shell with cement:

1. Expose the acetabulum widely.
2. Recognize the areas of structural bone deficiency, and define the normal hip centre with a standard reamer.
3. With the trial component in place, choose the most appropriately shaped and sized augment to fill the defect and support the trial.
4. Ream the segmental defect gently to better contain the augment. Fine adjustment of this fitting could be achieved using morselized allograft impacted into the remote defecits that the augment cannot reach.
5. Fasten the augment to the acetabular defect with screws.
6. Impact morcellized bone graft into any remaining cavities before the shell is implanted.
7. Fill the contact area of the cup, and the augment with cement to eliminate any micromovement between them during ingrowth.
8. Tamp the porous metal shell in place.
9. Introduce additional screws through the cup into the ilium if needed.

With time, osseointegration is achieved between the component bone and augment bone.

Augments can be used in various combinations and orientations. There are available sizes and a small variation of thicknesses that may fit into the defects. Face to face or one over the other augment are some of the most frequent combinations. It is advisable that the TM interface should always be protected by a layer of cement.

19.1.5 Advantages

- **The customized reconstruction** based on the modularity in the size and shape of the available augments that can be used in many combinations and orientations to reconstruct the defect [11, 14].

- **The maximised contact with** the host bone [1].
- **The potential restoration of the hip centre to near** normal [13, 14].
- The mechanical backing and the increased stability to the cup [15].
- **The salvage of the bone stock.** The addition of an augment in the roof may lessen the need for reaming expansion to the minimum necessary [1]. Reaming in the AP dimension to implant a jumbo cup, in type IIIA defects often results in greater bone loss along the anterior column.
- **The advantages related to the material**. Porous trabecular metal augments composed of tantalum have theoretical advantages over conventional porous metals such as titanium, including:
  (a) **The high coefficient of friction** [16] that improves the initial augment stability to the host bone especially in the presence of a poor bone stock [11, 17]. TM provides **primary stability** at the time of the procedure and allows an in-depth bony ingrowth leading to a secondary biologic fixation [18, 19].
  (b) **The highly porous architecture** with a distinguished 3D porosity (70–80%) [9, 16, 20] and the profoundly interconnected pores, resembling the structure of the trabecular bone [21, 22], maximize the degree of **biologic fixation** with significantly greater degree of ingrowth and shear strength [22–24] when compared with the conventional implants [1].
  (c) **The elastic modulus of TM is closer to that of subchondral bone** compared to other implant materials [20]. The TM elasticity is reported to be 3GPa but that of titanium and chrome cobalt 110–205 GPa, respectively [18]. The latter improves the load-directed bone remodeling and helps to minimise stress shielding adjacent to the cup [11, 18, 25].
  (d) **The preservation of the structural stability** of TM over time. A structural allograft can absorb over time, leading to eventual acetabular component instability [25].
  (e) **The honeycomb architecture of TM** that enables the surgeon to drill through the acetabular shells and augments and place screws without undermining the strentgh of the component [25].

19.1.6 Disadvantages

- The inability to restore the bone stock for a future revision [1]
- The potential for debris generation at the shell-augment interface
- The potential for fatigue failure
- The lack of long-term studies concerning the effects of tantalum metal debris on the surrounding soft tissue and the wear rate of the liner [1, 17]

19.1.7 Published Results

Several cohort studies are presenting short- to midterm follow-up of patients undergoing revision THA with TM shell and augments [1, 3, 10–15, 25–29]. These are usually retrospective but also prospective [10, 27] case series comprised of 13–263 patients. The mean follow-up ranged from 28 to 106 months. These studies, however, are non-homogenized. They include patients with different preoperative diagnoses, and different types of bone defects, from Paprosky types IIA to IIIB with pelvic discontinuity that were treated using TM acetabular cups with or without TM augments. The sample size of patients in these studies managed with TM shells and augments ranged from 8 to 72.

Seven studies reported homogenized groups of patients treated with TM shells and augments [1, 11, 13–15, 27, 28]. They are comprised of 28–55 patients that were followed at a mean of 34 to 110 months. Although the revision for any reason was reported from 87.7 to 96%, the results for aseptic loosening were better. At the longest follow-up study, Whitehouse et al. [12] reported 92% survival rate at 10 years in 53 revision THAs with TM cup and augments used for the treatment of IIA–IIIB Paprosky defects. Grapiollo et al. [14] also demonstrated 92.8% survival rate at five years, for 55 revision hip arthroplasties, 42 IIIA and 13 IIIB Paprosky defects managed with TM shells and augments.

Mid-term results have been quite promising, with a low rate of aseptic loosening, improvement in the clinical scores and restoration of the centre of rotation of the hip. Literature supports that they are superior to the structural or morselized contained allografts and bilobed components [1, 13, 14]. To our knowledge, there are no prospective trials, however, comparing TM cup augment revision to other forms of acetabular reconstruction for Paprosky type IIIA/IIIB defects. Longer follow-up is certainly required.

19.1.8 Complications

The rate of reported complications is varying. The exact percentage of complications is difficult to calculate due to the non-homogenized nature of studies. Instability (dislocations), infections, aseptic loosening, nerve injuries, and heterotopic ossification are the most common complications [1, 11, 14]. In the group of homogenized cohorts reporting revisions of TM cups and augments, the rate of complications ranged from 3.5 up to 25% [1, 11, 13–15, 27, 28]. Interestingly Guido Grapiollo et al. [14] reported 11% heterotopic ossification out of 55 revision hip arthroplasties managed with TM cups and augments. None of the patients, however, required further revision for heterotopic ossification removal. Gaizo et al. [11] also showed that 19% of patients suffering from IIIA and IIIB Paprosky defects required additional surgery for infection, periprosthetic fractures, loosening, and dislocations. This high percentage of complications was mainly attributed to the complexity of these types of revision THAs.

19.2 Case Title: Revision THA Acetabulum Paprosky Type IIIA. ARMD with Metallosis with Severe Periacetabular Osteolysis and Co-Cr Levels >7 μg/L

E. Kenanidis and E. Tsiridis

19.2.1 Demographics

Age: 79
Sex: Male
BMI: 28

19.2.2 Relevant Past Medical History

Principal pathologies: Pain, inability to walk, limitation of ROM, non-weight bearing on the right side

Previous surgical procedures: Bilateral THAs 10 (right) and 15 (left) years back using uncemented proximally coated and cylindrically tipped stems and XLP poly in metal shell back in the acetabulum

Medication: Antihypertensives, NSAIDs

History of presenting complaint: Pain, inability to walk, and dysfunction of the right hip

19.2.3 Clinical Examination

Symptoms: Pain and functional Trendelenburg due to the inability to bear weight on the left

Range of motion: Flexion: 70; extension: 0; internal/external rotation very painful and limited; abduction: 25; adduction painful and impossible

Specific tests: Unable to perform on the right

Main disability: Inability to walk

Scoring if available: HHS: 60

Neurovascular evaluation: Intact

19.2.4 Preoperative Radiological Assessment/Imaging (Fig. 19.1)

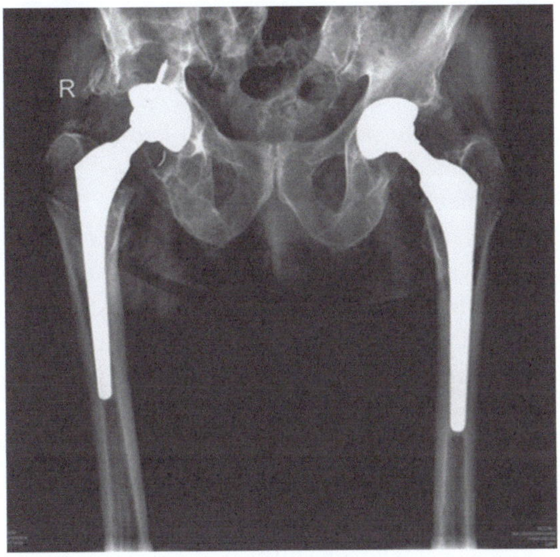

Fig. 19.1 Right THA acetabular component loose with severe osteolysis at the roof and the ischial tuberosity. Bobble-shaped roof osteolysis is typical of the polyethylene debris-related osteolysis. Also, the small wire fragment adjacent to the teardrop indicated that the marking wire of the polyethylene wass broken; thus, the head rubs against the metal liner. It is expected that some degree of metallosis and ARMD will be present

19.2.5 Preoperative Planning

Diagnosis: Osteolysis and need for acetabular revision with some augmentation to support the socket (Fig. 19.1).

Possible treatment options: This is an uncontained defect Paprosky type IIIA that requires solid reconstruction with augments and revision trabecular metal shell to press fit the periphery of the acetabulum.

Chosen treatment method: Exclusion of an infection via biochemical testing and joint aspiration. The tap sample was negative for microorganisms. ESR was elevated; the CRP was normal with WCC normal. Cobalt and chromium serum levels were just below seven μg/L; the patient was having, however, symptoms; the diagnosis of ARMD with extensive hard and soft tissue local destruction was suspected. Tantalum augment 54 mm by 10 mm thickness and bone graft, jumbo shell tantalum size 68 mm, and a liner size 59 mm with cement with a 32 mm diameter head.

Selection of implants if applicable and rational: Trabecular metal augments and shell for better bone integration. A solid allograft could also do for the reconstruction of the uncontained defect.

Expected difficulties: Stable reconstruction of the acetabular defect. Coordination of the augment placement and the acetabular shell insertion.

Strategies to overcome difficulties: Variability of augments to match the defect.

Templating: Performed preoperatively.

19.2.6 Surgical Note

With the patient in lateral decubitus position, a posterior approach of the hip was used. The joint was aspirated again but no fluid could be extracted easily. Entering the joint a creamy fluid dark colored came through confirming the diagnosis of metallosis and ARMD. Extensive removal of the affected tissues led to the exposure of the lateral pelvic aspect with the acetabulum easily viewed. Six tissue samples were sent for microbiology and biopsy to detect ALVAL. The stem was stable, and decision was made to leave it in situ. The femoral head was removed easily to allow access and better visualisation of the acetabulum. The femoral part of the joint was then moved anteriorly in front of the anterior acetabular wall, and the acetabulum was exposed. The implant was holding well from the screws; however, the bone all around it was severely compromised and eroded. The liner was removed using a liner elevator, and the shell was exposed. The screws were removed and the cup carefully extracted utilising the explant device (Zimmer). The defect was detected and was large enough to justify the use of a large augment to the roof. Reaming of the defected roof to shape it to the size of the appropriate augment and to remove the debris and the scar tissue until exposure of bleeding cancellous bone occurred. Then attention was turned to the acetabulum below. The teardrop and transverse ligament were identified, and concentric reaming started to bring the reamer up to 66 mm. Full tantalum revision socket goes up to 68 mm; thus, the reaming was stopped and the acetabular defect was reconstructed using dummy implants. A roof wedge tantalum augment 54 mm by 10 mm thickness and bone graft used to reconstruct the roof. The augment was inserted tightly and then stabilized with 2.6 mm screws through the augment screw holes. The dummy socket was again tested below the inserted augment and was measured 66 mm. To allow some distraction and better fitting, a jumbo shell tantalum size 68 mm was elected. One mix of Palacos cement was prepared and was applied in the interface between the augment and the shell. The 68 mm shell was then inserted tightly, and the cement was scrapped off the interface quickly. Then several long screws were passed through the shell to the augment to the bone of the roof for interdigitating stability. Using the diamond-tipped speed burr, extra screw holes were opened up against the roof and extra screws inserted including an iliac screw below. The appropriate HXLP size 59 mm (Zimmer) was cemented in place with a 32 mm inner diameter for the appropriate ceramic head to be used. Fresh frozen allograft filled the ischial defect and the upper part of the femoral metaphysis that was mildly osteolyzed. Stability and leg length were found satisfactory (Fig. 19.2).

19.2.7 Intraoperative Challenges

Challenges and solutions: Coordination of the roof augment and the shell insertion with the cement interface and screw insertion and stabilization.

Unanticipated problems and solution: Increasing the acetabular reaming to a jumbo size must be resisted when the fit to the anterior and posterior is good. The roof must be addressed separately and reconstructed. Increasing the reaming size may risk fracture of the walls that will compromise the acetabular integrity severely.

Thorough description of decision-making, including the reason for the final decision: Uncemented reconstruction was elected for the acetabular part as there is good evidence that trabecular metal shell can fit tightly into compromised acetabular defects and allow bone ingrowth. For the roof part of the reconstruction, a solid fresh frozen allograft could do the job as the defect is uncontained and the solidity is important for early stability. Trabecular augments can do the same, as it can be filled with morselized fresh frozen allograft or occasionally can be combined with a solid part of allograft if the defect is not concentric.

19.2.8 Postoperative Radiographs (Fig. 19.2)

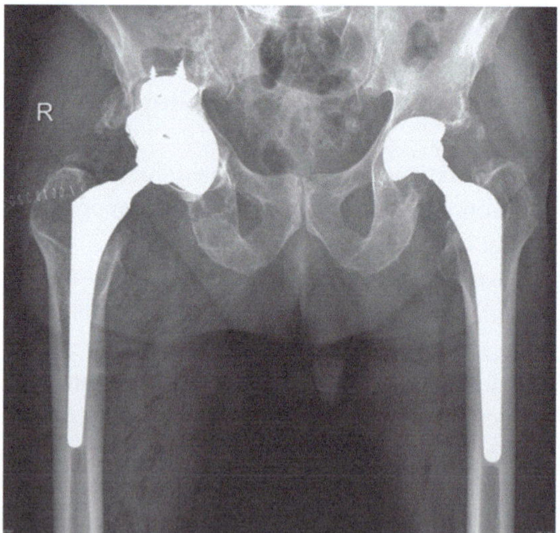

Fig. 19.2 Acetabular reconstruction using tantalum augment and shell. Screws through the shell and the augment up to the iliac wing. Jumbo-sized shell with good fit to the periphery of the acetabulum down to the teardrop maintaining the leg length equality to the contralateral side

19.2.9 Postoperative Management

Chemoprophylaxis and anticoagulant treatment period: Cefuroxime 750 mg (one dose preoperatively and two doses postoperatively), vancomycin 500 mg (one dose preoperatively and two doses postoperatively), and LMWH during hospitalization then rivaroxaban 10 mg for 30 days.

Gait/limb loading until full loading: Partial weight bearing for eight weeks and then as tolerated.

19.3 Case Title: Acetabular Augment for a Paprosky Type IIIA Acetabular Defect

Pedro Dantas, Vasco Mascarenhas, and Sérgio Gonçalves

19.3.1 Demographics

Age: 67 years
Sex: Male
BMI: 23.4

19.3.2 Relevant Past Medical History

Principal pathologies: Bilateral developmental hip dysplasia.

Previous surgical procedures: Left total hip replacement in 1999, which was revised three years later, due to loosening and osteolysis (bone allograft and a 56 mm cup with screws). Re-revision after two months due to migration (Muller ring with a cemented socket). Right total hip replacement in 1998. Right femoral shaft fracture operated (ORIF) at the age of 45; healed with valgus and shortening deformity.

Medication: Pazolan.

History of presenting complaint: The patient was referred with left hip pain for the last two years with progressive shortening of the limb. The pain increases with walking, which has only been possible using two crutches for the last year. Unable to bear weight and put on socks on the left side. The patient does not mention swelling or reddishness around the hip.

19.3.3 Clinical Examination

Symptoms: Pain with weight bearing, flexion, and rotation of the left hip. Right hip has slight pain with flexion and internal rotation. Left thigh muscle atrophy. Bilateral posterolateral surgical scars from previous surgeries.

Range of motion: Left hip: flexion 100°, extension 0°, abduction 30°, adduction 35°, internal rotation 30°, external rotation 40°. Flexion and rotation were painful.

Specific tests: Left lower limb shortening of 3 cm. Left Trendelenburg test positive.

Main disability: Unable to bear weight and walk without crutches.

Scoring: Harris Hip Score preoperatively—19.

Neurovascular evaluation: No changes.

19.3.4 Preoperative Radiological Assessment/Imaging (Figs. 19.3, 19.4, and 19.5)

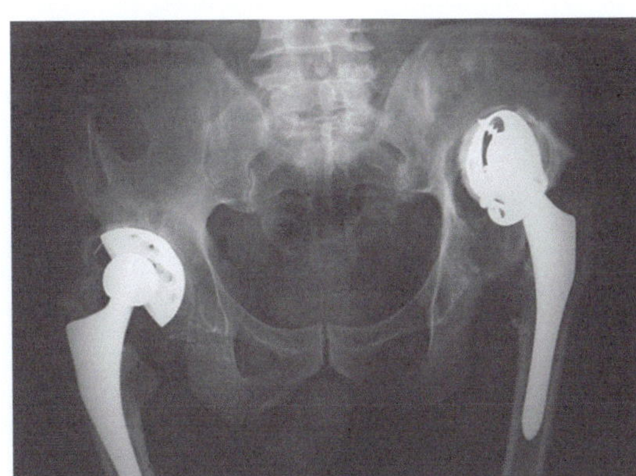

Fig. 19.3 AP pelvis x-ray. Loose Muller ring cup with superolateral hip centre migration greater than three cm. There is a destruction of the superior rim, but the Kohler's line is intact (Paprosky type IIIA acetabular defect). Apparently, the anterior column is deficient, but the CT scan shows that it is relatively preserved

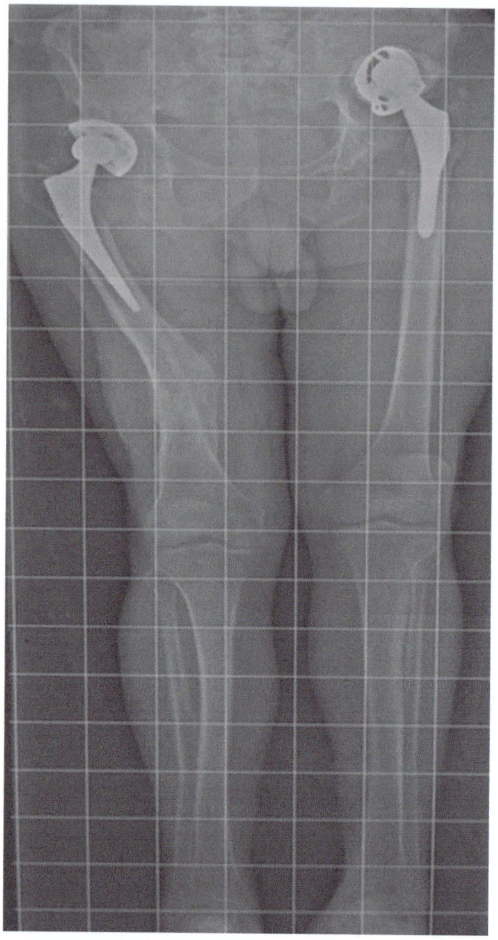

Fig. 19.4 Standing AP XR of both lower extremities. Valgus and shortening deformity of the right femur (2 cm shorter than the left femur)

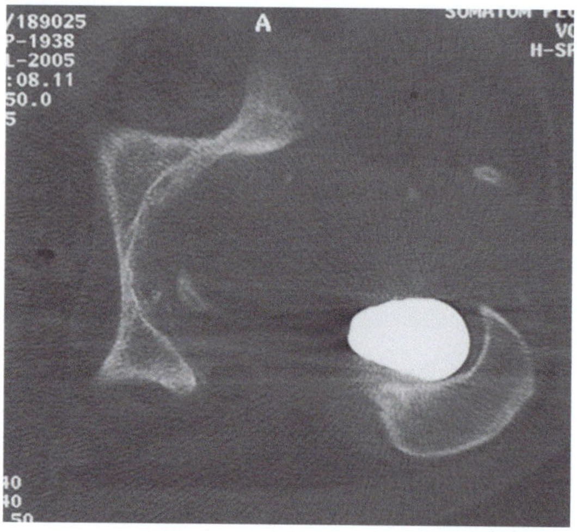

Fig. 19.5 Left hip CT scan. There is a posterior column deficiency with preservation of the anterior column and acetabular floor

Other: Blood leukocyte count and differential were normal, C-reactive protein 0.35 mg/dL, and erythrocyte sedimentation rate 12 mm/h. Left hip aspiration under x-ray control—clear fluid with a low count of leukocytes and cultures with no microbial growth.

19.3.5 Preoperative Planning

Diagnosis: Aseptic loosening of left Muller ring with proximal migration and loose acetabular cup on the right side. According to the Paprosky classification, this is a type IIIA acetabular defect with superior bone loss; the medial wall is relatively preserved, and the cup has migrated superolaterally (Figs. 19.3, 19.4 and 19.5).

Possible treatment options: Trabecular metal cup and augments, jumbo acetabular components, impaction bone grafting, structural allografts, acetabular cages, bilobed acetabular components, and high placement of the hip centre of rotation.

Chosen treatment method: Trabecular metal hemispherical cup in the native acetabulum and a superior augment.

Selection of implants if applicable and rational: Trabecular metal revision cup and augments. Non-cemented primary femoral stem and a distal fixation revision stem (if proximal fixation is not possible or in the case of a femoral osteotomy to remove the stem).

Expected difficulties: Poor stability of a hemispherical cup with lack of superior support. There is a high hip centre on the left side, defined as being more than 35 mm above the inter-teardrop line. We would expect difficulty in bringing the femur down and need to revise an ingrown uncemented femoral stem. A subtrochanteric shortening osteotomy may be needed if we cannot manage to bring the femur down or in case of sciatic nerve tension.

Strategies to overcome difficulties: An augment can be used to support the acetabular shell and achieve stability. Soft tissue release, a femoral revision to lower the centre of rotation, and a subtrochanteric femoral shortening osteotomy.

Templating: In the preoperative templating, we aimed to restore the hip centre of rotation, and an augment was necessary to support the cup superiorly.

19.3.6 Surgical Note

Patient's position: Right lateral decubitus.

Type of anesthesia: General anesthesia.

Surgical approach: Posterior approach.

Main steps: Two grams of cefazolin was given after taking intraoperative tissue cultures.

Reconstruction techniques: Progressive reaming was done in the native acetabulum until reaching the anterior and posterior columns. The intraoperative stability with a hemispherical cup was poor. A trial cup component and different trial augments were placed in the posterosuperior defect to simulate the reconstruction and access component sizes and stability. Reaming of the superior defect according to the planned size of the augment was performed. With the trial cup in place, the hemispherical trabecular metal augment was fixed with screws, and morselized fresh frozen bone allograft was used to fill the fenestrations and cavitary defects. A thin layer of cement was carefully applied in the augment-cup union to avoid extravasation of cement to the bone-implant interface. The tantalum revision cup was impacted, and additional screws were placed through the shell to enhance primary stability. The polyethylene liner was cemented. It was not possible to reduce the hip after capsular release, so the femoral stem was removed. Sciatic nerve tension was accessed after reduction with the trial femoral component and a non-cemented stem with a more profound sitting was implanted. The largest femoral head was used to reduce the risk of dislocation (Fig. 19.6).

19.3.7 Intraoperative Challenges

Unanticipated problems and solution: A possible infection, which would need a component removal, debridement, and a spacer. Trochanteric osteotomy may be necessary for stem removal and a subtrochanteric femoral shortening osteotomy if we are not able to bring the femur down or in case of sciatic nerve tension.

Thorough description of decision-making, including the reason for the final decision: The trial cup was stable in the true acetabulum with the superior augment. The hip reduction was possible with the trial stem with a more profound sitting and was stable for the tested ROM.

19.3.8 Postoperative Radiographs (Fig. 19.6)

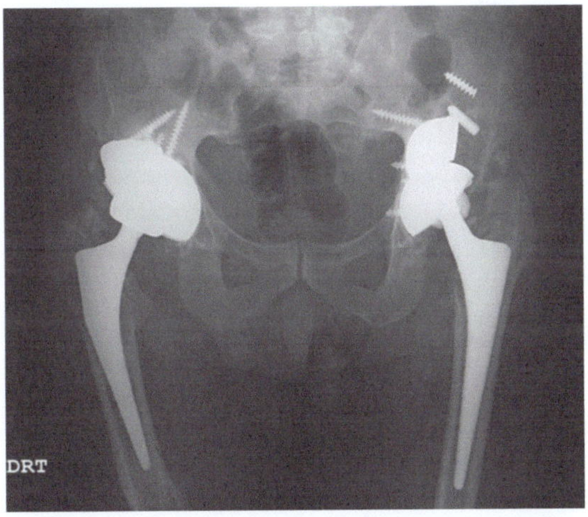

Fig. 19.6 Pelvis X-ray at 9.5 years after revision of left THR and six years after revision of right hip replacement with the same technique. There is a radiolucency in DeLee and Charnley zone 3 which has not progressed, and there is no evidence of implant migration. 2) Acetabular revision on the right hip with the same technique was carried out 4.5 years later

19.3.9 Postoperative Management

Chemoprophylaxis and anticoagulant treatment period: Enoxaparin 40 mg SC for four weeks

Gait/limb loading until full loading: Partial weight bearing with two crutches for twelve weeks

19.3.10 Follow-Up and Complications

Acetabular revision on the right hip with the same technique was carried out 4.5 years later. The high-riding trochanter raises some concern of impingement and instability. A stem with more offset could be used to decrease the risk of impingement.

Scoring: Harris Hip Score at 9.5 years follow-up—86.

19.3.11 Discussion

Advantages of the applied method: Most of the acetabular defects are elliptical, with the antero-posterior dimension smaller than the superior-inferior dimension. If the defect is small, reaming can be used to create a spherical cavity without compromising the anterior and posterior column support, and a standard hemispherical cup can be used. This solution can be used in the vast majority of acetabular revisions with favorable survivorship [30]. For more severe defects like the Paprosky type IIIA, the stability of the cup is questionable [11]. In this type of defect, a cementless acetabular fixation usually needs a superior buttress for primary implant stability. For segmental defects, the augment replaces part of the missing column and gives support to the hemispherical cup. This allows a lowering of the hip centre and placement of the cup in the anatomical location. With augments, it is possible to use a hemispherical revision cup in Paprosky type IIB and IIIA defects [11, 31]). There are different shapes and sizes for the augments, and their modularity is used for adaptation to the morphology and size of the defect. Another advantage is the possibility of customizing and adjusting the reconstruction intraoperatively. The use of a metal with high porosity like tantalum can increase the bone ingrowth potential, especially in cases of limited host bone contact, and the high coefficient of friction can increase primary stability [11]. The metal augments are a better option for the reconstruction of segmental defects compared to the structural allograft, with a lesser risk of fracture and bone reabsorption.

Disadvantages of the method: In the case of a cavitary defect, the bone allograft is the best option, and the use of an augment inadvisable because of the risk of wall fracture during component impaction. Cement used between the cup and the augment may penetrate the bone-implant interface interfering with the bone ingrowth. The implant should be in direct contact with host bone to allow ingrowth; this is not possible if the implant is only in contact with bone allograft. At present, it is not possible to define a minimum area of bone-implant contact to allow bone ingrowth and secondary stability. In younger patients, we should consider other techniques that restore the bone stock. The possibility of micro movements and metal wear between the cup and augment is also a concern. The long-term results of this technique are still unknown.

Alternative evidence-based techniques for the case: In uncontained defects, impaction bone grafting with rim meshes has the advantage of bone stock reconstruction, but there is a risk of bone reabsorption and cup migration in the case of massive bone loss. The revascularization and remodeling of structural bone allografts are associated with a high complication rate, with bone collapse and component loosening, mainly if they provide most of the support for the component. There is also a concern about possible disease transmission with allografts. Acetabular reconstruction cages have the advantage of bridging the ilium and the ischium and can be used if the posterior wall is missing and in the case of pelvic discontinuity. Their implantation is technically difficult, and the main disadvantage is the lack of bone ingrowth, and mechanical failure at the midterm follow-up. Other alternatives are bilobed acetabular components and high placement of the hip centre of rotation.

Why is the chosen technique better for this case? This technique permits the restoration of the migrated hip centre, and the augment gives superior support for cup stability.

Indications and contraindications for your technique: When implant stability and correction of the hip center is not possible with a standard revision cup due to the absence of superior support. With the acetabular distraction technique, this type of implant can be used in the case of chronic pelvic discontinuity. In cases where press-fit fixation is impossible to achieve, even with augments, other reconstruction strategies should be used.

Learning curve and how to manage complications: The use of augments is technically less demanding than the reconstruction cages and structural allografts.

Level of evidence concerning the superiority of this method against others: Porous cups and acetabular augments have shown reliable and durable results for reconstruction in the case of major bone defects (Paprosky types II and III) at midterm follow-up [11, 12].

19.4 Case Title: Revision of Paprosky IIIB Defect with Massive Bone Loss

Michael J. Feldstein, Matthew S. Austin, and William J. Hozack

19.4.1 Demographics

Age: 68 years old
Sex: Female
BMI: 32

19.4.2 Relevant Past Medical History

Principal pathologies: Rheumatoid arthritis, non-insulin-dependent diabetes mellitus, MI, DVT, CVA, HTN, HLD, GI bleed, SCFE, left TKA infection status post two-stage reimplantation.

Previous surgical procedures: IVC filter, SCFE pinning, removal of SCFE hardware.

Medication: Coumadin, Nexium, glipizide, gabapentin, leflunomide, atorvastatin, hydrochlorothiazide, metoprolol, verapamil, lisinopril.

History of presenting complaint: This is the case of a patient with a history of slipped capital femoral epiphysis that initially had a left total hip arthroplasty in 1985 at the age of 39 for degenerative joint disease and acetabular protrusio secondary to rheumatoid arthritis. This total hip replacement functioned well for 25 years until it was revised in 2010 for aseptic loosening of the acetabular shell. At the time of her first revision in 2010, she was found to have a Paprosky type IIC defect, and this was revised with bone grafting and placement of a large cup with six screws and an eccentric liner, while the femoral component was left in place. In 2013, she presented to the clinic with left hip pain and mechanical failure of the acetabular component. Radiographs and CT scan revealed a Paprosky type IIIB defect of the acetabulum with a >3 cm superior migration of the hip centre, ischial osteolysis, and violation of Kohler's line with obliteration of the teardrop (Fig. 19.7).

19.4.3 Clinical Examination

Symptoms: Groin pain, feeling of instability of the hip.

Range of motion: Limited exam secondary to hip pain.

Specific tests: ESR: 63 mm/h; CRP: 1.24 mg/dL; hip aspiration was performed revealing a negative gram stain; no growth from cultures, 108 WBCs and 55% PMNs.

Main disability: Ambulatory dysfunction.

Neurovascular evaluation: Sensation and motor intact distally. Palpable pulses distally.

19.4.4 Preoperative Radiological Assessment/Imaging (Figs. 19.7, 19.8, and 19.9)

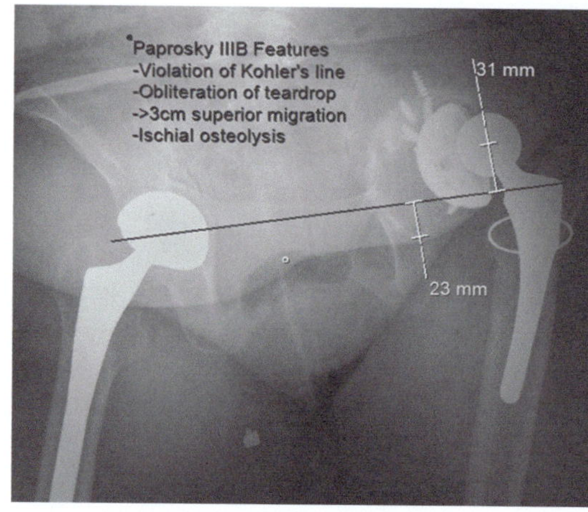

Fig. 19.7 Paprosky type IIIB defect with a failed acetabular cup. The horizontal line is the superior obturator line. From this, the level of superior migration and ischial osteolysis can be measured. The ischial involvement is greater than 15 mm indicating severe osteolysis. Kohler's line has been disrupted, and there is severe lysis of the teardrop. Although difficult to measure because the cup has failed, superior migration of the center of rotation of the femoral head is greater than 3 cm

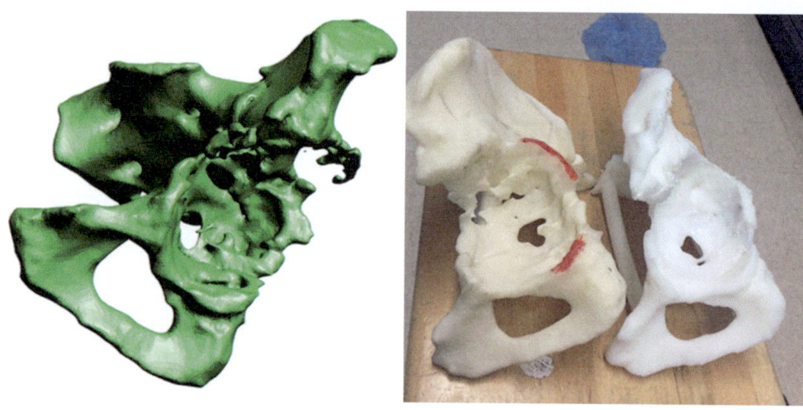

Fig. 19.8 3D CT reconstruction

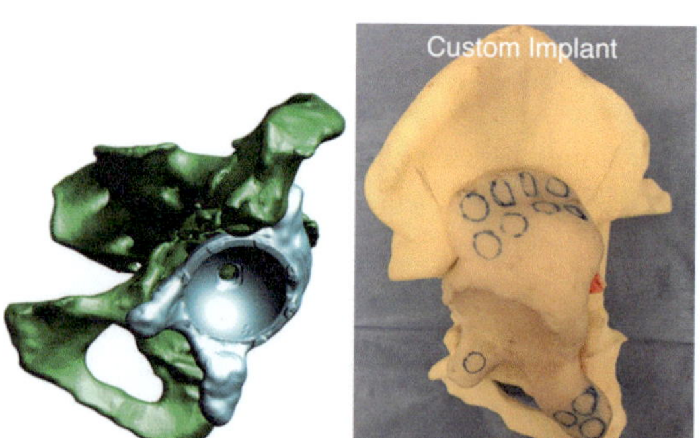

Fig. 19.9 Custom implant design

3D reconstructions of the pelvis were obtained for evaluation of the defect and custom implant design. The 3D CT and 3D printed models further highlight characteristics of the IIIB defect seen on X-ray. The medial wall of the acetabulum has been violated, and the anterior column is deficient. There is also an erosion of bone superiorly into the ilium as well as ischial bone erosion.

Three-dimensional models were used to create a custom triflange implant that can anchor to the ilium, ischium, and pubis to bridge the defect. This type of implant is especially useful in pelvic discontinuity.

19.4.5 Preoperative Planning

Diagnosis: Aseptic failure of revision total hip arthroplasty with Paprosky type IIIB acetabular defect (Fig. 19.7).

Possible treatment options: Cementless jumbo cup, cementless jumbo cup with augments, cup-cage construct, custom triflange cage.

Chosen treatment method: Custom triflange cage.

Selection of implants if applicable and rational: Custom triflange cage was chosen to provide maximum stability of the construct given the severe bone loss (Figs. 19.8 and 19.9).

Expected difficulties: Pelvis could convert to pelvic discontinuity during reaming. Custom cage may not fit well if there are intraoperative changes to anatomy or further progression of bone loss preoperatively.

Strategies to overcome difficulties: Must have equipment (pelvic reconstruction hardware) ready to treat discontinuity should this occur. If the custom implant does not fit, convert to acetabular porous metal augments that can be used to provide support for a cementless cup against host bone.

Templating: Radiographs and CT were used for pre-op planning and templating. A 3D printed pelvis model can be very useful for templating implants as the three-dimensional nature of the defect makes templating from images alone difficult. A 3D model was used to design the custom implant and to develop a backup construct (Figs. 19.8, 19.9 and 19.10).

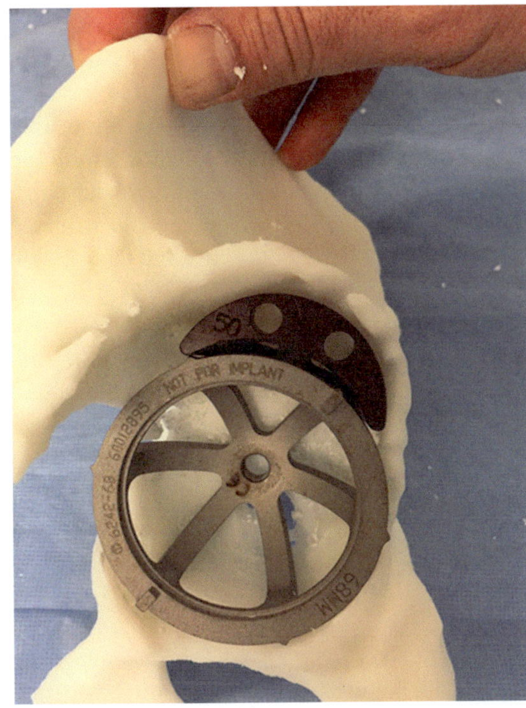

Fig. 19.10 The final implant used had been templated as a backup preoperatively. A 3D printed model was generated from the CT and was then reamed for placement of the jumbo cup with augment. The augment fills the superior defect while the jumbo cup fills in the medial and inferior defects

19.4.6 Surgical Note

Patient's position: Supine on a regular table.
Type of anesthesia: Spinal.
Surgical approach: Direct lateral.

Main steps: A modified anterolateral gluteus medius splitting approach was made to the left hip. There was no overt evidence of infection seen. The femoral component was exposed. The femoral head component was disimpacted and removed. The femoral stem was checked and noted to be in good position and stable and therefore, it was maintained. Attention was then turned to the acetabular component, which was grossly loose. There was a massive amount of bone loss encountered, and a Paprosky type IIIB defect was confirmed. An attempt was made to insert the custom cage; however, there was not a proper fit, and this was abandoned. The remaining acetabulum was reamed to accept a size 78 mm jumbo porous metal shell. The superior acetabular defect was augmented with an augment measuring 50 × 10 mm with two screws providing fixation. The acetabulum was then bone grafted with a combination of cancellous allograft and demineralized bone matrix. The acetabular cup was impacted into place, and three screws were utilized for supplemental fixation. The interface between the acetabular component and the augment was then cemented. A 36, 0-degree liner was utilized. Trial and final reduction of the hip revealed excellent leg length, stability, and range of motion. The incision was copiously irrigated at multiple points during the case and the incision was closed in layers (Fig. 19.11).

Reconstruction techniques: Reamers were used to reshape the pelvis for the jumbo revision porous metal cup. Augments were utilized and screws for acetabular fixation. A custom cage was attempted but was aborted because it did not fit.

19.4.7 Intraoperative Challenges

Challenges and solutions: The custom cage implant did not fit well. This was anticipated, and jumbo cups with augments were available. A good fit was achieved using a jumbo cup with screws for augmentation and a superior augment.

Thorough description of decision-making, including the reason for the final decision: The fit of the custom implant was inadequate due to continued bone loss since the CT that it was based upon had been taken. Both cages and augments were available as a backup. Because a 3D pelvis had been constructed to design the custom implant, this was also used to develop a backup construct consisting of a cementless jumbo cup and porous metal augment (Fig. 19.10). After reaming the model to size the cup and fitting the appropriate size and shape augment, the construct appeared to be stable. The final implant was chosen for this IIIB defect case and was based upon this preoperative "practice" run.

19.4.8 Postoperative Radiographs (Fig. 19.11)

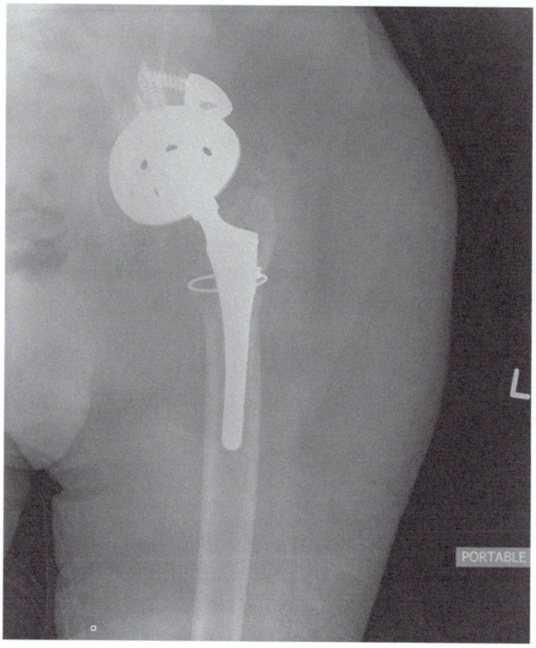

Fig. 19.11 AP of left hip post-op with jumbo cup and augment. Note that one broken screw was retained from the prior surgery

19.4.9 Postoperative Management

Chemoprophylaxis and anticoagulant treatment period: Perioperative antibiotics including vancomycin and cephalexin. The patient was on Coumadin preoperatively for a history of a thromboembolic disease, and this was restarted postoperatively.

Gait/limb loading until full loading: The patient was limited to toe-touch weight bearing (10% of body weight on the reconstructed side) for twelve weeks with hip precautions for six weeks.

19.4.10 Follow-Up and Complications

The revision became infected one month postoperatively and returned to the operating room for irrigation and debridement, removal of all hardware including the femoral components, and antibiotic spacer placement. The spacer was eventually replaced with another jumbo cup, and the femur had to be revised to a revision modular stem. This became infected, and the patient underwent irrigation and debridement and is now on chronic antibiotic suppression.

19.4.11 Discussion

Advantages of the applied method: The advantages of large porous metal cups are that they are technically straightforward, and once ingrown they provide a stable construct that will be anchored to both columns. They also maximize contact with host bone, reduce the need for bone grafting, and help normalize the hip center of rotation. Porous metal augments facilitate the fixation of the cementless cup when there is not enough circumferential bone. These augments are an alternative to traditional allograft reconstruction of severe acetabular bone loss.

Disadvantages of the method: The disadvantages of using large cups are that they may not have an adequate initial fixation in massive bone loss cases and may not become osseointegrated. If there is a pelvic discontinuity, this technique may not work unless a distraction technique is utilized.

Alternative evidence-based techniques for the case: Custom triflange components can help with fixation and bridging of defects, especially if there is a concern for discontinuity, but have the disadvantage of a potential mismatch between the implant and the bone stock found intraoperatively. This was the case here, as there was an additional bone loss from the time the CT scan was obtained and the surgical reconstruction. Modular cup, cage constructs, and cup-cage constructs have also been described. These provide extra modularity and more points of fixation, but have the disadvantage of requiring multiple interfaces, may require cement, and pose their own unique technical challenges.

Why is the chosen technique better for this case? In this case, the custom implant did not fit, but a jumbo cup and augment had good fixation after reaming and screw fixation with augments.

Indications and contraindications for your technique: The indications for jumbo cup with augment use are Paprosky type II and III defects that can be reamed to create a circumferential socket, with the aid of augments, that will provide adequate fixation for the hemispherical cup. If a good press fit cannot be obtained intraoperatively with the cup alone, augments or a cage should be used to aid fixation. In cases of pelvic discontinuity, alternative techniques must be added, for example, plating of the fracture or expansion osteotomy of the discontinuity.

Learning curve and how to manage complications: One advantage of jumbo cup use is that the technique is straightforward and similar to the placement of a standard cup.

Level of evidence concerning the superiority of this method against others: Most evidence for the use of jumbo cups or custom implants are level IV studies [32–34].

19.5 Case Title: Acetabular Augment for Acetabular Bone Deficiency

William L. Griffin

19.5.1 Demographics

Age: 80 years
Sex: Female
BMI: 27

19.5.2 Relevant Past Medical History

Principal pathologies: Infected THA with femoral and acetabular bone loss.

Previous surgical procedures: Multiple previous THAs with loss of abductors and recurrent dislocations. Currently with MRSA deep infection.

Other: Relatively healthy for age of 80 years.

History of presenting complaint: Presents with a draining wound and well-fixed cementless components with a constrained liner due to absent abductor mechanism (Fig. 19.12). Treated with Prostalac and six weeks of IV antibiotics (Fig. 19.13). At the 6-week point, the patient sustained a ground level fall with an acetabular fracture and displacement of the acetabular Prostalac (Fig. 19.14).

19.5.3 Clinical Examination

Symptoms: Pain, shortening of the right THA. Prior Trendelenburg gait, now unable to mobilize.

Range of motion: Painful ROM.

Specific tests: ESR and CRP were elevated, and hip aspiration revealed MRSA infection. After IV antibiotic treatment, CRP and ESR had improved but remained elevated. Aspiration of the hip was negative for infection.

Neurovascular evaluation: Intact.

19.5.4 Preoperative Radiological Assessment/Imaging (Figs. 19.12, 19.13, and 19.14)

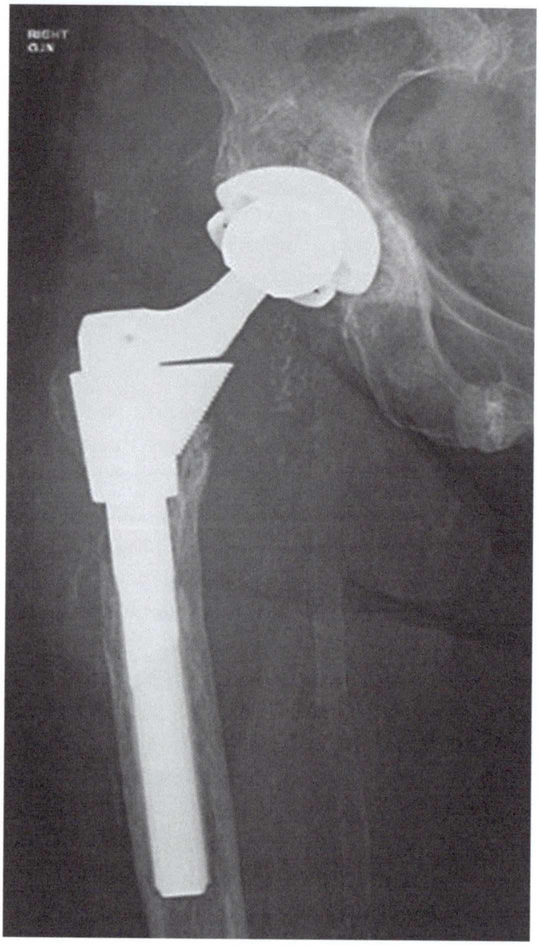

Fig. 19.12 AP X-ray right THA with well-fixed components and severe osteoporosis with healed inferior pubic ramus fracture

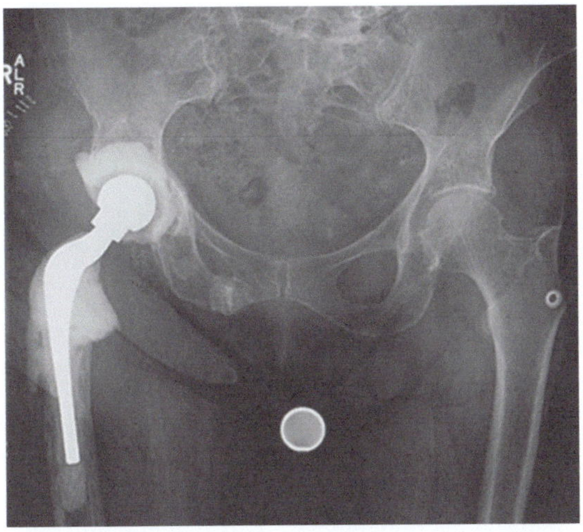

Fig. 19.13 AP pelvis X-ray after conversion to Prostalac and debridement of nonviable bone

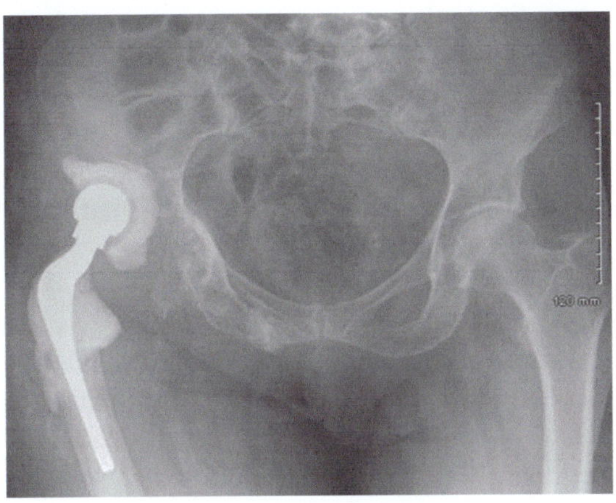

Fig. 19.14 AP pelvis X-ray: 6 weeks into antibiotic treatment of MRSA infection. Patient falls and fractures acetabulum with displacement of the acetabular Prostalac component

19.5.5 Preoperative Planning

Diagnosis: Treated MRSA infection of the right THA with acute acetabular fracture and patient now unable to mobilize due to pain (Fig. 19.14).

Possible treatment options: Infection workup to ensure that the infection has been treated adequately. Reimplant with acetabular augments for deficient acetabular rim and distal femoral fixation for femoral bony deficiency.

Chosen treatment method: Cementless acetabular fixation with a highly porous augment reconstruction of the superior rim and a modular Wagner revision stem for distal femoral fixation.

Expected difficulties: Severe osteoporosis and bone loss of the acetabulum and femur.

Strategies to overcome difficulties: Cementless high porous augment to buttress the superior rim of the acetabulum. Distal fixation of the femoral component to accommodate severe bone loss.

19.5.6 Surgical Note

Patient's position: Lateral.
Type of anesthesia: General.
Surgical approach: Posterior.

Main steps: (1) Prostalac removal. (2) Preparation of the anatomic acetabulum with reamers to determine the cup size. (3) Size acetabular rim defect and use reamers to size defect and prepare a smooth surface. (4) Place augment with provisional pins with the trial cup in place. (5) Add screws to augment. (6) Apply cement to the augment and impact acetabular component. (7) Prepare femur and insert stem (Figs. 19.15 and 19.16).

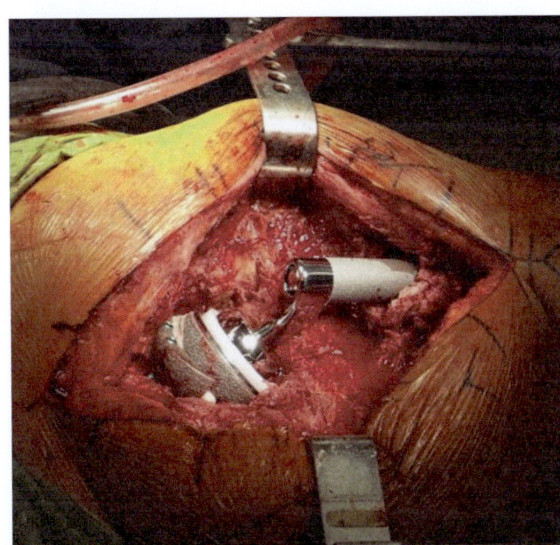

Fig. 19.15 Intraoperative view of the acetabular rim defect and augment with cement at the component interface. Modular Wagner femoral revision stem with severe proximal femoral bone loss

19.5.7 Intraoperative Challenges

Challenges and solutions: Need to anticipate the loss of acetabular rim bone and have appropriate implants available. Poor bone quality required very delicate reaming of the acetabulum and the rim defect.

19.5.8 Postoperative Radiographs (Fig. 19.16)

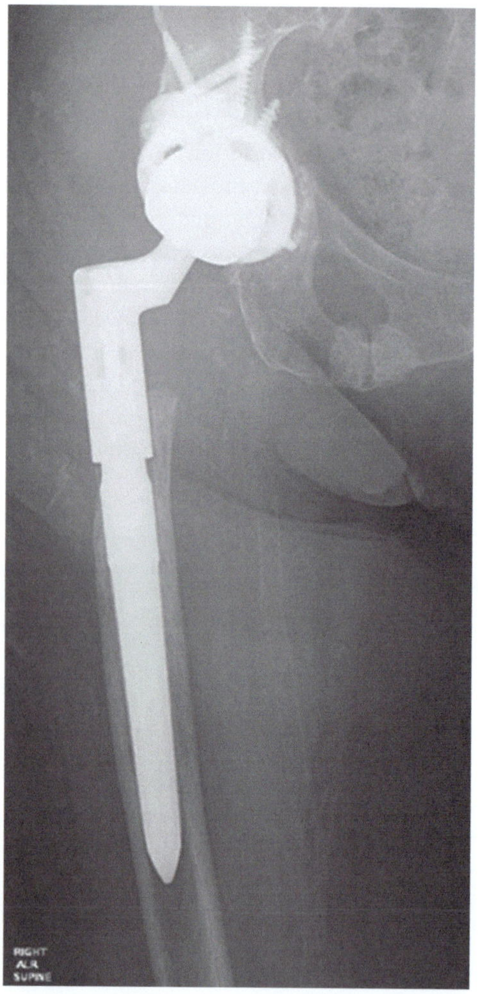

Fig. 19.16 Post-op AP pelvis X-ray: The acetabular component in anatomic position with superior acetabular augment and multiple screw fixation. Distal fixation of the modular Wagner revision stem and the use of a large unconstrained head to prevent dislocation of this abductor-deficient hip and avoid impingement and traction forces on this precarious fixation of the acetabular component

19.5.9 Postoperative Management

Chemoprophylaxis and anticoagulant treatment period: Standard DVT prophylaxis for high-risk patients (Coumadin × 4 weeks)

Gait/limb loading until full loading: Dislocation precautions and touchdown weight bearing for six weeks

19.5.10 Discussion

Why is the chosen technique better for this case? There are a number of techniques to address acetabular bone deficiencies. This defect could have been managed with a structural allograft, a cemented cage reconstruction, a cup-cage construct, or a custom triflange component. Morselized allograft or impaction grafting techniques would not have provided sufficient rim support in this case. With the recent infection, the use of allograft is worrisome for recurrent infection. The small size of the patient limits the effectiveness of a cup-cage construct in this particular case because a smaller cup would not allow for a large head to help prevent dislocation.

Level of evidence concerning the superiority of this method against others: Several publications have documented reliable fixation at midterm follow-up with the use of acetabular augments, and the use of modular Wagner revision stems in the face of severe bone loss [12, 35, 36].

19.6 Case Title: The Use of Acetabular Augments for Revision Total Hip Arthroplasty

Savyasachi C. Thakkar and James D. Slover

19.6.1 Demographics

Age: 71 years old
Sex: Male
BMI: 37

19.6.2 Relevant Past Medical History

Principal pathologies: Osteolysis and mechanical failure of total hip prosthesis.

Previous surgical procedures: Left total hip arthroplasty, left tibia open reduction internal fixation and skin grafting, right ankle open reduction internal fixation.

Medication: Multivitamins, Aleve.

Other: Obesity, former smoker (quit at the age of 61 years).

History of presenting complaint: Patient presented to the clinic with activity-related left hip pain for approximately one year. The patient also complained of night pain. The patient did not complain of instability.

19.6.3 Clinical Examination

Symptoms: Activity-related left hip/proximal thigh pain, limb length discrepancy

Range of motion: Flexion 90°, internal rotation 0°, external rotation 30°

Specific tests: Antalgic gait, left limb shorter than right limb by 2 inches

Main disability: Activity-related pain

Scoring: Lower extremity functional scale—29/80

Neurovascular evaluation: Intact distal pulses, sensory-motor exam normal in all nerve distributions

19.6.4 Preoperative Radiological Assessment/Imaging (Figs. 19.17, 19.18, and 19.19)

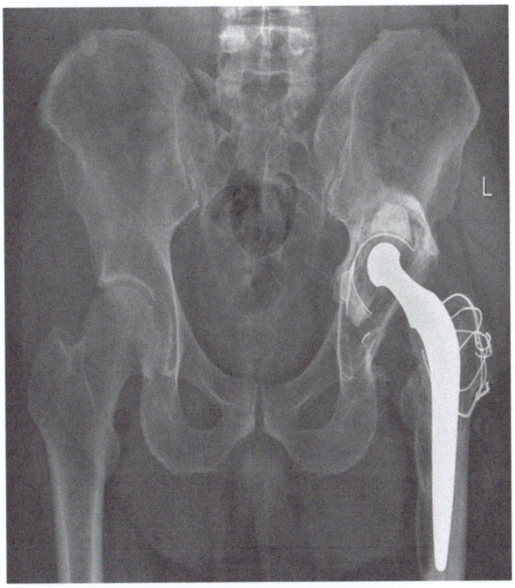

Fig. 19.17 Anteroposterior pelvis radiograph depicting a cemented total hip arthroplasty with eccentricity of the femoral head in the polyethylene liner

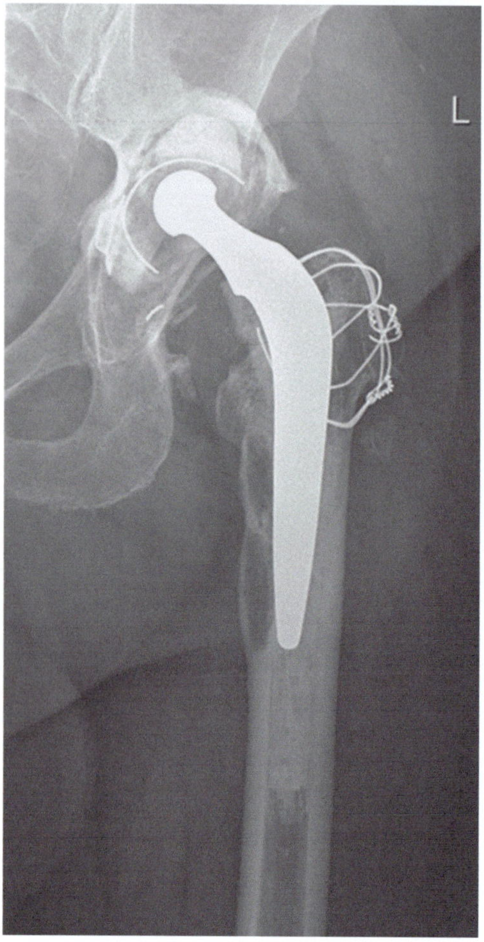

Fig. 19.18 Anteroposterior radiograph of the left hip showing osteolytic defects in the medial proximal femoral cortex

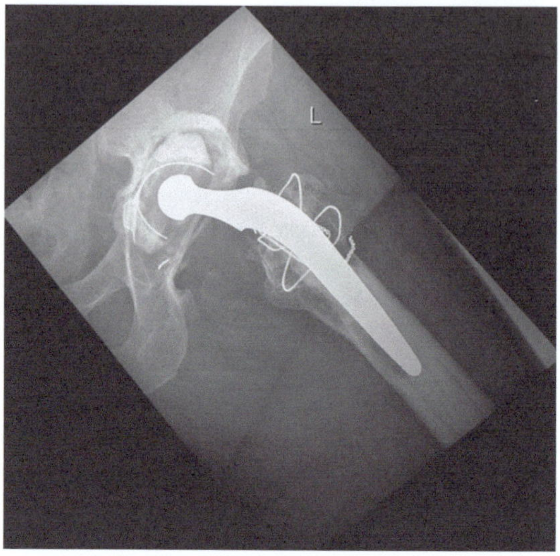

Fig. 19.19 Lateral radiograph of the left hip showing osteolytic defects in the posterior proximal femoral cortex *Other*: Interventional radiology-guided aspiration of the left hip joint fluid showed no organisms on gram stain and gram-negative cultures

19.6.5 Preoperative Planning

Diagnosis: Left total hip arthroplasty wear and aseptic loosening (Figs. 19.17, 19.18 and 19.19)

Possible treatment options: Acetabular component—hemispherical porous-coated shell, jumbo shell, oblong shell, impaction bone grafting, structural allograft, porous tantalum cups and augments, porous tantalum cup-cage construct. Femoral component—proximally coated femoral implants, fully coated stems, revision monolithic/modular stems

Chosen treatment method: Acetabulum—porous tantalum cup with an augment. Femur—revision fully coated modular stem

Selection of implants if applicable and rational: Acetabulum—Zimmer highly porous cup with acetabular augment to account for the acetabular bony defect. Femur—Stryker Restoration Modular stem with cobalt-chrome head to account for the femoral bony defect

Expected difficulties: Sciatic nerve entrapment in scar tissue. Gaining adequate exposure to components, fixation of implants, managing acetabular and femoral bone loss

Strategies to overcome difficulties: Extensile posterior approach, appropriate implant extraction instruments, performing an extended trochanteric osteotomy (ETO) to aid in removal of implants, access to revision implants, augments, bone graft, plates, cables

Templating: Acetate prints

19.6.6 Surgical Note

Patient's position: Lateral decubitus

Type of anesthesia: General endotracheal anesthesia

Surgical approach: Posterior

Main steps:

1. Identified and protected sciatic nerve.
2. Obtain adequate exposure to femoral and acetabular components.
3. Obtain tissue for frozen sample and intraoperative tissue culture for microbiological analysis.
4. Remove acetabular component and cement mantle.
5. Ream acetabulum.
6. Augment placed to buttress acetabular roof defect.
7. Bone graft impacted into native acetabulum floor.
8. Acetabular cup placed along with dome screws.
9. Cement at the cup-augment interface.
10. Perform extended trochanteric osteotomy to gain access to cement mantle and femoral component.
11. Extract femoral component.
12. Guide wire placed in the femur for sequential reaming.
13. Proximal reaming performed.
14. Trial components placed and intraoperative range of motion and stability assessed.
15. Final components placed.
16. Trochanteric osteotomy repaired using a plate, cerclage cables, and allograft strut.
17. Vancomycin powder and betadine irrigation.
18. Sequential layered complex closure.
19. Intraoperative X-rays.

Reconstruction techniques: Acetabulum—augment buttress, morcellized bone grafting, porous tantalum shell. Femur—modular revision stem, trochanteric plate, cerclage cables (Figs. 19.20 and 19.21).

19.6.7 Intraoperative Challenges

Challenges and solutions: Access to the components—extensile posterior approach and extended trochanteric osteotomy. Filling acetabular defect—impaction bone grafting, trabecular metal augment, and trabecular metal shell. Filling femoral defect—modular conical diaphyseal fitting stem

Unanticipated problems and solution: Excessive scar tissue around neurological structures—intraoperative neurological monitoring. Acetabular cement mantle—Moreland instruments. Femoral cement mantle and component extraction—extended trochanteric osteotomy

Thorough description of decision-making, including the reason for the final decision:

1. Positioning and approach—since the patient had undergone the index surgery with a posterior approach to the hip, the same approach was utilized and extended as necessary to obtain adequate exposure. The sciatic nerve was identified, and we did not note significant scar tissue around the nerve. We were also able to use the piriformis and external rotators to protect the nerve intraoperatively. We did not feel the need to have intraoperative neurological monitoring for the sciatic nerve.
2. Tissue samples—we decided to send tissue samples for frozen section and microbiological analysis especially to detect acute inflammation. Since the results were negative for acute inflammation, we decided to proceed with the revision surgery. Alternatively, we would have performed a two-stage revision with antibiotic spacer placement.
3. Acetabulum—once the acetabular components were removed, the bony void was classified as a Paprosky type IIIB defect, and we found that an appropriately sized trabecular metal augment could be used to buttress the roof of the acetabulum. Also, a porous tantalum multi-hole shell with impaction bone grafting was selected to achieve stability of the acetabular component.
4. Femur—since the patient had a long-stem cemented femoral component, we elected to perform an extended trochanteric osteotomy to gain access to the cement mantle and to aid in the extraction of the femoral component. We also elected to use a trochanteric plate with several cerclage cables and an allograft strut to augment stability for the revision femoral component. A modular femoral revision component that gave primary diaphyseal fixation was chosen due to severe proximal femoral bone loss secondary to osteolysis.

19.6.8 Postoperative Radiographs (Figs. 19.20 and 19.21)

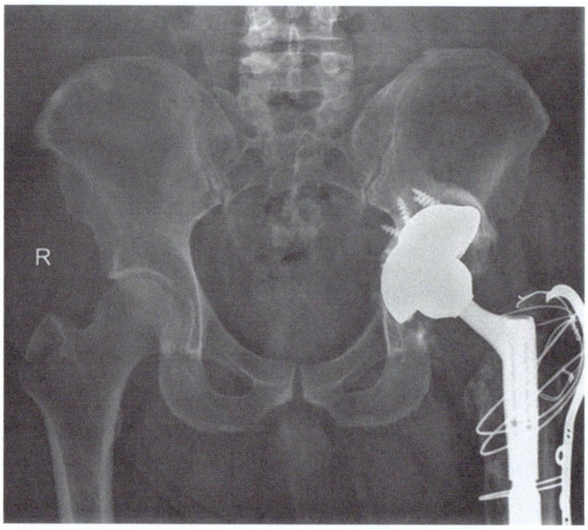

Fig. 19.20 Anteroposterior pelvic radiograph depicting a porous tantalum cup and augment with multiple screws and a uncemented modular revision femoral stem supported by an allograft strut and a trochanteric plate with cerclage cables

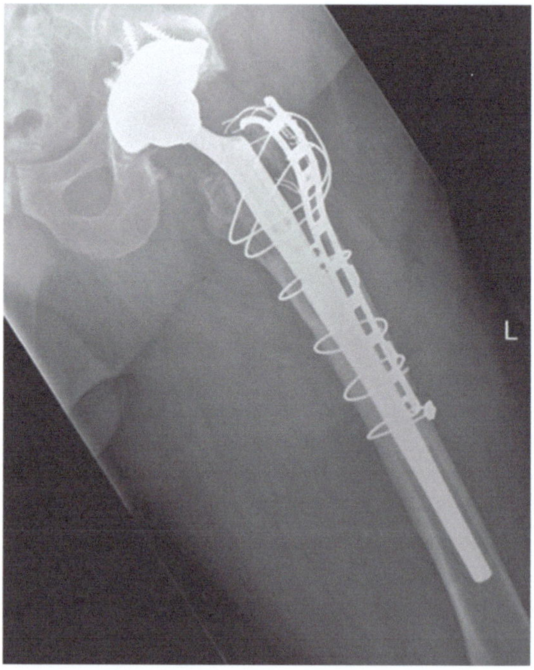

Fig. 19.21 Lateral radiograph of the left hip demonstrating a fully coated uncemented modular revision stem, trochanteric plate, cerclage cables, and porous tantalum cup with an augment

19.6.9 Postoperative Management

Chemoprophylaxis and anticoagulant treatment period: Aspirin 325 mg by mouth twice daily for four weeks postoperatively.

Gait/limb loading until full loading: 25–50% partial weight bearing on the operative limb for six weeks postoperatively with subsequent progression to full weight bearing.

19.6.10 Follow-Up and Complications

No complications were noted postoperatively.

19.6.11 Discussion

Advantages of the applied method: Porous tantalum cups have a high volumetric porosity (75–85%) and high frictional characteristics that make them conducive to biological fixation with extensive bony ingrowth. They are safe and biocompatible and have a modulus of elasticity (3 MPa) similar to that of subchondral bone to allow better physiologic load transfer and a higher endurance limit, yield strength, and ultimate strength. In acetabular revisions, porous tantalum cups have shown encouraging early results, and porous tantalum augments may serve as a structural bone graft substitute. Another advantage is that modularity of components to match bony defects results in a minimal need to remodel the host bone.

Disadvantages of the method: Porous tantalum cups and augments have limitations including notch sensitivity, brittleness, and the lack of host bone stock restoration. They are also expensive to use and may not be readily available universally to the arthroplasty surgeon.

Alternative evidence-based techniques for the case: Contained acetabular defects—standard cemented/uncemented primary-type cup with morcellized bone graft or impaction grafting with mesh and a cemented cup. Global contained defects can be treated with morcellized bone graft protected by reconstruction cage contact and a cemented cup. Uncontained acetabular defects—high hip center arthroplasty, oblong or eccentric cups, jumbo cups, minor/major column structural allografts, reconstruction cages/custom-made triflange cups, and porous tantalum cup-cage constructs.

Why is the chosen technique better for this case? Our patient had a Paprosky type IIIB acetabular defect which means that the columns are no longer supportive; there is a superomedial migration of the femoral head with teardrop lysis, and there is a rim defect from the 9 o'clock to 5 o'clock position. Also, based on the Saleh and Gross classification and based on the actual bone stock remaining at final reaming after implant/cement/debris removal, our patient had a type III defect—uncontained segmental defect involving less than 50% of the acetabulum and one column. Treatment strategies for Paprosky type IIIB defects are focused on restoring the superior support for a hemispherical cup with minimal removal of host bone. Options include high hip center arthroplasty, oblong/eccentric cups, jumbo cups, minor structural allograft, or porous tantalum cups and augments. High hip center arthroplasty has several biomechanical disadvantages related to abductor function. Hip stability may also be compromised due to bony impingement and small femoral head dictated by a small cup. High-offset femoral components are often used which may increase the bending moment on the stem and lead to loosening. Oblong/eccentric cups are technically challenging to place, and special reamers are often required making component position difficult to obtain. Simultaneous restoration of an appropriate hip center of rotation, contact on host bone, and proper version and inclination can be difficult. Jumbo cups, on the other hand, include the sacrifice of a large amount of host bone and can lead to soft tissue impingement especially of the iliopsoas. Minor structural allografts, even though are a very good alternative for porous tantalum cups and augments, are not universally available and do have a potential for disease transmission and the possibility of late graft resorption and collapse. Porous tantalum cups and augments have shown very good early results for type III defects, 96.4–98% survivorship at 1–4 years. In case of our patient with limited bone stock and already compromised soft tissue function from injury-related complications leading to a THA, porous tantalum cups and cages seemed to be the best option for reconstruction [37–39].

Indications and contraindications for your technique: Indications—Paprosky type IIIB acetabular defect, revision acetabular surgery. Contraindications—infection, pelvic discontinuity [37–39].

Learning curve and how to manage complications: These cases are best managed by a fellowship-trained adult reconstruction surgery who is familiar with the use of various options to manage acetabular and femoral bone loss in cases of revision surgery.

Level of evidence concerning the superiority of this method against others: IV.

19.7 Case Title: Acetabular Revision Following Two-Stage Exchange

Julie Shaner and Javad Parvizi

19.7.1 Demographics

Age: 71 years
Sex: Male
BMI: 26.2

19.7.2 Relevant Past Medical History

Principal pathologies: Non-insulin-dependent diabetes, hypertension, deep venous thrombosis.

Previous surgical procedures: Right total hip arthroplasty 2008, left total hip arthroplasty 2011, inferior vena cava filter (Fig. 19.22).

Medication: Januvia, atenolol, Tylenol, Coumadin.

History of Presenting Complaint: 71-year-old male with primary left THA in 2011 evaluated in the emergency room four years after index procedure for L THA dislocation. Described having several months of nagging left hip pain and two weeks of acutely worse and progressive left groin pain exacerbated by weight bearing for which he was taking Tylenol PRN. Laboratory values included ESR 49 mm/h and CRP 19 mg/L. An aspiration of the left hip showed 80,000 neutrophils and a differential of 92%.

19.7.3 Clinical Examination

Symptoms: Acute left anterior groin and pelvic pain and inability to bear weight on the left lower extremity.

Range of motion: The patient was unable to perform an active hip range of motion secondary to pain, subluxation, and dislocation of the hip with passive range of motion.

Main disability: Acute on chronic left groin pain and inability to bear weight on left lower extremity.

Neurovascular evaluation: Sensation intact to light touch over bilateral superficial and deep peroneal and tibial nerve distributions. Palpable, albeit weak, pulses bilaterally. Motor function intact with the exception of weak abduction.

19.7.4 Preoperative Radiological Assessment/Imaging (Figs. 19.22, 19.23, and 19.24)

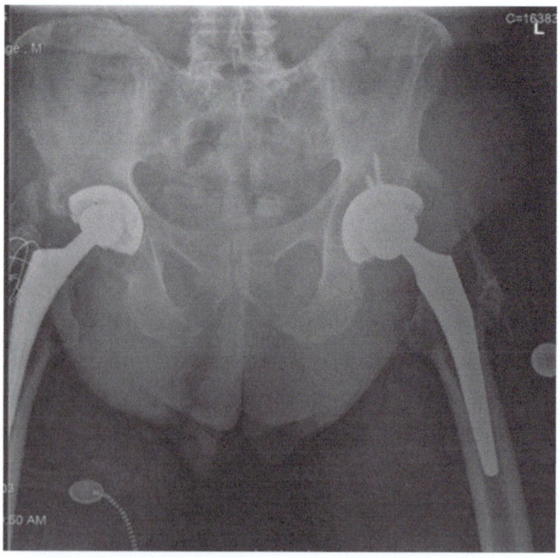

Fig. 19.22 Most recent routine follow-up PA pelvis, prior to emergency department presentation. Evidence of significant femoral peritrochanteric and pelvic periacetabular osteolysis

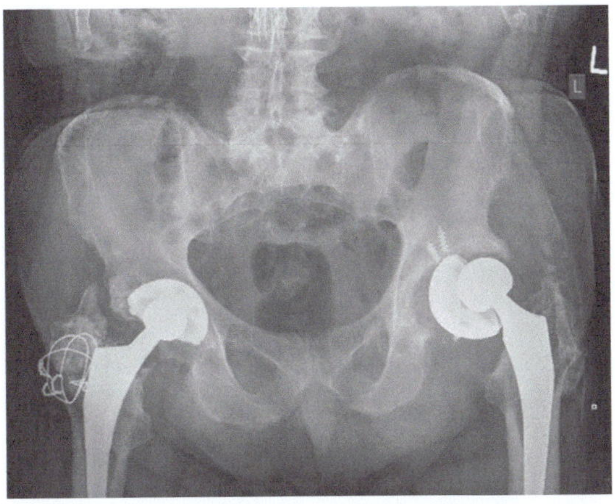

Fig. 19.23 AP pelvis taken in the emergency room; loose cup, with cup and head dislocation. Redemonstration of proximal femoral and periacetabular osteolysis

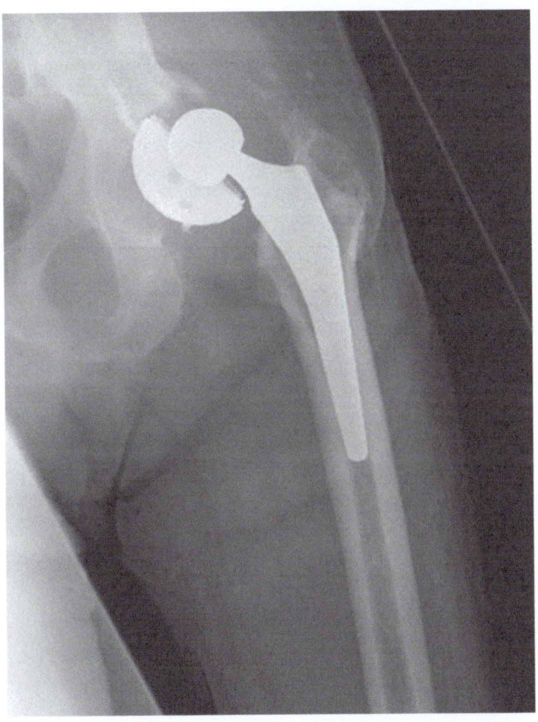

Fig. 19.24 AP left hip in the emergency room; loose cup, with cup and head dislocation. Redemonstration of proximal femoral and periacetabular osteolysis. Presence of heterotopic ossification and retained broken screw fragments in the posterosuperior acetabulum

19.7.5 Preoperative Planning

Diagnosis: Dislocated left total hip arthroplasty secondary to septic loosening and suspected corrosion and trunnionosis of the femoral stem (Figs. 19.23 and 19.24).

Possible treatment options: One-stage exchange versus two-stage exchange with an antibiotic spacer followed by revision total hip arthroplasty with acetabular reconstruction with either hemispheric cup, antiprotrusio cage, custom pelvic reconstruction, or structural allograft to address areas of deficiency.

Chosen treatment method: Two-stage exchange followed by revision THA with a press-fit hemispherical cup with screw fixation and periacetabular buttress plate.

Expected difficulties: Acetabular bone loss involving the posterior wall and fractured medial wall detected at the time of explantation and spacer insertion.

Strategies to overcome difficulties: Have multiple implants available at the time of surgery including hemispheric jumbo-sized cups and cages along with bone graft. Also, have instruments available to assist with the extraction of components and screw fragments. Need to plan for possible difficulty in removing a well-fixed femoral stem including removal instruments and fixation cables if an extended trochanteric osteotomy is required.

19.7.6 Surgical Note

Patient's position: Supine.
Type of anesthesia: Spinal.
Surgical approach: Utilization of the prior lateral incision and direct lateral approach.

Main steps: The cement spacer was removed. The acetabulum and femur were examined. The acetabulum was found to have a deficiency of the posterior wall, and there was a fracture of the medial wall that was detected at the time of spacer implantation. The acetabulum was gently reamed. Attention was then turned to the femur. The canal was debrided and irrigated.

Reconstruction techniques: A hemispherical socket was placed; however, in the presence of posterior wall deficiency, a buttress augment was utilized to support the socket. The cup was fixed with multiple screws, and demineralized bone matrix was placed behind the acetabulum. The augment and the acetabular components were adjoined with the use of cement (Figs. 19.25 and 19.26).

19.7.7 Intraoperative Challenges

Challenges and solutions: Posterior wall deficiency was resolved with tantalum trabecular metal buttress augmentation of the hemispherical cup.

Unanticipated problems and solution: Deficient bone stock led to challenges in securing buttress augment. This was resolved with application of cement to adjoin the cup and the augment. The cup was also secured with multiple points of fixation.

Thorough description of decision-making, including the reason for the final decision: Acetabular reaming revealed sufficient bone stock such that it was decided to avoid further bone loss associated with reaming to accommodate a jumbo-sized cup. It was decided to address posterior wall deficiency separately with a posterior buttress. A porous-coated multi-hole tantalum cup was selected as it was anticipated; multiple points of fixation would be needed to secure the cup. It was decided that porous tantalum offered the best potential for bone ingrowth and reduced chance of periprosthetic infection. Structural allograft was avoided due to an increased risk of recurrent infection and associated risk of bone resorption and collapse.

19.7.8 Postoperative Radiographs (Figs. 19.25 and 19.26)

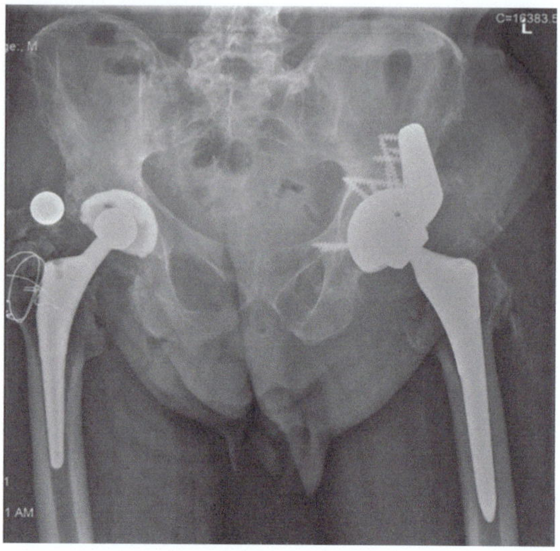

Fig. 19.25 AP pelvis with juxtaposed right-sided primary total hip arthroplasty with press-fit cup without additional screw fixation. Left side with cementless cup secured with multiple points of fixation. Trabecular metal augment functioning as a buttress to the cup

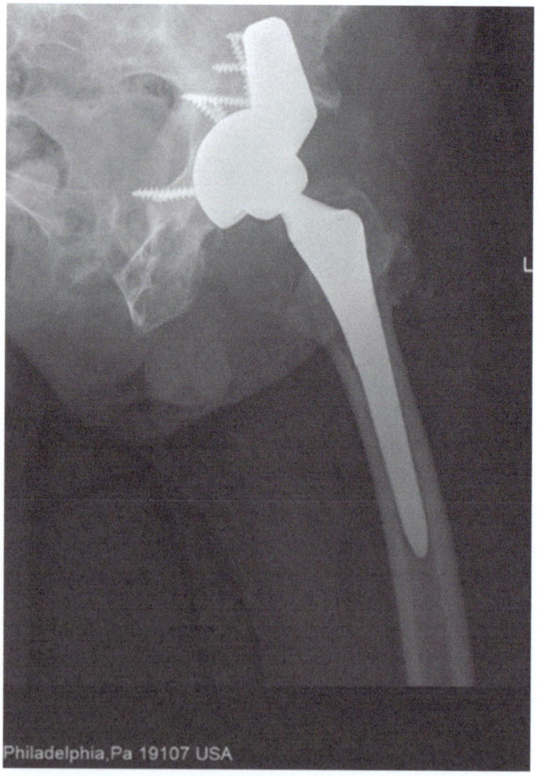

Fig. 19.26 Frog-leg lateral with redemonstration of the cementless cup with multiple points of screw fixation and trabecular metal augment

19.7.9 Postoperative Management

Chemoprophylaxis and anticoagulant treatment period: The patient was started on Coumadin post-op because of having had a history of prior DVTs.

Gait/limb loading until full loading: The patient was made toe-touch weight bearing for six weeks post-op.

19.7.10 Follow-Up and Complications

The patient has done well postoperatively except for developing a large hematoma because of uncontrolled anticoagulation. His INR was 8.5 at one point. The hematoma required evacuation. There have been no subsequent complications.

19.7.11 Discussion [27, 40–42]

Advantages of the applied method: The selected method of treatment offered the greatest preservation and potential restoration of host bone and biologic fixation. The increased elasticity and coefficient of friction of tantalum metal are associated with enhanced initial fixation and faster biologic fixation. This method also permits restoration of a normal hip center.

Disadvantages of the method: A disadvantage to this method of treatment includes the utilization of two discrete components lacking provisions for direct fixation to one another, therefore requiring supplemental means of adjoinment. In this setting, cement was used to adjoin the cup and the augment and may allow an additional interface for failure.

Alternative evidence-based techniques for the case: An alternative method of reconstruction would be using an antiprotrusio cage or a cup-cage construct.

Why is the chosen technique better for this case? Using a routine sized cup and an augment preserved host bone and allowed for potential restoration of bone stock with supplemental bone grafting. The use of an augment allows selection of sizes and shapes to address present defects specifically. It avoids creating a high hip center as can occur with the utilization of jumbo cups. And as opposed to using a structural allograft, the selected reconstruction is technically less difficult and without the risk of associated complications.

Indications and contraindications for your technique: Bone stock such that there is a minimum of 50% host bone contact is required to use a hemispherical cup. Augments are best applied in the setting of contained defects. Pelvic discontinuity would be a contraindication to hemispheric cup use.

References

1. Abolghasemian M, Tangsataporn S, Sternheim A, Backstein D, Safir O, Gross AE. Combined trabecular metal acetabular shell and augment for acetabular revision with substantial bone loss: a mid-term review. Bone Joint J. 2013;95-B:166–72.
2. Teeter MG, Naudie DDR, Howard JL, McCalden RW, MacDonald SJ. Do revision total hip augments provide appropriate modularity? Can J Surg. 2015;58(1):54–7.
3. Nehme A, Lewallen DG, Hanssen AD. Modular porous metal augments for treatment of severe acetabular bone loss during revision hip arthroplasty. Clin Orthop Relat Res. 2004;429:201–8.
4. Issack PS. Current concepts review use of porous tantalum for acetabular reconstruction in revision hip arthroplasty. J Bone Joint Surg Am. 2013;95:1981–7.
5. Sporer SM, Bottros JJ, Hulst JB, et al. Acetabular distraction: an alternative for severe defects with chronic pelvic discontinuity. Clin Orthop Relat Res. 2012;470:3156–63.
6. Brown NM. The revision hip arthroplasty acetabular distraction an alternative approach to pelvic discontinuity in failed total hip replacement. Bone Joint J. 2014;96-B(11 Suppl A):73–7.
7. Sheth NP. Management factorials in total hip arthroplasty acetabular distraction an alternative for severe acetabular bone loss and chronic pelvic discontinuity. Bone Joint J. 2014;96-B(11 Suppl A):36–42.
8. Ballester Alfaro JJ, Sueiro Fernandez J. Trabecular metal buttress augment and the trabecular metal cup-cage construct in revision hip arthroplasty for severe acetabular bone loss and pelvic discontinuity. Hip Int. 2010;20(S7):119–27.
9. Steven Borland W, et al. Use of porous trabecular metal augments with impaction bone grafting in management of acetabular bone loss early to medium-term results. Acta Orthop. 2012;83(4):347–52.

10. Weeden SH. The use of tantalum porous metal implants for Paprosky 3A and 3B defects. J Arthroplast. 2007;22(6 Suppl. 2):151–5.
11. Del Gaizo DJ. Tantalum augments for Paprosky IIIA defects remain stable at midterm follow up. Clin Orthop Relat Res. 2012;470:395–401.
12. Whitehouse MR. Continued good results with modular trabecular metal augments for Acetabular defects in hip Arthroplasty at 7 to 11 years. Clin Orthop Relat Res. 2015;473:521–7.
13. Fernandez-Fairen M, Murcia A, Blanco A, Merono A, Murcia A Jr, Ballester J. Revision of failed total hip arthroplasty acetabular cups to porous tantalum components: a 5-year follow-up study. J Arthroplast. 2010;25(6):865–72.
14. Grappiolo G, Loppini M, Longo UG, Traverso F, Mazziotta G, Denaro V. Trabecular metal augments for the Management of Paprosky Type III defects without pelvic discontinuity. J Arthroplast. 2015;30:1024–9.
15. Lingaraj K. The management of severe acetabular bone defects in revision hip arthroplasty using modular porous metal components. J Bone Joint Surg (Br). 2009;91-B:1555–60.
16. Cohen R. A porous tantalum trabecular metal: basic science. Am J Orthop. 2002;31:216–7.
17. Flecher X, Paproskyb W, Grillo JC, Aubaniaca JM, Argensona JN. Do tantalum components provide adequate primary fixation in all acetabular revisions? Orthop Traumatol Surg Res. 2010;96:235–41.
18. Levine B, la Valle CJ, Jacobs JJ. Applications of porous tantalum in total hip arthroplasty. J Am Acad Orthop Surg. 2006;14:646.
19. Meneghini RM, Meyer C, Buckley CA, et al. Mechanical stability of novel highly porous metal acetabular components in revision total hip arthroplasty. J Arthroplast. 2010;25:337.
20. Christie MJ. Clinical applications of trabecular metal. Am J Orthop. 2002;31:219–20.
21. Bobyn JD, Pilliar RM, Cameron HU, Weatherly GC, Kent GM. The effect of porous surface configuration on the tensile strength of fixation of implants by bone ingrowth. Clin Orthop Relat Res. 1980;149:291–8.
22. Bobyn JD, Poggie RA, Krygier JJ, Lewallen DG, Hanssen AD, Lewis RJ, Unger AS, O'Keefe TJ, Christie MJ, Nasser S, Wood JE, Stulberg SD, Tanzer M. Clinical validation of a structural porous tantalum biomaterial for adult reconstruction. J Bone Joint Surg Am. 2004;86(Suppl 2):123–9.
23. Bobyn JD, Stackpool GJ, Hacking SA, Tanzer M, Krygier JJ. Characteristics of bone ingrowth and interface mechanics of a new porous tantalum biomaterial. J Bone Joint Surg (Br). 1999;81-B:907–14.
24. Hacking SA, et al. Fibrous tissue ingrowth and attachment to porous tantalum. J Biomed Mater Res. 2000;52:631.
25. Van Kleunen JP, Lee GC, Lementowski PW, Nelson CL, Garino JP. Acetabular revisions using trabecular metal cups and augments. J Arthroplast. 2009;24(6 suppl):64–8.
26. Moličnik A. Porous tantalum shells and augments for acetabular cup revisions. Eur J Orthop Surg Traumatol. 2014;24:911–7.
27. Siegmeth A, Duncan CP, Masri BA, Kim WY, Garbuz DS. Modular tantalum augments for acetabular defects in revision hip arthroplasty. Clin Orthop Relat Res. 2009;467:199–205.
28. Sporer SM, Paprosky WG. The use of a trabecular metal acetabular component and trabecular metal augment for severe acetabular defects. J Arthroplast. 2006;21(6 suppl 2):83–6.
29. Sporer SM, Paprosky WG. Acetabular revision using a trabecular metal acetabular component for severe acetabular bone loss associated with a pelvic discontinuity. J Arthroplast. 2006;21(6 suppl 2):87–90.
30. Park DK, Della Valle CJ, Quigley L, Moric M, Rosenberg AG, Galante JO. Revision of the acetabular component without cement. A concise follow-up, at twenty to twenty-four years, of a previous report. J Bone Joint Surg Am. 2009;91(2):350–5.
31. Camacho A, Pinto F, Almeida R, Dantas P, Amaral L. Resultados da utilização de implantes de tântalo poroso em cirurgia de revisão acetabular. Rev Port Ortop Traum. 2013;21(1):17–25.
32. von Roth P, Abdel MP, Harmsen WS, Berry DJ. Uncemented jumbo cups for revision total hip arthroplasty: a concise follow-up, at a mean of twenty years, of a previous report. J Bone Jt Surg. 2015;97:284–7. doi:10.2106/JBJS.N.00798.
33. Chen AF, Hozack WJ. Component selection in revision total hip Arthroplasty. Orthop Clin North Am. 2014;45:275–86. doi:10.1016/j.ocl.2014.03.001.
34. Sheth NP, Nelson CL, Springer BD, Fehring TK, Paprosky WG. Acetabular bone loss in revision total hip arthroplasty: evaluation and management. J Am Acad Orthop Surg. 2013;21:128–39. doi:10.5435/JAAOS-21-03-128.
35. Klatte TO, Kendoff D, Sabihi R, Kamath AF, Rueger JM, Gehrke T. Tantalum acetabular augments in one-stage exchange of infected total hip arthroplasty: a case-control study. J Arthroplasty. 2014;29(7):1443–8.
36. Restrepo C, Mashadi M, Parvizi J, Austin MS, Hozack W. Modular femoral stems for revision total hip arthroplasty. Clin Orthop Relat Res. 2011;469(2):476–82.
37. Dahl B, McNeely C, Robinson BS, Maloney WJ, Paprosky WG, Ries MD, Saleh KJ. Acetabular reconstruction in revision total hip arthroplasty: maximizing function and outcomes in protrusio and cavitary defects. Instr Course Lect. 2014;63:219–25.
38. Pope D, Blankenship S, Jones G, Robinson BS, Maloney WJ, Paprosky WG, Ries MD, Saleh KJ. Maximizing function and outcomes in acetabular reconstruction: segmental bony defects and pelvic discontinuity. Instrc Course Lect. 2014;63:187–97.
39. Long WJ, Noiseux NO, Mabry TM, Hanssen AD, Lewallen DG. Uncemented porous tantalum acetabular components: early follow-up and failures in 599 revision total hip arthroplasties. Iowa Ortho J. 2015;35:108–13.

40. Deirmengian GK, Zmistowski B, O'Neil JT, Hozack WJ. Management of acetabular bone loss in revision total hip arthroplasty. JBJS Am. 2011;93(19):1842–52.
41. Tokarski AT, Novack TA, Parvizi J. Is tantalum protective against infection in revision total hip arthroplasty? Bone Joint J. 2015;97-B(1):45–9.
42. Jafari SM, Bender B, Coyle C, Parvizi J, Sharkey PF, Hozack WJ. Do tantalum and titanium cups show similar results in revision hip arthroplasty? Clin Orthop Relat Res. 2010;468(2):459–65.

Cup-Cage Technique

20

Eustathios Kenanidis, Eleftherios Tsiridis, Alan J. Highcock, Allan E. Gross, Xavier Flecher, Cameron K. Ledford, Joseph M. Statz, and Robert T. Trousdale

20.1 Current Concepts

E. Kenanidis and E. Tsiridis

The Cup-Cage is a relatively new technique that provides a viable option for the treatment of the complex, severe acetabular defects and the pelvic discontinuity [1]. A porous trabecular metal acetabular shell (titanium and tantalum) and a bridging ilioischial cage are used to achieve mechanical construct stability and biologic fixation of the acetabular shell [2]. It was first presented at the 2007 annual meeting of American Association of Orthopaedic Surgeons [3, 4].

20.1.1 Objective

The technique aims to bring back the continuity of the acetabulum by grafting the bone defects and improving the contact of the remaining viable bone to component surfaces with ingrowth potential, getting into mechanical stability [1].

An acetabular trabecular metal shell (+/− a porous metal augment) is fixed to the host bone [1]. The acetabular shell is an osteoconductive material that bridges the acetabular defect and not the actual shell to articulate with the femoral head. An antiprotrusio cage then is placed in the shell and fixed with screws to the ilium and ischium and with cement to the acetabular shell [1, 2]. The cage provides the initial stabilisation of the discontinuity and the load relief to the acetabular component thereby allowing time for biologic fixation of the porous non-cemented shell (+/− augment) to the host bone for a long-term stability [1, 2, 5]. The cage and any other nonbiological fixations usually fail after a few years due to fatigue [5].

E. Kenanidis, M.D., Ph.D., M.Sc. (✉)
Academic Orthopaedic Unit, Aristotle University Medical School, Thessaloniki, Greece

E. Tsiridis, M.D., Ph.D., F.A.C.S., F.R.C.S.
Academic Orthopaedic Unit, Papageorgiou General Hospital, Aristotle University Medical School, Thessaloniki, Greece
e-mail: etsiridis@doctors.org.uk

A.J. Highcock, F.R.C.S. (T&O)
Wirral University Teaching Hospital, Wirral, UK
e-mail: alan.highcock@nhs.net

A.E. Gross, M.D., F.R.C.S.C., O.Ont.
Division of Orthopaedic Surgery, Mount Sinai Hospital, University of Toronto, Toronto, Canada
e-mail: AGross@mtsinai.on.ca

X. Flecher, M.D., Ph.D.
Department of Orthopaedics and Traumatology Unit, Hospital Nord, Marseille, France

Aix Marseille Univ, APHM, CNRS, ISM, Sainte-Marguerite Hospital, Institute for Locomotion, Marseille, France

C.K. Ledford, M.D. · J.M. Statz, M.D. · R. T. Trousdale, M.D.
Mayo Clinic, Rochester, MN, USA
e-mail: Cameron.Ledford@hcahealthcare.com; Statz.Joseph@mayo.edu; trousdale.robert@mayo.edu

E. Tsiridis (ed.), *The Adult Hip - Master Case Series and Techniques*,
https://doi.org/10.1007/978-3-319-64177-5_20

20.1.2 Indications [2, 6]

- Paprosky types IIIA and IIIB bone loss
- Pelvic discontinuity

20.1.3 Surgical Technique [7]

1. Assess and prepare the acetabulum:
   - Expose the acetabulum widely, debride it from the fibrous tissue, define all borders, and evaluate the bone stock.
   - Gently ream the acetabular defect with hemispherical reamers till bleeding of the host bone.
   - Assess the acetabulum for the need of structural allograft or TM augments [7].
   - Impact the bone allograft mixed with any autograft from reaming into the contained defects, and reconstruct the uncontained defects with structural allografts or TM augments [5].
   - Identify the size and shape of the TM augments and Revision Shell to be used using trial components.
2. Implant the shell (± augments) [7]:
   - Firstly, insert the TM augments into the defects. Secure them using screws and allograft. Then the trial TM acetabular shell is inserted. A minimum of a 2 mm space should be allowed between the TM shell and augment to protect the interface with PMMA cement. Select the shell, and mix the PMMA. Apply the PMMA first, and protect the interface between the TM surfaces. Insert the TM shell at 4–6 min or when the cement is viscous enough to stay in place. Insert screws long enough through the screw holes to bypass the TM augment. Extra screw holes can be created using diamond-tipped speed burrs in any place selected for insertion as the roof of the shell or the ischial tuberosity.
3. Prepare the ischial notch for the inferior flange:
   - Identify the ischium, and make a cleft with a small osteotome to receive the inferior flange of the cage.
   - This will reduce the risk of screw fracture, cage migration and sciatic nerve injury [1]
4. Shape the cage:
   - Contour the cage by hand properly.
   - The superior flanges are regularly bent towards the ilium, and the inferior flange is inserted into the ischium cleft.
   - Occasionally, the shaping of the cage is not so simple resulting in a lateralisation of the whole construct. In this case the lower part of the cage, i.e. the ischial flange, can be cut away from the cage using a cutting speed tool.
5. Implant the cage:
   - When the appropriate shape of the cage is achieved, it is implanted firstly in the ischial notch then securely seated in the shell, and lastly, its superior flange is placed against the lateral portion of the ilium.
   - Insert screws through the existing holes in the dome and into the TM Revision Shell (+/−) as well as in the superior flange of the cage.
6. Insert the acetabular liner:
   - Apply PMMA cement into the dome of the cage, and pressurise it against the construct using a third-generation cementing technique.
   - Assure that the cement passes through the cage holes to fill gaps between the cage and the shell.
   - Insert the Polyethylene Revision Shell liner. This liner is specially designed to fit the TM shell by the manufacturer or is customarily selected by the surgeon, i.e. in case a constrained liner is cemented in place. The polyethylene liner is cemented into the cage with the appropriate inclination and version independent of the position of the cage.

20.1.4 Advantages

- The achievement of mechanical stability via the cage protection and biologic fixation via the TM fixation.
- The stiffness of fixation for a pelvic dissociation is supported to be similar to a combined cage and posterior column plate [8]. In a recent biomechanical study, Gilliland et al. [8] showed that the addition of a TM shell to the cage could distract the defect or the disconti-

nuity, thereby increasing the vertical stability of the construct relatively. The TM shell promotes bone ingrowth on both sides of the discontinuity, acting as a bridge and an osteoconductive graft.

20.1.5 Disadvantages

- Technically demanding technique
- The unexplored long-term tribological effects of the metal-on-metal surfaces of the construct
- The unknown consequence of the PMMA interference between TM surfaces, TM shell and cage, HXLP and TM/cage construct

20.1.6 Published Results

There is limited information in the literature for this new technique. Few papers providing level IV evidence are currently available [1, 3, 5, 7, 9, 10]. These are retrospective case series of 19–77 patients with a mean follow-up from 26 to 82 months (range 12–135) dealing with pelvic discontinuity and Paprosky type III/IV acetabular defects.

Satisfactory midterm results have been reported from centres of excellence; however, these cannot be generalized [1, 5, 7, 9, 10].

Albogashemian et al. [5] reported the midterm results at a mean of 82 months of a cohort of 26 patients that were treated with cup-cage technique for pelvic discontinuity. The early results of this cohort have been reported previously [7]. He showed that the 7-year survivorship for any reason and aseptic loosening was 87.2%. He also compared the results of this cohort with 19 patients with pelvic discontinuity treated with cages alone at a previous period. Although several differences existed between the two cohorts (chronologic periods, selection bias), they were comparable as far as the mean amount of contact with bleeding host bone was concerned. There was statistical significant greater seven-year survivorship for any reason of the cup cage (87.2%) compared with cage group alone (49.9%) (p = 0.009) and a trend towards significance for aseptic loosening (87.2% vs 60.9%, p = 0.076). At the lastest follow-up, there were comparable HHS between groups (76.3 vs. 77.6, $p = 0.958$) [5].

Amenabar et al. [1] reported encouraging midterm results for a group of 67 patients with Gross types III and IV defects treated with cup-cage technique. The mean follow-up was 74 months (24–135). They [1] demonstrated a 5-year survival rate with revision for any cause of 93% and a 10-year survival rate of 85%. There was no difference in the survival for any reason between Gross types III and IV defects; however, the risk of aseptic loosening in Gross type IV was greater. They supported that cup-cage technique had better results than ilioischial rings and cages alone and comparable to other recent methods for the treatment of pelvic discontinuity (triflange, acetabular distraction with TM cups) [1].

In another shorter follow-up period study, Rogers et al. [10] reported 86.3% survival for any reason at eight years for 42 cup-cage reconstructions.

Although these short to midterm outcomes are encouraging, giving evidence of a viable option for the treatment of complicated acetabular defects and pelvic discontinuity, they do not provide sufficient data to predict the long-term outcomes of the technique.

20.1.7 Complications

- The rates of complications in the studies varied. Instability was the most common complication followed by infection. Peroneal nerve injury was also reported.
- The rate of complications was reported up to 12%. Amenabar et al. [1] supported that the high complication rate (12%) of their series was mainly attributed to the nature of these complex procedures managed with several previous surgeries. The previously reported complication rate for complex acetabular revisions treated with TM with or without augments ranged from 5% to 20%, and in series treating pelvic discontinuities, from 16% to 29% [1].
- Radiographic migration of the cup cages was also reported [1]. Amenabar et al. [1] reported 4/67 such cases. This was seen in the ischial flange, was not progressive and was not related to aseptic loosening.

20.2 Case Title: Cup-Cage Reconstruction for Severe Acetabular Bone Loss

A.J. Highcock and A.E. Gross

20.2.1 Demographics

Age: 57
Sex: Female
BMI: 28.7

20.2.2 Relevant Past Medical History

Principal pathologies: Hypertension

Previous surgical procedures: Right THR 1994 for mild hip dysplasia (type I)

Medication: Amlodipine, Tylenol

History of presenting complaint: No prodromal hip symptoms. Three-week history of sudden onset acute, severe, right-sided groin pain with radiation into the posterior buttock. Rapid deterioration from unaided ambulation to using two crutches and is unable to weight bear through the right hip. Significant nocturnal symptoms

20.2.3 Clinical Examination

Symptoms: Buttock and groin pain with all ROM. Severely antalgic gait

Range of motion: Flexion to 40°, no internal or external rotation—all limited by pain

Specific tests: Trendelenburg positive. Unable to assess abductor strength. Hip provocative text positive. ESR 34 and CRP <5

Main disability: Unable to weight bear through the right hip, even to transfer. Using two crutches to mobilize

Neurovascular evaluation: Intact

20.2.4 Preoperative Radiological Assessment/Imaging (Figs. 20.1 and 20.2)

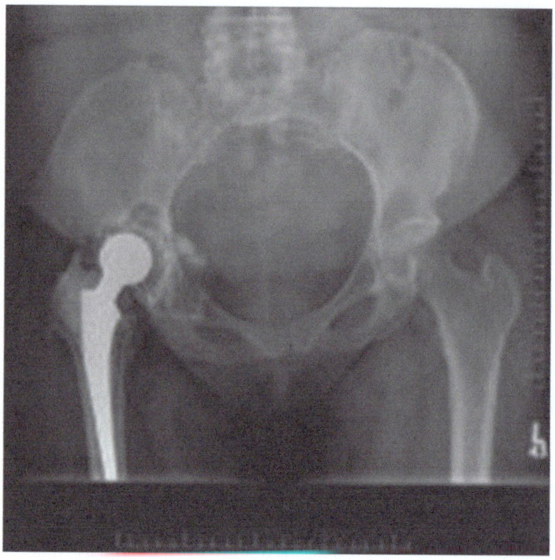

Fig. 20.1 AP right hip: Loose cemented cup with iliac and ischial osteolysis

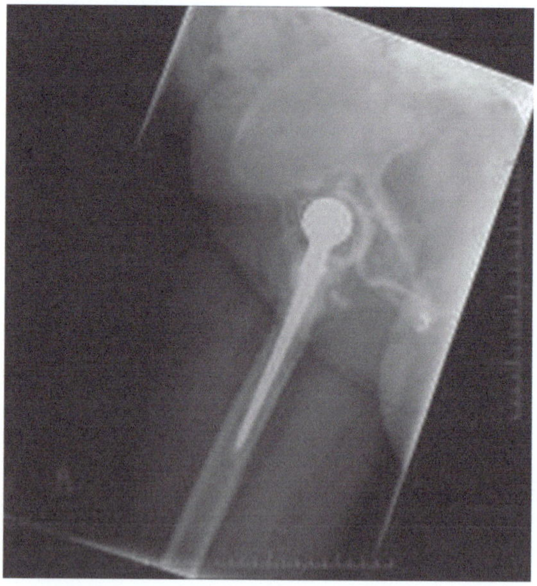

Fig. 20.2 Lateral right hip: Extent of iliac and ischial osteolysis demonstrated

20.2.5 Preoperative Planning

Diagnosis: Aseptic loosening of cemented acetabular cup with severe osteolysis ilium and ischium (Figs. 20.1 and 20.2)

Possible treatment options: Cup-cage reconstruction, structural allograft with rigid cage and cemented liner, CTAC (custom triflange acetabular component) and jumbo cup reconstruction

Chosen treatment method: Cup-cage reconstruction

Selection of implants if applicable and rational: (1) Zimmer trabecular metal acetabular shell—to maximize bone ingrowth where host bone contact is expected to be <50%. (2) Zimmer TM acetabular revision cage—with flanges for securing into host ilium and ischium. (3) 36 mm internal diameter 10-degree elevated rim liner. Longevity highly cross-linked polyethylene—maximising head size and rim to increase stability and highly cross-linked to minimize wear debris

Expected difficulties: (1) Severe iliac and ischial osteolysis. (2) Potential pelvic discontinuity. (3) Well-fixed monobloc stem. (4) Shortening proximally with tight abductors

Strategies to overcome difficulties: (1 and 2). Cup-cage construct. (3 and 4). Extended trochanteric osteotomy for stem removal, abductor length and function

Templating: Preoperative planning for the length of the extended trochanteric osteotomy and cup cage (Fig. 20.3)

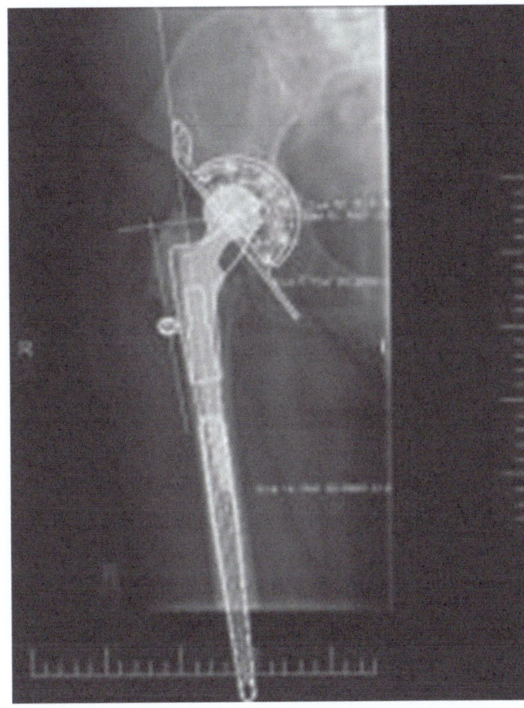

Fig. 20.3 Templating for trabecular metal shell, TM acetabular revision cage, ZMR and length of extended trochanteric osteotomy

20.2.6 Surgical Note

Patient's position: Lateral decubitus.

Type of anaesthesia: General.

Surgical approach: Extended trochanteric osteotomy.

Main steps: 12 cm ETO—posterior to anterior, lateral one-third of the femur. Proximally in the interval between gluteus minimus and piriformis, bevelled distally. Stem and cement mantle excised from the femur with cement osteotomes. ETO allows excellent exposure of the acetabulum and pelvis; therefore acetabulum is addressed at this juncture. Acetabular cup and cement and fibrous tissue are completely excised. Assessment of bone defects and pelvic discontinuity before reconstruction with the cup-cage construct (see below). After acetabular reconstruction, titanium diaphyseal modular taper stem (ZMR) is used to reconstruct femur. The rationale for this stem is twofold; firstly, the ETO precludes any metaphyseal press-fit stem or cementation with pressurization into the proximal canal; secondly, the modularity allows accurate restoration of leg length and offset. Once definitive stem is inserted, the trial reduction was performed with trial acetabular liner, femoral body and femoral head to ensure the appropriate degree of combined inclination and version to maximize stability and fine-tuning of leg length, prior to cementation of the definitive liner. Definitive implants inserted after correction of leg length, cup version and inclination and offset are confirmed. The ETO was reduced, ensuring correct length and tension of hip abductors, and secured with three cerclage wires (Figs. 20.4 and 20.5).

Reconstruction techniques: This technique maximizes the host bone contact with a porous trabecular metal shell, grafts the central defect and uses a cage to stabilize the ilium to the ischium. The acetabular defect is reamed by hemispherical reamers until contact is made with the bleeding bone, any defect is filled with packed morsellized bone allograft, and an absorbable gelatin compressed sponge (e.g. Gelfoam®) may be required on the floor of the defect to contain the packed graft. The acetabular defect is sized for a trabecular metal acetabular component for adequate scratch fit and 2–3 mm of distraction if pelvic discontinuity is present. The trabecular metal cup is inserted in a more open and retroverted manner, than the native acetabulum, to allow access to the ischium and ilium for the respective flanges of the cage. At least two screws with good purchase, each aiming at the posterior column or the acetabular dome, are inserted to improve the cup stability. The cage is appropriately sized and secured to the ischium through a slot made in the ischium and to the outer table of the ilium with minimum two bicortical screws. The polyethylene liner is cemented into the cage with an appropriate degree of version and inclination to maximize stability and the cement used to interdigitate the cup-cage construct [7, 11].

20.2.7 Intraoperative Challenges

Challenges and solutions: After excision of the cup, cement, fibrous and osteolytic tissue, there was a pelvic discontinuity, significant central defect and uncontained superior defect (type V acetabular defect—Gross classification). The cup-cage technique allows grafting of central defects with morsellized allograft; if containment is required medially, an absorbable gelatin compressed sponge is a useful adjunct. Where proximal and anterior migration of the acetabular cup has occurred, the hip abductors can be scarred and shortened; failure to address this can lead to several potential complications—shortening leg length, an irreducible hip intraoperatively or an unstable hip. A trochanteric slide, either in isolation or incorporated into the ETO, allows accurate restoration of leg length and offset while maintaining hip abductor function once the slide/ETO has healed.

Thorough description of decision-making, including the reason for the final decision: Decision for ETO and its advantages for stem removal, preservation of the hip abductors, and facilitation of trochanteric slide as discussed in the preoperative planning. Additionally, it facilitates excellent exposure of the acetabulum—particularly where exposure of the ilium and ischium will be required. The cup-cage reconstruction has several advantageous aspects in this case—(1) the tantalum acetabular shell has excellent scratch-fit and bone ingrowth properties and both beneficial where host bone stock is deficient. (2) The cage secures the construct, whilst bone ingrowth occurs and is flexible enough to prevent complications associated with large, rigid constructs in the periacetabular bone loss. (3) Facilitates bone grafting of central defects. (4) Modular system allows 'fine-tuning' to address individual defect encountered.

20.2.8 Postoperative Radiographs (Figs. 20.4 and 20.5)

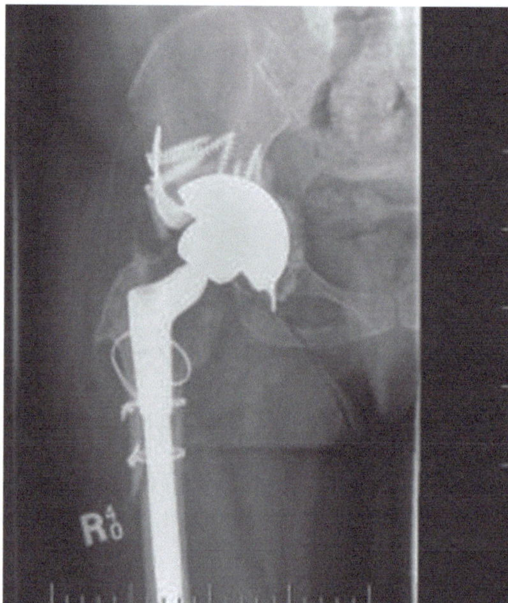

Fig. 20.4 Post-op anteroposterior radiograph: Medial allograft, cup cage and ETO with modular tapered femoral stem

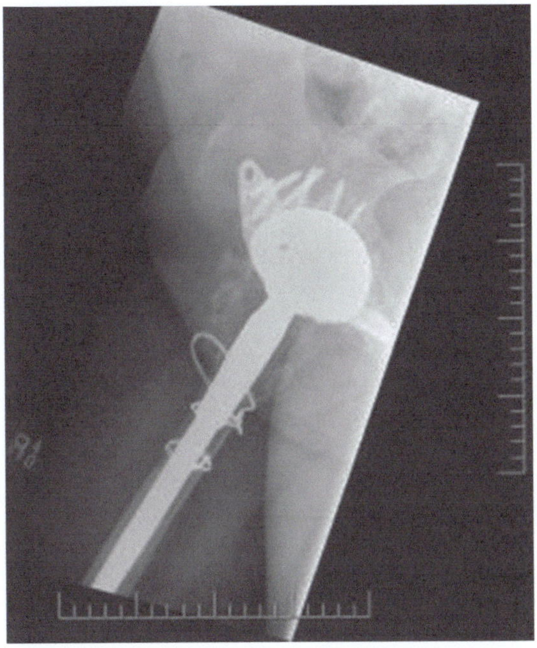

Fig. 20.5 Post-op lateral radiograph: Flanges of the cage engaging into the ischium and secured to the ilium

20.2.9 Postoperative Management

Chemoprophylaxis and anticoagulant treatment period: Enoxaparin for five weeks.

Gait/limb loading until full loading: Touch-toe four weeks, 50% four weeks and then full weight bearing. This allows for osteo-integration of the trabecular metal cup and tapered femoral stem.

20.2.10 Follow-Up and Complications

No post-op complications. Initial thigh pain observed in first 2 weeks, related to restoration of leg length.

20.2.11 Discussion

Advantages of the applied method: Our preferred treatment option in a significant acetabular bone loss and/or pelvic discontinuity is the cup-cage reconstruction. This technique incorporates elements of the acetabular distraction technique with the scratch-fit highly porous acetabular shell whilst having the added advantage of bridging the host ischium and ilium. It facilitates bone grafting of cavitary defects, and also this technique can be used with augments or structural allografts if there is an associated segmental defect.

Disadvantages of the method: Complication rates, particularly with the cage, associated with this technique were relative frequent with its early use [12]. These were, in part, owing to the technical difficulty of the procedure and lack of osseous integration of the cage. Most frequently sciatic nerve injury was associated with securing the inferior flange of the cage to the top of the ischium. This has led to the senior author (AEG) recommending slotting the inferior flange into the ischium rather than laying it on top.

Alternative evidence-based techniques for the case: Triflange reconstruction with a CTAC (custom triflange acetabular component) and jumbo hemispherical cup.

Why the is chosen technique better for this case? CTACs, by their very nature, have distinct time to manufacture and cost disadvantages, without demonstrably improved survivorship over cup-cage reconstruction [13]. Increasing the defect to accommodate a jumbo hemispherical cup has two disadvantages over the cup-cage reconstruction: firstly, reaming of host bone compounds acetabular bone loss and, secondly, raising the hip centre—which the senior author would not endorse as a basic philosophy.

Indications and contraindications for your technique: Indications—Gross classification type IV and type V acetabular defects with significant acetabular bone loss and pelvic discontinuity.

Learning curve and how to manage complications: A surgeon must be proficient in the technique of using a cage. Loosening of the construct is usually managed by a cage reconstruction with a more rigid type of cage, e.g. Burch-Schneider cage.

Level of evidence concerning the superiority of this method against others: III.

20.3 Case Title: Acetabular Revision 'Cup-Cage Techniques'

Xavier Flecher

20.3.1 Demographics

Age: 73
Sex: Female
BMI: 23

20.3.2 Relevant Past Medical History

Previous surgical procedures: Left hip—shelf arthroplasty 1962, THA 1985. Right hip THA 1989

Medication: Painkiller

Other: Rehabilitation

History of Presenting Complaint: Progressive groin pain over the last five years. Limping

20.3.3 Clinical Examination

Symptoms: Left groin pain for two years. Walk with two crutches for one year.

Range of motion: The range of motion was severely decreased (flexion 45, abduction 0).

Main disability: Leg length discrepancy close to 20 mm. Abductor muscle strength were quite sound (4/5). Two previous approaches: one Smith Petersen and one posterior approach.

Scoring: Harris Hip Score, 42.

Neurovascular evaluation: Normal.

20.3.4 Preoperative Radiological Assessment/Imaging (Figs. 20.6 and 20.7)

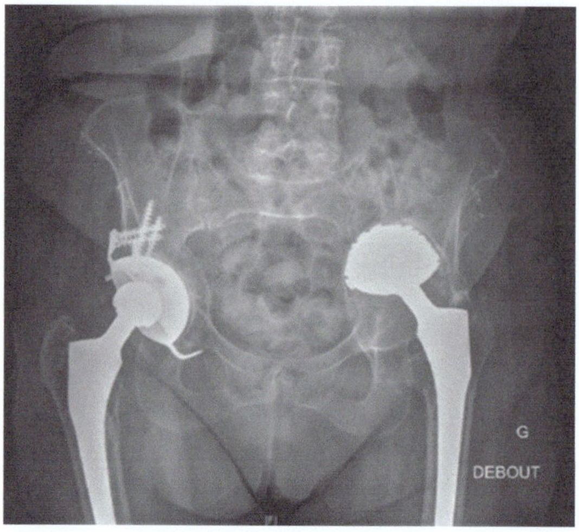

Fig. 20.6 Preoperative AP view of the pelvis

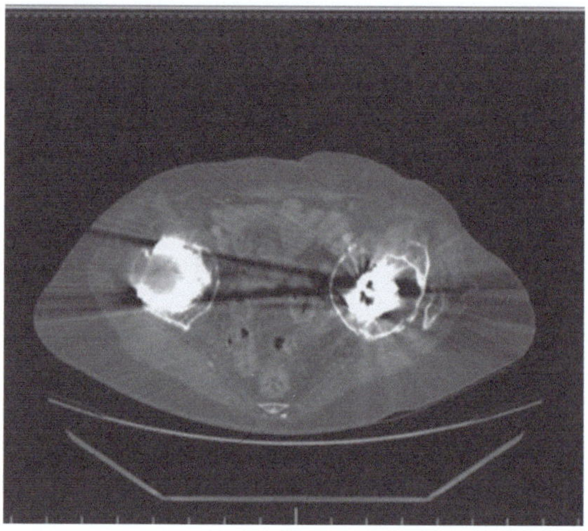

Fig. 20.7 CT scan with arteriography

20.3.5 Preoperative Planning

Diagnosis: Isolated aseptic cup loosening with acetabular protrusion (Paprosky IIIB) (Figs. 20.6 and 20.7).

Possible treatment options: Impaction grafting with a cage, massive allograft with a cage, a dedicated cage is an antiprotrusio cage (i.e. Burch-Schneider), cup-cage construct with porous tantalum components.

Chosen treatment method: Cup-cage construct with porous tantalum components.

Selection of implants if applicable and rational: Porous hemispheric tantalum-made cup with screws protected by a Burch-Schneider ring. Cementation of a UHMWPE Liner.

Expected difficulties: The joint access, the cup removal, a possible vascular injury and lengthening.

Strategies to overcome difficulties: Extended trochanteric osteotomy may be used if the access to the joint is impossible.

20.3.6 Surgical Note

Patient's position: Lateral.

Type of anaesthesia: General.

Surgical approach: You may use any approach for hip revision. The posterior approach, however, is the best one to assess the posterior column that is mandatory to achieve the reconstruction in this case.

Main steps: Posterior approach to the joint and luxation. Femoral head and cup removal. The foramen obturator has to be found to locate the appropriate hip centre. Reaming of the cup to reach two points of contact with the ischium and the ilium. Find the proper size of the cup using a trial. The trial needs to be stable by pushing gently with a tool or fingers. If not, then use a bigger one. The dedicated final component is then impacted and if possible fixed with screws. Prepare of the ischium with an osteotome to receive the Burch-Schneider ring with the appropriate inclination and anteversion. Use of multiples screws in the acetabular roof. Then cement of a liner in 15–20° of anteversion and 40° of inclination with the maximum possible inner diameter to avoid instability. Reduction of the femoral component with a femoral head trial (Fig. 20.8).

Reconstruction techniques: Cup-cage construct.

20.3.7 Intraoperative Challenges

Challenges and solutions: Obtain a stable fixation of the tantalum-made cup whilst remaining possible the insertion of the ring in the right position.

Unanticipated problems and solution: Instability of the hip or inability to achieve a hip reduction. It can be managed by restoring the hip centre as close to normal as possible. A femoral release can also be performed to lengthen the limb. If the reduction remains impossible, then consider femoral stem revision.

20.3.8 Postoperative Radiographs (Fig. 20.8)

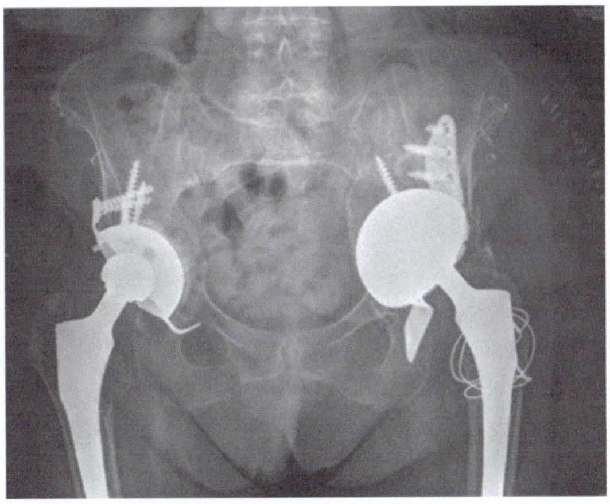

Fig. 20.8 Pelvis AP view

20.3.9 Postoperative Management

Chemoprophylaxis and anticoagulant treatment period: Low molecular weight heparin for a month

Gait/limb loading until full loading: Partial weight bearing with two crutches for six weeks

20.3.10 Follow-Up and Complications

Scoring: Harris Hip Score: 84.

20.3.11 Discussion

Advantages of the applied method: Bone ingrowth. No graft resorption. Postoperative weight bearing allowed.

Disadvantages of the method: More expensive. Short to midterm follow-up available only.

Alternative evidence-based techniques for the case: Impaction grafting, bulk allograft protected by an antiprotrusio ring, cementless high hip cup and cementless jumbo cup.

Why is the chosen technique better for this case? No graft resorption. Postoperative weight bearing allowed.

Indications and contraindications for your technique: No contraindication. The best indication is the implant loosening with protrusion (Paprosky IIIB or IIC) associated with a pelvic discontinuity.

Learning curve and how to manage complications: Its' a modular system. Primary stability is mandatory as for any other cementless fixation. Gain this by using porous metal augmentation and screws.

Level of evidence concerning the superiority of this method against others: Few retrospective studies on limited number of patients (level 4). Some non-comparative prospective monocentric or multicentre studies. Two recent meta-analyses [1, 5, 14].

20.4 Case Title: Acetabular Revision (Cup-Cage Techniques)

Cameron K. Ledford, Joseph M. Statz, and Robert T. Trousdale

20.4.1 Demographics

Age: 77
Sex: Female
BMI: 32

20.4.2 Relevant Past Medical History

Principal pathologies: Rheumatoid arthritis, hyperlipidaemia

Previous surgical procedures: (1) Left primary total hip arthroplasty (THA) 25 years previously; (2) left revision THA (acetabulum only) 1 month previously

Medication: Imuran, atorvastatin

History of presenting complaint: 77-year-old female status post recent revision left THA for osteolysis and aseptic loosening one month prior presented with an extreme left hip pain, difficulty ambulating and subjective 'looseness' of the prosthesis

20.4.3 Clinical Examination

Symptoms: Pain, crepitation with both passive and active hip range of motion

Range of motion: Extension-flexion, 0–90; internal-external rotation, 10–20; abduction-adduction, 15–30

Specific tests: Positive Stinchfield test

Main disability: Difficult weight bearing and ambulation

Neurovascular evaluation: Intact (including motor function of the sciatic and femoral nerve, sensibility throughout the lower extremity dermatomes and palpable distal pulses)

20.4.4 Preoperative Radiological Assessment/Imaging (Figs. 20.9 and 20.10)

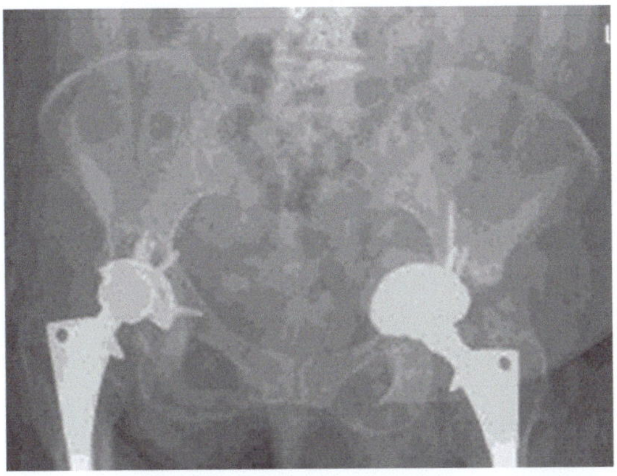

Fig. 20.9 AP Pelvis radiograph—bilateral THA with migration of the left acetabular component superomedially

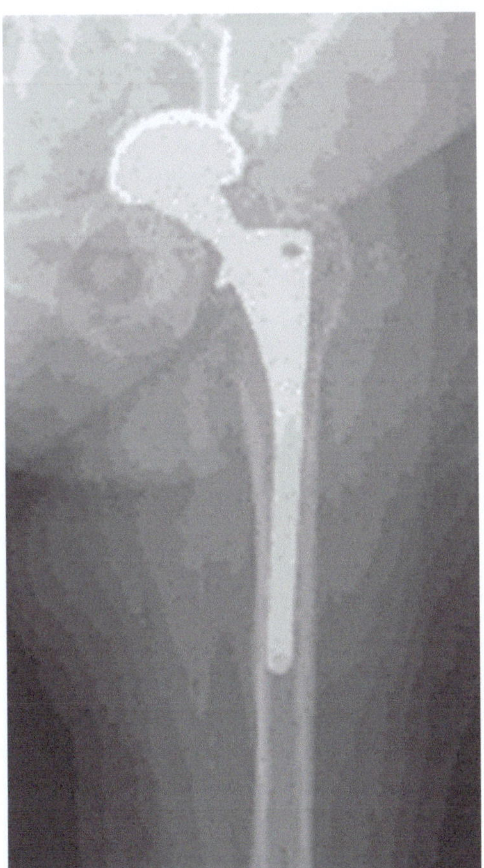

Fig. 20.10 Lateral left hip radiograph—redemonstration of migrated acetabular component with intact femoral stem without gross lucency or subsidence

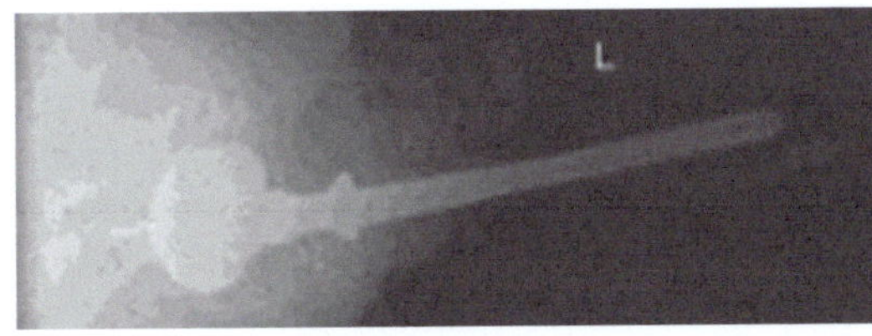

Fig. 20.11 Cross-table lateral left hip radiograph—acetabular component has flipped into retroversion with marked posterior bone loss

20.4.5 Preoperative Planning

Diagnosis: Pelvic discontinuity with severe acetabular bone loss (Paprosky acetabular bone loos classification, IIIb) (Figs. 20.9, 20.10 and 20.11)

Possible treatment options: Uncemented reconstruction (acetabular column plating with bulk structural allograft and/or highly porous metal (tantalum) implants with modular augments), 'cup-cage' reconstruction, custom (triflange) implants and acetabular distraction technique

Chosen treatment method: Cup-Cage reconstruction.

Selection of implants if applicable and rational: Large (jumbo) highly porous metal cup and corresponding spanning ilioischial cage to allow for mechanical construct stability whilst trying to achieve biological fixation of the acetabular shell

Expected difficulties: Fixation of the cup secondary to poor bone quality (rheumatoid disease, age and prior surgeries)

Strategies to overcome difficulties: Large (jumbo) highly porous metal cup for distraction fit into defect and multiple screw fixation in intact ischial bone

20.4.6 Surgical Note

Patient's position: Lateral decubitus position on the peg board

Type of anaesthesia: General endotracheal anaesthesia with regional nerve (psoas) catheter placed for postoperative pain control

Surgical approach: Standard posterior approach to hip

Main steps: (1) Removal of acetabular component and debridement of maximal tissue. (2)

Inspection of bone loss/pelvic discontinuity. (3) Reaming acetabulum to ensure host bone contact. (4) Bone grafting with allograft cancellous chips. (5) Implantation of jumbo highly porous metal cup so that there is a slight distraction of discontinuity to maximize fixation. (6) Placement of multiple screws to secure cup to intact host bone. (7) Place cage into the acetabular cup and secure with screws to the socket as well the ilium. (8) Trial accordingly to restore leg length and soft-tissue tension (Figs. 20.12 and 20.13).

Reconstruction techniques: Bone grafting, implanting jumbo highly porous metal cup, securing cage construct into cup and host bone and restoring hip centre, length and stability with construct (including cup cage and femoral head size/length).

20.4.7 Intraoperative Challenges

Challenges and solutions: Challenge, poor/minimal host bone with pelvic discontinuity; solution, utilizing large cup to distract the discontinuity to maximize bony contact/fixation, placing multiple screws into most supportive area of host bone and protecting cup through implantation of cage.

Unanticipated problems and solution: Problem, restoring hip stability; solution, utilizing dual mobility construction (by cementing dual mobility cup into the protrusio cage followed by placement of dual-mobility articulation).

Thorough description of decision-making, including the reason for the final decision: Multiple anatomical issues to consider including the pelvic discontinuity, poor bone quality and severe bone loss. The cup-cage construct affords management of both the discontinuity and the acetabular bone loss (cup and bone graft), whilst the cage provides the initial stability/fixation of pelvis in the setting of poor bone quality.

20.4.8 Postoperative Radiographs (Figs. 20.12 and 20.13)

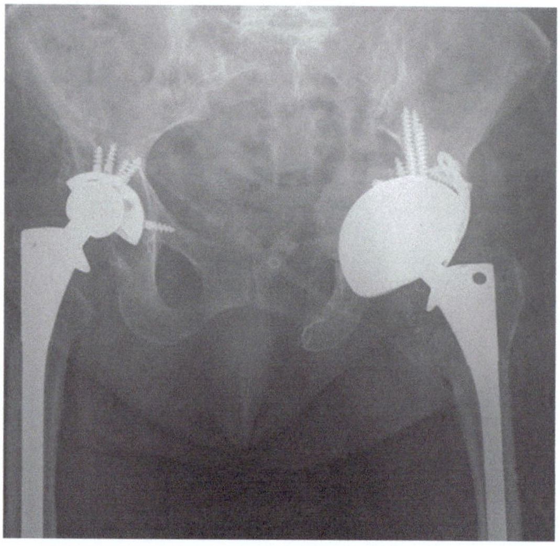

Fig. 20.12 AP Pelvis radiograph—revision THA components including jumbo acetabular cup and corresponding acetabular cage with multiple screw fixation of both (not as well visualized is the dual mobility articulation previously described); note hip centre has been restored, and medial defect bone grafted with morsellized allograft

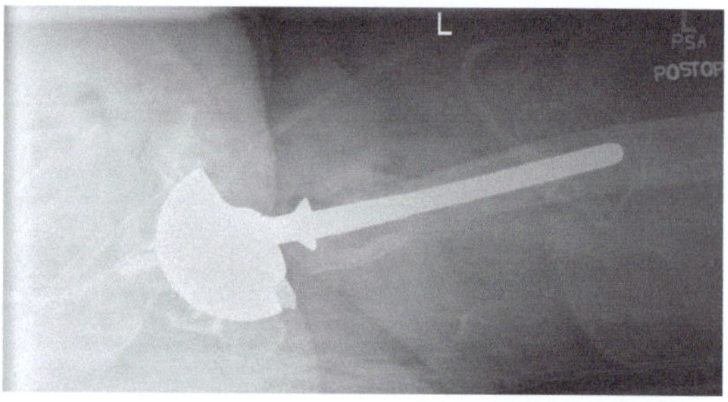

Fig. 20.13 Cross-table lateral hip radiograph—revision THA components with appropriate anteversion

20.4.9 Postoperative Management

Chemoprophylaxis and anticoagulant treatment period: Mechanical compressive devices during inpatient hospitalization with low-dose warfarin (goal INR 1.7–2.2) for six weeks

Gait/limb loading until full loading: Toe-touch weight bearing with a maximum of 30 pounds on operative extremity for six weeks followed by progression to weight bearing as tolerated after that.

20.4.10 Follow-Up and Complications

No complication.

20.4.11 Discussion

Advantages of the applied method: Revision surgery of acetabular components can be challenging because the surgeon must often manage acetabular defects and/or pelvic discontinuity. The cup-cage construct is a viable option because of its ability to provide a cup with a potential for biological fixation and a cage to provide initial stability and protection from biomechanical forces acting upon the cup. Assuming bone ingrowth of the highly porous metal cup, the entire construct has a documented 5-year survival rate from any revision of 93% with potential for long-term stability [1].

Disadvantages of the method: Aside from the complex challenge of evaluating acetabular bone loss and/or pelvic discontinuity, the 'cup cage' is technically difficult requiring careful preoperative planning and implementation of multiple advanced reconstruction techniques including bone grafting, implanting a large cup, securing a cage and restoring hip biomechanics. Although midterm survival rates are encouraging, long-term studies are needed to understand the potential longevity of the construct fully.

Alternative evidence-based techniques for the case: A variety of options are available during revision for severe acetabular defects including uncemented reconstruction (acetabular column plating with bulk structural allograft and/or highly porous metal (tantalum) implants with modular augments), 'cup- cage' reconstruction, custom (triflange) implants and acetabular distraction technique [2]. Pelvic discontinuity was traditionally addressed with the use of ilioischial cages; however, mid- to long-term failure rates were relatively high because of limited biological fixation. It may be difficult or impossible to achieve stability with the sole use of highly porous metal implants if the acetabular defect is large, bone quality is poor, there is limited host bone contact or there is a pelvic discontinuity. Newer techniques such as the use of custom triflange implants and acetabular reconstruction techniques are novel approaches to complex problems and have demonstrated <5% aseptic loosening revision rate at midterm [13, 15].

Why is the chosen technique better for this case? The cup-cage reconstruction provides initial mechanical stability with potential for long-term biological fixation in an otherwise healthy, active patient. Furthermore, there are perhaps more intraoperative flexibility/options for grafting and fixation than other newer techniques.

Indications and contraindications for your technique: Indications—severe acetabular bone loss (Paprosky IIIA and IIB) and pelvic discontinuity when stable fixation cannot be obtained through the use of highly porous cup and augments; contraindications, active infection.

Learning curve and how to manage complications: As with all complex acetabular revisions, the learning curve is long and requires progressive steps to maximize the chances of success including thoughtful preoperative planning, adequate surgical exposure, evaluation of bone loss and areas for potential fixation, limited postoperative weight bearing and careful follow-up. Complications inherent to such advanced reconstructions include infection, dislocation and sciatic nerve injury [1]. Acute infection may be treated with debridement and liner exchange, whereas surgeon and patient may decide to utilize suppression in the face of chronic infection. Dislocation has been treated with a larger femoral head or constrained liner or dual mobility component cemented into the cage as was utilized in this case example. Sciatic nerve palsy is best managed with observation and ankle-foot orthosis unless an initial irritant to the nerve is identified.

Level of evidence concerning the superiority of this method against others: Level IV.

References

1. Amenabar T, Rahman WA, Hetaimish BM, Kuzyk PR, Safir OA, Gross AE. Promising mid-term results with a cup-cage construct for large Acetabular defects and pelvic discontinuity. Clin Orthop Relat Res. 2016;474(2):408–14.
2. Sheth NP, Nelson CL, Springer BD, Fehring TK, Paprosky WG. Acetabular bone loss in revision Total hip Arthroplasty: evaluation and management. J Am Acad Orthop Surg. 2013;21:128–39.
3. Noiseux M, Lewallen DB, Kellet C, Gross AE. Results of a porous coated cup-cage construct in complex revision surgery with severe bone loss. Paper presented at the 2007 Annual Meeting of American Association of Orthopaedic Surgeons, San Diego, CA.
4. Pulido L, Rachala SR, Cabanela ME. Cementless acetabular revision: past, present, and future revision total hip arthroplasty: the acetabular side using cementless implants. Int Orthop. 2011;35:289–98.
5. Abolghasemian M, et al. The challenge of pelvic discontinuity cup-cage reconstruction does better than conventional cages in mid-term. Bone Joint J. 2014;96-B:195–200.
6. Deirmengian GK, Zmistowski B, O'Neil JT, Hozack WJ. Current concepts review Management of Acetabular Bone Loss in revision Total hip Arthroplasty. J Bone Joint Surg Am. 2011;93:1842–52.
7. Kosashvili Y, et al. Acetabular revision using an anti-protrusion (ilio-ischial) cage and trabecular metal acetabular component for severe acetabular bone loss associated with pelvic discontinuity. J Bone Joint Surg (Br). 2009;91-B:870–6.
8. Gililland JM, Anderson LA, Henninger HB, Kubiak EN, Peters CL. Biomechanical analysis of acetabular revision constructs: is pelvic discontinuity best treated with bicolumnar or traditional unicolumnar fixation? J Arthroplast. 2013;28:178–86.
9. Ballester Alfaro JJ, Sueiro Fernandez J. Trabecular metal buttress augment and the trabecular metal cup-cage construct in revision hip arthroplasty for severe acetabular bone loss and pelvic discontinuity. Hip Int. 2010;20(Suppl 7):S119–27.
10. Rogers BA, et al. The reconstruction of Periprosthetic pelvic discontinuity. J Arthroplast. 2012;27(8):1499–1506.e1.
11. Ballester Alfaro JJ, Sueiro FJ. Trabecular Metal buttress augment and the Trabecular Metal cup-cage construct in revision hip arthroplasty for severe acetabular bone loss and pelvic discontinuity. Hip Int. 2010;20(Suppl. 7):119.
12. Goodman S, Sastamoinen H, Shasha N, Gross A. Complications of ilio-ischial reconstruction rings in revision total hip arthroplasty. J Arthroplasty. 2004;19:436–46.
13. Taunton MJ, Fehring TK, Edwards P, Bernasek T, Holt GE, Christie MJ. Pelvic discontinuity treated with custom triflange component: a reliable option. Clin Orthop Relat Res. 2012;470:428.
14. Flecher X, Paprosky W, Grillo JC, Aubaniac JM, Argenson JN. Do tantalum components provide adequate primary fixation in all acetabular revisions? Orthop Traumatol Surg Res. 2010;96(3):235–41.
15. Sporer SM, Bottros JJ, Hulst JB, Kancherla VK, Moric M, Paprosky WG. Acetabular distraction: an alternative for severe defects with chronic pelvic discontinuity? Clin Orthop Relat Res. 2012;470:3156–63.

21 Custom Triflange Implant

Eustathios Kenanidis, Eleftherios Tsiridis, Aldo M. Riesgo, and Ran Schwarzkopf

21.1 Current Concepts

E. Kenanidis and E. Tsiridis

Triflange implant is a custom-designed implant for the treatment of severe bone loss in revision hip arthroplasty [1]. It consists of titanium, porous- or hydroxyapatite-coated acetabular component with ilial, ischial, and pubic flanges [1]. The latter provides areas of contact and screw fixation with the ilium, ischium, and pubis for initial rigid stability. Typically the larger ilial flange has two rows of 3–4 screw holes. The ischial flange has between 4 and 6 holes whether the smallest pubic has no holes [1] (Fig. 21.1).

E. Kenanidis, M.D., Ph.D., M.Sc. (✉)
Academic Orthopaedic Unit, Aristotle University Medical School, Thessaloniki, Greece

E. Tsiridis, M.D., Ph.D., F.A.C.S., F.R.C.S. (✉)
Academic Orthopaedic Unit, Papageorgiou General Hospital, Aristotle University Medical School, Thessaloniki, Greece
e-mail: etsiridis@doctors.org.uk

A.M. Riesgo, M.D.
Department of Orthopaedic Surgery, Cleveland Clinic Florida, Weston, FL, USA
e-mail: Aldo.Riesgo@nyumc.org

R. Schwarzkopf, M.D., M.Sc.
Adult Reconstructive Division, NYU Knee Center, Department of Orthopaedic Surgery, NYU Langone Health Orthopaedic Hospital, Hospital for Joint Diseases, New York, NY, USA

21.1.1 Objective

The triflange implant aims to span a critical acetabular defect and obtain fixation to the ilium, ischium and pubis with the three flanges [1]. Following a primary rigid stability of the implant, the host bone achieves biologic fixation through the implant coating [1].

21.1.2 Indications

1. Severe acetabular defects (Paprosky 3B) [1]
2. Pelvic discontinuity [1]
3. Previously failed reconstruction with cage or porous metal construct augments [2]
4. Insufficient bone stock to reconstruct using other means [2].

21.1.3 Preoperative Planning [1]

- The surgeon has to:
    1. Order the flange to the manufacturer based on CT imaging preoperatively
    2. Take into account the waiting time for the construction and availability of the custom implant (often 4–8 weeks)

E. Tsiridis (ed.), *The Adult Hip - Master Case Series and Techniques*,
https://doi.org/10.1007/978-3-319-64177-5_21

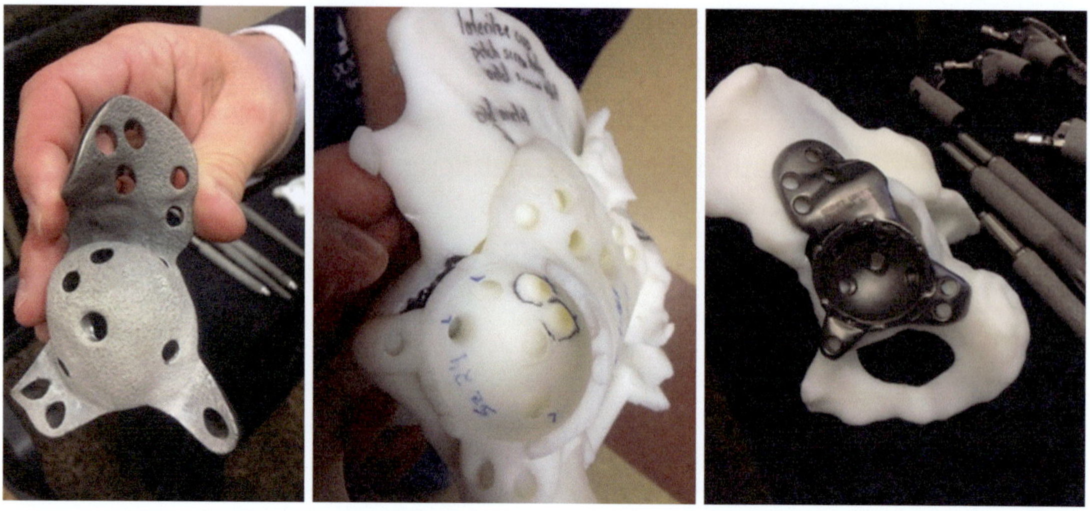

Fig. 21.1. A typical try-flange demonstration. The pelvic and triflange models were created using 3D printing, and the original implant was tested on it before surgery

21.1.4 Surgical Technique [1]

(a) Expose the ischium, ilium, and pubis widely to obtain an adequate view. You may also need to perform a trochanteric osteotomy.
(b) Intraoperatively typically you will have the implant prototype and a 3D hemipelvis model with the predefined areas of bone removed to permit the evaluation of the perfect implant position.
(c) Begin fixation from the ischial flange.
(d) Secure the implant with approximately 9–15 screws.
(e) Use lateralized, elevated or constrained options of polyethylene liners to achieve appropriate hip length, soft tissue tensioning, and stability.

21.1.5 Advantages

1. Restoration of the native hip center [1].
2. Reasonably straightforword surgical technique with no need to shape, fit, or fix the implant [3].
3. The initial provided rigid stability that is mediated through anatomical loading redistribution gives the opportunity to the host bone to achieve biological fixation through the implant coating [1].
4. A viable solution for difficult acetabular reconstructions involving severe bone loss or pelvic discontinuity.
5. Fit individualized to each patient [2].

21.1.6 Disadvantages

1. The complexity of the preoperative planning process [1]
2. The time required for the device manufacturing [1]
3. The requirement of a perfect pre-op design as the implant cannot be modified intraoperatively [2]

Options after failure of triflange component: constrained liner, tripolar, Girdlestone arthroplasty

21.1.7 Published Results

A limited number of papers providing level IV evidence is presently available [2–12]. These are retrospective case series with sample size ranging from 19 to 78 patients and a mean follow-up of 31 to 123 months. Long-term data are still missing. The type of defects treated is usually Paprosky type IIIA and B and pelvic discontinuity. The reported rate of aseptic loosening ranged from 0 to 11.5%. Revision for any reason was reported from 0 to 35% [2–12]. Revision rate was greater in studies where pelvic discontinuity was treated [5, 7].

To our knowledge, there are no prospective comparative trials of custom triflange revision to other forms of reconstruction for the treatment of Paprosky 3A/3B acetabular defects.

In one of the longest follow-up studies, Barlow et al. [4] studied retrospectively 63 patients treated with the triflange implant. He reported 85% survival rate at a mean follow-up of 4.3 years. He also supported that triflange tend to lateralize the hip center by approximately 1 cm. The lateralization was almost 2 cm in the small subset of failed custom triflange acetabular components. They supported that medializing the hip center in triflange components improve ingrowth and survivorship.

The rates of complications in the studies varied. Instability was the most common complication ranging from 0 to 30% and infection from 0 to 8% [2–12]. Injury to the superior gluteal and sciatic nerves was also described. In some studies migration of the implant was reported up to 14% [5, 6, 9].

Taunton et al. [5] studied retrospectively 57 patients with pelvic discontinuity treated with the triflange implant. In a cost comparison with other techniques, the authors reported similar overall costs comparing a triflange with a trabecular metal cup-cage construct.

21.2 Case Title: Custom Triflange Acetabular Component for Bone Loss in Infection

Aldo M. Riesgo and Ran Schwarzkopf

21.2.1 Demographics

Age: 77 years old
Sex: Female
BMI: 32

21.2.2 Relevant Past Medical History

Principal pathologies: Hypertension, osteoporosis, colon cancer in remission

Previous surgical procedures: Right total hip arthroplasty 2010, revision right total hip arthroplasty 2010, partial colectomy 2002

Medication: Metoprolol, Vitamin D

Other: Allergies—penicillin

History of presenting complaint: A 77-year-old female presenting with two weeks of wound drainage. Four years earlier, the patient underwent a primary right total hip arthroplasty (THA). In the immediate postoperative period, she sustained a prosthetic dislocation and acetabular cup failure and had revision surgery of the acetabular component. The patient was without complaints since revision surgery. She presented to us with a few months of a draining sinus from her surgical wound area.

21.2.3 Clinical Examination

Symptoms: Pain with ambulation, purulent wound drainage from the sinus tract located at the surgical wound.

Range of motion: Limited secondary due to pain.

Specific tests: Elevated CRP and ESR, correlating with the diagnosed periprosthetic joint infection (PJI). Draining sinus is a major criterion, and sufficient, for the diagnosis of PJI.

Main disability: Limited ambulation distance and purulent drainage from a sinus tract.

Neurovascular evaluation: Extremity sensorimotor exam within normal limits.

21.2.4 Preoperative Radiological Assessment/Imaging (Figs. 21.2, 21.3, and 21.4)

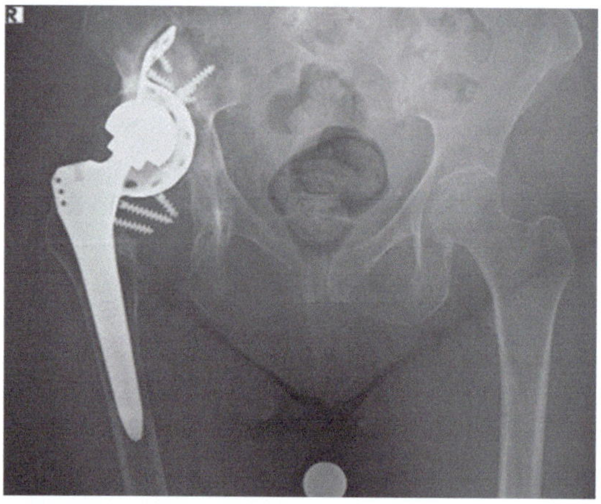

Fig. 21.2. AP pelvis radiograph—we can see the failed acetabular cage

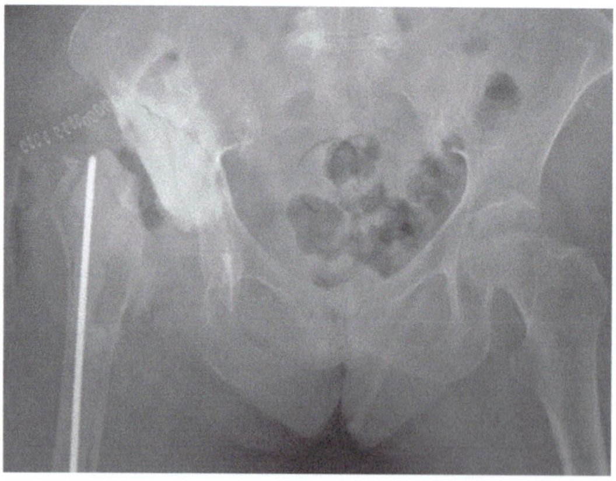

Fig. 21.3. AP pelvis—following explant of acetabular and femoral components and placement of antibiotic non-articulating spacer with significant superolateral bone loss

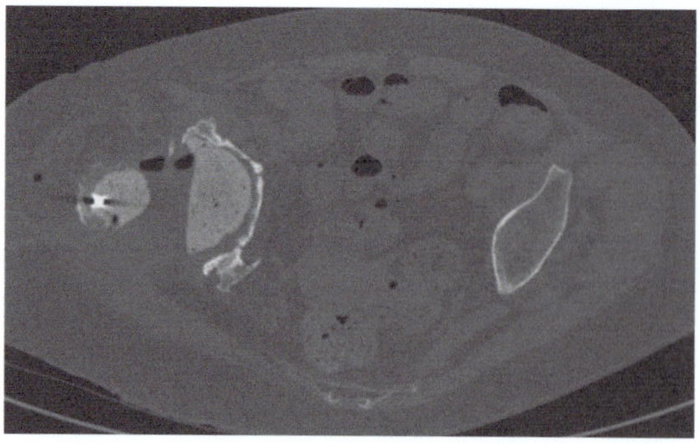

Fig. 21.4. CT axial—assessment of massive bone loss with possible pelvic discontinuity

21.2.5 Preoperative Planning

Diagnosis: Periprosthetic joint infection with a failed acetabular cage and femoral stem.

Possible treatment options: Staged exchange arthroplasty with temporary antibiotic spacer followed by allograft-cage construct, jumbo porous cup, cup-cage construct, or custom triflange acetabular component with a modular femoral stem.

Chosen treatment method: Staged exchange arthroplasty with a non-articulating antibiotic spacer for 12 weeks followed by custom triflange acetabular component and a modular femoral component.

Selection of implants if applicable and rational: Custom triflange acetabular implant matched to patient's specific bony defects with direct contact of porous surfaces. In comparison to an off-the-shelf malleable acetabular cage, the custom triflange allows for rigid fixation and healing of discontinuity with biological fixation of the implant. Furthermore, the triflange construct allows multiple locking screws with a preplanned trajectory. Modular femoral stem allows for independent diaphyseal fixation where there is improved bone stock and selection of proximal body to maximize version, leg length, and offset for optimal joint stability and mechanics.

Expected difficulties: Removal of a well-ingrown stem and acetabular cage with minimal bone loss. Eradication of periprosthetic infection. A custom acetabular triflange is not readily customizable to unexpected bone loss that is encountered intraoperatively. Unanticipated mismatch to patient's remaining bone stock. Restoration of hip center.

Strategies to overcome difficulties: Careful removal of the infected implant. Attention to balancing between debridement of fibrous tissue and scaring without removal of host bone is paramount. Curettage and sharp debridement to remove minimal bone. Proper antibiotic treatment. Sterilized hemipelvis model can assist during the second-stage reimplantation of the custom triflange by identifying areas that need further bony work, i.e., burring away unanticipated ridges or bony overgrowth since initial CT scan was performed.

Templating: CT scan with 3 mm axial slices and 3D reconstructions used to build the one-to-one model of hemipelvis (Fig. 21.4). Cup, liner, and head size determined for maximal stability and optimal wear. The option to include constrained liner should always be available given the high rate of prosthetic dislocation reported in prior series of complex THA revision.

21.2.6 Surgical Note

Patient's position: Lateral decubitus position with hip positioner.

Type of anaesthesia: Spinal anaesthesia with sedation.

Surgical approach: Posterolateral approach utilizing the prior incision.

Main steps: (1). Exposure, (2). Explant of the spacer, (3). Debridement, (4). Preparation of the bony surfaces, (5). Positioning of the custom triflange, (6). Screw placement, (7). Preparation of the femur and trial reduction.

Reconstruction techniques: A posterior approach to the hip using prior incision. The sciatic nerve was identified leading into the greater sciatic notch and protected throughout the operation. The posterior pseudocapsule was incised, and cement spacer visualized. The gluteus maximus tendon was released to facilitate exposure. The acetabular spacer was removed without difficulty using osteotomes. The femoral spacer left into protecting the femur from fracture during retraction while preparing the acetabulum. Subperiosteal elevation of the gluteus medius and minimus was performed of the ilium with care to not injure the superior gluteal neurovascular bundle existing from the greater sciatic notch. Ischium exposed with careful elevation of the quadratus femoris and hamstring origin as needed since the sciatic nerve nearby. All excess fibrous tissue was removed to expose all bony surfaces. The hemipelvis model was referenced, and all excess bone ridges were removed using a burr. A healed shell of medial bone was encountered and gently reamed to a bleeding bone surface to facilitate biologic fixation. Similar preparation of bony surfaces was performed using a burr. The cancellous allograft was used to fill in any defects in the medial wall. Iliac flange fixation with screws was performed first, then followed by ischial and pubic flanges supported by the "home-run" screws through the acetabular dome. The press-fit hemispherical liner was inserted. Femoral preparation began with removal of the cement around the lateral shoulder. The Steinman pin was identified, and the femoral cement spacer removed en bloc. Before reaming of the femoral canal, prophylactic cerclage cables were placed around the diaphysis. Canal preparation with reamers was performed, and final trial size was inserted. An intraoperative XR confirmed the position of the trial component. Excellent distal fixation was obtained in the diaphysis. Additional cerclage cables were inserted to reduce fracture risk around the stem, ensuring excellent contact with porous surfaces. Reduction of prosthesis and trialing confirms adequate stability and leg length.

21.2.7 Intraoperative Challenges

Challenges and solutions: Limiting bone loss during implant removal. Debridement should be cautious, and bone removal should be restricted to template hemipelvis.

Unanticipated problems and solution: The severe amount of scarring around the sciatic nerve. Careful dissection and identifying the sciatic nerve in its entire length.

Thorough description of decision-making, including the reason for the final decision: Prophylactic diaphyseal cerclage cables were placed to minimize the risk of iatrogenic fracture during stem insertion. Excellent fit in the diaphysis had been obtained. Stem design relies on diaphyseal fit for stability and fixation. The size of the proximal body should ensure bony contact and does not need to be press-fit.

21.2.8 Postoperative Radiographs (Figs. 21.5 and 21.6)

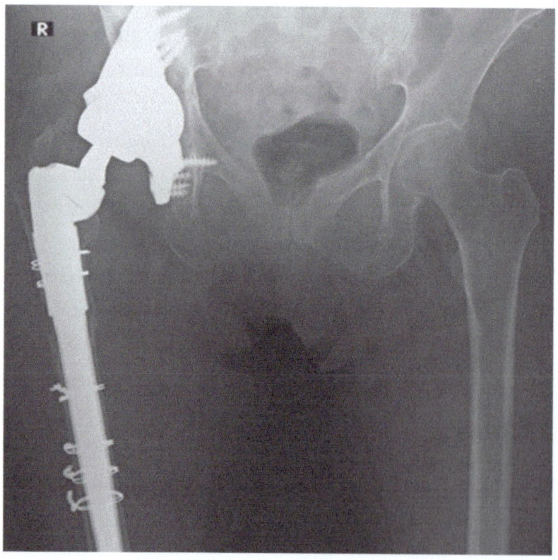

Fig. 21.5. AP pelvis—Postoperative custom triflange with excellent bony contact

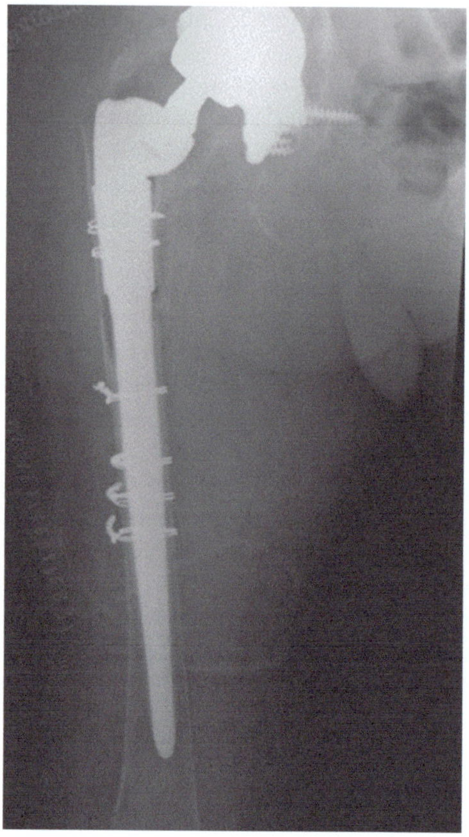

Fig. 21.6. AP femur—Modular femoral stem with cerclage cables

21.2.9 Postoperative Management

Chemoprophylaxis and anticoagulant treatment period: Coumadin treatment for an INR range of 1.8–2.3 and sequential compression devices for four weeks.

Gait/limb loading until full loading: Partial weight bearing for six weeks with gradually increased weight bearing to full weight bearing by twelve weeks.

21.2.10 Follow-Up and Complications

There were no postoperative complications.

21.2.11 Discussion

Advantages of the applied method: Custom triflange acetabular components allow for an implant designed for massive acetabular bone loss and pelvis dissociation that can restore the joint center and allow for socket position as referenced from 3D imaging [13]. Immediate component stability. This method allows for the ultimate customization based on the patient's bone stock and pelvic deformity.

Disadvantages of the method: There is limited intraoperative flexibility if an unexpected situation is encountered. For example, if a further bone loss occurs during bony preparation, the custom acetabular component is limited in further adaptability. Since the custom implant is fabricated from a CT scan of the patient's pelvis, this scenario is fortunately rarely encountered with meticulous technique during exposure and preparation. In addition, previous studies have reported a high (approximately 20%) hip dislocation rate for custom triflange acetabular components. Significant exposure of the gluteal fossa on the outer surface of the ilium may lead to iatrogenic damage of the abductors and/or superior gluteal neurovascular bundle. Another disadvantage of this method is the time and cost factored in fabricating the custom implant, which can take up to four weeks.

Alternative evidence-based techniques for the case: When massive acetabular bone loss is encountered, several authors have also reported similar results with tantalum metal cup-cage constructs. The costs of both treatment alternatives are comparable.

Why the chosen technique is better for this case? This patient had significant bone loss of both acetabular columns and had already failed a standard acetabular cage construct.

Indications and contraindications for your technique: Indications for custom triflange acetabular component include massive acetabular bone loss with or without pelvic discontinuity where immediate stability is desired.

Learning curve and how to manage complications: Complex acetabular revisions are best managed by those surgeons skilled and experienced with revision arthroplasty. Exposure and bony preparation are technically demanding, but the use of a custom triflange based on 3D CT scan helps to make this technique reproducible for the skilled arthroplasty surgeon. The custom implant may help to lessen learning curve compared to other constructs for acetabular reconstruction.

Level of evidence concerning the superiority of this method against others: Level IV and V evidence.

References

1. Goodman GP, Engh CA Jr. Acetabular revision. The custom triflange cup. Build it and they will come. Bone Joint J. 2016;98-B(1 Suppl A):68–72.
2. Berasi CC IV, Berend KR, Adams JB, Ruh EL, Lombardi AV Jr. Are custom triflange acetabular components effective for reconstruction of catastrophic bone loss? Clin Orthop Relat Res. 2015;473:528–35.
3. Christie MJ, Barrington SA, Brinson MF, Ruhling ME, DeBoer DK. Bridging massive acetabular defects with the triflange cup: 2- to 9-year results. Clin Orthop Relat Res. 2001;393:216–27.
4. Barlow BT, Oi KK, Lee Y-y, Carli AV, Choi DS, Eng M, Bostrom MP. Outcomes of custom flange acetabular components in revision total hip arthroplasty and predictors of failure. J Arthroplast. 2016;31:1057–64.
5. Taunton MJ, Fehring TK, Edwards P, et al. Pelvic discontinuity treated with custom triflange component: a reliable option. Clin Orthop Relat Res. 2012;470:428–34.
6. Holt GE, Dennis DA. Use of custom triflanged acetabular components in revision total hip arthroplasty. Clin Orthop Relat Res. 2004;429:209–14.
7. DeBoer DK, Christie MJ, Brinson MF, Morrison JC. Revision total hip arthroplasty for pelvic discontinuity. J Bone Joint Surg Am. 2007;89-A:835–40.
8. Joshi AB, Lee J, Christensen C. Results for a custom acetabular component for acetabular deficiency. J Arthroplast. 2002;17:643–8.
9. Wind MA Jr, Swank ML, Sorger JI. Short-term results of a custom triflange acetabular component for massive acetabular bone loss in revision THA. Orthopedics. 2013;36:260–5.
10. Colen S, Harake R, De Haan J, et al. A modified custom-made triflanged acetabular reconstruction ring (MCTARR) for revision hip arthroplasty with severe acetabular defects. Acta Orthop Belg. 2013;79:71.

11. Foster S, Chaudhary H, Assenmacher B. Intrapelvic cementless component extraction with immediate triflange acetabular reconstruction using the retroperitoneal approach. J Arthroplast. 2009;24:323.e1.
12. Paprosky WG, O'Rourke M, Sporer SM. The treatment of acetabular bone defects with an associated pelvic discontinuity. Clin Orthop Relat Res. 2005;441:216–20.
13. Schwarzkopf R, Ihn HE, Ries MD. Pelvic discontinuity: modern techniques and outcomes for treating pelvic disassociation. Hip Int. 2015;25(4):368–74.

22 Cement-in-Cement Acetabular Revision

Eustathios Kenanidis, Eleftherios Tsiridis, Eric Swanton, and William Farrington

22.1 Current Concepts

E. Kenanidis and E. Tsiridis

The CiC technique for the femur is well established. Several biomechanical studies [1–3] support the bonding between the old and the new cement and case series provide the good medium- to long-term results [4–10]. Acetabular CiC revision is less well recognised with limited indications [11].

22.1.1 Objective

The CiC technique is an alternative option for revision of a cemented cup. A well-fixed acetabular cement mantle that is both radiologically and intraoperatively assessed is a prerequisite to performing this procedure [12]. The procedure aims to minimise the risk of cement removal during revision THA and to contribute to the long-term acetabular shell stability.

22.1.2 Indications

There are limited indications of the technique.

The following have been proposed [11]:

1. The removal of a worn or mal-orientated cemented acetabular component
2. The removal of a well-fixed cemented acetabular component to change the orientation or size of the cup or change to constrained to manage recurrent dislocation (the most frequent)
3. The removal of a well-fixed cemented acetabular component to change the size or orientation of the cup at the time of a femoral revision

22.1.3 Requirements and Contraindications

- A well-fixed acetabular-cement mantle both radiologically and intraoperatively is a standard prerequisite for the CiC acetabular technique.
- Septic revision is a contraindication [9].

E. Kenanidis, M.D., Ph.D., M.Sc. (✉)
Academic Orthopaedic Unit, Aristotle University Medical School, Thessaloniki, Greece

E. Tsiridis, M.D., Ph.D., F.A.C.S., F.R.C.S. (✉)
Academic Orthopaedic Unit, Papageorgiou General Hospital, Aristotle University Medical School, Thessaloniki, Greece
e-mail: etsiridis@doctors.org.uk

E. Swanton, M.D. · W. Farrington, M.B.B.S., F.R.C.S., F.R.A.C.S.
North Shore Hospital, Auckland, New Zealand

E. Tsiridis (ed.), *The Adult Hip - Master Case Series and Techniques*,
https://doi.org/10.1007/978-3-319-64177-5_22

22.1.4 The Surgical Procedure [11]

- Remove the worn or mal-orientated cemented acetabular component without damaging the cement mantle.
- Remove it as piecemeal; do not use osteotomes.
- If it is not loose at the cement-prosthesis interface, then use standard acetabular reamers [13] to ream away the polyethylene implant in the same way as in a primary THR.
- Place damp gauze swabs around the acetabulum and lavage regularly to avoid the escape of polyethylene fragments into the soft tissues.
- Stop reaming when the polyethylene is still 1 mm to 2 mm thick.
- Recognise and remove the wire markers on the periphery of the implant.
- Use an elevator or osteotome to lever out the polyethylene from the underlying cement.
- Scrutinize the cement mantle to confirm adequate fixation and to check for any damage. If it is loose or damaged, use an alternative fixation method.
- If the internal diameter of the mantle is adequate, retain the ridges of cement made by the grooves of the polyethylene to improve fixation to the new cement.
- If the diameter of the original component is small, expand the mantle with a power burr to accommodate the new cup. Then make other shallow pits in the mantle to enhance the bond with the new cement.
- Do not penetrate the pits into the bone to avoid bleeding and the risk of contamination of blood between the layers of cement.
- Clean and dry the interface and add the new cement early to achieve maximum shear strength.
- Cement the new component into the old mantle.

22.1.5 Advantages

1. Simpler and straightforward technique as there is no need to remove the entire cement mantle.
2. Less-time consuming procedure.
3. Preservation of bone stock and reduction of blood loss.
4. Earlier postoperative full-weight-bearing mobilisation.
5. Reduce the possibility of fracture during the cement removal.
6. Position the cup in the preferred orientation to increase stability.

22.1.6 Disadvantages

1. Improper method for the acetabular revisions with compromised cement mantle. Ensure the integrity of the original cement mantle both pre- and intraoperatively.
2. Contamination of the cement-cement interface by blood and marrow fat may act as a stress riser, facilitating the formation of fatigue cracks in the cement [3].

22.1.7 Published Results

Data concerning the effectiveness of the acetabular CiC technique are limited. In the only so far published study, Brogan et al. [11] described the technique and reported the outcome of 60 acetabular CiC revisions in 59 patients. The indication in the majority of patients (77%) was recurrent dislocation; however, in 20% of them, the CiC technique was used as a complement to femoral revision. At the last follow-up, almost half of the patients had died. Survival rate was 100% for aseptic loosening and 92.2% for revision for any reason at 5 years. There were, however, two revisions for aseptic loosening at 6.9 and 7.7 years, an infection, four recurrent dislocations and a disarticulation of a constrained liner.

22.2 Case Title: Cement-in-Cement Acetabular Revision

Eric Swanton and William Farrington

22.2.1 Demographics

Age: 79
Sex: Female
BMI: 28

22.2.2 Relevant Past Medical History

Principal pathologies: Polyethylene wear with aseptic loosening and osteolysis around acetabular and femoral component.

Previous surgical procedures: Left hip hemiarthroplasty after #NOF 1996, Revision left hip to cemented total hip replacement 1997 (15 years previously).

Medication: Metoprolol, simvastatin, aspirin.

Other: Ischaemic heart disease.

History of presenting complaint: This 79-year-old patient initially sustained a fractured neck of femur 16 years previously which was treated with a cemented hemiarthroplasty. This was subsequently revised to a cemented total hip replacement a year later, due to groin pain from acetabular cartilage erosion. She managed well and was pain-free for several years until she presented to us with increasing groin and lateral-sided hip pain. There were no constitutional symptoms and no history of wound problems with her previous procedures.

22.2.3 Clinical Examination

Symptoms: Groin and lateral-sided hip pain

Range of motion: 100 degrees flexion, internal rotation 20 degrees, external rotation 40 degrees

Specific tests: Leg length equal, poor active hip abduction, positive Trendelenburg test and gait, pain over greater trochanter to palpation

Main disability: Hip pain with a reduced walking distance

Neurovascular evaluation: Unremarkable

22.2.4 Preoperative Radiological Assessment/Imaging (Figs. 22.1 and 22.2)

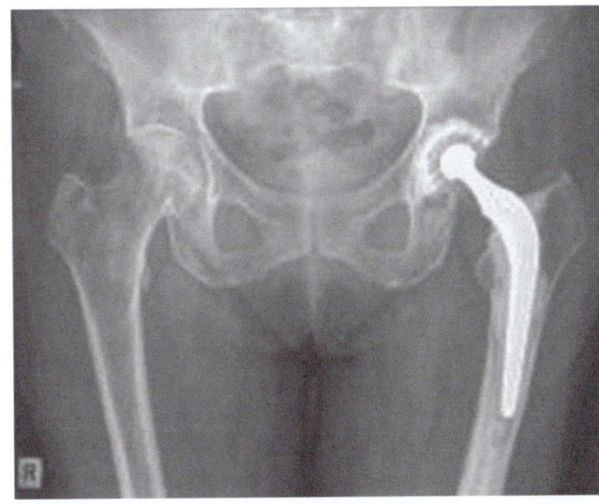

Fig. 22.1 Preoperative AP pelvis

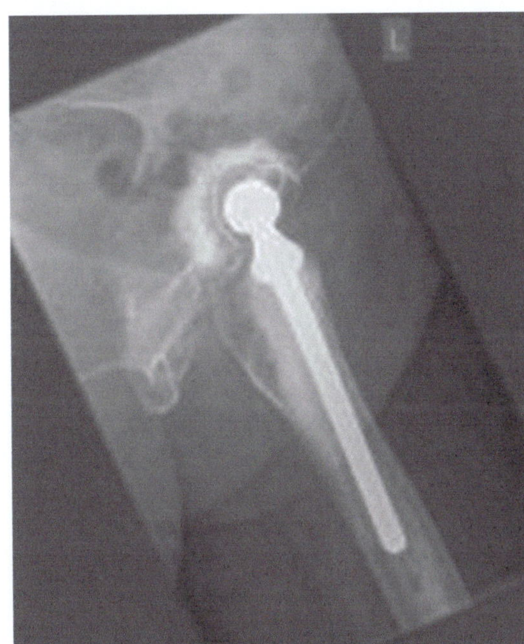

Fig. 22.2 Preoperative lateral left hip

22.2.5 Preoperative Planning

Diagnosis: The polyethylene wear was resulting in osteolysis and some early loosening of both components, combined with abductor dysfunction from two previous hip procedures (Figs. 22.1 and 22.2)

Possible treatment options: (1). Non-surgical treatment with hip strengthening physio. The latter had been tried for over a year with no success. (2). Surgical options; acetabular revision: (A) Uncemented acetabular component—this would entail removal of all acetabular cement, subsequent reaming and fixation of an uncemented shell. (B) Cemented acetabular component—this could require removal of all the old cement and re-cementing with or without impaction grafting using allograft bone or, as in this case, removing only the loose parts of the cement mantle and re-cementing with a cement-in-cement technique. Femoral revision: (1) Leave component in situ if stable intraoperatively. (2) Use cement-in-cement revision (as in this case). (3) Remove the femoral stem and cement and revise with impaction grafting of allograft bone and a cemented stem. (4) Remove the femoral component and cement and revise with uncemented prosthesis (proximal or distal fit).

Chosen treatment method: Cement-in-cement revision of acetabular and femoral components.

Selection of implants if applicable and rational: A 52 mm outer diameter cemented cup with flange (rimfit—Stryker) was used on the acetabular side (similar in size to the outer diameter of the old cup). By carefully matching the outside diameter of the new cup to the old cup, minimal cement reaming is required to seat the new cup. The flange provides cement containment and pressurisation as the periphery of the acetabulum can be slightly irregular. A 36 mm inside diameter was chosen to reduce the risk of post-op dislocation given the abductor dysfunction. The femoral component was a cemented 44 mm offset short revision stem (125 mm, Exeter, Stryker) that restored the patient's offset and leg length and fitted comfortably into the old cement mantle after removal of the femoral component. The cement-in-cement technique leaves the well-fixed cement mantle intact, which reduces blood loss, fracture risk and surgical time.

Expected difficulties: The exposure of the cement–bone interface at the acetabular rim and the femoral neck must be adequate to assess the state of the bone–cement interface and fixation of the components. The stability of the joint can be more challenging when the abductor mechanism is severely compromised. A periprosthetic fracture risk is high with thin osteolytic bone.

Strategies to overcome difficulties: Exposure, stability, fixation.

Exposure. The posterior approach allows an extensile option both proximally and distally as well as a good view circumferentially around the acetabulum and femoral neck for cement interface assessment. It also enables abductor repair and reconstruction. The gluteus maximus tendon was released which allows exposure of the femoral component with less tension on the femur and less risk of a femoral fracture.

Stability. In-cement cup revision enables orientation of the cup in any plane within the new cement mantle to achieve optimal positioning. Its orientation is independent to its fixation. In contrast, an uncemented shell in the revision situation may require a compromised final position to attain adequate bone fixation. A cemented constrained option is also available if needed. Cemented fully constrained components fare is significantly better than their uncemented rivals. On the femoral side, the use of a modular cemented stem (e.g. Exeter) with multiple offset options (both stem and head) allows for appropriate tensioning of the abductor's muscles and reduces impingement. The anteversion of the femoral component within the cement mantle can be altered by burring the inner margins of the existing mantle. The use of a larger head size (in this case from a 22.5 mm to a 36 mm diameter) also helps improve stability.

Fixation. There are three interfaces for fixation which require assessment and preparation:

(a) Original bone–cement interface—This is assessed on the preoperative X-rays (presence of progressive lytic lines and osteolysis) and intraoperatively (a scalpel blade should not be able to penetrate between the bone and cement—if it does the interface in this region is not adequate, and the cement here should be removed).
(b) New bone–cement interface (where previous cement has been removed)—The osteolytic tissue requires removal with curettage back

to a cancellous bone structure to allow the new cement to adequately penetrate this bone.

(c) Cement–cement interface—The previous cement mantle is commonly burred on the inside to remove any fibrous membrane that may have developed here. This allows direct contact between the 'old and new' cement. The structural strength at this interface is by chemical bonding of the new methyl methacrylate to the previous cement. It has proven to be a firm bond and has not shown evidence of failure. There are theoretical concerns with differing iso-elasticity at this junction when using cement of different ages. However, this does not appear to cause a clinical problem in its many years of use.

Templating: The ideal acetabular component position is calculated from standard AP images with reference points being the teardrop and ilioischial line. The teardrop marks the inferior edge of your perfect cup position and the ilioischial line the medial border of your cement mantle. Templating, therefore, allows you to appreciate how much extra cement should be added or removed to avoid improper positioning of the hip center.

22.2.6 Surgical Note

Patient's position: Lateral decubitus.

Type of anaesthesia: Spinal plus general anaesthetic plus local infiltration (LIA).

Surgical approach: Posterior approach. The incision through the previous surgical scar was extended slightly proximally and distally into normal tissue. It allowed identification of the layers more easily. There was over 50% detachment of gluteus medius and minimus tendon from the greater trochanter which was the cause of the abductor dysfunction. The latter required reconstruction/repair using intraosseous sutures at the time of closure and was the most likely cause of the patients lateral-sided hip pain. The original procedure of a hemiarthroplasty following the neck of femur fracture had been performed through a Hardinge approach. The posterior structures were attached but were scarred as expected from the posterior approach of the first revision (hemiarthroplasty to THR). The gluteus maximus tendon was released before the hip dislocation and was also repaired at the time of closure.

Main steps: Acetabular exposure—This was obtained with gluteus maximus release, excision of scar tissue and removal of the femoral component (removal of the shoulder of cement with osteotomes/burr was performed cautiously and completely to prevent fracture of the greater trochanter). Stem removal was easily performed after this. To enable inspection of the bone–cement interface of the proximal femur, 2mm of the femoral neck was resected with a saw. Some small areas of cement were removed proximally, but there was no removal of cement below the lesser trochanter, so the femur was suitable for an "in-cement" revision too. Cup removal—The existing polyethylene cup showed considerable wear. It was not loose within the acetabulum. It was removed by reaming out with small reamers, and when down to a thin shell, it could be levered out of the cement mantle with a Kochers. Acetabular preparation—The cement mantle was inspected. It was 'loose/unsupported' in Zone 1 (Charnley and De Lee) superolaterally but was well fixed medially. The unsupported cement in Zone 1 was removed using a combination of nibblers and a 5 mm burr. There was osteolytic tissue behind it, that was removed with a small curette down to the cancellous bone. The burr was used around the inside of the cement surface and to create holes in the old cement mantle and the cancellous bone in Zone 1. Trial cups were inserted to determine appropriate sizing. This trial was repeated with the final cup to ensure optimal seating possible with the flange. The 'cement spacers' on the outside of the cup medially were removed to avoid lateralisation of the hip center. The socket was lavaged and then dried with hydrogen-peroxide-soaked swabs. One mix of simplex cement was inserted and pressurised before inserting the cup (Figs. 22.3 and 22.4).

Reconstruction techniques: These are outlined in the section above.

22.2.7 Intraoperative Challenges

Challenges and solutions: As detailed above.

Unanticipated problems and solution: No.

Thorough description of decision making, including the reason for the final decision: The indication for revision was for lateral-sided hip pain, most likely due to the abductor dysfunction, as well as groin pain due to some osteolysis from polyethylene wear and possible loosening of the components. Surgical treatment of only the abductor condition may not have fully addressed her symptoms and would have exposed her to further surgery of hip revision in the near future. Thus, a combined procedure was performed. An abductor dysfunction/detachment is not an unusual finding at revision surgery, especially when the primary procedure was performed through a Hardinge approach. The reattachment of the gluteal tendons can require significant time to perform well. This should be figured into the time for the surgery, as prolonged procedures have increased the risk of infection. 'In-cement' revision has the advantage of less blood loss than when removing the whole cement mantle, as the underlying bone surface is not exposed. The latter can significantly reduce blood loss in the revision situation and avoid the need for transfusion, as was the case with this patient. There is also less risk of fracture. Removal of well-fixed cement is time-consuming, and there is a significant risk of fracture. Residual bone can also be inadvertently removed. If well-fixed cement can be left in situ, these risks are mitigated. In our case, while the Zone 1 cement was 'loose/unsupported' due to underlying osteolysis, the cement medially was well fixed. Removal of this well-fixed cement would have increased blood loss and risked fracture and may have resulted in unnecessary bone removal. The patient is elderly (aged 79) with ischaemic heart disease. She has a normal BMI (28) and weighs only 62 kg. Her lifestyle is not high demand. The reasoning behind my decisions, non-surgical treatment had failed to improve her symptoms over the last year. A combined abductor repair and revision THR would address all her current symptoms, and she should not require further surgery in the future. The 'cement-in-cement' technique on both the femoral and acetabular side was highly likely to be technically possible and unlikely to require conversion to a much more extensive procedure. This technique would keep surgical time and blood loss to a minimum, reducing the risk of transfusion, infection and fracture. She was at increased risk of post-op dislocation (2nd revision, abductor detachment, elderly), so the optimal component positioning and the reattachment of the abductors would be important and a large femoral head size desirable.

22.2.8 Postoperative Radiographs (Figs. 22.3 and 22.4)

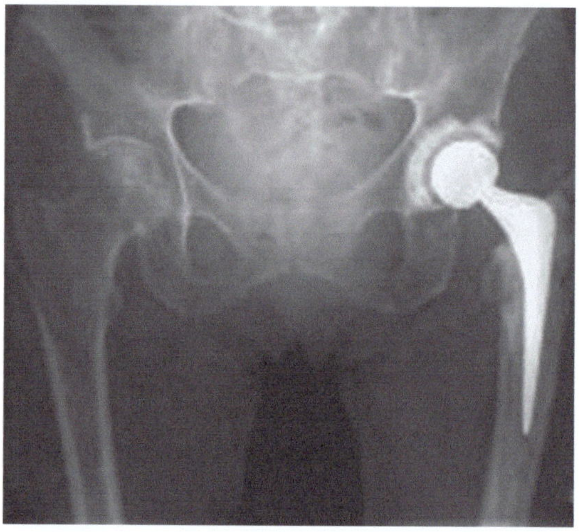

Fig. 22.3 AP pelvis taken 3 years post-op

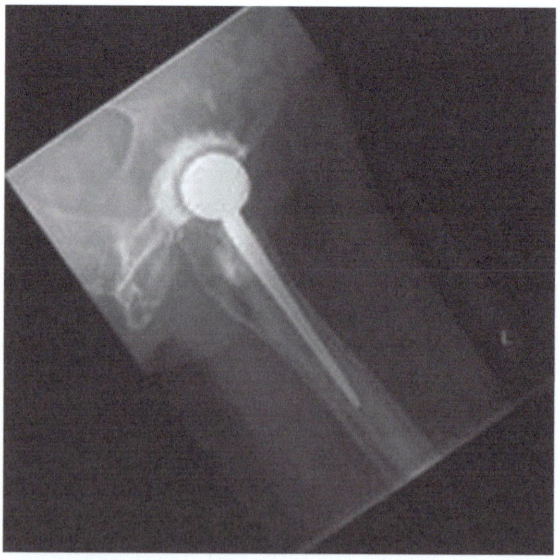

Fig. 22.4 Lateral left hip taken 3 years post-op

22.2.9 Postoperative Management

Chemoprophylaxis and anticoagulant treatment period: Mechanical prophylaxis with foot pumps as an in-patient with TED stockings after discharge for 4 weeks. Chemical prophylaxis was with aspirin.

Gait/limb loading until full loading: Partial weight bearing for 6 weeks on crutches to protect the abductor repair.

22.2.10 Follow-Up and Complications

The patient made an uneventful recovery and was discharged on crutches to protect the abductor repair at day 5 post-op. She did not require a blood transfusion. She completed 6 weeks on crutches before starting physiotherapy. She has had no complications with the surgery and remains pain-free three years later. She walks unaided, lives independently and continues to drive. She is pleased with the result of her operation and would recommend it for someone else in a similar situation.

22.2.11 Discussion

Advantages of the applied method: Straightforward and simple to perform without a prolonged surgical time. It minimises the iatrogenic damage of fracture and the inadvertent bone loss during extraction of components. Significantly reduced blood loss (often less than a primary THR). It allows positioning of the cup in whichever orientation the surgeon wishes to maximise stability. Can be used for revision of the femur, acetabulum or both.

Disadvantages of the method: Requires previously cemented components where the cement–bone interface is predominantly intact/well fixed. This may not be the case in an advanced revision setting due to progressive osteolysis and loose cement.

Alternative evidence-based techniques for the case: These all involve removal of the entire cement mantle. Revision can then be cemented (with or without bone grafting) or uncemented with a variety of options.

Why the chosen technique is better for this case? Most of the cement mantle remained well fixed with minimal osteolysis.

Indications and contraindications for your technique: Indications—cemented acetabular revisions; can be complete or partial cement-in-cement revision, where either the entire mantle is intact or only part of it remains well fixed. (1) On-table cup revision for mal-placement of a cup during a primary THR. (2) Revision of the socket for recurrent dislocation—to change cup orientation and upsize femoral head diameter. (3) Revision to a cemented constrained liner for recurrent dislocation. (4) Revision for cup wear/damage with no osteolysis (e.g. 3rd body wear). This technique is contraindicated where the bone cement interface is not well fixed, or there are large segmental defects.

Learning curve and how to manage complications: A reasonable learning curve is required for this technique, and it should be performed by a hip surgeon experienced in the use of cemented THR's and revision surgery. Complications are similar to that of a primary cemented THR. Accurate assessment of the cement–bone interface is essential to prevent early failure in unsuitable cases.

Level of evidence concerning the superiority of this method against others: There is little high-level evidence on acetabular cup revision. This is due to the considerable heterogeneity between patients, surgical technique for the primary as well as the revision procedure, the variety of components revised and their indications for revision. Brogan et al. [11] from the Exeter group published their 60 cement-in-cement acetabular revisions over an average of 8.5 years. The survival rate at five years was 92.2% for re-revision of any cause, which is comparable to that of uncemented cups. Kremers et al. [14] from the Mayo Clinic published their registry data regarding long-term follow-up of uncemented acetabular components. The five-year survivorship for any reason also was 92%. A paper from the Norwegian registry reported a reduced re-revision rate for uncemented vs cemented acetabular components. However, this was in comparison to cemented revisions without allograft and did not group in-cement revision separately. It has been shown that re-cementing after complete removal of the cement mantle can reduce the shear strength of this interface to 20%. The cement–cement interface created by cement-in-cement revision, however, does not seem to create a significantly weakened interface. It has been demonstrated that strong chemical bonding occurs between the old and new cement. Li et al. [1] have suggested that the presence of blood and bone marrow in the interface can reduce the shear strength by 85%. Rudol et al. [3] however, demonstrated that unless a substantial amount of highly viscous fluid is trapped within the interface, the shear strength of the interface remains close to that of a monoblock of cement. This is irrespective of whether a roughened surface is created. When one considers the reduced surgical time, blood loss and iatrogenic damage, along with the preservation of bone stock by leaving existing well-fixed cement in situ, we believe this is an important technique a hip surgeon should consider in this situation.

References

1. Li PL, Ingle PJ, Dowell JK. Cement-within-cement revision hip arthroplasty; should it be done? A biomechanical study. J Bone Joint Surg Br. 1996;78:809–11.
2. Weinrauch P, Bell C, Wilson L, Goss B, Lutton C, Crawford R. Shear properties of bilaminar polymethylmethacrylate cement mantles in revision hip joint arthroplasty. J Arthroplast. 2007;22:394–403.
3. Rudol G, Wilcox R, Jin Z, Tsiridis E. The effect of surface finish and interstitial fluid on the cement-in-cement interface in revision surgery of the hip. J Bone Joint Surg Br. 2011;93(2):188–93.
4. Duncan WW, Hubble MJW, Howell JR, et al. Revision of the cemented femoral stem using a cement-in-cement technique: a five- to 15-year review. J Bone Joint Surg (Br). 2009;91(5):577.
5. te Stroet MAJ, Moret-Wever SG, de Kam DCJ, Gardeniers JWM, Willem Schreurs B. Cement-in-cement femoral revisions using a specially designed polished short revision stem; 24 consecutive stems followed for five to seven years. Hip Int. 2014;24(5):428–33.
6. Hubble M, Patten A, Duncan W, Howell J, Timperley AJ, Gie G. Cement in cement femoral revision with the exeter hip. J Bone Joint Surg (Br). 2006;88(Supp)
7. Stefanovich-Lawbuary NS, Parry MC, Whitehouse MR, Blom AW. Cement in cement revision of the femoral component using a collarless triple taper: a midterm clinical and radiographic assessment. J Arthroplast. 2014;29:2002–6.
8. Quinlan JF, O'Shea K, Doyle F, et al. In-cement technique for revision hip arthroplasty. J Bone Joint Surg (Br). 2006;88(6):730.
9. Goto K, Kawanabe K, Akiyama H, Morimoto T, Nakamura T. Clinical and radiological evaluation of revision hip arthroplasty using the cement-in-cement technique. J Bone Joint Surg (Br). 2008;90:1013–8.
10. Lampropoulou Adamidou KI, Tsiridis EE, Kenanidis EI, HArtofylakidis GC. The outcome of 69 recemented hip femoral prostheses performed by one surgeon 22-40 years ago. J Arthroplast. 2016;31(10):2252–5.
11. Brogan K, Charity J, Sheeraz A, Whitehouse SL, Timperley AJ, Howell JR, Hubble MJW. Revision total hip replacement using the cement-in-cement technique for the acetabular component technique and results for 60 hips. J Bone Joint Surg Br. 2012;94:1482–6.
12. Hodgkinson JP, Shelley P, Wroblewski BM. The correlation between the roentgenographic appearance and operative findings at the bone-cement junction of the socket in Charnley low friction arthroplasties. Clin Orthop Relat Res. 1988;228:105–9.
13. Sabboubeh A, Al KM. A technique for removing a well-fixed cemented acetabular component in revision total hip arthroplasty. J Arthroplast. 2005;20:800–1.
14. Kremers HM, Howard JL, Loechler Y, Schleck CD, Harmsen WS, Berry DJ, Cabanela ME, Hanssen AD, Pagnano MW, Trousdale RT, Lewallen DG. Comparative long-term survivorship of uncemented acetabular components in revision total hip arthroplasty. J Bone Joint Surg Am. 2012;94(12):e82-1–8.

23 Jumbo Sockets

Eustathios Kenanidis, Fares E. Sayegh, Eleftherios Tsiridis, Eduardo García-Cimbrelo, Eduardo García-Rey, Mohammad Shahid, and Andrew R. J. Manktelow

23.1 Current Concepts

E. Kenanidis, F. E. Sayegh, and E. Tsiridis

The so-called jumbo cups are oversized shells that are used for the acetabular reconstruction [1]. The dimensions of jumbo cups are not precise. In the western countries, they are usually defined as cups 62 mm or larger in females or 66 mm or larger in males [2]. They are approximately 10 mm larger than the diameter of the native acetabulum used in primary THA or the contralateral normal acetabulum [1, 3]. There are also national demographic variations [4]. The jumbo cups for the Asians have been defined to be of an outside diameter of 64 mm for men and 60 mm for women [4].

23.1.1 Objective

These oversized cementless sockets are used to reconstruct moderate but not severe acetabular bone deficiencies in revision THA [1]. The cup is usually fixed with multiple screws, 360 degrees around the socket. Cancellous allograft is often employed for the remaining contained defects or protrusion situations.

There are two principal objectives:

1. The achievement of initial stability
   – The stability is also enhanced by the combination of the large socket with a thick plastic liner and large head size that reduces the rate of dislocation.
2. The increase of the total surface area of the implant- bone contact that promotes the biological fixation
   – Careful reaming, however, is indicated to:
   (a) Remove the less bone that is needed.
   (b) Redistribute it to the areas of bone defect.
   (c) Avoid removal of crucial bone from the posterior and medial wall or roof.

E. Kenanidis, M.D., Ph.D., M.Sc.
Academic Orthopaedic Unit, Aristotle University Medical School, Thessaloniki, Greece

E. Tsiridis, M.D., Ph.D., F.A.C.S., F.R.C.S. (✉)
F.E. Sayegh, M.D., Ph.D. (✉)
Academic Orthopaedic Unit, Papageorgiou General Hospital, Aristotle University Medical School, Thessaloniki, Greece
e-mail: etsiridis@doctors.org.uk; fsayegh@auth.gr

E. García-Cimbrelo, M.D., Ph.D. · E. García-Rey, M.D., Ph.D.
Hospital Universitario La Paz-Idi Paz, Madrid, Spain

M. Shahid, B.Sc., M.B.B.S., F.R.C.S.
Worcestershire Acute Hospitals NHS Trust, Worcester, UK
e-mail: shahidm99@doctors.org.uk

A.R.J. Manktelow, B.Sc., M.B.B.S., F.R.C.S.
Nottingham University Hospitals NHS Trust, Nottingham, UK
e-mail: a.mank@btinternet.com

E. Tsiridis (ed.), *The Adult Hip - Master Case Series and Techniques*,
https://doi.org/10.1007/978-3-319-64177-5_23

23.1.2 Indications

- They are usually used successfully for moderate but not severe acetabular bone deficiencies [1].

23.1.3 Contraindications

Their use is unpredictable in:

- Severe acetabular defects as Paprosky type IIIB where the superolateral acetabulum and the posterior column are entirely lacking and primary 3-point stability may not be possible [5].
- Compromised bone biology as in the acetabular defects in irradiated bone [5].

23.1.4 Advantages

1. It is considered a technically straightforward reconstruction technique. The acetabulum is prepared by reaming to a large hemisphere as in the primary THA [6, 7].
2. There is no need for extensive allografting and augmenting as the socket usually fills the bone deficiencies [5–7].
3. The increased contact area between the implant and the host bone promotes the bone in growth and stability (biological fixation) [6].
4. It improves hip biomechanics. This technique restores the centre of hip rotation closer to normal, translating it more laterally and inferiorly [6, 7].

23.1.5 Disadvantages

1. The limited bone-stock restoration with the excessive reaming.
2. The difficulties in large, oblong bone deficiencies as it may lead to extensive reaming of the anterior or posterior column or superior placement of the cup [8, 9].
3. The probability of proximal cup position that is correlated with increased risk of dislocation and impingement. The following high hip centre is associated with abnormal hip biomechanics, instability, leg discrepancy and suboptimal outcomes [7–9].
4. The possible complication of iliopsoas impingement and groin pain after revision THA when the anterior edge of the cup protrudes beyond the anterior wall. There is 14 and 26 times increased the risk for persistent postoperative pain and anterior iliopsoas impingement, respectively, when the implanted jumbo cups are >6 mm than the native femoral head [10].
5. The compromised initial fixation when there are limited screw fixation options due to poor pelvic bone stock [11].
6. This technique is not an option of treatment in severe bone defects as Paprosky type IIIB and the irradiated bone due to the unpredictable bone integration [5].

23.1.6 Literature

Several papers providing level IV evidence are presently available [1–7, 12–17]. These are retrospective case series of 17 to 196 patients [5, 14] with a mean follow-up from 4 to 20 years. Most studies, however, have included small numbers of patients at short- to intermediate-term follow-up [4, 13, 14, 16, 17]. It is difficult to directly compare the results of these studies because of a lack of consistency in the definition of jumbo components, the differences in acetabular bone deficiency, the differences in the duration of follow-up and the lack of survivorship data with the use of the three endpoints (aseptic, any reason and complication).

The porous jumbo cup acetabular revision with supplemental screw fixation was proven to be a viable reconstructive technique with good to excellent intermediate- and long-term outcomes. Paprosky types I to IIIA acetabular defects are usually managed. There are also reports including a limited number of type IIIB acetabular defects [5–7]. The reported prosthesis survival for any reason ranged from 79.8 to 96% [5, 7]. When the aseptic loosening was considered as the endpoint, the survival ranged from 82.8 to 98% [2, 7]. There were favourable results in the patients with a moderate but not a severe bone loss. Paprosky type IIIB defects are considered as contraindications for this technique.

The Mayo group reported the long-term results at a mean follow-up of 20 years (10–27 years) of 89 patients treated with jumbo sockets [6]. Almost half of the patients have died at the last follow-up. Paprosky types II to IIIA were mainly reconstructed. They demonstrated that the 20-year survivorship for any acetabular revision was 83% and for aseptic loosening 88%. Younger age was a significant predictor for revision [6].

In the greatest reported sample size, Gustke et al. [5]reported mid- to long-term results of 196 jumbo cups used in revision THA of 186 patients. The most usual types of acetabular defects were II to IIIA; however, eight type IIIB deficiencies were also reconstructed. The survival of jumbo cups was 98% at 4 years and 96% at 16 years. The overall percentage of complications was 6.4%.

To the best of our knowledge, no prospective trials are comparing jumbo cups to other forms of acetabular reconstruction.

23.1.7 Complications

- Varying rates of complications in the studies. Instability and septic and aseptic loosening were most frequently reported.
- Instability, however, was the most common complication, ranging up to 21% [13]. In one of the initial jumbo cohort studies, Dearborn et al. [13] showed 21% dislocation rate in 24 revision THAs. Lachiewicz et al. [7] reported 9.3% dislocation rate in 129 revision THAs. In this study, however, a femoral head size ≥32 mm was associated with a significantly lower risk of dislocation compared with smaller sizes.
- The reasons for the increased risk of dislocation seem to be rather multifactorial and are probably related to [7]:
  1. The surgical approach and dissection
  2. The number of prior revisions
  3. The amount of bone loss
  4. Femoral head size
- Clinical, radiological and simulation studies [5, 8, 9] demonstrated a hip centre elevation despite the placement of the cup at the inferior acetabulum. An increase in femoral head length may be needed to compensate with this complication.
- The possible protrusion of the anterior edge of the jumbo cup has been reported to increase the risk of iliopsoas impingement and groin pain [10].

23.1.8 Conclusion

Jumbo socket is a viable solution in types I and II Paprosky defects. Careful reaming is the key to success to avoid damage to the anterior or posterior wall. Elevation of the centre of rotation is unavoidable especially when the native socket compared to the implanted component has a difference of more than 10 mm in diameter. Large heads up to 36 mm can compensate for the latter and at the same time increase stability. It is crucial for the early in growth of the socket to stabilise the component with many and long screws. If possible put screws in the ischial and pubic bone and long screws >25 mm to the roof. If an allograft is used to fill the contained defects, use impaction grafting principles, i.e. large croutons up to 1 cm and tight impacted fresh frozen allograft washed before impaction, and never use reamers to smoothen the impacton grafting surface.

23.2 Case Title: Re-revision Socket Using Jumbo Revision TA Socket and Constrained Cemented Liner

E. Kenanidis and E. Tsiridis

Spinal fusion and hip revision in a high hip centre using an XLP cemented liner and a PLAD (posterior lip augmentation device by DePuy) to compensate for the abductor insufficiency or absence. Short limb by at least 3 cm (Fig. 23.1).

Re-revision using jumbo 68 mm TA revision shell (all tantalum by Zimmer) and five screws for extra stability. The centre of rotation moved down lengthening the leg, and a constrained liner (Stryker) was cemented in the shell to compensate for the missing abductors. The constrained liner has a lateralized profile that further lengthens the hip; thus, eventually the leg length recovered fully.

23.3 Case Title: Revision Socket Using Jumbo Acetabular Component

E. Kenanidis and E. Tsiridis

Jumbo socket revision on the right for acetabular component aseptic loosening. Simultaneous stem revision to a cemented double-tapered long stem (C-stem DePuy) (Fig. 23.2)

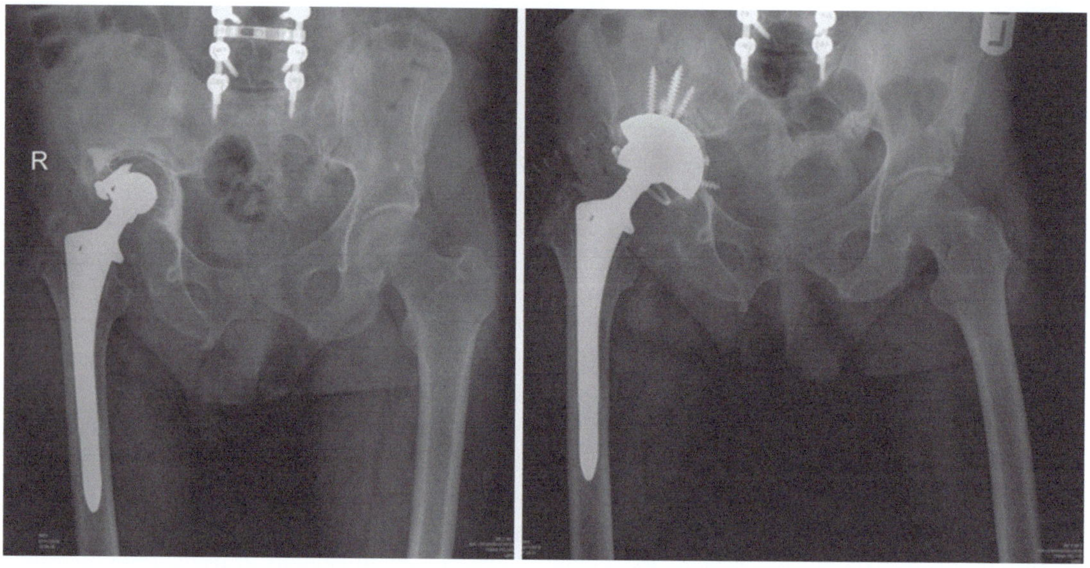

Fig. 23.1 Preoperative x-ray (*left*) and postoperative x-ray of the first day (*right*)

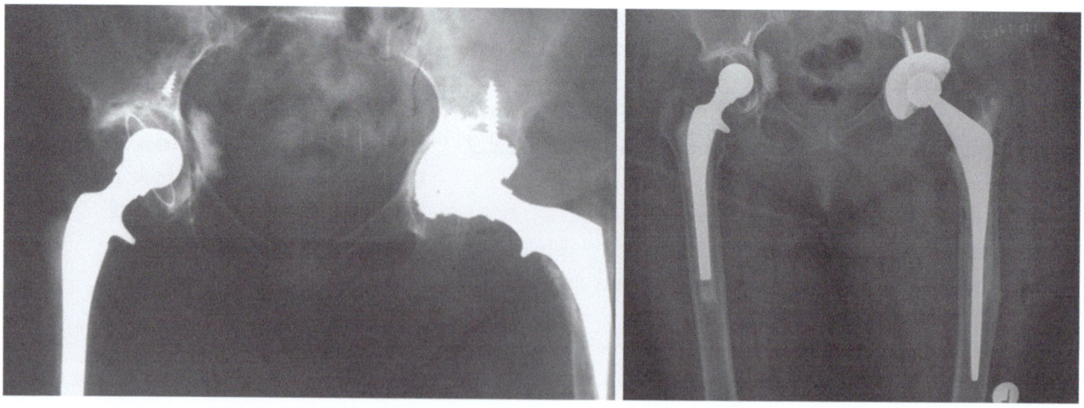

Fig. 23.2 Preoperative (*left*) and postoperative x-ray right hip revision of the first day (*right*)

23.4 Case Title: Jumbo Socket Revision

Eduardo García-Cimbrelo and Eduardo García-Rey

23.4.1 Demographics

Age: 46
Sex: Male
BMI: 30

23.4.2 Relevant Past Medical History

Principal pathologies: Bilateral avascular necrosis of both femoral heads.

Previous surgical procedures: Uncemented total hip replacement on the left side in 2003 and right side in 2009.

History of presenting complaint: Groin pain during physical activities for the last year. The patient is a heavy labour worker.

23.4.3 Clinical Examination

Symptoms: Groin pain during the last 4 months, even on daily activities such as squatting, putting on his shoes and walking for 20 min.

Range of motion: Limitation of hip flexion at 90° and internal rotation at 10°.

Specific tests: Straight leg rising in supine position.

Main disability: Pain during daily activities.

Scoring: 3-2-2 Merle D'Aubigne and Postel scale.

Neurovascular evaluation: Normal

23.4.4 Preoperative Radiological Assessment/Imaging (Fig. 23.3)

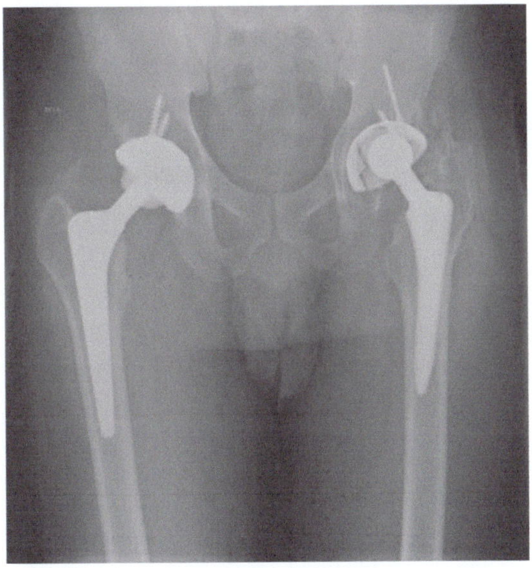

Fig. 23.3 *Left hip*: Evident polyethylene wear without any loosening sign. *Right hip*: Uncemented alumina-on-alumina total hip replacement

23.4.5 Preoperative Planning

Diagnosis: Left hip pain secondary to polyethylene wear (Fig. 23.3).

Possible treatment options: Acetabular revision surgery.

Chosen treatment method: Extra-large uncemented acetabular component.

Selection of implants if applicable and rational: Metal trabecular acetabular component and highly cross-linked polyethylene liner due to high activity level and young age.

Expected difficulties: The removal of the previous implant and the definite bone defect.

Strategies to overcome difficulties: The use of specific instruments to remove previous cup such as Explant (Zimmer) to avoid bone loss.

23.4.6 Surgical Note

Patient's position: Lateral decubitus.

Type of anaesthesia: Spinal.

Surgical approach: Posterolateral.

Main steps: Following the surgical approach, removal of the heterotopic ossification, fibrous tissue and metallosis due to the excessive polyethylene wear. Then removal of the screws and use of the Explant system to remove the previous implant and cleaning of all membrane from the bone.

Reconstruction techniques: Cavitary acetabular bone defect less than 30%. Reaming up to 59 mm until bleeding starts and insertion of a 60 mm Continuum cup (Zimmer), two screws and highly cross-linked polyethylene liner of 32 mm (Figs. 23.4 and 23.5).

23.4.7 Intraoperative Challenges

Challenges and solutions: The bone loss during removal of the previous cup and a small medial wall defect of 3 cm.

Unanticipated problems and solution: Use of the Explant system.

Thorough description of decision-making, including the reason for the final decision: Planned surgery could result in a minimal bone loss during extraction of the old cup.

23.4.8 Postoperative Radiographs (Figs. 23.4 and 23.5)

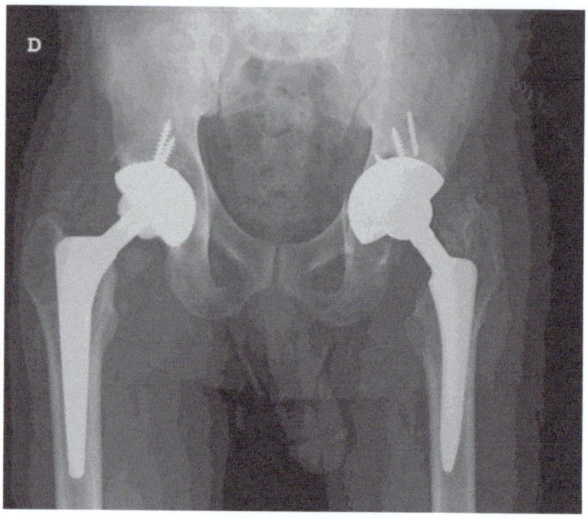

Fig. 23.4 Immediate postoperative radiograph. Please note the position of the acetabular component and the radiolucent gap in De Lee and Charnley zone 2

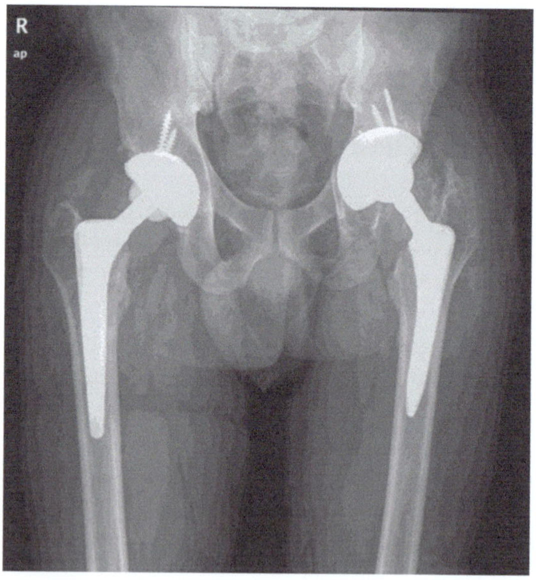

Fig. 23.5 Radiograph at 5 years after surgery showing complete osseointegration of the new cup

23.4.9 Postoperative Management

Chemoprophylaxis and anticoagulant treatment period: Subcutaneous low-weight heparin for six weeks.

Gait/limb loading until full loading: The patient was encouraged to walk with partial weight-bearing using two crutches during the first six postoperative weeks. Use of a cane until three months.

23.4.10 Follow-Up and Complications

Scoring: 6-6-5 Merle-D'Aubigne and Postel scale.

23.4.11 Discussion

Advantages of the applied method: Excellent bone osseointegration rates in small acetabular bone defects.

Disadvantages of the method: Another technique may be needed in major bone defects.

Alternative evidence-based techniques for the case: Acetabular impaction bone grafting.

Why is the chosen technique better for this case? Small bone defect, young and active patient.

Indications and contraindications for your technique: Large uncemented cups provide good results in hip revision surgery for small defects. An alternative technique may be necessary for larger defects.

Learning curve and how to manage complications: The surgical technique is similar to the most conventional uncemented contemporary acetabular components. The introduction of newer technology than porous-coated cups, such as trabecular metal may improve the results of this challenging management. In revision surgery, the use and combination of trabecular metal cups with or without augments may be very useful in many difficult cases; however, the bone loss remains the major limitation despite the excellent osseointegration that can be observed in hips without pelvic discontinuity [18–20].

Level of evidence concerning the superiority of this method against others: Excellent osseointegration signs can be found on the radiographs. Registry and large series show results at least as good as other standard techniques.

23.5 Case Title: Revision of the Acetabulum Using a Jumbo Cup

M. Shahid and A.R.J. Manktelow

23.5.1 Demographics

Age: 67
Sex: M
BMI: 37.5

23.5.2 Relevant Past Medical History

Principal pathologies: Haemochromatosis for which the patient had a previous venesection, gout and benign prostatic hyperplasia.

Previous surgical procedures: Right total hip replacement in 2001, left total knee replacement in 2003 and bilateral ankle replacements in 2013 and 2015.

Medication: Allopurinol, tamsulosin, atorvastatin, lansoprazole and naproxen.

History of presenting complaint: This 69-year-old gentleman presented to our clinic with right buttock and groin pain for the last six months. He had a right cemented total hip replacement performed in May 2001 for osteoarthritis. Prior to this, he had no problems with the hip.

23.5.3 Clinical Examination

Symptoms: Right groin and buttock pain.

Range of motion: On examination, he had an antalgic gait. He had significant pain in his right groin and restricted hip movements.

Specific tests: Blood tests showed a normal ESR, CRP and white cell count.

Main disability: His level of mobility was decreasing.

Neurovascular evaluation: The patient had a good dorsalis pedis and posterior tibial pulse. The sciatic nerve function was intact.

23.5.4 Preoperative Radiological Assessment/Imaging (Figs. 23.6, 23.7, and 23.8)

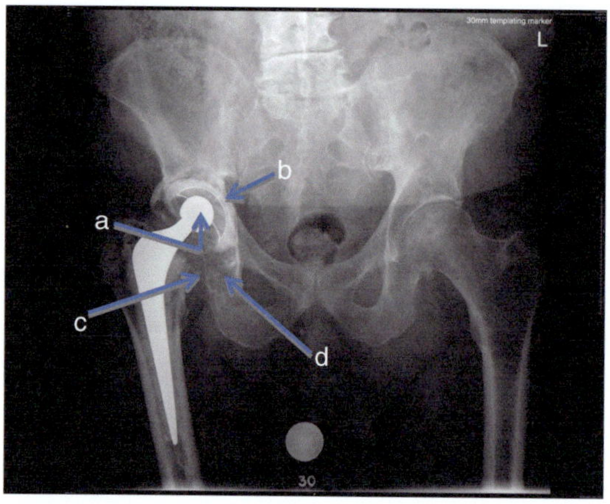

Fig. 23.6 AP plain radiograph showing the proximal migration of the femoral head (**a**), involvement but no disruption of Kohler's line (**b**), ischial (**c**) and teardrop lysis (**d**)

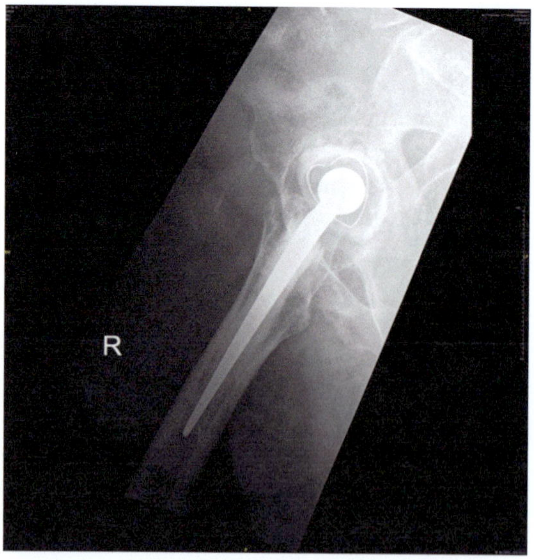

Fig. 23.7 Lateral radiograph of the hip joint showing loosening around the cup

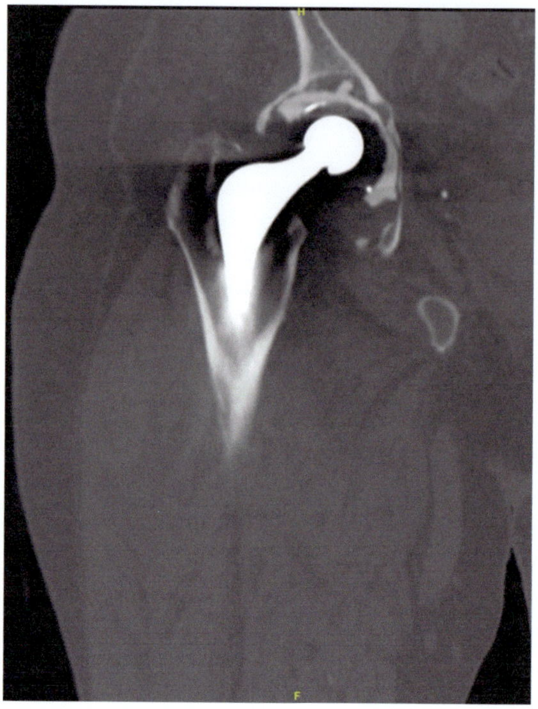

Fig. 23.8 Coronal CT view confirming the plain radiograph findings

23.5.5 Preoperative Planning

Diagnosis: Aseptic loosening of the acetabular component of a right total hip replacement (Figs. 23.6, 23.7 and 23.8).

Chosen treatment method: Revision of the acetabulum with a jumbo cup and a 'cement-in-cement' technique revision of the femoral component.

Selection of implants if applicable and rational: When relevant it is important to obtain the operation note for the index procedure as a part of the preoperative planning. In this case, the components used were an Opera (Smith and Nephew) cup (OD 47 mm ID 26 mm), 26 mm diameter CoCr, metal Exeter (Stryker) femoral head and Exeter (Stryker) femoral stem (No 2, 44 offset) (Fig. 23.7).

Instrumentation and implants required: Acetabulum—With regard to acetabular reconstruction, in addition to our standard instrumentation, we ensured that the TMARS (Trabecular Metal Acetabular Revision System—

Zimmer Biomet) was available. This system comprises a fully porous Trabecular Metal ™ revision shell, TM augments and buttresses, with the availability of the 'cup cage' construct. This provides the full inventory of options to deal with the bone loss predicted via the classification of the defect as well as any unexpected bone loss at surgery.

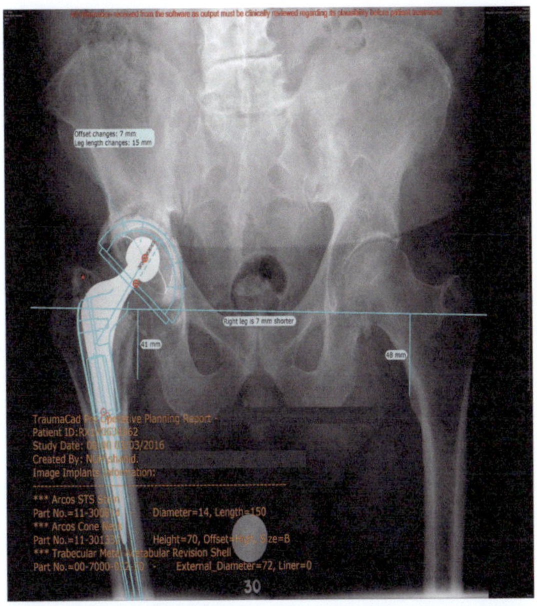

Fig. 23.9 Templating using the ARCOS and TMARS systems

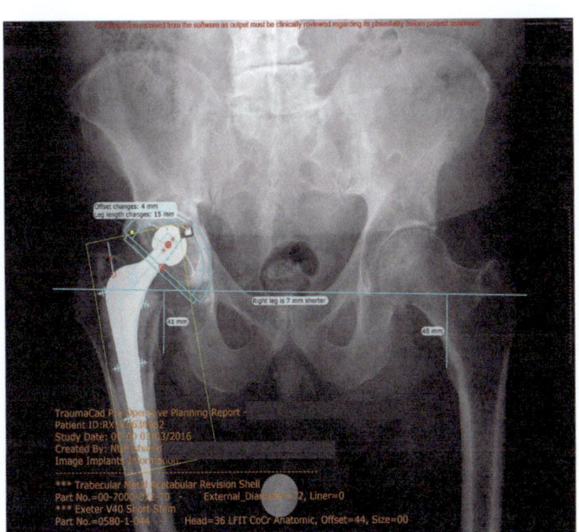

Fig. 23.10 Templating using the Exeter and TMARS systems

A femoral head was ordered to be used as allograft if required.

Femur: On the femoral side, Exeter 44, sizes 0, 1 and 2, stems alongside the 'short' 44 offset and 125 mm Exeter stems were arranged. This would allow a 'cement-in-cement' femoral revision. In case the existing stem was stable, or we were unable to extract it, then compatible Stryker heads (28, 32 and 36) were available.

(It is important to note that some Exeter stems pre-2001 have a different taper (non-V40 taper) to the current V40 stems (12/14)). An uncemented modular femoral revision system (ARCOS—Zimmer Biomet) in this case was available. The OSCAR cement removal system was available in theatre as was the Midas Rex Burr. This would allow the cement mantle to be freshened or indeed removed if the bone stock or the residual cement mantle was unsuitable for a 'cement-in-cement' revision.

Expected difficulties: (1) The potential for worse than expected bone loss found at the time of surgery. (2) Unable to perform 'cement-in-cement' revision. (3) An intraoperative femoral fracture.

Strategies to overcome difficulties: (1) The versatility of the TMARS system to deal with more bone loss than anticipated. (2) and (3) An uncemented modular femoral revision system available.

Templating: Using the TraumaCad® (Brainlab) system, we templated the acetabulum using the TMARS system and also the femoral side using both the ARCOS and Exeter systems (Figs. 23.9 and 23.10).

23.5.6 Surgical Note

Patient's position: Patient was in the lateral position with the pelvis positioned carefully and securely supported.

Type of anaesthesia: Spinal using heavy Marcaine and diamorphine. Antibiotics and tranexamic acid (1 g) were given at induction (flucloxacillin 2 g and gentamicin 200 mg).

Surgical approach: Posterior approach through the old incision. Main steps: The existing scar was used and extended proximally and distally. The fascia lata was incised. The sciatic nerve was identified and protected. An aspiration of the hip joint was performed. The piriformis was incised, and then this, along with the short external rotators and capsule, was elevated as a single flap. The gluteus maximus insertion was incised to improve access and to prevent undue tension on the sciatic nerve. The hip was dislocated easily. The femoral component was reviewed. The alignment was sound, and the stem was well fixed. However, to facilitate acetabular exposure and to allow us to utilise a larger head and a new V40 trunnion, the existing femoral component was removed. The cement mantle was intact within the proximal metaphysis and above the lesser trochanter. The socket was exposed with a circumferential release and with the femur transposed supero-anteriorly. Soft tissue samples were sent for microbiology. The existing polyethylene cup was loose. The component was removed initially using small curved osteotomes to loosen the implant-cement interface. Then the cement itself was cleared, with hand instruments and under direct vision, to reduce the possibility of additional bone loss. Careful debridement of all membranous debris was performed. Small cement plugs in the acetabulum were removed, being careful to avoid additional bone loss.

Acetabular reconstruction: The acetabulum was reamed sequentially at the desired hip centre. Reamer size was progressively increased towards the anteroposterior dimensions of the acetabulum. As anterior and posterior contact is approached, care must be taken not to lose the bone unnecessarily. In this case, we were able to ream sequentially until AP and SI dimensions were identical, thus achieving circumferential contact. We eventually reamed to 72 mm, and a trial for a 72 mm component was used to assess contact and stability. Similarly, reverse reaming can be used both to improve the structural integrity of the host bone and to allow the reaming to be used to fill minor bone defects (Fig. 23.11). Subsequently, a 72 mm trabecular metal-backed titanium modular acetabular cup (Fig. 23.12) was positioned, aligned carefully and impacted into the acetabulum. Using the alignment rod, we oriented it with 25° anteversion and 45° inclination (Fig. 23.13). Careful consideration must be given to the orientation of the socket to ensure that the screw holes are aligned with sound host bone. Once the socket was impacted with a good 'press fit', additional stability, to facilitate ingrowth, was achieved with a posterosuperior screw into the ilial bar. Where possible, it is often helpful to place short screws inferiorly, into the ischium or pubis, to gain better initial stability, as was done in this case. Secure initial implant stability is essential to facilitate bony ingrowth and improve the chance of long-term implant survival. In this instance, while initial fixation of the hemispherical component was sound, in light of the poor bone quality and limited availability, additional stability was achieved

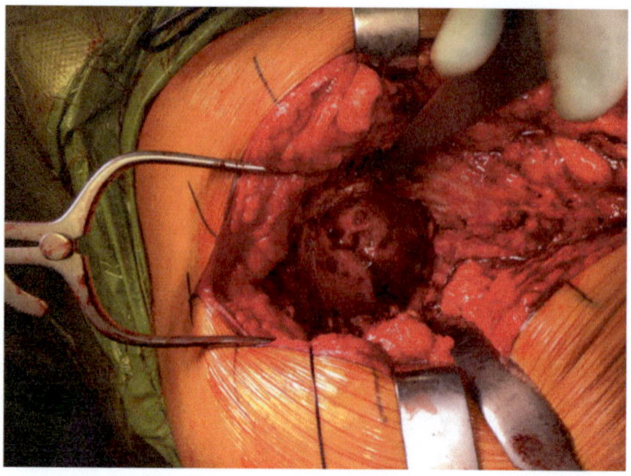

Fig. 23.11 Reamed acetabulum showing circumferential bone

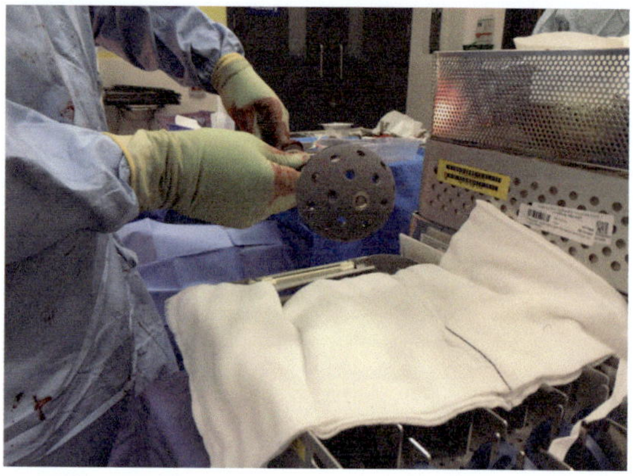

Fig. 23.12 Jumbo cup. Size 72 mm porous-coated Trabecular metal. Multihole Continuum socket (Zimmer, In 46580, USA)

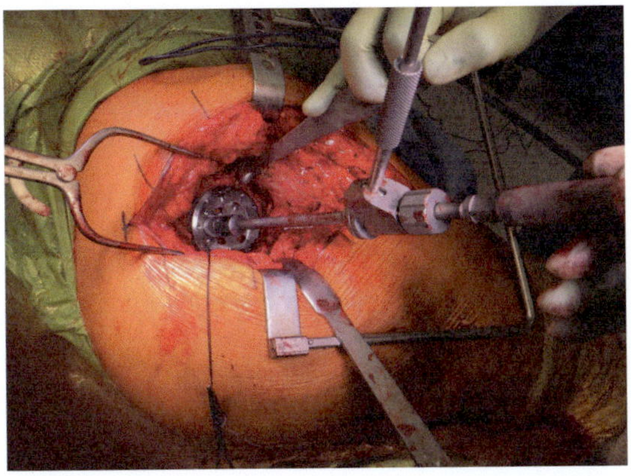

Fig. 23.13 Insertion of the cup with the use of alignment guide to ensure accurate placement

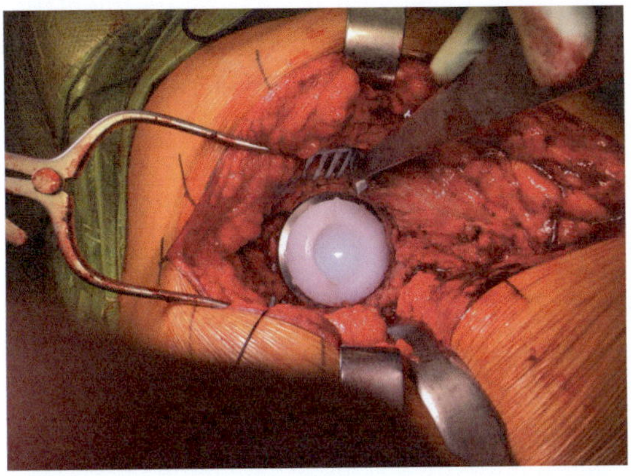

Fig. 23.14 Insertion of the 36 mm elevated highly crossed linked polyethylene liner (Zimmer, In 46580, USA)

with three screws inserted. A 36 mm highly crossed-linked polyethylene cup with a lipped liner was inserted. Care is taken to ensure locking mechanism is soundly engaged (Fig. 23.14).

Femoral reconstruction: Attention was now turned to the femur. A 'cement-in-cement' technique was used to achieve a sound femoral reconstruction. This was done using a slightly smaller stem (Exeter V40, 44 No 1) rather than the short 125 mm Exeter stem, as the patient was fairly well built. After trialling with various head options, the +5 mm–36 mm ceramic head (Biolox Delta, Stryker Orthopaedics) was the most stable and restored the biomechanics of the hip. It is important to achieve a sound soft tissue repair when closing the soft tissues. The short

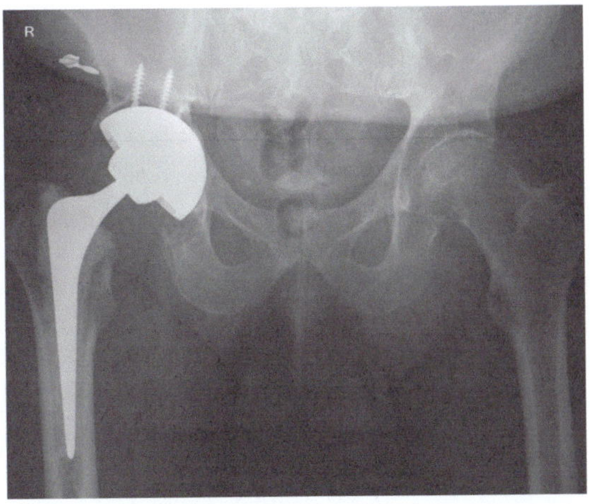

Fig. 23.15 AP pelvis post surgery. The stem and acetabulum are in an ideal position. The centre of rotation, offset and leg lengths are restored

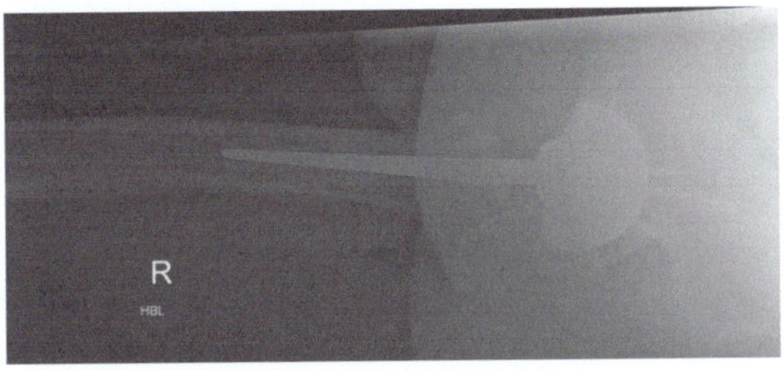

Fig. 23.16 Cross table lateral showing the cup in good alignment and the stem centrally down the femoral shaft

external rotators were attached with numerous 1 Vicryl sutures. A drain was placed just underneath the fascia lata, which was closed with a PDS suture. Deep and superficial fat was closed with 1 and 2-0 Vicryl, respectively. Clips were applied to the skin and a pressure dressing was applied (Figs. 23.15 and 23.16).

23.5.7 Intraoperative Challenges

Challenges and solutions: (1) Exposure: Careful soft tissue release is required in revision surgery to optimise exposure. The femoral stem was removed initially to obtain a circumferential exposure of the acetabulum (2) Implant removal: Care must be taken to avoid anything that could further compromise bone stock. Implants must be removed carefully after good exposure and with judicious use of appropriate instrumentation. (3) Characterisation of bone loss and reconstruction is required: the final decision of the correct option in reconstruction can only be done after the implant has been removed and residual bone quality, location and structural integrity have been established. (4) Reconstructive technique: For good results using a 'jumbo cup', it is important that a sound peripheral contact of the component on the host bone is achieved. The aim will be to establish anteroposterior (AP) contact and supero-inferior (SI) contact simultaneously without excessive or unnecessary loss of anteroposterior bone stock. If AP contact is achieved well in advance of SI, contact consideration must be given to an alternative technique, such as a posterior-superior TM augment to provide rim support.

23.5.8 Postoperative Management

Chemoprophylaxis and anticoagulant treatment period: Low-molecular-weight heparin for four weeks. While we do not use mechanical thromboprophylaxis routinely, the patient was mobilised rapidly allowing full weight-bearing to reduce the risk of thromboembolism.

Gait/limb loading until full loading: 50% Partial weight-bearing for four weeks and then weight-bearing as tolerated.

23.5.9 Follow-Up and Complications

No postoperative complications reported.

23.5.10 Discussion

Acetabular reconstruction is a major challenge in revision hip surgery. The initial goal is to achieve circumferential exposure of the acetabulum. This will facilitate safe removal of the existing implant without 'iatrogenic' bone loss. After successful implant removal, the surgeon can make a final assessment, 'characterising' bony deficiency, assessing the bone availability and quality, to determine the most appropriate reconstructive technique.

The central concept is to reconstitute structural support for an acetabular component, at the correct centre of rotation, while doing all possibility to maintain or improve bone stock. The 'jumbo' acetabular component is frequently utilised in acetabular revision surgery with an extensive bone loss. These are defined to have a minimum diameter of 62 mm in women and 66 mm in men or to be 10 mm larger than the contralateral acetabulum [2]. Advantages include a larger surface area which increases contact with the host bone and so enhances biological integration with a reduced need for bone grafting. Biological integration occurs even without full bony contact. There is also the ability to restore the centre of hip rotation using these cups [21].

Using a 'jumbo modular socket' provides a simple, reliable and versatile technique for acetabular reconstruction. It allows a variety of bearing surface options, specifically enabling relatively large head sizes to be used to minimise the risk of dislocation. Similarly, modular sockets provide the potential to deal with any future complications, without revising the components. Excellent mid- and long-term outcomes have been reported with this technique: 93% survival at 8 years [2], 100% survival at 7 years [13], 97% survival at 10 years and 83% survival at 15 years [7]. The most recent study demonstrated 98% survivorship at 4 years and 96% at 16 years and a significant increase in Harris Hip Scores [5]. However, it is important to note that while clinical results regarding high survivorship are reassuring, the technique does not fully restore bone stock. Therefore, its use should perhaps be concentrated in cases in which further acetabular revision is unlikely to be required. In younger patients, bone grafting or other options to maintain or improve bone stock should be considered. There are numerous options available for acetabular reconstruction [22]. The surgeon confronting such cases needs to feel comfortable with many options and to be flexible enough to deal with unexpected difficulties. However, with regard to the predictability of what the surgeon is likely to encounter, we feel that the Paprosky classification is very useful providing a reliable mechanism by which the pattern of bone loss and likely reconstruction required can be predicted from a careful evaluation of a plain AP radiograph [23]. The four important parameters to classify acetabular defects and guide treatment are the proximal migration of the femoral head, ischial lysis, teardrop lysis and disruption of Kohler's line. Proximal migration of the hip centre indicates loss of superior supportive acetabular bone. When this is more than 3 cm, then a significant bone loss can be anticipated. Teardrop and ischial lysis suggest a lack of acetabular structural integrity antero-inferiorly and postero-inferiorly, respectively. When Kohler's line is intact, in the presence of acetabular migration, it is likely that the surgeon will find suitable antero-medial support but deficient acetabular bone postero-superiorly. Typically, the surgeon will be able to address this by using options to reconstitute postero-superior rim support, in what is likely to be a type IIIA defect.

A specific concern for a jumbo socket technique in this type IIIA defect is that the surgeon will 'run out 'of antero-posterior bone by increasing the reamer size, before achieving supero-inferior contact. In this scenario, the available bone stock can be compromised, and useful AP structural support lost, in the search for a circumferential contact that is not truly 'available'. In these situations, once AP contact is established and with a significant residual superior defect, a decision should be taken, at that time and before any additional bone is lost with further expansive reaming, to use an alternative option to fill the residual superior defect, thus reconstituting structural support.

Increased complexity is associated with defects where Kohler's line has been disrupted, in association with proximal migration (a type IIIB defect). In this circumstance, the surgeon is likely to encounter additional bone loss and deficient structural support antero-medially and antero-superiorly. This pattern of bone loss raises the possibility of pelvic discontinuity. In this circumstance, more complex reconstruction is likely to be required.

In the case described above, the preoperative films show less severe proximal migration with an intact Kohler's line, however, with some inferior bone loss. In this circumstance, and with a relatively large acetabulum, it was possible to 'ream up' the socket to make AP and SI dimensions identical and achieve circumferential contact and fixation. As such, a jumbo option was a relatively straightforward reconstruction.

References

1. Patel JV, Masonis JL, Bourne RB, Rorabeck CH. The fate of cementless jumbo cups in revision hip arthroplasty. J Arthroplast. 2003;18(2):129–33.
2. Whaley AL, Berry DJ, Harmsen WS. Extra-large uncemented hemispherical acetabular components for revision total hip arthroplasty. J Bone Joint Surg Am. 2001;83:1352.
3. Gustke KA. Jumbo cup or high hip center is bigger better? J Arthroplast. 2004;19(4 Suppl):1.
4. Fan CY, Chen WM, Lee OK, Huang CK, Chiang CC, Chen TH. Acetabular revision arthroplasty using jumbo cups: an experience in Asia. Arch Orthop Trauma Surg. 2008;128(8):809.
5. Gustke KA. Use of jumbo cups for revision of acetabular with large bony defects. J Arthroplast. 2014;29: 199–203.
6. Philipp von Roth MD. Uncemented jumbo cups for revision total hip arthroplasty a concise follow-up, at a mean of twenty years, of a previous report. J Bone Joint Surg Am. 2015;97:284–7.
7. Lachiewicz PF. Fixation, survival, and dislocation of jumbo acetabular components in revision hip arthroplasty. J Bone Joint Surg Am. 2013;95:543–8.
8. Nwankwo CD. Do jumbo cups cause hip center elevation in revision THA? A radiographic evaluation. Clin Orthop Relat Res. 2014;472:2793–8.
9. Chima Nwankwo BS. Do jumbo cups cause hip center elevation in revision THA? A computer simulation. Clin Orthop Relat Res. 2014;472:572–6.
10. Odri GA, Padiolleau GB, Gouin FT. Oversized cups as a major risk factor of postoperative pain after total hip arthroplasty. J Arthroplast. 2014;29(4):753.
11. Faizan A, Black BJ, Fay BD, Heffernan CD, Ries MD. Comparison of head center position and screw fixation options between a jumbo cup and an offset center of rotation cup in revision total hip arthroplasty: a computer simulation study. J Arthroplast. 2016;31:307–11.
12. Hendricks KJ. Revision of failed acetabular components with use of so-called jumbo noncemented components a concise follow-up of a previous report. J Bone Joint Surg Am. 2006;88-A(3):559–63.
13. Dearborn JT, Harris WH. Acetabular revision arthroplasty using so called jumbo cementless components: an average 7-year follow-up study. J Arthroplast. 2000;15:8–15.

14. Wedemeyer C, Neuerburg C, Heep H, von Knoch F, von Knoch M, Loer F, Saxler G. Jumbo cups for revision of acetabular defects after total hip arthroplasty: a retrospective review of a case series. Arch Orthop Trauma Surg. 2008;128(6):545–50.
15. Harold W. Rees revision total hip arthroplasty without bone graft of high-grade acetabular defects. J Arthroplast. 2012;27(1):41–7.
16. Jasty M. Jumbo grafts and morselized graft. Orthop Clin North Am. 1998;29:249.
17. Obenaus C, Winkler H, Girtler R, Huber M, Schwagerl W. Extra-large press-fit cups without screws for acetabular revision. J Arthroplast. 2003;18:271–7.
18. García-Cimbrelo E. Porous-coated cementless acetabular cups in revision surgery: a 6- to 11- year follow-up study. J Arthroplasty. 1999;14:397–406.
19. Mohaddes M, Rolfson O, Kärrholm J. Short-term survival of the trabecular metal cup is similar to that of standard cups used in acetabular revision surgery. Acta Orthop. 2015;86:26–31.
20. Abolghasemian M, Tangsataporn S, Sternheim A, Backstein D, Safir O, Gross AE. Combined trabecular metal acetabular shell and augment for acetabular revision with substantial bone loss: a mid-term review. Bone Joint J. 2013;95-B:166–72.
21. Lachiewicz PF, Watters TS. The jumbo acetabular component for acetabular revision: curtain calls and caveats. Bone Joint J. 2016;98-B(1 Suppl A): 64–7.
22. Bloch B, O'Hara L, ARJ M. A practical approach to acetabular reconstruction in revision hip surgery. Orthopaedics and Trauma. 2015;29(2):117–26.
23. Paprosky WG, Perona PG, Lawrence JM. Acetabular defect classification and surgical reconstruction in revision arthroplasty. A 6-year follow-up evaluation. J Arthroplasty. 1994;9(1):33–44.

24 Trabecular Metal Shells for Revision (Porous Tantalum or Trabecular Titanium)

Eustathios Kenanidis, Ioannis Nakopoulos, Eleftherios Tsiridis, Alan J. Highcock, Allan E. Gross, Adolph V. Lombardi Jr., Dean J. Marshall, and Kristian Stahl Otte

24.1 Current Concepts

E. Kenanidis, I. Nakopoulos, and E. Tsiridis

Porous tantalum (PT) shells are used in the acetabular revision reconstruction with major bone loss (Paprosky types 2 and 3) [1]. PT obtains immediate stability and long-term fixation on the compromised host bone due to its favourable mechanical properties. PT augments also are excellent alternative to allograft bone for filling large bone defects.

24.1.1 Structure of Porous Tantalum Shells [1]

1. The **modular PT shell** has a titanium inner surface, an outer coating of porous tantalum and a locking mechanism for a modular polyethylene liner.
2. The **revision PT shell** allows for cementation of the polyethylene liner.
3. There is opportunity to drill holes through the revision PT shell to optimize the fixation with screws.

E. Kenanidis, M.D., Ph.D., M.Sc. (✉)
I. Nakopoulos, M.D.
Academic Orthopaedic Unit, Aristotle University Medical School, Thessaloniki, Greece

E. Tsiridis, M.D., Ph.D., F.A.C.S., F.R.C.S. (✉)
Academic Orthopaedic Unit, Papageorgiou General Hospital, Aristotle University Medical School, Thessaloniki, Greece
e-mail: etsiridis@doctors.org.uk

A.J. Highcock, F.R.C.S. (T&O)
Wirral University Teaching Hospital, Wirral, UK
e-mail: alan.highcock@nhs.net

A.E. Gross, M.D., F.R.C.S.C., O. Ont.
Division of Orthopaedic Surgery, Mount Sinai Hospital, Toronto, ON, Canada

University of Toronto, Toronto, ON, Canada
e-mail: AGross@mtsinai.on.ca

A.V. Lombardi, Jr, M.D., F.A.C.S.
Joint Implant Surgeons, Inc., New Albany, OH, USA

Department of Orthopaedics, The Ohio State University Wexner Medical Center, Columbus, OH, USA

Mount Carmel Health System, Columbus, OH, USA
e-mail: LombardiAV@joint-surgeons.com

D.J. Marshall, D.O.
Spectrum Orthopaedics, North Canton, OH, USA
e-mail: MarshallDJ@joint-surgeons.com

K.S. Otte, M.D.
Section of Hip and Knee Arthroplasty, Department of Orthopaedic Surgery, Hvidovre University Hospital, Hvidovre, Denmark
e-mail: Peter.Henrik.Gebuhr@regionh.dk; niels.kristian.stahl.kristensen.otte@regionh.dk

E. Tsiridis (ed.), *The Adult Hip - Master Case Series and Techniques*,
https://doi.org/10.1007/978-3-319-64177-5_24

24.1.2 Biomechanics

PT has beneficial mechanical properties for revision acetabular reconstruction (see also TM augments introduction). PT has:

1. Two to three times greater porosity than cobalt chromium and titanium mesh. This enables a higher bone and fibrous in growth potential that is valuable in cases of limited host bone [2, 3].
2. Similar modulus of elasticity to the subchondral bone. This facilitates physiologic load transfer from the implant to the host bone, minimizing stress shielding and preserving the bone stock [4].
3. Greater yield and ultimate strength than the subchondral bone. This enables the tantalum augments to have less risk of fracture and graft resorption than the structural allograft [5].
4. High coefficient of friction. This permits superior implant stability compared with traditional cementless designs, necessary when structural support is lacking [6].

24.1.3 Disadvantages

1. PT has greater cost than titanium mesh-coated component.
2. Long-term follow-up studies are not yet available.

24.1.4 Literature

There are multiple studies [3, 7–21] with excellent early and midterm survivorship results in major acetabular defect revision. These are retrospective and prospective case series, usually mixed cohorts with different Paprosky classification. Although PT is used in Paprosky type 2 and 3 defects, in some cohorts, it has also been used for type 1 defects [14]. The sample size of these studies ranges from 15 to 827 patients demonstrating short- to midterm results. Overall reported survival rate ranges from 88 to 98% [3, 7–21].

In one of the largest series reported from the Finnish National Arthroplasty, Skytta et al. [7] reported a 3-year survivorship for aseptic loosening of 98% in 827 PT acetabular revisions.

In a retrospective midterm comparative study [14], 214 HA-coated titanium cups were compared with 81 porous tantalum cups following revision THA. The majority of cases had minor bone deficiencies. There was no difference in the overall mechanical failure rate at midterm follow-up. In the major bone deficiency group, however, the titanium cups had greater but non-significant numbers of lucent zones around the cup and twofold but non-significant higher incidence of failure rate ($p = 0.27$). The pattern of failure of the two cups in this series was different. Eighty percent of the tantalum cups that failed did so within the first 6 months, whilst 82.3% of the titanium cups that failed did so after 6 months from the revision surgery.

In a recent systematic review, Beckman et al. [22] compared the rate of acetabular component loosening following revision THA using reinforcement rings (Ganz, Muller, Burch-Schneider) and TM cups, shells and augments. There were only case series and no RCTs. Between 2005 and 2010, one of the three most commonly used reinforcement rings was used for 1541 patients whether TM in 1959 revision THA. The mean follow-up period of the TM was 3.7 years smaller than this of the rings (5.7). The failure rate of the TM components was significantly lower than the yearly failure rate observed in different revision rings (1.9% vs 12.3%, OR = 0.326, $p = 0.002$). The overall TM loosening rate for Paprosky type 3A and 3B defects was 2.5%, and it was significantly lower than those of rings and cages (2.5% vs 14.0%, OR= 0.259, $p = 0.002$). TM showed also better results for the treatment of pelvic discontinuity; however, the number of patients treated was limited. Forty-two patients suffering from pelvic discontinuity were treated with TM. Although the follow-up period was greater for the rings compared to TM and no randomized comparative study existed, TM was considered a better treatment option for any moderate- to high-grade acetabular defect.

Tokarski et al. [18] supported that tantalum was more beneficial than titanium for acetabular components in revision THA. In a midterm retrospective comparative review, Ta group had significantly lower incidence of failure (4.4%) compared with Ti group (9.9%) ($p < 0.001$). Ta group had non-significantly lower incidence of infection (2.9%) than Ti group (5%) ($p = 0.105$). Among the 144 hips (64 Ta, 80 Ti) for which revision had been performed for infection, Ta group had a lower failure due to a subsequent infection (3.1%) compared to Ti group (17.5%) ($p = 0.006$). The authors supported that Ta is more protective against infection. This protective effect was attributed to the (1) higher potential to the osseointegration of Ta that obliterates any dead space, (2) possibly different topographical three-dimensional structure of the surface of Ta that may make difficult for organisms to access and colonize and (3) possible specific charge transfer of Ta or its surface characteristics that are hostile to infecting organisms.

24.1.5 Complications

Varying rates of complications. Instability was the most common complication, with an incidence reaching 13% [10]. Other complications included infection and periprosthetic fractures [3, 7–21].

24.2 Case Title: Revision of Acetabular Component Using Jumbo Trabecular Metal Tantalum-Backed Shell

E. Kenanidis and E. Tsiridis

24.2.1 Demographics

Age: 69
Sex: Female

24.2.2 Relevant Past Medical History

Principal pathologies: Arterial hypertension.

Previous surgical procedures: Primary THA (right hip) in 2004 and hysterectomy in 1992.

24.2.3 Preoperative Radiological Assessment/Imaging (Fig. 24.1)

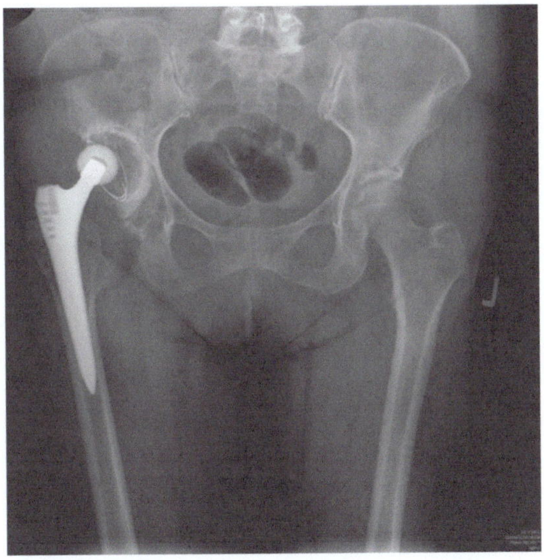

Fig. 24.1 AP x-ray of the right hip demonstrates that the polyethylene liner is destroyed

24.2.4 Preoperative Planning

This is a loosely cemented socket with a stable stem (Fig. 24.1). The acetabular defect appears contained, so it can be classified as Paprosky type 2 or 3A. A 3D reconstruction CT scan would be advisable before the surgery for the proper assessment of the defect and its containment.

Possible treatment options: Include jumbo sockets if concentric reaming could be achieved or a combination of a roof tantalum trabecular metal augment and a trabecular metal-backed socket underneath.

Chosen treatment method: Continuum Acetabular System Zimmer shell 60 mm, four cancellous bone screws 6.5 mm (2 × 20 mm, 1 × 25 mm, 1 × 30 mm) and polyethylene liner Zimmer 28 mm.

24.2.5 Surgical Note

Patient's position: Lateral decubitus.

Type of anaesthesia: General.

Surgical approach: Mini posterior.

Relatively easy removal of the cemented acetabulum using revision chisels all around the cement-bone interface. The polyethylene was worn out dorsally with plastic deformation of the inner surface and crack propagation to the posterior aspect of it. The residual defect was contained though it had an oval shape. Gradual reaming was then commenced, up until size 59 mm in diameter, and a 60 mm trial was inserted to check for conduct and shell stability. A 60 mm diameter implant, trabecular metal component for better gripping, and also integration was chosen to be inserted. To achieve an excellent fit and stability, however, three screws were inserted dorsally for the initial stability of the construct. We then elected to retain the ceramic head from the previous procedure as the taper of the in situ stem was not matching the current designs. The femoral stem, in this case, did not prohibit visualization of the socket, and the procedure was easily done by pushing the whole femur with the head on in front of the anterior wall. This is not, however, the case in every revision procedure, and sometimes it is important to remove the femoral component to access the acetabulum. An additional reason for retaining the in situ femoral implant was the absolute stability of the implant and its good bonding to the surrounding cortexes (Figs. 24.2 and 24.3).

24.2.6 Postoperative Radiographs (Figs. 24.2 and 24.3)

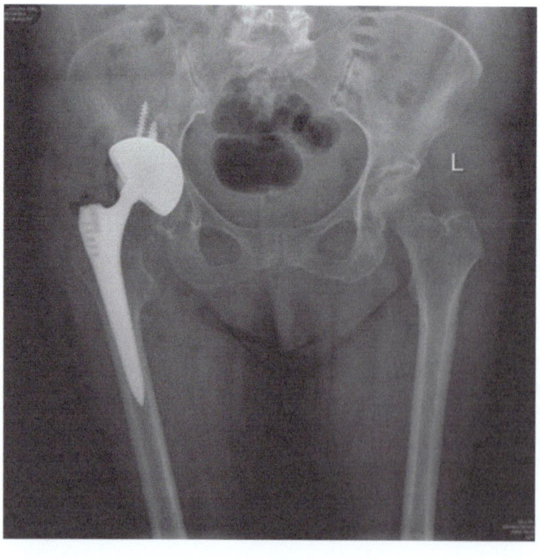

Fig. 24.2 AP of the right hip first day

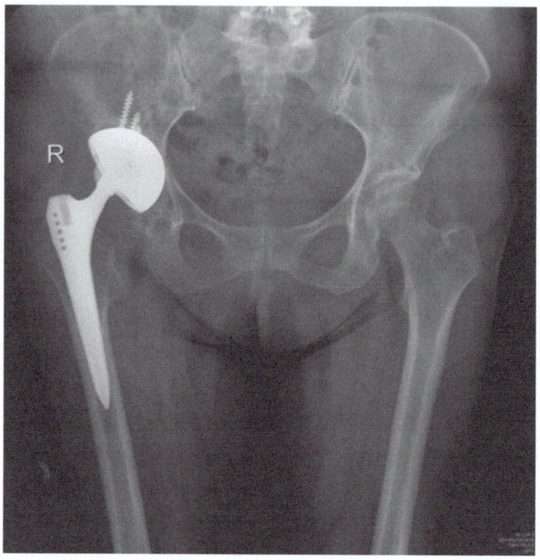

Fig. 24.3 AP of the right hip third month

24.2.7 Postoperative Management

Chemoprophylaxis and anticoagulant treatment period: Vancomycin 500 mg (one dose preoperatively and two doses postoperatively), cefuroxime 750 mg (one dose preoperatively and two doses postoperatively) and enoxaparin 1 × 1 for 35 days.

Gait/limb loading until full loading: Partial weight bearing for four weeks and then as tolerated.

24.3 Case Title: TA Socket Revision for a Screw-Type Loose Acetabular Component

E. Kenanidis and E. Tsiridis

The preoperative radiograph shows a loose acetabular component (Fig. 24.4). The Muller-type prosthesis was used with a screw-type acetabular component. The latter type of acetabular prosthesis creates a trapezoidal deformity with an immense medial bone loss when it gets loose. For the above reasons, a Ta socket was elected for the revision, to achieve the optimal interdigitation and bone ingrowth to the revision shell (Fig. 24.4).

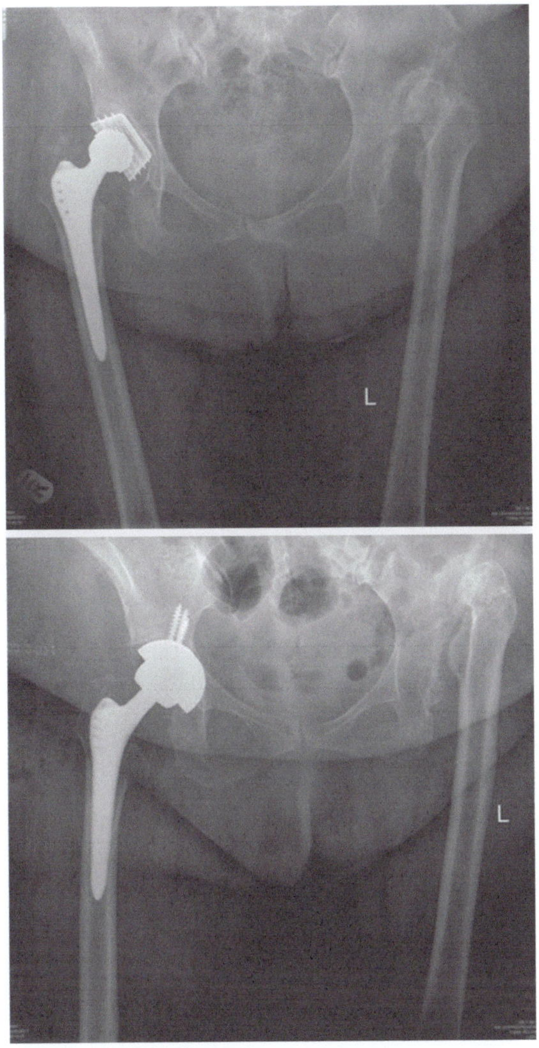

Fig. 24.4 Preoperative x-ray of the right hip (*above*) and postoperative x-ray of the first day (*below*)

24.4 Case Title: Trabecular Metal Tantalum Shell Revision

A.J. Highcock and A.E. Gross

24.4.1 Demographics

Age: 77
Sex: Female
BMI: 27.3

24.4.2 Relevant Past Medical History

Principal pathologies: Previous right-sided DDH, thalassaemia, hypertension and hypothyroidism.

Previous surgical procedures: Right Chiari pelvic osteotomy in 1981 and right primary total hip replacement with shelf autograft in 1994.

Medication: Amlodipine, Tylenol.

History of presenting complaint: High-functioning total hip arthroplasty for 21 years. Several months history of a gradual onset increasing right groin pain. Exacerbated by ambulation and relieved, but not eliminated, by rest. Shortening of 1 cm in the right leg noted—previously no leg length discrepancy.

24.4.3 Clinical Examination

Symptoms: Groin pain with ambulation. Mild antalgic gait with a cane.

Range of motion: Flexion 90 degrees, IR 10 degrees and ER 35 degrees—all limited by pain.

Specific tests: Trendelenburg positive.

Main disability: Pain and difficult ambulation.

Neurovascular evaluation: Intact.

24.4.4 Preoperative Radiological Assessment/Imaging (Figs. 24.5, 24.6, and 24.7)

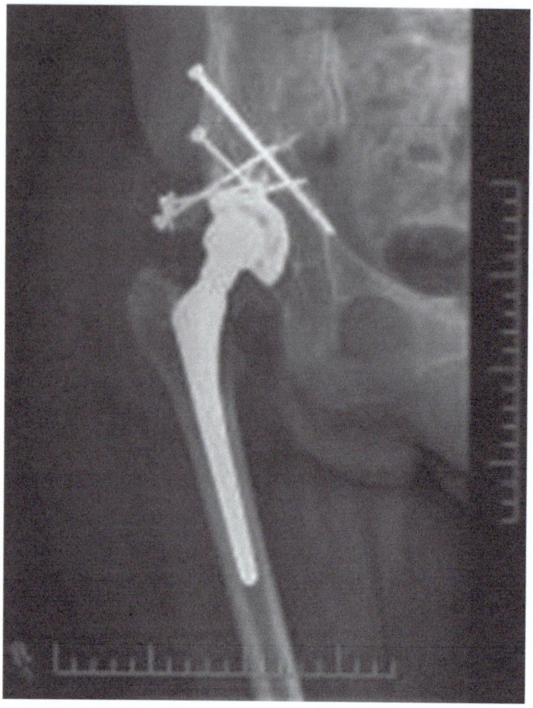

Fig. 24.5 Anteroposterior radiograph of the right hip: loose uncemented cup with previous shelf autograft and iliac screws from Chiari pelvic osteotomy. Evidence of metal debris secondary to backside wear between loose cup and graft screws

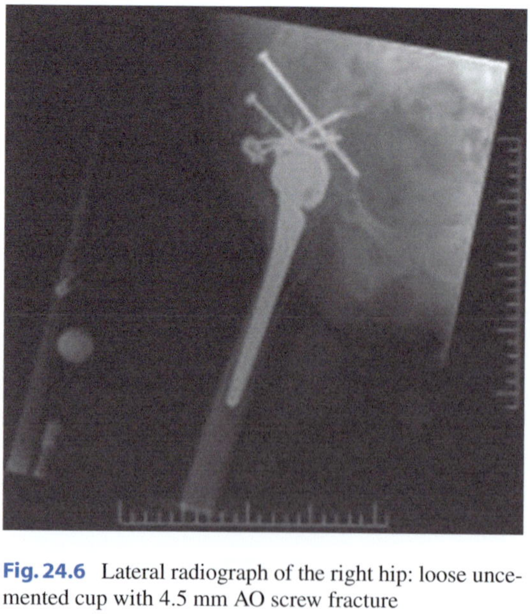

Fig. 24.6 Lateral radiograph of the right hip: loose uncemented cup with 4.5 mm AO screw fracture

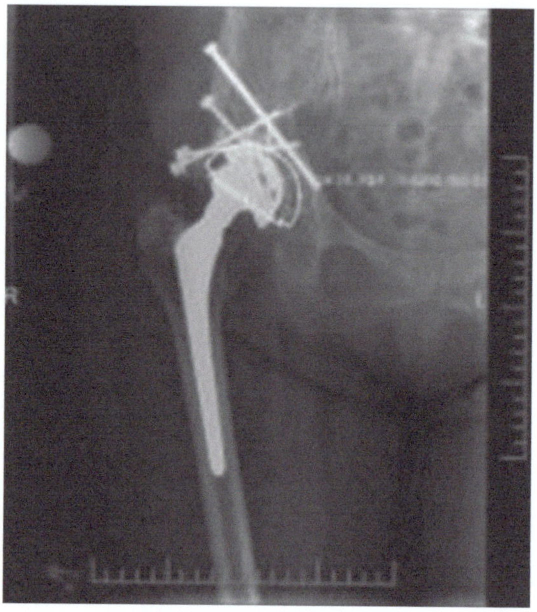

Fig. 24.7 Templating for trabecular metal cup

24.4.5 Preoperative Planning

Diagnosis: Aseptic loosening of uncemented acetabular cup. Previous shelf autograft and broken screw in acetabular dome (Figs. 24.5 and 24.6).

Possible treatment options: Trabecular metal tantalum cup, cemented cup ± impaction bone grafting, jumbo hemispherical cup, traditional porous, grit-blasted or hydroxyapatite-coated uncemented shell.

Chosen treatment method: Trabecular metal tantalum cup.

Selection of implants if applicable and rational: (1) Zimmer trabecular metal multihole cup. (2) Trilogy highly cross-linked 10 degree elevated liner.

Expected difficulties: (1) Sufficient host bone contact. (2) Adequate scratch fit of uncemented cup. (3) Fractured screw in acetabular dome. (4) Screws in ileum may prevent adequate reaming.

Strategies to overcome difficulties: (1) and (2) Tantalum acetabular shell. (3) Small trephines and bone osteotomes available. (4) AO large fragment screwdriver available.

Templating: Preoperative planning for tantalum TM shell size and restoration of hip centre and leg length. Stem appeared well fixed, stem (Osteonics) and relevant taper (C-taper) are identified and the appropriate femoral heads for potential head exchange are made available (Fig. 24.7).

24.4.6 Surgical Note

Patient's position: Lateral decubitus.

Type of anaesthesia: General.

Surgical approach: Through the previous approach—transgluteal.

Main steps: Previous transgluteal approach, abductors found to be healed and well attached. Therefore, a transgluteal approach was reused. Significant metallosis was noted, and thorough synovectomy was performed before and after the hip dislocation. An external outrigger was inserted into the iliac crest and leg length measured before the dislocation. Hip is dislocated and cup grossly loose and easily removed. The broken screws were removed from the acetabulum. The cup was medialized and expanded to a size 58. The shelf autograft was found to be fully incorporated providing an excellent superior bone quality. The cup was reamed to the bleeding bone circumferentially. Type 2 (contained) bone defect was identified within the floor of the acetabulum which extended into the pelvis. This defect was grafted with reamings from the acetabulum, a size 58 (line-to-line) multihole tantalum shell was inserted and fixation augmented with three screws. Following the excision of the osteophytes, a size 36/58 with 10-degree liner is inserted with the lip anterosuperior. Attention was then turned to the femur. The femur had evidence of osseointegration with excellent fixation. Therefore, head exchange only to a 36 mm head. Hip reduced and leg length, offset, stability and component position checked with trial implants, prior to definitive implantation (Figs. 24.8 and 24.9).

Reconstruction techniques: Highly porous trabecular metal tantalum cups have osseous integration via bony ingrowth which, once achieved, provides solid structural support for the acetabular component. The high coefficient of friction provides the excellent initial scratch fit of the shell. The multihole option allows for supplemental screw fixation whilst bone ingrowth occurs where host bone contact is limited or in the revision scenario—as with this case. Modular or cemented liners are available; cemented liners may be used if the cup orientation and inclination require fine-tuning after implantation of the shell.

24.4.7 Intraoperative Challenges

Challenges and solutions: There were two fractured screws within the acetabulum after the primary acetabular shell was removed. The head and shank of the screws were removed with an AO large fragment screwdriver. The thread of the broken screws was removed utilizing a narrow bone osteotome to delineate the screw shaft from the surrounding bone and a vice grip to engage the shaft. The screw thread could then be reversed and removed.

Unanticipated problems and solution: The type 2 contained defect extended through the medial wall of the acetabulum. To address this, the floor had to be contained with an absorbable gelatin compressed sponge (e.g. Gelfoam) before bone grafting into the defect. In this case, the acetabular reamings were utilized for the graft; however, if insufficient reamings are obtained, they could be combined with morsellised allograft to create an auto-allograft composite. Metallosis from backside wear of the screw and the previous shell was identified intraoperatively. A thorough debridement of the synovium was performed. This is crucial to limit the potential for third body wear at the metal-on-poly articulation.

Thorough description of decision-making, including the reason for the final decision: In this revision setting, the potential problems were adequate initial press fit of the revision acetabular component and osseointegration of the acetabular shell, given the previous shelf autograft. Trabecular metal tantalum shells address both of these issues, with a high coefficient of friction for initial scratch fit, ability to augment any fixation with supplemental screws and excellent osseointegration demonstrated in multiple studies. The availability of modular trabecular metal augments to address any unexpected bone defects heightens the versatility of the system, particularly in the acetabular revision scenario.

24.4.8 Postoperative Radiographs (Figs. 24.8 and 24.9)

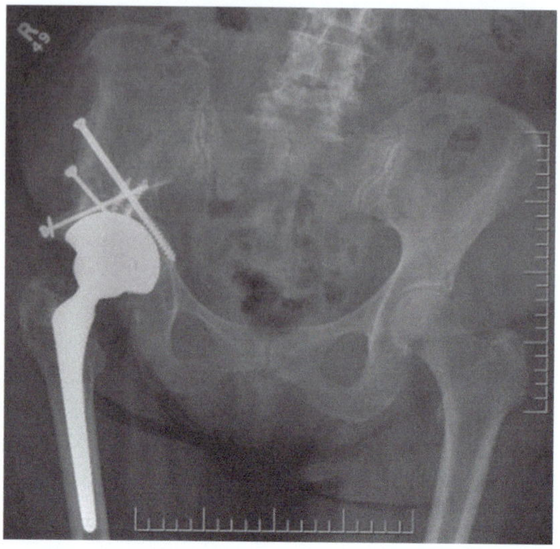

Fig. 24.8 Post-op anteroposterior radiograph: medial bone grafting, trabecular metal shell and retention of the stem

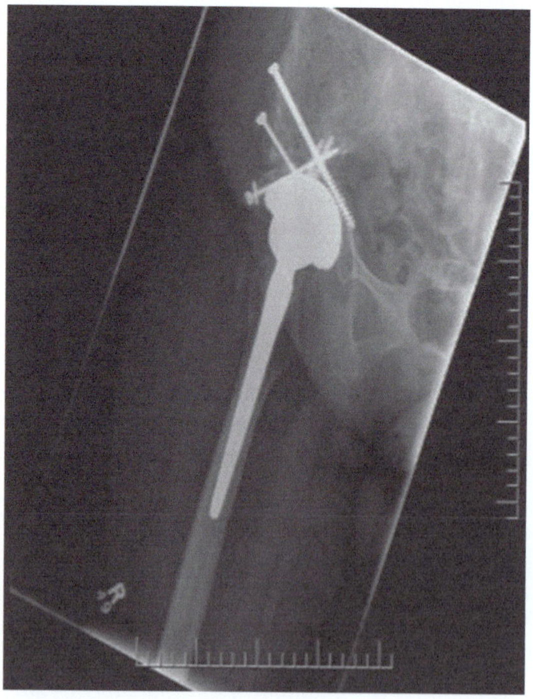

Fig. 24.9 Post-op lateral radiograph: trabecular metal shell with screw augmentation

24.4.9 Postoperative Management

Chemoprophylaxis and anticoagulant treatment period: Enoxaparin for five weeks. Intravenous antibiotics for five days followed by oral antibiotics for further five days.

Gait/limb loading until full loading: Full weight bearing. The scratch fit and screw augmentation allow initial stability, even with full weight bearing while osseointegration of the trabecular metal shell occurs.

24.4.10 Follow-up and Complications

No post-op complications.

24.4.11 Discussion

Advantages of the applied method: (1) Excellent osseous integration of porous trabecular metal shells, even into the previous autograft. (2) The excellent initial scratch fit of the TM shell and potential to augment initial fixation with screws allow for full weight bearing immediately postoperatively, whilst osseointegration occurs in the initial 6–12 weeks postoperatively. (3) Trabecular metal augments add modularity to the system to simultaneously address acetabular defects that were present.

Disadvantages of the method: Cost—tantalum trabecular metal shells are currently more expensive than conventional porous, titanium grit blasted or hydroxyapatite-coated shells.

Alternative evidence-based techniques for the case: Traditional uncemented shells, cemented cups and jumbo hemispherical cups.

Why is the chosen technique better for this case? Trabecular metal shell has impressive osseointegration, with studies demonstrating an integration of the cups with as little as 50% bleeding host bone contact without structural support with augments or allografts [11]. Although less expensive, conventional porous grit blasted or hydroxyapatite-coated uncemented cups require a minimum 70% host bone contact and, even then, have inferior long-term integration and survival. Cemented acetabular cups in the revision scenario are a recognized option; however, the cement interdigitation into the native acetabulum in revision procedures is poorer than in the primary setting, owing to sclerotic and/or cavitary nature of the host bone. Longevity of cemented cups in the revision scenario is a concern. The excellent reported results with trabecular metal shells from multiple centres [23], alongside results at our institution [24], are such that the senior author recommends their use in most acetabular revisions.

Indications and contraindications for your technique: Indications: Majority of acetabular revisions are primary THA with >30% uncontained defect. Contraindication: Large contained or uncontained bone defect making it impossible to stabilize cup at correct anatomic level—requires augmentation of fixation, e.g. cup cage. Greater than 50% uncover age of the acetabulum—requires structural support with allograft, autograft or trabecular metal augments.

Learning curve and how to manage complications: Minimal learning curve. Technical skills are similar to other uncemented cup systems.

Level of evidence concerning the superiority of this method against others: II.

24.5 Case Title: Tantalum Revision Cups in Cup Sockets

Adolph V. Lombardi Jr and Dean J. Marshall

24.5.1 Demographics

Age: 90 years old
Sex: Male
BMI: 25.8 kg/m^2

24.5.2 Relevant Past Medical History

Principal pathologies: The mechanical complication of total hip arthroplasty with aseptic loosening of the acetabular component.

Previous surgical procedures: Right total hip arthroplasty in 1995, left total hip arthroplasty in 2005 and right total knee arthroplasty in 2014.

Medication: Metoprolol 25 mg, lisinopril/HCTZ 20/12.5 mg, amlodipine besylate 5 mg, warfarin sodium 2.5 mg, timolol 5 mL, 0.5%, Xalatan 2.5/0.005%, multivitamin and fish oil.

History of presenting complaint: Pain in the right hip and thigh with difficulty ambulating and loss of range of motion over one month period.

24.5.3 Clinical Examination

Symptoms: Anterior thigh pain present on the right. The patient is unable to put on socks or shoes on the right. The patient walks with a limp and must use a wheeled walker for ambulation. The patient is only able to ambulate indoors.

Range of motion: Right hip—Flexion 60–79 degrees, abduction 0–29 degrees, internal rotation 0–29 degrees, external rotation 0–29 degrees and adduction 0–29 degrees; no fixed flexion deformity is noted.

Specific tests: X-rays were taken of the right hip. Infection work up was performed with laboratory analysis and joint aspiration. All laboratory analysis was within normal limits, and joint aspirate was negative for any growth on culture.

Main disability: Pain and limitation of the right hip causing disability.

Scoring if available: Harris Hip Score of the right hip:28.

Neurovascular evaluation: Patient has a full neurovascular function with appropriate motor control.

24.5.4 Preoperative Radiological Assessment/Imaging (Figs. 24.10 and 24.11)

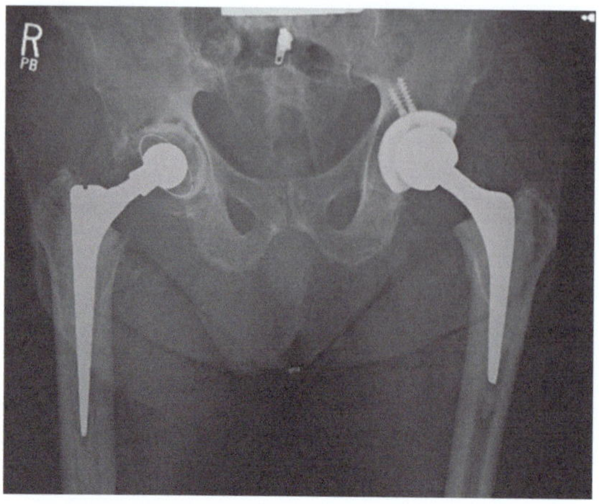

Fig. 24.10 AP of the pelvis—radiolucencies present in all zones around the acetabular component. Femoral component appears satisfactory

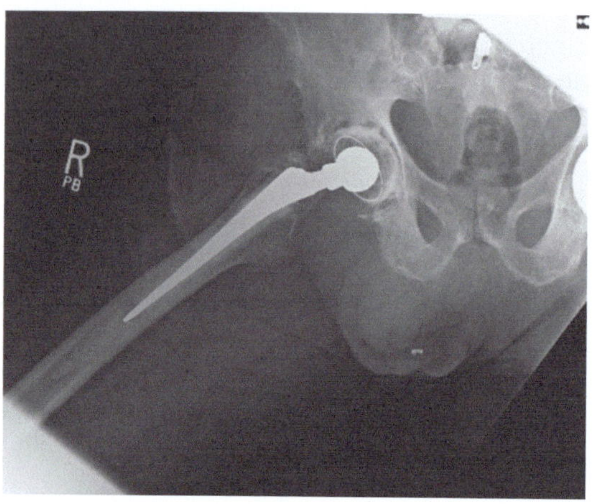

Fig. 24.11 Lateral right hip—radiolucencies present around the acetabular component

24.5.5 Preoperative Planning

Diagnosis: Mechanical complication of right total hip arthroplasty—aseptic loosening of the acetabular component (Figs. 24.10 and 24.11).

Possible treatment options: With patient's advanced age, continued conservative management and activity modification were discussed as a possible treatment. Revision right total hip arthroplasty of the acetabulum was also offered. Options for revision include placement of a porous metal cup, placement of a porous metal cup with augmentation using allograph bone or porous metal and utilization of a cup - cage construct or a custom triflange component.

Chosen treatment method: Revision right total hip arthroplasty with a modular exchange of the femoral head/neck attachment and revision of the acetabular component employing the use of a porous metal tantalum cup.

Selection of implants if applicable and rational: Tantalum cementless press-fit acetabular cup with screw fixation, ultra-high-molecular-weight polyethylene lipped liner and new femoral head/neck. This was chosen as the method of treatment for this patient due to its efficacy in acetabular reconstruction [25].

Expected difficulties: Gaining access to the acetabulum whilst leaving the femoral stem in place; management of any unexpected bone loss present in the acetabulum.

Strategies to overcome difficulties: Meticulous dissection and release of scar tissue to mobilize the femur. Instruments were available if the femoral stem needed to be removed via osteotomy. Allograft bone, augments and cup cage constructs were made available for any unexpected acetabular bone loss.

24.5.6 Surgical Note

Patient's position: Right lateral decubitus.

Type of anaesthesia: General anaesthesia with spinal.

Surgical approach: Direct lateral (Hardinge) approach.

Main steps: Patient was prepped and draped in sterile fashion. A portion of previous surgical incision was used, and dissection was carried down to the underlying tensor fascia lata. The tensor fascia lata was incised creating a myofascial sleeve. The vastus lateralis was elevated in continuity with the inferior fibres of the gluteus medius and minimus. The hip was dislocated and head/

neck disimpacted. The femoral component was found to be well fixed. The periacetabular scar was removed, and the acetabular component was grossly loose. The component was removed as well as all surrounding cement. Once the acetabulum was exposed and no extensive bone loss was encountered, reaming was performed until a 64 mm, tantalum cup was able to be impacted with a good press fit. The reaming was done line to line as implant has a peripheral flare. Five 6.5 mm screws were then placed. In revision surgery, unlike primary cases, screws are placed where the bone is present. This is done very carefully as we are cognizant of the safe zones. A high-walled liner was used for added stability. A 36 mm head was chosen, and after trailing a +10 mm option was chosen to re-establish leg lengths and stability. The gluteus medius and minimus were re-approximated to the-ir insertion, and all other layers were closed after irrigation. Local injection and vancomycin were used. A drain was placed before closure (Figs. 24.12 and 24.13).

Reconstruction techniques: Cementless press-fit acetabular revision with a tantalum cup.

24.5.7 Intraoperative Challenges

Challenges and solutions: No specific challenges were encountered. Mobilization of the femur with the femoral stem in place was done with care to provide good exposure of the acetabulum. There was no significant bone loss present needing augmentation or grafting. There were no acetabular rim defects, and the cup was able to be placed in proper position.

Unanticipated problems and solution: There were no unanticipated problems.

Thorough description of decision-making, including the reason for the final decision: The patient, in this case, has a minimal bone loss and was graded as a Paprosky type 1 defect. Tantalum cups have emerged as a reliable treatment in revision surgery with minor to severe bone loss (Paprosky type 2 and type 3) in several published reports. Mechanical properties of tantalum are ideal for immediate stability and fixation and have outperformed titanium and cobalt chrome cups in revision arthroplasties. For these reasons, the use of a cementless press-fit tantalum cup was made for the acetabular revision.

24.5.8 Postoperative Radiographs (Figs. 24.12 and 24.13)

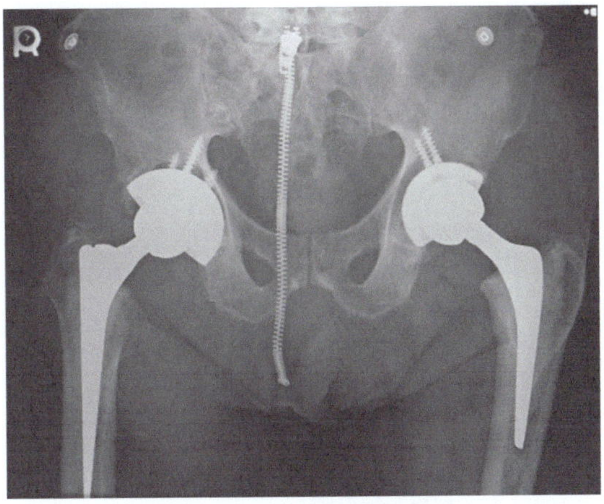

Fig. 24.12 AP of the pelvis—satisfactory placement and alignment of acetabular component and screws without radiolucencies. Femoral component well fixed and unchanged

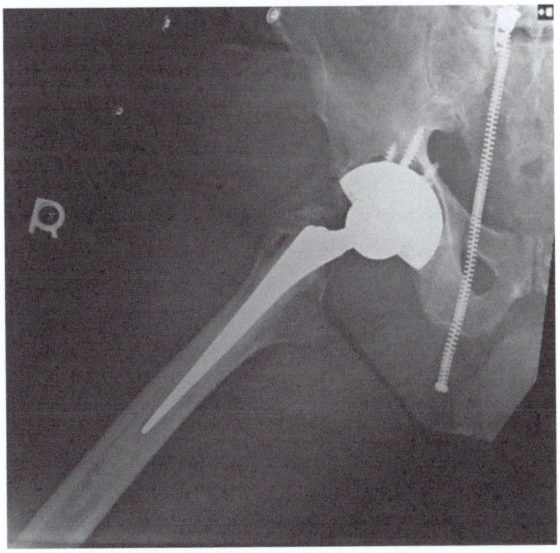

Fig. 24.13 Lateral right hip—satisfactory placement and alignment of acetabular component and screws without radiolucencies. Femoral component well fixed and unchanged

24.5.9 Postoperative Management

Chemoprophylaxis and anticoagulant treatment period: Patient was placed on a low-molecular-weight heparin and warfarin until INR was therapeutic, and then low-molecular-weight heparin was discontinued.

Gait/limb loading until full loading: Patient was made a touch-down weight bearing until 2-week follow-up. The patient was then able to progress weight bearing by 25% per week until full weight bearing.

24.5.10 Follow-up and Complications

No complications were encountered.

Scoring if available: Harris Hip Score right hip:84.

24.5.11 Discussion

Advantages of the applied method: The advantage of this treatment is the ability to gain fixation with a cementless press-fit tantalum cup, thus conserving the host bone. Porous metal tantalum cups have also shown to outperform more traditionally used titanium and cobalt chrome cups in revision surgery [1]. The biomechanical properties of tantalum show a high coefficient of friction, increased porosity and better-matched modulus of elasticity compared to titanium or cobalt chrome [1]. This allows for greater stability, bony ingrowth and bone conservation and makes these cups a great option for revision of the acetabulum [1]. In this patient, his pattern of bone loss was minimal, and the use of a tantalum cup also avoids the need for revision with using a high hip centre technique or other implants such as cup cage or triflange constructs. These techniques and implants have been shown to have long-term complications and problems such as altered hip biomechanics and dislocation [1]. There have been several published reports of tantalum cup use in revision being superior to the use of other materials [1]. There is also a large series from Skytta et al. that retrospectively reviewed 827 acetabular revisions using tantalum cups. Results showed 98% survivorship when aseptic loosening was used as the end point for revision [7]. This data supports and defines the advantage of using tantalum cups for use in acetabular revision.

Disadvantages of the method: In this case, we can find no specific disadvantages to the use of a tantalum cup. Tantalum has been shown to outperform titanium and cobalt chrome cups clinically in revision acetabular surgery, and with superior fixation, tantalum provides a good option for this case [1]. If there was more extensive bone loss and compromise of supporting structures, the tantalum cup alone may be insufficient. Allograft or porous metal augmentation may be an option to use with the tantalum cup. Other constructs could be considered as well. Fletcher et al. published a series of 23 acetabular revisions using tantalum cups with and without augments for major bone loss during acetabular revision surgery. They found good results with the use of these implants as an alternative to cages and allografts [25].

Alternative evidence-based techniques for the case: Alternative evidence-based techniques for this case could include the use of titanium or cobalt chrome cups, jumbo hemispherical cups, off the shelf cages or a custom triflange component. These options have failed to show superior results in the latest review [1]. Jumbo cups, cup cage constructs or custom triflange components would likely be unnecessary in this patient with minimal bone loss. The use of titanium or cobalt chrome cups may have been used as an alternative, but their results when compared to tantalum have been shown to be inferior [1].

Why is the chosen technique better for this case? Placement of a tantalum cup has shown to be better for several reasons. Tantalum cups have outperformed other materials such as titanium and cobalt chrome in cases of acetabular revision [1]. There was minimal bone loss present, and the use of a jumbo hemispherical cup was unnecessary. These cups can disrupt column support and sacrifice host bone stock. The tantalum cup has been shown to be better than off the self-cages because they have very little bony ingrowth potential and are likely to fail in the first decade [1]. Custom triflange components have a high rate of dislocation compared to tantalum cups, as well as needing a CT scan and delay in treatment until component can be manufactured [1].

Indications and contraindications for your technique: Indications for the use of a tantalum cup, in this case, would be an aseptic loosening of the acetabular component with a minor bone loss. A tantalum cup will gain stable fixation with improved potential for bony ingrowth compared to titanium or cobalt chrome cups [1]. Contraindications could be in a case of significant bone loss in which augmentation or other methods of more stable fixation might be needed. In the case, that augmentation would be deemed necessary, good results can be expected when used with a tantalum cup as an alternative to a cage construct [25].

Learning curve and how to manage complications: There is not a significant learning curve for this specific case as reaming, and placement of this type of cup are very similar to the placement of a primary acetabular cup. Principles of proper version and abduction should be followed as the placement of any acetabular implant.

Level of evidence concerning the superiority of this method against others: There are several studies supporting the use of tantalum cups for revision of the acetabulum. Most studies are retrospective, but there are several prospective studies as well. The majority of the literature found for this review is level II and III.

24.6 Case Title: Acetabular Revision Using Tantalum Augments

Kristian Stahl Otte

24.6.1 Demographics

Age: 76
Sex: Male
BMI: 24

24.6.2 Relevant Past Medical History

Principal pathologies: Ischaemic heart disease. Pacemaker.

Previous surgical procedures: Uncemented right hip arthroplasty in 1995. Cemented cup revision in 2006. Cemented revision of both components in 2007.

Medication: Carvedilol, furosemide and aspirin.

History of presenting complaint: Never pain-free after last hip revision in 2007. During the last 3 months, accelerating pain is observed.

24.6.3 Clinical Examination

Symptoms: Pain in the right hip both at rest and weight bearing. Only able to walk with two crutches. A 2 cm leg length shortening.

Range of motion: Unable to evaluate because of pain.

Main disability: Impaired walking.

Neurovascular evaluation: Normal.

24.6.4 Preoperative Radiological Assessment/Imaging (Figs. 24.14 and 24.15)

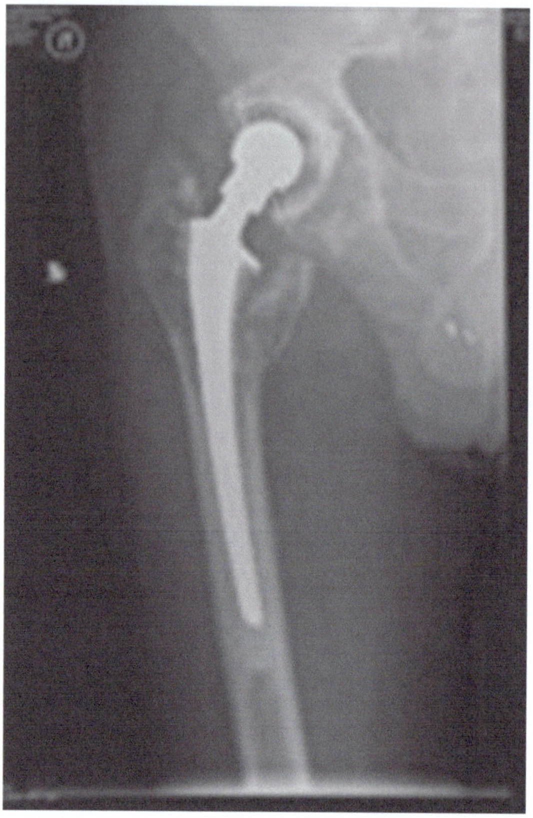

Fig. 24.14 Loose cup, gross osteolysis, mild ischial lysis and tear drop not intact, but Kohler's line seems to be intact. A <2 cm—but close to—proximal migration of the cup. Type 2B to C defect. Femoral component seems well fixed although with some lysis proximally

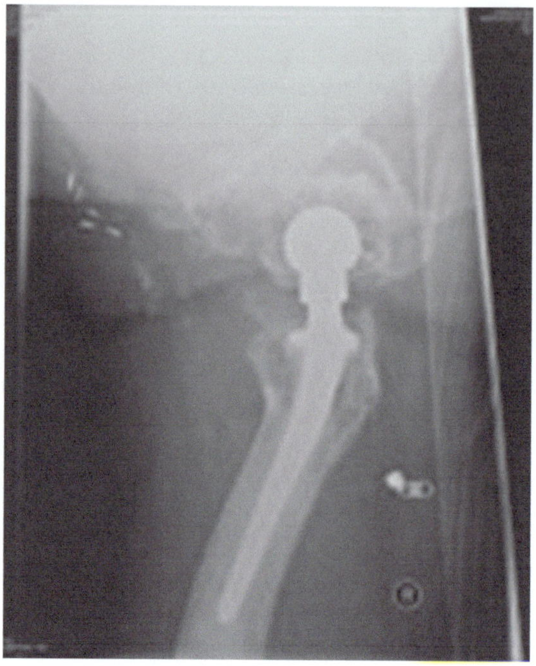

Fig. 24.15 Loose displaced cup

24.6.5 Preoperative Planning

Diagnosis: Loose acetabular component. Type 2B to C defect. Femoral component is well fixed confirmed by negative scintigram although with some proximal osteolysis (Figs. 24.14 and 24.15).

Possible treatment options: Bone grafting and cemented cup using the Sloof technique. Bone grafting, eventually a structural graft and an uncemented cup. Bone grafting, tantalum augments and tantalum cup.

Chosen treatment method: Bone graft, tantalum cup and tantalum augment.

Selection of implants if applicable and rational: A large defect and a possible posterior defect might leave you with a non-contained defect, and bone grafting alone will not give a stable and durable reconstruction. A tantalum augment will give sufficient support for the cup.

Expected difficulties: Quality of remaining bone stock and quality of the anterior and especially the posterior wall.

Strategies to overcome difficulties: The full sentiment of augments is available including cup cage solution.

24.6.6 Surgical Note

Patient's position: Decubitus.

Type of anaesthesia: Epidural.
Surgical approach: Posterior.

Main steps: After exposure testing of the femoral component. Clearing of all acetabular membranes. Assessing of acetabular defect. Reconstruction of the acetabulum. Cup insertion (Figs. 24.16 and 24.17).

Reconstruction techniques: Tantalum augment is positioned where it is most stable and giving adequate support for the tantalum cup. Fixation of the augment with two screws. Bone grafting using impaction technique and finally retrograde reaming. Cementation of the cup against augment and fixation with two screws.

24.6.7 Intraoperative Challenges

Challenges and solutions: Large acetabular defect proximally, the large defect of the posterior wall and very thin anterior wall. Defects with bone grafted. A 20 mm tantalum augment posteriorly.

Unanticipated problems and solution: None.

Thorough description of decision-making, including the reason for the final decision: As the defect was not contained in combination with a large posterior defect, augmentation was mandatory. Bone grafting with impaction technique gave—combined with the augment—a very stable primary fixation of the cup, and no further reconstruction was needed.

24.6.8 Postoperative Radiographs (Figs. 24.16 and 24.17)

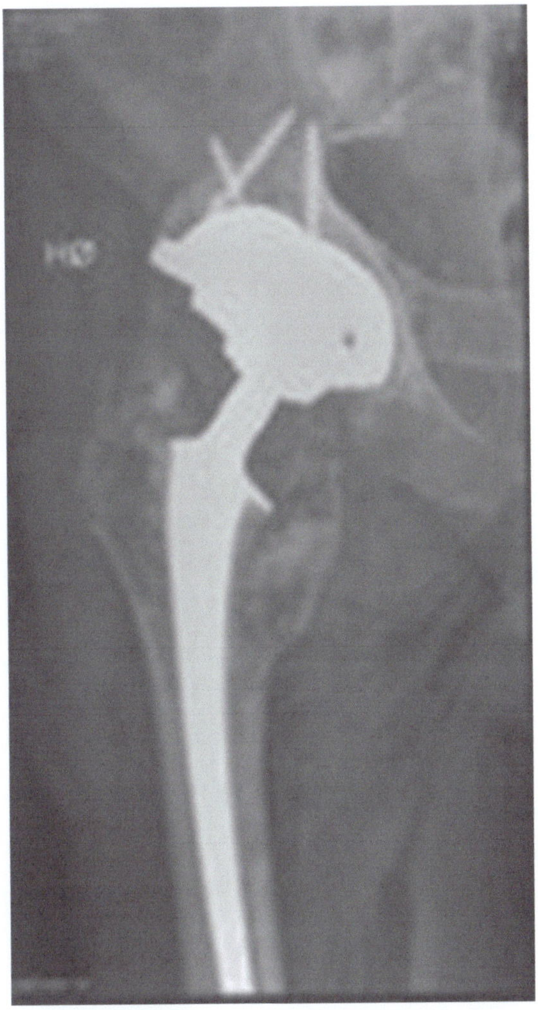

Fig. 24.16 The proximal defect of bone grafted and posterior defect treated with tantalum augment fixated with two screws. The hip centre restored to normal

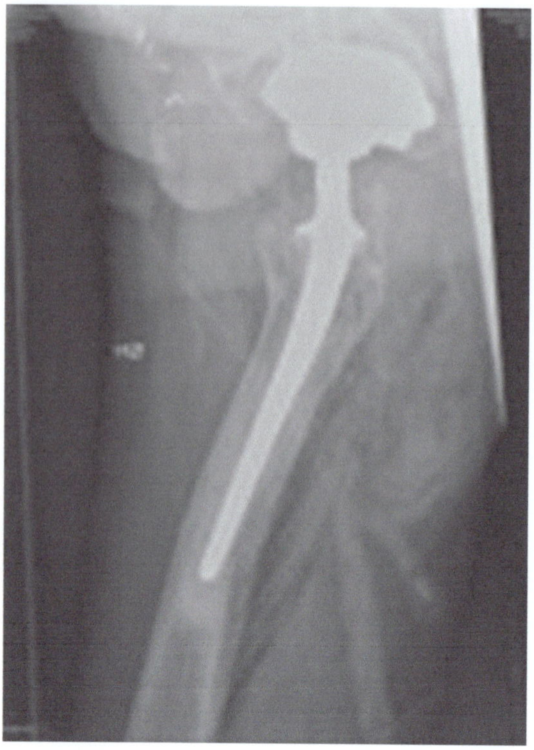

Fig. 24.17 Augment positioned proximally and posteriorly

24.6.9 Postoperative Management

Chemoprophylaxis and anticoagulant treatment period: Cefuroxime IV preoperatively and for five days postoperatively until negative cultures. DVT prophylaxis: rivaroxaban for five weeks.

Gait/limb loading until full loading: Full weight bearing.

24.6.10 Follow-up and Complications

No postoperative complications. Pain-free at one-year follow-up, no limp and no walking aids.

24.6.11 Discussion

Advantages of the applied method: This technique gives a rigid reconstruction of the acetabulum and a solid fixation of the cup.

Disadvantages of the method: Rigid stability of the augment is mandatory and can be difficult to obtain.

Alternative evidence-based techniques for the case: Bone grafting and cemented cup using the Sloof technique.

Why is the chosen technique better for this case? The augment gives you the excellent primary stability of the cup allowing bony ingrowth into the tantalum augment and tantalum cup.

Indications and contraindications for your technique: Type 2 and 3 defects. Active infection is a contraindication regarding bone grafting.

Learning curve and how to manage complications: Truly there is a learning curve as with every technique especially regarding placing and rigid fixation of the augment. All types of augments need to be available in the OR including a cup/cage solution should a complication occur intraoperatively or if the defect is larger than expected.

Level of evidence concerning the superiority of this method against others: IV [26, 27]

References

1. Paul S. Issack current concepts review use of porous tantalum for acetabular reconstruction in revision hip arthroplasty. J Bone Joint Surg Am. 2013;95:1981–7.
2. Bobyn JD, Stackpool GJ, Hacking SA, Tanzer M, Krygier JJ. Characteristics of bone ingrowth and interface mechanics of a new porous tantalum biomaterial. J Bone Joint Surg Br. 1999;81(5):907–14.
3. Malkani AL, Price MR, Crawford CH 3rd, Baker DL. Acetabular component revision using a porous tantalum biomaterial: a case series. J Arthroplast. 2009;24(7):1068–73.
4. Meneghini RM, Ford KS, McCollough CH, Hanssen AD, Lewallen DG. Bone remodeling around porous metal Cementless acetabular components. J Arthroplast. 2010;25(5):741–7.
5. Levine BR, Sporer S, Poggie RA, Della Valle CJ, Jacobs JJ. Experimental and clinical performance of porous tantalum in orthopedic surgery. Biomaterials. 2006;27(27):4671–81.
6. Meneghini RM, Meyer C, Buckley CA, Hanssen AD, Lewallen DG. Mechanical stability of novel highly porous metal acetabular components in revision total hip arthroplasty. J Arthroplast. 2010;25(3):337–41.
7. Skytta ET, Eskelinen A, Paavolainen PO, Remes VM. Early results of 827 trabecular metal revision shells in acetabular revision. J Arthroplast. 2011;26(3):342–5.

8. Kosashvili Y, Safir O, Backstein D, Lakstein D, Gross AE. Salvage of failed acetabular cages by nonbuttressed trabecular metal cups. Clin Orthop Relat Res. 2010;468(2):466–71.
9. Kim WY, Greidanus NV, Duncan CP, Masri BA, Garbuz DS. Porous tantalum uncemented acetabular shells in revision total hip replacement: two to four year clinical and radiographic results. Hip Int. 2008;18(1):17–22.
10. Lachiewicz PF, Soileau ES. Tantalum components in difficult acetabular revisions. Clin Orthop Relat Res. 2010;468(2):454–8.
11. Lakstein D, Backstein D, Safir O, Kosashvili Y, Gross AE. Trabecular metal cups for acetabular defects with 50% or less host bone contact. Clin Orthop Relat Res. 2009;467(9):2318–24.
12. Sternheim A, Backstein D, Kuzyk PR, Goshua G, Berkovich Y, Safir O, Gross AE. Porous metal revision shells for management of contained acetabular bone defects at a mean follow-up of six years: a comparison between up to 50% bleeding host bone contact and more than 50% contact. J Bone Joint Surg Br. 2012;94(2):158–62.
13. Davies JH, Laflamme GY, Delisle J, Fernandes J. Trabecular metal used for major bone loss in acetabular hip revision. J Arthroplast. 2011;26(8):1245–50.
14. Jafari SM, Bender B, Coyle C, Parvizi J, Sharkey PF, Hozack WJ. Do tantalum and titanium cups show similar results in revision hip arthroplasty? Clin Orthop Relat Res. 2010;468(2):459–65.
15. Molicnik A. Porous tantalum shells and augments for acetabular cup revisions. Eur J Orthop Surg Traumatol. 2014;24:911–7.
16. Weeden SH. The use of tantalum porous metal implants for paprosky 3A and 3B defects. J Arthroplast. 2007;22(6 Suppl):2.
17. Clement RGE. Trabecular metal use in paprosky type 2 and 3 acetabular defects: 5-year follow-up. J Arthroplast. 2016;31(4):863–7.
18. Tokarski T. Is tantalum protective against infection in revision total hip arthroplasty? Bone Joint J. 2015;97-B:45–9.
19. Batuyong ED. Outcome of porous tantalum acetabular components for paprosky type 3 and 4 acetabular defects. J Arthroplast. 2014;29:1318–22.
20. Flechera X. Do tantalum components provide adequate primary fixation in all acetabular revisions? Orthop Traumatol Surg Res. 2010;96:235–41.
21. Unger AS. Evaluation of a porous tantalum uncemented acetabular cup in revision total hip arthroplasty clinical and radiological results of 60 hips. J Arthroplast. 2005;20(8):1002–9.
22. Beckmann NA. Loosening after acetabular revision: comparison of trabecular metal and reinforcement rings. A systematic review. J Arthroplast. 2014;29:229–35.
23. Siegmeth A, Duncan CP, Masri BA, Kim WY, Garbuz DS. Modular tantalum augments for acetabular defects in revision hip arthroplasty. Clin Orthop Relat Res. 2009;467:199–205.
24. Abolghasemian M, Tangsataporn S, Sternheim A, Backstein D, Safir O, Gross AE. Combined trabecular metal acetabular shell and augment for acetabular revision with substantial bone loss A mid-term review. Bone Joint J. 2013;95(2):166–72.
25. Fletcher X, Sporer S, Paprosky W. Management of severe bone loss in acetabular revision using a trabecular metal shell. J Arthroplasty. 2008;23(7):949–55. Epub 2008 Mar 04
26. Gehrke T, Bangert Y, Schwantes B, Gebauer M, Kendoff D. Acetabular revision in THA using tantalum augments combined with impaction bone grafting. Hip. Int. 2013;23(4):359–65.
27. Sporer SM, Paprosky WG. The use of trabecular metal acetabular component and trabecular metal augment for severe acetabular defects. J Arthroplasty. 2006;21(6 suppl 2):83–6.

25 Instability (INS)/Dislocation (DISL)

Eustathios Kenanidis, Eleftherios Tsiridis,
Nathanael Heckmann, Braden McKnight,
Lawrence D. Dorr, Emmanuel Gibon,
and Stuart B. Goodman

25.1 Current Concepts

E. Kenanidis and E. Tsiridis

(a) **Epidemiology**
   - The incidence ranges from 0.2 to 7% for primary and 5 to 25% for revision THA [1–3].
   - INS is the third reason of revision THA following loosening and infection but the first reason of early revision. Greater than 50% of DISLs occur within three months postoperatively [4, 5].
   - The risk of recurrence following the first episode is estimated up to 33% [4].

(b) **Types** [4–7]
   1. **Early dislocation** [6, 7]
      - It occurs during the first 3–6 postoperative months.
      - It is the most common type (50–70%).
      - The inadequate healing and other preoperative risk factors are the main reasons.
      - It has a better prognosis with a lower rate of recurrence.
      - Usually nonoperative treatment.
   2. **Intermediate** [6]
      - It occurs between the six months and five years postoperatively.
      - The older age, muscular laxity, and cognitive impairment are the main reasons.
   3. **Late dislocation** [6, 7]
      - It occurs more than five years postoperatively.
      - It usually has a multifactorial etiology.
      - It has a higher rate of recurrence.
      - Frequently involves operative treatment.

E. Kenanidis, M.D., Ph.D., M.Sc. (✉)
Academic Orthopaedic Unit, Aristotle University Medical School, Thessaloniki, Greece

E. Tsiridis, M.D., Ph.D., F.A.C.S., F.R.C.S. (✉)
Academic Orthopaedic Unit, Papageorgiou General Hospital, Aristotle University Medical School, Thessaloniki, Greece
e-mail: etsiridis@doctors.org.uk

N. Heckmann, M.D. • B. McKnight, M.D., B.S.
Department of Orthopaedic Surgery, Keck School of Medicine of USC, Los Angeles, CA, USA

L.D. Dorr, M.D.
USC, Los Angeles, CA, USA
e-mail: lawrence.dorr@med.usc.edu

E. Gibon, M.D., Ph.D.
Department of Orthopaedic Surgery, Stanford University, Stanford, CA, USA

S.B. Goodman, MD, PhD, FRCSC, FACS
Department of Orthopaedic Surgery and (by Courtesy) Bioengineering, Stanford University Medical Center Outpatient Center, Redwood City, CA, USA
e-mail: goodbone@stanford.edu

E. Tsiridis (ed.), *The Adult Hip - Master Case Series and Techniques*,
https://doi.org/10.1007/978-3-319-64177-5_25

(c) **Risk Factors**
   1. **Patient's** [5]
      (a) **Neuromuscular and cognitive disorders** [5, 8]
         – Muscular dystrophy, dementia, alcoholism, Parkinson, MS, etc.
         – Muscle weakness, imbalance, and inability to comply with activity restriction
      (b) **Age** [9, 10]
         – It is not definitely considered an independent risk factor [5].
         – Muscle weakness, frailty, propensity to fall, and lack of adherence to the postoperative protocol that follows the older age are the main reasons.
      (c) **Posttraumatic/prior hip surgery and history of fracture**
      (d) **Other underlying diseases (osteonecrosis, inflammatory arthritis, DDH)** [11]
      (e) **Patient noncompliance with activity restrictions**
   2. **Surgical** [5]
      (a) **Surgical approach**
         – Although the posterior approach was considered an independent risk factor of dislocation at the past [11], the meticulous repair of the soft tissue and the use of large heads lessened the risk [10]. A meta-analysis [12] found that the dislocation rates of posterior approach with and without repair were 0.49 and 4.46%, respectively, and 8.21 times the greater relative risk for the posterior approach without soft tissue repair than with soft tissue repair [12]. Goldstein [13] et al. and Pellici [14] et al. reported a decrease in the dislocation rate with the posterior capsule repair from 4.8 to 0.7% in 1515 patients and from 4.1 to 0%, respectively.
         – A recent meta-analysis [15] involving 13,203 primary THAs found dislocation rates of 1.27% for trans-trochanteric, 3.23% for posterior (2.03% with capsular repair), 2.18% for anterolateral, and 0.55% for the direct lateral approach. There were, however, only four prospective studies that did not have sufficient power to reach statistical significance [15].
      (b) **Soft tissue tensioning** [4, 5]
         – Meticulous reconstruction of the posterior joint capsule and short external rotators lessened the dislocation risk [14].
         – Non-healing of the soft tissue following revision THA increases the risk.
         – Trochanteric nonunion increases sixfold the risk of dislocation.
         – Abductor deficiency [16].
      (c) **Restoration of the offset** [3, 4]
         – Less offset limits the soft tissue tensioning and increases the dislocation risk.
      (d) **Restoration of the leg length** [17]
      (e) **Component positioning** [18]
         – It is the most common cause of instability [5, 19].
         – The cup safe zone of abduction is 40 ± 10 and anteversion is 15–20 (± 5–10). It is also affected by the orientation of the pelvis and the body position [4, 5, 20, 21].
         – Risk factors for malpositioning are the low-volume surgeons, the obesity, and the minimal approaches [17, 19].
         – A femoral stem false positioning (inadequate offset, length, and version on the femoral side) is another reason.
         – An uncombined version of the cup and stem and the effect of pelvic tilt [22].
         – The X-rays are more suitable for the inclination than anteversion measurement. Different CT protocols have been proposed, but they lack standardization [4].

- The femoral anteversion is easier to measure on a CT by evaluating the angle between the femoral neck and the axis of posterior condyles [22].

(f) **Impingement**
- The femoral neck comes into contact during ROM with the liner or cement, an osteophyte, or heterotopic ossification creating torque and dislocation.
- The medial placement of the femoral component and the cup is another reason.
- The increased head-neck ratio decreases possibility.

(g) **Head size** [18]
- Larger head advantages: increased head/neck ratio, avoidance of a skirted component, and increased jump distance because the head sits deeper in the shell and allows greater range of subluxation before dislocation occurs [5, 16, 23, 24].

(h) **Liner profile**
- Neutral liners increased risk than posteriorly elevated (however posteriorly elevated increase time of neck impingement and liner wear so not uniformly recommended).

(i) **Surgeon experience**
- A higher dislocation rate was reported among surgeons who perform < 30 THAs yearly [5].

Treatment

Primary THA: first dislocation

Patient assessment [5, 10]

1. History (of dislocation and surgical note)
2. Physical examination (LLD, ROM, neurovascular integrity)
3. Infection exclusion (CRP, ESR, aspiration, culture)
4. Imaging (AP X-rays, CT) to detect cup orientation, eccentric wear, the possibility of liner dissociation, osteophytes, bone quality and integrity, femoral offset, subsidence, angulation, anteversion (difficult) component geometry (including head-to-neck ratio), osteolysis, and component loosening
5. The time of dislocation is crucial for the underlying reason. When a dislocation occurs following weeks or months, think soft tissue tension (including muscle weakness and inadequate capsular healing and scarring), component malposition, infection, or patient noncompliance. For late dislocations (> 1 year) think stretching of the soft tissues or polyethylene wear

Closed reduction: spica
- With sedation to prevent damage to the implant.
- In case of well-positioned and stable implant [3].
- 6–12 weeks spica (its use is based on small series [3]).
- The use is extremely patient dependent [25], as even the most compliant have difficulties.
- Almost two-thirds have effective treatment in this way.

Indications for operative management
1. Recurrent dislocation >2 times
2. Chronic dislocation
3. Irreducible dislocation
4. Soft tissue tension
5. Impingement
6. Malposition of components (one of the primary causes)

Recurrent dislocation
- Identify the cause to have a better chance of successful management [26].
- Assess the patient using the previously mentioned steps for primary DISL.
- Revision seems to be more effective for component malpositioning, infection, and abductor insufficiency.

- However, none of the available surgical procedures can uniformly solve the problem of instability [6].
- In case of multifactorial cause, the treatment is less obvious.

The available surgical options [5, 6]

1. Component revision
2. Modular component exchange (acetabular liner and the femoral head)
3. Bipolar arthroplasty (motion between the femoral head and the acetabular liner and also between the acetabular liner and the native acetabular cavity)
4. Dual mobility arthroplasty
5. Use of a larger femoral head
6. Soft tissue reinforcement
7. Advancement of the greater trochanter
8. Use of a constrained liner
9. Posterior lip augmentation device (PLAD)

1. **Revision arthroplasty/component revision**
   - Reasonable solution for patients with component malpositioning, a primary cause of recurrent dislocation [6].
   - There are difficulties in identifying the malposition preoperatively.
   - The plain X-rays offer limited information (see above) [6].
   - CT is mainly used to evaluate the cup position [27].
   - Assess also a possible LLD or abductor insufficiency.
   - Most accurate information intraoperatively [6].
   - A suboptimal position of a component may not lead to revision in frail patients where you can accept it with revision to a constraint liner.
   - Parvizi et al. [28] reported that component malpositioning was the primary cause of instability in a series of patients treated for hip instability. In a previous report, Morrey et al. [29] showed that cup reorientation was successful at approximately 80% in the treatment of hip instability.
2. **Modular component exchange**
   - In selected patients exchange of the acetabular liner with an elevated liner and the femoral head with a greater femoral head or other modular options as increasing the length of the neck [6, 30].
   - Prerequisite: well-positioned and well-fixed acetabular and femoral components, no significant abductor weakness and a sufficient acetabular cup to allow for an adequate thickness of polyethylene (a minimum of 4 mm) to be used with larger head [6].
   - It requires a meticulous surgical technique to avoid complications as the failure of the modular interface attributed to detachment of the femoral head from the trunnion, dislodgment of the polyethylene liner from the shell, and asymmetrical rotation of the polyethylene liner [6].
   - There are small cohort studies in the literature evaluating the efficacy of modular component exchange in the treatment of recurrent instability [30–35]. These are usually studies of less than 50 patients (13–48) reporting midterm results (4.7–5.8 years). Several studies reported a reasonable success of this method ranging from 45 to 76% [30–35]. Toomey et al. [32] showed that ten from thirteen patients were successfully treated with modular component exchange for recurrent dislocation; these patients had been carefully selected from a larger cohort of patients. In a retrospective cohort study, Bivijj et al. [31] also demonstrated a reasonable overall success rate of 73% in 48 patients treated for hip instability with 4.7 years of follow-up. However, in other studies, the reported results were not favorable. Earl et al. [33] reported that 16 from 29 patients (55%) experienced redislocation and 9 (31%) repeated dislocations following modular component exchange surgery to treat instability. Isolated liner exchange was one of the most significant factors of failure in a series of 156 hips treated for instability [34].

3. **Use of large heads**
   - The majority of the studies are focused on the efficacy of large heads on the primary THA stability and wear debris volume.
   - The beneficial effect of the large heads has also been demonstrated in revision THA. In a prospective randomized study, Garbuz et al. [36] compared the dislocation rate following revision THA between two groups that received large head 36 or 40 mm vs. standard head 32-mm treatment. During the first five postoperative years, the rate of dislocation was significantly lower in the large head group (1.1%) compared to the standard head group (8.7%). This beneficial effect of large heads is disputed in the absence of abductor mechanism. Kung et al. [37] supported that the use of 36-mm femoral heads at revision THA diminished dislocation rate (0%) only for the group that has intact abductors. The combination of large heads and abductor deficiency resulted in 33% dislocation rate. The use of large femoral heads (32 mm) combined with a capsular repair following revision THA with posterior approach also resulted in significantly less dislocation rate (2.7%) than the use of smaller heads (28 mm) without capsular repair [38].

Advantages

1. Increased ROM [39]
2. Increased jump distance [39]

Disadvantages

1. Possible increased production of volumetric wear for heads > 36 mm combined with the thinner polyethylene liner (improved with highly cross-linked poly)
2. Disadvantages of the large MoM or Cer/Cer (unexpected pain, pseudotumor, squeaking, etc.)

Indications [39]

Primary total hip arthroplasty
Revision total hip arthroplasty for recurrent instability
Resurfacing arthroplasty
Young age
High-demand patients
Advanced age
Mental confusion
Hip dysplasia
Neuromuscular disability

Contraindications [39]

Absent abductors

Published results

There are not plenty of studies dealing with the efficacy of large heads to treat the instability following revision hip arthroplasty [40–43]. These are usually small sample size studies following patients for short term to midterm [40–43]. Amstutz et al. [40] evaluated a cohort of 135 THA where large femoral heads of 36 mm were used. Twenty nine of them were revisions for recurrent dislocation. Only one of them redislocated at 12.5 years postoperatively. Beaule et al. [41] also evaluated the effect of a jumbo femoral (40–50 mm) bipolar or unipolar head for the management of 12 patients that had undergone a mean of four prior revision THAs and suffered from recurrent dislocation. There was only one further dislocation immediately postoperatively.

Two other studies evaluated the possibility of the femoral head size to be an independent risk factor of dislocation following revision THA [42, 43]. Jo et al. [42] demonstrated that the cumulative risk of redislocation was 34.5% at fifteen years in a group of patients that were retrospectively evaluated following revision THA. Among others a femoral head size <36 mm was recognized as independent risk factor for redislocation. In another retrospective study [43], the femoral head <32 mm was found to be an independent risk factor for redislocation following revision THA, increasing almost fourfold the risk.

4. **Polyethylene lip augmentation (PLAD)**

It is a horseshoe piece of ultrahigh-molecular-weight polyethylene bearing with a partial or complete metal-backing plate [4, 44] that is used to augment the acetabulum posteriorly. The device is fixed with five predrilled self-tapping screws 4.5 mm in diameter and 25 mm in length [44]. The contoured inner curve provides congruency with the head of the femoral component whether the metal-backing plate mechanical strength.

Objective/indication

PLAD is alternatively used to treat recurrent dislocation in patients and stable implants and minimal intervention [44].

Prerequisite

Stable prosthesis

Advantages (compared to revision THA) [45, 46]

- Less operating time
- Less intraoperative blood loss and need for transfusion
- Shorter length of hospital stay

Disadvantages

- It is recommended only for Charnley/Charnley Elite cemented acetabular components and cannot be used to augment metal-backed cementless acetabular prostheses [44].
- Impingement of the neck on the PLAD and dislocation or increased stresses [47].
- Failure of the device through breakage of screws [48, 49].
- Weakening of the polyethylene by the screw trajectories.

Published results

A limited number of studies demonstrated the efficacy of PLADs in the management of recurrent dislocation following THA [44–51]. These are usually retrospective studies with small sample size, less than 30 patients [45–51] except of McConway study [44]. The mean follow-up of studies ranged from 2 to 7 years. PLADs were found effective in the treatment of recurrent dislocation usually demonstrating less than 10% dislocation rate.

In the greatest in sample size and follow-up study, Mc Conway et al. [44] reported 1.6% redislocation rate in 310 revision Charnley/Charnley Elite THAs with PLADs at a mean of 6.9 years of follow-up.

5. **Constrained liners (CL)**

General

CL is a device that locks the head into the acetabular cup and resists dislocation. The CL has a smaller diameter than the mating head; however, the reduction of the head within the liner is accomplished through a mechanical expansion of the inner diameter of the rim. An external metal ring is then attached to the liner to prevent it from re-expanding and secures the articulation.

Indications

They are used as salvage treatment method under challenging cases [52]:

1. Recurrent hip dislocation following THA due to abductor deficiency [6, 53]
2. Recurrent hip dislocation following THA of unknown etiology and elderly patients with well-fixed components [6, 53]
3. Patients with neurological impairment [6, 53]
4. Failed previous operative treatment [6, 53]
5. Multidirectional intraoperative instability [6, 53]

A low-demand patient with impaired soft tissue that has either a well-fixed cup suitable for a constrained liner or adequate bone stock for maximal screw fixation of a constrained cup is considered an ideal candidate [4, 6, 53].

Contraindications [39]

1. Prophylaxis for potential dislocations
2. High-demand patients
3. Acute dislocation
4. Dislocation due to component loosening or malposition
5. Acute infection
6. Skeletal immaturity
7. Neurologic spasticity

Surgical technique/important notes [6]

1. Proper preparation of the liner.
2. Correct sizing of the component.

3. Use of the optimal cementing technique with 2 mm of cement mantle. The newly inserted constrained liner must be seated within the shell while simultaneously trying to prevent it from bottoming out.
4. When you intend to cement a previous cup, you must make sure it is secured and well positioned:
   - Evaluate with a CT preoperatively.
   - Intraoperatively you will need full exposure, removal of the former liner, and all placed screws to assess cup position and fixation.
   - Be sure that the cup is great enough to accommodate an adequate cement mantle around the constrained liner.

Advantages

- There is the possibility of de novo implantation or cementation of a CL in another positioned cup for revision of a well-fixed and well-positioned acetabular component [54].
- The cementation in another positioned cup technique decreases operation time and blood loss and also does affect the acetabular bone stock.

Disadvantages

1. Loss of ROM following mechanical prevention of dislocation [39].
2. A possible impingement, especially with flexion and internal rotation, can damage the liner and transfer increased forces to the bone-cement and the liner-shell interface or the locking mechanism that leads to loosening and implant failure [6, 39].

Mechanisms of CL failure

Cooke et al. [55] proposed four different mechanisms of failure of a constraint liner:

1. Type I failure concerns the bone-prosthesis interface. It is promoted by the inadequate screw fixation of the cementless shell before inserting the CL.
2. Type II failures are related to the liner-locking mechanism that are up to 50% of failures in some studies [56]. To reduce the incidence when cementing the constrained liner into the cementless shell, fully seat the liner into the cup and roughen the surface of the poly lightly to enhance the bond with cement.
3. Type III failure concerns the femoral head-locking mechanism. It is promoted from component-component or component-bone impingement.
4. Type IV refers to the complete dissociation of the pelvis. In that a case is use of a constrained liner in combination with a cage.

In a retrieval study of 57 CL, Noble et al. [56] demonstrated that the failure of the locking liner ring and loosening of the acetabular cup are the primary causes of mechanical failure of the constrained liners.

Published results

Several papers evaluating the survival and the efficacy of CL to prevent dislocation following revision THA are currently available [54, 57–74]. These are mainly retrospective case series of small sample size ranging from 17 to 166 patients. In the study of Berend et al. [66], although 755 CL were examined, only 129 patients suffered from recurrent dislocation. The mean follow-up of these studies ranged from two to ten years. Patients included in these studies were treated for recurrent dislocation or they were at great risk for dislocation. The reported risk for redislocation ranged from 0 to 29%.

In a review of 15 long-term studies, Williams et al. [53] reevaluated 1.199 CL for a mean of 51 months of follow-up. The mean rate of dislocation was 10%, and the mean reoperation rate for reasons other than dislocation was 4%. However, in a recent study, Clave et al. [58] evaluated 166 CL; 73% of them suffered from recurrent dislocation. The mean follow-up was 6.2 years. Ten-year survival for any reason was 89%, for noninfectious reasons 92%, and redislocation 99%.

Carter et al. 2011 [34] reported that 20% of constrained liners used to solve the instability in 56 revision THAs have also failed.

6. **Unconstrained tripolar cups or dual mobility cups (DMC)**
   Dual mobility cup concept was first developed by Bousquet (1974) [75]. There are currently many available designs worldwide that are used for primary and revision THA [76]. They are also referred as unconstrained tripolar cups and mobile-bearing hips.

Objective

DMC are composed by [77]:

1. A cemented or press-fit metal-polished acetabular component.
2. A large standard or highly cross-linked polyethylene head that articulates and is freely mobile concerning the metallic cup in a large-diameter articulation.
3. A smaller 22- or 28-mm femoral head that is coupled but mobile with the polyethylene.

These two points of articulations increase the range of movement and jump distance and are used to decrease the risk of dislocation.

Indications

- These are ambiguous.
- They are considered a salvage procedure for treating recurrent dislocation. They are increasingly used, however, in primary THA.
- Many surgeons consider that these are an alternative to constrained components in select patients with recurrent dislocation.

Advantages

Although the basic science studies are scarce [76], the DMC have the following benefits:

(a) Greater in vitro range of motion to impingement compared to conventional components of the same diameter femoral head [78]
(b) Greater stability and range of motion
(c) Simplification of revisions as they are compatible with 28- and 22.2-mm femoral heads and may not need a femoral stem exchange or they are possibly fixed by cement to cages when acetabular reconstruction is needed
(d) Opportunity to improve hip centering and further decrease the risk of instability with cages and cement

Disadvantages

(a) The possible impingement of the femoral neck or the femoral component itself against the large outer polyethylene bearing due to excessive ROM.
(b) The intraprosthetic dislocation. This is a dislocation of the femoral head and the liner and must be differentiated from the classic dislocation of the liner and the cup. Although the exact reason is uncertain, an extensive fibrosis at the large articulation, cup loosening, the surface topography of the femoral neck, and the design of the mobile liner are considered potential causes [79].
(c) The possible paucity of the movement of the outer smaller articulation after replacement of the postoperative hematoma with fibrous tissue [76].
(d) The possibility of increased wear rates following excessive ROM [76]. These cups are not subjected to the same traction forces as constrained liners and might therefore not have a higher risk of aseptic loosening than conventional cups [11].

The aseptic loosening incidence, however, is not well studied in the literature.

Published results

Several papers dealing with the efficacy of DMC to prevent dislocation following revision THA are currently available [1, 71, 80–91]. These are mainly retrospective case series of 29–228 patients; many patients, however, were treated with DMC for another than recurrent dislocation reasons [82, 84]. The mean follow-up of these studies ranged from 2 to 8 years. The majority however of these studies have included small numbers of patients for a short-term follow-up [86, 87, 89]. Patients included were usually at great risk for dislocation due to the increased number of prior revisions that they had undergone. There were favorable results as far as the redislocation was concerned. The reported risk for redislocation ranged from 0 to 5.5% [80, 87].

In one of the greatest reported sample size and follow-up time, Merti et al. [81] retrospectively evaluated 180 revision THA with recurrent instability. Redislocation occurred at 4.8% of patients at a mean follow-up of 8 years. The reported survival was 92.6% at the same time. A higher rate of dislocation was reported for patients that have undergone multiple earlier revisions or in case of greater trochanter nonunion (and may advocate repair of GT or constrained liner use).

Information from the Swedish Hip Arthroplasty Register [11] demonstrated 228 reconstructions with DMC for recurrent instability. The reported survival for any reason was 94% and for redislocation 99% at a mean of 2 years of follow-up. The age between 50 and 59 years compared to 75 years and previous revision surgery increased the risk for subsequent re-revision at 5 and 1.7 times, respectively.

Complications

- Reported complications in these studies included heterotopic ossification, aseptic loosening, infection fractures, groin pain, and intraprosthetic dislocations.
- The rate of intraprosthetic dislocations ranges in different studies of revision THA, but it is low (0–3.7% [78, 81]).

7. **Soft tissue reinforcement and trochanteric advancement**

These are less frequently used surgical procedures for the management of recurrent dislocation at revision THA.

Indications

- Not well defined
- Patients with well-fixed and positioned components
- Patients that are poor candidates for previous treatment options

Disadvantages

- Variability in outcome
- Technically demanding procedures

(a) **Soft tissue reinforcement**

These procedures usually involve augmentation of the deficient posterior capsule (capsulorrhaphy) and capsular plication or enhance an insufficient abductor mechanism with Achilles tendon allograft, fascia lata, or synthetic ligament [92–96].

There are some studies, mainly of previous decades with a small number of patients and good reported results in selected patients. Van Warmendarm et al. [92] reported 7/8 patients treated for recurrent hip dislocation and good postoperative ROM at a mean of 5 years of follow-up. In another study [93] 16 from 18 patients suffering from recurrent posterior dislocation were managed with reinforcement of abductors with the fascia lata.

(b) **Restoration of soft tissue tensioning and elimination of impingement**

This involves restoration of the femoral offset (easier with modular implants) or lateralized liner, restoration of LLD, and resection of any bony or other type of impingements.

(c) **Greater trochanter advancement**

It is a method that is very seldom in use only when there is a proximal migration of an ununited trochanter after a trochanteric osteotomy [97, 98]. It uses hook plates to lower the greater trochanter (by 18 ± 6 mm) and increase abductor tension and their lever arm and THA stability. The most serious complication is nonunion. It proposed limited weight bearing with two forearm crutches for four months.

25.2 Case Title: Revision Using PLAD Device for Recurrent Dislocation

E. Kenanidis and E. Tsiridis

Octogenarian with muscle weakness due to chronic Parkinson's disease. She sustained two early consecutive dislocations; the hip was found unstable due to muscle weakness regardless of the excellent orientation of the components, and a PLAD device was added to the socket for protection (Fig. 25.1).

25.3 Case Title: Dislocation Following Total Hip Arthroplasty in a Patient with Decreased Pelvic Motion (A Case Report)

Nathanael Heckmann, Braden McKnight, and Lawrence D. Dorr

25.3.1 Abstract

This case report illustrates the importance of including the spinopelvic motion in planning the cup position for total hip replacement (THR) in some patients. A singular inclination and anteversion position of the cup for all patients, and even just using the Lewinnek safe zone, is a cause for complications. This case report emphasizes the importance of personalizing the cup position, which is important in 15% of patients.

25.3.2 Introduction

The pelvis shifts posteriorly when a patient changes postural position from standing to sitting. An acetabular cup is fixed to the pelvis so it too changes its angles as the pelvis moves. Only recently have surgeons learned to incorporate this knowledge into planning cup position for an individual patient undergoing THR [99, 100]. Total hip replacement has done well in the past because the necessity for precision in cup placement is required for only 15% of patients and is critical for 5%. Precision in acetabular cup position is crucial in patients with low pelvic incidence and those with a sacral tilt change between standing and sitting of $\leq 10°$ (very stiff spinopelvic construct). This stiff construct requires special attention to cup position no matter the pelvic incidence but is especially critical with a low pelvic incidence. Our recent research has expanded our

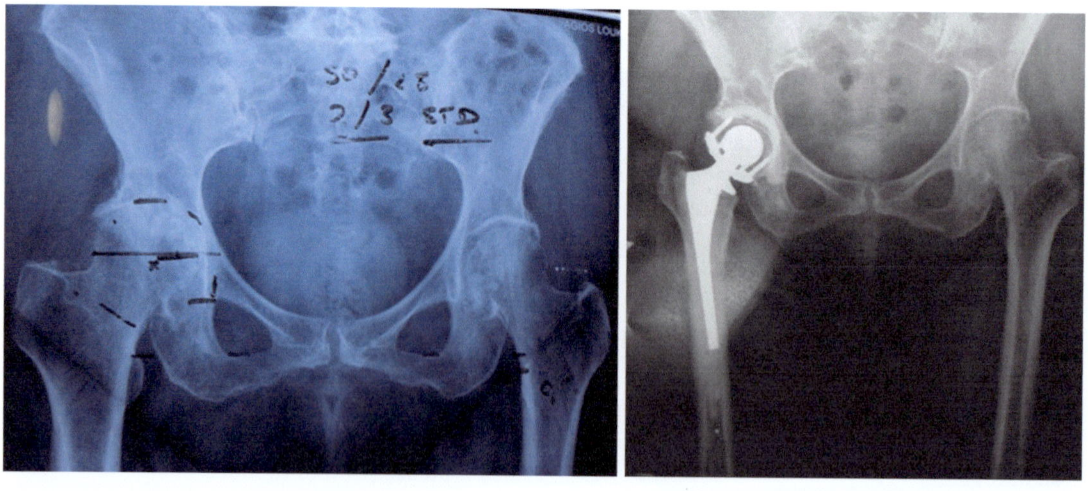

Fig. 25.1 Preoperative x-ray (*left*) and postoperative x-ray of the right hip demonstrating the PLAD device in a patient with Parkinson disease (*right*)

understanding of the interrelationship between the spine-pelvis-hip construct and hip stability.

When studying the connection of spinopelvic motion and hip position, there are "new" terms for the hip surgeon to learn (though familiar to the spine surgeon) (Figs. 25.2 and 25.3). Pelvic incidence (PI) is the static morphologic measurement of pelvic width, and its importance to hip surgery is the position of the hip joint relative to the spine—the hip joint moves anteriorly as PI increases. In arthritis patients, we found normal PI = 50°–60°, low PI ≤ 49°, and high PI ≥ 61°. Sacral tilt (ST), called sacral slope (SS) by some, is a measure of the dynamic motion of the spinopelvic junction. It can be used as a measure of pelvic stiffness, and the normal motion is a change between standing and sitting of 13°–27°. Therefore, a stiff pelvis has motion of 12° or less and a flexible one has 28° or more. As such, we use ST exclusively as a measure of pelvic motion. The absolute normals (as compared to the above-listed change between standing and sitting) are 40° ± 5° for standing and 20° ± 7° for sitting.

Ante-inclination is the term we coined for the change in sagittal position of the cup as the pelvis tilts. This sagittal position of the acetabular cup is affected by both acetabular inclination and anteversion [100]. It changes from standing to sitting according to the cup position achieved at surgery and the stiffness of the pelvis. The normal values for ante-inclination are 35° ± 10° while standing and 53° ± 9° while sitting.

The sacral acetabular angle (SAA) is the angle formed by the intersection of the lines of ante-inclination of the acetabulum and the superior end plate of the sacrum. It is a sum of the absolute sacral tilt number and ante-inclination and is measured in both standing and sitting though the SAA value in both of these postural positions remains unchanged [101]. The normal value is 74° ± 9°. Pelvic femoral angle (PFA) is a measure of the angle of the femur to the pelvis (from the S1 vertebra) and is also measured in both the standing and sitting position. The mean standing PFA is 174° ± 9° and for sitting is 125° ± 10°.

The importance of cup inclination and anteversion at the time of surgery is the effect of these two angles on ante-inclination, particularly when the patient sits. If the ante-inclination is low, the patient is at risk of impingement with hip flexion while sitting. The patients at the highest risk of impingement are those with low pelvic incidence and decreased spinopelvic motion. An ante-inclination of 70° or more with sitting

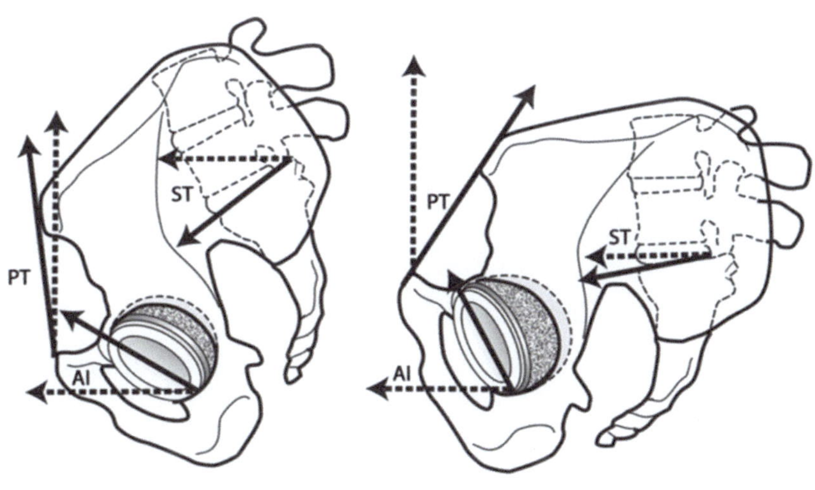

Fig. 25.2 Ante-inclination (AI), sacral tilt (ST), and pelvic tilt (PT). AI increases with the posterior pelvic tilt of sitting; ST decreases as the spine straightens with pelvic posterior tilt; PT increases but the quantitative difference between PT standing and sitting and ST standing and sitting is quantitatively the same (Modified with permission from: Kanawade V, Dorr LD, Wan Z. Predictability of Acetabular Component Angular Change with Postural Shift from Standing to Sitting Position. *J Bone Joint Surg Am*. 2014;96(12):978–986.)

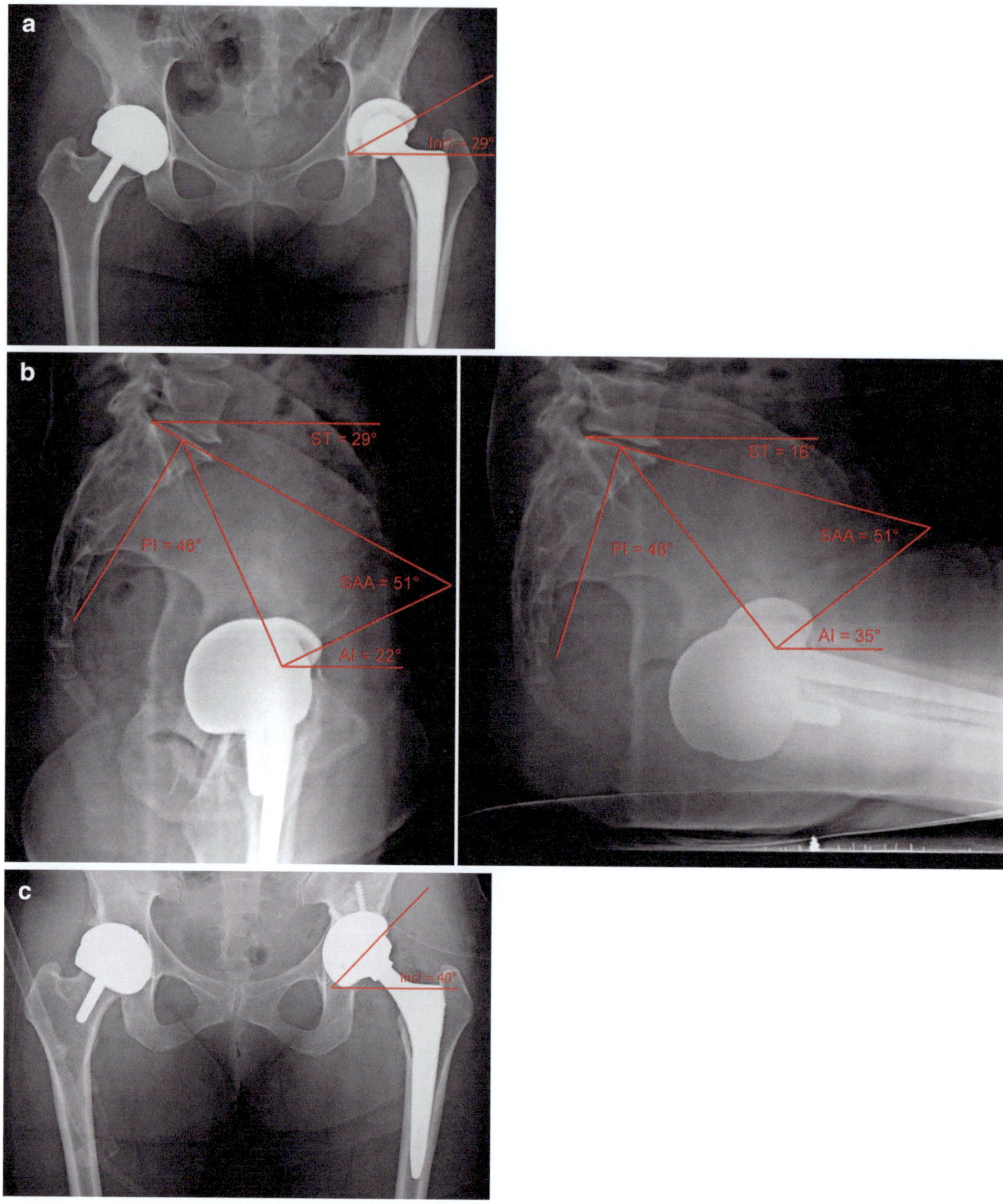

Fig. 25.3 (**a**) Postoperative AP pelvis of primary left hip replacement. Cup inclination is 29° and anteversion is 17°. (**b**) Standing postoperative lateral spinopelvic X-rays show PI of 48°, sacral tilt of 29°, cup ante-inclination (AI) of 22° (low normal AI is 25°), and sacral acetabular angle (SAA) of 51° (low normal SAA is 65°). (**c**) Sitting lateral spinopelvic X-ray: AI = 35° (low normal sitting AI is 44°), and SAA is the same sitting and standing (51°). (**d**) AP pelvis postoperative revision of left cup. Computer navigation inclination was 43° and anteversion 17° with inclination on X-ray of 40°. Offset was increased to provide clearance in flexion. (**e**) Standing lateral spinopelvic X-ray postoperative revision: ST = 36°, AI = 34°, and SAA = 70° (all within normal). (**f**) Sitting lateral spinopelvic X-ray postoperative revision: ST = 19°, AI = 51°, and SAA = 70° (all within normal)

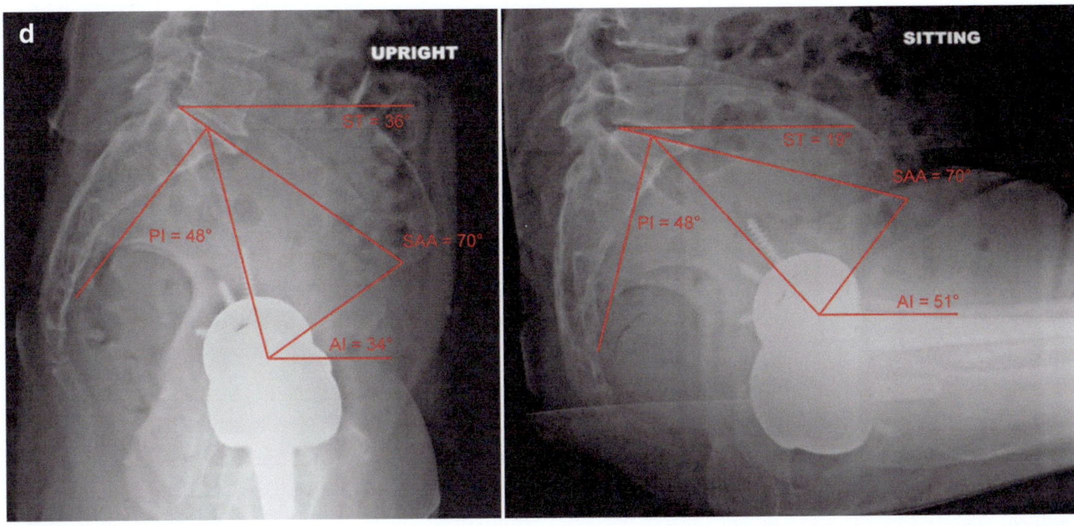

Fig. 25.3 (continued)

increases the threat of dropout dislocation, particularly if there is any shortening of the hip length or hip offset. Excessively high ante-inclination usually occurs in patients with high pelvic incidence and flexible spinopelvic motion. This subset of patients is usually women and is one reason why women have a higher rate of dislocation; the second reason is that women are the gender who have the greater incidence of low pelvic incidence which is the PI that has the greatest risk for impingement.

25.3.3 Case Report

A 52-year-old woman presented to our clinic with worsening left hip pain over the past few months. Prior to her left hip symptoms, she was an active ballet dancer who exercised regularly. One year earlier, she underwent an arthroscopic hip procedure because of a labral tear in her left hip but noted only transient symptom relief. She had a surface replacement for her right hip 5 years previously but was not satisfied with her outcome so she desired conventional hip replacement for her left hip. Her left hip had 120° of flexion, 40° of external rotation, 20° of internal rotation, 40° of abduction, and 20° of adduction. This was relatively stiff for her because she had been a very flexible ballet dancer, and her right surface replacement had a range of motion of 140° flexion, 50° of external rotation, 30° of internal rotation, 70° of abduction, and 20° of adduction. Radiographs showed osteolysis in zone II of the acetabulum of her right surface replacement (Fig. 25.3a).

The AP pelvis following her left total hip replacement is shown in Fig. 25.3a. In Fig. 25.3b, c, the sagittal standing and sitting radiographs of her lower lumbar spine/pelvis/hip/proximal femur had the following measurements: pelvic incidence was 48° (low PI), ST change from standing to sitting was 23° (normal motion), standing pelvic femoral angle was 180°, and sitting was 120°. Her sitting ante-inclination was 35° and her SAA was 51°, so both were very low, causing impingement with flexion of the hip. At the time of surgery, we were in the early stage of our research and did not understand the importance of cup position related to pelvic incidence. Prior research had suggested keeping the inclination lower in younger patients, especially women with dysplasia (30°–35°), which provided more medial compression loading on the acetabulum.

As such, during surgery her cup was placed with an inclination angle of 29° with 17° of anteversion. The acetabular positioning was done with computer navigation using the Orthosoft system (Zimmer, Warsaw, IN). At her 6-week follow-up appointment, the patient was thrilled with her results because she had complete resolution of her pain.

Approximately 3 months postoperatively, the patient dislocated while she was doing a deep squat during exercise with the femoral head, dislocating inferior to the acetabulum. The patient lived in another state so her hip was reduced in an emergency room and she returned 3 weeks later to our clinic. At that time, her pain from the dislocation had resolved, and she had good abduction strength to manual exam. Furthermore, there was no evidence of component loosening on plain films, so no intervention was performed at this time. However, the patient subsequently dislocated twice more and agreed to revision surgery.

By this time we understood the relationship between cup inclination and anteversion at the time of surgery with ante-inclination and sagittal acetabular angle during sitting. Therefore, during revision surgery her acetabular component was revised to 43° of inclination and 17° of anteversion (Fig. 25.3d). This resulted in an AI of 51° while sitting and an SAA of 70°, returning these values to normal (Fig. 25.3f). Following this surgery the patient has not had subsequent dislocation or symptoms of impingement.

25.3.4 Discussion

Dislocation occurred in this patient because the inclination of her acetabular cup at the primary operation was 29°. While this was at the low end of the Lewinnek safe zone [20], it resulted in a sitting AI of 35° and an SAA of 51°, and this cup position promoted impingement in this patient with a low PI. In the data from our research, the three causes of dislocation are a short hip which means a short hip length and/or offset or both, spinopelvic imbalance with resultant stiff pelvic motion during sitting as measured by an ST change between sitting and standing of less than 10 (this is particularly dangerous in patients with a low PI), and, thirdly, low inclination or anteversion in patients with a low pelvic incidence such as was present in this patient.

This patient illustrates why anterior-posterior (AP) plain radiographs have not been diagnostic for the cause of dislocation in all patients. In our experience, dislocation is caused by a leg length and/or offset reduced by 5 mm or more and patients with decreased spinopelvic mobility (ST change $\leq$ 10° with any PI is at risk; ST change $\leq$5°, we consider biological fusion). As such, the cup inclination and anteversion as measured on the AP pelvis radiograph will not be diagnostic for patients that dislocate for this reason, whereas a sitting and standing sagittal spine/pelvic/hip radiograph may be diagnostic. If these lateral X-rays show an AI of $\leq$40° or an SAA of $\leq$60°, the threat of impingement is high and is increased further if the PFA is < 115°. In these patients, dislocation is likely unless constraint is added to their articulation; the cup position is changed to have more inclination and anteversion or both. In primary operations we now use a dual mobility-type cup for those patients with a low PI and ST $\leq$10° and in patients with an ST change of $\leq$7° with any PI (in our hip replacements, this is no more than 10% of patients).

There are two other groups that require special attention to their cup position: patients with an unbalanced spine that is "stuck" in the sitting and standing positions. An unbalanced spine means that the spine motion is outside the normal range of ST change. Patients with a rigid unbalanced spine often have a pelvis with posterior tilt during standing (i.e., the pelvis assumes a seated position while standing) and are at risk for late anterior dislocation of the hip. For this reason in these patients, it is very important that the offset is increased to 5 mm to improve their clearance in extension and secondly to ensure that the posterior edge of the cup does not protrude above the posterior bone of the acetabulum. In the unbalanced and flexible group, the spine often flattens out (i.e., becomes kyphotic) with sitting, and the absolute sacral tilt can be 0°–5°. In these patients there can be a high ante-inclination of the cup, so these patients should have their cup placed near 37°–40° of inclination.

We support the safe zones published from the University of Iowa Laboratory (and winner of the Hip Society Award) that recommended inclination of 37°–47° and anteversion of 12°–22°. We would only change the anteversion to 15°–25°. We recognize that in patients who require special attention to their cup position, there is a safe zone with 10° margin. However, the 20° margin of the Lewinnek safe zones have historically worked because almost all patients with a normal PI or high PI will do well in this safe zone. This, of course, also explains why THR has done so well for so many through time.

In summary, we remind the reader that the most important technical aspects of THR are that the center of rotation of the cup is restored [102–104], the offset and hip length are restored within 5 mm on radiographs [105], and the cup be in the safe zones we described. We now believe there is no indication for a cup to be placed at an inclination of ≤ 35°. We believe that optimal combined anteversion is 30°–40°. We now know there are patients who need special cup position because of their spinopelvic anatomy and motion, as illustrated by this case report.

25.4 Case Title: THA Subluxation

Emmanuel Gibon and Stuart B. Goodman

25.4.1 Demographics

Age: 68
Sex: Male
BMI: 40.2

25.4.2 Relevant Past Medical History

Principal pathologies: angina, hypertension, convulsions, sleep apnea, anemia, diverticulosis, prostate issues, alcohol abuse, smoking, and depression.

Previous surgical procedures: bilateral total hip arthroplasty (THA), bilateral total knee arthroplasty (TKA), back surgery, and neck surgery (C5, C6, C7).

Medication: tamsulosin, trazodone, atenolol, diclofenac, simvastatin, lisinopril, and baby aspirin.

History of presenting complaint: the left THA has never been right since the surgery. The surgery was done in 2006, and the patient came to the clinic in 2013. He states that occasionally when he sits down, it feels like the hip is going to slip out. He also has a lot of groin pain. He does not trust the hip and has had several falls. He has pain in his back and along the side of the hip. He has difficulty with stairs, getting up from a chair, kneeling, squatting, getting into and out of a car, walking, and exercising. He has serious limitations and feels that his leg is weak. He uses a cane. He does limp on the left side as well. Preop workup showed CRP 1.1 and white blood cell 7900.

25.4.3 Clinical Examination

Symptoms: instability, left groin pain, left hip instability, and falls.

Range of motion: flexion 90°, IR 30°, ER 30° in flexion, IR neutral in extension, and ER 45° in extension.

Specific tests: hip flexion tends to elicit an apprehension sign and subluxation.

Main disability: left THA instability.

Neurovascular evaluation: sciatic and femoral nerves normal.

25.4.4 Preoperative Radiological Assessment/Imaging (Figs. 25.4 and 25.5)

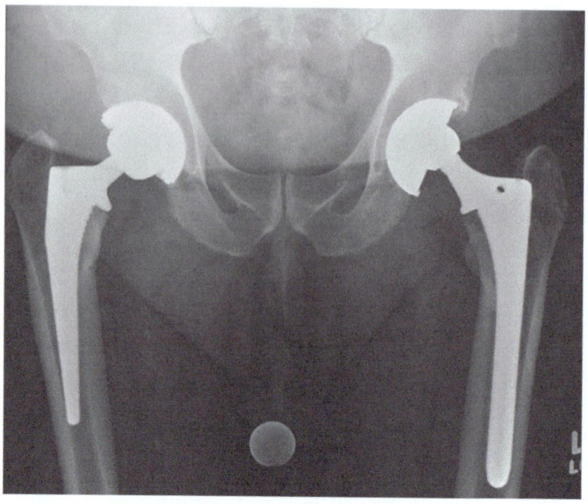

Fig. 25.4 Preoperative AP pelvis X-ray

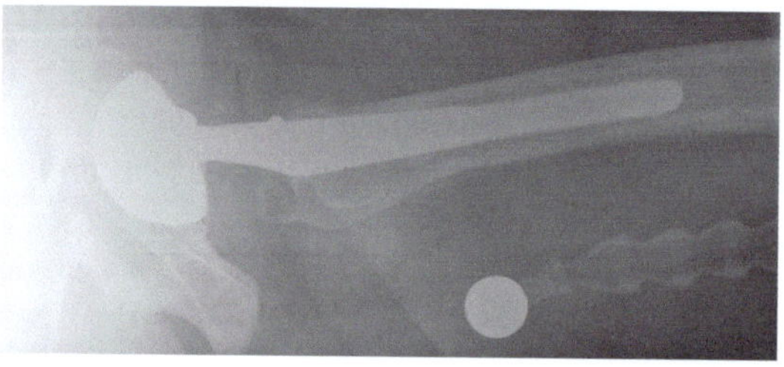

Fig. 25.5 Preoperative cross table view left hip X-ray

25.4.5 Preoperative Planning

Diagnosis: left failed total hip arthroplasty (Figs. 25.4 and 25.5).

Chosen treatment method: left total hip revision with cup, head, and liner exchange.

Selection of implants if applicable and rational: Zimmer Continuum shell, size 66; a 36-mm elevated liner; and a cobalt chrome 36 +3.5 head.

Expected difficulties: removing the implants and severe bone defects.

Strategies to overcome difficulties: use of the Explant system, possible bone allograft.

25.4.6 Surgical Note

Patient's position: lateral decubitus with the left hip facing up.

Type of anesthesia: general endotracheal anesthesia with a spinal.

Surgical approach: posterolateral approach.

Main steps: after the skin incision, the fascia layer was incised, and retractors were placed. There was dissection of the external rotators and the posterior capsule and then posterior dislocation of the hip. The soft tissue surrounding the neck and the head was cleared off. The head was dislodged from the neck. There was no evidence of trunnionosis. The stem was retracted off anteriorly. With the use of a combination of Aufranc gouges and the Explant system, the cup was dislodged with a minimal amount of bone loss that was mainly medial.

Reconstruction techniques: the soft tissue surrounding the acetabulum was cleared off, and the acetabulum was reamed from a 58 up to a 65. The final cup was then impacted, and the fixation was augmented with the use of three 6.5-mm screws. A neutral liner was impacted. A 36 +3.5 head was placed, and the hip was reduced (Figs. 25.6 and 25.7).

25.4.7 Intraoperative Challenges

Challenges and solutions: challenges are to obtain a stable, flexible hip. Solutions are to have a good acetabular fit and position, test the hip in all position, and use an elevated liner if necessary.

Unanticipated problems and solution: the hip was found to be stable in extension and ER but a little bit unstable in extension and IR and was subluxating posteriorly. All of the positions were verified as well as the acetabular version, the abduction angle, and the femoral position. It was decided that the patient would benefit from an elevated liner. The old liner was removed by drilling a hole and putting in a 6.5-mm screw. An elevated liner with the elevation centered posteriorly and superiorly was then inserted. A trial 36 +3.5 head was placed, and this time the hip was stable in flexion, in IR, in extension, and in ER. The trial head was removed and cleaned off the trunnion and impacted the real ball into place.

25.4.8 Postoperative Radiographs (Figs. 25.6, 25.7, and 25.8)

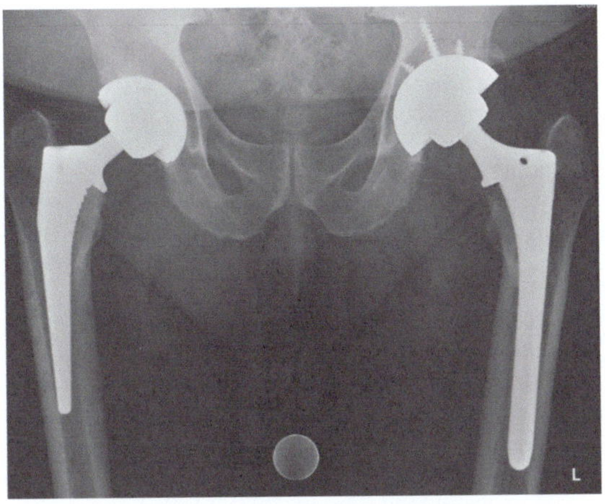

Fig. 25.6 Immediate postoperative AP pelvis X-ray

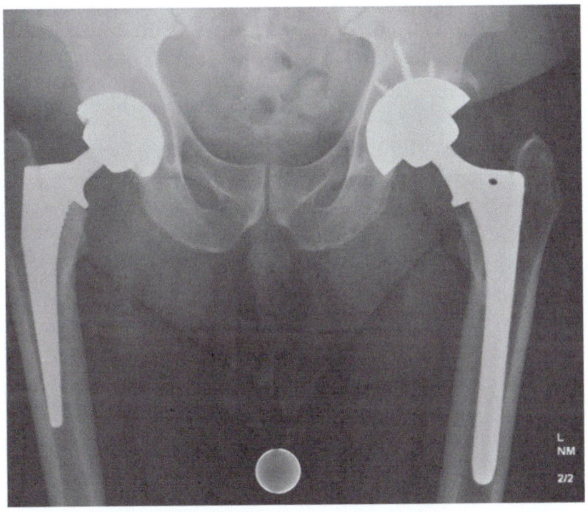

Fig. 25.7 AP pelvis X-ray at 1-year post-op

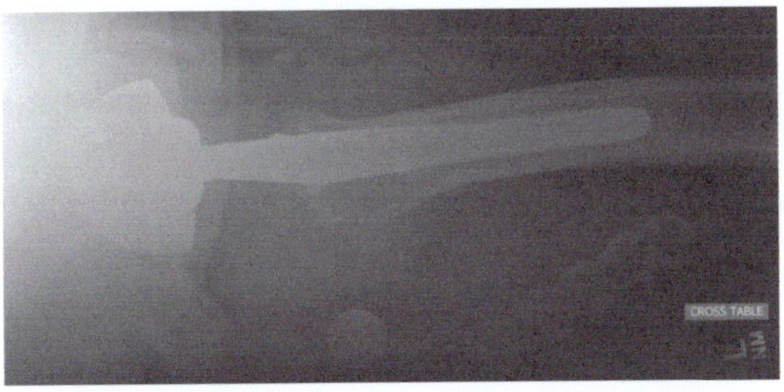

Fig. 25.8 Cross table view left hip at 1-year post-op

25.4.9 Postoperative Management

Chemoprophylaxis and anticoagulant treatment period: deep vein thrombosis prophylaxis included Lovenox, in addition to mechanical compression devices.

Gait/limb loading until full loading: patient was weight bearing as tolerated in an abduction brace.

25.4.10 Follow-Up and Complications

There were no complications. The cultures at surgery were negative.

25.4.11 Discussion

Advantages of the applied method: minimal bone loss, revision limited to the acetabular component, unconstrained liner, and large femoral head.

Disadvantages of the method: no control over the femoral stem position, impingement of the femoral component against the lip, increased polyethylene loading, and limitation of movement caused by the lip [106].

Alternative evidence-based techniques for the case: the use of a dual mobility cup [107].

Why is the chosen technique better for this case? the malposition is limited to the cup initially, and the hip is subluxating posteriorly.

Indications and contraindications for your technique: indications are hip instability due to cup malposition only and unidirectional instability. Contraindications are multidirectional instability.

Level of evidence concerning the superiority of this method against others: there is no superiority of this method against others.

References

1. Langlais FL, Ropars M, Gaucher F, Musset TH, Chaix O. Dual mobility cemented cups have low dislocation rates in THA revisions. Clin Orthop Relat Res. 2008;466:389–95.
2. Berend KR, Sporer SM, Sierra RJ, Glassman AH, Morris MJ. Achieving stability and lower-limb

length in total hip arthroplasty. J Bone Joint Surg Am. 2010;92:2737–52.
3. Patel PD, Potts A, Froimson MI. The dislocating hip arthroplasty. Prevention and treatment. J Arthroplast. 2007;22(4 Suppl):1.
4. Charissoux J-L, Asloum Y, Marcheix P-S. Surgical management of recurrent dislocation after total hip arthroplasty. Orthop Traumatol Surg Res. 2014;100:S25–34.
5. Cui Q. Instability after total hip arthroplasty. World J Orthop. 2012;3(8):122–30.
6. Parvizi J, Picinic E, Sharkey PF. Revision total hip arthroplasty for instability: surgical techniques and principles. J Bone Joint Surg Am. 2008;90(5):1134–42.
7. Pulido L, Restrepo C, Parvizi J. Late instability following total hip arthroplasty. Clin Med Res. 2007;5(2):139–42.
8. Jolles BM, Zangger P, Leyvraz PF. Factors predisposing to dislocation after primary total hip arthroplasty. A multivariate analysis. J Arthroplast. 2002;17:282–8.
9. Berry DJ, Von Knoch M, Schleck CD, Harmsen WS. The cumulative long-term risk of dislocation after primary Charnley total hip arthroplasty. J Bone Joint Surg Am. 2004;86:9–14.
10. Yun AG, Padgett D, Pellicci P, Dorr LD. Constrained acetabular liners: mechanisms of failure. J Arthroplast. 2005;20:536–41.
11. Hailer NP, Weiss RJ, Stark A, Kδrrholm J. Dual-mobility cups for revision due to instability are associated with a low rate of re-revisions due to dislocation 228 patients from the Swedish Hip Arthroplasty Register. Acta Orthop. 2012;83(6): 566–71.
12. Kwon MS, Kuskowski M, Mulhall KJ, Macaulay W, Brown TE, Saleh KJ. Does surgical approach affect total hip arthroplasty dislocation rates? Clin Orthop Relat Res. 2006;447:34–8.
13. Goldstein WM, Gleason TF, Kopplin M, Branson JJ. Prevalence of dislocation after total hip arthroplasty through a posterolateral approach with partial capsulotomy and capsulorrhaphy. J Bone Joint Surg Am. 2001;83(Suppl 2):2–7.
14. Pellicci PM, Bostrom M, Poss R. Posterior approach to total hip replacement using enhanced posterior soft tissue repair. Clin Orthop Relat Res. 1998;355:224–8.
15. Masonis JL, Bourne RB. Surgical approach, abductor function, and total hip arthroplasty dislocation. Clin Orthop Relat Res. 2002;405:46.
16. Wetters NG, Murray TG, Moric M, Sporer SM, Paprosky WG, Della Valle CJ. Risk factors for dislocation after revision total hip arthroplasty. Clin Orthop Relat Res. 2013;471:410–6.
17. Callaghan JJ, Heithoff BE, Goetz DD, et al. Prevention of dislocation after hip arthroplasty: lessons from long-term followup. Clin Orthop. 2001;393:157–62.
18. Barrack RL. Dislocation after total hip arthroplasty: implant design and orientation. J Am Acad Orthop Surg. 2003;11:89–99.
19. Werner BC, Brown TE. Instability after total hip arthroplasty. World J Orthop. 2012;3(8):122–30.
20. Lewinnek GE, Lewis JL, Tarr R, Compere CL, Zimmerman JR. Dislocations after total hip-replacement arthroplasties. J Bone Joint Surg Am. 1978;60:217–20.
21. Biedermann R, Tonin A, Krismer M, Rachbauer F, Eibl G, Stöckl B. Reducing the risk of dislocation after total hip arthroplasty the effect of orientation of the acetabular component. J Bone Joint Surg Br. 2005;87:762–9.
22. Dorr LD, Malik A, Dastane M, Wan Z. Combined anteversion technique for total hip arthroplasty. Clin Orthop Relat Res. 2009;467:119–27.
23. Triclot P, Gouin F, Richter D, Musset T, Bonnan J, Ollivier H, et al. Update'big-head': the solution to the problem of hip implant dislocation? Orthop Traumatol Surg Res. 2011;97S:S120–7.
24. Howie DW, Holubowycz OT, Midelton R. Large femoral heads decrease the inci-dence of dislocation after total hip arthroplasty. A randomised controlled trial. J Bone Joint Surg Am. 2012;94:1095–102.
25. Dewal H, Maurer SL, Tsai P, et al. Efficacy of abduction bracing in the management of total hip arthroplasty dislocation. J Arthroplast. 2004;19:733.
26. Salassa T, Hoeffel D, Mehle S, Tatman P, Gioe TJ. Efficacy of revision surgery for the dislocating total hip arthroplasty: report from a large community registry. Clin Orthop Relat Res. 2014;472(3):962–7.
27. Puri L, Lapinski B, Wixson RL, Lynch J, Hendrix R, Stulberg SD. Computed tomographic follow-up evaluation of operative intervention for periacetabular lysis. J Arthroplast. 2006;21(6 Suppl 2):78–82.
28. Parvizi J, Kim KI, Goldberg G, et al. Recurrent instability after total hip arthroplasty: beware of subtle component malpositioning. Clin Orthop Relat Res. 2006;447:60.
29. Morrey BF. Difficult complications after hip joint replacement. dislocation. ClinOrthop Relat Res. 1997;344:179–87.
30. Lombardi AV, Berend KR. Isolated acetabular liner exchange. J Am Acad Orthop Surg. 2008;16:243–8.
31. Biviji AA, Ezzet KA, Pulido P, Colwell CW. Modular femoral head and liner exchange for the unstable total hip arthroplasty. J Arthroplast. 2009;24:625–30.
32. Toomey SD, Hopper RH, McAuley JP, Engh CA. Modular component exchange for treatment of recurrent dislocation of a total hip replacement in selected patients. J Bone Joint Surg Am. 2001;83:1529–33.
33. Earll MD, Fehring TK, Griffin WL, Mason JB, McCoy T, Odum S. Success rate of modular component exchange for the treatment of an unstable total hip arthroplasty. J Arthroplast. 2002;17:864–9.
34. Carter AH, Sheehan EC, Mortazavi SM, Purtill JJ, Sharkey PF, Parvizi J. Revision for recurrent

instability: what are the predictors of failure? J Arthroplast. 2011;26(6 Suppl):46–52.
35. Lachiewicz PF, Soileau E, Ellis J. Modular revision for recurrent dislocation of primary or revision total hip arthroplasty. J Arthroplast. 2004;19(4):424–9.
36. Garbuz DS, Masri BA, Duncan CP, Greidanus NV, Bohm ER, Petrak MJ, et al. Dislocation in revision THA. Do large heads (36 and 40 mm) result inreduced dislocation rates in a randomised clinical trial? Clin Orthop Relat Res. 2012;470:351–6.
37. Kung PL, Ries MD. Effect of femoral head size and abductors on dislocation after revision THA. Clin Orthop Relat Res. 2007;465:170–4.
38. Hummel MT, Malkani AL, Yakkanti MR. Baker DL Decreased dislocation after revision total hip arthroplasty using larger femoral head size and posterior capsular repair. J Arthroplast. 2009;24(6 Suppl):73–6.
39. Van Sikes C, Lai LP, Schreiber M, Mont MA, Jinnah RH, Seyler TM. Instability after total hip arthroplasty treatment with large femoral heads vs constrained liners. J Arthroplast. 2008;23(7 Suppl):59–63.
40. Amstutz HC, Le Duff MJ, Beaulé PE. Prevention and treatment of dislocation after total hip replacement using large diameter balls. Clin Orthop Relat Res. 2004;429:108–16.
41. Beaulé PE, Schmalzried TP, Udomkiat P, Amstutz HC. Jumbo femoral head for the treatment of recurrent dislocation following total hip replacement. J Bone Joint Surg Am. 2002;84:256–63.
42. Jo S, Jimenez Almonte JH, Sierra RJ. The cumulative risk of re-dislocation after revision THA performed for instability increases close to 35% at 15 years. J Arthroplast. 2015;30(7):1177–82.
43. Yoshimoto K, Nakashima Y, Aota S, Kaneuji A, Fukui K, Hirakawa K, Nakura N, Kinoshita K, Naito M, Iwamoto Y. Re-dislocation after revision total hip arthroplasty for recurrent dislocation: a multicentre study. Int Orthop. 2017;41(2):253–8.
44. McConway J, O'Brien S, Doran E, Archbold P, Beverland D. The use of a posterior lip augmentation device for a revision of recurrent dislocation after primary cemented Charnley/Charnley Elite total hip replacement. Results at a mean follow-up of six years and nine months. J Bone Joint Surg Br. 2007;89:1581–5.
45. Charlwood AP, Thompson NW, Thompson NS, Beverland DE, Nixon JR. Recurrent hip arthroplasty dislocation: good outcome after cup augmentation in 20 patients followed for 2 years. Acta Orthop Scand. 2002;73(5):502–5.
46. Charlwood P, Thompson NW, Brown JG, Nixon JR. The Belfast Posterior Lip Augmentation Device (PLAD) in the management of recurrent posterior dislocation following primary total hip arthroplasty. J Bone Joint Surg Br. 2001;84-B(Suppl II):154.
47. Gie GA, Scott TD, Ling RS. Cup augmentation for recurrent hip replacement dislocation. J Bone Joint Surg Br. 1989;71-B:338.
48. Campbell D, Muthusamy K, Sturdee S, Finlayson D, Stone M. The posterior lip augmentation device for recurrent dislocation. J Bone Joint Surg [Br] 2001;84-B(Suppl II):154.
49. Williamson JB, Galasko CSB, Rowley DI. Failure of acetabular augmentation for recurrent dislocation after hip arthroplasty: report of 3 cases. Acta Orthop Scand 1989;60:676–7.
50. Schmidl S, Jakobs O, Guenther D, Lausmann C, Schoof B, Beckmann J, Gehrke T, Gebauer M. Effective prevention of recurrent dislocation following primary cemented Endo-MarkIII/SP2 total hip arthroplasty using a posterior lip augmentation device. Arch Orthop Trauma Surg. 2016;136(4):579–83.
51. Gholve PA, Lovell ME, Naqui SZ. Minimal surgical approach for recurrent hip dislocation using the posterior lip augmentation device for the Charnley hip arthroplasty. J Arthroplast. 2006;21(6):865–8.
52. Lombardi AV Jr. Constrained liners in revision: total hip arthroplasty an overuse syndrome: in opposition. J Arthroplast. 2006;21(4 Suppl 1):126–30.
53. Williams JT Jr, Ragland PS, Clarke S. Constrained components for the unstable hip following total hip arthroplasty: a literature review. Int Orthop. 2007;31:273.
54. Callaghan JJ, Parvizi J, Novak CC, et al. A constrained liner cemented into a secure cementless acetabular shell. J Bone Joint Surg Am. 2004;86:2206.
55. Cooke CC, Hozack W, Lavernia C, Sharkey P, Shastri S, Rothman RH. Early failure mechanisms of constrained tripolar acetabular sockets used in revision total hip arthroplasty. J Arthroplast. 2003;18:827–33.
56. Noble PC, Durrani SK, Usrey MM, Mathis KB, Bardakos NV. Constrained cups appear incapable of meeting the demands of revision THA. Clin Orthop Relat Res. 2012;470:1907–16.
57. Della Valle CJ, Chang D, Sporer S, Berger RA, Rosenberg AG, Paprosky WG. High failure rate of a constrained acetabular liner in revision total hip arthroplasty. J Arthroplast. 2005;20(7 Suppl 3): 103–7.
58. Clavé A, Maurer D, Tristan L, Dubrana F, Lefèvre C, Pandit H. Midterm survivorship of the Lefèvre constrained liner: a consecutive multisurgeon series of 166 cases. J Arthroplast. 2016;31(9):1970–8.
59. Chalmers BP, Arsoy D, Sierra RJ, Lewallen DG, Trousdale RT. High failure rate of modular exchange with a specific design of a constrained liner in high-risk patients undergoing revision total hip arthroplasty. J Arthroplast. 2016;31(9):1963–9.
60. Mäkinen TJ, Fichman SG, Rahman WA, Amenabar T, Safir O, Gross AE, Kuzyk PR. The focally constrained liner is a reasonable option for revision of unstable total hip arthroplasty. Int Orthop. 2016;40(11):2239–45.
61. Khoury JI, Malkani AL, Adler EM, Markel DC. Constrained acetabular liners cemented into

cages during total hip revision arthroplasty. J Arthroplast. 2010;25(6):901–5.

62. Shrader MW, Parvizi J, Lewallen DG. The use of a constrained acetabular component to treat instability after total hip arthroplasty. J Bone Joint Surg Am. 2003;85:2179–83.
63. Anderson MJ, Murray WR, Skinner HB. Constrained acetabular components. J Arthroplast. 1994;9: 17–23.
64. Goetz DD, Capello WN, Callaghan JJ, Brown TD, Johnston RC. Salvage of a recurrently dislocating total hip prosthesis with use of a constrained acetabular component: a retrospective analysis of fifty-six cases. J Bone Joint Surg Am. 1998;80:502–9.
65. Goetz DD, Bremner BR, Callaghan JJ, et al. Salvage of a recurrently dislocating total hip prosthesis with use of a constrained acetabular component. A concise follow-up of a previous report. J Bone Joint Surg Am. 2004;86:2419.
66. Berend KR, Lombardi AV Jr, Mallory TH, et al. The long-term outcome of 755 consecutive constrained acetabular components in total hip arthroplasty examining the successes and failures. J Arthroplast. 2005;20:93.
67. Shapiro GS, Weiland DE, Markel DC, Padgett DE, Sculco TP, Pellicci PM. The use of a constrained acetabular component for recurrent dislocation. J Arthroplast. 2003;18:250–8.
68. Karvonen M, Karvonen H, Seppänen M, Liukas A, Koivisto M, Mäkelä KT. Freedom constrained liner for the treatment and prevention of dislocation in total hip arthroplasty. Scand J Surg. 2017;106
69. Stanton DA, Bruce WJ, Goldberg JA, Walsh W. Salvaging unstable or recurrent dislocating total hip arthroplasty with the constrained acetabular component. J Orthop Surg. 2002;10(2):165–9.
70. Andersen AV, Kjersgaard AG, Solgaard S. Trilogy-constrained acetabular component for recurrent dislocation. ISRN Orthop. 2013;2013:629201.
71. Levine BR, Della Valle CJ, Deirmengian CA, Breien KM, Weeden SH, Sporer SM, Paprosky WG. The use of a tripolar articulation in revision total hip arthroplasty: a minimum of 24 months' follow-up. J Arthroplast. 2008;23(8):1182–8.
72. Knudsen R, Ovesen O, Kjaersgaard-Andersen P, Overgaard S. Constrained liners for recurrent dislocations in total hip arthroplasty. Hip Int. 2007;17(2):78–81.
73. Rady AE, Asal MK, Bassiony AA. The use of a constrained cementless acetabular component for instability in total hip replacement. Hip Int. 2010;20:434–9.
74. Zywiel MG, Mustafa LH, Bonutti PM, Mont MA. Are abductor muscle quality and previous revision surgery predictors of constrained liner failure in hip arthroplasty? Int Orthop. 2011;35(6):797–802. doi:10.1007/s00264-010-0962-3.
75. Farizon F, de Lavison R, Azoulai JJ, Bousquet G. Results with a Cementless alumina-coated cup with dual mobility: a twelve-year follow-up study. Int Orthop. 1998;22(4):219–24.
76. Lachiewicz PF, Watters TS. The use of dual-mobility components in total hip arthroplasty. J Am Acad Orthop Surg. 2012;20:481–6.
77. Ko LM, Hozack WJ. The dual mobility cup: what problems does it solve? Bone Joint J. 2016;98(1 Suppl A):60–3.
78. Guyen O, Chen QS, Bejui-Hugues J, Berry DJ, An KN. Unconstrained tripolar hip implants: effect on hip stability. Clin Orthop Relat Res. 2007;455:202–8.
79. Fabry C, Langlois J, Hamadouche M, Bader R. Intra-prosthetic dislocation of dual-mobility cups after total hip arthroplasty: potential causes from a clinical and biomechanical perspective. Int Orthop. 2016;40(5):901–6.
80. Guyen O, Pibarot V, Vaz G, Chevillotte C, Béjui-Hugues J. Use of a dual mobility socket to manage total hip arthroplasty instability. Clin Orthop Relat Res. 2009;467(2):465–72.
81. Mertl P, Combes A, Leiber-Wackenheim F, Fessy MH, Girard J, Migaud H. Recurrence of dislocation following total hip arthroplasty revision using dual mobility cups was rare in 180 hips followed over 7 years. HSSJ. 2012;8:251–6.
82. Philippot R, Adam P, Reckhaus M, et al. Prevention of dislocation in total hip revision surgery using a dual mobility design. Orthop Traumatol Surg Res. 2009;95(6):407–13.
83. Leiber-Wackenheim F, Brunschweiler B, Ehlinger M, Gabrion A, Mertl P. Treatment of recurrent THR dislocation using of a cementless dual-mobility cup: A 59 cases series with a mean 8 years follow-up. Orthop Traumatol Surg Res. 2011;97(1):8–13.
84. Simian E, Chatellard R, Druon J, Berhouet J, Rosset P. Dual mobility cup in revision total hip arthroplasty: dislocation rate and survival after 5 years. Orthop Traumatol Surg Res. 2015;101(5): 577–81.
85. Wegrzyn J, Tebaa E, Jacquel A, Carret JP, Béjui-Hugues J, Pibarot V. Can dual mobility cups prevent dislocation in all situations after revision total hip arthroplasty? J Arthroplast. 2015;30(4):631–40.
86. Saragaglia D, Ruatti S, Refaie R. Relevance of a press-fit dual mobility cup to deal with recurrent dislocation of conventional total hip arthroplasty: a 29-case series. Eur J Orthop Surg Traumatol. 2013;23(4):431–6.
87. Civinini R, Carulli C, Matassi F, Nistri L, Innocenti M. A dual-mobility cup reduces risk of dislocation in isolated acetabular revisions. Clin Orthop Relat Res. 2012;470(12):3542–8.
88. Jakobsen T, Kappel A, Hansen F, Krarup N. The dislocating hip replacement – revision with a dual mobility cup in 56 consecutive patients. Open Orthop J. 2014;8:268–71.
89. Plummer DR, Christy JM, Sporer SM, Paprosky WG, Della Valle CJ. Dual-mobility articulations for

patients at high risk for dislocation. J Arthroplast. 2016;31:131.

90. van Heumen M, Heesterbeek PJ, Swierstra BA, Van Hellemondt GG, Goosen JH. Dual mobility acetabular component in revision total hip arthroplasty for persistent dislocation: no dislocations in 50 hips after 1-5 years. J Orthop Traumatol. 2015;16(1):15–20.
91. Hamadouche M, Biau DJ, Huten D, Musset T, Gaucher F. The use of a cemented dual mobility socket to treat recurrent dislocation. Clin Orthop Relat Res. 2010;468(12):3248–54.
92. Van Warmerdam JM, McGann WA, Donnelly JR, Kim J, Welch RB. Achilles allograft reconstruction for recurrent dislocation in total hip arthroplasty. J Arthroplast. 2011;26:941–8.
93. Strømsøe K, Eikvar K. Fascia lata plasty in recurrent posterior dislocation after total hip arthroplasty. Arch Orthop Trauma Surg. 1995;114:292–4.
94. Lavigne MJ, Sanchez AA, Coutts RD. Recurrent dislocation after total hip arthroplasty: treatment with an Achilles tendon allograft. J Arthroplast. 2001;16:13–8.
95. McGann WA, Welch RB. Treatment of the unstable total hip arthroplasty using modularity, soft tissue, and allograft reconstruction. J Arthroplast. 2001;16:19–23.
96. Barbosa JK, Khan AM, Andrew JG. Treatment of recurrent dislocation of total hip arthroplasty using a ligament prosthesis. J Arthroplast. 2004;19:318–21.
97. Ekelund A. Trochanteric osteotomy for recurrent dislocation of total hip arthroplasty. J Arthroplast. 1993;8:629–32.
98. Kaplan SJ, Thomas WH, Poss R. Trochanteric advancement for recurrent dislocation after total hip arthroplasty. J Arthroplast. 1987;2:119–24.
99. Lazennec J-Y, Boyer P, Gorin M, Catonné Y, Rousseau MA. Acetabular anteversion with CT in supine, simulated standing, and sitting positions in a THA patient population. Clin Orthop Relat Res. 2011;469(4):1103–9. doi:10.1007/s11999-010-1732-7.
100. Kanawade V, Dorr LD, Wan Z. Predictability of acetabular component angular change with postural shift from standing to sitting position. J Bone Joint Surg Am. 2014;96(12):978–86. doi:10.2106/JBJS.M.00765.
101. Radcliff KE, Kepler CK, Hellman M, et al. Does spinal alignment influence acetabular orientation: a study of spino-pelvic variables and sagittal acetabular version. Orthop Surg. 2014;6(1):15–22. doi:10.1111/os.12090.
102. Inaba Y, Dorr LD, Wan Z, Sirianni L, Boutary M. Operative and patient care techniques for posterior mini-incision total hip arthroplasty. Clin Orthop Relat Res. 2005;441:104–14.
103. Dorr LD, Faugere MC, Mackel AM, Gruen TA, Bognar B, Malluche HH. Structural and cellular assessment of bone quality of proximal femur. Bone. 1993;14(3):231–42.
104. Karachalios T, Hartofilakidis G, Zacharakis N, Tsekoura M. A 12- to 18-year radiographic follow-up study of Charnley low-friction arthroplasty. The role of the center of rotation. Clin Orthop Relat Res. 1993;296:140–7.
105. Dastane M, Dorr LD, Tarwala R, Wan Z. Hip offset in total hip arthroplasty: quantitative measurement with navigation. Clin Orthop Relat Res. 2011;469(2):429–36.
106. Insull PJ, Cobbett H, Frampton CM, Munro JT. The use of a lipped acetabular liner decreases the rate of revision for instability after total hip replacement: a study using data from the New Zealand Joint Registry. Bone Joint J. 2014;96-B:884–8.
107. Epinette J-A, Béracassat R, Tracol P, Pagazani G, Vandenbussche E. Are modern dual mobility cups a valuable option in reducing instability after primary hip arthroplasty, even in younger patients? J Arthroplasty. 2014;29:1323–8.

26 Dual Mobility Cups

Eustathios Kenanidis, Eleftherios Tsiridis, Jacques Tabutin, and Pierre Marie Cambas

26.1 Current Concepts

E. Kenanidis and E. Tsiridis

Dual mobility cups are a new valuable option in treating and preventing dislocation in primary and revision THAs. In contrast with all alternative treatments, they do not compromise the implant durability and the clinical outcomes [1].

Since the initial concept design that was developed by Professor Gilles Bousquet and André Rambert in 1974, the DMCs have undergone several modifications and improvements in metallurgy, mechanics, and material [2]. Several cemented and uncemented designs with 22- and 28-mm femoral heads are now available both in Europe and in the USA.

E. Kenanidis, M.D., Ph.D., M.Sc. (✉)
Academic Orthopaedic Unit, Aristotle University Medical School, Thessaloniki, Greece

E. Tsiridis, M.D., Ph.D., F.A.C.S., F.R.C.S. (✉)
Academic Orthopaedic Unit, Papageorgiou General Hospital, Aristotle University Medical School, Thessaloniki, Greece
e-mail: etsiridis@doctors.org.uk

J. Tabutin, M.D. · P.M. Cambas, M.D.
Hospital of Cannes, Cannes, France
e-mail: j.TABUTIN@ch-cannes.fr

26.1.1 Objective

DMCs are composed by (Fig. 26.1) [3]:

1. A cemented or press-fit metal polished acetabular component
2. A large standard or highly cross-linked polyethylene head that articulates and is easily mobile concerning the metallic cup in a large-diameter articulation
3. A smaller 22- or 28-mm femoral head that is coupled but mobile with the polyethylene

The primary role of DMC design is to:

(a) Achieve an increased ROM until impingement occurs, mainly through increase of the head-to-neck ratio and the jump distance [3].
(b) Increase the stability of the joint.

This role is attained through the particular construct design of DMC, namely, the two different articulations:

1. The first articulation is a typical one between the femoral head and polyethylene, a hard on soft articulation.
2. The second one is non-typical, between the back of the polyethylene liner and the inner surface of the metallic acetabular shell.

E. Tsiridis (ed.), *The Adult Hip - Master Case Series and Techniques*,
https://doi.org/10.1007/978-3-319-64177-5_26

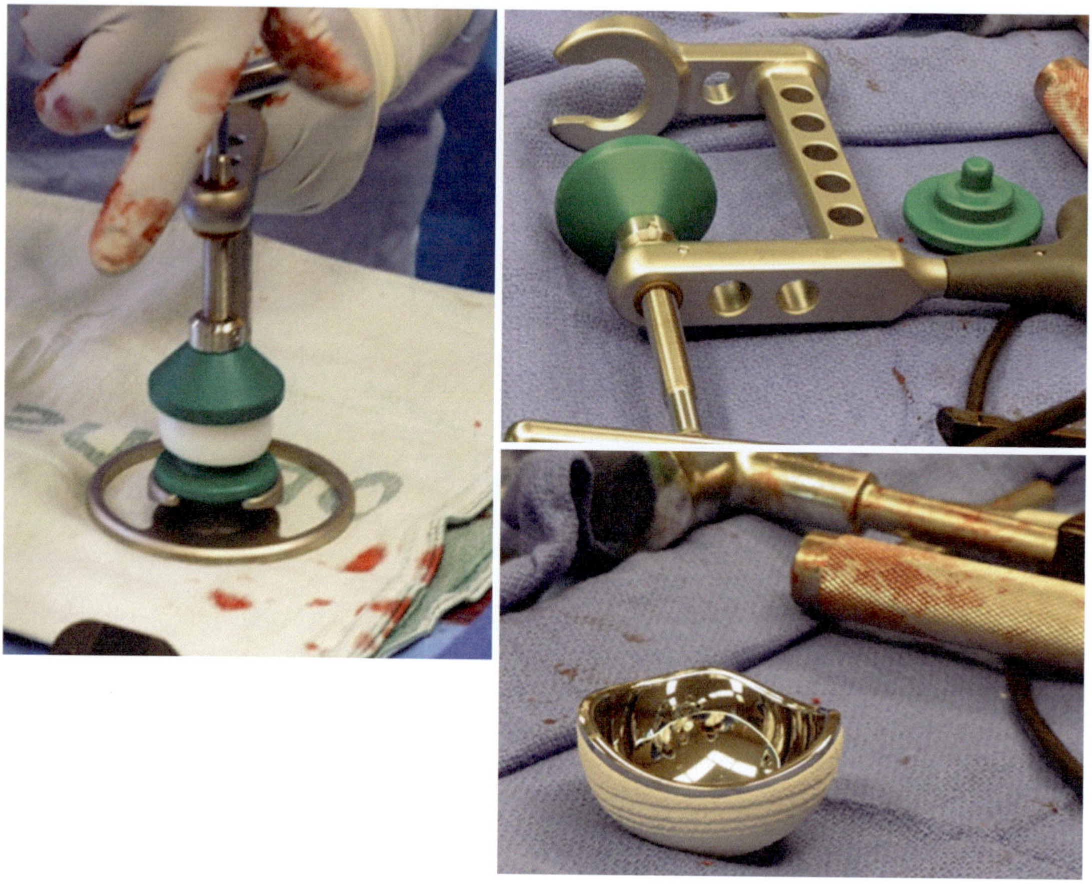

Fig. 26.1 Dual Mobility Socket Assembly

- The second articulation is "turned on"/activated when the femoral neck comes into contact with the rim of the polyethylene.
- It produces excessive efficient ROM till the femoral head impinges on the rim of the shell.

26.1.2 Indications

Although there are no absolute indications, DMCs are well-accepted treatment options in the following cases [1]:

1. Patients at high risk of dislocation undergoing primary or revision THA
   - Neuromuscular disorders
   - Cognitive impairment
   - Age >75 with a previous hip surgery
   - Revision THA
   - Primary THA for a femoral neck fracture
   - Primary THA for tumor resection
2. Treatment of recurrent instability (alternative to constrained components in select patients)

26.1.3 Contraindications

There are not enough data for the use of DMCs in younger people.

26.1.4 Advantages

Although the basic science studies are scarce [4] the DMCs have the following benefits:

(a) Greater in vitro range of motion to impingement compared to conventional components of the same diameter femoral head [5]

(b) Greater stability and range of movement
(c) Simplification of revisions as they are compatible with 28- and 22.2-mm femoral heads and may not need femoral exchange or they can be fixed by cement to cages when acetabular reconstruction is needed
(d) Opportunity to improve hip centering and further decrease risk of instability using cages and cement

26.1.5 Disadvantages

(a) The possible impingement of the femoral neck or the stem itself against the sizeable outer polyethylene bearing due to excessive ROM.
(b) The intraprosthetic dislocation. It is a dislocation of the femoral head and the polyethylene liner.
   - It has, as a result, the articulation of the head with the acetabular shell producing metal wear, metallosis, limping and limb shortening [6].
   - Although the exact reason is uncertain, extensive fibrosis at the large articulation, cup loosening, wear products, surface topography of the femoral neck, and the design of the mobile liner are considered potential causes [7, 8].
   - A radiographic characteristic is the "bubble sign" in x-rays [1].
   - The management depends on the time of diagnosis. The early diagnosis is treated with a liner exchange but the late due to wear products, with an acetabular and head revision [1].
(c) A potential lack of movement of the outer smaller articulation following the replacement of postoperative hematoma with fibrous tissue [4].
(d) The likelihood of increased wear rates due to the excessive ROM [4] and the thinner liner [9]. These cups are not subjected, however, to the same traction forces as constrained liners and might have a lower risk of aseptic loosening than conventional cups [10].Their aseptic loosening incidence, however, is not well studied in the literature.
   - The radiographic evaluation of PE wear can be difficult because of the inward position of the head within the cup and the cylindrical-spherical shape of the shell itself [11].

26.1.6 Published Results

26.1.6.1 Primary THA

Several papers reported the efficacy of DMCs in the treatment of primary total THA [2, 3, 9, 12–20]. These are prospective and retrospective case series of 106 to 2480 patients. The mean follow-up of these studies ranged from 2.3 to 22 years. Several implant designs were used with a femoral head diameter of 22.2- and 28-mm. There were favorable results as far as the dislocation was concerned. The reported risk of dislocation ranged from 0 to 1.1%. The rate of intraprosthetic dislocation ranged from 0 to 5.2%. The reported overall survival ranged from 74.5% to 99.6% [2, 3, 9, 12–20].

The studies are characterized from heterogeneity concerning the implant choice and the reported results. Several studies [2, 13, 15, 16, 20] published results of the use of the first-generation Bousquet cups (Novae®, Serf, Décines, France) with a 22.2-mm metal head and conventional polyethylene.

In the longest follow-up reported, Boyer et al. [20] demonstrated the survival of 240 primary THAs treated with PF modular femoral stem and a dual mobility Novae tripodal socket from 1985 to 1990. They reported 74% overall survival at 22 years' follow-up. No dislocation was reported; however, the main issue arrived was the cup failure.

Vielpaeu et al. [13] reported comparative data of two cohorts of primary THAs treated with first- and second-generation DMCs. The 15-year survival rate of the 437 hips treated with the first-generation Bousquet DMC was 84.4% with aseptic loosening to be the main reason of failure; only five dislocations were described. The 5-year survival rate of the second-generation cups (Novae E, SERF Company, Saint-Étienne, France) were 99.6% with no dislocation and mechanical failures reported.

In the greatest cohort so far reported, Combes et al. [14] supported that the DMCs are an excellent choice for patients with high risk of instability but should be avoided in younger people due to the risk of osteolysis. The 10-year survivorship of 2480 THAs was 93%. Dislocation rate was 0.6% and intraprosthetic dislocation rate 0.28%. Younger patients suffered more frequently from osteolysis and loosening.

Short-term studies demonstrated the utility of DMCs in the treatment of femoral neck fractures and prevention of dislocation. Adam et al. [21] reported 1.4% dislocation rate in 214 patients suffering from femoral neck fractures that were treated with DMC. The follow-up was for less than a year. Taracevicious et al. [22] further proved the utility of DCMs in the reduction of dislocation for patients with femoral neck fractures. In a prospective comparative study, DMCs were significantly more effective in the prevention of dislocation than conventional (single mobility) cemented acetabular components ($p = 0.01$).

DMCs have been reported to be efficient in the treatment of dislocation in various other pathologic conditions that are predisposing to dislocation as spastic disorders or tumors [23, 24]. Philippeau et al. [23] demonstrated lower dislocation rate for 71 patients treated with a DMC for primary bone tumors or metastases (overall 9.8%) than this reported in the literature.

26.1.6.2 Revision THA

Several papers, dealing with the efficacy of DMCs to prevent dislocation following revision THA, are currently available [10, 25–37]. These are mainly retrospective case series of 29 to 228 patients; many patients, however, were treated with DMC for another than a recurrent dislocation reason [28, 31]. The mean follow-up of these studies ranged from 2 to 8 years. The majority however of these studies have included small numbers of patients for a short-term follow-up [33, 34, 36]. The patients included were usually at great risk for dislocation due to an increased number of prior revisions. There were favorable results as far as the redislocation was concerned. The reported risk for redislocation ranged from 0 to 5.5% [25, 34].

In one of the largest reported sample size and follow-up time, Merti et al. [25] retrospectively evaluated 180 revision THAs with recurrent instability. Redislocation occurred at 4.8% of patients at a mean follow-up of 8 years. The reported survival was 92.6% at the same time. The higher rate of dislocation was reported for patients that have undergone multiple earlier revisions or in case of greater trochanter nonunion (and may advocate repair of GT or constrained liner use).

The Swedish Hip Arthroplasty Register [10] demonstrated 228 reconstructions with DMC for recurrent instability. The reported survival for any reason was 94% and redislocation 99% at a mean follow-up of 2 years'. The age between 50 and 59 years compared to 75 years and previous revision surgery increased 5 and 1.7 times the risk for subsequent re-revision, respectively.

26.1.7 Complications

- The reported complications in these studies included heterotopic ossification, aseptic loosening, infection fractures, groin pain, and intraprosthetic dislocations.
- The rate of intraprosthetic dislocations ranges in different studies of revision THA, but it is generally low (0–3.7% [5, 26]).

26.2 Case Title: Dual Mobility Cup (The Prosthetic Neck Must Be Smooth)

Jacques Tabutin and Pierre Marie Cambas

26.2.1 Demographics

Age: 89 years
Sex: Female
BMI: 25

26.2.2 Relevant Past Medical History

Principal pathologies: Hypertension, renal insufficiency.

Previous surgical procedures: Right THA 2002 (osteoarthritis) — left THA 2005 (osteoarthritis). Cementless total hip arthroplasty with dual mobility cups on both sides.

Medication: Atenolol, Triatec, and Tildiem.

History of Presenting Complaint: Two falls from height eight months and three months earlier that were treated by rest. There were no radiographs taken. Progressive pain and shortening.

26.2.3 Clinical Examination

Symptoms: Pain on motion, limping, two crutches.

Range of motion: 0.50.10.10.10.20.

Main disability: Loss of mobility.

Scoring if available: PMA 5 (1.3.1) HHS 24.

Neurovascular evaluation: Intact.

26.2.4 Preoperative Radiological Assessment/Imaging (Figs. 26.2 and 26.3)

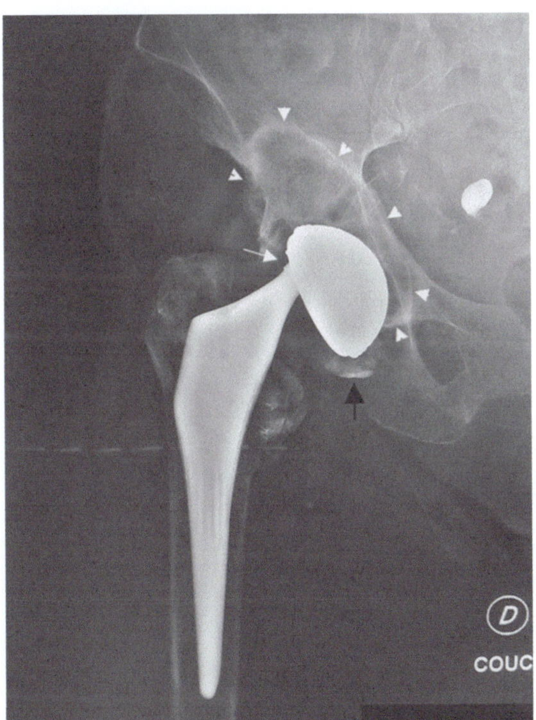

Fig. 26.2 Right hip AP view: well-fixed cup (*no lucent line*). Major supra- and periacetabular osteolyses (*white arrowheads*). Intra-prosthetic dislocation: the head is not centered in the cup and contacts it. Metal debris at the bottom (*black arrow*). The Morse taper is not covered by the 22-mm head (*white arrow*)

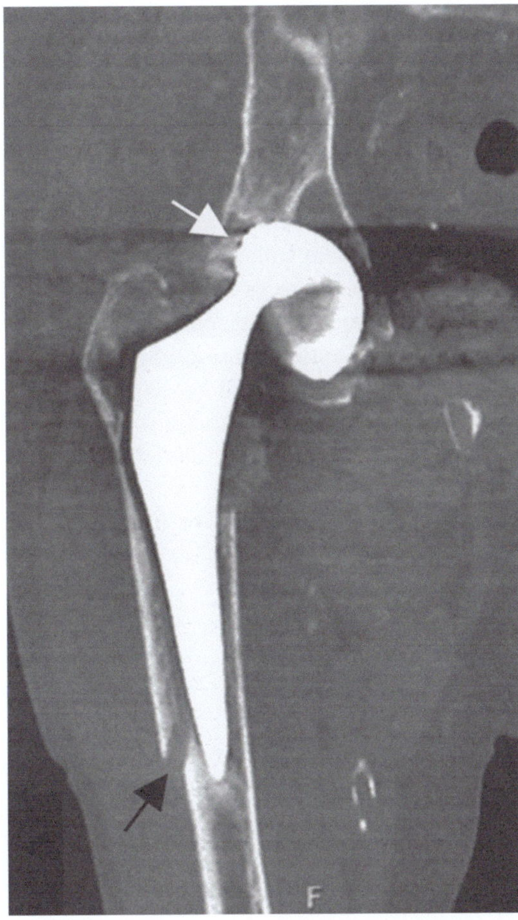

Fig. 26.3 Right hip CT scan coronal view. The head touches the metal cup (*white arrow*). Femoral periprosthetic fracture Vancouver B2, SOFCOT B3 (*black arrow*). Femoral osteolysis especially at the lesser trochanter

26.2.5 Preoperative Planning

Diagnosis: Femoral periprosthetic fracture, acetabular and femoral granuloma after an intraprosthetic dislocation of a dual mobility cup (Figs. 26.2 and 26.3).

Possible treatment options: Internal fixation of femur + cemented revision stem. Acetabular ring (Kerboull's or Burch-Schneider's) + allograft + cemented cup.

Chosen treatment method: Cementless bipolar revision + graft.

Selection of implants if applicable and rational: Dual mobility cup (to reduce the risk of instability in a revised elderly patient) + autograft ± bone substitutes (to deal with the large bone loss). Locked revision cementless stem to get primary stability.

Expected difficulties: The size of the proximal femoral bone loss. Large acetabular cavitary defect. Well-fixed metal cup.

Strategies to overcome difficulties: At the femur: revision stem with an oversized proximal part that was locked to get stability. At the acetabulum: explantation with curved thin chisels (Moreland's). Gentle reaming. Slightly oversized cup (diameter limited by anteroposterior dimensions of bony acetabulum). Filling of the cavitary bone defects (autograft + bone substitute).

Templating: A size of 60 or 61 for the cup should be correct. The size 8 revision stem fills the diaphysis.

26.2.6 Surgical Note

Patient's position: Lateral decubitus.

Type of anesthesia: General.

Surgical approach: Posterolateral.

Main steps: A careful soft tissue release of the hip with progressive capsulectomy. A hook under the femoral neck supported the dislocation. A distal capsulectomy was done as far as the psoas tendon to gain internal rotation. Easy stem implantation (loose), thorough capsulo-synovectomy. Cup explanation with Moreland's chisels (wear and scratches on the inner surface) (Fig. 26.4).

Reconstruction techniques: Careful acetabular reaming. Filling of bone defects with cancellous bone chips from the distal femur mixed with bone substitutes to increase the volume. Gentle reverse reaming. Press-fit cup (with a proximal screw and two studs as security). Gentle hand reaming of the femoral canal to bone contact. The revision trial stem was stable. The implanted stem was locked distally for security (Fig. 26.5).

26.2.7 Intraoperative Challenges

Challenges and solutions: Bone fragility managed with adequate release and gentle handling.

Unanticipated problems and solution: Excessive bone loss: adding of a bone substitute was necessary.

Thorough description of decision making, including the reason for the final decision: The revision stem was solid, but the fracture was not secured entirely; the latter was the reason of the distal locking. The cup was stable in press-fit but the poor bone quality required further fixation (screw and studs).

26.2.8 Postoperative Radiographs (Figs. 26.4 and 26.5)

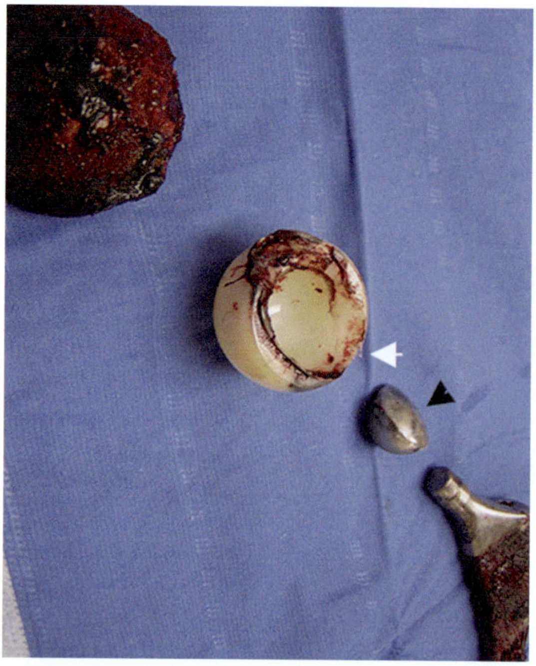

Fig. 26.4 The explant. The cup was well integrated (bone attached to the metal. The retention rim of the dual mobility polyethylene cup had a destruction (*white arrow*). Excessive damage and flattening of the metal head (*black arrow*). Almost no bone attached to the stem

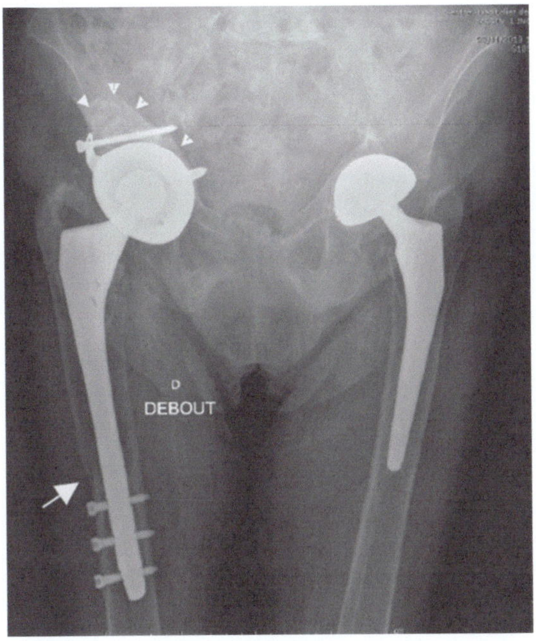

Fig. 26.5 AP pelvis at 3 postoperative years. The graft was incorporated at the acetabulum (*white arrow heads*). The cup was well-fixed (*no lucent line*). The femoral fracture was healed (*white arrow*). The revision stem was fixed with no lucency and cortical thickening at the locking pins level

26.2.9 Postoperative Management

Chemoprophylaxis and anticoagulant treatment period: Cefamandole lg/12 h 1 day. LMWH for 5 weeks.

Gait/limb loading until full loading: Progressive gain in the hip range of motion. At the fifth postoperative day the patient was able to seat in an armchair having 80° of flexion. No weight bearing during the first month and then progressive weight bearing. Full weight bearing at 6 weeks.

26.2.10 Follow-Up and Complications

Secondary fall at 4 months: a non-displaced contralateral pelvic fracture that was treated conservatively with rest.

Scoring: 4 years: PMA 6.6.4. HHS 86.

26.2.11 Discussion

1. The principal interest of this case is the estimation of the severity of damage that an intraprosthetic dislocation of a dual mobility cup may produce [38, 39]. The polyethylene cup turned distally, and the femoral ball came in contact with the metal cup and wore progressively, causing metallosis (seen on the radiography at the lower part of the joint) (Fig. 26.4). The osteolysis was due to the wear of the polyethylene rim (mainly supra-acetabular osteolysis). This process is dangerous because it progresses almost silently (apart from the shortening).

   The cause of an intraprosthetic dislocation is the loss of the retentive effect of the rim of the polyethylene cup. This is due to a progressive abrasion from a rough surface; in this case, this surface was the part of the Morse taper that was outside the metallic head. It points to a standard rule in the dual mobility cups that the prosthetic neck must be smooth (polished). No matte surface finish of a part of a Morse taper, or a collared head are acceptable.

   A technological mistake was done as a 28-mm-diameter head should have been used to cover the taper. The geometry of the taper was modified in 2005 by the industry, shortened to be fully covered by the metal head.

   We have had several such cases but this one was the worst and the most demonstrative. It shows that any technological option has drawbacks.
2. The indication of a dual mobility cup for the primary THA in an 80 years old lady was correct, reducing almost ten times the risk of instability. The severity of the produced damage was the result of the lack of radio-clinical follow-up and the wrong technological option.
3. Concerning the revision
   - The wear of the metal cup imposed the acetabular revision. The revised cup could

be cemented in an acetabular ring, either a Kerboull's with an obturator hook or a Burch-Schneider ring with screws. In both cases, the outer diameter might have been about 56 mm. A dual mobility cup might have been cemented in the ring. The other option was a slightly oversized press-fit cup (61 mm) with additional fixation due to the poor bone quality. A dual mobility option was preferred because it was a revision of an elderly lady.

- The grafting of the acetabulum was compulsory because of the extent of the bone loss. As the defect was cavitary, we favored cancellous bone chips from the distal femur that are easy to obtain with little morbidity. An iliac crest graft is preferred when a shape is needed, however, a loss of strength of the gluteus medius is possible.
- The removal of the femoral stem was easy because it was loose. In a younger patient, less than 60 years old, rebuilding the femur with cerclages and impaction grafting + a cemented stem would have been on option. In the elderly lady of our case with the almost healed fracture (no motion of the fracture site), bridging with a locked stem was simple, addressing at the same time the metaphyseal enlargement.

4. This case shows that the surgeon at the primary arthroplasty is responsible not only for the technique (posterolateral approach) and the indication (total hip arthroplasty with a dual mobility cup) but also for the technological aspect (uncovered taper) and for the radio-clinical follow-up: an earlier revision would have dealt less damages.

References

1. De Martino I, Triantafyllopoulos GK, Sculco PK, Sculco TP. Dual mobility cups in total hip arthroplasty. World J Orthop. 2014;5(3):180–7.
2. Farizon F, de Lavison R, Azoulai JJ, Bousquet G. Results with a cementless alumina-coated cup with dual mobility. A twelve-year follow-up study. Int Orthop. 1998;22:219–24.
3. Guyen O, Chen QS, Bejui-Hugues J, Berry DJ, An KN. Unconstrained tripolar hip implants: effect on hip stability. Clin Orthop Relat Res. 2007;455:202–8.
4. Lachiewicz PF, Watters TS. The use of dual-mobility components in total hip arthroplasty. J Am Acad Orthop Surg. 2012;20:481–6.
5. Fabry C, Langlois J, Hamadouche M, Bader R. Intraprosthetic dislocation of dual-mobility cups after total hip arthroplasty: potential causes from a clinical and biomechanical perspective. Int Orthop. 2016;40(5):901–6.
6. Mohammed R, Cnudde P. Severe metallosis owing to intraprosthetic dislocation in a failed dual-mobility cup primary total hip arthroplasty. J Arthroplast. 2012;27:493.e1–3.
7. Guyen O, Pibarot V, Vaz G, Chevillotte C, Béjui-Hugues J. Use of a dual mobility socket to manage total hiparthroplasty instability. Clin Orthop Relat Res. 2009;467(2):465–72.
8. Philippot R, Boyer B, Farizon F. Intraprosthetic dislocation: a specific complication of the dual-mobility system. Clin Orthop Relat Res. 2013;471:965–70.
9. Philippot R, Farizon F, Camilleri JP, Boyer B, Derhi G, Bonnan J, Fessy MH, Lecuire F. Survival of cementless dual mobility socket with a mean 17 years follow-up. Rev Chir Orthop Reparatrice Appar Mot. 2008;94:e23–7.
10. Nils P Hailer, Rődiger J Weiss, Andrı Stark, Johan Kδrrholm Dual-mobility cups for revision due to instability are associated with a low rate of re-revisions due to dislocation 228 patients from the Swedish Hip Arthroplasty Register. Acta Orthop. 2012;83(6):566–71.
11. Grazioli A, Ek ET, Rüdiger HA. Biomechanical concept and clinical outcome of dual mobility cups. Int Orthop. 2012;36:2411–18.
12. Leclercq S, Benoit JY, de Rosa JP, Euvrard P, Leteurtre C, Girardin P. Results of the Evora dual-mobility socket after a minimum follow-up of five years. Rev Chir Orthop Reparatrice Appar Mot. 2008;94:e17–e22.
13. Vielpeau C, Lebel B, Ardouin L, Burdin G, Lautridou C. The dual mobility socket concept: experience with 668 cases. Int Orthop. 2011;35:225–30.
14. Combes A, Migaud H, Girard J, Duhamel A, Fessy MH. Low rate of dislocation of dual-mobility cups in primary total hip arthroplasty. Clin Orthop Relat Res. 2013;471:3891–900.
15. Lautridou C, Lebel B, Burdin G, Vielpeau C. [Survival of the cementless Bousquet dual mobility cup: Minimum 15-year follow-up of 437 total hip arthroplasties]. Rev Chir Orthop Reparatrice Appar Mot. 2008;94:731–39.
16. Philippot R, Adam P, Farizon F, Fessy MH, Bousquet G. [Survival of cementless dual mobility sockets: ten-year follow-up]. Rev Chir Orthop Reparatrice Appar Mot. 2006;92:326–31.

17. Bouchet R, Mercier N, Saragaglia D. Posterior approach and dislocation rate: a 213 total hip replacements case-control study comparing the dual mobility cup with a conventional 28-mm metal head/polyethylene prosthesis. Orthop Traumatol Surg Res. 2011;97:2–7.
18. Hamadouche M, Arnould H, Bouxin B. Is a cementless dual mobility socket in primary THA a reasonable option? Clin Orthop Relat Res. 2012;470:3048–53.
19. Bauchu P, Bonnard O, Cyprès A, Fiquet A, Girardin P, Noyer D. The dual-mobility POLARCUP: first results from a multicenter study. Orthopedics. 2008;31.
20. Boyer B, Philippot R, Geringer J, Farizon F. Primary total hip arthroplasty with dual mobility socket to prevent dislocation: a 22-year follow-up of 240 hips. Int Orthop. 2012;36:511–18.
21. Adam P, Philippe R, Ehlinger M, Roche O, Bonnomet F, Molé D, Fessy MH. Dual mobility cups hip arthroplasty as a treatment for displaced fracture of the femoral neck in the elderly. A prospective, systematic, multicenter study with specific focus on postoperative dislocation. Orthop Traumatol Surg Res. 2012;98: 296–300.
22. Tarasevicius S, Busevicius M, Robertsson O, Wingstrand H. Dual mobility cup reduces dislocation rate after arthroplasty for femoral neck fracture. BMC Musculoskelet Disord. 2010;11:175.
23. Philippeau JM, Durand JM, Carret JP, Leclercq S, Waast D, Gouin F. Dual mobility design use in preventing total hip replacement dislocation following tumor resection. Orthop Traumatol Surg Res. 2010; 96:2–8
24. Sanders RJ, Swierstra BA, Goosen JH. The use of a dual-mobility concept in total hip arthroplasty patients with spastic disorders: no dislocations in a series of ten cases at midterm follow-up. Arch Orthop Trauma Surg. 2013;133:1011–16.
25. Mertl P, Combes A, Leiber-Wackenheim F, Fessy MH, Girard J, Migaud H. Recurrence of dislocation following total hip arthroplasty revision using dual mobility cups was rare in 180 hips followed over 7 years. HSSJ. 2012;8:251–6.
26. Langlais FL, Ropars M, Gaucher F, Musset T, Chaix O. Dual mobility cemented cups have low dislocation rates in THA revisions. Clin Orthop Relat Res. 2008;466(2):389–95.
27. Philippot R, Adam P, Reckhaus M, et al. Prevention of dislocation in total hip revision surgery using a dual mobility design. Orthop Traumatol Surg Res. 2009;95(6):407–13.
28. Leiber-Wackenheim F, Brunschweiler B, Ehlinger M, Gabrion A, Mertl P. Treatment of recurrent THR dislocation using of a cementless dual-mobility cup: a 59 cases series with a mean 8 years follow-up. Orthop Traumatol Surg Res. 2011;97(1):8–13.
29. Levine BR, Della Valle CJ, Deirmengian CA, Breien KM, Weeden SH, Sporer SM, Paprosky WG. The use of a tripolar articulation in revision total hip arthroplasty: a minimum of 24 months' follow-up. J Arthroplast. 2008;23:1182–8.
30. Simian E, Chatellard R, Druon J, Berhouet J, Rosset P. Dual mobility cup in revision total hip arthroplasty: dislocation rate and survival after 5 years. Orthop Traumatol Surg Res. 2015;101(5):577–81.
31. Wegrzyn J, Tebaa E, Jacquel A, Carret JP, Béjui-Hugues J, Pibarot V. Can dual mobility cups prevent dislocation in all situations after revision total hip arthroplasty? J Arthroplast. 2015;30(4):631–40.
32. Saragaglia D, Ruatti S, Refaie R. Relevance of a press-fit dual mobility cup to deal with recurrent dislocation of conventional total hiparthroplasty: a 29-case series. Eur J Orthop Surg Traumatol. 2013;23(4):431–6.
33. Civinini R, Carulli C, Matassi F, Nistri L, Innocenti M. A dual-mobility cup reduces risk of dislocation in isolated acetabular revisions. Clin Orthop Relat Res. 2012;470(12):3542–8.
34. Jakobsen T, Kappel A, Hansen F, Krarup N. The dislocating hip replacement – revision with a dual mobility cup in 56 consecutive patients. Open Orthop J. 2014;8:268–71.
35. Plummer DR, Christy JM, Sporer SM, Paprosky WG, Della Valle CJ. Dual-mobility articulations for patients at high risk for dislocation. J Arthroplast. 2016;31:131–5.
36. van Heumen M, Heesterbeek PJ, Swierstra BA, Van Hellemondt GG, Goosen JH. Dual mobility acetabular component in revision total hip arthroplasty for persistent dislocation: no dislocations in 50 hips after 1-5 years. J Orthop Traumatol. 2015;16(1):15–20.
37. Hamadouche M, Biau DJ, Huten D, Musset T, Gaucher F. The use of a cemented dual mobility socket to treat recurrent dislocation. Clin Orthop Relat Res. 2010;468(12):3248–54.
38. Mohammed R, Cnudde P. Severe metallosis owing to intraprosthetic dislocation in a failed dual-mobility cup primary total hip arthroplasty. J Arthroplasty. 2012;27:493.e1–3.
39. Lecuire F, Benareau I, Rubini J, Basso M. Intra-prosthetic dislocation of the Bousquet dual mobility socket [In French]. Rev. Chir Orthop Reparatrice Appar Mot. 2004;90:249–55.

Reinforcement Rings and Cages

27

Eustathios Kenanidis, Eleftherios Tsiridis, Thiago Aguiar, Luís Melo Tavares, Pedro Dantas, Rashid Tikhilov, Igor Shubnyakov, Alexey Denisov, Fritz Thorey, Volodymyr Filippenko, Volodymyr Mezentsev, Mandus Akonjom, Georgios Petsatodis, and Filon Agathangelidis

27.1 Current Concepts

E. Kenanidis and E. Tsiridis

Reinforcement rings and cages are implants used in revision THA when the remaining bone stock is deficient. They span the bone defect and act as a scaffold while protecting morcellized or structural allograft during the bone remodelling phase [1]. The use of cages has been reduced over time following the mechanical failure of cages and the introduction of newer techniques of trabecular metal components [1].

27.1.1 Objective

The cages are usually fixed securely but "non-biologically" to ischium and ilium with the maximum number of screws to provide short-term mechanical stability to the cup liner. At the same time, they transfer the load to the peripheral host bone protecting morcellized and structural grafts from excessive forces, during the bone remodelling phase [1, 2]. During this period, bone grafting remodels, supports, and bridges areas of bone loss to achieve long-term fixation. Failure of graft incorporation leads to eventual cage fatigue and construct failure [2, 3].

E. Kenanidis, M.D., Ph.D., M.Sc. (✉)
Academic Orthopaedic Unit, Aristotle University Medical School, Thessaloniki, Greece

E. Tsiridis, M.D., Ph.D., F.A.C.S., F.R.C.S. (✉)
Academic Orthopaedic Unit, Papageorgiou General Hospital, Aristotle University Medical School, Thessaloniki, Greece
e-mail: etsiridis@doctors.org.uk

T. Aguiar, M.D.
Hospital Curry Cabral, Lisbon, Portugal

Hospital SAMS, Lisbon, Portugal

L.M. Tavares, M.D. • P. Dantas, M.D.
Hospital Curry Cabral, Lisbon, Portugal

R. Tikhilov, M.D., Ph.D. • I. Shubnyakov, M.D., Ph.D.
A. Denisov, M.D., Ph.D.
Vreden Russian Research Institute of Traumatology and Orthopedics, Saint Petersburg, Russia

F. Thorey, M.D., Ph.D.
ATOS Hospital Heidelberg, Heidelberg, Germany
e-mail: fritz.thorey@atos.de

V. Filippenko, M.D. • V. Mezentsev, M.D., Ph.D.
M. Akonjom, M.B.B.Ch., M.D., F.I.C.S.
Department of Joint Pathology, Sytenko Institute of Spine and Joint Pathology, Kharkiv, Ukraine

G. Petsatodis, M.D., Ph.D. • F. Agathangelidis, M.D., Ph.D.
First Department of Orthopaedics, Papanikolaou General Hospital, Aristotle University of Thessaloniki, Thessaloniki, Greece

E. Tsiridis (ed.), *The Adult Hip - Master Case Series and Techniques*,
https://doi.org/10.1007/978-3-319-64177-5_27

27.1.2 Types

There are usually two types of reinforcement rings and cages:

1. Roof reinforcement ring (RRR): these are small devices used in the mild bone loss to protect the superior acetabular dome [1] and to provide stable fixation for the polyethylene liner [4]. Segmental acetabular integrity should always be ensured before using this device [4]. An uncemented porous cup is now usually preferred instead of RRR [5].
2. Ilioischial antiprotrusio cage (APC): These are greater devices than RRR that extend from the ilium to the ischium and protect the entire acetabulum [1, 6]. They have been used for more complex acetabular reconstructions than RRR. In severely combined defects or pelvic discontinuity (PD), the cage is implanted with allograft [6]. Various types are available.

27.1.2.1 The Burch-Schneider (BS) Antiprotrusio Cage

It was originally designed by Burch (1974) and later modified by Schneider (1975) to manage protrusion acetabuli [2]. Its latest form consists of a hemispherical shell that holds a polyethylene inlay, a proximal flange angled 22° posteriorly with respect to the middle of the shell and a distal nose. It has a shell size variability and numerous anchorage holes for screws in the shell, flange, and nose.

It is indicated for the reconstruction of large acetabular floor and roof defects (the rim and the cranio-lateral border of the acetabulum) and severe acetabular deficiency including PD [7]. It bridges the acetabular defect using a proximal flange to the ilium and a distal nose to the ischium.

Success with the cage is dependent on the surgical technique used [8]. Some technical considerations of the cage are the following:

- BS must be adjusted to the bone and vice versa by smoothing any bone irregularities and removal of the osteophytes [8].
- BS requires three-point fixation: the inferior flange must be slotted into the ischial tuberosity before fixation to permit a more medialized, horizontal placement of the cage. The superior flange must be fixed with at least three screws to the ilium and the third point to the middle of the acetabulum.

27.1.2.2 The Ganz Ring

It is also known as acetabular RRR with a hook that is used since 1989 [9]. It is indicated for acetabular floor or cavitary defects and smaller defects of the lateral border of the acetabular rim [10]. Prerequisite for its use is an intact inferior part of the acetabulum (incisura acetabuli) for anchoring the hook [10].

27.1.2.3 The Mueller Acetabular Reinforcement Ring

It was designed since 1976, and it is available in many sizes. It is indicated only for cavitary defects [4]. It is stably fixed to host bone with cancellous screws, and the polyethylene cup is fixed with cement within the ring and where it can be freely positioned in appropriate anteversion and inclination [11].

27.1.3 Indications

(a) Revision THA with inadequate bone stock, massive bone loss, or PD [5].
(b) Indications depend on cage type.
   1. RRR are used in smaller mainly contained defects.
   2. APC is used in more complex acetabular reconstruction when the bone loss severity and the geometry of loss do not favour a stable biologic fixation of an uncemented porous socket. In cases where the graft supports ≥50% of the acetabular component, APC is needed to span bone defect, to protect the graft, and provide structural stability [5, 12].
(c) Intact acetabular walls, no matter how thin, and an intact ischial tuberosity are prerequisite for their use. Deficiencies of the walls or the anterior and posterior columns do not support the cage leading to early failure [8]. In such cases, the cage must be used with structural allografts to relieve excessive stress.

(d) They need adequate support by host bone or allograft depending on the characteristics of the defects. Smaller defects could be packed with particulate graft, but in global, superior, posterior wall or posterior column bone loss, it is necessary to use structural allograft [5, 8].

27.1.4 Contraindications

- Deficiencies of the medial wall and protrusion acetabuli are definite contraindications for the RRR [12].

27.1.5 Advantages

- The primary advantage of an RRR is the capacity to cement and support a cemented cup in any position independently of the ring position [1, 13].
- APC span bone defects, distribute load, protect large bone grafts from overstress, and resist early migration [13].
- APC help to restore the appropriate centre of hip rotation and support the polyethylene cemented cup [12].
- Possible use of APC in greater defects (Paprosky III A and B), massive defects, and even PD [7, 8].
- APC help to restore the bone stock through protection of bone graft during acetabular revision [13].The new bone stock is often able to facilitate the re-revisions even with an uncemented component [14].

27.1.6 Disadvantages

- Historically the standard cages lack porous or bioactive coating that does not allow osseointegration/biologic fixation which increases the risk of fatigue failure and loosening [15, 16]. The new generation cages are designed and manufactured with ingrowth surfaces although the impact of this design feature on the failure rate has yet to be determined [2, 3].
- The risk of infection and disease transmission with allograft use [12].
- The limited number of available sizes of BS; newer, however, designs have better versatility [12].
- The BS cage usually needs a wide exposure to the supra-acetabular part of the ilium. This increases the risk of the superior gluteal nerve injury and postoperative limping [5, 7].
- The prolonged postoperative delay in weight bearing to reduce overloading on the cage and prevent possible graft resorption and cage migration [12].
- The cementation of a polyethylene liner limits the ability to perform a trial reduction and choose the appropriate liner to enhance the stability of the hip.
- Difficult surgical technique.
- An extremely rare complication is the transection of the sciatic nerve by migration of an acetabular metal frame support [17].

27.1.7 Published Results

There a lot of studies in the literature demonstrating satisfactory mid- to long-term results of rings or cages in revision THA [4, 11, 18–41]. The rates of success of cage reconstruction have been conflicting, ranging from 69 to 100% [2]. These studies are case series with a very mixed group of patients, variable pathology, and bone loss. This makes any comparison between them difficult; there is also no RCT comparing different methods and implants.

In a recent systematic review, Beckman et al. [42] compared the rate of loosening of the acetabular component following revision THA with reinforcement rings (Ganz, Mueller, Burch-Schneider) to Trabecular Metal (TM) cups, shells, and augments for a 20-year period between 1992 and 2012. There were only case series and no RCTs. 1541 patients had an acetabular revision with reinforcement rings, 479 a Burch-Schneider ring, 235 a Ganz ring, and 827 a Mueller ring. The mean follow-up and rate of loosening were 5.1 years and 12.3% for Burch-Schneider rings, 7.5 years and 7.7% radiographic loosening for Ganz rings, and 5.5 years and 7.5% for Mueller rings. The failure rate of the TM components was lower than the yearly failure rate observed in different revision rings (OR = 0.326, $p = 0.002$). 369 revision THAs with a mean follow-up period of 6.3 years were performed with reinforcement rings in more severe Paprosky IIIa and IIIb cases. The loosening rate per year was 14.0%, significantly greater than 2.6% that was for TM (OR=0.259, $p = 0.002$). The same was also true for the treatment of PD; however, the sample size was very limited. One should take into consideration, however, that the follow-up period was greater for the rings compared to TM.

The reported mechanical failure rate of BS ranges between 0 and 15% and radiographic loosening from 0 to 24% at midterm follow-up [2]. The varying results in different series relate to different selection criteria for the use of antiprotrusio cages and perhaps also to surgical technique and various types of bone grafts used to fill pelvic deficiencies.

Recent studies report more homogenous samples [2, 7, 8, 10, 12, 13, 43, 44]. Regis et al. [12] reported long-term results of 71 BS cages (BSCs) combined with bulk allografts for the treatment of type IIIa and b defects in revision THA. Total survival rate was 87.5% at a mean of 11.7 years. Regis supported that the increased reported high failure rate of BSCs is related to the poor surgical technique (achievement of initial stability of the device and tight impaction of the graft, together with additional screw fixation of the cage to viable ilium promoting new bone formation). Regis et al. [2] also reported the cumulative survival rates of 97 BSCs at a mean of 14.6 years. The cumulative survival rates with removal for any reason or X-ray migration of the cage and aseptic or radiographic loosening were 80.0% and 84.6%, respectively. The use of Burch-Schneider cage and bulk allografts was an effective technique for the treatment of pelvic discontinuity. Regis et al. [7] reported 72.2% survival rates of PDs treated with BSCs at 16.6 years with acetabular revision for any reason, radiographic loosening, or unhealing of the discontinuity. Alrumaih et al. [8] recently reported midterm results of 33 revision THAs with BS cage; there were nine IIIA defects and twenty four type IV defects. The cumulative failure rate was 15.1% at a mean of 6.19 years.

27.2 Case Title: Burch-Schneider Cage and Morselized Allograft for a Paprosky Type 3 B Acetabular Defect

Thiago Aguiar, Luís Tavares, and Pedro Dantas

27.2.1 Demographics

Age: 60 years
Sex: Female
BMI: 22,48

27.2.2 Relevant Past Medical History

Principal pathologies: Rheumatoid arthritis.

Previous surgical procedures: Right total hip replacement in 1993 which was revised fifteen years later (2008) due to acetabular cup loosening and osteolysis (press-fit acetabular cup with screws). The patient was sent to our institution for re-revision two years later (2010) due to acetabular cup loosening and migration. Right total knee replacement in 1994 and left total knee replacement in 2006.

Medication: Naproxen, leflunomide, deflazacort, tocilizumab, risedronate sodium, calcium carbonate + cholecalciferol.

History of presenting complaint: The patient was referred with severe right hip pain for the last two years with an inability to walk without two crutches and progressive shortening of the limb. Muscle weakness and incapacity to bear weight on the right side. The patient denies fever, swelling, or inflammatory signs around the hip.

27.2.3 Clinical Examination

Symptoms: Excruciating pain with weight bearing, pain with flexion, and rotations of the right hip. Right limb muscle atrophy, especially in the thigh. Right posterolateral surgical scars from previous surgeries. Knees unchanged. Straight midline scars from previous knee surgeries.

Range of motion: Right hip: flexion 40°; extension 0°; abduction 10°; adduction 0°; internal rotation 5°; external rotation 5°. Hip mobilization was very painful.

Specific tests: Right lower limb shortening of three cm.

Main disability: Unable to bear weight and walk without crutches. Right hip pain.

Scoring if available: Harris Hip Score preoperatively: 20.75.

Neurovascular evaluation: No changes.

27.2.4 Preoperative Radiological Assessment/Imaging (Figs. 27.1, 27.2, and 27.3)

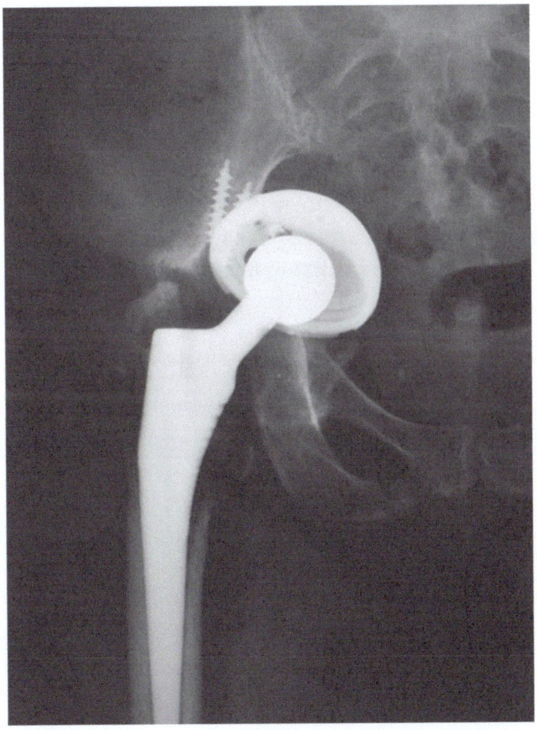

Fig. 27.1 AP hip X-Ray (sent with the patient). Loose acetabular cup, broken screws, and superomedial cup migration. There is an interruption of Kohler's line

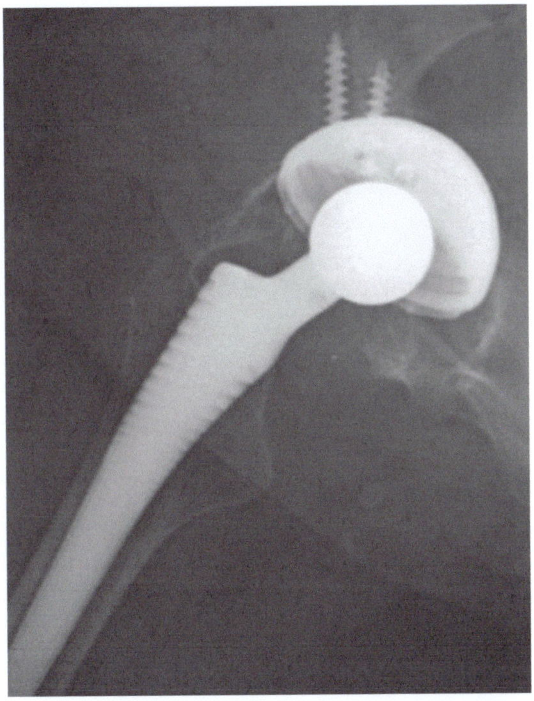

Fig. 27.2 Oblique Judet view X-Ray (sent with the patient). Loose acetabular cup, broken screws, and supermedial cup migration. There is an interruption of Kohler's line

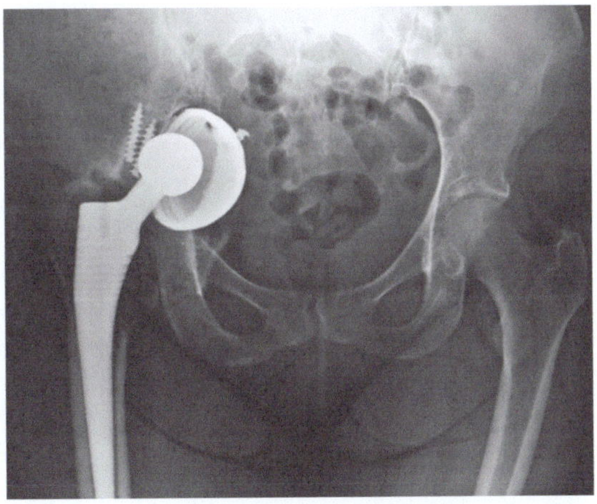

Fig. 27.3 AP Pelvis X-Ray (in our institution). Loose right acetabular cup with breakage of the screws. There is a bone loss and further endopelvic cup migration with apparent destruction of the rim and interruption of Kohler's line (Paprosky type 3 B acetabular defect)

Others: Blood leukocyte count and differential were normal, C- reactive protein 0.1 mg/dL, and erythrocyte sedimentation rate 5 mm/h. Left hip aspiration under X-Ray control—clear fluid with a low count of leukocytes and cultures with no microbial growth.

27.2.5 Preoperative Planning

Diagnosis: Aseptic loosening of the right acetabular cup. According to the Paprosky classification, this is a type 3 B acetabular rim defect from 9 am to 5 pm and superomedial cup migration (endopelvic protrusion) (Figs. 27.1, 27.2 and 27.3). High risk of occult pelvic discontinuity.

Possible treatment options: Acetabular reconstruction cages, trabecular metal cup and augments, hemispherical jumbo, structural and/or morselized bone grafting, combined methods. Posterior column osteosynthesis in case of pelvic discontinuity.

Chosen treatment method: Acetabular reconstruction cage and morselized allograft.

Selection of implants if applicable and rational: Burch-Schneider cage, morselized allograft, cemented primary acetabular cup, and compatible femoral heads (the stem taper was identified in the previous surgical notes). Additionally, column reconstruction plates if the pelvic discontinuity is confirmed and the acetabular cage fixation isn't enough.

Expected difficulties: Careful exposure and removal of the acetabular cup to avoid further bone damage and major vascular bleeding—iliac vessels proximity. In the presence of an intraoperative pelvic discontinuity, we would expect a possible need for additional fixation. The acetabular floor is unable to support the implant, so it must be fixed to the ileum and ischium.

Strategies to overcome difficulties: When a plain X-ray reveals a massive acetabular bone deficiency with endopelvic protrusion of the cup, we routinely perform a preoperative CT angiography to define the vascular location and assess the need of a laparotomic approach isolating the iliac vessels before component removal. If the pelvic discontinuity is detected intraoperatively (CT scan didn't show it preoperatively) and if the acetabular cage fixation isn't sufficient, we will use column reconstruction plate(s).

Templating: In the preoperative templating, we aimed to restore the hip centre of rotation.

27.2.6 Surgical Note

Patient's position: Left lateral decubitus.

Type of anesthesia: General anesthesia.

Surgical approach: Posterior approach.

Main steps: Two grams of cefazolin was given after taking intraoperative tissue cultures.

Reconstruction techniques: The acetabulum was exposed to the cup and the surrounding scar tissue careful removal, trying to avoid any neurovascular lesion. The gluteus medius and minimus were elevated from the superior acetabulum with care to avoid injury to the superior gluteal nerve, so the superior flange of the cage can subsequently be attached. Osteophytes were removed from the circumference of the acetabulum to adequate cage position. Acetabular progressive reaming was used to debride the acetabulum until bleeding from cancellous bone occurs. In this case and because of the medial defect, the periosteum/scar tissue from the acetabular floor must be retained to act as osteoinduction and avoid cement penetration and graft migration. Different trial cages were inserted (to access component size and stability), and the amount of necessary bone graft was determined. After preparation of the descending branch of the ischium, the morselized fresh-frozen bone allograft was used to fill the acetabular defects. The bone graft was impacted by a trial cup and reverse reaming. The Burch-Schneider cage was prepared (adapted to the anatomic situation) and applied in a usual manner (first, the inferior flange is tapped into the ischium until the inferior part is close to the teardrop with subsequent medialization and superior flange fixation into the ilium with screws). Afterwards, the remaining gaps of the acetabular floor were filled with bone allograft, and a thin layer of cement was applied to the cage for the final cementing of the polyethylene cup (Figs. 27.4 and 27.5).

27.2.7 Intraoperative Challenges

Challenges and solutions: Difficulty in removing the cup without any neurovascular lesion. Attention to the proper filling of the defect and allograft bone impaction. When applying the cage, it is important to avoid breaking the ischium.

Unanticipated problems and solution: A possible infection, which would need a component removal, debridement, and a spacer. Extended trochanteric osteotomy may be necessary for stem removal.

Thorough description of decision making, including the reason for the final decision: The option for the Burch-Schneider cage and morselized bone allograft was due to the uncertainty of achieving stability with trabecular metal components and the impossibility of restoring the bone stock in a still young patient.

27.2.8 Postoperative Radiographs (Figs. 27.4 and 27.5)

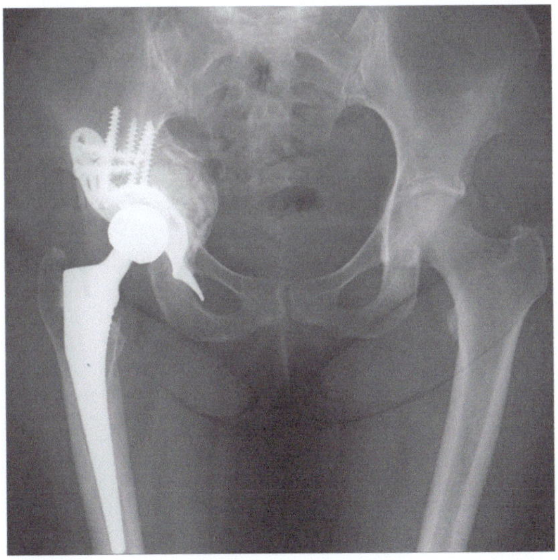

Fig. 27.4 Pelvis X-ray four years after re-revision of right THR. No radiologic evidence of loosening, implant migration, or any sign of fatigue fracture of the cage and/or screws can be observed. Bony incorporation has occurred. The inferior flange was slotted into the ischium with some protrusion to the obturator foramen

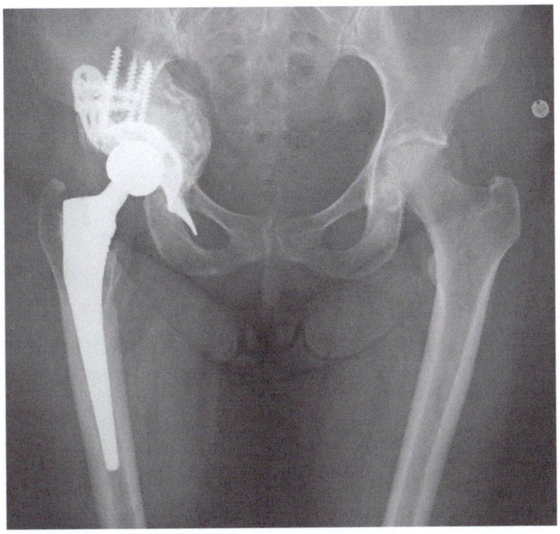

Fig. 27.5 Pelvis X-ray five years after re-revision of right THR. Presence of a cage fracture (after a fall) without any migration or change in orientation

27.2.9 Postoperative Management

Chemoprophylaxis and anticoagulant treatment period: Enoxaparin 40 mg SC for one month.

Gait/limb loading until full loading: Partial weight bearing with two crutches for eight weeks.

27.2.10 Follow-up and Complications

Cage fracture after a fall documented by X-ray. After the incident, the patient gradually returned to its previous state without any complaint. This fracture raises some concerns about a possible fatigue fracture without any relationship with the previous fall. Some authors concluded that fracture of the cage or breakage of the screws without continuing migration or change in orientation of the cage should not be defined as a failure.

Scoring: Harris Hip Score at five years' follow-up—87.2

27.2.11 Discussion

Advantages of the applied method: The goals are to obtain a primary fixation, to restore the normal hip mechanics, and to reconstitute the bone stock, providing a durable long-term fixation of the acetabular components [7, 45]. The use of a cage partially protects the grafted bone from excessive loading during incorporation and remodeling processes [42, 45, 46]. Following these principles, we can aim to fulfil our objectives. Also in the presence of an occult pelvic discontinuity, this system could be a good solution [7, 46]. Thereby this option can be used with favorable survivorship in the more severe defects like Paprosky type 3A and 3 B or in the presence of a pelvic discontinuity [46]. For segmental defects, some authors defend the use of structural and morselized bone grafting while others advocate the use of a well-impacted morselized graft [46]. There is a high complication rate (bone collapse and loss of support) with the use of structural bone allografts. Therefore, a close fit between the graft and the residual acetabulum, in addition to a good mechanical anchorage of the cage to the host bone, is critical to the successful outcome of the reconstructive procedure [7, 45, 46].

Disadvantages of the method: The major concern with standard acetabular cages is the lack of a porous coating for bone ingrowth [7]. Consequently, the potential for long-term biological fixation through osseointegration is not predictable [7]. Cement used for cup fixation may penetrate in the bone-cage interface interfering with bone graft remodeling and incorporation [7, 46]. However, the potential risk of interdigitating with the bone graft could lead to an increased stability of the cup-cage-bone system [7]. There is also a concern about possible disease transmission with allografts. An additional limitation is the a need for a wide exposure of the supra-acetabular ilium, involving the risk to injury of the superior gluteal nerve. Moreover, cages may require a prolonged delay in weight bearing to reduce overloading on the cage (fatigue fracture) and prevent possible graft reabsorption and cage migration [7, 42, 45, 46].

Alternative evidence-based techniques for the case: Undoubtedly, trabecular metal components provide an attractive alternative for complex acetabular pelvic reconstructions, but only short-term to midterm results are currently available [7, 42, 46]. The possibility of micromovements and metal wear between the cup and augment is also a concern. In younger patients, we should consider other techniques that restore the bone stock.

Why is the chosen technique better for this case? This procedure permits the reestablishment of the hip biomechanics and leads to a bone stock restoration in a still young patient, who may require another intervention in the future.

Indications and contraindications for your technique: Severe defects like Paprosky type 3A and 3B or in the presence of a pelvic discontinuity. In cases that we aim for a major bone stock restoration. When a standard revision cup with/without augments cannot be used due to the lack of stability/press fit.

Learning curve and how to manage complications: The use of reconstruction cages and allografts is technically more demanding than the trabecular metal components.

Level of evidence concerning the superiority of this method against others: Using a Burch-Schneider cage can be considered as a reliable procedure to manage acetabular deficiencies and appears to be able to successfully restore vital bone stock at long-term follow-up [7, 42, 45, 46].

27.3 Case Title: Acetabular Revision "Reinforcement Rings"—Long-Term Result of the Burch-Schneider Cage Use

Rashid Tikhilov, Igor Shubnyakov, and Alexey Denisov

27.3.1 Demographics

Age: 55
Sex: Female
BMI: 31

27.3.2 Relevant Past Medical History

Principal pathologies: Hip arthritis.

Previous surgical procedures: In 1991, using the Russian uncemented hip implant "Phenix" with ceramic-on-polyethylene bearing surfaces, the primary total hip arthroplasty was performed. The first revision of the acetabulum component occurred three years later due to severe osteolysis. A cemented cup was implanted with cement filling bone defects. The patient subsequently underwent three further revisions, each using cement fixation of the acetabulum. Two years have passed from the last revision.

Medication: NSAIDs.

27.3.3 Clinical Examination

Symptoms: Permanent groin pain during activity and intermittent pain at rest.

Range of motion: Flexion 70°, extension 0°, external rotation 20°, internal rotation 0°, adduction 20°, abduction 0°.

Specific tests: Trendelenburg's sign.

Main disability: Walking with two crutches, inability to walk up the stairs, unable to work.

Scoring if available: Harris Hip Score: 32 points.

Neurovascular evaluation: There were no neurovascular problems.

27.3.4 Preoperative Radiological Assessment/Imaging (Figs. 27.6, 27.7, and 27.8)

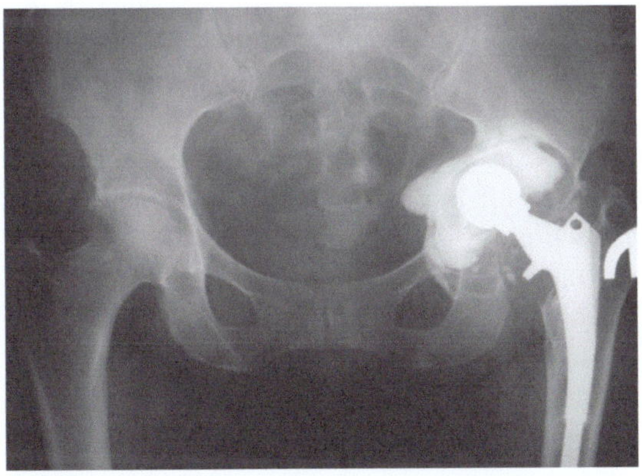

Fig. 27.6 The anterior view X-ray of the pelvis demonstrates the joint prosthesis with aseptic loosening of the acetabular component—type 3B bone Paprosky defect. Superomedial migration, centre of acetabulum is >3 cm above the obturator line osteolysis, medial protrusion of the bone cement, violation of Kohler's line

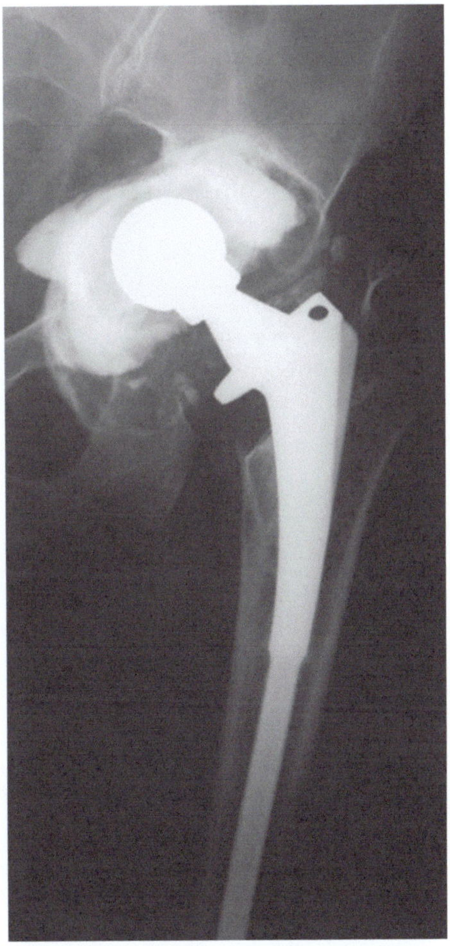

Fig. 27.7 The anterior view X-ray of the left hip jointshowing a continuous radiolucent line

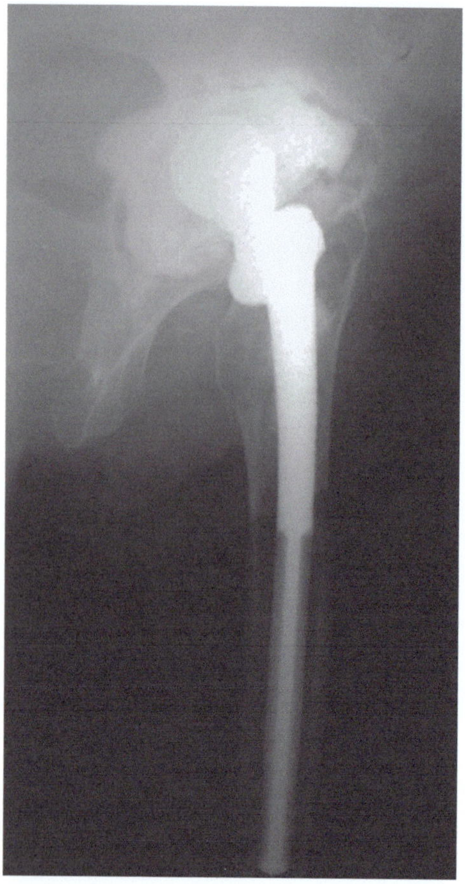

Fig. 27.8 Lateral view X-ray of the left hip joint demonstrating the defect that is more than one-half of circumference, located between 9 o'clock and 3 o'clock

27.3.5 Preoperative Planning

Diagnosis: Aseptic loosening of the cemented cup, Paprosky defect of the acetabulum type IIIB (Figs. 27.6, 27.7 and 27.8).

Possible treatment options: Revision arthroplasty using jumbo cup or reinforcement device. In 2005, there was no possibility for TRM system.

Chosen treatment method: Burch-Schneider Cage.

Selection of implants if applicable and rational: In young patients, the use of morselized allograft with Burch-Schneider Cage promotes restoration of bone; it allows the next revision to restore the correct anatomical level with a cementless cup.

Expected difficulties: Insufficient bone stock.

Strategies to overcome difficulties: Reconstruction of the surrounding supporting structures and insertion of the Burch-Schneider cage.

Templating: determining the approximate size of the cage.

27.3.6 Surgical Note

Patient's position: Lateral decubitus position and stabilizing the pelvis with a central sacral pad and two anterior pads against the iliac crests and above the anterior superior iliac spines. The supine position may not allow for full access to the acetabulum.

Type of anesthesia: Spinal anesthesia and neuroleptanalgesia. Spinal anesthesia provides excellent muscular relaxation and results in less blood loss.

Surgical approach: Direct lateral approach.

Main steps: Soft tissue release; dislocation and removal of the head of the femoral component; removal of the acetabular implant with the cement mantle and the membrane; evaluation of the defect; the ilium, dome, the anterior and posterior columns are examined; impaction of the morcellized allograft; using a trial cup and determining the size of the cage and contouring flanges; insertion of the cage and screws fixation carried out; implantation of the cemented cup; reduction of the femoral head and evaluation of the range of motions; closing of the wound.

Reconstruction techniques: After removal of the unstable implant and debridement, bone autograft is used. The morcellized bone is impacted to support the cage. Impaction is carried out using reverse reaming. The diameter of the final reamer determines the outer diameter of the Burch-Schneider cage. Cage insert in the correct position, the positioning of the cemented acetabular component, and insertion of the head of the endoprosthesis (Figs. 27.9 and 27.10).

27.3.7 Intraoperative Challenges

Challenges and solutions: The presence of the femoral component obstructs the removal of the acetabulum component and the reconstruction.

Unanticipated problems and solution: No.

27.3.8 Postoperative Radiographs (Figs. 27.9 and 27.10)

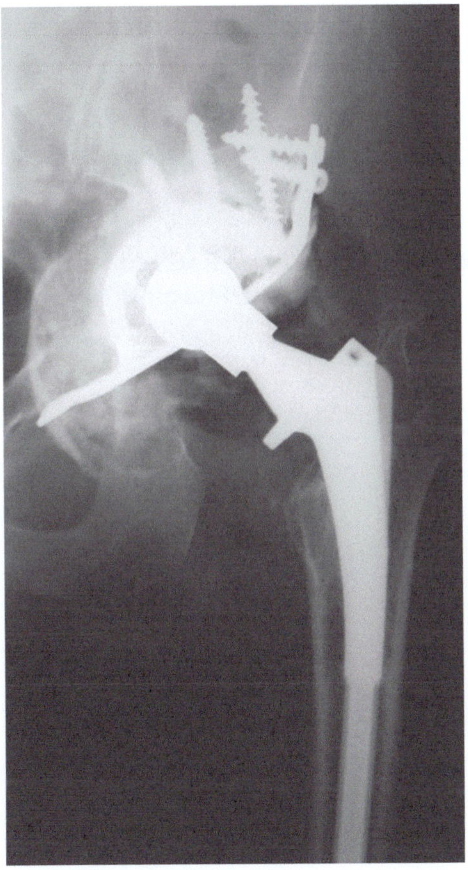

Fig. 27.9 Postoperative radiograph after acetabular reconstruction using a BS cage and a cemented socket

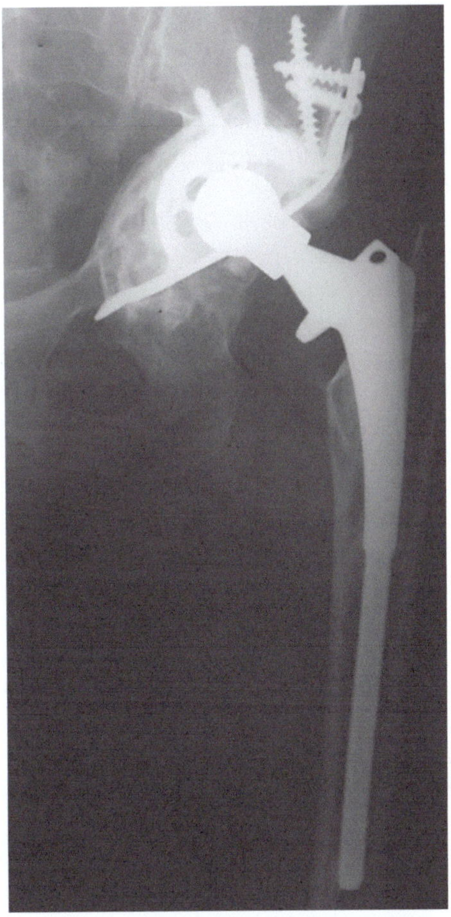

Fig. 27.10 Radiograph of the same patient 10 years postoperatively, showing the remodeling of the allograft and no migration of the BS cage

27.3.9 Postoperative Management

Chemoprophylaxis and anticoagulant treatment period: Cefazolin three days, LMWHs (Clexane ten days), and warfarin three weeks MHO (1.3–1.5).

Gait/limb loading until full loading: Walking with crutches for 1.5 months with no weight bearing.

27.3.10 Follow-Up and Complications

There were no complications.

Scoring: at 10 years HHS: 82 points.

27.3.11 Discussion [2, 8, 10]

Advantages of the applied method: The cage promotes restoration of the bone; it allows the next revision to reconstruct the correct anatomic level with a cementless cup.

Disadvantages of the method: The cage has a limited life span, because of no biologic fixation—osteointegration impossible, only mechanical fixation with screws.

Alternative evidence-based techniques for the case: TM cup with augments is another option for many types of defects. The TM cup with augment uses the oblong cup principle (of filling the defect), but since the augment is separate from the cup, one can place the cup independently.

Why is the chosen technique better for this case? In a younger, higher demand patient, this may be a better choice.

Indications and contraindications for your technique: Large contained defects—contained defects involving the entire acetabulum requiring a device that spans from ilium to ischium, used with morcellized allograft bone. Uncontained defects involving more than 50% of the acetabulum. The cage can be used in conjunction with a structural allograft. Pelvic discontinuity—a cage is used to bridge the discontinuity. A graft may also be necessary. If the cage does not stabilize the discontinuity, a plate can be used with the cage. Cages can be used in irradiated bone and also allow the use of a constrained cup.

Learning curve and how to manage complications: Use of this surgical technique only by experienced surgeons.

Level of evidence concerning the superiority of this method against others: Expert opinion.

27.4 Case Title: Acetabular Revision "Reinforcement Rings"

Fritz Thorey

27.4.1 Demographics

Age: 76
Sex: female
BMI: 22.15

27.4.2 Relevant Past Medical History

Principal pathologies: Cup loosening.

Previous surgical procedures: Total Hip Arthroplasty in 2007.

Medication: Painkiller

History of presenting complaint: Since the primary THA there was no improvement of complaints.

27.4.3 Clinical Examination

Symptoms: Pain, limitations in walking and ADL, pressure pain in the groin, and the major trochanter.

Range of motion: Flexion/extension 80-10-0°, internal/external rotation 10-0-10°.

Main disability: Severe pain during walking.

Scoring if available: VAS for pain: 6; Harris Hip Score: 39 (without sections 2 and 3); HOOS: 39.4 (subscales, symp: 40%; pain: 47.5%; function: 48.5%; sports: 0%; QOL: 18.75%).

Neurovascular evaluation: Normal.

27.4.4 Preoperative Radiological Assessment/Imaging (Figs. 27.11, 27.12, and 27.13)

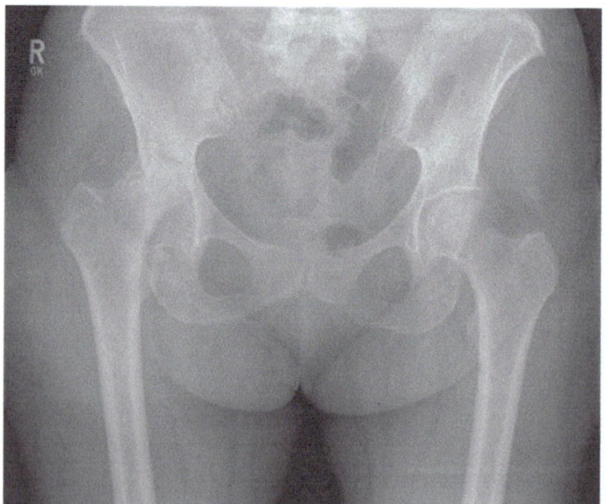

Fig. 27.11 Preoperative pelvic X-ray

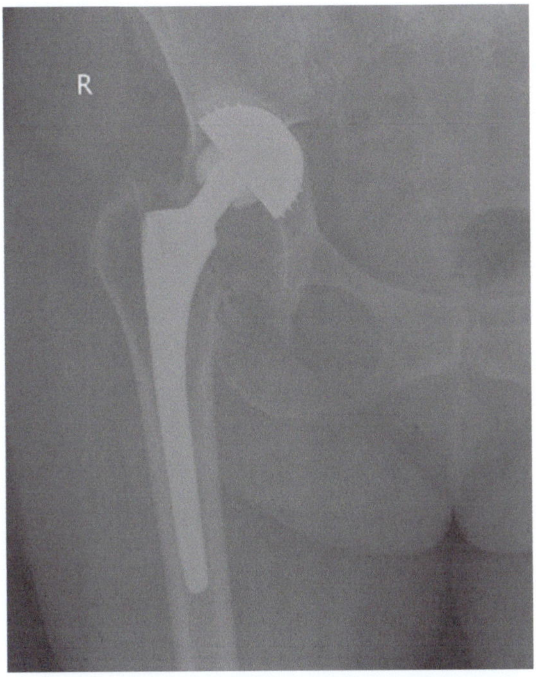

Fig. 27.12 AP X-ray eight years after the primary THA

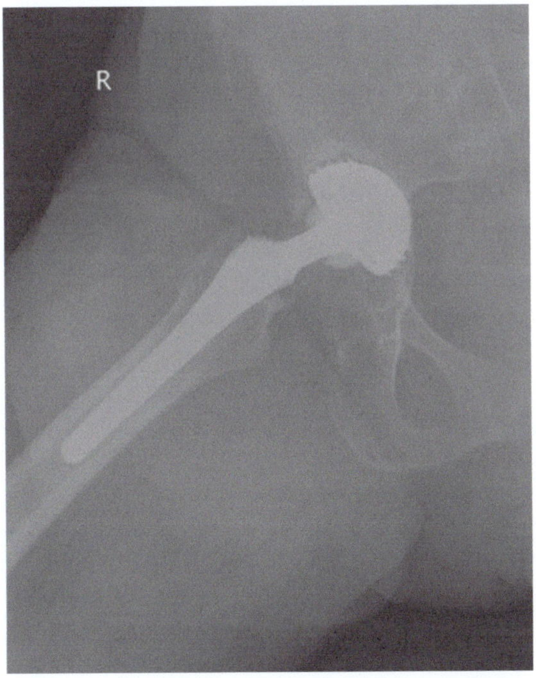

Fig. 27.13 Lateral X-ray eight years after the primary THA

27.4.5 Preoperative Planning

Diagnosis: Cup loosening with protrusion (Figs. 27.12 and 27.13).

Possible treatment options: Revision of the cup.

Chosen treatment method: Revision of the cup with allograft impaction grafting.

Selection of implants if applicable and rational: Primary cup, in case of bone deficiency a revision cage or jumbo cup.

Expected difficulties: Bone deficiency at the acetabular side.

Strategies to overcome difficulties: Availability of different revision cages and bone bank.

Templating: Templating with a revision and a primary cup.

27.4.6 Surgical Note

Patient's position: Supine.

Type of anesthesia: General anesthesia.

Surgical approach: Modified lateral transgluteal.

Main steps: Mobilization of the proximal femur, visualization of the cup, and acetabular defect.

Reconstruction techniques: Impaction grafting with bone chips on the acetabular side (Figs. 27.14 and 27.15).

27.4.7 Intraoperative Challenges

Challenges and solutions: Careful debridement of the deep bone defect to reconstruct the acetabulum, fixation of the revision cage.

Unanticipated problems and solution: None were found; a possible problems might be the loss of the medial wall (Paprosky IIIa/b).

Thorough description of decision making, including the reason for the final decision: Deep bone defect and mild loss of anterior and posterior wall, a revision cage was chosen.

27.4.8 Postoperative Radiographs (Figs. 27.14 and 27.15)

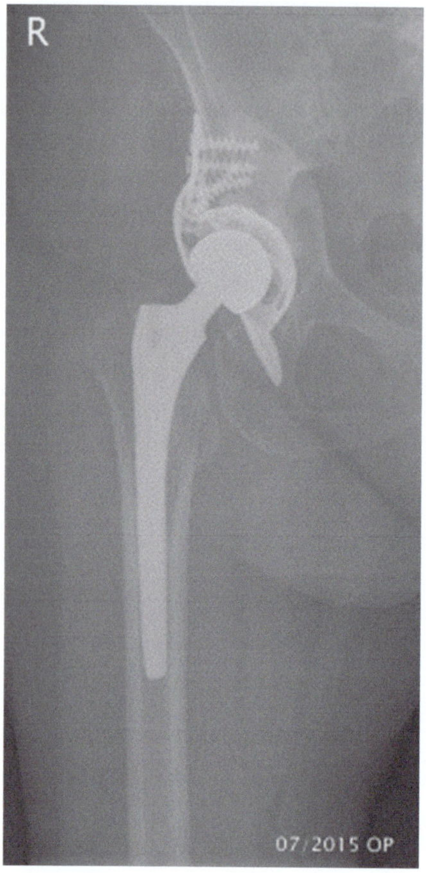

Fig. 27.14 AP view showed the reconstruction of the bone defect and reconstruction of the centre of rotation to the original position

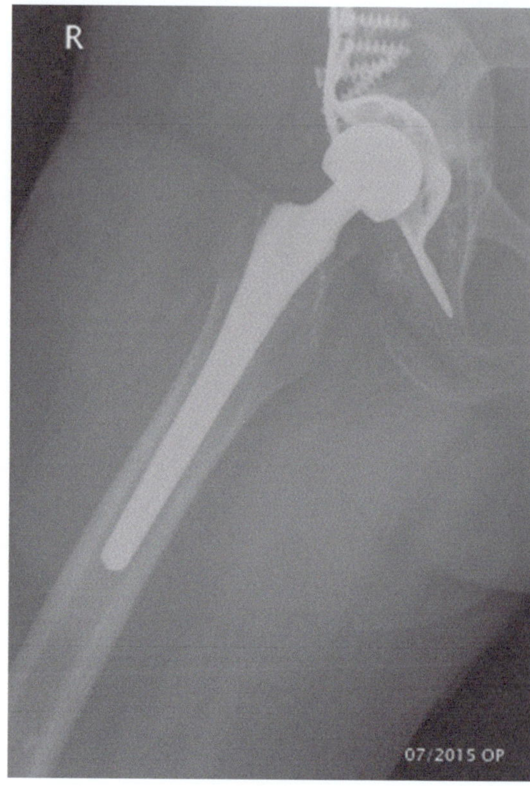

Fig. 27.15 Axial view showed the correct position of all implants

27.4.9 Postoperative Management

Chemoprophylaxis and anticoagulant treatment period: Xarelto for four weeks, antibiotics for seven days.

Gait/limb loading until full loading: Weight bearing as tolerated from the first postoperative day.

27.4.10 Follow-Up and Complications

No complications.

Scoring: VAS for pain: 1; Harris Hip Score: 89 (without sections 2 and 3).

27.4.11 Discussion [7, 13, 45]

Advantages of the applied method: Good primary stability, compression of impaction grafting.

Disadvantages of the method: None.

Alternative evidence-based techniques for the case: Reconstruction of the bone defect with trabecular metal.

Why is the chosen technique better for this case? Based on the age of the patient and the bone defects, this is the better reconstruction treatment.

Indications and contraindications for your technique: Age of the patient, bone stock and defects.

Learning curve and how to manage complications: Longer learning curve due to the technique of impaction grafting and implantation of revision cage.

27.5 Case Title: Acetabular Revision for Paprosky-3B Acetabular Defect

Volodymyr Filippenko, Volodymyr Mezentsev, and Mandus Akonjom

27.5.1 Demographics

Age: 60
Sex: Female
BMI: 35.6

27.5.2 Relevant Past Medical History

Principal pathologies: Aseptic loosening and instability of the left uncemented acetabular cup with protrusion into the pelvis.

Previous surgical procedures: Uncemented primary THA three years ago.

Medication: Analgesics and NSAID's, antibiotics, and anticoagulants.

Others: Obesity and peripheral vascular disease (varicose veins) of both lower extremities.

History of presenting complaint: five months after the primary THA, the patient presented with left groin pain, limping, and leg length discrepancy with pelvic obliquity. The pain was mild and initially bearable but gradually became severe three months later; pain was said to be relieved at rest and aggravated with ambulation. She noticed increased difficulty with weight bearing on the affected limb and ambulated with the aid of crutches. There was no history of fever, anorexia, nausea, weakness, or weight loss.

27.5.3 Clinical Examination

Symptoms: Moderate pain, leg length discrepancy of 30 mm, Trendelenburg's gait, postsurgical scar on the lateral thigh, abductor muscles weakness, and pelvic obliquity.

Range of motion: Extension/flexion 0/15/70, abduction/adduction 0/0/10, external rotation/internal rotation 15/0/15.

Specific tests: CBC-T/D: within normal; serum electrolyte, urea, and creatinine: normal; CRP: negative; ESR: 8 mm/h; aspiration: negative; ECG, CT, contrast angiography, Doppler USS: all within normal limits.

Main disability: Pain, limping, inability to bear weight, pelvic obliquity.

Scoring if available: VAS: 5, HHS: 30.

Neurovascular evaluation: All major lower limb nerves (sciatic, femoral, obturator, and superior gluteal) and vessels were intact.

27.5.4 Preoperative Radiological Assessment/Imaging (Figs. 27.16 and 27.17)

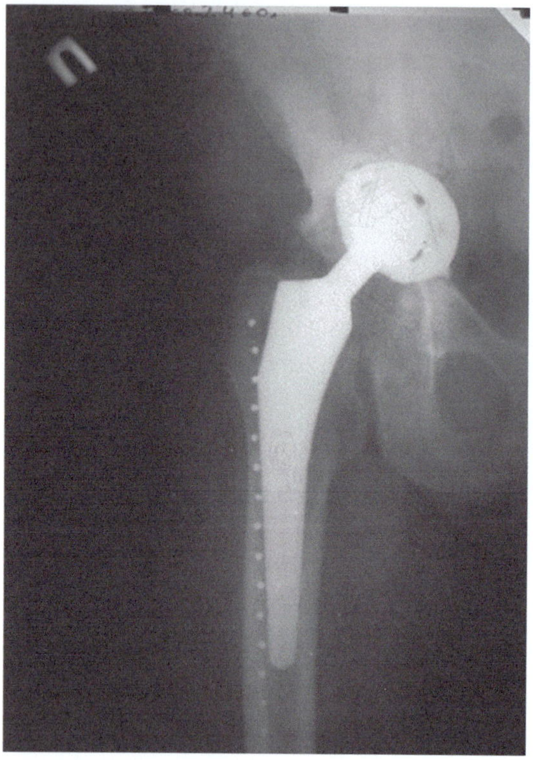

Fig. 27.16 AP X-ray view of the right hip showing uncemented implant with migration into the pelvis and Paprosky type IIIb defect

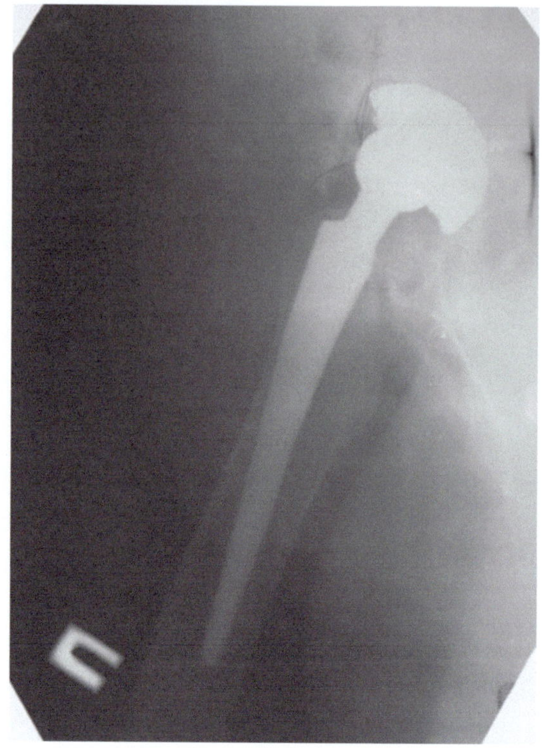

Fig. 27.17 Lateral X-Ray view of the right hip showing protrusion of the prosthetic cup into the pelvis

27.5.5 Preoperative Planning

Diagnosis: Aseptic loosening and instability of the uncemented acetabular cup of the right hip with protrusion (Figs. 27.16 and 27.17).

Possible treatment options: Revision THA with (1) acetabulum reconstruction with reinforcement cage and bone grafting, (2) cementless or cemented cup with bone grafting, (3) cup cage and acetabular reconstruction, (4) trabecular metal cup with augments.

Chosen treatment method: Reconstruction of acetabular defects with reinforcement cage and bone grafting.

Selection of implants if applicable and rational: Restoration of the hip rotation centre, secure mechanical support on ilium and ischium, reliable incorporation of cancellous graft, mechanical protection for structural graft, and restoration of bone stock for later revision were the rational for our choice of Burch-Schneider cage.

Expected difficulties: Difficulty in reconstructing acetabular bone defect (Paprosky type 3b) due to significant bone loss and poor bone quality.

Strategies to overcome difficulties: Preparing cancellous and structural allografts for reconstructing acetabular bone defects (cavitary, segmental, combined).

Templating: Manual templating was done with AP and lateral radiographs using standard templates supplied by the manufacturers.

27.5.6 Surgical Note

Patient's position: Lateral decubitus.

Type of anesthesia: Spinal anesthesia.

Surgical approach: Direct lateral approach.

Main steps: Through a direct lateral approach, a midline incision of about fifteen cm, beginning three cm above the greater trochanter was made and the tissues dissected to the right hip joint. The fibrous tissue and capsule were incised, and the prosthetic cup was removed after dislocating the femoral head. Paprosky type 3b acetabular defect was visualized intraoperatively. The segmental defects of the medial wall of the acetabulum were filled with structural allografts and impacted and reamed to prepare the bed for the cage. The allografts were from two femoral heads. Cavity defects of superior and anterior walls of the acetabulum were filled with morcellized bone grafts. Next was the insertion of the Burch-Schneider cage with the attachment of proximal flange at the ilium and distal flange at the ischium. The proximal flange of the cage was held in place with five screws. We inserted a cemented cup into the cage and reduced the femoral head into its anatomical position (Figs. 27.18 and 27.19).

Reconstruction techniques: The segmental defect of the medial wall of the acetabulum of 2.5 cm in diameter was reconstructed using allograft from the femoral head which was reamed to permit cage insertion. cavitary defects of the superior and anterior walls of the acetabulum were filled by morcellized bone grafts. The inferior flange of Burch-Schneider cage was first attached to the ischium and the superior flange attached to the ilium with five screws under intraoperative X-ray control.

27.5.7 Intraoperative Challenges

Challenges and solutions: There was a difficulty with the acetabular exposure because we were not revising the stem; using, however, an extended approach we overcome this difficulty. Dislocating the prosthetic head from the acetabular cup was another challenge due to the protrusion. An extensive resection of fibrous tissues and the capsule with partial resection of the iliopsoas and abductors were carried out to facilitate dislocation. The bone defect of acetabulum intraoperatively was greater than what was anticipated preoperatively. We had to use additional allograft to reconstruct the segmental defect.

Unanticipated problems and solution: There was no unanticipated problem encountered during this procedure.

Thorough description of decision making, including the reason for the final decision: Intraoperatively we decided to use six screws to achieve adequate fixation and stability of the cage.

27.5.8 Postoperative Radiographs (Figs. 27.18 and 27.19)

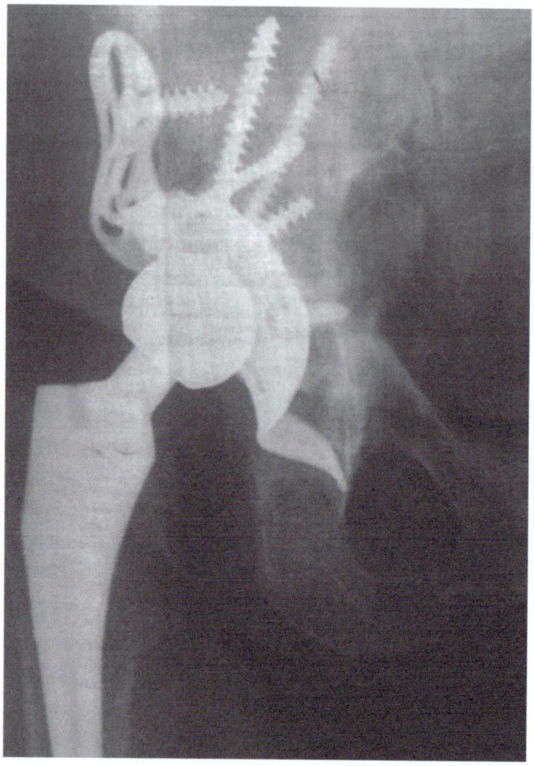

Fig. 27.18 AP postoperative view after revision THA on right hip with Burch-Schneider cage showing the restoration of the bone stock and hip rotation centre

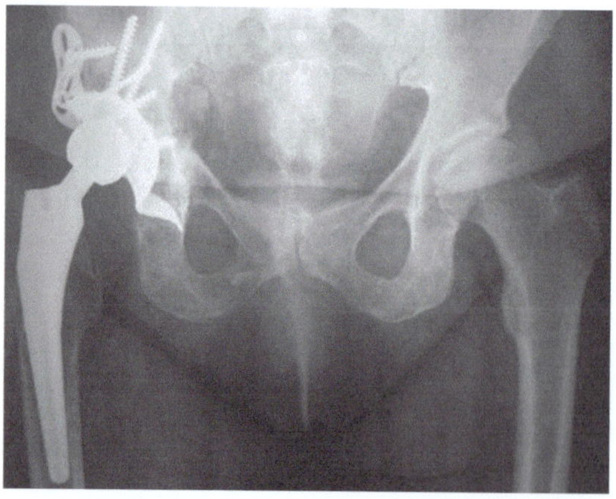

Fig. 27.19 AP view six years after revision THA on right hip demonstrating the stable implant, no osteolysis around the cage and the allograft incorporation with the restoration of bone stock

27.5.9 Postoperative Management

Chemoprophylaxis and anticoagulant treatment period: Ceftazidime 1000 mg twice daily for seven days, Clexane 40 mg once daily for thirty five days postoperatively, celecoxib 200 mg once daily for seven days, one unit of whole blood.

Gait/limb loading until full loading: Patient was on restricted weight bearing with crutches for six months before commencing full weight bearing. During this period, there was limited hip flexion and adduction until full weight bearing.

27.5.10 Follow-Up and Complications

Report of postoperative complications and their management (i.e., recurrent dislocation): There was a postoperative hematoma which was aspirated and covered with antibiotic prophylaxis. Follow-up was at an interval of 3, 6, and 12 months and subsequently yearly.

27.5.11 Discussion [12, 47, 48]

Advantages of the applied method: Restoration of hip rotation centre, secure mechanical support on ilium and ischium, reliable incorporation of cancellous graft, mechanical protection for structural graft, restoration of bone stock.

Disadvantages of the method: Wide exposure increases neurovascular risks, the potential for decreased abductor function and limp, mechanical construct, dependent on multiple screws for long-term fixation, loosening, or breakage at repeated loads. Mechanical fixation, rather than biologic fixation, as there is lack of porous coating for bone growth. The potential for osseointegration is not predictable.

Alternative evidence-based techniques for the case: (1) acetabulum reconstruction with reinforcement cage and bone grafting, (2) cementless or cemented cup with bone grafting, (3) cup cage and acetabular reconstruction, and (4) trabecular metal cup with augments.

Why is the chosen technique better for this case? This technique increases the chance of biological restoration of bone stock. The use of the Burch-Schneider cage enables the surgeon to achieve secure fixation of the flanges to the ilium and ischium, and it protects extensive acetabular bone graft by transferring some of the load from the acetabulum to the ilium and the ischium.

Indications and contraindications for your technique: At present, the cage is indicated for the revision arthroplasty with large acetabular floor or roof defects, acetabular destruction by metastases, and acetabular fractures when immediate weight bearing is desired, following Girdlestone. Contraindications for this procedure are Paprosky type I and II acetabular bone defects.

Learning curve and how to manage complications: This procedure has a steep learning curve and should only be undertaken by experienced surgeons who practice in centres with high-volume surgery.

Level of evidence concerning the superiority of this method against others: Level III evidence.

27.6 Case Title: Acetabular Revision Using a Cementless Cup with a Hook and Flanges

Georgios Petsatodis and Filon Agathangelidis

27.6.1 Demographics

Age: 42
Sex: Female
BMI: 26

27.6.2 Relevant Past Medical History

Principal pathologies: Developmental dysplasia of the right hip.

Previous surgical procedures: Cementless total hip arthroplasty four months ago.

Medication: None.

History of presenting complaint: The patient experienced intermittent hip pain since the age of eighteen. She presented to our outpatient clinic complaining of night pain and inability to walk even short distances without excruciating pain. She underwent cementless total hip replacement. Four months postoperatively, the acetabular component failed, and the patient was admitted to our department to undergo a revision hip arthroplasty.

27.6.3 Clinical Examination

Symptoms: Hip pain and unable to fully weight bear.

Range of motion: Flexion 0-40°, adduction 0°, and abduction 10°.

Main disability: Unable to fully weight bear without pain.

Neurovascular evaluation: Neurovascular status of the involved right lower extremity was intact.

27.6.4 Preoperative Radiological Assessment/Imaging (Figs. 27.20, 27.21, and 27.22)

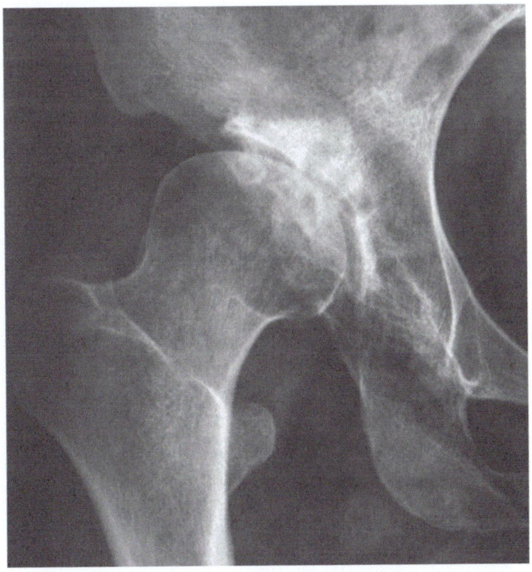

Fig. 27.20 Anterolateral radiograph of the right hip. Osteoarthritis secondary to developmental hip dysplasia

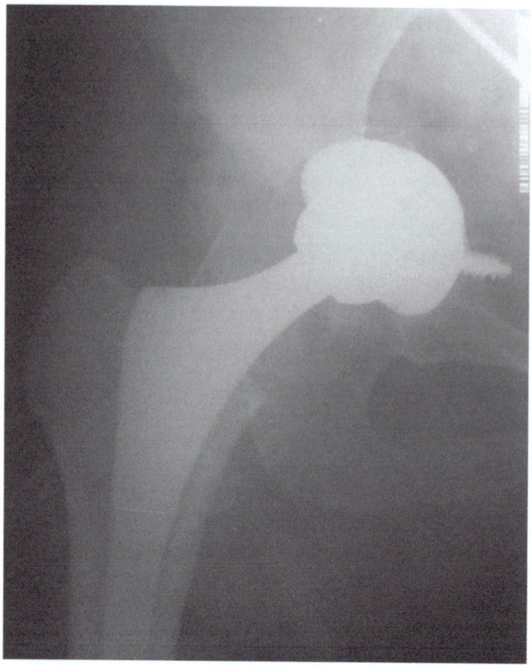

Fig. 27.21 Postoperative anterolateral radiograph: cementless total hip arthroplasty

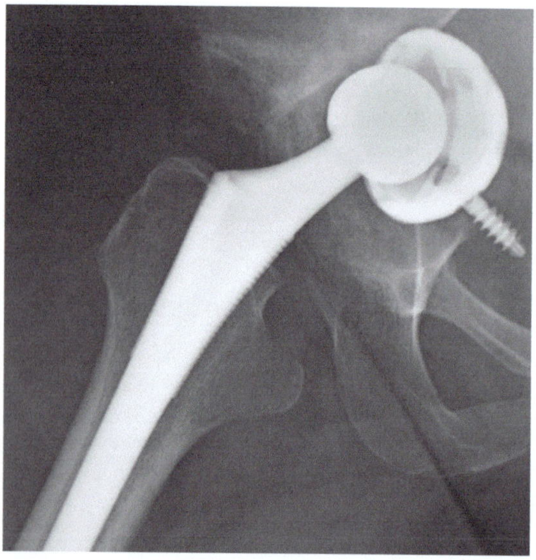

Fig. 27.22 Anterolateral radiograph four months postoperatively: failure of the acetabular component

27.6.5 Preoperative Planning

Diagnosis: Failure of the acetabular component of cementless total hip replacement (Figs. 27.20, 27.21 and 27.22).

Possible treatment options: Revision total hip arthroplasty.

Chosen treatment method: Revision total hip arthroplasty.

Selection of implants if applicable and rational: (1) Trabecular metal acetabular revision system, (2) porous titanium-hydroxyapatite flanged revision cup, and (3) Burch-Schneider antiprotrusio cage.

Expected difficulties: Insufficiency of the anterior wall that would make implantation of a press-fit cup difficult.

Strategies to overcome difficulties: Intraoperative availability of various revision systems ranging from trabecular metal revision cup to antiprotrusio cage. A freeze-dried femoral head allograft was also available.

27.6.6 Surgical Note

Patient's position: Lateral decubitus.

Type of anesthesia: General anesthesia.

Surgical approach: Anterolateral Hardinge's approach.

Main steps: Surgical approach, dislocation, removal of the acetabular cup, grafting of the acetabular floor, and implantation of the flanged revision cup.

Reconstruction techniques: Following the removal of the acetabular cup, there was a defect which was classified as IIC according to the Paprosky classification. The rim was intact but with a weak anterior wall. The previous cup migrated medial to Kohler's line, and as a result, there was a significant medial wall defect. We used a freeze-dried femoral head as a structural allograft. Using an oscillating saw, a four to five millimeters slice was cut from the largest diameter of the head. This was used to cover the medial wall defect. We prepared the acetabulum by reaming progressively up to 56 mm and paying attention to push the reamer posteriorly since the anterior wall was insufficient. Using a bone mill, the remains of the femoral head were morselized and impacted around the structural graft at the acetabular floor. A flanged revision cup was implanted (Hilock Rev., Symbios, Switzerland)

and supported by four screws, two through the flange and two through the superior part of the cup. A highly cross-linked polyethylene liner was used with an elevated lip placed posteriorly (Figs. 27.23 and 27.24).

27.6.7 Intraoperative Challenges

Challenges and solutions: The first challenge was to remove the cup without causing neurovascular damage. In our case, the failure occurred briefly following the index surgery. In chronic cases, we have been using a CT angiography to ascertain the proximity of the cup to the pelvic blood vessels. The second challenge was to estimate the acetabular deficiency and use an implant which would provide primary stability with the minimum surgical trauma. We also had to take into account the young age of our patient which warrants that any implant used will need revision in the future.

Thorough description of decision making, including the reason for the final decision: Our case involved a young patient with a dysplastic hip. We planned the revision surgery, making sure that a wide range of implants was available. The best-case scenario would be a trabecular metal cup and the worst an antiprotrusio cage. Since we had a young and active patient, we aimed for an implant which would provide enough primary stability with minimal surgical trauma. Intraoperatively the defect was classified as IIC according to Paprosky, with a large medial wall defect and a weak anterior wall. Therefore, a press-fit hemispherical implant would not be a safe option. Fortunately, the rim was intact, and there was no need for a cage. The final decision included a porous-coated flanged revision cup which had the benefit of excellent primary stability. We also reconstructed the acetabular floor. The combination of the grafting technique with a porous-coated cup is a biomechanically friendly option. The primary stability provided by the flanges and the screws promotes bony incorporation of the cup. Furthermore, over time the bone graft undergoes revascularization and remodeling, and we believe that it provides secondary stability to the cup and adequate bone bed for a revision when needed in the future.

27.6.8 Postoperative Radiographs (Figs. 27.23 and 27.24)

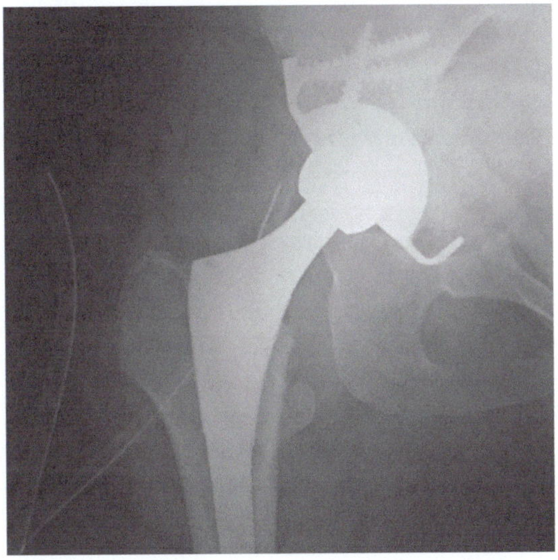

Fig. 27.23 Anteroposterior radiograph of the right hip following the revision surgery

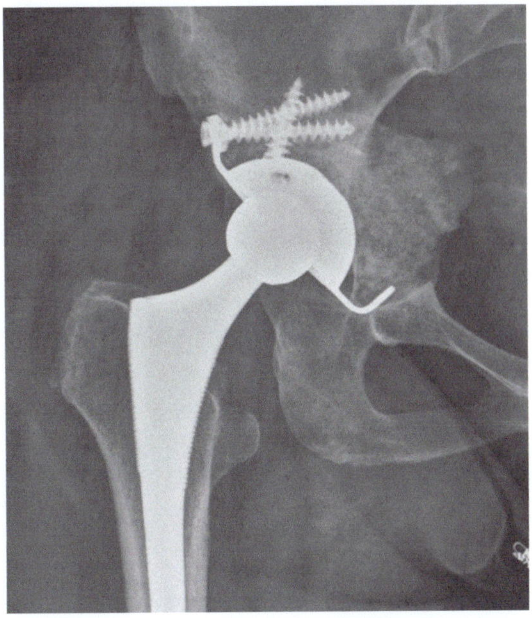

Fig. 27.24 Anteroposterior radiograph of the right hip six months postoperatively. Note the medial wall reconstruction and incorporation of the bone grafts

27.6.9 Postoperative Management

Chemoprophylaxis and anticoagulant treatment period: Intravenous cefuroxime and amikacin 48 hours perioperatively and 45 days of 4500 units of tinzaparin once daily.

Gait/limb loading until full loading: Partial weight bearing with crutches for two months.

27.6.10 Discussion

Cemented cups in acetabular revision have been linked to unacceptably high failure rates in the mid and long term [6]. Current treatment strategies involve options ranging from uncemented hemispheric reconstruction to antiprotrusio cage. The final decision depends mainly on the assessment of acetabular bone loss [1, 49]. In our case, we were prepared to use a wide range of implants if necessary. Intraoperatively, the bone defect was classified as a largely contained defect of the medial wall. A large trabecular metal cup could also have been used, but we preferred an acetabular component with an ischium hook and two iliac flanges. This design is relatively new, and there are few reports in the literature with promising results [50]. We have used this type of implant to treat defects up to IIIC according to Paprosky classification, and we agree that the midterm outcome is very good. Primary stability is warranted by the use of screws until osseointegration occurs. The bone defects in all our cases were reconstructed using allografts either structural, morselized, or a combination of both, and there were no instances of bone resorption. We assume that this is due to the primary stability and porous coating this cup design offers.

Level of evidence concerning the superiority of this method against others: Level IV.

References

1. Sheth NP, Nelson CL, Springer BD, Fehring TK, Paprosky WG. Acetabular bone loss in revision total hip arthroplasty: evaluation and management. J Am Acad Orthop Surg. 2013;21:128–39.
2. Regis D. Acetabular reconstruction with the Burch-Schneider antiprotrusio cage and bulk allografts: minimum 10-year follow-up results. Biomed Res Int. 2014;9:194076.
3. Deirmengian GK, Zmistowski B, O'Neil JT, Hozack WJ. Management of acetabular bone loss in revision total hip arthroplasty gregory. J Bone Joint Surg Am. 2011;93:1842–52.
4. Starker M, Kandziora F, Jager A, Kerschbaumer F. Acetabular reconstruction using acetabular reinforcement rings. Orthopade. 1998;27:366–74.
5. Daniel J. Berry antiprotrusio cages for acetabular revision. Clin Orthop. 2004;420:106–12.
6. Pulido L, Rachala SR, Cabanela ME. Cementless acetabular revision: past, present, and future revision total hip arthroplasty: the acetabular side using cementless implants. Int Orthop. 2011;35:289–98.
7. Regis D, Sandri A, Bonetti I, Bortolami O, Bartolozzi P. A minimum of 10-year follow-up of the Burch-Schneider cage and bulk allografts for the revision of pelvic discontinuity. J Arthroplast. 2012;27(6):1057–1063.e1.
8. Ilyas I, Alrumaih HA, Kashif S, Rabbani SA, Faqihi AH. Revision of type III and type IVB acetabular defects with Burch–Schneider antiprotrusio cages. J Arthroplast. 2015;30:259–64.
9. Gill TJ, Siebenrock K, Oberholzer R, Ganz R. Acetabular reconstruction in developmental dysplasia of the hip: results of the acetabular reinforcement ring with hook. J Arthroplast. 1999;14(2):131–7.
10. Ewers A, Spross C, Ebneter L, Külling F, Giesinger K, Zdravkovic V, Erhardt J. 10-year survival of acetabular reinforcement rings/cages for complex hip arthroplasty. Open Orthop J. 2015;9:163–7.
11. Schlegel UJ, Bitsch RG, Pritsch M, Clauss M, Mau H, Breusch SJ. Mueller reinforcement rings in acetabular revision outcome in 164 hips followed for 2–17 years. Acta Orthop. 2006;77(2):234–41.
12. Regis D, Magnan B, Sandri A, Bartolozzi P. Long-term results of anti-protrusio cage and massive allografts for the management of periprosthetic acetabular bone loss. J Arthroplast. 2008;23(6):826–32.
13. Angles AC-MF, Tramunt C, Casanova X. Burch-Schneider antiprotrusio cage for acetabular revision: a 5- to 13-year follow-up study. Hip Int. 2010;20(Suppl 7):S112–8.
14. Abolghasemian M, SadeghiNaini M, Tangsataporn S, Lee P, Backstein D, Safir O, Kuzyk P, Gross AE. Reconstruction of massive uncontained acetabular defects using allograft with cage or ring reinforcement an assessment of the graft's ability to restore bone M. Abolghasemian, stock and its impact on the outcome of re-revision. Bone Joint J. 2014;96:319–24.
15. Paprosky W, Sporer S, O'Rourke MR. The treatment of pelvic discontinuity with acetabular cages. Clin Orthop Relat Res. 2006;453:183–7.
16. Sembrano JN, Cheng EY. Acetabular cage survival and analysis of factors relatedto failure. Clin Orthop Relat Res. 2008;466:1657–65.

17. Ruatti S, Grimaldi M, Saragaglia D. Section of the sciatic nerve by a metal acetabulum reinforcement ring: a literature review through one case. Eur J Orthop SurgTraumatol. 2012;22(Suppl 1):S117–20.
18. Berry DJ, Muller ME. Revision arthroplasty using an anti-protrusio cage for massive acetabular bone deficiency. J Bone Joint Surg Br. 1992;74(5):711.
19. Rosson J, Schatzker J. The use of reinforcement rings to reconstruct deficient acetabula. J Bone Joint Surg Br. 1992;74(5):716.
20. Zehntner MK, Ganz R. Midterm results (5.5–10 years) of acetabular allograft reconstruction with the acetabular reinforcement ring during total hip revision. J Arthroplast. 1994;9(5):469.
21. Levai JP, Boisgard S. Acetabular reconstruction in total hip revision using a bone graft substitute. Early clinical and radiographic results. Clin Orthop Relat Res. 1996;330:108.
22. Garbuz D, Morsi E, Gross AE. Revision of the acetabular component of a total hip arthroplasty with a massive structural allograft. Study with a minimum five-year follow-up. J Bone Joint Surg Am. 1996;78(5):693.
23. Schatzker J, Wong MK. Acetabular revision. The role of rings and cages. Clin Orthop Relat Res. 1999;369:187.
24. Bohm P, Banzhaf S. Acetabular revision with allograft bone. 103 revisions with 3 reconstruction alternatives, followed for 0.3–13 years. Acta Orthop Scand. 1999;70(3):240.
25. van der Linde M, Tonino A. Acetabular revision with impacted grafting and a reinforcement ring: 42 patients followed for a mean of 10 years. Acta Orthop Scand. 2001;72(3):221.
26. Winter E, Piert M, Volkmann R, et al. Allogeneic cancellous bone graft and a Burch- Schneider ring for acetabular reconstruction in revision hip arthroplasty. J Bone Joint Surg Am. 2001;83(6):862.
27. Goodman S, Saastamoinen H, Shasha N, et al. Complications of Ilioischial reconstruction rings in revision total hip arthroplasty. J Arthroplast. 2004;19(4):436.
28. Ilchmann T, Gelzer JP, Winter E, et al. Acetabular reconstruction with the Burch- Schneider ring: an EBRA analysis of 40 cup revisions. Acta Orthop. 2006;77(1):79.
29. Ochs BG, Schmid U, Rieth J, et al. Acetabular bone reconstruction in revision arthroplasty: a comparison of freeze-dried, irradiated and chemically-treated allograft vitalised with autologous marrow versus frozen non-irradiated allograft. J Bone Joint Surg Br. 2008;90(9):1164.
30. Gaiani L, Bertelli R, Palmonari M, et al. Total hip arthroplasty revision in elderly people with cement and Burch-Schneider anti-protrusio cage. La Chirurgiadegli organi di movimento. 2009;93(1):15.
31. Siebenrock KA, Trochsler M, Sadri H, et al. Hooked roof cup in revision of difficult loose hip prosthesis cups. Results after a minimum of 10 years. Der Orthopade. 2001;30(5):273.
32. Eggli S, Muller C, Ganz R. Revision surgery in pelvic discontinuity: an analysis of seven patients. Clin Orthop Relat Res. 2002;398:136.
33. Gerber A, Pisan M, Zurakowski D, et al. Ganz reinforcement ring for reconstruction of acetabular defects in revision total hip arthroplasty. J Bone Joint Surg. 2003;85(12):2358.
34. Capone A, Setzu V, Ennas F, et al. Ganz reinforcement rings in acetabular revision: indications and medium-term results. La Chirurgiadegliorgani di movimento. 2004;89(2):107.
35. Uchiyama K, Takahira N, Fukushima K, et al. Radiological evaluation of allograft reconstruction in acetabulum with Ganz reinforcement ring in revision total hip replacement. J Orthop Sci. 2010;15(6):764.
36. Korovessis P, Spastris P, Sdougos G, et al. Acetabular roof reinforcement rings. Clin Orthop Relat Res. 1992;283:149.
37. Gurtner P, Aebi M, Ganz R. The acetabular roof cup in revision arthroplasty of the hip. Z Orthop Ihre Grenzgeb. 1993;131(6):594.
38. Pascarel X, Liquois F, Chauveaux D, et al. The use of Muller acetabular rings in revision surgery of total hip prosthesis. Apropos of 141 cases with a minimal 5-year follow-up. Rev Chir Orthop Reparatrice Appar Mot. 1993;79(5):357.
39. Dihlmann SW, Ochsner PE, Pfister A, et al. Analysis of migration of screwed acetabular components following revision arthroplasty of the hip joint. Results of single-image roentgen analysis. Z Orthop Ihre Grenzgeb. 1994;132(4):286.
40. Stockl B, Beerkotte J, Krismer M, et al. Results of the Muller acetabular reinforcement ring in revision arthroplasty. Arch Orthop Trauma Surg. 1997;116(1-2):55.
41. Panski A, Tauber C. Acetabular supporting ring in total hip replacement. Arch Orthop Trauma Surg. 1997;116(4):233.
42. Beckmann NA, Weiss S, Klotz MCM, MatthiasGondan SJ, Bitsch RG. Loosening after acetabular revision: comparison of trabecular metal and reinforcement rings. A systematic review. J Arthroplast. 2014;29:229–35.
43. Symeonides PP, Petsatodes GE, Pournaras JD, Kapetanos GA, Christodoulou AG, Marougiannis DJ. The effectiveness of the Burch-Schneider antiprotrusio cage for acetabular bone deficiency five to twenty-one years' follow-up. J Arthroplast. 2009;24(2):168–74.
44. Pieringer H, Auersperg V, Bfhler N. Reconstruction of severe acetabular bone-deficiency the Burch-Schneider antiprotrusio cage in primary and revision total hip arthroplasty. J Arthroplast. 2006;21(4):489–96.
45. Kawanabe K, Akiyama H, Goto K, Maeno S, Nakamura T. Load Dispersion effects of acetabular reinforcement devices used in revision total hip arthroplasty. J Arthroplasty. 2011;26(7):1061–6.

46. Akiyama H, Yamamoto K, Tsukanaka M, Kawanabe K, Otsuka H, So K, Goto K, Nakamura T. Revision total hip arthroplasty using a Kerboull-type acetabular reinforcement device with bone allograft. J Bone Joint Surg Br. 2011;93:1194–200.
47. Rogers BA, Whittingham-Jones PM, Mitchell PA, Safir OA, Bircher MD, Gross AE. The reconstruction of periprosthetic pelvic discontinuity. J. Arthroplasty. 2012;27(8):1499–506.
48. Korzh NA, Filippenko VA, Mezentsev VA, Bondarenko SE. Reconstruction of acetabular defects in revision total hip arthroplasty. "Ars Medica" Traumatology and Orthopaedics. 2010;9(29):415–7.
49. Lachiewicz PF, Soileau ES. Fixation, survival, and dislocation of jumbo acetabular components in revision hip arthroplasty. J Bone Joint Surg Am. 2013;95(6):543–8.
50. Kim KC, Ha YC, Kang BJ, Lee YK, Ji HM, Koo KH. Use of cementless acetabular component with a hook and iliac flanges in revision arthroplasty for massive acetabular defect. J Orthop Sci. 2012;17(1):18–24.

28 Periprosthetic Infection: Revision Arthroplasty

Eustathios Kenanidis, Iakovos Vlastos, Fares E. Sayegh, Eleftherios Tsiridis, Rihard Trebše, Luigi Zagra, Eleonora Caboni, and Gösta Ullmark

28.1 Current Concepts

E. Kenanidis, I. Vlastos, F. E. Sayegh, and E. Tsiridis

It is a severe complication of Total Joint Arthroplasty (TJA) with laborious management [1]. The main characteristics of the disease that compromise the treatment are:

1. The heterogeneity of the disease concerning:
   (a) Species and sensitivity of the bacteria involved among countries and hospitals
   (b) Patient's characteristics
   (c) Lack of uniform classification
   (d) The timing of infection and local tissue presentation
   (e) Diagnosis of the disease
   (f) Creation of a universally effective treatment protocol
2. The existing studies:
   (a) Lack of high-quality prospective randomized studies [2].
   (b) Studies are mainly focused on the time free of infection but not to the functional improvement and mechanical failure [3].
   (c) The recent meta-analyses are based on data of low-quality previous studies where the virulence of microbes was different [3].

28.1.1 Incidence

- Remained invariable during the last decades [1, 4].
- 0.3–2.9% of primary THA performed [5, 6].
- The third most common reason of failure after primary and the first of revision THAs [1, 7, 8].
- Infection rate is greater during the first two postoperative years than later [1, 9].

E. Kenanidis, M.D., Ph.D., M.Sc. (✉) I. Vlastos, M.D.
Academic Orthopaedic Unit, Aristotle University Medical School, Thessaloniki, Greece

E. Tsiridis, M.D., Ph.D., F.A.C.S., F.R.C.S. (✉)
F.E. Sayegh, M.D., Ph.D.
Academic Orthopaedic Unit, Papageorgiou General Hospital, Aristotle University Medical School, Thessaloniki, Greece
e-mail: etsiridis@doctors.org.uk;
e-mail: fsayegh@auth.gr

R. Trebše, M.D., Ph.D.
Valdoltra Orthopedic Hospital, Ankaran, Slovenia
e-mail: Rihard.Trebse@ob-valdoltra.si

L. Zagra, M.D. · E. Caboni, M.D.
Hip Department, Istituto Ortopedico Galeazzi IRCCS, Milan, Italy
e-mail: luigi.zagra@fastwebnet.it

G. Ullmark, M.D., Ph.D.
Uppsala University, Uppsala, Sweden

Department of Orthopaedic, Gävle hospital, Gävle, Sweden
e-mail: gosta.ullmark@regiongavleborg.se

E. Tsiridis (ed.), *The Adult Hip - Master Case Series and Techniques*,
https://doi.org/10.1007/978-3-319-64177-5_28

28.1.2 Definition of Periprosthetic Joint Infection (PJI)

Aiming to homogenize and make a precise diagnosis of PJI infection, the workgroup of Musculoskeletal Infection Society [10] evolved criteria that were revised by the International Consensus Meeting on PJI [11] and accepted by the Centers for Disease Control [12]. Based on them at least one of the following criteria must be met [1]:

1. Two positive periprosthetic (tissue or fluid) cultures with isolated organism.
2. A sinus tract that communicates with the implant.
3. Three of the ensuing minor criteria must be met:
   (a) Raised CRP and ESR
   (b) Increased synovial WBC count or ++ change on leukocyte esterase test strip
   (c) Raised synovial fluid polymorphonuclear neutrophil percentage (PMN%)
   (d) Positive histological analysis of periprosthetic tissue
   (e) A single positive periprosthetic (tissue or fluid) culture

28.1.2.1 The Following Criteria in Biomarkers Define Acute and Chronic PJI [1]

For acute PJI using of ESR is considered not applicable. Acute PIJ is characterized by CRP serum >100 mg/mL, synovial WBC > 10.000 cells/μL, synovial polymorphonuclear neutrophils >90%, and synovial leukocyte esterase test ++.

Chronic PJI: ESR > 30 mm/h., CRP serum >10 mg/mL, synovial WBC > 3.000 cells/μL, synovial polymorphonuclear neutrophils >80%, and synovial leukocyte esterase test +.

28.1.3 Diagnosis [1, 5]

No single test has 100% sensitivity and specificity for PJI diagnosis [5]. A diagnostic algorithm introduced by the American Academy of Orthopaedic Surgeons [13] and adapted by Parvizi [1] follows.

28.1.3.1 First Step [1]

Begin with history, physical examination and hip X-rays. Possible related to PJI information may be:

(a) History of extended hip pain or stiffness, previous PJI or current bacteremia, many prior hip procedures, immunodeficiency diseases as diabetes mellitus, inflammatory arthropathy, undernourishment, psoriasis, or chronic venous stasis.
(b) The physical examination may reveal increased temperature, redness or irritation of the wound, discharge of trauma, or even dehiscence.
(c) The radiographic evaluation may show focal osteolysis, bone destruction or loosening of a previous well-fixed implant, subperiosteal reactions, or intracortical sinus tract. They are considered positive for PJI especially within the first five postoperative years.

28.1.3.2 Second Step

Evaluate serum ESR and CRP [1]. They have high sensitivity (95–96%) but low specificity for PJI diagnosis [13, 14]. Multiple factors influence their measured levels as the age, the sex, other inflammatory comorbidities, the first postoperative weeks, and the different laboratory methods employed for their evaluation [11, 13]. False-negative ESR and CRP may hide PJI with low-virulence organisms such as *Propionibacterium acne* or coagulase-negative *Staphylococcus aureus* [1].

28.1.3.3 Third Step (Joint Aspiration)

Perform joint aspiration [1] to:

(a) Evaluate synovial biomarkers
(b) Culture

It is not considered necessary for patients with pathognomonic signs as a sinus tract or low-risk patients with normal serological tests. It may be repeated in case of negative initial results but high clinical suspicion [1].

Revision surgery, rheumatoid arthritis, diabetes, obesity, poor nutrition, the immunosuppressive diseases and drugs, and the presence of infective skin lesions are considered risk factors for PJI. In a recent systematic review, Donna

Urquhart et al. [15] supported that the severe pre-existing illness and the longer duration of surgery are independent risk factors for deep infection after primary THA. Conflicting evidence arose for the older age and limited evidence for the number of comorbidities, the condition of trauma, the greater nosocomial infections surveillance risk index, the low income, and the lower surgeon volume.

28.1.3.4 Biopsy [1]

- It is the gold standard for PJI diagnosis with culture.
- Three to five samples of fluid or periarticular tissue are necessary.
- Preoperative arthroscopic or open sampling during revision surgery could be done.
- Swab cultures from the wound or periprosthetic tissues are not recommended.

28.1.3.5 Synovial Fluid Taken from Aspiration Should Be Evaluated

1. **Synovial WBC count and PMN%** [16, 17] (see above)
2. **Synovial biomarkers**
   (a) **Leukocyte esterase (LE)**
   - An enzyme secreted by activated neutrophils.
   - Reported sensitivity and specificity for PJI are 81–93% and 87–100%, respectively [18].
   - LE levels are affected by elevated synovial protein and glucose levels [1].

   (b) **Alpha-defensin**
   - A peptide secreted by human cells and attached to the pathogen's cell wall.
   - Reported sensitivity and specificity for PJI 100% [15].
   - May play an essential role in the evaluation of PJI in the future.
3. **Culture (the gold standard/with biopsy)**
   - The routine time of culture incubation is five days [1].
   - More extended incubation up to two weeks significantly increases yields [19, 20].
   - When low-virulence organisms are suspected, it can be extended up to twenty-one days.
   - In high-risk patients think about fungal or acid-fast bacillus infection.
   - Keep the patient off antibiotics for at least two weeks prior to culture [21].

28.1.3.6 Histological Analysis

- Evaluates the number of PMN/high-power field (HPF) in periprosthetic tissues [22].
- >5–10 PMN per HPF in at least five HPF is a minor diagnostic criterion [22].
- Sharp dissection instead of cautery is recommended for histological analysis.

28.1.4 Imaging

- It has restricted role in the diagnosis.
- The AAOS guidelines cannot recommend in favor or against MRI and CT for diagnosis of PJI (the presence of metal artifacts) [13].
- The most cost-effective and accurate modality of nuclear imaging has not been defined [1].
- Bone scans have very low sensitivity and specificity even when white cell labelling with indium or other agents are used [23].

28.1.5 Classification

Introduced by Tsukayama [24] and further modified [25]. The treatment, however, is not always based on these classifications. The pathogen, the patient, and the local tissue characteristics are also important to determine the outcome [3].

1. **Acute perioperative infection** [26]
   - Acute inflammation caused by perioperative bacterial contamination.
   - Onset: <4–6 weeks [25]/up to three months after surgery.
   - Origin of contamination: (a) Intraoperative, the airways of the surgeons and the skin of the patient. (b) Postoperative, a urinary tract infection (hematogenous) and microlesions from the urinary catheter, a postoperative hematoma, and wound healing disturbance
   - Typical bacteria involved: *Staphylococcus* (*aureus*, *epidermidis*) and *E. coli*

   - Clinical presentation: Fever, chills, sweating, and swollen and red wound
   - Diagnosis: Challenging to differentiate between superficial and deep infection
   - Treatment: Implant salvage (debridement and long-term antimicrobial therapy)
2. **Delayed periprosthetic infection or late chronic infection** [26]
   - Inflammation caused by slow-growing bacteria.
   - Onset: 4 weeks—2 years/never following four years.
   - Origin: Intraoperative contamination by slow-growing bacteria that form the biofilm.
   - Typical bacteria involved: *Streptococcus epidermidis*, *Propionibacterium acnes*, *Peptostreptococcus* spp., and *Corynebacterium* spp.
   - Clinical presentation: Chronic infection, aseptic loosening, and slight pain in projection to the joint.
   - Diagnosis: More complex. There is usually mild elevation of the markers and often negative cultures.
   - Treatment options: (a) One- or two-stage exchange of the prosthesis, thorough debridement and antibiotic therapy delivered systemically and locally with impregnated spacers, and (b) long-term antimicrobial treatment.
3. **Late hematogenous periprosthetic infection or late acute infection** [26]
   - Acute infection close to a previously well-functioning implant
   - Onset: Usually >2 years postoperatively
   - Origin: Hematogenous infection following infection of another organ like pneumonia, urosepsis, dental manipulation, and urinary tract infection
   - Typical bacteria involved: *Staphylococcus aureus*, streptococci, and gram (−) bacteria
   - Clinical presentation: Free of symptoms for some years and then acute onset of symptoms (fever, chills, sweating, red and swollen skin, sometimes a sinus)
   - Treatment options: Implant salvage (rapid debridement and long-term antimicrobial therapy) in the early phase and then one- or two-stage treatment
4. **Unexpected positive culture results in what was thought to be an aseptic revision** [3]

28.1.6 Treatment Options

1. **Suppression therapy**
   - It is only recommended when the surgery is contraindicated (limited life expectancy, serious comorbidities, patient that refuses to undergo revision) [2].
   - Limited literature [1].
   - Trebse et al. [27] reported 96% survival for twenty four patients with infection for less than one year, a stable prosthesis (hip, knee, or internal device) and no sinus track.
2. **Debridement and implant retention**
   - It is indicated for an acute infection (stages I and III), a stable and well-aligned prosthesis, an antibiotic-susceptible organism, and a sufficient soft tissue coverage [2, 28].
   - It involves a thorough debridement, lavage and the exchange of the modular parts of the implant.
   - Reported efficacy 36–73% [2, 29].
   - Lack of I and II level and comparative studies (difficulties to conclude).
   - It has a higher efficacy in acute infection with short duration of symptoms, following a quick initiation of treatment (<1 month), and not antibiotic-resistant bacterium [2].
   - Combination therapies seem more beneficial [2].
   - The proper duration of antibiotic administration is unknown [2].
   - In one of the largest series, Byren et al. [29] evaluated 112 cases (52 THA) retrospectively that treated PJI with debridement, microbiological sampling, early intravenous antibiotics, and a mean of 1.5 years antibiotic therapy. Eradication of infection was reported in 78–89% for 1–3 years. More than six weeks duration of antibiotic therapy was not critical to the outcome, but there was an increased risk

for treatment failure for less than 3–4 months therapy.
- Estes et al. [30] reported two-stage debridement protocol in twenty patients (4 THA and 16 TKA) with acute PJI that were treated with initial debridement, retention of prosthesis and placement of antibiotic-impregnated cement beads, and second debridement with removal of the beads and six weeks of intravenous and a variable course of oral antibiotics. Control of the infection was managed in 18/20 cases.

3. **One-stage revision**
   - It is a single-stage revision followed by fourteen days of intravenous antibiosis and orally for three months.
   - Various techniques are used based on the surgeon experience. Thorough debridement, closure of the dead space, and the bacterial colonization are very important.
   - This technique has the best outcome and may be considered in the immune-competent patients and no serious comorbidities with a healthy soft tissue envelope suffering from an acute infection caused by a single, gram-positive organism sensitive to first-line antibiotics [2].
   - Contraindications: Polymicrobial infections, resistant or anaerobic or unknown organisms, patient with serious comorbidities, sepsis, MRSA, and other highly resistant microorganisms as pseudomonas, soft tissue compromise [31, 32].
   - Advantages: Lower perioperative risk, no exposure to spacer associated risks, financial benefits, lower cost, and maintenance of the function of patient [2, 3].
   - Disadvantages: Risk of recurrent infection.
   - Reported rates free of infection range between 70 and 90% [2, 3, 31].
   - It was reported and used for cementing but also uncemented techniques.
   - In a previous review, Jackson and Schmalzried [32] reported 83% survival rate for 1299 infected THAs treated with one-stage revision at a mean follow-up of 4.9 years. (1) The absence of postoperative wound complications, (2) the good general health, (3) the sensitive *Staphylococcus* or *Streptococcus* spp., and (4) an organism sensitive to the antibiotic in the cement were found as good prognostic factors.
   - Recent studies on one stage for uncemented or hybrid THAs usually with particulate bone grafts reported survival of 82–93% at midterm follow-up [33–35].
4. **Two-stage revision** [2]
   - The gold standard of treatment.
   - For the late chronic and delayed initiation of therapy in the acute infection [2, 3].
   - >90% of success are usually reported [32, 36]. The recorded success ranged from 87.7 to 95% [2, 32, 36, 37]. Luu et al. [37] in a systematic review reported 11% risk of the recurrence of infection for following a two-stage revision in 544 patients.
   - Principles of the two-stage technique [2]:

   (a) Remove all implants and the cement.
   (b) Debride the nonviable or infected soft tissues and bone, the synovial membrane, irrigate, and ream the medullary canal.
   (c) Insert an antibiotic-impregnated cement beads or spacer in the dead space.
   (d) Provide systemic antibiotics for six weeks (in most centers) based on the sensitivities of microbes from intra- or preoperative cultures.
   (e) Continue oral antibiotic administration for up to three months and then following antibiotic holiday of at least two weeks check CRP/ESR for trend.
   (f) If these markers are negative, then proceed to the second stage. If they remain elevated or there are clinical signs of persistent infection, repeat the aspiration.
   (g) There are no cutoff values of ESR and CRP to confirm the eradication of the infection. The actual values may never return to absolute normality, but when the trend is to go down and then stabilize without fluctuation at a relatively low level, and the wound looks good and healed, then reimplantation is advised. The delay

of reimplanatation till markers return to normal compromises the functional result.

(h) Second procedure: Repeat the aspiration before implantation
   1. If the contamination exists, then implant a spacer again or think about resection arthroplasty
   2. If not, proceed to reimplantation (at 6–12 weeks/depends on many factors)

– This technique is not unique, and there are many variables that concern the type, the duration of antibiosis, the dead space management, and the time of reimplantation.

– The two-stage technique is related with an increased morbidity and mortality, soft tissue changes, a functional deficit after reimplantation, a potential toxicity associated with the high doses of antibiotics used over a relatively extended period, and acute kidney injury [37]. Although multifactorial, Luu et al. [37] in a systematic review reported 4.8% incidence of acute kidney injury and speculated a possible connection with aminoglycoside contained spacers. One, however, must keep in mind that patients undergoing two-stage revision THA often have more comorbidities.
– Comparable results between cemented and uncemented techniques.

28.1.6.1 Duration of the Antibiotic Therapy Between Stages

– There is no consensus.
– Various treatment protocols have been reported [38–41].
– Most orthopaedic units use 4–6 weeks of intravenous antibiotics ± oral antibiotics for months.
– A prolonged intravenous therapy is proposed for the MRSA and if immunosuppression, a poor soft tissue envelope, or a large sinus exists [5].
– The duration of therapy usually depends on:
  • The patient's medical profile
  • The virulence of the microbe, i.e., MRSA difficult to eradicate with short-term antibiotics
  • Need to check the trend of ESR and CRP reduction
  • Must have a two-week antibiotic holiday, and then check again for markers
  • The clinical evaluation of the soft tissue envelope
  • The radiographic evaluation of the bone resorption
  • The aspiration prior to the second stage

28.1.6.2 Comparison of the Effectiveness of One- to Two-Stage Revision

– Several systematic reviews and meta-analyses [2, 42–46] are supporting no difference in the reoccurrence of infection following one- or two-stage method.
– Engesæter et al. [45] using data from 1987 to 2009 of the Norwegian Arthroplasty demonstrated that the two-stage revision has the higher survival and the lesser chance for re-revision compared with one stage and other methods of revision.
– Leonard et al. [42] analyzed nine poor quality nonrandomized studies comparing one- and two-stage revision. The groups had differences in the baseline characteristics. There was a trend toward a better functional result for one-stage method, but this must be evaluated with caution due to the methodological quality of the studies.
– In a more recent meta-analysis, Kunutsor et al. [43] compare the effectiveness of existing prospective and retrospective cohort studies for one- and two-stage revision and found similar reinfection rates of 8.2 vs. 7.9% respectively.
– Lange et al. [44] compared 36 studies of either one- or two-stage treatment, none of which was randomized or comparative. The risk of re-revision for infection was lower for two stage (10.45 vs. 13.1%).
– These studies [2, 42–46] have major methodological concerns, and they are not considered as definite. They are based on low-quality studies usually prospective comparative studies but no RCTs; they have methodological differences and no consensus on definitions of outcome such as reinfection. Also, there are usually preoperative differences in patient's characteristics between the groups of patients that are treated with the one or the other method.

28.1.6.3 Proposed Surgical Treatment Algorithm [1]

Decide to remove or preserve the implant based on the chronicity of the infection, the fixation of the implant, the microbe resistance, and the soft tissue envelope.

- An acute PJI < 4 weeks in a patient with a stable and aligned prosthesis, an antibiotic-susceptible organism, and a sufficient soft tissue coverage can be managed with debridement, implant retention and antibiotic therapy.
- When PJI > 4 weeks of symptoms (biofilm formation), choose one- or two-stage exchange arthroplasty.

28.1.6.4 Spacers

1. Static: Block or beads of antibiotic-impregnated cement left within the dead space following implant removal [2].
2. Articulating or dynamic [5]
   (a) Monoblock: Antibiotic cement prosthesis supported by a metal endoskeleton/scaffold (either ready or manufactured by the surgeon on a suitable metal rod)

   Handmade [5]
   - Resemble unipolar hemiarthroplasty.
   - They have low cost.
   - They are easy to fashion but have design inconsistencies.
   - In small series, infection eradication of 89–100% [47, 48].

   Custom molded
   - They have a more consistent form.
   - Limited size.
   - 96–100% effectiveness [49, 50].
   - Slightly greater risk of dislocation and fracture.

   Prefabricated
   - They have limited sizes.
   - Predetermined the dose and antibiotic and cannot be tailored to patient's infection.
   - In some studies, dislocation of 0–16% [51, 52].

   (b)Conventionally metal on poly prostheses with antibiotic-loaded cement (PROSTALAC – prosthesis with antibiotic-loaded acrylic cement/or other conventional stems). Different methods of construction.

28.1.6.5 Advantages [2]

1. Local delivery of antibiotics.
2. Maintain limb length and soft tissue tensioning.
3. Easier reimplantation.
4. Improves patient function and prevents bone loss.

28.1.6.6 Disadvantages [2]

1. Due to the unknown release of antibiotics and the variety of bacteria involved, the routine use of vancomycin and carbapenem increases the resistance of bacteria.
2. New potential complications
   - Spacer fracture or dislocation. Jung et al. [53] reported 17% dislocations and 10% fractures with handmade single-size spacer used.
   - Difficulty in removal, migration.
   - Allergic reactions and acute renal failure. Jung et al. [53] reported 2 and 6%, respectively.

28.1.6.7 Articulating Spacers

- They offer range of head size and length [2, 54, 55].
- More mechanically stable with the known concentration of antibiotics [2].
- Spacers using a femoral component as endoskeleton seem to have other advantages [2]:
  1. Superiority at restoring offset and leg length
  2. Tailoring of antibiotics to the infecting organism
  3. Superior functional results and allows longer periods of use before the exchange
  4. Joint stability and early mobilization

Disadvantages: Possible colonization of the exposed articulating surfaces [2]

28.1.6.8 Antibiotic Concentration in Spacers

- The optimal dosage of antibiotic/40 g cement has not been determined.
- In PJI infections, we use only high concentration > 3.6 g of powdered antibacterial, respectively, per 40 g of bone cement.

- Antibiotic should be no more than 10% of the cement used to maintain mechanical integrity.
- Tobramycin, gentamicin, and vancomycin are the most commonly used.
- Vancomycin gained popularity because it is effective against MRSA and MRSE.
- In the systematic review of Iarikov et al. [56], it was found that although the addition of antibacterial drugs to interim antibacterial cement spacers (ACSs) is considered to be standard of care for surgical revision in prosthetic joint infections (PJIs), this is not supported by the literature. There were no randomized trials to compare either ACSs with different concentrations of antibacterials or ACSs with or without antibacterials. There were 20 publications with spacer loaded mostly with vancomycin and aminoglycosides (1–4 gr), but they were uncontrolled, and no association was found with antibacterial load and effectiveness. So their additional benefit to systematic antibiotic therapy was questionable.

28.2 Case Title: Two-Stage Revision for MRSA Infection Using Articulating Spacer

E. Kenanidis and E. Tsiridis

MRSA infected cemented bipolar hemiarthroplasty. Articulated spacer using long Exeter cemented stem and a prophylactic cerclage wire. Second-stage Exeter cemented stem and socket with PLAD for stability. The cemented option was elected to maintain antibiotic delivery throughout the revision process. The articulated spacer (Fig. 28.1) was removed.

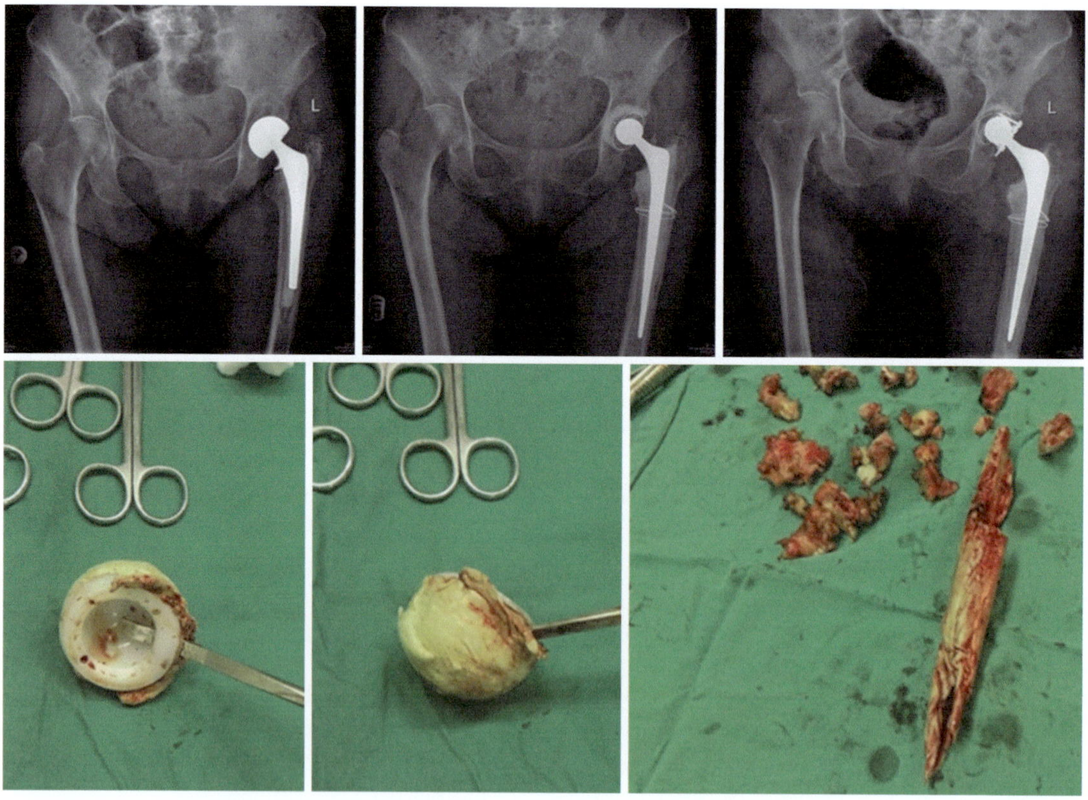

Fig. 28.1 (Upper row): X-ray of the cemented bipolar hemiarthroplasty (left), the articulating spacer with a long cemented Exeter stem (middle) and the second-stage cemented Exeter stem with PLAD (right). (Lower row): polyethylene and parts of cement removed during the operations

28.3 Case Title: Two-Stage Replacement of Chronic Prosthetic Hip Infection Due to *Escherichia coli*

Rihard Trebše

28.3.1 Demographics

Age: 82
Sex: Female
BMI: 30

28.3.2 Relevant Past Medical History

Principal pathologies: Left prosthetic joint infection, right hip osteoarthrosis

Previous surgical procedures: Primary THR 1984, first revision 2004 (femoral component), second revision 2006 (both components)

Medication: Aspirin, pantoprazole, lercanidipine, mirtazapine, alprazolam

Other: History of CVI, juvenile rheumatoid arthritis, arterial hypertension, depression, allergic to metamizole

History of presenting complaint: After the last revision in 2006, she has been doing fine. Seven months before the presentation, she developed a fistula on the right side without fever, and moderate pain judged 4 out of 10 on the visual analogue scale. Together with the development of the fistula, the right hip became painful as well due to end-stage degeneration.

28.3.3 Clinical Examination

Symptoms: Pain 4/10, decreased walking ability

Range of motion: Flexion 100^{0}, retroflexion 0^{0}, abduction 30^{0}, adduction 30^{0}, internal rotation 20^{0}, external rotation 30^{0}

Main disability: Chronic discharge

Scoring if available: HHS 28

Neurovascular evaluation: Normal.

28.3.4 Preoperative Radiological Assessment/Imaging (Figs. 28.2 and 28.3)

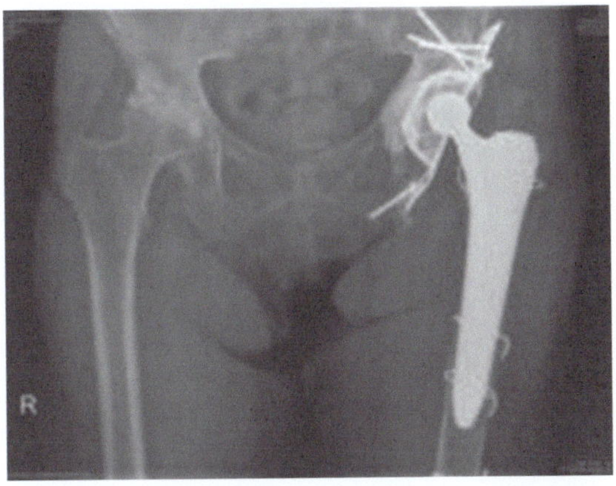

Fig. 28.2 X-ray before the first step. Suboptimally positioned but stable Burch-Schneider ring with a cemented cup, loose screw not in contact with the implant, and stable femoral cementless tapered femoral component. Severe bone loss in the metaphyseal and proximal diaphyseal region

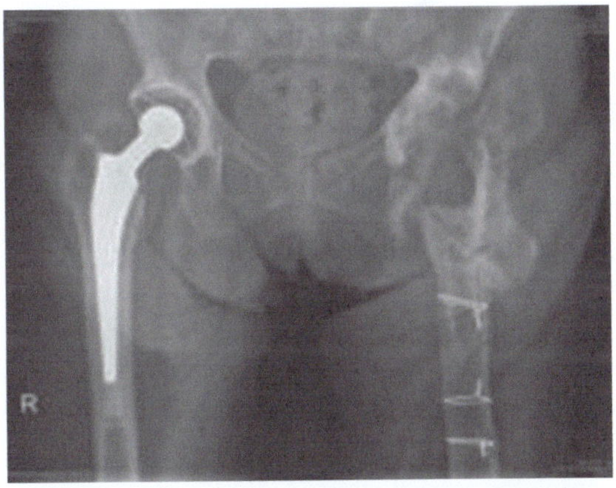

Fig. 28.3 X-ray before the second step: Trochanteric malunion in Girdlestone situation before the second step reimplantation

28.3.5 Preoperative Planning

Diagnosis: Hematogenous infection of the left prosthetic hip (Fig. 28.2)

Possible treatment options: One-stage replacement, two-stage replacement

Chosen treatment method: Two-stage replacement

Selection of implants if applicable and rational: During the first stage, the application of an antibiotic-loaded cement spacer was considered but was not used because the pathogen was not identified before the surgery and due to risky medical condition of the patient before removal of the prosthesis (Fig. 28.3). The second stage was unpredictable, and the possibility to end with the spacer in situ with a patient unfit for second-stage replacement was imminent. For the second stage, a press-fit cup and diaphyseal fixating tapered rectangular stem were selected with a hooked plate with cables for reduction and osteosynthesis of the malunited greater trochanter and proximal femur.

Expected difficulties: Before the first stage, we expected the possibility to fracture the proximal femur during explantation of well-fixed stem due to severe bone loss. Before the second stage, difficulties with achieving appropriate leg length and reduction of the malunited proximal femur were anticipated.

Strategies to overcome difficulties: Since the osteosynthesis of the fractured proximal femur was not performed, we decided to use a Thomas-like brace to ease ambulation. An appropriate length hooked plate with cables was ordered for secure osteosynthesis of the greater trochanter during the second stage. A 3D CT scan was performed before the second stage of the planning of the surgical approach and correct execution of the osteotomies.

Templating: We templated another Burch-Schneider ring with the cemented cup, and a revision tapered quadrangular femoral component.

28.3.6 Surgical Note

Patient's position: Supine

Type of anesthesia: Spinal

Surgical approach: Distally extended direct lateral approach for both steps

Main steps: First stage, before proceeding with the surgery, 10 mL of methylene blue was injected through the fistula opening, and the full range of motion was performed to spread the dye around the pseudo-synovial cavity around the hip. After excision of the scar and the fistula, the fascia was opened and dissected from the underlying tissue. Direct lateral approach was performed to expose the capsule that was dissected from the surrounding tissues anteriorly, superiorly, and medially. The capsule was then excised in all regions but in the posterior part. After dislocation of the femoral component, the interval between the strongly fixed implant and the bone was developed with thin chisels and K wires. Despite careful work, the bone started to fissurize in the weakest region before the stem was out. During the extraction of the stem, the fracture completed. The ball head of the prosthesis and the stem were placed in sterile container with physiological solution and were immediately sonicated. The surgery proceeded with dissection and removal of the posterior capsule. The cemented liner was then chiselled out and the screws removed. The well-fixed ring was then levered out. The acetabular cavity was cleared from cement and debris till the healthy bone bed was achieved. The capsulectomy was nearly completed besides in the most medial part where a sinus protruded deep into the pelvis through the obturator foramen in the region of the acetabular ligament. During debridement of that region, the remaining free screw was found. The complete debridement of the sinus was not considered possible, so we judged the debridement uncomplete, and we decided not to perform the osteosynthesis of the fracture to avoid leaving foreign material in an incompletely debrided cavity. The cerclage wires were well distal to the level of the procedure, so we decided not to remove them. The debridement of the femoral canal was then completed. The wound was then lavaged with copious amounts of saline and closed in layers over a suction drain (Fig. 28.3).

Second step reimplantation: After skin incision, the fascia was prepared and dissected from the underlying tissues and freed to allow suturing at the end. A long distal subvastus approach to femoral diaphysis well distal to the fracture line was performed and advanced to the lateral part of the greater trochanter and continuing short into the abductors to visualize the acetabulum. The acetabular cavity was then cleared of the soft tissues, and tissue biopsies were taken for microbiological and histological analysis.

Reconstruction techniques: The most important is the optimal visualization of the deformed proximal femur, which is the best accomplished through the distally extended direct lateral approach which allows full visualization without compromising trochanter muscles; if there is no need for an extended approach to the acetabulum as in this case where the approach to acetabulum is rather straightforward with an easy reconstruction. The second important point is to implant first the socket then the revision stem and only after that to secure as distal as possible the trochanteric fragment to the construct with a strong hooked plate and wires to allow good gait and function after the second step (Fig. 28.4).

28.3.7 Intraoperative Challenges

Challenges and solutions: During the first step, the most critical challenge is to remove all the unfunctional fibrous tissue all around the artificial hip and to remove all parts of the components. For the soft tissue removal, it is essential to use methylene blue to systematically remove all the infected tissue.

Unanticipated problems and solution: Leg length restoration may be particularly challenging during a second step when there is no spacer. The best option is to implant the larger trial implant with the shortest trial head with the trial acetabulum. The slightly forced range of motion exercises is commenced, and gradually the muscles stretch and a longer head is implantable. The exercises can be repeated several times, and only rarely it is not possible to achieve the correct leg length.

Thorough description of decision-making, including the reason for the final decision: For chronic fistulating PJI, the only option is a two-stage approach. *Escherichia coli* PJI is not very well documented due to their relative rarity. Despite biofilm antibiotics such as fluoroquinolones are usually active against *E. coli*, the long-term outcomes of PJI with this pathogen treated with a less invasive approach such as one-stage replacement are not known.

28.3.8 Postoperative Radiographs (Fig. 28.4)

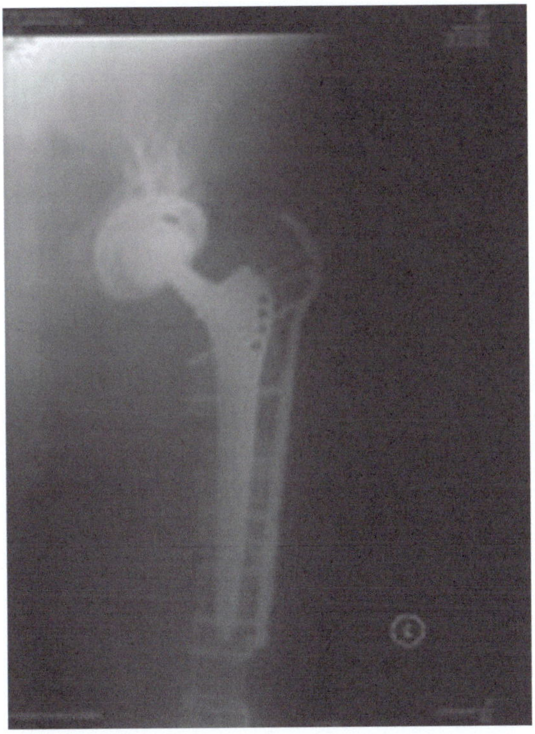

Fig. 28.4 Radiograph of the patient after second-stage reimplantation

28.3.9 Postoperative Management

Chemoprophylaxis and anticoagulant treatment period: After the first-stage explantation and debridement, the patient receives ciprofloxacin 400 mg bid i.v. for eight days continuing with the same antibiotic 750 mg bid orally till the end of the 12th postoperative week. After the second-stage implantation, the antibiotics were administrated till the cultures proved negative at the seventh postoperative day. After both procedures, low molecular weight heparin was administrated subcutaneously till the 35th postoperative day.

Gait/limb loading until full loading: After the first step, the patient was bound to a wheelchair because of simultaneous end-term osteoarthritis of the right hip and the Girdlestone situation in the left hip. After the right hip was operated on with an arthroplasty between the stages, she became ambulatory with crutches. After the second step, she learned to walk with two crutches gradually reducing to one stick.

28.3.10 Follow-Up and Complications

After discharge when still on ciprofloxacin, she developed a mild *Clostridium difficile* diarrhea which was treated successfully with the addition of metronidazole for one week with no other side effect. She was able to complete the antibiotic treatment as planned.

Scoring: At the last follow-up, the HHS was 68, with no pain (1/10 on the visual analogue scale). She was ambulating with one stick.

28.3.11 Discussion [28, 57, 58]

Advantages of the applied method: A two-stage protocol is the safest method for chronic fistulating PJI. With the avoidance of the use of painful articulating spacer, the possibility to end with a patient not fit for the second stage was circumvented. The addition of vancomycin in the spacer wound does not add a lot to the sterilization of the bone bed since vancomycin is not appropriate for gram negatives.

Disadvantages of the method: The length of the leg would be more easily achieved during the second step if a spacer would have been applied with all the shortcomings.

Alternative evidence-based techniques for the case: There are in my opinion no other well-documented techniques for cases where an optimal debridement is not possible due to the intrapelvic extension of the infected sinuses.

Why is the chosen technique better for this case? The chosen technique allows for the most secure infection eradication in this particular setting with the potential of a good functional result.

Indications and contraindications for your technique: There is nearly no contraindication to this technique, but I must stress the importance of tailoring the treatment protocol for patients with a PJI relative to their infection particularities like bone stock availability, age, immune status, infecting agent general health, and preferences. So, this technique is only suitable for some chronic fistulating infection and all chronic infections due to difficult-to-treat organisms.

Learning curve and how to manage complications: The learning time for these procedures is long. The problem is to learn how to radically enough remove the infective tissues in the first step. In the second step, the approach and the removal of the scar are very difficult to master particularly for those not frequently engaged with revision surgery. As for other procedures, high volumes of revisions are the cue for repeatability and reproducibility of the results. Clinical pharmacologist should be an essential part of the team for bone infections to help with overcoming complications related to long and toxic antibiotic regimens after these surgeries.

Level of evidence concerning the superiority of this method against others: There are no randomized and nearly no controlled studies in this field. The best we have is Level III.

28.4 Case Title: One-Stage Replacement for Treatment of a Prosthetic Hip Infection Due to *Staphylococcus epidermidis*

Rihard Trebše

28.4.1 Demographics

Age: 55
Sex: Female
BMI: 28

28.4.2 Relevant Past Medical History

Principal pathologies: Developmental hip dysplasia.

Previous surgical procedures: Shelf plasty at the age of four, THR 2012.

Medication: No medications.

Other: No comorbidities.

History of Presenting Complaint: She has had developmental dysplasia of both hips with shelf plasties bilaterally during childhood. During 2012 she has been operated on the right hip due to increased degeneration of the dysplastic hip. A threaded cementless cup and a metaphyseal fixed cementless stem were implanted. After the surgery, she never felt well with gradually increasing pain and difficulties with ambulation. During the preoperative evaluation, an aspiration was performed growing *Staphylococcus epidermidis* sensitive to all tested antibiotic but penicillin. The diagnosis of a prosthetic hip infection was confirmed.

28.4.3 Clinical Examination

Symptoms: Hip pain judged 8 out of 10 on the visual analogue scale. Limited weight bearing. Walking ability limited to 500 m

Range of motion: Normal

Main disability: Continuous pain

Scoring if available: HHS 48

Neurovascular evaluation: Normal

28.4.4 Preoperative Radiological Assessment/Imaging (Figs. 28.5, 28.6, and 28.7)

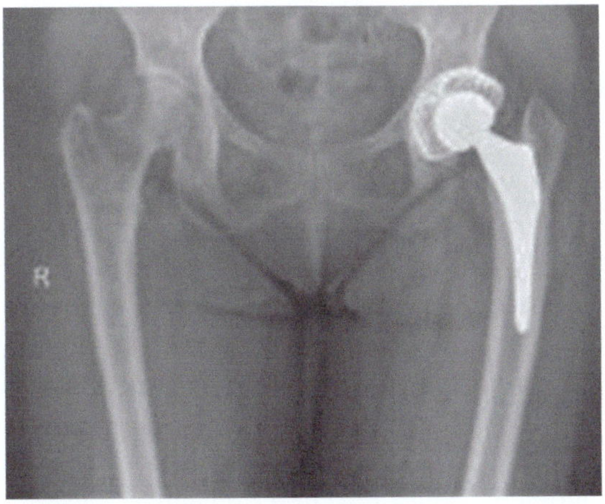

Fig. 28.5 Cementless THR of the left hip. No osteolytic lesions

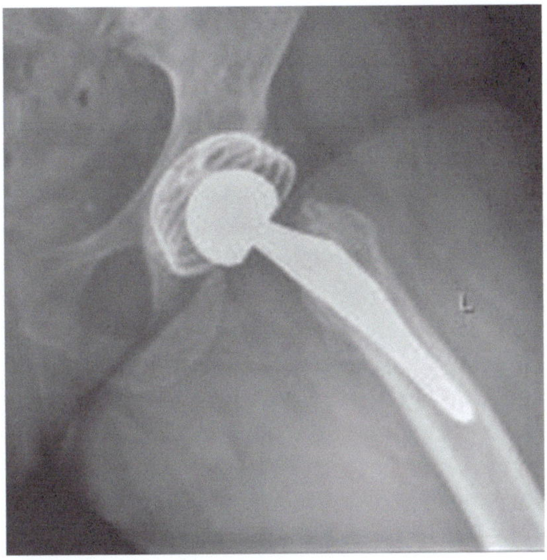

Fig. 28.6 Axial view of the left prosthetic hip

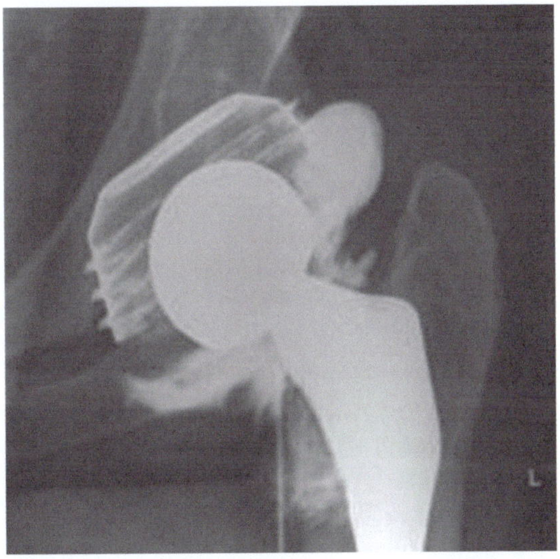

Fig. 28.7 Preoperative arthrography and needle aspiration. The contrast is not filling the interface between implant and the bone indicating a stable implant

28.4.5 Preoperative Planning

Diagnosis: Left prosthetic hip infection (Figs. 28.5, 28.6 and 28.7)

Possible treatment options: One-stage revision, two-stage revision

Chosen treatment method: One-stage revision

Selection of implants if applicable and rational: Due to a shallow acetabulum with dysplastic but preserved acetabular columns and roof, a

Muller ring with a cemented cross-linked polyethylene liner was selected. Antibiotic-loaded cement provided additional protection against recurrence of infection. Before reaming the femoral canal, a cerclage wire was placed to prevent eventual fracture, and a diaphyseal fixed rectangular tapered stem was implanted.

Expected difficulties: Dysplastic hips present difficulties with exposure to a higher risk for trochanter fracture. Primarily a press-fit cup was expected, but intraoperatively the acetabular bone ring was not good enough for a safe press-fit socket implantation.

Strategies to overcome difficulties: To avoid fractures, forceful maneuvers and improve exposure for debridement a distally extended direct lateral approach were selected. A Muller ring was implanted to avoid insufficient stability of a press-fit socket.

Templating: As seen in Fig. 28.8, the templating was performed for a primary acetabular component; intraoperatively a Muller ring was selected instead.

28.4.6 Surgical Note

Position: Supine, hip slightly protruding over the edge of the table

Type of anesthesia: Spinal

Surgical approach: Distally extended direct lateral approach

Main steps: Since the primary implantation was performed through a posterior approach, a new incision line more laterally was selected. A direct lateral distally extended approach starting from the posterior aspect of the origin of the vastus lateralis continued proximally over the trochanter ending approximately 3 cm into the abductors. After the complete exposure of the anterior, superior, and inferior capsule, an aspiration was performed to release the pressure in the capsule and to sample the synovial fluid which was immediately exanimated under the microscope showing 38×10^9/mL cells with 83% of neutrophils confirming the septic nature of the failure. After that, we injected 5 mL of methylene blue in the capsule and moved the joint through the range of motion allowing the dye to spread to all parts of the capsule. Then the capsule was excised completely, leaving no blue parts behind. The synovial cavity extended around the proximal femur but did not protrude into the pelvis, so complete removal was possible. The muscles and tendon attachment were not destroyed by the inflammatory process. The joint was then dislocated. With a thin chisel the interface between the femoral component and the bone was disrupted and the well-fixed femoral component was gently removed. The liner was dislodged from the socket and the bony interface between the threaded acetabular component was chiselled. The implant was then unscrewed with the appropriate tool. All the components were sonicated, and the sonicate was sent for microbiological analyses and tissue samples were sent for microbiology as well, and one was sampled for histological analysis. The acetabulum was then reamed, but the rim was thin and instead of a press-fit implant, Muller ring was screwed in, and a cross-linked liner was cemented in the ring with an antibiotic-loaded cement. Then we placed a cerclage around proximal femur to allow for machine reaming of the canal, and a cementless rectangular stem was implanted and the hip reduced.

Reconstruction techniques: Careful removal of the existing implants. Removal of the capsule and all the necrotic and fibrous tissues leaving all muscles tendons and bones. A reinforcement ring was selected for acetabular reconstruction. The good bone stock allowed for primary femoral replacement (Fig. 28.9).

28.4.7 Intraoperative Challenges

Challenges and solutions: The primary challenge in one-stage replacement is the removal of the infected soft masses till healthy tissue is exposed. Methylene blue injected in the capsule improves the discrimination between healthy and infected tissues. Cerclage wire efficiently prevents cracks during the preparation of the medullary canal.

Unanticipated problems and solution: The capsule extended all around the proximal femur making the complete excision dangerous and complex. An additional exposure of the retro femoral region was necessary to remove the capsule in that region.

Thorough description of decision-making, including the reason for the final decision: The possibility of the complete removal of infected tissues together with the good quality bone and residual functional soft tissues and a known low-virulence organism susceptible to rifampicin allowed the selection of the less invasive one-stage replacement of the infected prosthetic hip.

28.4.8 Postoperative Radiographs (Fig. 28.9)

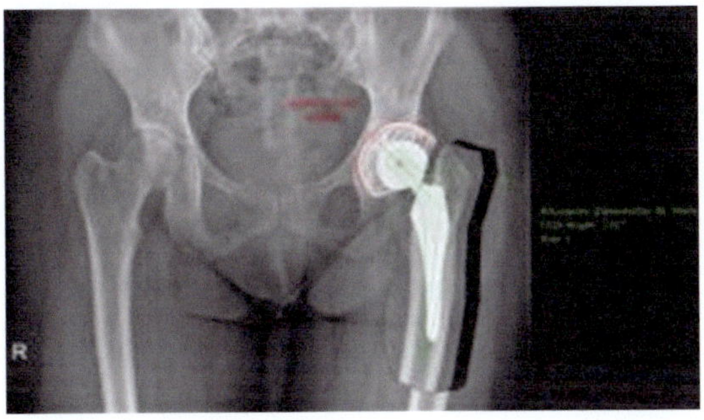

Fig. 28.8 Templating of the revision

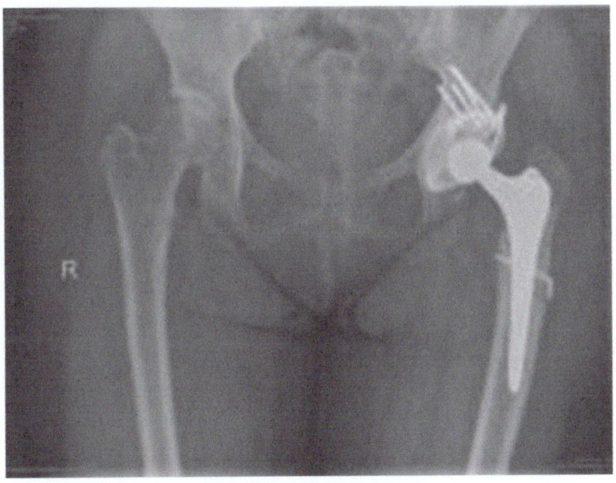

Fig. 28.9 Postoperative X-ray with the appropriate center of the rotation and femoral offset

28.4.9 Postoperative Management

Chemoprophylaxis and anticoagulant treatment period: Anti-staphylococcal intravenous penicillin together with oral rifampicin (after the wound dried) were administrated for fourteen days and then switched for a combination of oral ciprofloxacin 750 mg bid and rifampicin 450 mg bid for additional ten weeks. The patient received thirty five days of low molecular weight heparin subcutaneously.

Gait/limb loading until full loading: Full weight bearing was allowed as tolerated.

28.4.10 Follow-Up and Complications

There was no postoperative complication.

Scoring: HHS after three months was 75, pain 3 out of 10.

28.4.11 Discussion [43, 59, 60]

Advantages of the applied method: The main advantage is only one surgical step and good functional recovery with low operative morbidity.

Disadvantages of the method: One-step revisions have in general a slightly lower rate of infection eradication.

Alternative evidence-based techniques for the case: Due to long-lasting low-grade infection debridement and retention as a potential alternative was not an option.

Why is the chosen technique better for this case? In this case, with a low-virulence pathogen susceptible to rifampicin, good soft tissues and good general health better functional result without compromising the eradication rate was the reason for selection of the one-stage technique.

Indications and contraindications for your technique: Good soft tissues, preoperatively known low-virulence organism, and no fistula limit are the indications for this technique. Difficult to treat organisms, polymicrobial flora, poor condition of soft tissues. Unfeasibility of a radical soft tissue debridement and the need to debride functional tissue are the contraindication for the technique.

Learning curve and how to manage complications: Long learning curve is expected for mastering appropriate soft tissue debridement. The implantation of revision implants is usually easy. Explantation of well-fixed components can be very frustrating and may cause bone fractures, particularly if appropriate tools are not available.

Level of evidence concerning the superiority of this method against others: Only a few controlled studies are available so the level of evidence is mainly III.

28.5 Case Title: "Two-Stage Revision of an Infected THA"

Luigi Zagra and Eleonora Caboni

28.5.1 Demographics

Age: 51
Sex: M
BMI: 29.92

28.5.2 Relevant Past Medical History

Principal pathologies: Smoker (5–10/day), HBV+, HCV+, HDV+

Previous surgical procedures: Tonsillectomy

Medication: Methadone

Other: Drug addict in the past

History of Presenting Complaint: 1998 Left THA. 2002 Two-stage revision for septic loosening (*Staphylococcus aureus*). 2013 recurrence of fistula (negative cultures). 2014 painful hip with clear X-ray signs of loosening of the stem

28.5.3 Clinical Examination

Symptoms: Painful hip. Walking is possible only with two crutches.

Range of motion: Severe limitation of ROM due to pain

Specific tests: Swelling of the thigh (the fistula is closed for few months)

Main disability: Pain and severe walking limitation

Neurovascular evaluation: No neurovascular lesions detected.

28.5.4 Preoperative Radiological Assessment/Imaging (Figs. 28.10, 28.11, and 28.12)

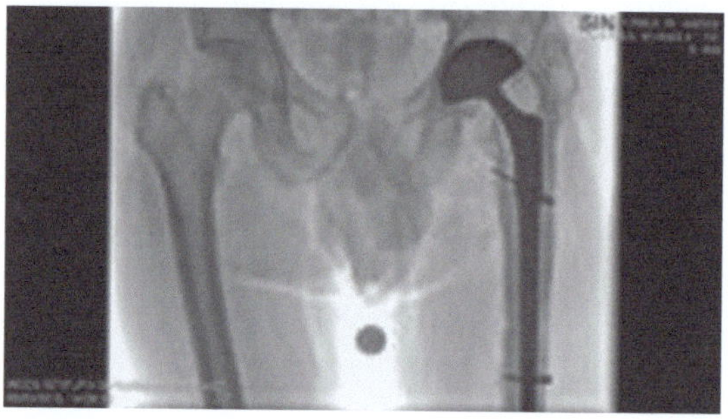

Fig. 28.10 Preoperative AP X-rays of the pelvis showing the loosening of the stem

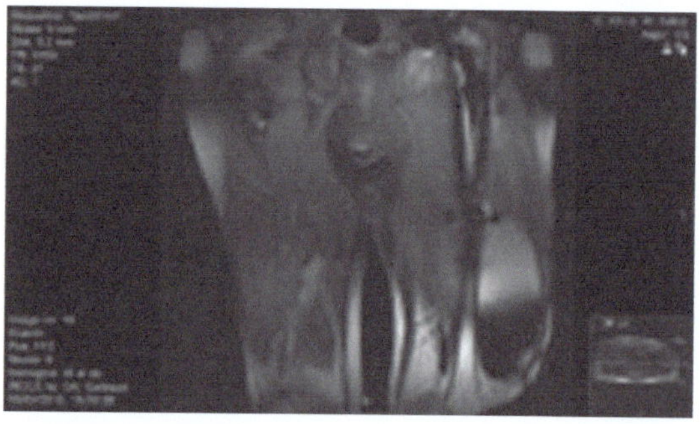

Fig. 28.11 MARS MRI showing huge fluid collection from the joint extending distally along the thigh until the proximal aspect of the knee

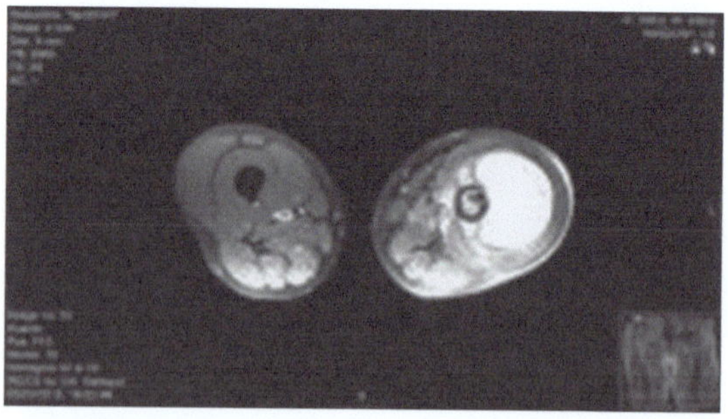

Fig. 28.12 MARS MRI showing huge fluid collection from the joint extending distally along the thigh until the proximal aspect of the knee

Other: CRP 5.88 mg/dl (0–0.5), ESR 80

28.5.5 Preoperative Planning

Diagnosis: Recurrence of late infection THA (Figs. 28.10, 28.11 and 28.12)

Possible treatment options: (1) One-stage revision, (2) two-stage revision with or without antibiotic-loaded spacer, and (3) implant removal

Chosen treatment method: Two-stage revision with custom-molded spacer prepared in the operating room

Selection of implants if applicable and rational: Custom-molded spacer prepared in the operating room in the first-stage and cementless THA in the second stage (primary or revision implant)

Expected difficulties: Stage one, removal of the stable cup and the devices. Aggressive debridement of all septic tissues extending distally in the thigh and the femur. Stage two, reliable primary stability with the less invasive implant

Strategies to overcome difficulties: Stage one, availability of explant instrumentation for the removal of the cup. Careful evaluation of the extension of the septic tissues according to pre-op MRI. Availability of long spacer with the possibility of using cement with the addition of antibiotics, according to the bacteria isolated during the previous revision in 2002. Stage two, availability of high-porosity titanium cup for primary stability and revision stem in case of need of fixation in the distal femur. Intraoperative histology and leukocytes esterase

Templating: To evaluate the stem length and the size and the size of the cup

28.5.6 Surgical Note

Patient's position: Right lateral decubitus

Type of anesthesia: General

Surgical approach: Posterolateral approach, extended distally

Main steps: Stage one, ten samples for culture including tissues prior to antibiotic prophylaxis administration. Easy removal of the stem and removal of the cup by explant instrumentation. Aggressive debridement of internal devices, soft tissues, and fluid collection. Cleaning of all bone surfaces and preparation of custom-molded spacer with gentamycin and clindamycin loaded cement with the addition of vancomycin (Fig. 28.13). Stage two, removal of the spacer. Intraoperative histology and leukocyte esterase (both negative for infection). Insertion of a primary cementless THA (Fig. 28.14)

Reconstruction techniques: Reaming of the acetabulum and preparation of the proximal femur with the rasps. Insertion of a high-porosity titanium cup with cross-linked polyethylene and Zweymuller stem with 36 mm ceramic head, XL neck

28.5.7 Intraoperative Challenges

Challenges and solutions: Eradication of the infection and management of a large femur after previous surgeries

Unanticipated problems and solution: During the first stage, the antibiotic treatment was based to the old cultures that were later on confirmed by the new ones.

Thorough description of decision-making, including the reason for the final decision: The use of a custom-molded spacer gave the possibility, during stage one, of a reliable stability in a very large femoral canal after the removal of a long revision stem. The second stage was performed after six months, two months of antibiotic therapy, and normal CRP.

28.5.8 Postoperative Radiographs (Figs. 28.13 and 28.14)

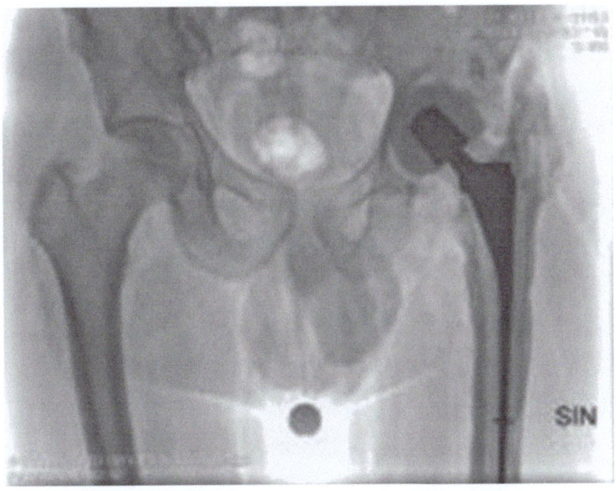

Fig. 28.13 Stage two preoperative AP X-rays of the pelvis showing the spacer

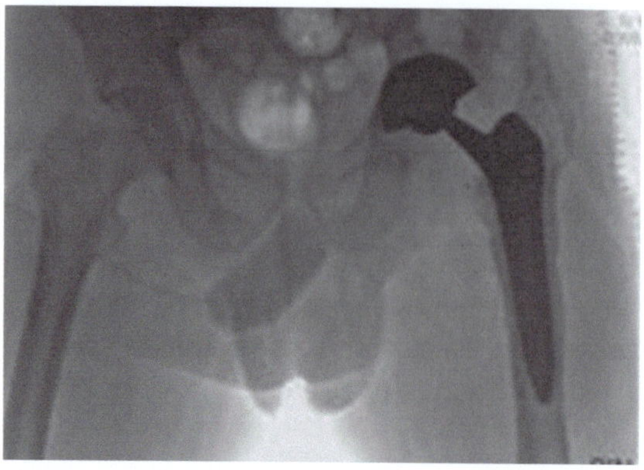

Fig. 28.14 Stage two postoperative AP X-rays of the pelvis

28.5.9 Postoperative Management

Chemoprophylaxis and anticoagulant treatment period: Nadroparin calcium 0.6 mL 1 fl/day for five weeks from the surgery as protocol. Stage one: vancomycin + piperacillin/tazobactam for two weeks, then cefazolin for one month, and levofloxacin for two months (according to intraoperative cultures positive for *Staphylococcus aureus*). Stage two: Prophylaxis with vancomycin for three days and doxycycline for two weeks until the final result of the intraoperative cultures (negative)

Gait/limb loading until full loading: The patient walked with two crutches and partial weight bearing until the second stage of surgery. Partial weight bearing with crutches for three months after the second stage.

28.5.10 Follow-Up and Complications

No complications

28.5.11 Discussion [42, 61, 62]

Advantages of the applied method: Management of the infection with good functional recovery

Disadvantages of the method: Two surgeries compared to the one-stage revision.

Alternative evidence-based techniques for the case: One-stage revision

Why is the chosen technique better for this case? Two-stage technique: Because we had no clear evidence of the microorganism responsible for the recurrence of the late infection, due to the negative cultures. The patient was a drug abuser so he can be considered as high risk for persisting infection and immunodeficiency. The infection was extended in all thighs with a huge fluid collection. Custom-molded spacer: because of the large canal with the extension of bone loss in the distal part of the femoral shaft due to the loosening of the previous revision stem.

Indications and contraindications for your technique. Indications: Late infection in a patient with a possibility of further surgeries (stage two). Contraindications: No active patient at risk for a second surgery. In this case, implant removal (Girdlestone procedure) can be the treatment of choice.

Learning curve and how to manage complications: Quite easy and reproducible technique. In case of recurrence of infection, need for further surgery to eradicate the infection

Level of evidence concerning the superiority of this method against others: Level III

28.6 Case Title: Prosthetic Loosening and Severe Pain

Gösta Ullmark

28.6.1 Demographics

Age: 30
Sex: Female
BMI: 20.5

28.6.2 Relevant Past Medical History

Principal pathologies: Healthy

Previous surgical procedures: Pelvic fracture by a car accident treated by open reduction and internal fixation at 2003 in Armenia. Secondary osteoarthritis in the right hip treated by a cemented THA in 2005 in Armenia. Surgery for a minor "fibroma" in the right thigh in 2010. The patient arrived in Sweden in 2012.

Medication: None

History of Presenting Complaint: The patient has always had some pain in the hip after the accident and also following THA. She had more pain during last week, and pain in rest. Some continuing pain since the last surgery. She was able to walk with two crutches

28.6.3 Clinical Examination

Symptoms: Some pain in the groin

Range of motion: Saggital 80°, rotation 40°, abduction and adduction 30°

Specific tests: Pain when lifting the leg and when laying on the back

Main disability: Constant hip pain, more pain when moving or standing on the leg.

Scoring if available: Walking with crutches

Neurovascular evaluation: Normal

28.6.4 Preoperative Radiological Assessment/Imaging (Figs. 28.15 and 28.16)

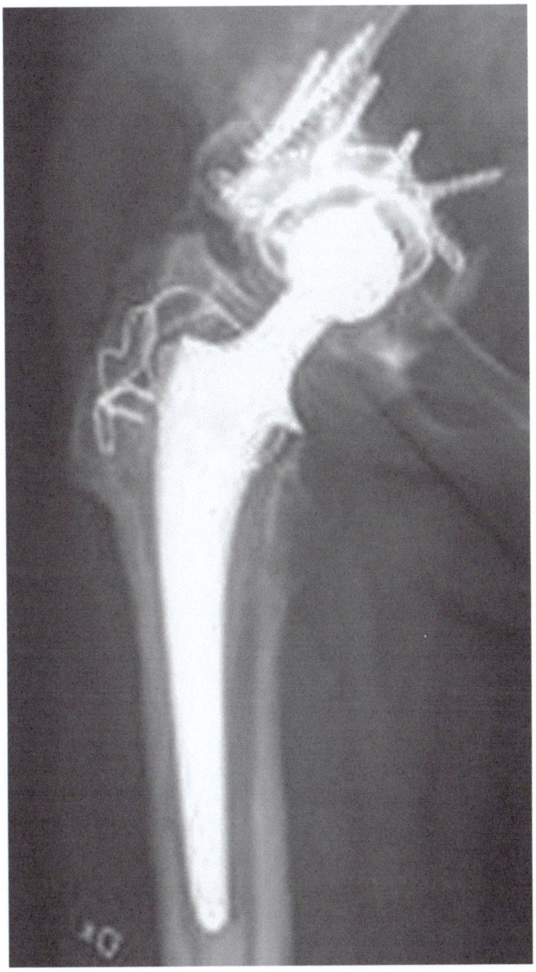

Fig. 28.15 Preoperative frontal view showing the cup and the stem loosening. Migration of the cup, the mesh, and the screws into the pelvis

Other. Blood tests: Hemoglobin is low (108 g/L), WBC is normal (8.2), sedimentation rate is slightly increased (26 mm), and CRP is slightly increased (6.0 mg/L). Body temperature is normal.

28.6.5 Preoperative Planning

Diagnosis: Prosthetic loosening and a cavitary bone defect of the acetabular floor. Suspicious for periprosthetic infection (Figs. 28.15 and 28.16)

Possible treatment options: (1) One-stage procedure with a revision to an uncemented prosthesis with titanium augments in the acetabulum and a cup stabilized by screws. (2) One-stage procedure with a revision to impaction bone grafting (IBG) using metal mesh or augments to restore segmental acetabular defects before graft impaction. (3) A two-stage procedure. The first stage involves the extraction of the prostheses, all the cement, the screws, the metal mesh and performing a synovectomy

Chosen treatment method: The first stage of a two-stage procedure has been previously mentioned with the insertion of an antibiotic containment cement spacer (Figs. 28.17 and 28.18). The second-stage of the surgical procedure involves the restoration of the cavitary acetabular bone

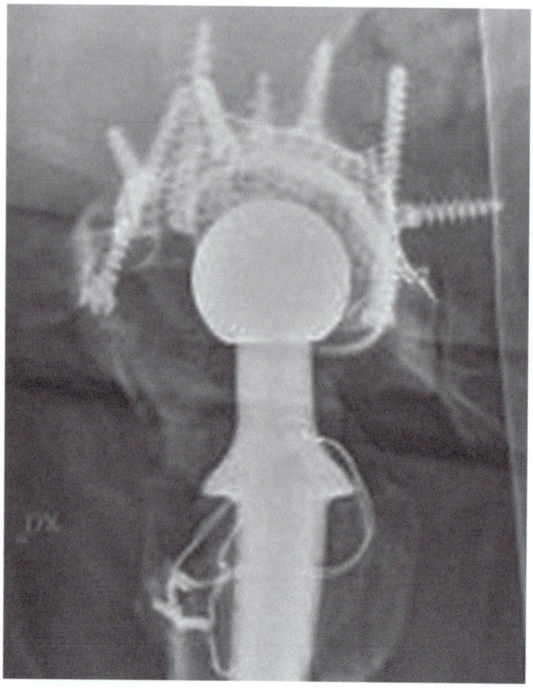

Fig. 28.16 Preoperative lateral view

defect, IBG, and cementing prosthetic components

Selection of implants if applicable and rational: A variety of revision instruments is needed as the Titanium Acetabular Graft Cup and Acetabular Rim Mesh, the Lubinus SP II stem and the Lubinus cup (Waldemar Link, Hamburg, Germany).

Expected difficulties: Risk for damaging blood vessels in the pelvis when extracting the screws

Strategies to overcome difficulties: Preoperatively, a balloon catheter was inserted in the ipsilateral arteria iliaca communis [63]. The balloon could be filled during surgery to stop any blood flow.

28.6.6 Surgical Note

Patient's position: Lateral decubitus position

Type of anesthesia: General anesthesia

Surgical approach: Posterolateral approach

Main steps: The surgical procedure included five intra-operative biopsies for bacteria culturing before antibiotic treatment. Extraction of the prosthesis, cement, screws, mesh, and cerclage wire is followed by synovectomy. The casting of a cement spacer containing gentamicin and vancomycin. Insertion of the spacer, reduction of the joint, and closing the wound. Repair of the segmental acetabular defects. IBG and cementing the poly cup. The femur was graft impacted, and a 170 mm Lubinus SP II stem was cemented. During the reduction procedure, a distal femoral fracture occurred.

Reconstruction techniques: Repair of the segmental acetabular floor defect by titanium mesh from the inside of the Acetabulum. The lateral wall defect of the acetabulum was repaired from the outside by screwing a 0.8 mm titanium acetabular rim mesh (Waldemar Link, Hamburg, Germany). Bone graft from fresh-frozen femoral heads was morselized in a milling machine (Howex, Gävle, Sweden). The bone chips were fat reduced by washing in warm saline solution. Impaction Bone Grafting using dedicated acetabular impactors (Waldemar Link, Hamburg, Germany) using the meshes as a counter hold for the sturdy impaction. After impaction, a 1 mm thin perforated titanium graft cup from the same supplier was inserted inside the acetabulum, on top of the impacted graft bed to further compress and stabilize the graft bed by screws. After that, the poly cup was cemented inside the graft cup. The femur was impacted by dedicated graft impaction instruments (Waldemar Link, Hamburg, Germany) [64]) adapted to the 170 mm Lubinus SP II stem followed by cementing the stem (Figs. 28.19 and 28.20).

28.6.7 Intraoperative Challenges

Unanticipated problems and solution: The sciatic nerve is lying prominently in the wound. The joint is firmly bound by fibrous tissue. Thereby it was difficult to dislocate. During the joint reduction, a distal femoral fracture occurred. The fracture was openly reduced and fixated by a plate with screws distally and cables in the upper part.

Thorough description of decision-making, including the reason for the final decision: The sciatic nerve is carefully marked and protected. Fibrous tissue surrounding the joint is thoroughly cut away to enable dislocation.

28.6.8 Postoperative Radiographs (Figs. 28.17, 28.18, 28.19, and 28.20)

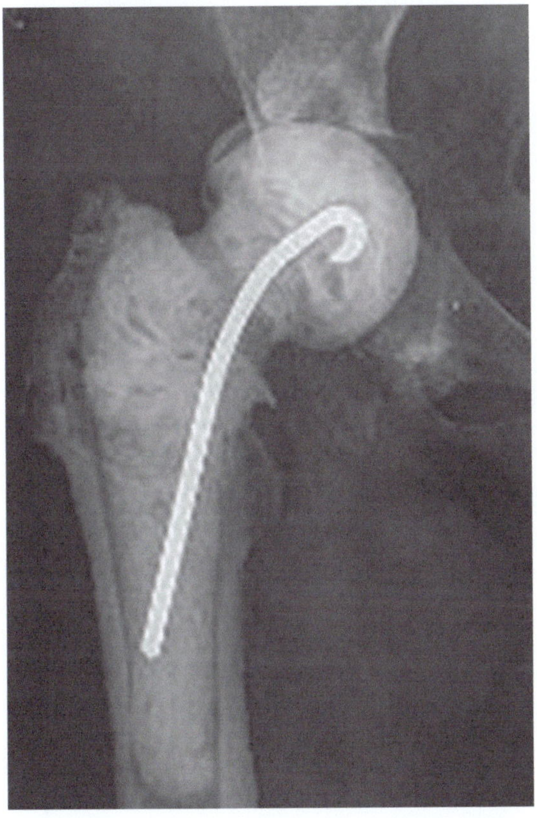

Fig. 28.17 Frontal view after the first-stage procedure with the cement spacer inserted

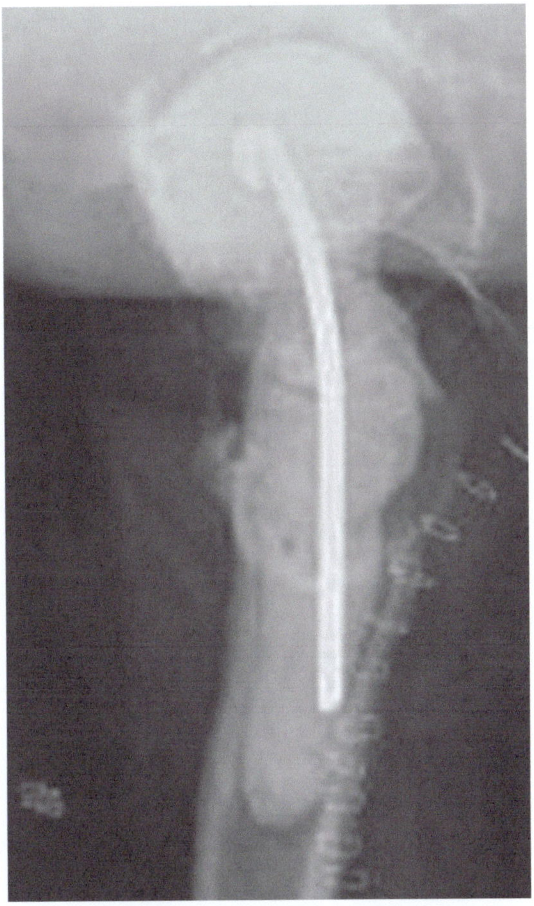

Fig. 28.18 Lateral view after the first-stage procedure with the cement spacer inserted

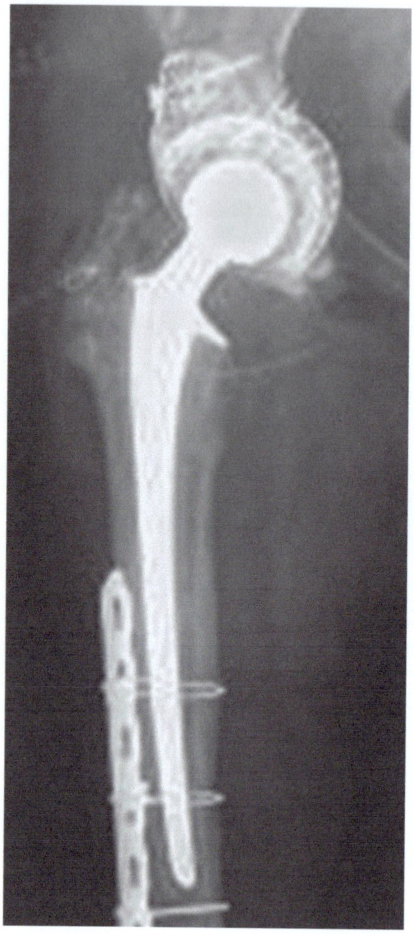

Fig. 28.19 Frontal view after the second step of the procedure

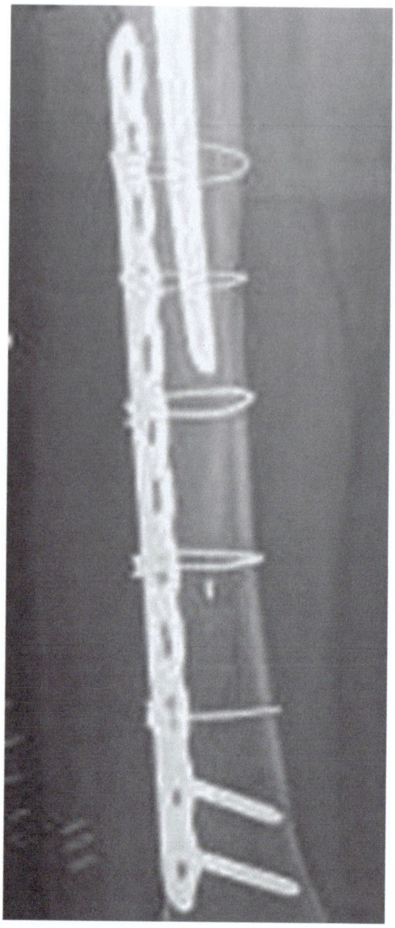

Fig. 28.20 Frontal view of reduced femur fracture and plate after the second step of the procedure

28.6.9 Postoperative Management

Chemoprophylaxis and anticoagulant treatment period: The bacteria cultures showed a coagulase-negative *Staphylococcus* with partial resistance to antibiotics. The antibiotic treatment included clindamycin 300 mg orally three times per day, plus rifampicin 450 mg orally once a day until ten days prior to the second-stage procedure. Anticoagulant treatment by injection of 5000 IE LMWHs per day for thirty days.

Gait/limb loading until full loading: Walking with crutches with partial weight bearing until the second-stage surgical procedure. Planning for stage two surgery: Antibiotic treatment for seven weeks followed by two weeks of antibiotic-free period. After that, the stage two surgery was planned for.

Scoring: At seven months follow-up after the second surgical procedure, the patient had no pain and she was walking without support. Radiography showed healed fracture and unchanged position and appearance of prosthetic components and meshes. After that, the patient moved back to Armenia.

28.6.10 Discussion

Advantages of the applied method: The two-stage procedure has somewhat better results of treating a long-lasting periprosthetic infection. The method of IBG enables the restoration of a normal hip center of rotation and it is the only technique able to restore the bone, lost secondary to osteolysis, by new living bone [65].

Disadvantages of the method: You need access to bone graft, graft impaction instruments, and you need to have learned the IBG method.

Alternative evidence-based techniques for the case: An uncemented distal anchoring femoral component. Uncemented cup with titanium augments and holes for screws together with some structural or particulated bone graft. Alternatively, a cup cage in the acetabulum, some additional bone graft and a cemented cup

Why is the chosen technique better for this case? The IBG method allows for a free and anatomical correct placement of the hip rotation center. The method of IBG using dedicated graft impaction instruments results in a much better graft healing compared to using structural graft. Graft healing is inferior if a particulate graft is inserted without impaction by dedicated impaction instrument. When using a cage in combination with particulate bone graft, the graft bed is mainly not loaded after surgery. Loading of a graft bed is a major stimulus for bone healing.

Indications and contraindications for your technique: Indication is any revision THA when osteolysis is present in the femur or the acetabulum. High age is not a contraindication since graft healing is not shown to be dependent to age. Infection is neither a contraindication. Studies of revision have shown similar incidence of persistence and recurrent infection when using IBG or not. Contraindication is an insufficient support for the graft bed and/or the prosthetic components. That is the femur either an insufficient repaired cortical defect in the calcar region or pronounced cortical weakening in the stem tip region. Some of those relative contraindications may be overcome by repair using mesh and cerclage wires, a longer stem or a complimentary plate. For the acetabulum, the critical issue is enough stable repair of major segmental defects. A large segmental defect in the direction of load requires a sufficient stable metal repair as counter hold both for the impaction procedure and for forces acting through the joint during the first postoperative period, before bone healing is established.

Learning curve and how to manage complications: Education and training is an absolute condition for starting IBG. The method is not difficult but slightly different from many regular orthopedic methods. Complications are mainly the same as for other revision methods. Revision of a former IBG-treated hip is often easier accomplished compared to when other revision methods have been used.

Level of evidence concerning the superiority of this method against others: The IBG method in combination with cemented prosthetic components have widespread clinical use for 40 years. Many studies of both long time clinical, radiological, biomechanical, histological, and PET results have been published from all over the world.

References

1. Enayatollahi MA, Parvizi J. Diagnosis of infected total hip arthroplasty. Hip Int. 2015;25(4):294–300.
2. Senthi S, Munro JT, Pitto RP. Infection in total hip replacement: meta-analysis. International Orthopaedics. 2011;35:253–60.
3. Karachalios T, Koutalos A, Komnos G. Management strategies for infected total hip arthroplasty. A critical appreciation of problems and techniques. Hip Int. 2014;24(Suppl 10):S44–S4.
4. Pivec R, Johnson AJ, Mears SC, Mont MA. Hip arthroplasty. Lancet. 2012;380(9855):1768–77.
5. Kuzyk PRT, Dhotar HS, Sternheim A, Gross AE, Safir O, Backstein D. Two-stage revision arthroplasty for management of chronic periprosthetic hip and knee infection: techniques, controversies, and outcomes. J Am Acad Orthop Surg. 2014;22:153–64.
6. Kurtz S, Ong K, Lau E, Mowat F, Halpern M. Projections of primary and revision hip and knee arthroplasty in the United States from 2005 to 2030. J Bone Joint Surg Am. 2007;89(4):780–5.
7. Bozic KJ, Kurtz SM, Lau E, Ong K, Vail TP, Berry DJ. The epidemiology of revision total hip arthroplasty in the United States. J Bone Joint Surg Am. 2009;91(1):128–33.
8. Jafari SM, Coyle C, Mortazavi SMJ, Sharkey PF, Parvizi J. Revision hip arthroplasty: infection is the most common cause of failure. Clin Orthop Relat Res. 2010;468(8):2046–51.
9. Ong KL, Kurtz SM, Lau E, Bozic KJ, Berry DJ, Parvizi J. Prosthetic joint infection risk after total hip arthroplasty in the Medicare population. J Arthroplast. 2009;24(6):105–9.
10. Parvizi J, Zmistowski B, Berbari EF, et al. New definition for Periprosthetic joint infection: from the workgroup of the musculoskeletal infection society. Clin Orthop Relat Res. 2011;469(11):2992–4.

11. Zmistowski B, Della Valle C, Bauer TW, et al. Diagnosis of Periprosthetic joint infection. J Arthroplast. 2014;29(2):77–83.
12. CDC - ACH Surveillance for Surgical Site Infection (SSI) Event - NHSN. http://www.cdc.gov/nhsn/acute-care-hospital/ssi/. Accessed 07 Mar 2015.
13. Della Valle C, Parvizi J, Bauer TW. American Academy of Orthopaedic Surgeons. et al. Diagnosis of periprosthetic joint infections of the hip and knee. J Am Acad Orthop Surg. 2010;18(12):760–70.
14. Ghanem E, Antoci V Jr, Pulido L, Joshi A, Hozack W, Parvizi J. The use of receiver operating characteristics analysis in determining erythrocyte sedimentation rate and C-reactive protein levels in diagnosing periprosthetic infection prior to revision total hip arthroplasty. Int J Infect Dis. 2009;13(6):e444–9.
15. Urquhart DM, Hanna FS, Brennan SL, Wluka AE, Leder K, Cameron PA, Graves SE, Cicuttini FM. Incidence and risk factors for deep surgical site infection after primary total hip arthroplasty: a systematic review. J Arthroplast. 2010;25(8):1216–22.
16. Schinsky MF, Della Valle CJ, Sporer SM, Paprosky WG. Perioperative testing for joint infection in patients undergoing revision total hip arthroplasty. J Bone Joint Surg Am. 2008;90(9):1869–75.
17. Cipriano CA, Brown NM, Michael AM, Moric M, Sporer SM, Della Valle CJ. Serum and synovial fluid analysis for diagnosing chronic periprosthetic infection in patients with inflammatory arthritis. J Bone Joint Surg Am. 2012;94(7):594–600.
18. Parvizi J, Jacovides C, Antoci V, Ghanem E. Diagnosis of periprosthetic joint infection: the utility of a simple yet unappreciated enzyme. J Bone Joint Surg Am. 2011;93(24):2242–8.
19. Deirmengian C, Kardos K, Kilmartin P, et al. The alpha-defensin test for periprosthetic joint infection outperforms the leukocyte esterase test strip. Clin Orthop Relat Res. 2015;473(1):198–203.
20. Schäfer P, Fink B, Sandow D, Margull A, Berger I, Frommelt L. Prolonged bacterial culture to identify late periprosthetic joint infection: a promising strategy. Clin Infect Dis. 2008;47(11):1403–9.
21. Shahi A, Deirmengian C, Higuera C, et al. Premature therapeutic antimicrobial treatments can compromise the diagnosis of late periprosthetic joint infection. Clin Orthop Relat Res. 2015;473(7):2244–9.
22. Tsaras G, Maduka-Ezeh A, Inwards CY, et al. Utility of intraoperative frozen section histopathology in the diagnosis of periprosthetic joint infection: a systematic review and metaanalysis. J Bone Joint Surg Am. 2012;94(18):1700–11.
23. Diaz-Ledezma C, Lamberton C, Lichstein P, Parvizi J. Diagnosis of periprosthetic joint infection: the role of nuclear medicine may be overestimated. J Arthroplast. 2015;30(6):1044–9.
24. Tsukayama DT, Estrada R, Gustilo RB. Infection after total hip arthroplasty. A study of the treatment of one hundred and six infections. J Bone Joint Surg Am. 1996;78:512–23.
25. Toms AD, Davidson D, Masri BA, Duncan CP. The management of peri-prosthetic infection in total joint replacement. J Bone Joint Surg Br. 2006;88:149–55.
26. Krismer M. Definition of infection. Hip Int. 2012;22(Suppl 8):S2–4.
27. Trebse R, Pisot V, Trampuz A. Treatment of infected retained implants. J Bone Joint Surg Br. 2005;87(2):249–56.
28. Zimmerli W, Trampuz A, Ochsner PE. Prosthetic-joint infections. N Engl J Med. 2004;351(16):1645–54.
29. Byren I, Bejon P, Atkins BL, Angus B, Masters S, McLardy-Smith P, Gundle R, Berendt A. One hundred and twelve infected arthroplasties treated with 'DAIR' (debridement, antibiotics and implant retention): antibiotic duration and outcome. J Antimicrob Chemother. 2009;63:1264–71.
30. Estes CS, Beauchamp CP, Clarke HD, Spangehl MJ. A two-stage retention débridement protocol for acute Periprosthetic joint infections. Clin Orthop Relat Res. 2010;468:2029–38.
31. Chen AF, Heller S, Parvizi J. Prosthetic joint infections. Surg Clin North Am. 2014;94(6):1265–81.
32. Jackson WO, Schmalzried TP. Limited role of direct exchange arthroplasty in the treatment of infected total hip replacements. Clin Orthop Relat Res. 2000;381:101–5.
33. Rudelli S, Uip D, Honda E, Lima ALLM. One-stage revision of infected total hip arthroplasty with bone graft. J Arthroplast. 2008;23:1165–77.
34. Winkler H, Stoiber A, Kaudela K, Winter F, Menschik F. One stage uncemented revision of infected total hip replacement using cancellous allograft bone impregnated with antibiotics. J Bone Joint Surg Br. 2008;90:1580–5.
35. Yoo JJ, Kwon YS, Koo KH, Yoon KS, Kim YM, Kim HJ. One-stage cementless revision arthroplasty for infected hip replacements. Int Orthop. 2009;33:1195–201.
36. Camurcu Y, Sofu H, Buyuk AF, Gursu S, Kaygusuz MA, Sahin V. Two-stage cementless revision total hip arthroplasty for infected primary hip arthroplasties. J Arthroplast. 2015;30:1597–601.
37. Luu A, Syed F, Raman G, Bhalla A, Muldoon E, Hadley S, Smith E, Rao M. Two-stage arthroplasty for prosthetic joint infection a systematic review of acute kidney injury, systemic toxicity and infection. J Arthroplast. 2013;28:1490–8.
38. Stockley I, Mockford BJ, Hoad-Reddick A, Norman P. The use of two-stage exchange arthroplasty with depot antibiotics in the absence of long-term antibiotic therapy in infected total hip replacement. J Bone Joint Surg Br. 2008;90(2):145–8.
39. Whittaker JP, Warren RE, Jones RS, Gregson PA. Is prolonged systemic antibiotic treatment essential in two-stage revision hip replacement for chronic gram-positive infection? J Bone Joint Surg Br. 2009;91:44–5.
40. McKenna PB, O'Shea K, Masterson EL. Two-stage revision of infected hip arthroplasty using a short-

ened postoperative course of antibiotics. Arch Orthop Trauma Surg. 2009;129:489–94.

41. Hsieh PH, Shih CH, Chang YH, Lee MS, Shih HN, Yang WE. Two-stage revision hip arthroplasty for infection: comparison between the interim use of antibiotic-loaded cement beads and a spacer prosthesis. J Bone Joint Surg Am. 2004;86:1989.
42. Leonard HAC, Liddle AD, Burke O, Murray DW, Pandit H. Single- or two-stage revision for infected total hip arthroplasty? A systematic review of the literature. Clin Orthop Relat Res. 2014;472:1036–42.
43. Kunutsor SK, Whitehouse MR, Blom AW, Beswick AD. INFORM team Re-infection outcomes following one- and two-stage surgical revision of infected hip prosthesis: a systematic review and meta- analysis. Plos One. 2015; doi:10.1371/journal.pone.0139166.
44. Lange J, Troelsen A, Thomsen RW, Søballe K. Chronic infections in hip arthroplasties: comparing risk of reinfection following one-stage and two-stage revision: a systematic review and meta-analysis. Clin Epidemiol. 2012;4:57–73.
45. Engesæter LB, Dale H, Schrama JC, Hallan G, Lie SA. Surgical procedures in the treatment of 784 infected THAs reported to the Norwegian Arthroplasty register. Acta Orthop. 2011;82(5):530–7.
46. Beswick AD, Elvers KT, Smith AJ, Gooberman-Hill R, Lovering A, Blom AW. What is the evidence base to guide surgical treatment of infected hip prostheses? Systematic review of longitudinal studies in unselected patients. BMC Med. 2012;10(1):18.
47. Yamamoto K, Miyagawa N, Masaoka T, Katori Y, Shishido T, Imakiire A. Clinical effectiveness of antibiotic-impregnated cement spacers for the treatment of infected implants of the hip joint. J Orthop Sci. 2003;8(6):823–8.
48. Barrack RL. Rush pin technique for temporary antibiotic-impregnated cement prosthesis for infected total hip arthroplasty. J Arthroplast. 2002;17(5): 600–3.
49. Durbhakula SM, Czajka J, Fuchs MD, Uhl RL. Spacer endoprosthesis for the treatment of infected total hip arthroplasty. J Arthroplast. 2004;19(6):760–7.
50. Hsieh PH, Chen LH, Chen CH, Lee MS, Yang WE, Shih CH. Two-stage revision arthroplasty for infection with a custom made, antibiotic-loaded, cement prosthesis as an interim spacer. J Trauma. 2004;56(6):1247–52.
51. Pattyn C, De Geest T, Ackerman P, Audenaert E. Preformed gentamicin spacers in two-stage revision hip arthroplasty: functional results and complications. Int Orthop. 2011;35(10):1471–6.
52. D'Angelo F, Negri L, Binda T, Zatti G, Cherubino P. The use of a preformed spacer in two-stage revision of infected hip arthroplasties. Musculoskelet Surg. 2011;95(2):115–20.
53. Jung J, Schmid NV, Kelm J, Schmitt E, Anagnostakos K. Complications after spacer implantation in the treatment of hip joint infections. Int J Med Sci. 2009;6(5):265–73.
54. Scharfenberger A, Clark M, Lavoie G, O'Connor G, Masson E, Beaupre LA. Treatment of an infected total hip replacement with the PROSTALAC system. Part 1: infection resolution. Can J Surg. 2007;50:24–8.
55. Hofmann AA, Goldberg TD, Tanner AM, Cook TM. Ten year experience using an articulating antibiotic cement hip spacer for the treatment of chronically infected total hip. J Arthroplast. 2005;20:874–9.
56. Iarikov D, Demian H, Rubin D, Alexander J, Nambiar S. Choice and doses of antibacterial agents for cement spacers in treatment of prosthetic joint infections: review of published studies. Clin Infect Dis. 2012;55(11):1474–80.
57 Trebše R. The diagnostic protocol for evaluation of periprosthetic joint infection. Hip Int. 2012;22(Suppl. 8):S25–35.
58 Sendi P, Frei R, Maurer TB, Trampuz A, Zimmerli W, Graber P. Escherichia coli variants in periprosthetic joint infections: diagnostic challenges with sessile bacteria and sonication. J Clin Mic. 2010;48:1720–5.
59 Zahar A, Gehrke TA. One stage revision for infected total hip arthroplasty. Orthop Clin North Am. 2016;47(1):11–8.
60 Ilchmann T, Zimmerli W, Ochsner PE, Kessler B, Zwicky L, Graber P, Clauss M. One stage revision of infected hip arthroplasty. Outcome of 39 consecutive hips. Int Orthop. 2016;40(5):913–8.
61 Wolf M, Clar H, Friesenbichler J, Schwantzer G, Bernhardt G, Gruber G, Glehr M, Leithner A, Sadoghi P. Prosthetic joint infection following total hip replacement: results of one-stage versus two-stage exchange. Int Orthop. 2014;38(7):1363–8. doi:10.1007/s00264-014-2309-y.
62 van Diemen MP, Colen S, Dalemans AA, Stuyck J, Mulier M. Two-stage revision of an infected total hip arthroplasty: a follow-up of 136 patients. Hip Int. 2013;23(5):445–50. doi:10.5301/hipint.5000049.
63 Ullmark G, Hovelius L, Strindberg L, Wallner A. Reduced bleeding through temporary balloon occlusion in hip and knee revision surgery. Acta Orthop Scand. 2000;71(1):51–4.
64 Ullmark G, Hallin G, Nilsson O. Impacted corticocancellous allografts and cement for femoral revision of total hip arthroplasty using Lubinus and Charnley prostheses. J Arthroplasty. 2002;17(3):325–34.
65 Ullmark G, Obrant KJ. Histology of impacted bonegraft incorporation. J Arthroplasty. 2002;17(2):150–7.

29 Revision THA Post Resurfacing Arthroplasty

Eustathios Kenanidis, Eleftherios Tsiridis, and Klaus-Peter Günther

29.1 Current Concepts

E. Kenanidis and E. Tsiridis

Femoral neck fracture and aseptic loosening of either the acetabular or femoral component are the most frequent indications of revision of the Hip Resurfacing Arthroplasty HRA. Among others, infections and metallosis, with or without adverse local tissue reactions (ALTRs), are additional revision reasons (Fig. 29.1) [1]. Several risk factors have been implicated; however, their role is not fully understood. Female sex is considered as a risk factor for HRA revision as a result of the smaller implant size used [1]. Older people have a worse bone quality that further increase the risk for revision [2, 3]. A small component size and malpositioning, have also been recognised as risk factors [4].

Although the revision of an HRA is considered a straightforward procedure, this is not always true. Several factors as the time, the extent (femoral, acetabular, or both) of revision and the selection of implants need further evaluation.

29.1.1 Evaluation of the Painful SRA [5]

- Take a comprehensive history.
- Make a thorough physical examination.
- Evaluate of the implant stability.
  - Use serial radiographs to identify any differences of implant position, radiolucent lines around implants, or reactive sclerosis.
  - Use a bone scan or metal artifact reduction magnetic resonance imaging scan.
  - It was supported that the single-photon emission computed tomography (SPECT/CT) has higher specificity and sensitivity when compared with a bone scan to detect aseptic loosening [6].
- Exclude infection.
  - Count ESR and CRP. Notice, however, that these tests may be chronically elevated, due to a secondary reaction to the metal debris [7].
  - Aspire the joint and culture of the incoming fluid. Order a manual cell count as the presence of metal ions can distort the automatic cell count [8].
- Evaluate the presence of metal debris or ALTRs as potential sources of pain.

E. Kenanidis, M.D., Ph.D., M.Sc. (✉)
Academic Orthopaedic Unit, Aristotle University Medical School, Thessaloniki, Greece

E. Tsiridis, M.D., Ph.D., F.A.C.S., F.R.C.S. (✉)
Academic Orthopaedic Unit, Papageorgiou General Hospital, Aristotle University Medical School, Thessaloniki, Greece
e-mail: etsiridis@doctors.org.uk

K.-P. Günther, M.D.
University Center of Orthopaedics and Traumatology, University Medicine at Technische Universität Dresden, Dresden, Germany
e-mail: Peter.Guenther@uniklinikum-dresden.de; Klaus-Peter.Guenther@uniklinikum-dresden.de

E. Tsiridis (ed.), *The Adult Hip - Master Case Series and Techniques*,
https://doi.org/10.1007/978-3-319-64177-5_29

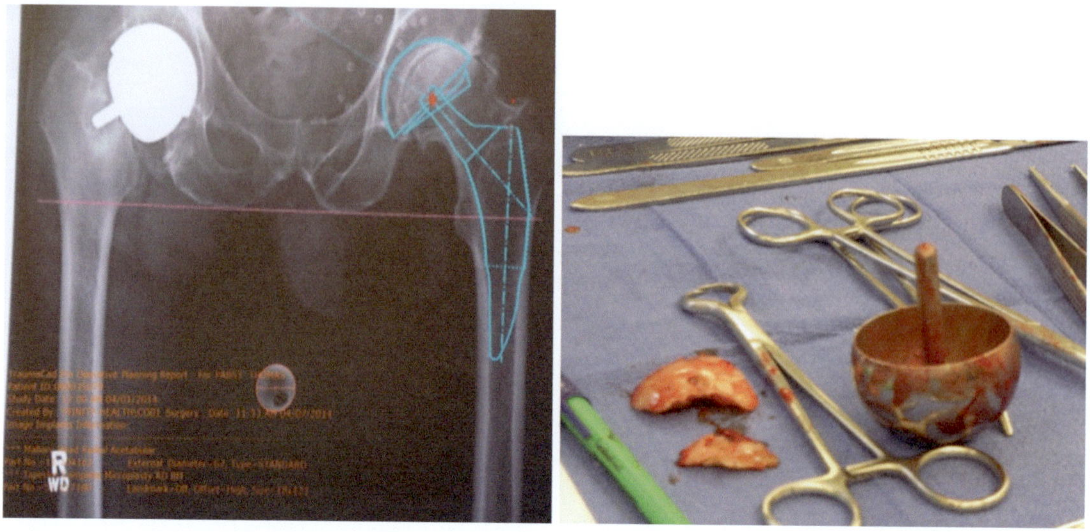

Fig. 29.1 A failed resurfacing arthroplasty due to neck absorption and Aseptic Lymphocytic Vasculitis Associated Lesions (ALVAL). The removal of the implant was easy. The bone was debrided until the healthy bleeding bone was exposed in the femoral metaphysis. Revision to a standard uncemented THA was performed

- Count the serum cobalt or chromium levels; the absolute threshold of concern, however, has not been fully defined. A level of ≥7 parts per billion is considered a threshold of concern.
- Use an ultrasound, CT, or MRI artifact reduction to find ALTRs or pseudotumors. They may be present in both asymptomatic and symptomatic patients, whether or not metal ion levels are elevated [9].
- If they are symptomatic, recognize the size and relationship of a pseudotumor to the neighboring anatomic structures before undertaking revision surgery [10].

29.1.2 Potential Surgical Revision Options [5]

There are multiple options when planning for revision of a painful HRA.

1. Infection
   - The gold standard treatment is the two-stage exchange (removal of all prior implants + aggressive debridement + cement loaded spacer) [11].
   - Six-week course of the proper intravenous antibiotics and monitor of inflammatory markers. Discontinue antibiotics for at least 2 weeks and then perform a synovial fluid analysis and culture and evaluate the serum metal ion level before reimplantation.
   - Single-stage explantation, for a selected patient population
   - Implant choice: primary or revision components due to bone loss and compromised quality of bone and soft tissues.
2. Isolated femoral revision and retention of a well-fixed acetabular shell

   Indications [5, 12, 13]

   (a) Femoral neck fracture

   (b) Aseptic loosening

   (c) Metallosis with femoral stem malposition

   Advantages
   - Less operative time and less technically demanding.
   - Preservation of the acetabular bone stock.
   - Maintain the hip stability using a large-diameter femoral head.

   Disadvantages
   - Possible implant mismatch.
   - In case of revision to a stemmed MoM, the potential source of metal ions is maintained.
   - Increased polyethylene wear if a dual mobility bearing is used.

Implant options

- Conversion to a stemmed MoM with a primary (or revision) femoral component with a large-diameter metal femoral head (concerns regarding MoM, THA, and corrosion-related complications).
- Use a primary (or revision) femoral component with a dual mobility femoral head, with a smaller-diameter femoral head within a larger, polyethylene outer bearing to convert any metal resurfacing procedure with a secure acetabulum to a polyethylene metal bearing (not FDA approved/concerns exist including implant mismatch/coverage angles and edge loading that can lead to subsequent polyethylene wear).

3. Isolated acetabular revision with retention of the well-fixed femoral component
   - It is not widely supported (lack of long-term follow-up studies)

   Indications [5, 12, 13]

   (a) Osteolysis
   (b) Malposition
   (c) Impingement

   Implant options

   – Thorough debridement + grafts + screws with a greater acetabular shell. Concerns exist for ongoing wear from metal ions.

   (d) Conversion to THA
   – It is the primary option in the setting of femoral or acetabular component failure

Indications

(a) Infection
(b) Fracture
(c) Metallosis
(d) Loosening

Advantages

- Lack of concern for implant mismatch
- Elimination of the primary sources of metal ion production and use of ceramic or Oxinium femoral heads or even ceramic-on-ceramic implants

Potential drawbacks

- A possible loss of bone stock secondary to removal of the implants
- Inferior stability given the smaller femoral head often utilized in THA

29.1.3 Technical Considerations [5, 14]

(a) Identify the anatomic relationships of a pseudotumor. The natural surgical landmarks can be distorted [13]. A thorough debridement of metal debris and inflammatory soft tissue is needed.

(b) Understand the potential extent of the soft tissue damage that has occurred from an aggressive pseudotumor and its impact on the hip stability and function.
   - You may need bone grafting along with supplemental fixation in the case of extensive acetabular osteolysis.
   - Preoperatively assess the strength of abductor, and be ready for additional stability options (dual mobility or constrained acetabular liner, transfer of the gluteus maximus, or Achilles tendon allograft [15]).

(c) In the case of isolated femoral revision, dislocate the hip, remove the head, and perform femoral neck osteotomy with a reciprocating saw blade around the femoral stem of the resurfacing component [14]. Proceed for femoral preparation as for a primary THA. Use large-diameter cobalt chrome head with a modular neck or a dual mobility implant to achieve a reduction.

(d) In the case of an isolated acetabular revision, proceed with an extensive capsular release to dislocate the hip, remove the femoral head, and position appropriately the femur to enable acetabular exposure. Use specific devices to remove the acetabular shell with minimal bone loss efficiently.

29.1.4 Outcomes of Conversion of HRA to THA

There are several case series reporting short- to mid-term results of HRA revision [12–14, 16–24]. These are usually retrospective cohort studies of less than 100 patients. There are also results from two registries. These studies, however, are not homogenised; they have differences concerning the indication for revision, the implant choice, as well as the type of revision (femoral, acetabular or both).

The results of revisions to THA were more consistent. In a retrospective review, Su et al. [13] evaluated 55 HRA revisions at a mean follow-up of 2.3 years. Mechanical reasons and adverse tissue reactions were the main revision reasons. Fourteen revisions were only femoral, four only acetabular and thirty seven both acetabular and femoral. Although the overall results were sufficient, the postoperative clinical scores differ based on the indication for revision. The mean postoperative HHS was significantly lower in patients revised for unexplained pain than for mechanical reasons (femoral neck fracture or implant loosening) (86.9 vs. 99; $p = 0.029$).

Revision of a part of an HRA has been associated with mixed clinical results. In a previous study, Ball et al. [12] compared the clinical and radiological outcomes of 21 HRA revisions with 64 primary THAs that had been performed during the same time period by the same surgeon. 18 out of 21 HRA revisions involved the femoral-sided only. The mean follow-up was almost four years. There was no significant difference between the groups about the operative time, blood loss, complication rates, postoperative clinical scores studied, and the quality of component fixation. There had been no instances of aseptic loosening in both groups and no dislocations after conversion of an HRA.

Pritchett et al. [16] reported the results of 90 single component revisions (76 acetabular and 14 femoral) for adverse soft tissue reactions. The decision for revision was based on clinical criteria, mainly pain, effusion, and instability. The acetabular-only revisions in patients with a femoral head component size ≤45 mm were made with a polyethylene acetabular revision prosthesis whether in those with a head size of ≥46 mm with a metal acetabular revision prosthesis of the same manufacturer as the primary prosthesis. A dual mobility polyethylene femoral head was utilised for all femoral-sided revisions. Revision was successful in 87 of the 90 (97%) procedures with a clinical improvement of all patients at a mean of 61 months. There was only one infection. The authors postulated that for some patients, it is more important to try saving the HRA than revising to THA in an attempt to maintain the advantages of HRA.

There are very limited other literatures on acetabular-only revision following HRA with unfavorable results [1, 2, 5]. De Steiger et al. [17] reported the results of 397 revisions of primary HRA for reasons other than infection out of 12.000 HRA performed between 1999 and 2008 in the Australian registry. After excluding infection, the major reason for revision of primary resurfacing hip arthroplasty was a fracture of the femoral neck (43%), followed by loosening/lysis (32%), metal sensitivity (7%), and pain (6%). The most common type of revision was a femoral-only revision (62%), followed by acetabular and femoral (29%) and acetabular only (9%). Twenty four revisions underwent further revision for loosening ($n = 9$), infection ($n = 6$), and dislocation ($n = 4$). The cumulative 5-year re-revision rate was 9% (20% of the acetabular-sided-only revisions, 7% rate of the femoral-sided revisions, and 5% for revision of both acetabulum and femur). The acetabular-only revision had a higher risk of re-revision than femoral-only revision (HR = 3 (1.2–10), $p = 0.02$); however, there was no statistically significant difference when compared to acetabular and femoral revision.

Complete revision of HRA to THA demonstrated different clinical outcomes in studies. Sandiford et al. [14] found significantly postoperative increased clinical results of 25 patients undergoing conversion of HRA to THA, similar to revision of THA. Twenty were revisions of both components and five of the femoral components. The mean follow-up was 12 years and 7 months. The indications for revision included pain, mechanical factors, and infection. The quality of life of patients was significantly improved. All patients were revised to ceramic-on-ceramic bearing couples. Wong et al. [20] in a recent registry-based study of 882 HRA revisions, reported that the 10-year cumulative re-revision rate following previous HRA revision was 26%. They reported no difference in re-revision rates and clinical outcomes between the acetabular-sided, femoral-sided, or combined acetabular- and femoral-sided (conversion to THA) cohorts. Eswaramoorthy et al. [21] supported that the clinical outcomes in patients undergoing conversion of HRA to THA were significantly worse when compared with patients undergoing primary HRA.

Reports on clinical outcomes following HRA revision for complications associated with metal wear are also confusing. Pritchett et al. [16] reported 97% success rate at mid-term results of 90 acetabular revisions for ALTRs reactions following the primary HRA. Grammatopoulos et al. [18], however, supported that HRA revision for pseudotumor was significantly worse than other reasons, and primary THA also has significantly higher major complication rate.

29.2 Case Title: Revision of a Failed HIP Resurfacing Arthroplasty with Pelvic Osteolysis

Klaus-Peter Günther

29.2.1 Demographics

Age: 60 years
Sex: Female
BMI: 28.7

29.2.2 Relevant Past Medical History

Principal pathologies: No comorbidities.

Previous surgical procedures: Hip resurfacing arthroplasty (HRA) 10 years previously.

Medication: No relevant medication.

History of presenting complaint: Groin pain and increasing abductor weakness in the last 12 months.

29.2.3 Clinical Examination

Symptoms: Painful hip flexion, abductor tenderness.

Range of motion: Flexion/extension 95°-0°-0°, Abd/Add 30°-0°-10°, ER/IR 30°-0°-0°.

Specific tests: Trendelenburg sign negative, marked elevation of whole blood cobalt concentration (75 μg/L).

Main disability: Painful limping after 15–20 min walking distance.

Neurovascular evaluation: Intact.

29.2.4 Preoperative Radiological Assessment/Imaging (Figs. 29.2, 29.3, and 29.4)

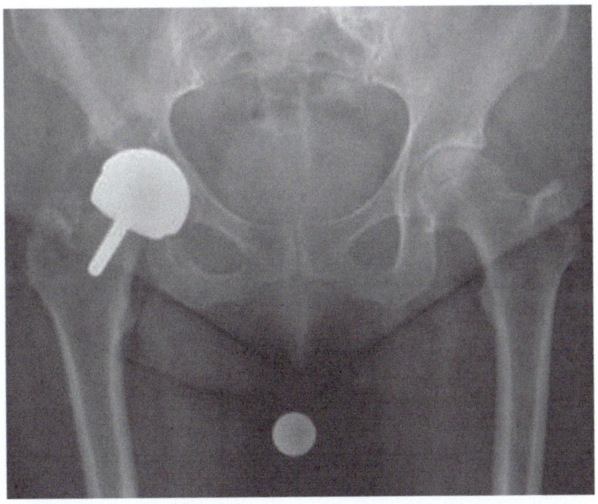

Fig. 29.2 An anteroposterior pelvis radiograph shows well-seated HRA with an extensive periacetabular osteolysis

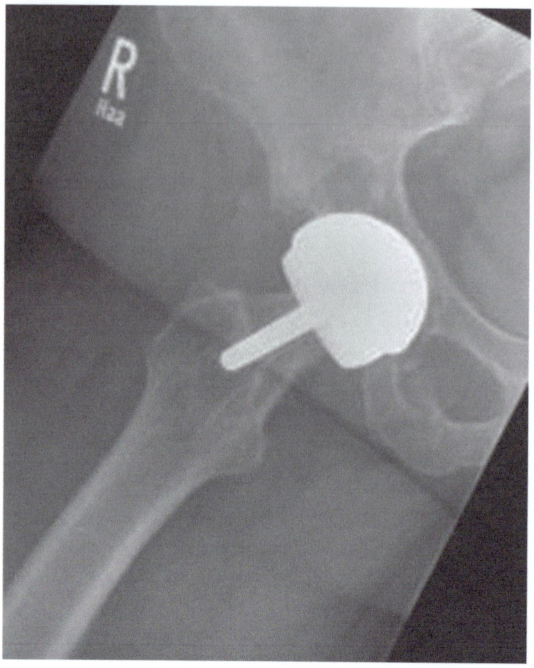

Fig. 29.3 Lateral view shows femoral neck thinning

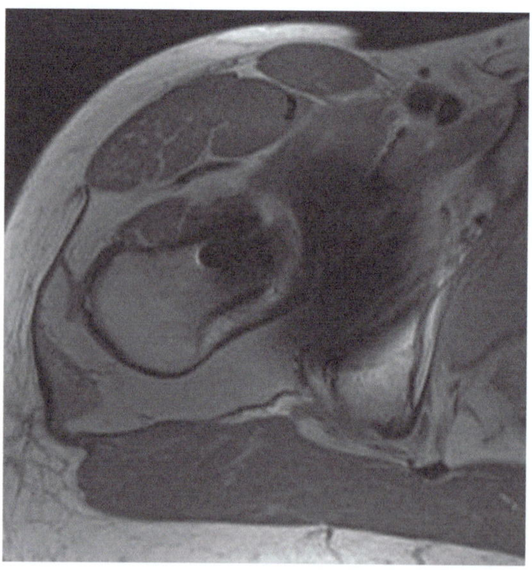

Fig. 29.4 Hip MRI shows large pseudobursa with fluid collection posterior to the greater trochanter

29.2.5 Preoperative Planning

Diagnosis: Failed HRA with adverse reaction to metal debris (ARMD) (Figs. 29.2, 29.3 and 29.4).

Possible treatment options: [25] Femoral and acetabular revision with HRA removal, conversion to conventional femoral stem and revision acetabular component with bone grafting of the defect [20], conversion of the femoral component to a conventional stem with size-matched dual mobility liner, and retaining acetabular HRA component.

Chosen treatment method: [25].

Selection of implants if applicable and rational: Due to the large pelvic bone defect, an acetabular revision with impaction of bone allograft or even a metallic wedge may be indicated. Depending on the remaining vital host bone, uncemented press-fit revision cups or cemented liners in combination with reinforcement rings and/or cages can be appropriate. For femoral revision of failed HRA, all conventional stem designs are usually appropriate. In case of expected postoperative instability (abductor damage), dual mobility cups can support a stable reconstruction.

Expected difficulties: [25] Soft tissue destruction ("pseudotumor" with abductor damage, destruction of external rotator cuff and capsule) with risk of instability [20], bone destruction due to metallosis [26], elevated postoperative complication rate (i.e., infection, instability), and inferior functional results due to soft tissue destruction.

Strategies to overcome difficulties: Preoperative patient information about the elevated surgical risk to avoid dissatisfaction, availability of the appropriate revision instruments (i.e., curved cup extraction chisels), bone allograft, variety of acetabular revision implants (uncemented revision cups as well as reinforcement rings/cages, dual mobility cups).

Templating: Preoperative templating of standard femoral stem and uncemented as well as cemented revision cups with reinforcement ring.

29.2.6 Surgical Note

Patient's position: Lateral position.

Type of anesthesia: General anesthesia.

Surgical approach: Posterior approach.

Main steps: Incision of skin, subcutaneous tissue, and fascia lata, positioning of Charnley retractor, careful retraction of sciatic nerve, and identification of the pseudobursa/pseudotumor. Tenotomy of the piriformis and the short external rotators together with the posterior joint capsule if possible (in severe ARMD, the posterior soft tissue structures often have severe damage). Dislocation of the femoral head by internal rotation and partial femoral neck osteotomy around the small stem of the femoral component. Complete the osteotomy with a chisel and remove of the femoral component together with the remaining bone. Acetabular exposure with Hohmann retractors by positioning the femur anteriorly to the acetabulum. Extensive soft tissue debridement (removal of as much pseudotumor tissue as possible around the cup and stem and along the psoas tendon toward the inner pelvic surface). Repeat pulse lavage. Acetabular preparation with careful exposure of the implant rim. Develope a plane in the bone prosthesis interface with various thin chisels. Use the Explant Acetabular Cup Removal System (Zimmer, Warsaw Indiana) with short and long curved blades to remove the cup. The final removal of the cup is achieved through numerous circular movements of the blades until circumferential clearance is achieved. Careful assessment of the acetabular socket to identify any kind of cysts and defects together with the removal of all granulation tissue and metal debris. Prepare the inner surface of the acetabulum with a maximum of 1–2 sequential hemispherical reamers (matching the size of the removed implant) just to expose the surface of intact host bone. Fill the bone defects with allogeneic cryopreserved grafts (if extensive global erosion of the acetabulum with attenuation or destruction of relevant supporting structures is present, reconstruction may require application of metal wedges). Application of the acetabular trial components to identify the appropriate implant and select either a press-fit uncemented cup or an augmentation with reinforcement device/cage depending on size and quality of the remaining host bone. Final implantation of the acetabular component (in case of impaired stability due to extensive soft tissue destruction a dual mobility liner is recommended). Exposure of the proximal femur with internal rotation and adduction of the leg. Elevation of the femur with Hohmann retractors and conventional femoral preparation. Trial reduction and stability testing, final offset, and implant selection. Following the final femoral stem and head application (non-metal bearing), the external rotators and posterior capsule are attached to the proximal femur if possible (Fig. 29.5).

29.2.7 Intraoperative Challenges

Challenges and solutions: [25] Variability of the soft tissue destruction due to metal debris (large fluid collections and pseudotumors): Radical debridement and extensive removal of the pathologic tissue, separate exposure of inner pelvic wall and large vessels if necessary [20]. Danger of postoperative instability due to the soft tissue destruction: choice of dual mobility cups [26]. Impaired acetabular bone stock with partial fixation of stable cup. Careful removal of the acetabular HRA monoblock through the application of Explant Acetabular Cup Removal System (Zimmer, Warsaw, Indiana) (Fig. 29.6)—with short and long curved blades at the plane of bone prosthesis interface of the cup [4]. In case of large acetabular bone defects due to the initial over-reaming with HRA and consecutive metallosis restore the bone stock (bone grafting whenever possible) and prefer application of reinforcement rings/cages instead of large uncemented cups.

Thorough description of decision making, including the reason for the final decision: Selection of the final implants according to the type and size of soft tissue and the bone defect.

29.2.8 Postoperative Radiographs (Figs. 29.5 and 29.6)

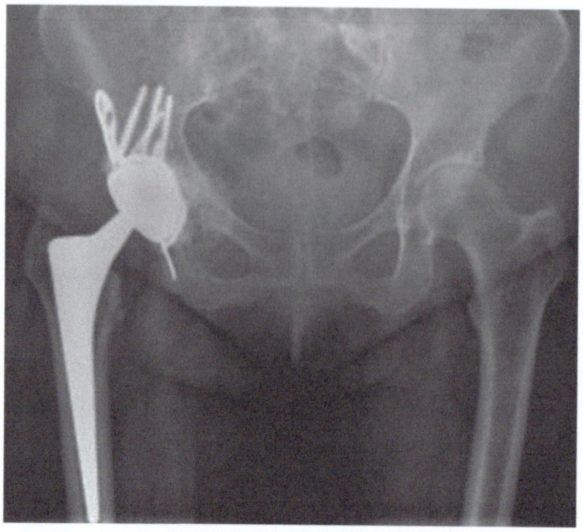

Fig. 29.5 Postoperative anteroposterior pelvis radiograph shows a Burch-Schneider antiprotrusio cage with extensive cancellous bone grafting and a dual mobility cup together with a conventional uncemented femoral stem. Restored offset and no relevant leg length discrepancy

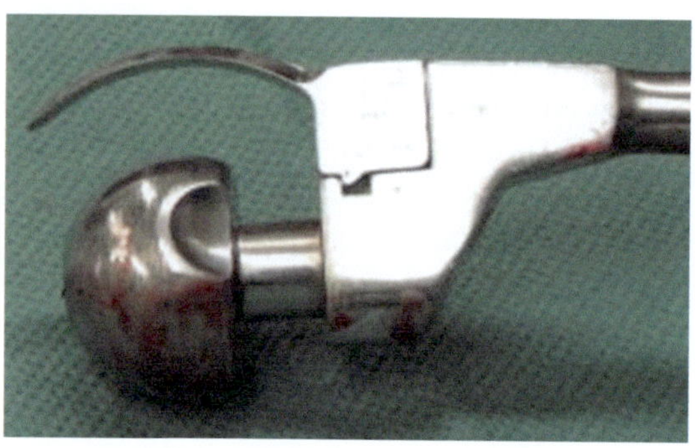

Fig. 29.6 Explant Acetabular Cup Removal System (Zimmer, Warsaw Indiana)

29.2.9 Postoperative Management

Chemoprophylaxis and anticoagulant treatment period: Perioperative antibiotics (cefuroxime 1.5 g for 24 h, DVT prophylaxis with rivaroxaban over four weeks, prevention of heterotopic bone formation with ibuprofen 3 × 50 mg over two weeks postoperatively.

Gait/limb loading until full loading: Six-week partial weight bearing (20 kg).

29.2.10 Follow-Up and Complications

Uneventful postoperative rehabilitation.

29.2.11 Discussion

Advantages of the applied method: The main advantage of the used technique is the bony reconstruction of the osteolytic areas and the possibility to keep the size of the revision implant as small as the original HRA or even smaller. Reconstruction of the bone stock is a prerequisite for the mostly young patients to facilitate later reinterventions.

Disadvantages of the method: Necessary availability of appropriate revision instruments and several uncemented/cemented revision implants including reinforcement rings/cages as well as a bone graft to adequately reconstruct the acetabular side.

Alternative evidence-based techniques for the case: Alternative methods (uncemented jumbo cups and conversion of femoral component to conventional stem with size-matched dual mobility liner and retaining acetabular HRA component) are also not evidence-based.

Why is the chosen technique better for this case? Better choice is the bone reconstruction and complete removal of metal-containing implants.

Indications and contraindications for your technique: The procedure is indicated if the acetabular osteolysis warrants extensive bone grafting or the initial size of the HRA was too large to convert it to an uncemented revision cup with even larger diameter. Contraindication would be a well implanted and small initial HRA cup without significant bone destruction.

Learning curve and how to manage complications: Appropriate knowledge of revision surgery with experience in the application of bone grafts and reinforcement rings/cages is necessary to reduce the learning curve.

Level of evidence concerning the superiority of this method against others: Level IV.

References

1. Carrothers AD, et al. Birmingham hip resurfacing: the prevalence of failure. J Bone Joint Surg. 2010;92(10):1344–50.
2. Prosser GH, et al. Outcome of primary resurfacing hip replacement: evaluation of risk factors for early revision. Acta Orthop. 2010;81(1):66–71.
3. Gross TP, Liu F. Risk factor analysis for early femoral failure in metal-on-metal hip resurfacing arthroplasty: the effect of bone density and body mass index. J Orthop Surg Res. 2012;7:1.
4. Langton DJ, et al. The effect of component size and orientation on the concentrations of metal ions after resurfacing arthroplasty of the hip. J Bone Joint Surg (Br). 2008;90(9):1143–51.
5. Haynes JA, Stambough JB, Barrack RL, Nam D. Conversion of a failed hip resurfacing arthroplasty to total hip arthroplasty: pearls and pitfalls. Curr Rev Musculoskelet Med. 2016;9:103–11.
6. Arican P, et al. The role of bone SPECT/CT in the evaluation of painful joint prostheses. Nucl Med Commun. 2015;36(9):931–40.
7. Walter LR, et al. Distribution of chromium and cobalt ions in various blood fractions after resurfacing hip arthroplasty. J Arthroplast. 2008;23(6):814–21.
8. Wyles CC, et al. Utility of synovial fluid aspirations in failed metal on-metal total hip arthroplasty. J Arthroplast. 2013;28(5):818–23.
9. Kwon YM, et al. Lymphocyte proliferation responses in patients with pseudotumors following metal-on-metal hip resurfacing arthroplasty. J Orthop Res. 2010;28(4):444–50.
10. Nam D, Barrack RL, Potter HG. What are the advantages and disadvantages of imaging modalities to diagnose wear-related corrosion problems? Clin Orthop Relat Res. 2014;472(12):3665–73.
11. Sharma AK, et al. Two-stage exchange for infected resurfacing arthroplasty: use of a novel cement spacer technique. J Arthroplast. 2011;26(6):976.
12. Ball ST, Le Duff MJ, Amstutz HC. Early results of conversion of a failed femoral component in hip resurfacing arthroplasty. J Bone Joint Surg Am. 2007;89(4):735–41.
13. Su EP, Su SL. Surface replacement conversion: results depend upon reason for revision. Bone Joint J. 2013;95(11 Suppl A):88–91.
14. Sandiford NA, Muirhead-Allwood SK, Skinner JA. Revision of failed hip resurfacing to total hip arthroplasty rapidly relieves pain and improves function in the early post-operative period. J Orthop Surg Res. 2010;5:88.
15. Whiteside LA. Surgical technique: gluteus maximus and tensor fascia lata transfer for primary deficiency of the abductors of the hip. Clin Orthop Relat Res. 2014;472(2):645–53.
16. Pritchett JW. One-component revision of failed hip resurfacing from adverse reaction to metal wear debris. J Arthroplast. 2014;29:219–24.
17. de Steiger RN, Miller LN, Prosser GH, Graves SE, Davidson DC, Stanford TE. Poor outcome of revised resurfacing hip arthroplasty 397 cases from the Australian joint replacement registry. Acta Orthop. 2010;81(1):72–6.
18. Grammatopoulos G, Pandit H, Kwon YM, Gundle R, McLardy-Smith P, Beard DJ, Murray DW, Gill HS. Hip resurfacings revised for inflammatory pseudotumour have a poor outcome. J Bone Joint Surg. 2009;91(8):1019–24.
19. Schmidutz F, Wanke-Jellinek L, Jansson V, Fottner A, Mazoochian F. Revision of hip resurfacing arthroplasty with a bone-conserving short-stem implant: a case report and review of the literature. J Med Case Rep. 2012;6:249.
20. Wong JM, et al. What is the rerevision rate after revising a hip resurfacing arthroplasty? Analysis from the AOANJRR. Clin Orthop Relat Res. 2015;473(11):3458–64.
21. Eswaramoorthy VK, Biant LC, Field RE. Clinical and radiological outcome of stemmed hip replacement after revision from metal-on-metal resurfacing. J Bone Joint Surg. 2009;91(11):1454–8.
22. De Smet KA, Van Der Straeten C, Van Orsouw M, et al. Revision of metal-on-metal hip resurfacing: lessons learned and improved outcome. Orthop Clin North Am. 2011;42:259.
23. de Haan R, Campbell PA, Su EP, De Smet KA. Revision of metal-on-metal resurfacing arthroplasty of the hip: the influence of malpositioning of the components. J Bone Joint Surg Br. 2008;90:1158–63.
24. Garrett SJ, Bolland BJ, Yates PJ, Gardner EM, Latham JM. Femoral revision in hip resurfacing compared with large-bearing metal-on-metal hip arthroplasty. J Arthroplast. 2011;26:1214–8.
25. Sandiford NA, Muirhead A, Skinner J. Revision of the well-fixed Birmingham Hip Resurfacing acetabular component–results using a novel device. Acta Orthop Belg. 2012;78:49–54.
26. Günther KP, Stiehler M. Revision in metal-on-metal hip arthroplasty: current knowledge. In: Bentley G, editor. European Instructional lectures, vol. Vol. 15. Berlin, Heidelberg: Springer; 2015. p. 143–51.

30 Revision of Metal on Metal THA

Eustathios Kenanidis, Eleftherios Tsiridis, Luigi Zagra, and Eleonora Caboni

30.1 Current Concepts

E. Kenanidis and E. Tsiridis

- MoM THAs were considered to have biological and biomechanical benefits compared to conventional MoP THAs [1].
- The proposed advantages of MoM THAs were the reduction of the occurrence of the polyethylene wear disease (aseptic loosening) and the hip dislocation using large-diameter femoral head components [2].
- However, several concerns emerged from the reported higher failure rates of MoM implants that have been attributed to a spectrum of findings termed as adverse reaction to metal debris.

30.1.1 Reported Survival of MoM Implants

- Several clinical series have reported good survivorship, especially for specific MoM designs. Neumann et al. [3] demonstrated 98% for the stem, and 96% for the cup 10-year follow-up for 100 THAs with Lubrimet (Smith and Nephew) MoM hip artrhoplasty. Engh et al. [4] also reported 98% survivorship and 0.3% rate of local reaction to the MoM bearing surface at a minimum 5-year follow-up for 126 patients treated with large-head MoM articulations and stated that this implant has comparable results to other bearing surfaces. Barret et al. [5] published 97.0% overall survivorship at five years for 779 large-diameter MoM THAs and only seven revisions for an adverse reaction to metallic debris.
- However, many other clinical studies and registries have reported higher than expected early failure rates and inferior midterm results [6, 7]. The National Joint Registry of England and Wales [6] demonstrated a high failure rate for MoM implants related to the head size, reaching 5·1% for 52-mm head at five years in men aged 60 years. Bolland et al. [8] showed cumulative survival rate 89.6% at five years for 199 hybrid MoM THAs whether Langton et al. [9] emphasised sharp differences in the rates of failure of various designs.

E. Kenanidis, M.D., Ph.D., M.Sc. (✉)
Academic Orthopaedic Unit, Aristotle University Medical School, Thessaloniki, Greece

E. Tsiridis, M.D., Ph.D., F.A.C.S., F.R.C.S. (✉)
Academic Orthopaedic Unit, Papageorgiou General Hospital, Aristotle University Medical School, Thessaloniki, Greece
e-mail: etsiridis@doctors.org.uk

L. Zagra, M.D. · E. Caboni, M.D.
Hip Department, Istituto Ortopedico Galeazzi IRCCS, Milan, Italy
e-mail: luigi.zagra@fastwebnet.it

E. Tsiridis (ed.), *The Adult Hip - Master Case Series and Techniques*,
https://doi.org/10.1007/978-3-319-64177-5_30

- Increasing evidence exist also that at medium-term follow-up, the survivorship for cementless stemmed MoM THA is inferior to that for MoP THA [10] and that MoM implants have higher revision rates than ceramic on polyethylene [11].
- A recent meta-analysis has demonstrated an increased risk of mortality and morbidity for patients undergoing MoM THA compared to non-MoM THAs [12]. In another current meta-analysis Lee et al. [13] showed that MoM implants were associated with higher revision rate than CoC for any reason (odds ratio = 2.39, $p = 0.046$) and periprosthetic joint infection (odds ratio = 6.21, $p = 0.015$) after cementless THA.

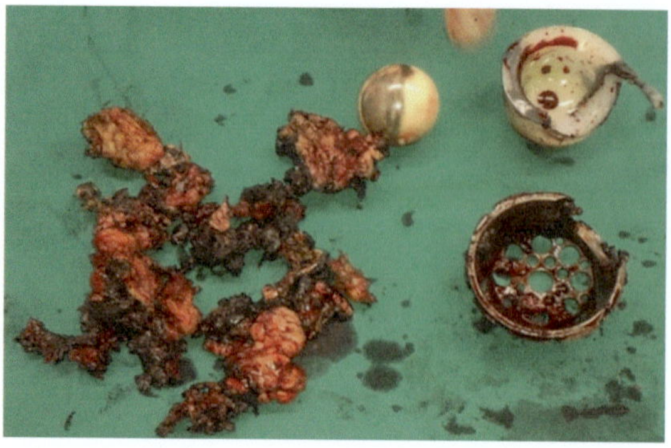

Fig. 30.1 Typical severe poly and metal shell erosion. The femoral head was ceramic, however, at some point, the ceramic surface was scraped off the head exposing the metal substrate which caused advanced ALVAL, part of which is demonstrated in the specimen

30.1.2 Unique Modes of Failure of MoM THAs

- The wear, corrosion, and mechanical factors such as fretting and third body wear produce metal debris mainly constituted of cobalt and chromium [14].
- Metal particles are considerably smaller, and their total number is two orders of magnitude higher than that found with conventional metal-on-polyethylene bearings [15, 16]. The latter is the primary reason for the increased biological activity of metal particles [17].
- Metal wear debris is phagocytosed by macrophages and transferred in lysosomes, where they are subject to corrosion, producing high intracellular levels of ions and causing cell death [17].
- The phagocytosis of metal particles may impair the osteoblastic activity of the cell and even cause DNA damage and genomic instability [17, 18].
- Hip metal particles and ionic wear debris are released into the periprosthetic tissues and transported systemically throughout the body [19].
    1. Systemic effects
        - The significance of high systemic metal ion concentrations still is not fully understood.
        - Cases of cardiac, endocrine, neurological, and dermatological complications have been reported [20] that are usually improved following the removal of the implant.
    2. Local tissue reactions
        - These are variously named, as adverse local tissue reactions (ALTRs) or adverse reaction to metal debris (ARMD) (Fig. 30.1). The term aseptic lymphocytic vasculitis-associated lesions (ALVAL) refers to the discrete histological findings linked with MoM bearings due to the perivascular lymphocytic infiltration of local tissue [4, 7].
        - The local tissue reactions have been attributed to the release of metal particles into the periprosthetic space, involving areas of macroscopic necrosis bounded by perivascular lymphocyte-dominated inflammation [21], corrosive osteolysis, large, sterile hip effusions, and periprosthetic solid and cystic large infiltrative soft-tissue masses (i.e., pseudotumors) [22, 23].
        - The local tissue reactions have variable clinical presentations, causing pain, damage to the local bone and soft tissue, and instability of the prosthetic joint, and there is difficulty differentiated from pain caused by infection [24].

   - A recent study [25] demonstrated that the peri-implant pseudotumor tissue expressed two principal phenotypes, namely, macrophage-dominated and T-lymphocyte-dominated response and low percentages of B lymphocytes and granulocytes. The inflammatory response phenotype was heterogeneous, and the metal levels were an important predisposing factor. It was supported that higher metal levels caused cytotoxicity and tissue injury, and recruitment of macrophages, however, lower metal levels, triggered T-lymphocyte-dominated response, and is likely to reflect hypersensitivity reaction.
3. Pseudotumors
   - There are limited data in the literature.
   - The reported prevalence in symptomatic and asymptomatic MoM THAs is 0.1–69% [14, 26, 27].
   - The specific aetiology is unknown [14]. A delayed-type IV hypersensitivity reaction to metal ions has been suggested as a cause [28].
   - They may be cystic or solid.
   - The natural history of pseudotumors has not been delineated. It is supported that they have slow progression and require follow-up every year [29–31].
   - Pseudotumors may produce necrosis and compress nearby structures such as the iliac and femoral vessels and the sciatic nerve [14] and the surrounding muscles. Progressive muscle atrophy is considered a reason for revision to prevent permanent damage [32].
4. Mechanisms of failure that are specific to the MoM articulation include:
   (a) Aseptic loosening of the monoblock acetabular component.
   (b) Adverse local tissue reaction (ALTR) due to the delayed-type hypersensitivity-like reactions termed ALVAL with the formation of pseudotumor.
   (c) Extensive necrotic changes with significant soft-tissue damage.

- Liddle et al. [33] demonstrated five type of failure of MoM THAs, namely, conventional failure mechanisms, including infection and impingement (8/39), synovitis without significant disruption of soft tissue (14/39), cystic pseudotumor with significant soft-tissue disruption (6/39), extensive osteolysis (7/39), and solid pseudotumor (4/39).

30.1.3 Evaluation of a Painful MoM THA

- It is necessary to optimize the evaluation and management of patients with failed MoM.
- The decision to revise a MoM THA is multifactorial and should be based on objective clinical findings [1].
- There are several guidelines [34–37] for the management of MoM revision arthroplasties; however, there are many uncertainties at the moment.
- The evaluation is based on a thorough clinical history and physical examination, along with laboratory data and imaging.

1. A comprehensive history and physical examination
   - Common symptoms are groin pain, difficulty with stair climbing, clunking, catching, limited strength, and iliopsoas irritation.
2. Imaging
   (a) High-quality radiographs
      - Look for common reasons of THA failure, as loosening and lysis.
      - Presume iliopsoas impingement due to an excessively large femoral head size [38].
      - Evaluate the component position: although there are conflicting results, the high inclination [39] angle and anteversion of the cup, small head size, and discrete prosthesis designs have been considered as risk factors for the failure of MoM THAs [2]. In a retrospective review, Desy et al. [40] correlated high acetabular inclination directly with metal ion levels. Hart et al. [41] reported that the cup inclination (the greatest effect),

version angles, and gender influenced blood cobalt and chromium levels.

(b) The metal artifact reduction sequence MRI (MARS MRI)
   - It has outstanding sensitivity and specificity for the detection of both superficial and deep lesions and muscle atrophy [42, 43].

(c) Ultrasound
   - It is used to evaluate tendon abnormalities [42].

(d) Computed tomography
   - It is used to evaluate osteolysis with plain radiographs.

(e) Single-photon emission CT (SPECT-CT)
   - It has been recommended for patients with unexplained pain [44].

3. Metal ion levels
   - Controversy exists regarding the clinical significance of serum cobalt and chromium ion levels and their impact on THA surveillance [14].
   - The variability of laboratory methods for measuring metal ion levels in the blood is a disadvantage.
   - Metal ion levels following MoM remain elevated postoperatively for some time. Blood peak of cobalt levels is usually at six and chrome at nine post-op months [45]. Following the revision to another bearing material, the ion levels fall but do not return to the preoperative levels [46].
   - Blood cobalt and chrome levels are affected by (a) the material design, (b) the implant positioning [41, 47, 48] (studies, however, are for resurfacing MoM).
   - The metal ions level were double following an unexplained pain in well-functioning THA [49]. The presence of elevated ion levels makes more likely the revision of MoM, although patients with asymptomatic MOM hips and elevated ion levels have been observed. Raised metal ion levels have been correlated with increased wear and pseudotumor formation [50].
   - It is well established that less than seven parts per billion (ppb) metal ion levels are predictive of a well-functioning MOM THA after the initial run-in period [14]. This cutoff point, however, derived from research based on hip resurfacings [47] and it is not uniformly accepted in different reported guidelines.
4. Pseudotumors
   - There is a lack of evidence [14] concerning
   (a) The long-term natural history of pseudotumors
   (b) The need for revision secondary to pseudotumors
   (c) The outcome following revision surgery
   (d) The interpretation of MRI findings
   - The revision for a pseudotumor excision is associated with significant postoperative complications [51] and recurrence as high as 30% [14].
   - Absolute indication for revision is the presence of cystic or solid pseudotumors that are large enough to cause pressure necrosis or stretch of soft tissues.
   - Large pseudotumors with intrapelvic extensions along the psoas sheath or arising wholly within the pelvis may compress neurovascular structures, and multidisciplinary surgical approach with vascular surgeons is required.
5. **Osteolysis**: progressive osteolysis may be indication for early revision [52].
6. **Muscle atrophy**
   - Preoperative planning and imaging for revision of a failed MoM THA may underestimate the degree of soft-tissue abnormalities as severe abductor muscle atrophy and stripping of the tendinous attachment [33].
   - There is growing evidence supporting early revision of a failed MoM hip implant to prevent irreparable damage [14].
   - Progressive muscle atrophy has been associated with elevated metal ion levels [32].
   - Campbell et al. [53] supported that patients can expect a good outcome if their soft tissues remain intact.

30.1.4 Published Data

There are a limited number of articles evaluating the outcome of revision THA for failed MoM hip arthroplasty [24, 33, 54–59]. These are retrospective or prospective cohort studies of 9 to 102 patients undergoing revision for a failed MoM THA. The follow-up is also limited ranging from a mean of 12 to 45 months postoperatively.

Revision of the failed MOM hip must be unique. It usually, however, involves the exchange of the modular femoral head and cup in the presence of a well-fixed femoral stem or an isolated head and liner exchange in case of a well-fixed and well-positioned cup. Revision hip arthroplasty surgery for ALTR can be technically challenging as a result of bone and soft-tissue changes [56]. Thorough resection of necrotic tissue, metallosis is recommended [17]. These revision procedures are often associated with a high incidence of complications [54].

Munro et al. [54] reviewed the results of 32 failed MoM revisions with fiber metal-backed and porous tantalum cups. He reported a high overall complication rate (38%). Dislocation was reported in nine cases (28%) using 32-mm, 36-mm, and 40-mm heads and a non-constrained liner in all patients. Although no precise reason was found for this high dislocation rate, this was attributed to an extensive soft-tissue damage and weakness of the hip abductor muscles. The risk of dislocation is also amplified from the usual necessary downsizing of the femoral head component and the significant soft-tissue damage from the ARMD or infection. Variable dislocation rates have been reported in the other studies ranging from 0 to 19% [24, 33, 51]. Snir et al. [58] supported the use of dual-mobility for the revision of failed resurfacing and total MoM hip arthroplasties.

Munro et al. [54] proposed the use of porous tantalum instead of fiber metal acetabular shell for the revision of a failed MoM; no failure to ingrowth occurred in porous tantalum cups compared with four failures in fiber metal cups [54]. Satisfactory early-term results for revision THA after failed MoM hip arthroplasty using highly porous metal acetabular components was also reported in other studies [57].

Wyles et al. [24] reported 92% survival for 37 revised MoM THAs at 24–81 months postoperatively. Infection was the main reason of the high (8%) failure rate at the short term that was eradicated with a two-stage exchange. 2/3 of the patients revised for infection had ALVAL, and this was considered as a possible connection. Judd et al. [55] supported that there are difficulties in the preoperative diagnosis of infection in patients suffering from ALVAL. This overlap of signs, symptoms, and values with non-infected patients and presence of atypical pathogens was noticed especially in patients having a cystic pseudotumor [55].

In the largest cohort study reported, Liow et al. [56] demonstrated 88% survival following revision of 102 consecutive large-head MoM hip arthroplasties due to symptomatic pseudotumor at three years. 14% complication rate and 7% re-revision rate at 30-month follow-up was reported. The pre-revision radiographic loosening, solid lesions with abductor deficiency on MRI, and a high-grade intraoperative tissue damage were significantly associated with poorer revision outcomes and considered as risk factors. 3 of 102 patients (3%) demonstrated pseudotumor recurrence. All patients with dislocations and pseudotumor recurrence were found to have extensive tissue necrosis with grade 3 intraoperative tissue damage. The pseudotumor recurrence rate in other studies [33, 54, 59] was 3–18%. The precise etiology of ALTR recurrence after revision for symptomatic pseudotumor remains mostly unknown. It is likely to be multifactorial related to surgical (incomplete surgical debridement and inadequate removal), patient, or implant factors.

In a recent review, Penrose et al. [60] disputed the high prevalence of complications following revision of a failed MoM. Authors supported that there were no differences between the MoM and MoP isolated acetabular revisions in the incidence of 30-day local complications. There were no differences at two years between the MoM and MoP acetabular revisions in the incidence of dislocation, infection, or re-revision.

30.2 Case Title: Metal-on-Metal THA Revision Socket for ALVAL

E. Kenanidis and E. Tsiridis

Metal-on-metal THA large-head 46 mm on a metal liner. ALVAL with early pain, inability to walk and levels of Co and Cr >7 µg/L. MRI was positive for joint effusion and pseudotumor formation. Mild osteolysis of the proximal femur but a loosening of the acetabular component (Fig. 30.2).

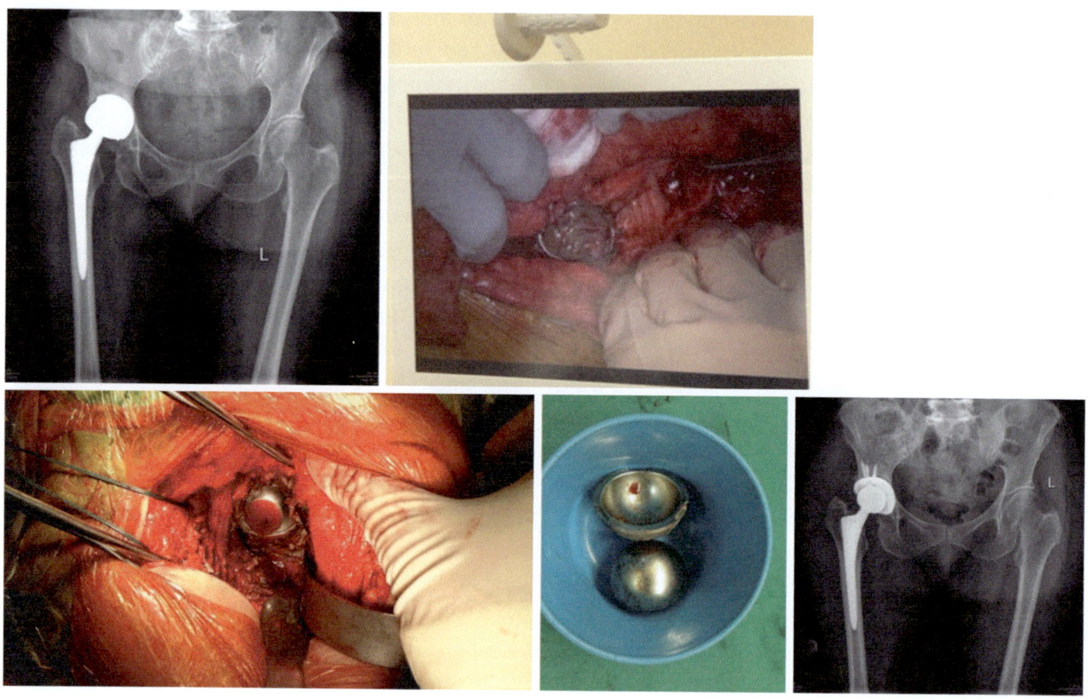

Fig. 30.2 Five figures depicting the preoperative MoM THA, intraoperative views of the cup, the revised metallic cup and head and the postoperative ceramic on poly THA

Easy revision of the loose socket to a larger revision shell with three stay screws and an HXLP on a ceramic 36-mm head. The taper of the stem in situ was intact and there was no need for grafting of the proximal femur (Fig. 30.2).

30.3 Case Title: Revision for ALVAL from Metal-on-Metal THA. The Pseudotumor Was Removed, the Stem Left In Situ as it Was Very Well Fixed and the Acetabular Component Was Revised to a Tantalum-Coated Shell with HXLP Poly and a Ceramic 36-mm Head (Fig. 30.3)

E. Kenanidis and E. Tsiridis

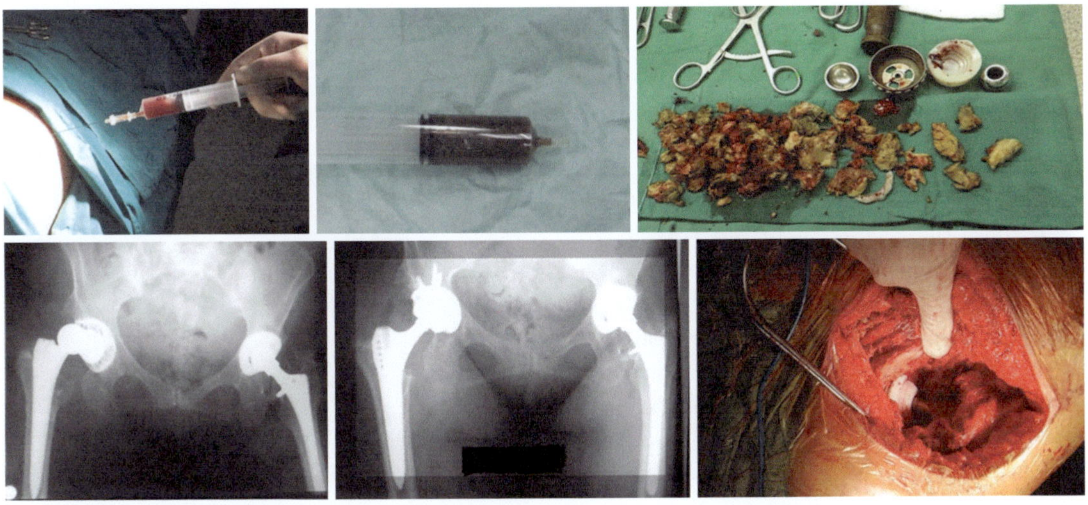

Fig. 30.3 Several figures demonstrating the preoperative joint aspiration and the dark-coloured aspirate, the implants and pseudotumor removed, the preoperative and postoperative x-ray as well as intraoperative view of the revised THA

30.4 Case Title: Hip Revision "MoM Revision"

Luigi Zagra and Eleonora Caboni

30.4.1 Demographics

Age: 63
Sex: F
BMI: 27.18

30.4.2 Relevant Past Medical History

Principal pathologies: Hypertension.

Previous surgical procedures: Tonsillectomy, appendicectomy, gastric banding in 1990, right THA in 2008, partial mastectomy in 2013.

Medication: Zofenopril 30 mg 1 cp/die, atenolol 50 mg 1cp/die, anastrozole 1 mg 1cp/die.

History of presenting complaint: 27/03/2007—left metal-on-metal THA with a large head. During the last 2 years, there was a mild pain with the feeling of local swelling not affecting the function and everyday life of the patient. One month and a half before the consultation, there was a sudden left hip pain, and limping. The patient was evaluated in another hospital, with the referred suspected diagnosis of metallosis, but without any further treatment nor exams out of standard X-rays and CT.

30.4.3 Clinical Examination

Symptoms: Left hip—groin and trochanteric pain, mainly on weight-bearing.

Range of motion: Painful hip, but full ROM.

Specific tests: Trendelenburg sign test + +..

Main disability: Severe limp.

Neurovascular evaluation: No neurovascular lesions detected.

30.4.4 Preoperative Radiological Assessment/Imaging (Figs. 30.4, 30.5, and 30.6)

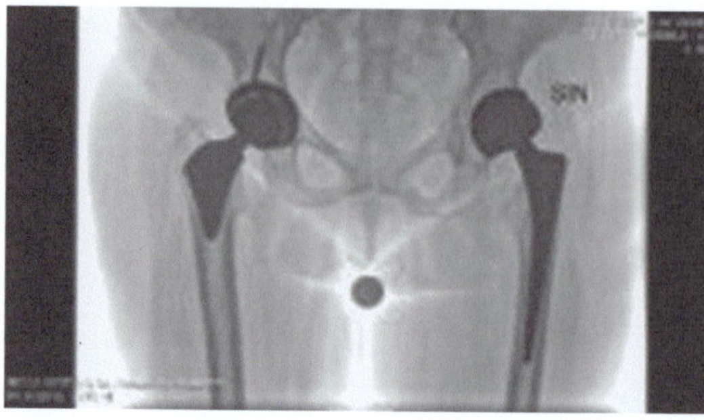

Fig. 30.4 Anteroposterior preoperative X-ray of the pelvis: the greater trochanter completely disappeared, osteolysis all around the socket and a fracture of the ischiopubic branch are visible

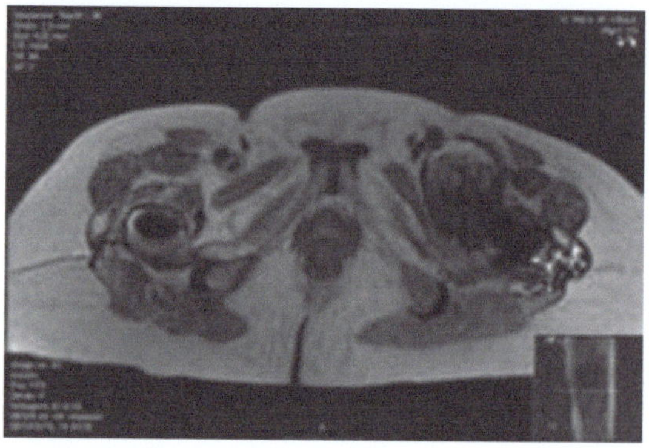

Fig. 30.5 MRI with MARS technique: anterior partially solid pseudotumor with fluid collection also extended to the trochanteric area

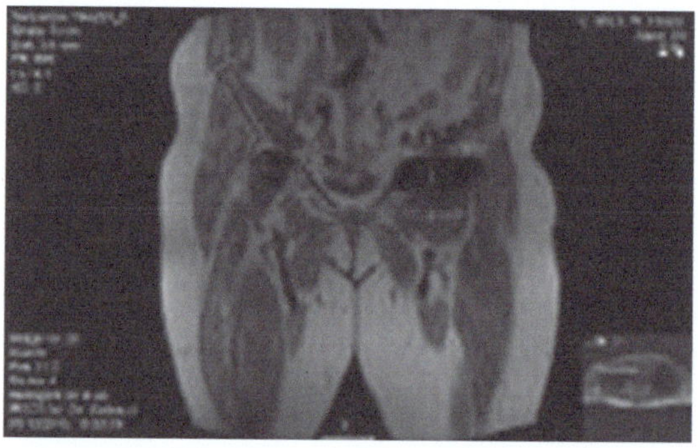

Fig. 30.6 MRI with MARS technique: the pseudotumor is extended along the iliac muscle inside the pelvis

Other: Blood metal ions—Co 88.4 mcg/L, Cr 41.0 mcg/L. CRP 5.3 mg/dL (0–0.5), ESR 57.

30.4.5 Preoperative Planning

Diagnosis: ARMD in left THA (Figs. 30.4, 30.5 and 30.6).

Possible treatment options: Full revision (cup and stem) or partial revision (only the cup).

Chosen treatment method: Revision of the cup and replacement of the head.

Selection of implants if applicable and rational: Aiming to avoid any metal, titanium cup with XLPE liner and ceramic head with titanium sleeve (Biolox Option).

Expected difficulties: The management of the soft tissues and bone stock, and the removal of the stable implant.

Strategies to overcome difficulties: Use of MRI to estimate the real extension of the pseudotumor and the muscle damages, CT scan to evaluate the bone stock, availability of bone graft, special instrumentation for removal of stable implants, availability of a ceramic head with the sleeve compatible with the previous cone in case of retaining of the stem.

Templating: Not necessary in this case.

30.4.6 Surgical Note

Patient's position: Right lateral decubitus.

Type of anesthesia: General anesthesia.

Surgical approach: Posterolateral approach.

Main steps: Careful removal of the pathological tissues that can be removed from this approach. Samples to rule out infection, removal with explant tool of the cup, removal of the head, evaluation of the cone and the stem stability.

Reconstruction techniques: Impaction grafting of morcellized bone from fresh frozen heads to fill the bone defects, high porosity titanium cup with two screws, cross-linked PE liner, 32-mm ceramic Biolox Option head with XL neck (Figs. 30.7 and 30.8). Repair of the few residual fibers of the gluteus medius and soft tissues with nonabsorbable sutures.

30.4.7 Intraoperative Challenges

Challenges and solutions: Soft-tissues damages—repair and tension of the tissues with the XL neck. Bone loss on the acetabular side: morcellized bone grafting to fill the defects. Severe bone loss of the greater trochanter: impossible to be addressed effectively.

Unanticipated problems and solution: None.

Thorough description of decision making, including the reason for the final decision: Uncemented cup and bone graft on the acetabular side because of reliable stability to the native bone. The stem was retained because it was stable and osseointegrated and to avoid major damage to the femur in the presence of slight damage to the cone.

30.4.8 Postoperative Radiographs (Figs. 30.7 and 30.8)

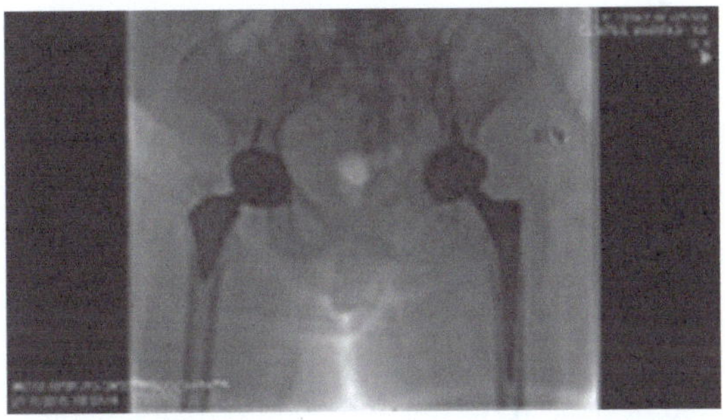

Fig. 30.7 Postoperative AP X-ray of the pelvis

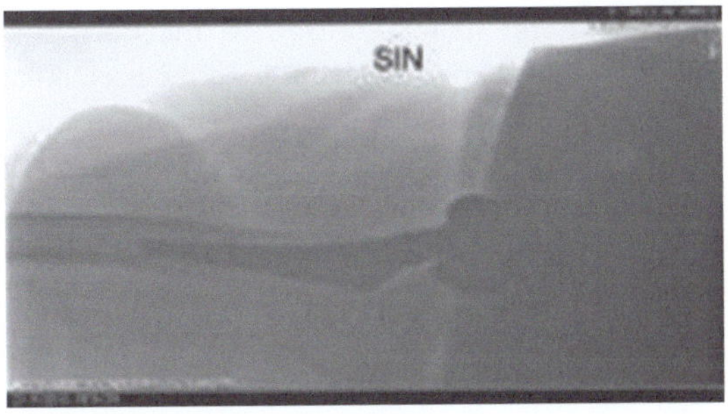

Fig. 30.8 Postoperative shoot-through lateral view X-rays of the hip

30.4.9 Postoperative Management

Chemoprophylaxis and anticoagulant treatment period: Nadroparin calcium 0.4 mL 1 fl/die 5 weeks postoperatively as protocol. Antibiotic prophylaxis with cefazolin 2 g.

Gait/limb loading until full loading: Partial weight-bearing with two crutches for four months.

30.4.10 Follow-Up and Complications

No reported complication.

30.4.11 Discussion

Advantages of the applied method: Restoring of the bone stock on the acetabular side and preserving of the osseointegrated stem.

Disadvantages of the method: Maintaining a cone that worked for some years and that was possibly involved in the metal problems.

Alternative evidence-based techniques for the case: Revision of both the cup and the stem, cemented impaction grafting of the implant on the acetabular side.

Why is the chosen technique better for this case: Less invasive procedure on the femoral side and of bone restoring and good primary stability on the acetabular side.

Indications and contraindications for your technique: Indications—well-fixed femoral components with no major damage to the cone and achieving good primary stability on the acetabular side with an acceptable hip centre position. Contraindications—major damages of the cone of the stem and major bone loss of the acetabular side.

Learning curve and how to manage complications: The technique is quite easy; the two possible complications of this case are an infection (that will need all the prevention and treatment of infected cases) and a dislocation (this could require the conversion to a dual mobility or to a constrained liner in case of instability).

Level of evidence concerning the superiority of this method against others: IV (there is no clear evidence of what is the best option for this type of cases) [61, 62].

References

1. Bolognesi MP, Ledford CK. Metal-on-metal total hip arthroplasty: patient evaluation and treatment. J Am Acad Orthop Surg. 2015;23(12):724–31.
2. Haddad FS, Thakrar RR, Hart AJ, Skinner JA, Nargol AV, Nolan JF, Gill HS, Murray DW, Blom AW, Case CP. Metal-on-metal bearings: the evidence so far. J Bone Joint Surg Br. 2011;93:572–9.
3. Neumann DR, Thaler C, Hitzl W, Huber M, Hofstädter T, Dorn U. Long-term results of a contemporary metal-on-metal total hip arthroplasty: a 10-year follow-up study. J Arthroplast. 2010;25:700–70.
4. Engh CA, Ho H, Engh CA. Metal-on-metal hip arthroplasty: does early clinical outcome justify the chance of an adverse local tissue reaction? Clin Orthop Relat Res. 2010;468:406–12.
5. Barrett WP, Kindsfater KA, Lesko JP. Large-diameter modular metal-on-metal total hip arthroplasty: incidence of revision for adverse reaction to metallic debris. J Arthroplast. 2012;27(6):976–83.
6. Smith AJ, Dieppe P, Vernon K, Porter M, Blom AW, on behalf of the National Joint Registry of England and Wales. Failure rates of stemmed metal-on-metal hip replacements: analysis of data from the National Joint Registry of England and Wales. Lancet. 2012;379:1199–20.
7. Korovessis P, Petsinis G, Repanti M, Repantis T. Metallosis after contemporary metal-on-metal total hip arthroplasty. Five to nine year follow-up. J Bone Joint Surg Am. 2006;88:1183–91.
8. Bolland BJ, Culliford DJ, Langton DJ, Millington JPS, Arden NK, Latham JM. High failure rates with a large-diameter hybrid metal-on-metal total hip replacement: clinical, radiological and retrieval analysis. J Bone Joint Surg Br. 2011;93:608–15.
9. Langton DJ, Jameson SS, Joyce TJ, Gandhi JN, Sidaginamale R, Mereddy P, Lord J, Nargol AVF. Accelerating failure rate of the ASR total hip replacement. J Bone Joint Surg Br. 2011;93:1011–6.
10. Varnum C, Pedersen AB, Mäkelä K, Eskelinen A, Havelin LI, Furnes O, Kärrholm J, Garellick G, Overgaard S. Increased risk of revision of cementless stemmed total hip arthroplasty with metal-on-metal bearings. Acta Orthop. 2015;86(4):491–7. https://doi.org/10.3109/17453674.2015.1023132.
11. Milosev I, Kovac S, Trebse R, Levasic V, Pisot V. Comparison of ten-year survivorship of hip prostheses with use of conventional polyethylene, metal-on-metal, or ceramic-on-ceramic bearings. J Bone Joint Surg Am. 2012;94:1756–63.
12. Pijls BG, Meessen JMTA, Schoones JW, Fiocco M, van der Heide HJL, Sedrakyan A, Nelissen RGHH. Increased mortality in metal-on-metal versus non-metal-on-metal primary total hip arthroplasty at 10 years and longer followup: a systematic review

and meta-analysis. PLoS One. 2016;11(6):e0156051. https://doi.org/10.1371/journal.pone.0156051.

13. Lee YK, Yoon BH, Choi YS, Jo WL, Ha YC, Koo KH. Metal on metal or ceramic on ceramic for cementless total hip arthroplasty: a meta-analysis. J Arthroplast. 2016;31(11):2637–2645.e1. https://doi.org/10.1016/j.arth.2016.04.01.
14. Berber R, Skinner JA, Hart AJ. Management of metal-on-metal hip implant patients: who, when and how to revise? World J Orthop. 2016;7(5):272–9.
15. Doorn PF, Campbell PA, Worrall J, Benya PD, McKellop HA, Amstutz HC. Metal wear particle characterization from metal on metal total hip replacements: transmission electron microscopy study of periprosthetic tissues and isolated particles. J Biomed Mater Res. 1998;42:103–11.
16. Brodner W, Bitzan P, Meisinger V, Kaider A, Gottsauner-Wolf F, Kotz R. Serum cobalt levels after metal-on-metal total hip arthroplasty. J Bone Joint Surg Am. 2003;85:2168–73.
17. Griffin JW, D'Apuzzo M, Browne JA. Management of failed metal-on-metal total hip arthroplasty. World J Orthop. 2012;3(6):70–4.
18. Lohmann CH, Schwartz Z, Köster G, Jahn U, Buchhorn GH, MacDougall MJ, Casasola D, Liu Y, Sylvia VL, Dean DD, Boyan BD. Phagocytosis of wear debris by osteoblasts affects differentiation and local factor production in a manner dependent on particle composition. Biomaterials. 2000;21:551–61.
19. Merritt K, Brown SA. Release of hexavalent chromium from corrosion of stainless steel and cobalt-chromium alloys. J Biomed Mater Res. 1995;29:627–33.
20. Prentice JR, Clark MJ, Hoggard N, Morton AC, Tooth C, Paley MN, Stockley I, Hadjivassiliou M, Wilkinson JM. Metal-on-metal hip prostheses and systemic health: a cross-sectional association study 8 years after implantation. PLoS One. 2013;8:e66186.
21. Campbell P, Ebramzadeh E, Nelson S, Takamura K, De Smet K, Amstutz HC. Histological features of pseudotumor-like tissues from metal-on-metal hips. Clin Orthop Relat Res. 2010;468:2321–7.
22. Bosker BH, Ettema HB, Boomsma MF, Kollen BJ, Maas M, Verheyen CCPM. High incidence of pseudotumour formation after large-diameter metal-on-metal total hip replacement: a prospective cohort study. J Bone Joint Surg Br. 2012;94:755–61.
23. Pandit H, Glyn-Jones S, Mclardy-Smith P, Gundle R, Whitwell D, Gibbons CLM, Ostlere S, Athanasou N, Gill HS, Murray DW. Pseudotumours associated with metal-on-metal hip resurfacings. J Bone Joint Surg Br. 2008;90:847–51.
24. Wyles CC, Van Demark RE III, Sierra RJ, Trousdale RT. High rate of infection after aseptic revision of failed metal-on-metal total hip arthroplasty. Clin Orthop Relat Res. 2014;472:509–16.
25. Paukkeri E-L, Korhonen R, Hämäläinen M, Pesu M, Eskelinen A, Moilanen T, Moilanen E. The inflammatory phenotype in failed metal-on-metal hip arthroplasty correlates with blood metal concentrations. PLoS One. 2016;11(5):e0155121. https://doi.org/10.1371/journal.pone.0155121.
26. Canadian Hip Resurfacing Study Group. A survey on the prevalence of pseudotumors with metal-on-metal hip resurfacing in Canadian academic centers. J Bone Joint Surg Am. 2011;93(Suppl 2):118–21.
27. Williams DH, Greidanus NV, Masri BA, Duncan CP, Garbuz DS. Prevalence of pseudotumor in asymptomatic patients after metal-on-metal hip arthroplasty. J Bone Joint Surg Am. 2011;93:2164–71.
28. Kwon YM, Thomas P, Summer B, Pandit H, Taylor A, Beard D, Murray DW, Gill HS. Lymphocyte proliferation responses in patients with pseudotumors following metal-on-metal hip resurfacing arthroplasty. J Orthop Res. 2010;28(4):444–50.
29. Almousa SA, Greidanus NV, Masri BA, Duncan CP, Garbuz DS. The natural history of inflammatory pseudotumors in asymptomatic patients after metal-on-metal hip arthroplasty. Clin Orthop Relat Res. 2013;471:3814–21.
30. Ebreo D, Bell PJ, Arshad H, Donell ST, Toms A, Nolan JF. Serial magnetic resonance imaging of metal-on-metal total hip replacements. Follow-up of a cohort of 28 mm Ultima TPS THRs. Bone Joint J. 2013;95-B:1035–9.
31. van der Weegen W, Brakel K, Horn RJ, Hoekstra HJ, Sijbesma T, Pilot P, Nelissen RG. Asymptomatic pseudotumours after metal-on-metal hip resurfacing show little change within one year. Bone Joint J. 2013;95-B:1626–31.
32. Berber R, Khoo M, Cook E, Guppy A, Hua J, Miles J, Carrington R, Skinner J, Hart A. Muscle atrophy and metal-on-metal hip implants: a serial MRI study of 74 hips. Acta Orthop. 2015;86:351–7.
33. Liddle AD, Satchithananda K, Henckel J, et al. Revision of metal-on-metal hip arthroplasty in a tertiary center: a prospective study of 39 hips with between 1 and 4 years of follow-up. Acta Orthop. 2013;84(3):237.
34. Kwon YM, Lombardi AV, Jacobs JJ, Fehring TK, Lewis CG, Cabanela ME. Risk stratification algorithm for management of patients with metal-on-metal hip arthroplasty: consensus statement of the American Association of Hip and Knee Surgeons, the American Academy of Orthopaedic Surgeons, and the hip society. J Bone Joint Surg Am. 2014;96:e4.
35. Epstein M, Emri I, Hartemann P, Hoet P, Leitgeb N, Martinez L, Proykova A, Rizzo L, Rodriguez-Farre E, Rushton L, Rydzynski K, Samaras T, Testai E, Vermeire T, Case C, Dekant W, De Jong W, Gunther K, Hensten A, Morlock M, Stea S, Van Der Straeten C, Verheyen C. The safety of Metal-on-Metal joint replacements with a particular focus on hip implants. 2014. http://ec.europa.eu/health/scientific_committees/emerging/docs/scenihr_o_042.pdf.
36. Hannemann F, Hartmann A, Schmitt J, Lützner J, Seidler A, Campbell P, Delaunay CP, Drexler H, Ettema HB, García-Cimbrelo E, Huberti H, Knahr K, Kunze J, Langton DJ, Lauer W, Learmonth I, Lohmann CH, Morlock M, Wimmer MA, Zagra L, Günther KP. European multidisciplinary consensus statement on the use and monitoring of metal-on-metal bearings for total hip replacement and hip resurfacing. Orthop Traumatol Surg Res. 2013;99:263–71.

37. Ludgate S, Haque F, Cacou C. Medical device alert: all metal-on-metal (MoM) hip replacements. 2012. http://www.mhra.gov.uk/home/groups/dtsbs/documents/medicaldevicealert/con155767.pdf.
38. Browne JA, Polga DJ, Sierra RJ, Trousdale RT, Cabanela ME. Failure of larger-diameter metal-on-metal total hip arthroplasty resulting from anterior iliopsoas impingement. J Arthroplast. 2011;26:978.e5–8.
39. Emmanuel AR, Bergin KM, Kelly GE, et al. The effect of acetabular inclination on metal ion levels following metal-on-metal hip arthroplasty. J Arthroplast. 2014;29(1):186.
40. Desy NM, Bergeron SG, Petit A, Huk OL, Antoniou J. Surgical variables influence metal ion levels after hip resurfacing. Clin Orthop Relat Res. 2011;469: 1635–1641.13.
41. Hart AJ, Skinner JA, Henckel J, Sampson B, Gordon F. Insufficient acetabular version increases blood metal ion levels after metal-on-metal hip resurfacing. Clin Orthop Relat Res. 2011;469:2590–7.
42. Siddiqui IA, Sabah SA, Satchithananda K, Lim AK, Cro S, Henckel J, Skinner JA, Hart AJ. A comparison of the diagnostic accuracy of MARS MRI and ultrasound of the painful metal-on-metal hip arthroplasty. Acta Orthop. 2014;85:375–82.
43. Garbuz DS, Hargreaves BA, Duncan CP, Masri BA, Wilson DR, Forster BB. The John Charnley award: diagnostic accuracy of MRI versus ultrasound for detecting pseudotumors in asymptomatic metal-on-metal THA. Clin Orthop Relat Res. 2014;472:417–23.
44. Berber R, Henckel J, Khoo M, Wan S, Hua J, Skinner J, Hart A. Clinical usefulness of SPECT-CT in patients with an unexplained pain in metal on metal (MOM) total hip arthroplasty. J Arthroplast. 2015;30:687–94.
45. Daniel J, Ziaee H, Pradhan C, McMinn DJ. Six-year results of a prospective study of metal ion levels in young patients with metal-on-metal hip resurfacings. J Bone Joint Surg Br. 2009;91:176–9.
46. Ball ST, Severns D, Linn M, Meyer RS, Swenson FC. What happens to serum metal ion levels after a metal-on-metal bearing is removed? J Arthroplast. 2013;28:53–5.
47. Hart AJ, Sabah SA, Bandi AS, Maggiore P, Tarassoli P, Sampson B, A Skinner J. Sensitivity and specificity of blood cobalt and chromium metal ions for predicting failure of metal-on-metal hip replacement. J Bone Joint Surg Br. 2011;93:1308–131.
48. Matthies AK, Henckel J, Cro S, Suarez A, Noble PC, Skinner J, Hart AJ. Predicting wear and blood metal ion levels in metal-on-metal hip resurfacing. J Orthop Res. 2014;32:167–74.
49. Hart AJ, Sabah SA, Sampson B, Skinner JA, Powell JJ, Palla L, Pajamäki KJ, Puolakka T, Reito A, Eskelinen A. Surveillance of patients with metal-on-metal hip resurfacing and total hip prostheses: a prospective cohort study to investigate the relationship between blood metal ion levels and implant failure. J Bone Joint Surg Am. 2014;96:1091–9.
50. Kwon YM, Ostlere SJ, McLardy-Smith P, Athanasou NA, Gill HS, Murray DW. "asymptomatic" pseudotumors after metal-on-metal hip resurfacing arthroplasty: prevalence and metal ion study. J Arthroplast. 2011;26:511–8.
51. Grammatopolous G, Pandit H, Kwon Y-M, Gundle R, McLardySmith P, Beard DJ, Murray DW, Gill HS. Hip resurfacings revised for inflammatory pseudotumour have a poor outcome. J Bone Joint Surg Br. 2009;91:1019–24.
52. Randelli F, Banci L, Favilla S, Maglione D, Aliprandi A. Radiographically undetectable periprosthetic osteolysis with ASR implants: the implication of blood metal ions. J Arthroplast. 2013;28:1259–64.
53. Campbell P, Shimmin A, Walter L, Solomon M. Metal sensitivity as a cause of groin pain in metal-on-metal hip resurfacing. J Arthroplast. 2008;23:1080–5.
54. Munro JT, Masri BA, Duncan CP, Garbuz DS. High complication rate after revision of large-head metal-on-metal total hip arthroplasty. Clin Orthop Relat Res. 2014;472:523–8.
55. Judd KT, Noiseux N. Concomitant infection and local metal reaction in patients undergoing revision of metal on metal total hip arthroplasty. Iowa Orthop J. 2011;31:59–63.
56. Liow MHL, Dimitriou D, Tsai T-Y, Kwon Y-M. Preoperative risk factors associated with poor outcomes of revision surgery for "Pseudotumors" in patients with metal-on-metal hip arthroplasty. J Arthroplast. 2016;31(12):2835–42.
57. Rahman WA, Amen T, Hetaimish BM, Safir OA, Kuzyk PR, Gross AE. Outcome of revision total hip arthroplasty in management of failed metal-on-metal hip arthroplasty. J Arthroplast. 2016;31(11):2559–63.
58. Snir N, Park BK, Garofolo G, Marwin SE. Revision of failed hip resurfacing and large metal-on-metal total hip arthroplasty using dual-mobility components. Orthopedics. 2015;38(6):369–74. https://doi.org/10.3928/01477447-20150603-04.
59. Rajpura A, Porter ML, Gambhir AK, Freemont AJ, Board TN. Clinical experience of revision of metal on metal hip arthroplasty for aseptic lymphocyte dominated vasculitis associated lesions (ALVAL). Hip Int. 2011;21:43–51.
60. Penrose CT, Seyler TM, Wellman SS, Bolognesi MP, Lachiewicz PF. Complications are not increased with acetabular revision of metal-on-metal total hip arthroplasty. Clin Orthop Relat Res. 2016;474(10):2134–42. https://doi.org/10.1007/s11999-016-4793-4.
61. Zagra L, Maccario C, Mondini A, Bianchi L. Treatment of failures related to articulation material in THA. A comprehensive algorithm of surgical options and open questions. Hip Int. 2014;24(Suppl 10): S48–57. https://doi.org/10.5301/hipint.5000170.
62. Lainiala O, Reito A, Elo P, Pajamäki J, Puolakka T, Eskelinen A. Revision of metal-on-metal hip prostheses results in marked reduction of blood cobalt and chromium ion concentrations. Clin Orthop Relat Res. 2015;473(7):2305–13. https://doi.org/10.1007/s11999-015-4156-6.

31 Trunnion Disease

Eustathios Kenanidis, Eleftherios Tsiridis, Luigi Zagra, Eleonora Caboni, Yale A. Fillingham, Darren R. Plummer, and Craig J. Della Valle

31.1 Current Concepts

E. Kenanidis and E. Tsiridis

The modularity of stems at the head-neck junction has certain advantages as the decrease of implant stock, the simplification of revision (option to retain the stem and perform head exchange), the adaptation of leg length and offset, and the use of alternative bearing options [1]. The main disadvantages, however, are the increase in fretting and crevice corrosion at the taper junction [2, 3]. Their contribution to implant failure is now increasingly recognized [4].

31.1.1 Pathogenesis

The head-neck junctions of femoral stems (Ti-6Al-4V or CoCr) resist to corrosion, forming a protective surface oxide layer through a process of self-passivation. Cyclic loading of the hip joint and the resulting oscillatory motions between the head and neck at the taper disrupt the passive oxide layer by fretting. The result is that the underlying metal is exposed and re-passivation occurs, but as the time passes, this ability is depleted and corrosion occurs [5].

Taper corrosion includes [6]:

1. Crevice corrosion due to local chemistry changes within crevices
2. Fretting that disintegrates the protective oxide layer on the taper

E. Kenanidis, M.D., Ph.D., M.Sc. (✉)
Academic Orthopaedic Unit, Aristotle University Medical School, Thessaloniki, Greece

E. Tsiridis, M.D., Ph.D., F.A.C.S., F.R.C.S.
Academic Orthopaedic Unit, Papageorgiou General Hospital, Aristotle University Medical School, Thessaloniki, Greece
e-mail: etsiridis@doctors.org.uk

L. Zagra, M.D.
Hip Department, Istituto Ortopedico Galeazzi IRCCS, Milan, Italy
e-mail: luigi.zagra@fastwebnet.it

E. Caboni, M.D.
Hip Department, Istituto Ortopedico Galeazzi IRCCS, Milan, Italy

Y.A. Fillingham, M.D.
Department of Orthopaedic Surgery, Dartmouth College, Geisel School of Medicine, Hanover, NH, USA

D.R. Plummer, M.D., M.B.A.
The Ohio State University Wexner Medical Center, Columbus, OH, USA

C.J. Della Valle, M.D.
Division of Adult Reconstruction, Rush University Medical Center, Chicago, IL, USA

E. Tsiridis (ed.), *The Adult Hip - Master Case Series and Techniques*,
https://doi.org/10.1007/978-3-319-64177-5_31

3. Galvanic corrosion due to the presence of mixed metal systems (Ti-6Al-4 V stems with CoCr heads)

Corrosion can produce by-products at the head-neck junction, mainly metal ions, that can migrate locally and systemically. Extensively corroded tapers can initiate a cascade of local macrophage or lymphocyte adverse events leading to necrosis of periprosthetic tissues, local synovitis, osteolysis, implant loosening, and early failure [7].

31.1.2 Etiology

This phenomenon is probably multifactorial in origin due to its rarity. A crucial limitation is that our data on taper corrosion are based on in vitro and retrieval studies [7]. In vitro studies, however, cannot precisely reproduce all the in vivo conditions, and retrieval studies usually involve analysis of clinically failed implants where corrosion was not the only cause of failure [8]. The heterogeneity of parameters that may be associated with taper corrosion as the bearing surfaces, head size, offset, stem type and alloy, and implant manufacturer is another difficulty in trunnion disease interpretation in the majority of studies [8]. The heterogeneous and non-validated description of corrosion (kind of corrosion/histological findings), the non-always-provided taper information, and the small sample sizes are further problems. Some parameters under investigation are the following:

31.1.2.1 Taper Design

There are no clear taper geometric parameters that influence corrosion [7]. Trunnions are now manufactured shorter, with a smaller diameter and a trapezoidal neck to reduce the head/neck ratio and the risk of dislocation; 12 mm/14 mm (proximal/distal diameter) trunnions replaced 14 mm/16 mm [9]. Not all "12/14" tapers, however, have the same cone angles, as this is also dependent on the trunnion length. For the equal posterior to the distal diameter, the cone angle increases with increased length [7]. The effect of the taper width and length on taper corrosion seems uncertain. It was supported that shorter, smaller tapers that enhance joint stability also result in increased fretting and corrosion [10]. A retrieval study [11], however, demonstrated the opposite that shorter, thinner tapers had lower fretting scores compared to longer, thicker tapers. Shorter trunnions that usually sit entirely within the bore increase edge loading and local stresses at its base and augment damage to the taper [9]. Narrower trunnions provide less surface area for the interference fit.

The effects of the cone angle and the angular mismatch at the taper junction on corrosion are uncertain. Nassif et al. supported that different taper angles had no relation to corrosion [11]. Parekh et al. reported that an angular mismatch up to 0.075 did not increase micromotion at the taper junction and corrosion [12]. Indeed, the effect of these parameters needs further clarification.

31.1.2.2 Head Material

Ceramic heads usually have less risk of corrosion than metal [13]. The hazard however of taper corrosion is alleviated but not eliminated by using ceramic heads. A retrieval study [8] supported that 50 alumina ceramic heads had lower but not entirely reduced corrosion scores than 50 matched CoCr heads on metal tapers. The safety of reimplantation of a ceramic head onto an unrevised femoral stem during revision has not been fully delineated. The possible damage of the trunnion during removal of the femoral head may act as a stress riser responsible for the initiation of a fracture in a newly implanted ceramic head and may increase the risk of wear production due to abnormal movements of the damaged taper [7]. Hannouche et al. [14] supported the reimplantation of alumina heads onto well-fixed titanium stems during revision THA; prerequisite was the inspection of only minor scratches on the taper and a stable fit of the newly implanted ceramic head on the taper.

31.1.2.3 Head-Neck Couple

Different coupling material combinations demonstrated different corrosion types in vitro studies [15, 16]; the results are not however sure for in vivo conditions. An in vitro study [16] following testing of various material coupling combinations, supported that the Ti-6Al-4 V/Ti-6Al-4 V couple showed the most significant surface damage under axial loading. In a retrieval study, Nassif et al. [11] demonstrated that titanium-titanium interfaces had the least amount of fretting compared to CoCr/CoCr and CoCr/titanium interfaces probably due to its ability to form a better interference fit via cold-welding. This better fit, however, may complicate dislodging the femoral head from the stem during revision surgery, damage the trunnion, or even lead to the revision of a (well-fixed) stem in case of impossible head detachment [17]. Other similar studies [6, 18] reported that different alloy pairing of the head and the stem damages more both the head and the taper than components of similar alloy pairing as the former is more susceptible to galvanic corrosion. In an another multicenter retrieval study, Goldberg et al. [6] demonstrated moderate to severe corrosion in 28% of heads of similar alloy couples compared to 42% of heads of mixed alloy couples.

31.1.2.4 Femoral Head Size

The use of larger heads decreased dislocation rate over time; it may, however, result in higher stresses at the femoral head-neck junction and increased corrosion [2, 9, 19]. A retrieval study [2] reported a significant increase in taper corrosion scores of 36 mm heads compared with 28 mm heads in metal-on-polyethylene THA, with CoCr alloy head and stem and 12/14 mm taper. The head size was not a reason of taper corrosion in all studies. In a retrieval study [20] of 100 taper junctions of metal-on-polyethylene articulations, 16% of the tapers had severe or moderate corrosion independent of femoral head size. Taper corrosion was most strongly correlated with the severity of the abrasive wear affecting the surface of the CoCr head, and the femoral head size was only a cofactor in predicting corrosion.

31.1.2.5 Others

The role of several other factors such as the body mass index, lateral offset, varus femoral stem positioning, longer necks, time since implantation, variance in the force of impaction and the vector of the applied force during the assembly of modular heads and contamination of the interface is also explored [6, 20]. The modern changes in taper designs and head-neck taper interface such as the use of taper sleeves to provide further modulation of neck length and offset and the circular machining ridges of current trunnions also require further investigation.

31.1.3 Diagnosis

The diagnosis of the trunnion disease is challenging. This is mainly attributed to the rarity of the phenomenon, the variety of clinical representation of the disease, and the absence of a specific diagnostic test. Taper corrosion is an infrequent cause of painful THA that is overdiagnosed. The actual incidence of clinically relevant taper corrosion seems to be low. Cooper et al. [21] reported that only 1.8% of revision MoP THAs performed were the result of complications arising from corrosion at the head-neck taper. There is a broad spectrum of taper corrosion, ranging from mild corrosion with no tissue reaction and little or no clinical implications to ALTRs with significant clinical effects. Diagnosis is often difficult unless important associated ALTRs occur. Increased serum cobalt and chromium levels, particularly a differential elevation of serum cobalt levels for chromium levels may be suggesting of the diagnosis [21, 22]. The hip aspiration to exclude infection provides the opportunity for joint fluid metal ion analysis. Ultrasound and metal artifact reduction magnetic resonance imaging (MRI) are also useful in the diagnosis.

31.1.4 Treatment

To prevent corrosion:

1. Use the appropriate femoral head material and size.
2. Clean and dry blood or fat of the taper surfaces before the engagement of the taper to avoid angular mismatch at the taper junction and ensure adequate interlocking of the taper [23, 24].

To treat a well-fixed stem that has trunnion damage:

1. Consider the potential benefits of revising against the potential morbidity associated with stem revision.
2. There is no well-accepted way to measure the trunnion damage. In practice, it is supported that the head and not the stem should be replaced when the trunnion has mild visible but not palpable defects and when interference fit can be achieved with the new head. The long-term consequence of this practice is unknown [25].
3. Ensure that the new femoral head implanted onto a trunnion is compatible with the design of the trunnion to avoid micromotion and corrosion [12]. Proximal to distal diameters of trunnions from different implants and companies may be identical; however, they may differ in dimensions, and cone angles [12, 26].

31.1.5 Published Results

In one of the recently reported systematic reviews, Carli et al. [27] analysed 24 studies that demonstrated clinically notable corrosion at the head-neck taper interface. These were studies with a limited sample size that did not provide always taper information and with a heterogeneous and non-validated description of corrosion. In the 776 THA reported cases with documented head-neck corrosion found at revision surgery, the patients had the clinical picture of aseptic loosening and unexplained thigh pain in the intermediate THA follow-up period. More than half of them were MoM THA. The combination of large femoral head sizes and small taper dimensions comprised the majority of published corrosion cases. The size however of the femoral head was not reported in more than half of the cases. The median head size of MoM THAs was 46 mm. 38.1% of the cases have the same metal alloy at the head-neck interfaces (CoCrMo on CoCrMo, or Ti6Al4V on Ti6Al4V), whether 61.9% were composed of different alloys (CoCrMo and Ti6Al4V). Revision to a ceramic head and ceramic/polyethylene liner was the most commonly utilised treatment. In the majority of cases, the trunnion was found intact (83.3%), and no stem revision was necessary. Coating precipitation, mixed alloy coupling, and head-neck modulus mismatch collectively appear to contribute to the destructive process.

31.2 Case Title: Hip Revision "Trunnion Disease Revision"

Luigi Zagra and Eleonora Caboni

31.2.1 Demographics

Age: 71
Sex: F
BMI: 23.05

31.2.2 Relevant Past Medical History

Principal pathologies: Diverticulosis, atrial fibrillation in 2002, hypertension, celiac disease, and Duhring disease.

Previous surgical procedures: None.

Medication: Irbesartan, dapsone, mesalazine, lorazepam.

Other: Allergy—amoxicillin, nickel.

History of presenting complaint: 2009 left THA with a cementless implant, 36 mm ceramic head (+0) on cross-linked polyethylene, modular stem with an exchangeable neck (130° long neck) (Fig. 31.1). 2012 cup revision following a diagnosis of cup loosening (tantalum cup with a cross-linked polyethylene liner and replacement of the head with a new 32 mm ceramic one, taper V40, + 4 mm) (Fig. 31.2).

31.2.3 Clinical Examination

Symptoms: Groin and thigh pain since the first surgery, no benefit after the previous revision.

Range of motion: Full ROM.

Main disability: Mild pain during walking with a limitation of walking distance.

Neurovascular evaluation: No neurovascular lesions detected.

31.2.4 Preoperative Radiological Assessment/Imaging (Figs. 31.1, 31.2, and 31.3)

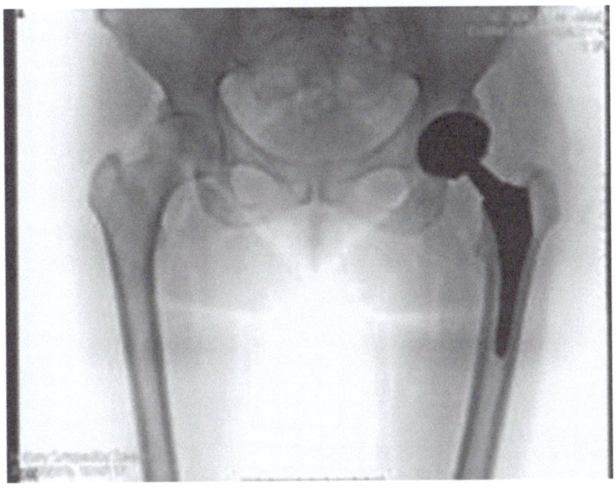

Fig. 31.1 X-rays 6 months after the primary THA

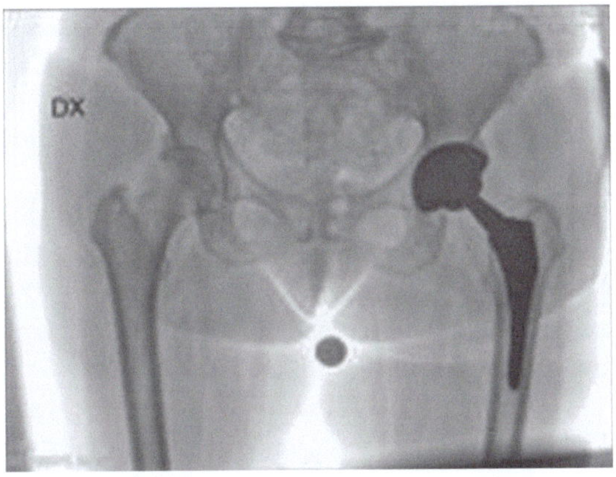

Fig. 31.2 Preoperative X-rays (3 years after cup revision)

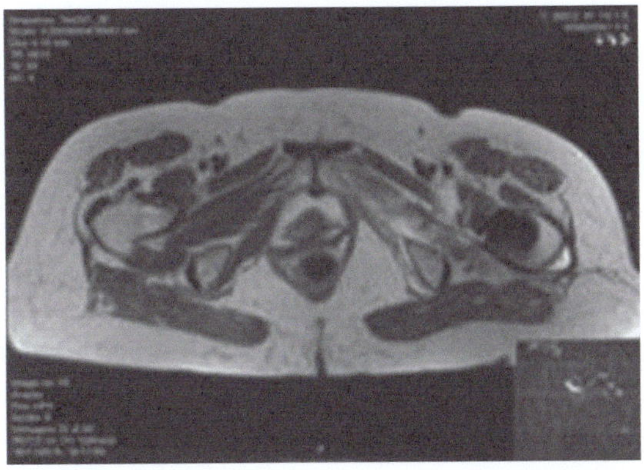

Fig. 31.3 MARS-MRI showing fluid collection inside the joint and surrounding the great trochanter

Other: Blood metal ions—Co 2.10 μg/L, Cr 7.0 μg/L, ESR 7.0 CRP 0.37 mg/dL (0–0.5). Joint aspiration = negative for infection.

31.2.5 Preoperative Planning

Diagnosis: Trunnion disease is coming from the neck modularity (the body of the stem is in titanium; the neck is in CoCr).

Possible treatment options: (1) Full revision (cup and stem). (2) Replacement of the modular neck with a titanium one. (3) Revision of the stem (removal of the stem with or without a transfemoral approach).

Selection of implants if applicable and rational: Monoblock stem for primary THA or revision stem.

Expected difficulties: Stable osseointegrated stem.

Strategies to overcome difficulties: Extended trochanteric osteotomy to remove the stem.

Templating: To plan the size and the length of the new stem.

31.2.6 Surgical Note

Patient's position: Right lateral decubitus.

Type of anesthesia: Blended.

Surgical approach: Posterolateral approach.

Main steps: Removal of the pathological tissues in the trochanteric area and from the joint (Fig. 31.3). Samples to rule out infection. Evaluation of the cup stability and orientation. Removal of the head and the neck, then with thin chisels removal of the bone at the interface of the body of the stem and the proximal part of the femur, and with proper instrumentation, quite an easy removal of the stem from the top.

Reconstruction techniques: Preparation of the proximal femur with rasps and insertion of an offset Zweymuller stem with a 32 mm ceramic head, medium neck (Figs. 31.4 and 31.5).

31.2.7 Intraoperative Challenges

Challenges and solutions: Removal of the stable stem with proper devices without opening the femur and use of an offset stem to improve soft tissues tension and joint stability.

Unanticipated problems and solution: Joint stability enhanced by the use of an offset stem.

Thorough description of decision making, including the reason for the final decision: The cup was in correct position, stable, and osseointegrated so it was preserved. The stem was any way removed, even if stable, because of the apparent evidence of fretting and corrosion at the level of the stem neck modularity.

31.2.8 Postoperative Radiographs (Figs. 31.4 and 31.5)

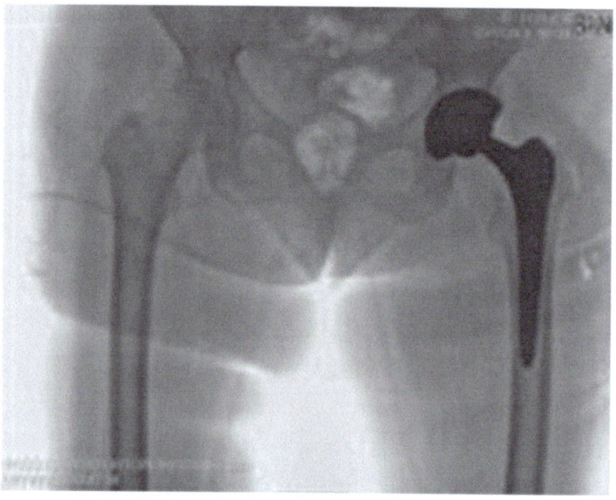

Fig. 31.4 Postoperative AP X-rays of the pelvis

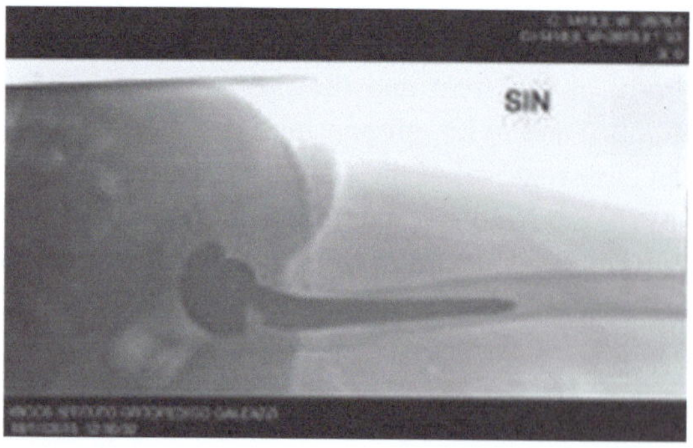

Fig. 31.5 Postoperative shoot-through lateral view X-rays of the hip

31.2.9 Postoperative Management

Chemoprophylaxis and anticoagulant treatment period: Nadroparin calcium 0.4 mL 1 fl/die five weeks from the surgery as protocol. Antibiotic prophylaxis with cefazolin 2 g.

Gait/limb loading until full loading: Partial weight bearing with two crutches for 3 months.

31.2.10 Follow-Up and Complications

No complication reported.

31.2.11 Discussion

Advantages of the applied method: Preserving of the stable cup and removal of the possible cases of metal ions debris, avoiding any metal modularity.

Disadvantages of the method: Preserving of the liner that already worked for 3 years.

Alternative evidence-based techniques for the case: No other evidence-based solutions.

Why is the chosen technique better for this case? Removal of the stem from the top gave the possibility of avoiding a long revision stem. The ceramic head without any modularity of the stem avoids risks of further trunnion problems.

Indications and contraindications for your technique: Indications: modular stems with the availability of proper instruments for the removal of exchangeable CoCr necks. Contraindications: stable stems with a distal osseointegration that requires an extended trochanteric osteotomy.

Learning curve and how to manage complications: The technique is quite easy; the two possible complications are an infection (that will need all the prevention and treatment of infected cases) and a dislocation (this could require the conversion to a dual mobility).

Level of evidence concerning the superiority of this method against others: IV (There is no clear evidence of what is the best option in this type of cases) [28–30].

31.3 Case Title: Corrosion at the Modular Head-Neck Taper in Metal-on-Polyethylene Total Hip Arthroplasty

Yale A. Fillingham, Darren R. Plummer, and Craig J. Della Valle

31.3.1 Demographics

Age: 68 years old
Sex: Female
BMI: 29.9

31.3.2 Relevant Past Medical History

Principal pathologies: Hypertension, hyperlipidemia, irritable bowel syndrome, cataracts.

Previous surgical procedures: Right total hip arthroplasty (Fig. 31.6), left total shoulder arthroplasty, tonsillectomy, appendectomy, and hysterectomy.

Medication: Benazepril, dicyclomine, hydrochlorothiazide, Metamucil, multivitamin, and supplements.

Other: Right total hip arthroplasty performed September 2008. Components used were cementless fully porous-coated stem and hemispherical acetabular cup with a metal-on-polyethylene bearing surface.

History of presenting complaint: The patient presented 3 years after a right total hip arthroplasty with progressive right groin pain and an increasing difficulty walking. Originally she had a period with a well-functioning hip but experienced worsening right hip symptoms over the past year. The workup of a painful total hip arthroplasty was initiated with serum inflammatory markers and metal levels. Results demonstrated elevated inflammatory markers with an erythrocyte sedimentation rate of 99 mm/h and C-reactive protein of 199.5 mg/L (laboratory normal reference <8 mg/L). Plain X-rays showed well-fixed components however there was an area that appeared similar to osteolysis in the area of the calcar (Fig. 31.7). Serum metal levels showed cobalt at 49.83 ng/mL (reference 0.15 ± 0.1 ng/mL) and chromium at 9.81 ng/mL (reference 0.12 ± 0.1 ng/mL). Aspirate analysis demonstrated a white blood cell count of 322 cell/uL and no growth of the culture. As a result of the elevated serum metal levels, a metal artifact reduction sequence-magnetic resonance scan (MARS-MRI) was obtained that demonstrated three well-circumscribed mass-like lesions arising from the region of the total hip arthroplasty with surrounding muscular oedema (Fig. 31.8).

31.3.3 Clinical Examination

Symptoms: Right groin pain

Range of motion: 80° of flexion, 20° of internal rotation, 30° of external rotation, and no flexion contracture

Specific tests: Reproducible groin pain with resisted straight leg raise

Main disability: Pain causing a coxalgic gait pattern

Neurovascular evaluation: Sensation intact throughout lower extremity, palpable pedal pulses.

31.3.4 Preoperative Radiological Assessment/Imaging (Figs. 31.6, 31.7, and 31.8)

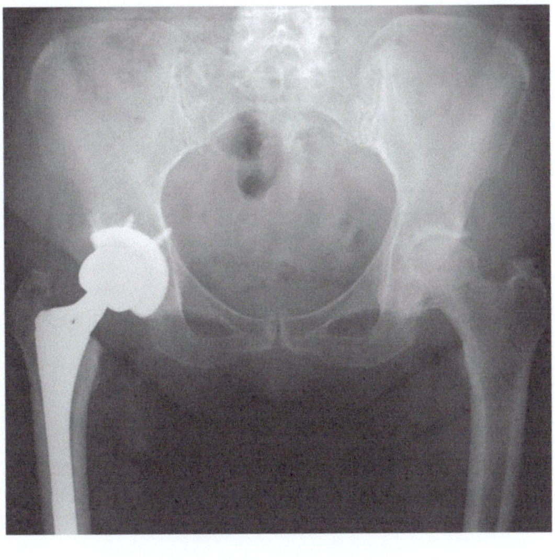

Fig. 31.6 AP pelvis is demonstrating the patient's right total hip arthroplasty six weeks after surgery

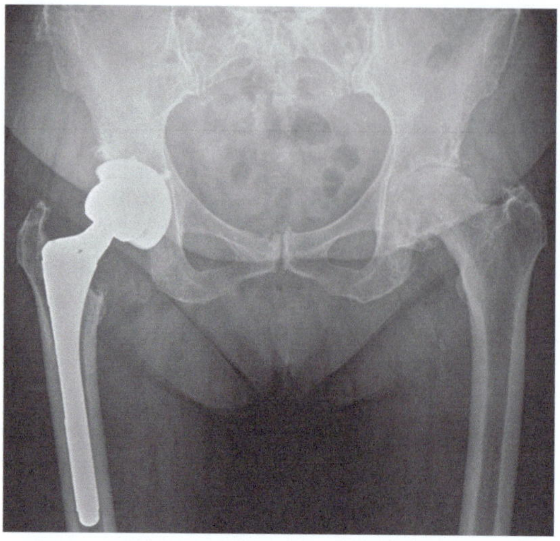

Fig. 31.7 AP pelvis three years postoperatively is showing a right total hip arthroplasty with well-fixed components. There is an area of what appears to be osteolysis in the calcar area

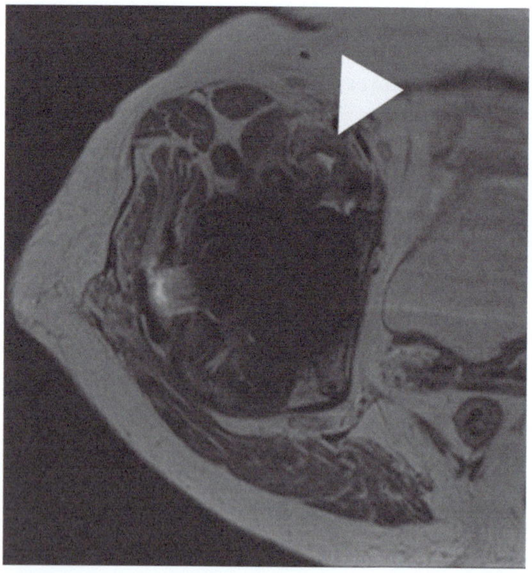

Fig. 31.8 Axial MARS-MRI is identifying the presence of a pseudotumor *(arrow)*

Other: It is important to recognize that for patients with a metal-on-polyethylene bearing, normal serum cobalt and chromium levels should be less than 1 ng/mL. This is a different and lower threshold than many surgeons use when evaluating a metal-on-metal bearings.

31.3.5 Preoperative Planning

Diagnosis: Adverse local tissue reaction secondary to taper corrosion at the modular head-neck junction.

Possible treatment options: Revision arthroplasty with metal femoral head, revision arthroplasty with ceramic femoral head (with or without titanium adapter sleeve), retention of well-fixed components, and revision of all components.

Chosen treatment method: Revision arthroplasty with ceramic femoral head and titanium adapter sleeve and retention of well-fixed femoral stem and cup.

Selection of implants if applicable and rational: Biolox delta ceramic femoral head with titanium adapter sleeve and highly cross-linked acetabular liner.

Expected difficulties: Potential for complexity in exposing the acetabulum with a well-fixed stem in place.

Strategies to overcome difficulties: Prepare for an extensile exposure or a trochanteric osteotomy if needed.

31.3.6 Surgical Note

Patient's position: Lateral decubitus

Type of anesthesia: Combined spinal epidural

Surgical approach: Posterior

Main steps: Removal of the cobalt-chromium head, synovectomy, gross cleaning of the Morse taper of the stem, exchange of acetabular liner, and placement of a titanium sleeve and ceramic head (Fig. 31.9).

Reconstruction techniques: Exposure of the cup by mobilizing the femur and retracting it anteriorly

31.3.7 Intraoperative Challenges

Challenges and solutions: Exposure of the acetabulum could be hard as explained above. Be ready to use a more extensive exposure or perform a trochanteric osteotomy if needed.

Thorough description of decision making, including the reason for the final decision: Our data suggest that when corrosion is present at the head-neck junction, the components can be retained assuming they are appropriately positioned and well fixed. The modular femoral head is exchanged to a ceramic head to remove the source of cobalt and chromium. A ceramic head with a titanium taper sleeve is preferred to mitigate the potential increased risk of ceramic head fracture when placed on a taper that has previously been used. The modular head and liner exchange is a far less morbid option than removing the stem, and our results suggest the resolution of symptoms and a return of the serum metal levels to normal levels postoperatively.

31.3.8 Postoperative Radiographs (Fig. 31.9)

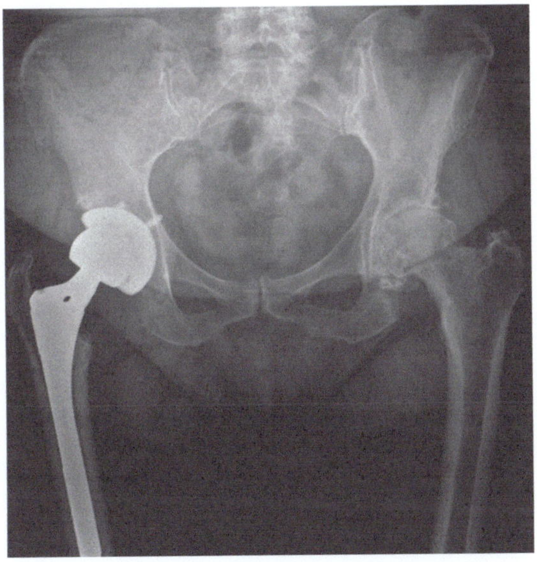

Fig. 31.9 AP pelvis obtained three weeks after surgery demonstrating retainment of the femoral stem and acetabular cup

31.3.9 Postoperative Management

Chemoprophylaxis and anticoagulant treatment period: Patient was placed on Coumadin for 3 weeks following the surgery.

Gait/limb loading until full loading: Patient had no postoperative weight-bearing restrictions.

31.3.10 Follow-Up and Complications

Patient experienced no postoperative complications. Her pain resolved, and the follow-up serum metal levels showed a cobalt of 0.71 ng/mL and chromium of 1.16 ng/mL.

31.3.11 Discussion

Advantages of the applied method: As described above, data from Cooper et al. [21] and Plummer et al. [31] suggest that in cases of head-neck corrosion with a metal-on-polyethylene bearing, a well-fixed stem can be retained, so long as the head is exchanged to a ceramic head. This technique avoids the morbidity of removing a well-fixed stem which, again, data from the sources above suggests is unnecessary. The only failures observed in our experience have been when a new cobalt-chromium alloy head was utilized at the time of revision, as opposed to a ceramic head. A titanium taper sleeve is preferred to decrease the potentially increased risk of ceramic head fracture if placed on a taper that has previously been used.

Disadvantages of the method: The primary drawback of the technique described is that with time, there is the possibility that corrosion could occur once again. The study by Plummer et al. [31], however, demonstrated no clinical failures when a ceramic head was utilized and the serum cobalt and chromium levels returned to less than 1 ng/mL, which is considered normal for patients with a metal-on-polyethylene bearing. The most common complication following revision total hip arthroplasty is dislocation, and the surgeon must ensure appropriate stability at the time of revision surgery. If the abductor musculature is damaged from the corrosion reaction, strong consideration should be given to using a dual mobility bearing or a constrained liner as large heads alone are associated with a higher risk of dislocation if the abductor musculature has been damaged or is incompetent.

Alternative evidence-based techniques for the case: Alternatives to the method utilized in this case include a complete revision of the femoral component; however, there is no data that we are aware of that has evaluated this strategy.

Why the chosen technique is better for this case: This method was preferred in this patient given the data reported by Plummer et al. [31]. An isolated exchange of the liner and head to a ceramic femoral head with a titanium taper sleeve is associated with a lower risk to the patient of most complications given the shorter operative time and decreased blood loss compared to a revision of the femoral stem.

Indications and contraindications for your technique: The primary indications for the revision method described include a painful total hip arthroplasty with evidence of taper corrosion, including common causes of pain such as osteolysis and infection, a modular total hip implant, elevated serum metal ion levels with a serum cobalt and chromium greater than 1 ng/mL, and advanced imaging significant for adverse local tissue reaction. Contraindication for the specific technique described included a loose femoral stem requiring revision of the stem or significant abductor muscle damage requiring a more constrained implant.

Learning curve and how to manage complications: As described, the most common expected complication is recurrent dislocation. To prevent this complication, we routinely use larger femoral head diameters and ensure that component positioning is acceptable. If damage to the abductor musculature is encountered, strong consideration should be given to using a dual mobility bearing or a constrained liner. If a dislocation does occur postoperatively, a CT scan is useful to confirm that the anteversion of the cup and stem are appropriate. If malposition is identified, a further revision to correct the malposition is warranted. If the patient had abductor damage and a dual mobility bearing or constrained liner was not utilized, a revision to one of these bearings will likely be required.

Level of evidence concerning the superiority of this method against others: Adverse local tissue reactions secondary to corrosion at the head-neck interface have been managed successfully in the short term with the method recommended, exchange of the modular head to a ceramic femoral head with a titanium adapter sleeve and retaining a well-fixed femoral component, thus altering the composition of the taper interface and removing a potential source of cobalt and chromium debris while minimizing morbidity. Studies have shown ceramic femoral heads confer an advantage in trunnion fretting, corrosion, and the subsequent development of adverse local tissue reactions (Plummer et al. [31]; Kurtz et al. [8]). Modular head exchange to a ceramic bearing has been shown to provide a rapid improvement in serum metal levels in the short term although longer follow-up will be necessary to confirm whether these encouraging early results are durable (Plummer et al. [31]).

References

1. Srinivasan A, Jung E, Levine BR. Modularity of the femoral component in total hip arthroplasty. J Am Acad Orthop Surg. 2012;20(4):214–22.
2. Dyrkacz RMR, et al. The influence of head size on corrosion and fretting behaviour at the head-neck interface of artificial hip joints. J Arthroplasty. 2013;28(6):1036–40.
3. Higgs GB, et al. Is increased modularity associated with increased fretting and corrosion damage in metal-on-metal total hip arthroplasty devices? A retrieval study. J Arthroplasty. 2013;28(8 Suppl):2–6.
4. Engh CA, et al. The surgical options and clinical evidence for treatment of wear or corrosion occurring with THA or TKA. Clin Orthop Relat Res. 2014;472(12):3674–86.
5. Sivakumar B, Kumar S, Sankara Narayanan TSN. Fretting corrosion behaviour of Ti–6Al–4V alloy in artificial saliva containing varying concentrations of fluoride ions. Wear. 2011;270(3-4):317–24.

6. Goldberg JR, Gilbert JL, Jacobs JJ, Bauer TW, Paprosky W, Leurgans S. A multicenter retrieval study of the taperinterfaces of modular hip prostheses. Clin Orthop Relat Res. 2002;401:149–61.
7. Hussenbocus S, Kosuge D, Solomon LB, Howie DW, Oskouei RH. Head-neck taper corrosion in hip arthroplasty. Biomed Res Int. 2015;2015:758123.
8. Kurtz SM, et al. Do ceramic femoral heads reduce taper fretting corrosion in hip arthroplasty? A retrieval study. Clin Orthop Relat Res. 2013;471(10):3270–82.
9. Langton DJ, Sidaginamale R, Lord JK, Nargol AV, Joyce TJ. Taper junction failure in large-diametermetal-on-metal bearings. Bone Joint Res. 2012;1(4):56–63.
10. Panagiotidou A, et al. Enhanced wear and corrosion in modular tapers in total hip replacement is associated with the contact area and surface topography. J Orthop Res. 2013;31(12):2032–9.
11. Nassif NA, et al. Taper design affects failure of large-head metal-on-metal total hip replacements. Clin Orthop Relat Res. 2014;472(2):564–71.
12. Parekh J, et al. Effect of angular mismatch tolerance on trunnion micro-motion in metal-onmetal THA designs. Bone Joint J. 2013;95(Suppl 34):261.
13. Hallab NJ, et al. Differences in the fretting corrosion of metal-metal and ceramicmetal modular junctions of total hip replacements. J Orthop Res. 2004;22(2):250–9.
14. Hannouche D, et al. Is there a risk in placing a ceramic head on a previously implanted trunion? Clin Orthop Relat Res. 2010;468(12):3322–7.
15. Duisabeau L, Combrade P, Forest B. Environmental effect on fretting of metallic materials for orthopaedic implants. Wear. 2004;256(7-8):805–16.
16. Swaminathan V, et al. Fretting corrosion of CoCrMo and Ti6Al4V interfaces. Biomaterials. 2012;33(22):5487–503.
17. Kop AM, et al. Proximal component modularity in THA—at what cost? An implant retrieval study. Clin Orthop Relat Res. 2012;470(7):1885–94.
18. Urban RM, et al. Are fretting and corrosion reduced in contemporary head/neck modular junctions?. In Proceedings of the ORS Annual Meeting, Poster No. 1050, 2012.
19. Moga I, et al. Trunnion surface damage in THR: MPE vsMOMarticulations. Bone Joint J. 2013;95(Suppl 34):140.
20. Moga M, et al. Variables influencing tribo-corrosion of modular junctions in metal-on polyethylene THR? In proceedings of the American academy of orthopedic surgeons annual meeting, Paper 614, 2014.
21. Cooper HJ, et al. Corrosion at the head-neck taper as a cause for adverse local tissue reactions after total hip arthroplasty. J Bone Joint Surg Am. 2012;94(18):1655–61.
22. Garbuz DS, et al. The John Charnley award: metal-on-metal hip resurfacing versus large-diameter head metal-on-metal total hip arthroplasty: a randomized clinical trial. Clin Orthop Relat Res. 2010;468(2):318–25.
23. Mroczkowski ML, et al. Effect of impact assembly on the fretting corrosion of modular hip tapers. J Orthop Res. 2006;24(2):271–9.
24. Rehmer A, et al. Influence of assembly procedure and material combination on the strength of the taper connection at the head-neck junction of modular hip endoprostheses. Clin Biomech. 2012;27(1):77–83.
25. Alexander J, et al. The effect of tribo-chemical damage on mechanical performance of TIAlV-CoCr taper junctions. In international society for technology in arthroplasty, Poster 2556, 2013.
26. Hernigou P, et al. One hundred and fifty years of history of the Morse taper: from Stephen a. Morse in 1864 to complications related to modularity in hip arthroplasty. Int Orthop. 2013;37(10):2081–8.
27. Carli A, Politis A, Zukor D, Huk O, Antoniou J. Clinically significant corrosion at the head-neck taper interface in total hip arthroplasty: a systematic review and case series. Hip Int. 2015;25(1):7–14.
28. Kwon YM, Fehring TK, Lombardi AV, Barnes CL, Cabanela ME, Jacobs JJ. Risk stratification algorithm for management of patients with dual modular taper total hip arthroplasty: consensus statement of the American association of Hip and Knee Surgeons, the American Academy of Orthopaedic Surgeons and the Hip Society. J Arthroplasty. 2014;29(11):2060–4. doi:10.1016/j.arth2014.07.029. Epub 2014 Jul 31
29. Walsh CP, Hubbard JC, Nessler JP, Markel DC. Revision of recalled modular neck rejuvenate and ABG femoral implants. J Arthroplasty. 2015;30(5):822–6. doi:10.1016/j.arth.2014.12.002. Epub 2014 Dec 5
30. Esposito CI, Wright TM, Goodman SB, Berry DJ. What is the trouble with trunnions? Clin Orthop Relat Res. 2014;472(12):3652–8. doi:10.1007/s11999-014-3746-z.
31. Plummer DR, Berger RA, Paprosky WG, Sporer SM, Jacobs JJ, Della Valle CJ. Diagnosis and management of adverse local tissue reactions secondary to corrosion at the head-neck junction in patients with metal on polyethylene bearings. J Arthroplast. 2016;31(1):264–8.

32 Acute and Chronic Pelvic Dissociation

Eustathios Kenanidis, Eleftherios Tsiridis, Michael Nogler, Neil P. Sheth, Christopher M. Melnic, Wayne G. Paprosky, Fritz Thorey, Stanislav Bondarenko, Volodymyr Filippenko, and Volodymyr Mezentsev

32.1 Current Concepts

E. Kenanidis and E. Tsiridis

Pelvic Dissociation (PD) is the loss of structural bone or fracture that separates completely the superior (ilium) from the inferior pelvis (ischiopubic segment) through the anterior and posterior columns of the acetabulum [1, 2]. It is a rare complication that ranges between 1 and 8% in revision THA series. Patients at risk are women, patients suffering from RA, and those with a history of radiation therapy [1].

The main causes of PD are the following [3]:

- Periprosthetic osteolysis in patients with THA (most common)
- Excessive acetabular reaming during primary THA (iatrogenic)
- Forced impaction of an uncemented shell during THA (iatrogenic)
- Trauma
- Infection
- Stress fracture

32.1.1 Types/Classification

There are two types of PD, acute (APD) and chronic (CPD) [1]. APD is usually iatrogenic (during acetabular component explantation,

E. Kenanidis, M.D., Ph.D., M.Sc. (✉)
Academic Orthopaedic Unit, Aristotle University Medical School, Thessaloniki, Greece

E. Tsiridis, M.D., Ph.D., F.A.C.S., F.R.C.S.
Academic Orthopaedic Unit, Papageorgiou General Hospital, Aristotle University Medical School, Thessaloniki, Greece
e-mail: etsiridis@doctors.org.uk

M. Nogler, M.D.
Orthopaedic Surgery, Innsbruck, Austria
e-mail: michael.nogler@professor-nogler.at

N.P. Sheth, M.D.
Orthopaedic Surgery, Pennsylvania Hospital, University of Pennsylvania, Philadelphia, PA, USA
e-mail: Neil.Sheth@uphs.upenn.edu

C.M. Melnic, M.D.
Massachusetts General Hospital, Boston, MA, USA

Newton-Wellesley Hospital, Newton, MA, USA

Harvard Medical School, Boston, MA, USA

W.G. Paprosky, M.D
Midwest Orthopaedics at Rush University, Chicago, IL, USA

Central DuPage Hospital—Northwestern University, Winfield, IL, USA
e-mail: wpaprosky@reagan.com

F. Thorey, M.D., Ph.D.
ATOS Hospital Heidelberg, Heidelberg, Germany
e-mail: fritz.thorey@atos.de

S. Bondarenko, M.D., Ph.D.
V. Filippenko, M.D.
V. Mezentsev, M.D., Ph.D.
Department of Joint Pathology, Sytenko Institute of Spine and Joint Pathology, Kharkiv, Ukraine

E. Tsiridis (ed.), *The Adult Hip - Master Case Series and Techniques*,
https://doi.org/10.1007/978-3-319-64177-5_32

acetabular preparation, or implant impaction) or traumatic whether CPD is mainly the result of periprosthetic osteolysis [3]. APD usually has a minimal gap between the hemipelves that can be compressed and a good healing potential. CPD, however, has fibrous tissue between the hemipelves that cannot be easily compressed and sclerotic and non-vascularized bone at the edge with poor healing potential [2].

AAOS [4] and Gross [5] classifications of acetabular defects include a category for PD. Berry's [6] modification of the original AAOS classification includes a subclassification of PD related to the efficacy of healing. The first subclass includes PD with cavitary or moderate segmental bone loss, the second PD with severe segmental loss or combined segmental and massive cavitary bone loss and the third PD with previously irradiated bone with or without bone loss. The first type heals more effectively than the other.

32.1.2 Preoperative Diagnosis and Evaluation

Preoperative diagnosis is based on the high degree of suspicion and needs careful preoperative assessment and planning. The following radiographs are recommended [3]:

1. A well-centred anteroposterior view of the pelvis.
2. Obturator and iliac oblique Judet views of the acetabulum [7, 8]. In a cadaveric study, oblique views, especially false-profile views, were more sensitive (79%) than standard views to detect PD [7].
3. Thin cut CT scan of the acetabulum. It is the most effective imaging tool to detect PD and monitor periprosthetic osteolysis preoperatively [9, 10]. Its use, however, is limited in patients with prosthetic implants due to metallic artifact [11].

The radiographic criteria on standard anteroposterior radiographs are not consistently reproducible [6]. Possible suspicious radiographic findings of PD are:

1. A visible fracture line through the pelvis [6].
2. The superior migration of the hip centre. Sporer et al. [12] supported that there is minimal PD probability if the hip centre has migrated <3 cm above the superior obturator line.
3. The translation/rotation of the inferior relative to the superior part pelvis.
4. An asymmetry of the obturator rings (indicates the three criteria) [6].
5. The interrupted Kohler line with medial translation of the inferior hemipelvis or medial protrusion of the implant [6].

In cases where PD is not preoperatively suspected, or it is caused intraoperatively, it may be presumed from visually assessed pathologic motion between the superior and inferior portions of the acetabulum after removal of the acetabular components. In CPD, however, where the bone loss is usually filled with fibrous tissue, this is of limited value.

32.1.3 Management

The management of PD is challenging. The absence of the accurate classification and radiological interpretation criteria, the selection of the appropriate implants and the high rate of surgical complications and mechanical failures compromise the management [2].

There are several treatment options of PD. The optimal surgical technique is still controversial, and the treatment should be individualized to the patients' needs [1]. The choice of treatment should be based on the:

1. Quality and quantity of the local bone
2. Quality of soft tissue
3. General health status
4. The type of the discontinuity (APD vs. CPD)

The aim of the current treatment options is the long-term stable fixation of the revision implants with or without healing of the discontinuity. They involve:

1. "Biologic" osseous consolidation of the pelvic ring

2. "Nonbiologic" bridging of the acetabular defect with osseointegratable implants [plates, uncemented cups (jumbo), acetabular cages (standard antiprotrusio cages, custom tri-flanged cages, or modular "cup-cage" constructs) with morcellized or massive structural bone grafts]

The outcome of reconstruction depends on:

1. The extent of bone loss associated with the discontinuity
2. The severity of osteopenia
3. The pelvic bone vascularity
4. The chronicity of discontinuity
5. The reconstruction technique

In APD or CPD patients with good osseous healing potential and minor bone deficiencies, usually, a good construct stability can be obtained. Compression can typically be applied, and successful healing is possible using plating of the anterior and/or posterior column, bone defect filling with allograft bone, and implantation of an antiprotrusio cage or a jumbo cup [1]. When at high risk of dislocation, a dual mobility cup may be cemented into the antiprotrusio cage.

In CPD with larger defects and little rim support, the bony ends are often avascular, and healing is unlikely. In these cases, a jumbo cup with trabecular metal augments to achieve cup stability or distraction techniques as the "cup cage" that bridge the defect can be useful [1, 2].

In more severe massive defects with little remaining dome, the bone reconstruction is more difficult [1–3]. In such situations jumbo cups or cup-cage constructs are likely to fail. Effective management with a custom triflange component is usually needed.

32.1.4 Published Results

Numerous case series of various treatment options with small sample size have been published [13–43]. Long-term studies involving adequate series of patients treated with specific surgical procedures and comparative studies are lacking.

32.1.4.1 Internal Fixation with Acetabular Reconstruction

Isolated plates seem not to be the perfect choice [13]. Internal fixation and acetabular reconstruction with non-custom reconstruction rings and cages are a better treatment option. Both of them reduce micromotion, enhance bone graft incorporation, and improve healing [1]. Dual plating of posterior and anterior columns [14] and plating of just the posterior or anterior column [15] or specific plates [16] have been described in the literature. Dual plating requires combined ilioinguinal pelvic and posterior surgical approaches [1, 2]. Reconstruction rings and cages are devices used to fix the ischium and ilium, bridging the area of significant acetabular bone loss or PD and protecting the extensive acetabular bone graft by transferring the load from the acetabulum to the ilium and the ischium. These implants provide good initial stability; however, the inability for biologic fixation at the cage-bone interface may compromise long-term success [1, 3, 17].

There are studies with short to midterm results of small number of patients suffering from PD treated with revision THA with internal fixation and reconstruction cages [13–18, 20–22]. The results were best in patients who did not have severe segmental acetabular bone loss [6]. Eggli et al. [14] evaluated seven patients with PD treated with dual plating, reinforcement cage, and bone allograft and autograft. There was one re-revision for aseptic loosening and another for screw removal. After a mean follow-up of 96 months, all acetabular components were stable, and the pelvic discontinuities had healed. Rogers et al. [18] also demonstrated that none out of eight patients treated with compression plating of the posterior column plating and an acetabular shell required revision after a mean follow-up of 34 months.

In a recent systematic review, Beckman et al. [19] found documentation in five studies [14, 15, 20–22] of the follow-up results in 37 patients with PD treated with reinforcement rings during revision THA. At a mean follow-up of 6.1 years, these patients had 30% rate of radiographic loosening of their acetabular components.

32.1.4.2 Porous Metal Components

Trabecular metal shells and augments demonstrated favourable results in the revision THA. They facilitate bony ingrowth and promote long-term stability of the implants via biologic fixation [2]. Porous trabecular metal shells can be used in revision THA of patients with PD alone or combination with augments [23–31], in the cup-cage technique [33, 35, 36], and the acetabular distraction technique [12, 32].

There are limited short- to medium-term data in the literature of patients with PD that were treated with porous trabecular metal shells alone. Sporer et al. [23] evaluated thirteen patients with PD that received tantalum components at revision THA; there were no revisions at a mean follow-up of 2.6 years. In the recent systematic review of Beckman et al. [19], 42 patients were found with pelvic discontinuities treated with Trabecular Metal components during revision THA in six publications [23–28]. At a mean follow-up of 2.9 years, the rate of radiographic loosening was 4.8%; this was significantly lower than in patients treated with reinforcement rings.

Several studies demonstrated the combination of trabecular metal shells and augments for the management of pelvic discontinuity [23, 29–31].

32.1.4.3 Acetabular Distraction with Porous Acetabular Cup

This is a recently reported difficult technique initially described by Paprosky [12]; it treats PD by compressing the non-union and achieving mechanical fixation. This is usually accomplished via expansion of the defect, use of porous tantalum components (hemispheric shell and porous metal augments), and creation of elastic recoil forces to compress the porous metal construct to achieve a stable construct. The strong pelvic "recoil" around the cup as a result of ligamentotaxis from the stout pelvic ligaments combined with the inherent material properties of the TM implant and the augments provides the initial stability to the construct. The subsequent bony ingrowth leads to the long-term biological fixation [12].

Surgical Technique: Short Description

- Use standard posterior approach.
- Remove the acetabular component.
- Debride the interposed tissue at the fracture sites to bleed.
- Identify areas of cavitary bone defects using a hemispherical reamer.
- A distraction device is anchored to the pelvis onto the anterior and posterior columns to expand the defect in cephalad-caudal direction.
- Fill any defect with trial augments and place an appropriately sized reamer for sizing.
- Remove the trial implants.
- Secure the augments into the host bone with screws.
- Ream till to make two contact points typically posteroinferior to anterosuperior.
- The correct cup size should catch in the acetabulum but also easily disengage.
- Coat with PMMA cement only the augment surface, impact the cup into place, and further secure it with screws.
- Release the distracting force, and the pelvis is allowed to recoil under ligamentotaxis to further secure the construct.
- Cement the liner into place.
- Use no significant weight on the extremity for twelve weeks, partial weight bearing for the next twelve weeks, and then full weight bearing.

There are limited midterm follow-up data currently available. Sporer et al. [12] reported good short-term results of a cohort of twenty patients with PD using the acetabular distraction technique; only one case required revision for aseptic loosening at nine months. At 4-year follow-up, four hips demonstrated the migration of the acetabular component but were clinically stable [32].

32.1.4.4 Cup-Cage Construct

It is another technique that provides a viable option for the treatment of complex, severe acetabular defects and pelvic discontinuity [33]. A porous trabecular metal acetabular shell and augments are used as the osteoconductive material that bridges the acetabular defect and not the actual shell to articulate with the femoral head. Then an antiprotrusio cage is placed in the shell and fixed with screws to the ilium and ischium and with cement to the acetabular shell [33]. The cage provides the initial mechanical stabilization of the discontinuity and load relief to the acetabular component, thereby allowing time for biologic fixation of the porous non-cemented shell (± augment) to the host bone for long-term stability [33–35]. The technique is fully described in the appropriate chapter.

There are also limited but encouraging short- and midterm outcomes for the treatment of PD in centres of excellence [33, 35, 36].

Abolghasemian et al. [35] demonstrated the midterm results of a previous cohort of twenty six patients [36] that was treated with cup-cage technique for PD; he compared the results of this cohort with nineteen patients with PD treated with cages alone for the same period. The cup-cage cohort demonstrated significant greater 7-year survivorship than the cage-alone group (87.2 vs. 49.9%, $p = 0.009$). Amenabar et al. [33] reported forty five cup-cages for the treatment of PD among 67 patients with Gross type IV and V undergoing revision THA. At a mean follow-up of 77 months, the revision rate for any reason was 9%. There were four revisions for aseptic loosening.

32.1.4.5 Custom Triflange Implants

Triflange implants are custom-made, porous-coated titanium alloy components for the treatment of severe bone loss and PD in revision hip arthroplasty [37]. They have an acetabular component with ilial, ischial, and pubic flanges for spanning the defect, initial fixation, and rigid stability to the host bone. These are personalized implants designed and manufactured based on a CT preoperative templating process. A drawback is the time for implant preparation that is up to several weeks or longer; an advantage is the relatively uncomplicated surgical technique [38]. The technique is fully described in the appropriate chapter.

There are limited but promising short- and midterm results of custom triflange components for the treatment of PD [37–41]. In a retrospective follow-up study, Taunton et al. [39] reported the results of fifty seven patients with PD treated with revision THA using a custom triflange acetabular component. At a mean of 65-month follow-up, there were three revisions of the triflange component, one for aseptic loosening and two for septic revisions. Thirty-seven (65%) were free of revision for any reason at the same time, and 49% were free of revision for any reason and free of any component migration and had a healed discontinuity. Ten of the patients demonstrated postoperative instability; the majority of them were treated with re-revision with constrained liner. DeBoer et al. [40] evaluated twenty patients with PD treated with revision at a mean follow-up of 123 months. There was no triflange removal and aseptic loosening; however, there were 30% of dislocations.

32.1.4.6 Complications

There are many methods available for the treatment of PD in revision THA; however, none of them are completely efficient. High complication rates of 25–80% have been reported [14, 15, 42]. The most frequent are dislocation, nerve injury, and infection. Dislocations remain the most common (from 0 to 40%) [13, 32]. The high number of previous operations with resultant tissue scars and defects, abductor weakness, extensive approaches, and cup orientation are the main risk factors for instability [1]. Some recommend the use of constrained liners or dual mobility cups in those patients at risk for dislocation but not as a routine use [1]. Deep infections have been reported to occur from 0 to 30% [13, 14]. The increased operative time, extensive tissue dissection, recurrent operations, and poor general patient health are considered as risk factors for deep infection. The incidence of aseptic loosening has been reported up to 44% for the treatment of PD with cages [43]. It is supported that there are improved results for aseptic loosening using custom triflanged [40] and trabecular metal components [32].

32.2 Case Title: Reinforcement Ring (Posterior Pelvic Plate) Acetabular Revision for Chronic Pelvic Dissociation

E. Kenanidis and E. Tsiridis

This is a dislocation caused by an unstable acetabular cemented implant due to chronic pelvic dissociation (Fig. 32.1). There is a great loss of bone stock, and the case is classified as Paprosky IV. Removing the cemented implant was very easy as there was no bonding between the bone and cement. This occurred with the minimal efforts; however, it is advisable not to pull hard the implants away from the pelvis regardless the suspected instability, as this may result in a lot of additional bone loss from the aggressive removal. The fracture of the posterior wall was then plated with a Matta plate system from the roof of the socket to the beginning of the ischium, to compensate for the pelvic dissociation from the back (Fig. 32.2). A cage was then applied, to compensate the medial wall and was hooked to the ischium and the ilium. The whole construct was secured with multiple screws through the roof of the cage and the iliac fin to add on stability and continuation of the dissociation. A cemented socket was then inserted into the cage at the proper orientation. Due to complete lack of greater trochanter and abductors, the stability of the hip joint was achieved using a PLAD (posterior lip augmentation device) secured firmly around the head-neck junction and spanning from the roof of the socket to the whole posterior wall of it. The femoral component—a monoblock Wagner revision stem—was left in situ, and only two wires were put around the proximal end of the bone around the prosthesis to maintain contact with a hope of osseointegration.

Figure 32.2.a. Intraoperative view of reconstruction. The Matta (Stryker) plate is placed on the posterior wall to stabilize the columnar fracture, and the cage supports the whole construct to the acetabulum. Figure 32.2.b. An intraoperative C-arm radiographic view of the reconstruction.

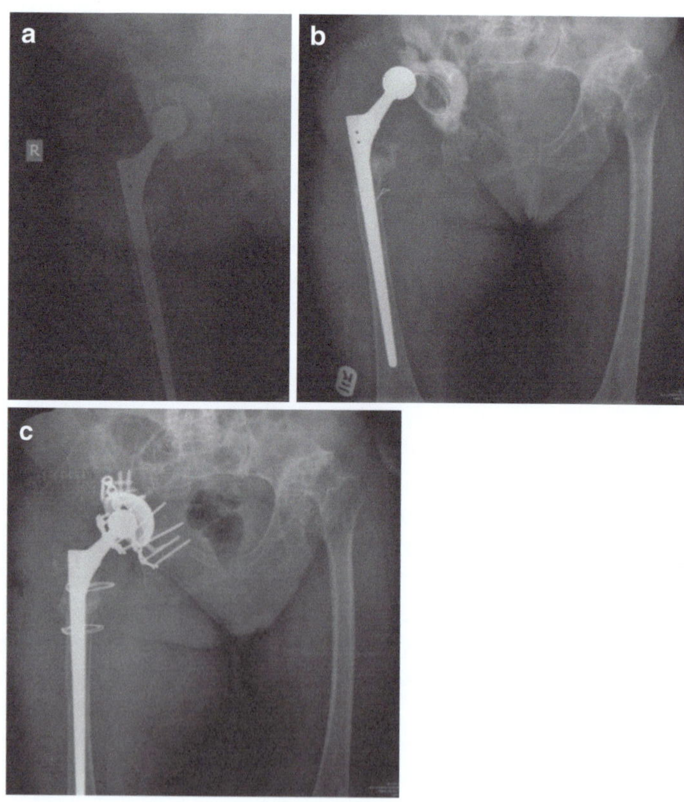

Fig. 32.1 (**a**) AP pelvic x-ray before and (**b**) after the THA dislocation (**c**) AP pelvic x-ray showing the final reconstruction

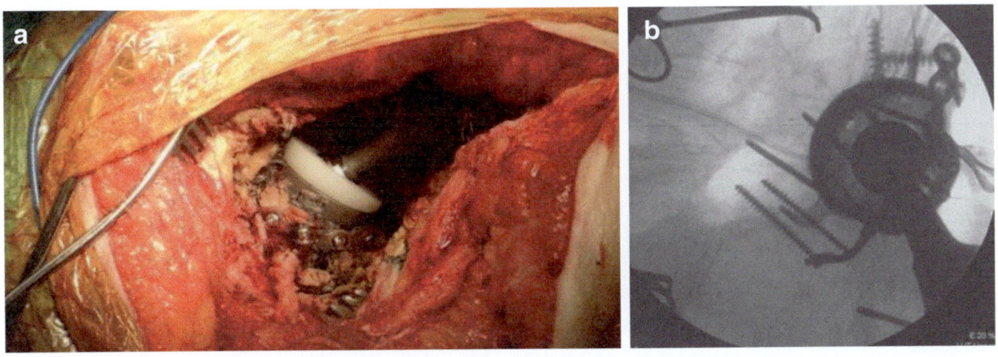

Fig. 32.2 (**a**) Intraoperative view of reconstruction. The Matta (Stryker) plate is placed on the posterior wall to stabilize the columnar fracture, and the cage supports the whole construct to the acetabulum. (**b**) An intraoperative C-arm radiographic view of the reconstruction

32.3 Case Title: Chronic Pelvic Dissociation Using Paprosky Distraction Technique

E. Kenanidis and E. Tsiridis

Removal of Heterotopic Ossification tension banding of the greater trochanter fracture and socket reconstruction is done using the Paprosky distraction technique. A full tantalum shell was used after removing the peripheral ring to distract the socket and a plate at the posterior wall to stabilize the posterior column. The TA socket was stabilized with five screws all around it, and HXLP socket was cemented into it with success (Fig. 32.3).

32.4 Case Title: Pelvic Discontinuity (Treated with Impaction Bone Grafting)

Michael Nogler

32.4.1 Demographics

Age: 73
Sex: Female
BMI: 29

32.4.2 Relevant Past Medical History

Principal pathologies: THA—Loose acetabular component

Previous surgical procedures: Cup revision

Medication: NSAID

History of presenting complaint: Patient presented with pelvic discontinuity following an insufficient attempt of cup reconstruction

32.4.3 Clinical Examination

Symptoms: Pain, unstable acetabular component

Range *of motion*: Fl

Main disability: Pain

Neurovascular evaluation: No relevant findings

32.4.4 Preoperative Radiological Assessment/Imaging (Figs. 32.4, 32.5, and 32.6)

32.4.5 Preoperative Planning

Diagnosis: Pelvic discontinuity as a result of cup revision attempt, insufficiently treated (Figs. 32.4, 32.5 and 32.6)

Possible treatment options: Posterior and anterior plating, structural grafting, cranial socket cup, and impaction bone grafting with cage enhancement

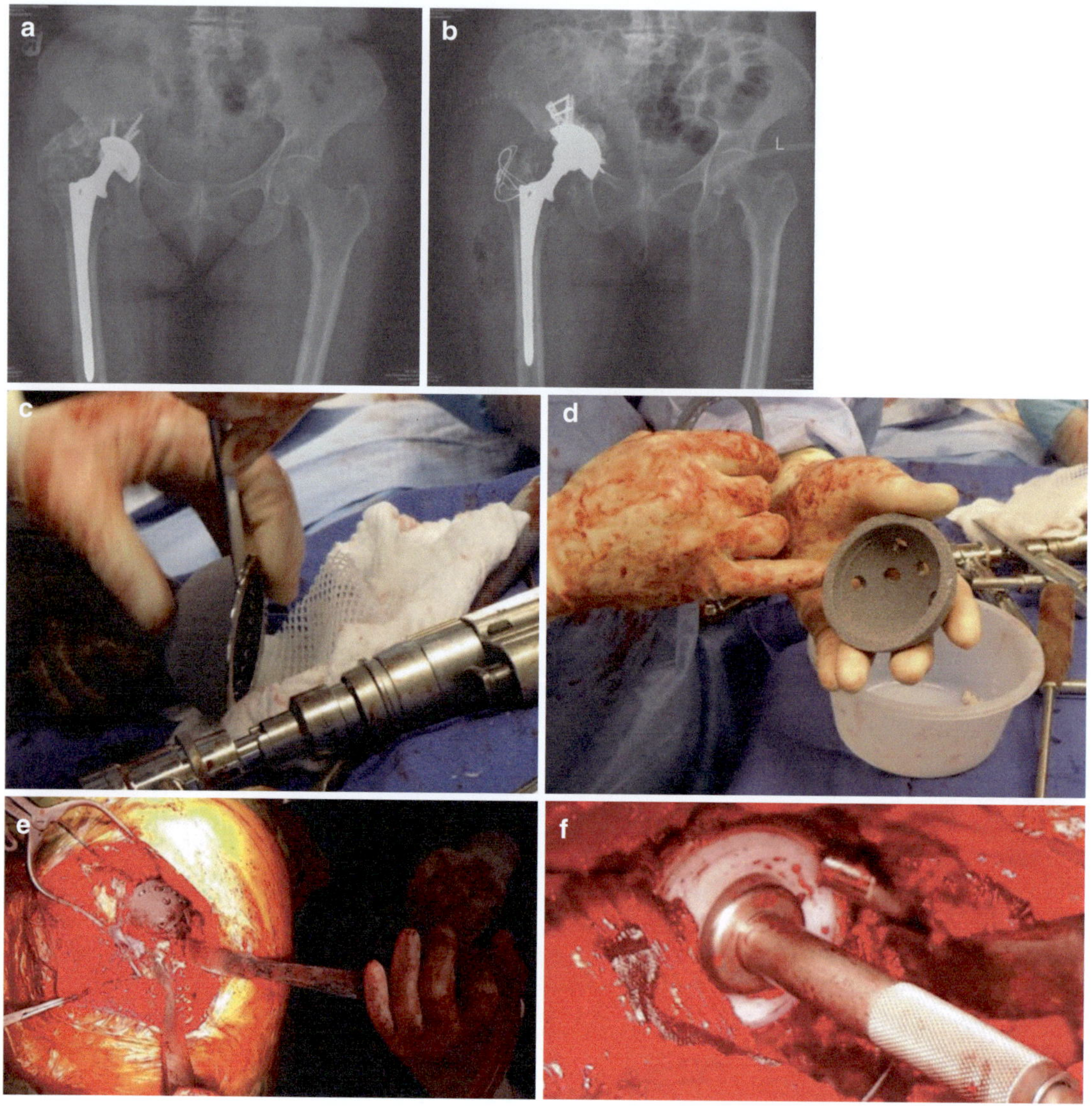

Fig. 32.3 (**a**) Preoperatrive AP pelvic X-ray. Brooker type 4 Heterotopic Ossification and chronic pelvis dissociation with severe osteolysis and fracture of the greater trochanter. (**b**) Postoperative AP pelvic X-ray showing the distraction reconstruction technique of the right hip. (**c-f**) Intraoperative photographs demonstrating (**c**) the full tantalum shell before and (**d**) after the removal of the peripheral ring. (**e**) The final implantation of the tantalum socket. (**f**) The cemented polyethylene in the cup

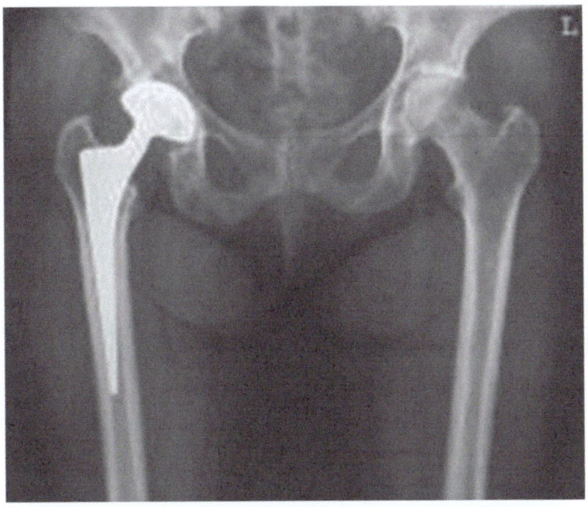

Fig. 32.4 AP pelvic x-ray showing the right THA before the cup revision

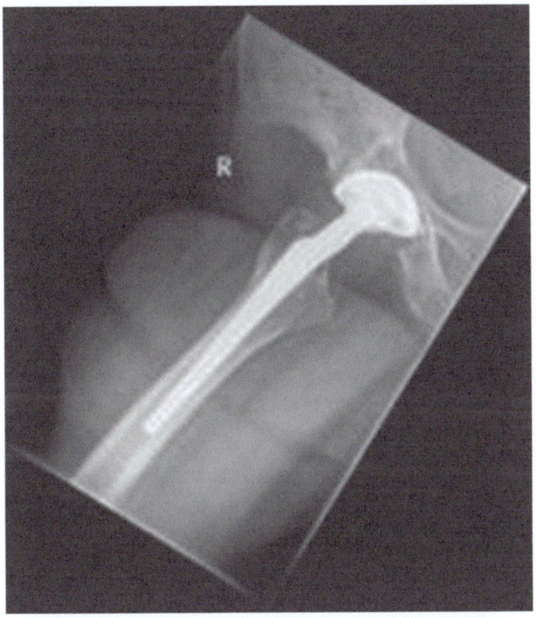

Fig. 32.5 Lateral hip x-ray of the right THA before cup revision

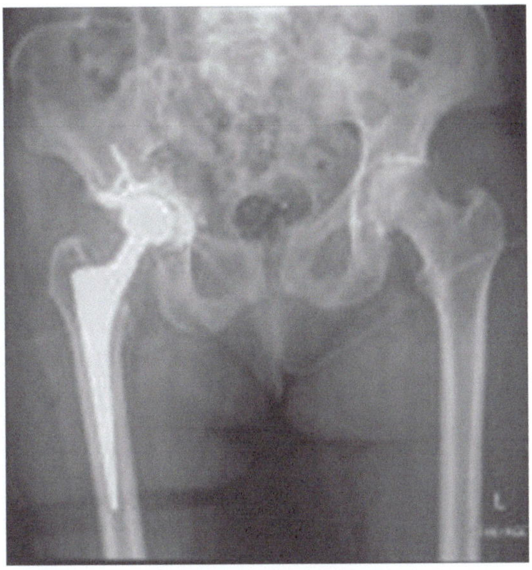

Fig. 32.6 AP pelvic x-ray demonstrating a complete pelvic discontinuity and a loose acetabular component following revision THA with an insufficient attempt to bridge the defect with a cage that is not connected to os ischium or pubis.

Chosen treatment method: Impaction bone grafting with cage enhancement

Selection of implants if applicable and rational: GAP II cup size 60 (Stryker, Kalamazoo, MI, USA) and a mesh for impaction bone grafting. Mueller PE cemented cup size 52 (Zimmer, Warsaw, Indiana, USA), Biolox head 32 mm (Ceramtec, Plochingen, Germany)

Expected difficulties: Non-union of the fracture, bone graft resorption

Strategies to overcome difficulties: Protection of the bone graft with metal reinforcement cage (GAP II)

32.4.6 Surgical Note

Patient's position: Supine

Type of anesthesia: General anaesthesia

Surgical approach: Direct anterior approach

Main steps: Cup and cement removal, mesh implantation, impaction bone grafting, augmentation ring placement, fixation with screws, and cementing in of a PE cup

Reconstruction techniques: The acetabular component and the cement were removed; a metal mesh was placed in the space between the two pelvic parts. The mesh was fixated with small screws and served as a scaffold for bone chips that were impacted into the mesh and remaining bone surfaces of ilium, ischium, and pubis. Then an augmentation ring with a distal hook was adjusted and put in place—making sure that the hook was inserted correctly into the notch. Afterwards, large screws were placed to fixate the cage to the ilium. After that, a PE cup was cemented in place into the cage. Several trial reductions with different head length followed; the final head was put on the trunnion of the stem and the joint was definitely reduced (Figs. 32.7 and 32.8).

32.4.7 Intraoperative Challenges

Challenges and solutions: Accurate implantation of the ring into the notch was performed under C-arm guidance.

Unanticipated problems and solution: None

Thorough description of decision-making, including the reason for the final decision: Impaction bone grafting is a method to reconstruct defects "biologically." With this bone can be regrown and provide more and better bone stock for the future. In this case, the patient had a complete discontinuity of the pelvis with a significant distance of the bone parts (>2 cm). The treatment of such cases is difficult and not highly successful. Plating the pelvis bears a high risk of plate failures due to the rigidity of the osteosynthesis and the high loads during walking. Alternatively, a cranial socket cup cut has been implanted. This would have given a functional THA but would not have addressed the discontinuity, thus creating an unstable pelvic ring. A reconstruction of the pelvic ring with bone regrowth and an eventually stable pelvis and stable THA is preferable. In close communication and consent with the patient, I decided to take this route of treatment.

32.4.8 Postoperative Radiographs (Figs. 32.7 and 32.8)

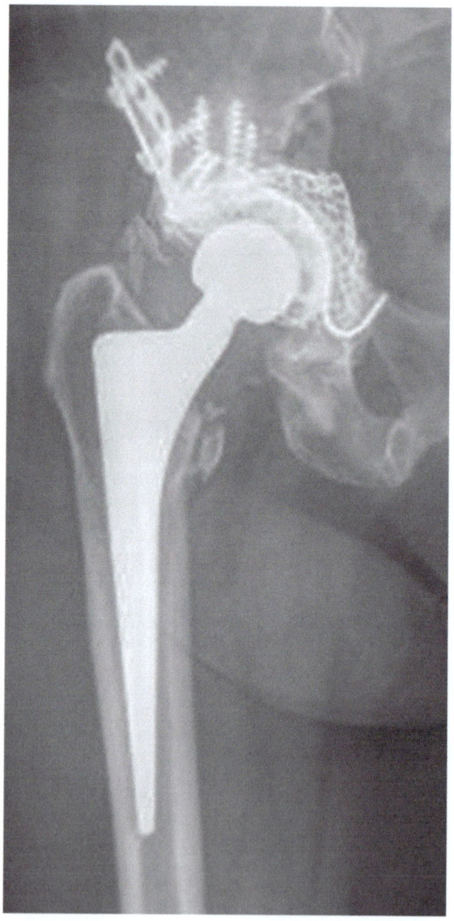

Fig. 32.7 AP hip x-ray at the third postoperative day

32.4.9 Postoperative Management

Chemoprophylaxis and anticoagulant treatment period: Ciprofloxacin 3 × 400 mg for one week, Lovenox 40 mg s.c. for three weeks

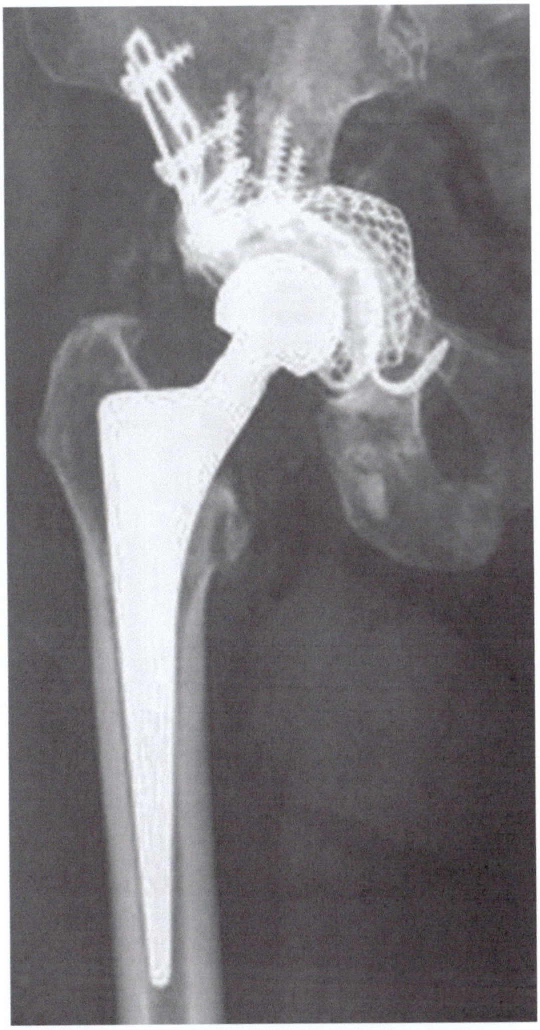

Fig. 32.8 AP x-ray at the fifth postoperative year

Gait/limb loading until full loading: Partial weight bearing (50% body weight) for six months, full loading afterward

32.4.10 Follow-Up and Complications

No postoperative complications occurred.

32.4.11 Discussion [2, 44, 45]

Advantages of the applied method: Regrowth of bone and reconstruction of pelvic continuity is possible through a small approach.

Disadvantages of the method: Long postoperative partial weight bearing.

Alternative evidence-based techniques for the case: Cranial socket cup, plating.

Why is the chosen technique better for this case? Pelvic continuity could be restored through the bone grafting.

Indications and contraindications for your technique: Pelvic discontinuities.

Learning curve and how to manage complications: As difficult as other reconstruction techniques. Experience with impaction bone grafting is required.

Level of evidence concerning the superiority of this method against others: Medium for this method in pelvic discontinuities, high for impaction bone grafting.

32.5 Case Title: Acetabular Revision (Acute Pelvic Dissociation)

Neil P. Sheth, Christopher M. Melnic, and Wayne G. Paprosky

32.5.1 Demographics

Age: 41
Sex: Female
BMI: 25

32.5.2 *Relevant Past Medical History Principal pathologies: History of developmental dysplasia of the left hip*

Previous surgical procedures: s/p left total hip arthroplasty (THA) with subtrochanteric femoral shortening osteotomy

Medication: None

History of presenting complaint: The patient is a 41-year-old female that is three weeks s/p left THA with a subtrochanteric femoral shortening osteotomy that was performed at an outside hospital. As per the patient, on postoperative day #2, she felt a sudden shortening of the left lower extremity. She was made touchdown weight bearing (10%), without new radiographs of the left hip being obtained, and was discharged and asked to follow-up in the outpatient clinic in two weeks. At the time of her clinic follow-up, an X-ray was obtained, and an acute pelvic discontinuity with acetabular component migration was recognized. The patient presented to clinic one week later on crutches for a second opinion.

32.5.3 Clinical Examination

Symptoms: Severe groin pain, left lower extremity shortening (3 cm), and an inability to bear weight on the left lower extremity.

Specific tests: Preoperative erythrocyte sedimentation rate and C-reactive protein values were 18 (0–20) and 4.4 (0–7.4), respectively, which were within normal values—the preoperative suspicion for a deep space infection was very low.

Main disability: Inability to ambulate.

Neurovascular evaluation: 5/5 motor strength in the distribution of the L4, L5, and S1 nerve roots and sensation intact to light touch in the distribution of the superficial and deep peroneal, saphenous, sural, and tibial nerves. There was a 2+ femoral, dorsalis pedis, and posterior tibial artery pulse.

32.5.4 Preoperative Radiological Assessment/Imaging (Figs. 32.9, 32.10, and 32.11)

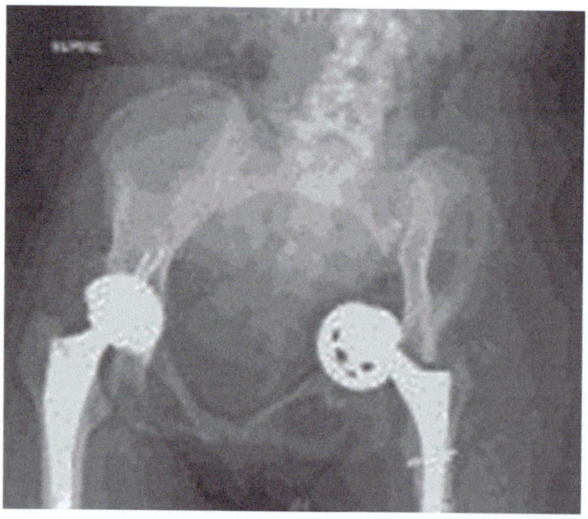

Fig. 32.9 AP pelvis X-rays demonstrating acute pelvic discontinuity with medial migration of the acetabular component beyond Kohler's line

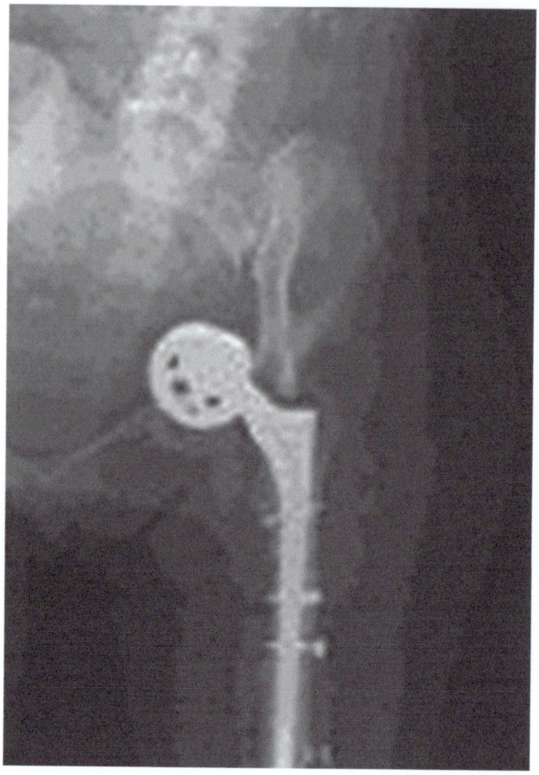

Fig. 32.10 AP hip X-ray depicting the acute pelvic discontinuity and cup migration. Note the minimally displaced femur fracture along the medial femoral cortex (*white arrow*) distal to the subtrochanteric osteotomy

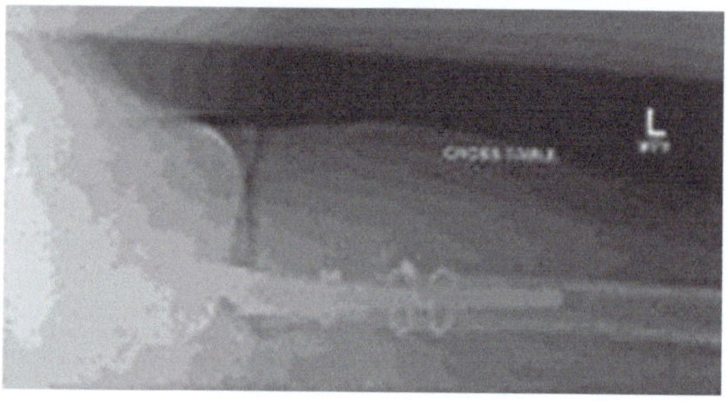

Fig. 32.11 A cross table lateral X-ray showing excessive anteversion of the acetabular shell and anterior subluxation of the femoral head

32.5.5 Preoperative Planning

Diagnosis: Aseptic loosening of the acetabular component with acute pelvic discontinuity (Figs. 32.9, 32.10 and 32.11).

Possible treatment options: Open reduction of the posterior column and revision THA—fixation of the discontinuity—plating of the posterior column must be performed to provide a stable pelvis for revision of the acetabular component.

Chosen treatment method: Open reduction internal fixation of the posterior column and revision THA.

Selection of implants if applicable and rational: Implants chosen—Synthes pelvic reconstruction plate, revision tantalum elliptical shell (Trabecular Metal, Zimmer, Warsaw, IN, USA), and acetabular augments for acetabular reconstruction (Trabecular Metal augments, Zimmer, Warsaw, IN, USA). The use of a tantalum revision shell allows for improved stress distribution to the remaining retroacetabular bone stock, placement of a cemented liner which creates a locked construct with all properly placed screws, fine-tuning of abduction and version by positioning of the cemented liner, and holes to be customized in the tantalum shell with a burr for additional screw fixation.

Expected difficulties: In the immediate postoperative period, surgical exposure can be challenging due to difficulty in accurately defining each tissue layer. Since the patient initially underwent a subtrochanteric femoral shortening osteotomy for presumed Crowe IV dysplasia, excessive lengthening of the limb may result in sciatic nerve palsy. Plate fixation of the posterior column also may be difficult due to the narrow nature of the posterior column and disuse osteopenia secondary to long-term weight bearing through the pseudoacetabulum.

Strategies to overcome difficulties: Wide surgical exposure with identification of the normal tissue that was not violated at the time of previous surgery is the most effective way to determine the appropriate tissue layer. In this setting, the sciatic nerve was dissected out to prevent iatrogenic injury and to determine the tension on the nerve once the hip centre was restored.

Templating: Digital templating of the acetabular component was performed to determine a "ball park" size of the component to be used. The revision acetabular shell was templated to a size 56 mm.

32.5.6 Surgical Note

Patient's position: Lateral decubitus position

Type of anesthesia: General anesthesia with an arterial line and Foley catheter placed prior to the start of the procedure

Surgical approach: A posterolateral approach with proximal extension into a Kocher- Langenbeck approach was utilized for appropriate exposure of the posterior column.

Main steps:

1. Wide posterolateral surgical exposure.
2. Posterior capsular approach with tagging of the capsule for later repair.
3. Two samples of pseudocapsule should be sent for final microbiology for aerobic and anaerobic culture.
4. Identify the sciatic nerve and understand its course.
5. Following sequential scar excision, dislocate the hip, remove the femoral head, and check the stability of the remaining femoral stem (stem was stable).
6. Placement of acetabular retractors for acetabular exposure (may require additional scar excision for complete exposure).
7. Following adequate acetabular exposure, the acetabular liner and two screws should be removed from the shell.
8. A "cup-out" (Zimmer, Warsaw, IN, USA) osteotome may be required for removal of the acetabular shell to prevent iatrogenic acetabular bone loss.
9. The proximal extent of the sciatic nerve should be dissected out as it courses into the greater sciatic notch.
10. The acetabulum should be cleared of any fibrous tissue with a Cobb elevator, and the acute discontinuity should be identified [now the reconstruction can be performed].

Reconstruction techniques: (1) The posterior column should be reduced with a fracture reduction clamp, and tentative plate placement on the column should be attempted. (2) In this case, two plates were used to plate the posterior column. (3) Following internal fixation of the posterior column, attention can be turned to the acetabular reconstruction. (4) The initial step for acetabular reconstruction is to determine the integrity of the anterosuperior (AS) and posteroinferior (PI) columns—in this case, both columns were intact. (5) A reamer should then be used in reverse to achieve an interference fit between the AS and PI columns. (6) When the reamer achieves a proper fit between the columns, it will disengage from the reamer handle and the reamer head can be used as a surrogate acetabular component. (7) In this case, a size 58 reamer was the correct size—a size 58 revision Trabecular Metal shell was used [this shell is elliptical and thus measures 60 mm at the periphery allowing for additional 1 mm peripheral "press fit"]. (8) There is a titanium ring at the edge of the revision shell—this ring is typically removed in order to get access to the periphery of the cup. (9) Once the ring is removed, a metal cutting burr should be used to drill additional holes into the cup, specifically at the periphery to allow for screw fixation into the ischium to avoid abduction failure of the final construct ["kickstand screw"]. (10) The acetabular component should be impacted with a bone tamp, and at least four good screws should be placed through the cup into host bone [five screws were placed in this case, but only three screws exhibited good purchase]. (11) An orange slice augment (50 × 10—Zimmer, Warsaw, IN, USA) was placed in the posterosuperior position for supplemental fixation and secured to host bone [a 30 mm and 25 mm screw were used in this case]. (12) Cement should be used to unitize all augments to the acetabular shell, which is done at the same time as cementing the final liner into the shell following trial reduction (Figs. 32.12 and 32.13).

32.5.7 Intraoperative Challenges

Challenges and solutions: The biggest challenge, in this case, is plating the posterior column due to disuse osteopenia as well as the narrow nature of the posterior column for this specific patient.

Unanticipated problems and solution: The posterior column bone stock exhibited significant disuse osteopenia as was anticipated in the preoperative planning phase. The intraoperative decision was made to dual plate the posterior column to provide additional support of the osteopenic bone.

32.5.8 Postoperative Radiographs (Figs. 32.12 and 32.13)

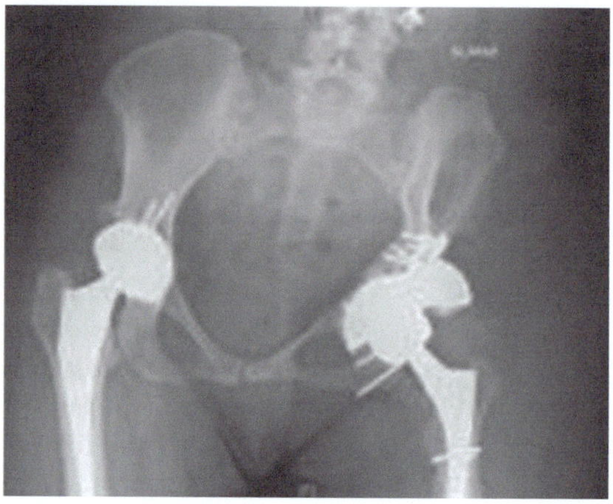

Fig. 32.12 Postoperative AP pelvis X-ray demonstrating plating of the posterior column and acetabular revision with use of a posterosuperior augment for supplemental fixation

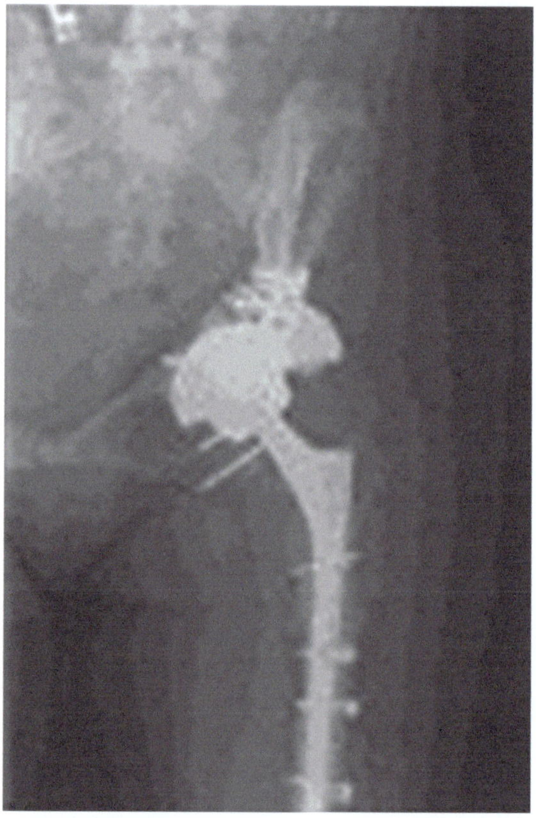

Fig. 32.13 Postoperative AP hip X-ray depicting the retained femoral component and restoration of the hip centre compared to the preoperative acetabular component position

32.5.9 Postoperative Management

Chemoprophylaxis and anticoagulant treatment period: The patient was placed on ASA 325 mg po bid × 6 weeks for DVT prophylaxis.

Gait/limb loading until full loading: The patient was made touchdown weight bearing (10%) for three months, followed by partial weight bearing (50%) for an additional six weeks. Serial X-rays demonstrating no change in component position allowed for weight bearing as tolerated at 4.5 months postoperatively.

32.5.10 Follow-Up and Complications

Report of postoperative complications and their management (i.e., recurrent dislocation): This patient has not had any postoperative complications. At this time, the patient is one year s/p the revision procedure.

32.5.11 Discussion [6]

Advantages of the applied method: Plating of the posterior column creates a stable pelvis, allowing for acetabular reconstruction.

Disadvantages of the method: There are no disadvantages of this method of reconstruction. Due to the acute nature of the pelvic discontinuity, posterior column plating is required prior to acetabular revision.

Alternative evidence-based techniques for the case: In the setting of severe acetabular defects, the use of acetabular allograft in conjunction with posterior column plating has resulted in favorable clinical outcomes [13].

Why is the chosen technique better for this case? The literature supports the use of a cementless device with posterior column plating as a superior technique with regard to addressing pelvic discontinuity [18].

Learning curve and how to manage complications: The learning curve associated with this procedure can be steep. As an arthroplasty surgeon, it can be helpful to have a trauma colleague to assist with posterior column plating. Following internal fixation of the posterior column, acetabular reconstruction adheres to standard revision principles.

Level of evidence concerning the superiority of this method against others: Plating of the posterior column in association with a cemented cup has exhibited high failure rate, but better results were seen when a cementless acetabular cup was used [6]. Steihl et al. demonstrated 80% (8/10) healing of the discontinuity when an acetabular allograft was used in conjunction with single or dual column plating [13]. More recently, Rogers et al. compression plated the posterior column in 8 patients with an acute pelvic discontinuity. At a mean follow-up of 34 months, all discontinuities had healed with none of the patients requiring a repeat revision [18].

32.6 Case Title: Acetabular Revision "Acute Pelvic Dissociation"

Fritz Thorey

32.6.1 Demographics

Age: 23
Sex: Male
BMI: 27.9

32.6.2 Relevant Past Medical History

Principal pathologies: Acetabular fracture after an accident in Saudi Arabia

Previous surgical procedures: Distraction, no osteosynthesis/plating for reconstruction

Medication: NSAID

History of presenting complaint: Increasing pain over twelve months after fracture

32.6.3 Clinical Examination

Symptoms: Limping, limited ROM, and severe pain

Range of motion: Flexion/extension 30-10-0°, no internal/external rotation

Main disability: Pain, walking not possible

Scoring: VAS for pain: 7; Harris Hip Score: 34 (without section 2 and 3)

Neurovascular evaluation: Normal

32.6.4 Preoperative Radiological Assessment/Imaging (Figs. 32.14, 32.15, and 32.16)

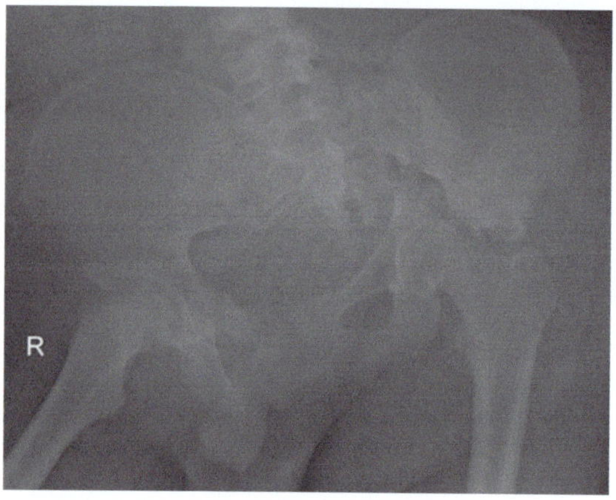

Fig. 32.14 Pelvic AP x-ray with protrusion of the acetabulum after fracture

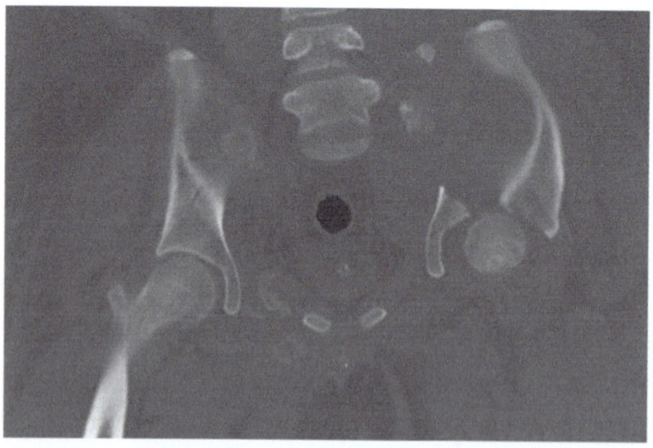

Fig. 32.15 CT scan to visualize the protrusion of the acetabular fracture

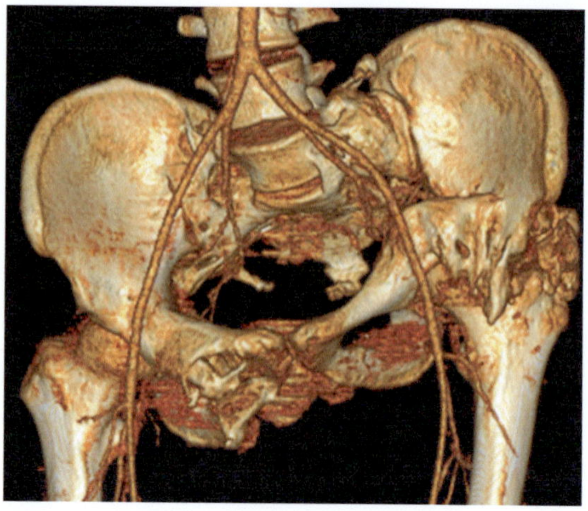

Fig. 32.16 CT scan with visualization of the vessels

32.6.5 Preoperative Planning

Diagnosis: Posttraumatic osteoarthritis with protrusion of the acetabulum after fracture (Figs. 32.14, 32.15 and 32.16)

Possible treatment options: First surgery with stabilization and trial to make a reposition of the acetabulum using a periacetabular osteotomy, resection of the non-union, augmentation with bone graft, and stabilization with osteosynthesis. Second surgery with partial removal of screws and THA using a revision cage, bone grafting, and primary femoral implant

Chosen treatment method: See above

Selection of implants if applicable and rational: Revision cup and primary stem

Expected difficulties: Difficult reposition of the fracture and placement of the cup

Strategies to overcome difficulties: Careful exposure of the acetabulum (cave, neurovascular structures)

Templating: Templating of a revision implant with reconstruction of the centre of rotation

32.6.6 Surgical Note

Patient's position: Supine

Type of anesthesia: General anesthesia

Surgical approach: Lateral transgluteal

Main steps: First surgery with stabilization and trial to make a reposition of the acetabulum using a periacetabular osteotomy, resection of the non-union, augmentation with bone graft, and stabilization with osteosynthesis (Fig. 32.17). Second surgery with partial removal of screws and THA using a revision cage, bone grafting, and primary femoral implant (Fig. 32.18)

Reconstruction techniques: Reposition of the fracture, impaction grafting intraoperative challenges

Challenges and solutions: Bone loss on medial wall with posteromedial instability

Unanticipated problems and solution: None

Thorough description of decision-making, including the reason for the final decision: Bone loss was reconstructed with impaction grafting and bone block. The anterior and posterior wall at the rim of the acetabulum were stable. Fixation of primary cup was possible.

32.6.7 Postoperative Radiographs

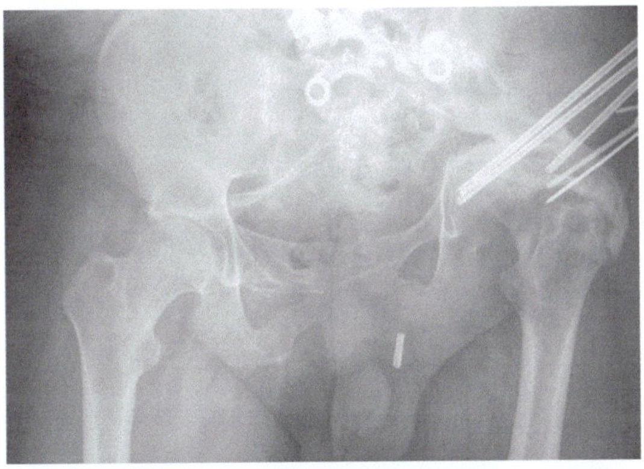

Fig. 32.17 AP x-ray view of the pelvis showing the partial reposition and osteosynthesis of the acetabular fracture

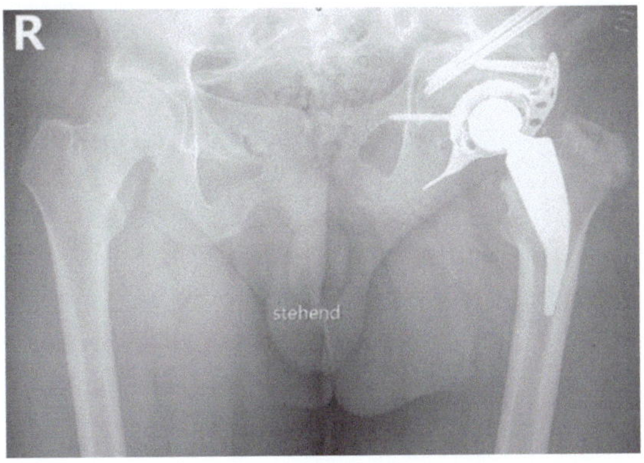

Fig. 32.18 AP x-ray view of pelvis showing the implantation of the revision cage with bone graft and femoral stem

32.6.8 Postoperative Management

Chemoprophylaxis and anticoagulant treatment period: Xarelto, antibiotics for four weeks

Gait/limb loading until full loading: weight bearing as tolerated

32.6.9 Follow-Up and Complications

No complication.

Scoring: VAS for pain: 2; Harris Hip Score: 83 (without section 2 and 3).

32.6.10 Discussion [46–48]

Advantages of the applied method: Reconstruction without reconstruction of the centre of rotation and allograft.

Disadvantages of the method: None.

Alternative evidence-based techniques for the case: Jumbo cups with trabecular metal.

Why is the chosen technique better for this case? For future revisions, there is still a good bone stock after allograft and impaction grafting.

Indications and contraindications for your technique: Indication for this technique is a sufficient stability of the acetabulum.

Learning curve and how to manage complications: Longer learning curve.

Level of evidence concerning the superiority of this method against others: Should only be used in cases with sufficient bone condition.

32.7 Case Title: Pelvic Dissociation Cage Technique

Stanislav Bondarenko, Volodymyr Filippenko, and Volodymyr Mezentsev

32.7.1 Demographics

Age: 49
Sex: Female
BMI: 31.2

32.7.2 Relevant Past Medical History

Principal pathologies: Aseptic instability of cemented acetabular cup of the right hip with protrusion into the pelvis

Previous surgical procedures: Cemented THA eleven years before the index procedure

Medication: Analgesics and NSAIDs, antibiotics, and anticoagulants

Other: Mild hypertension and obesity

History of presenting complaint: Right groin and lumbar pain worst with ambulation and improving at rest. A difficulty with weight bearing on the affected limb, which is aided with crutches. There was an associated right leg shorting and limping for three years before the index procedure. She experienced severe difficulty with sitting, and she was on pain medications which temporarily relieved her symptoms.

32.7.3 Clinical Examination

Symptoms: Severe pain, leg length discrepancy of 55 mm, Trendelenburg gait, pelvic obliquity, inability to sit, hypertrophic scar on the lateral thigh, ipsilateral lower limb muscle swelling and pallor with attempted weight bearing, quadriceps muscle hypertrophy, and abductor muscle weakness

Range of motion: Extension/flexion, 0/0/20; adduction/adduction, 0/0/0; external rotation/internal rotation, 40/40/0

Specific tests: ESR: 10mm/h; CRP: negative; CBC-T/D: normal; aspiration: negative; serum electrolyte, urea, and creatinine (within normal limit); ECG; CT; contrast angiography; Doppler USS

Main disability: Pain, limping, unable to bear weight, and difficulty in sitting down

Scoring if available: VAS: 9; HHS: 23

Neurovascular evaluation: The major lower limb nerves (sciatic, femoral, obturator, and superior gluteal nerves) were all intact.

32.7.4 Preoperative Radiological Assessment/Imaging (Figs. 32.19, 32.20, and 32.21)

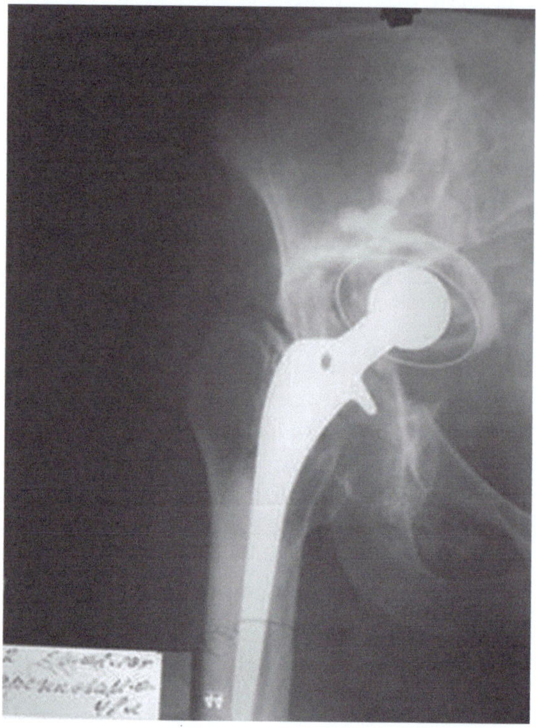

Fig. 32.19 AP X-ray view of right hip joint showing cemented implant with migration into the pelvis, associated with Paprosky 3b acetabular defect

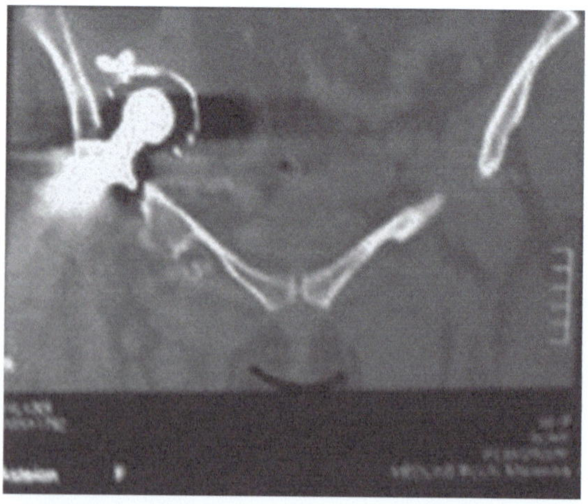

Fig. 32.20 Coronal CT view showing the implant and cement migration into the pelvis, the extent of osteolysis with pelvic dissociation

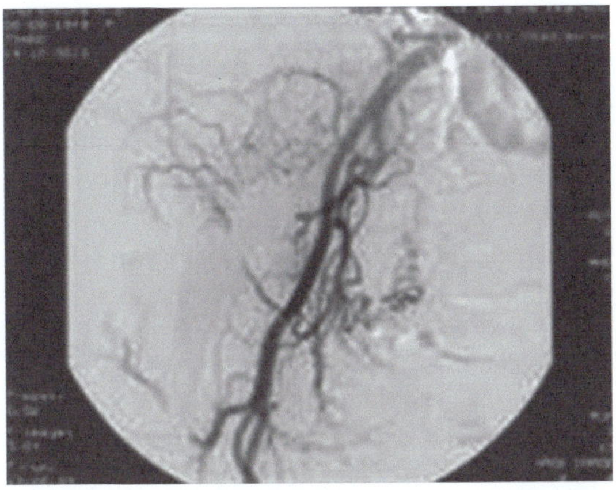

Fig. 32.21 Preoperative angiography scan shows the cemented implant migration into the pelvis and enables visualization of the acetabular cup and bone cement and its proximity relative to the vessels

32.7.5 Preoperative Planning

Diagnosis: Aseptic instability of the cup of cemented implant with protrusion into the pelvis and pelvic discontinuity (Figs. 32.19, 32.20 and 32.21).

Possible treatment options: Revision THA with (1) reconstruction of the acetabulum with reinforcement cage and bone grafting; (2) cementless/cemented cup with posterior ± anterior column plate fixation with bone grafting; (3) cup-cage and acetabular reconstruction; (4) distraction technique with augments; (5) triflanged components; and (6) combinations of the above.

Chosen treatment method: The reconstruction of the acetabulum with reinforcement cage and bone grafting.

Selection of implants if applicable and rational: The rationale for implant selection in this case was due to its proven efficacy for restoration of hip rotation centre, secure mechanical support on ilium and ischium, reliable incorporation of cancellous graft, mechanical protection for structural graft, and restoration of bone stock for later revision.

Expected difficulties: The expected difficulties encountered are with the extraction of cup and bone cement from the pelvic cavity which requires retroperitoneal approach with the help of a vascular surgeon to reduce risk of damage to vessels. Second difficulty is reconstructing severe acetabular bone defect (Paprosky type 3b) with pelvic discontinuity.

Strategies to overcome difficulties: The following were the strategies used to overcome difficulties: First we employed the assistance of a vascular surgeon who helped us mobilized the vessels while extracting the cup and cement. Secondly, the procedure was carried in two stages to decrease the risk of hemodynamic imbalance and effect of the prolonged anesthesia to the patient. Thirdly, creating conditions for recovery of a bone mass by reconstructing acetabular bone defects (cavitary, segmental, combined) using cancellous, structural allografts and ceramics.

Templating: Manual templating was done using AP and lateral radiographs. This is supplied by the implant manufacturers.

32.7.6 Surgical Note

Patient's position: For extraction of the cemented cup, the patient lied supine; for extraction of the stem, the patient was placed laterally; and for revision THA, the patient is positioned laterally.

Type of anesthesia: Spinal.

Surgical approach: Retroperitoneal for acetabular implant extraction, direct lateral for femoral implant extraction and revision THA.

Main steps: The first stage which is the extraction of the acetabular cup and bone cement involves an incision parallel to the right inguinal ligament. After incising the skin, subcutaneous tissue, and fat, the aponeurosis of the external oblique muscle was separated. We then proceeded between the internal oblique muscle and rectus abdominis, and the transverse acetabular ligament was visualized. The acetabular cup was covered with extensive fibrosis and in close proximity to the iliac vessels. After mobilizing the vessels, the capsule was resected and the cup and cement extracted. The second stage was the extraction of the stem with cement from the femur through a direct lateral approach. The wounds were closed. Twelve weeks after the implant extraction, a revision THA was performed through a direct lateral approach. The Paprosky type 3b acetabular defect with separation of anterior and posterior column (pelvic discontinuity) was visualized. Fibrosis within the zone of pelvic discontinuity was carefully excised. Segmental defects were filled with structural allografts from two femoral heads, and cavity defects were filled with morcellized bone grafts and granules of biphasic calcium phosphate ceramics. Next was the insertion of Bursch-Schneider cage with the attachment of the proximal flange at the ilium and the distal flange at the ischium. The proximal flange was in held in place with four screws. We inserted cemented cup in the cage. We then proceeded with the insertion of Wagner revision stem and the prosthetic femoral head. The femoral head was reduced into the acetabular cup and satisfactory range of motion was achieved. Three drainages were inserted at the level of the joint capsule, fascia, and subcutaneous fats. Wound was closed in three layers and patient mobilized to intensive care unit (Figs. 32.22 and 32.23).

Reconstruction techniques: We reconstructed the segmental defects with structural allografts (freeze-dried bone allografts) from bone bank requiring two femoral heads. They were adequately reamed, shaped, and sized to closely press-fit to the host bone. Cavity defects of the acetabulum were filled with granules of calcium phosphate ceramics and morcellized cancellous allograft before inserting the cage. We attached the inferior flange of Bursch- Schneider cage first at the ischium before proceeding to attach the superior flange with four screws.

32.7.7 Intraoperative Challenges

Challenges and solutions: The bone defect of acetabulum intraoperatively was greater than what was anticipated preoperatively. We had to use extra allograft to construct the segmental defect. The traction and dislocation of the limb was difficult due to the increased tone of the thigh muscles. In order to overcome this challenge, we performed partial resection of the short external rotators and iliopsoas tendon.

Unanticipated problems and solution: There was no unanticipated problems in this index case because we plan ahead of the procedure and ensured that the required instruments, materials, and personnel were available.

Thorough description of decision-making, including the reason for the final decision: Due to the anticipated intrapelvic bleeding, we invited a vascular surgeon who assisted in mobilizing the vessels during cup extraction. We staged the procedure to reduce the metabolic demands on the patient that comes with unduly prolonged operation time. We used porous biphasic ceramics as granules by a diameter of 4–6 mm with porosity of 40–70%, in which correlation hydroxyapatite/tricalcium phosphate proportions were 60:40; structure of ceramics consisted of pores through interconnective system of micro- (till 10 μm) and macropores (350–600 μm). Calcium phosphate ceramics are osteoconductive and resorbable, i.e., they provide a scaffolding for new bone formation.

32.7.8 Postoperative Radiographs (Figs. 32.22 and 32.23)

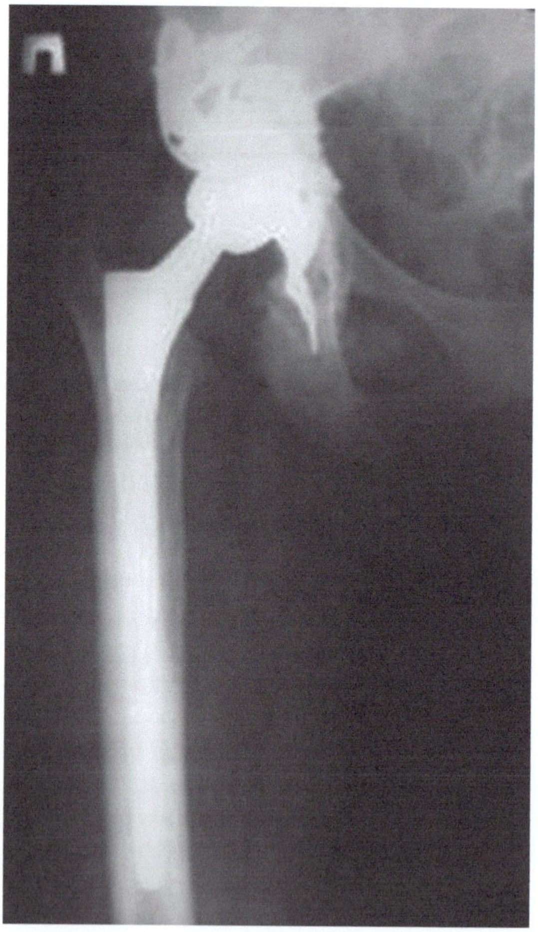

Fig. 32.22 AP view four years after revision THA on the right hip with Bursch-Schneider cage, the implant is stable, no loosening around the cage, allograft incorporation, there is the formation of bone-ceramic block and restoration of bone stock with the healing of discontinuity and no screw breakage

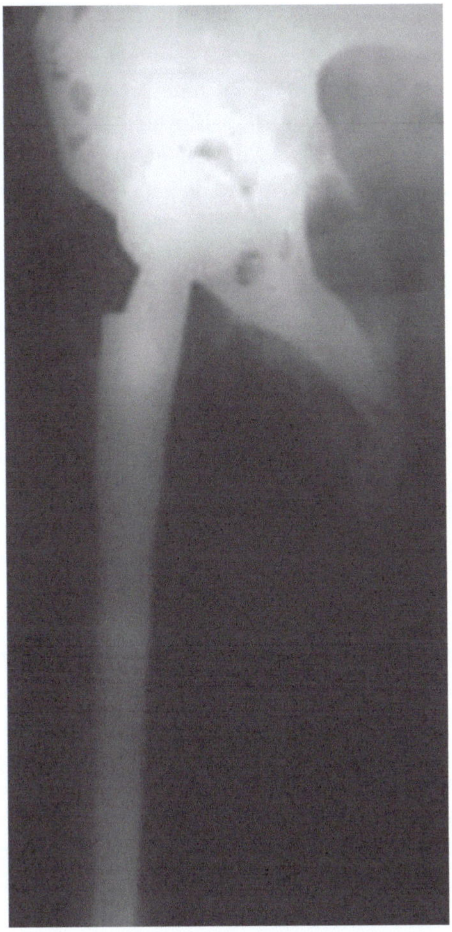

Fig. 32.23 Lateral view four years after revision THA on the right hip showing the formation of bone-ceramic block and restoration of bone stock with the healing of discontinuity and no screw breakage and no migration of reinforcement ring

32.7.9 Postoperative Management

Chemoprophylaxis and anticoagulant treatment period: Cefuroxime 750 mg twice daily for seven days, Clexane 40 mg once daily for 35 days postoperative, celecoxib 200 mg once daily for seven days, and blood transfusion with one unit.

Gait/limb loading until full loading: Patient was on restricted weight bearing with crutches for six months before commencing full weight bearing. During this period, there was limited hip flexion and adduction until full weight bearing.

32.7.10 Follow-Up and Complications

There were no postoperative complications for this case; the patient was followed up at an interval of 3, 6, and 12 months and subsequently yearly.

32.7.11 Discussion [18, 47, 49]

Advantages of the applied method: Restoration of hip rotation centre, secure mechanical support on the ilium and ischium, reliable incorporation of the cancellous graft, mechanical protection for the structural graft, and restoration of the bone stock.

Disadvantages of the method: Wide exposure increases neurovascular risks, the potential for decreased abductor function and limp, mechanical construct, dependent on multiple screws for long-term fixation, loosening, or breakage at repeated loads. Because it is a two-stage procedure, it requires longer treatment time, more expensive for the patient and labor intensive for the surgeons.

Alternative evidence-based techniques for the case: (1) Cementless/cemented cup with posterior ± anterior column plate fixation with bone grafting, (2) cup-cage and acetabular reconstruction, (3) distraction technique with augments, and (4) triflanged components.

Why is the chosen technique better for this case? The use of the Burch-Schneider cage enables the surgeon to achieve secured fixation of the flanges to the ilium and ischium, and it protects extensive acetabular bone graft by transferring some of the load from the acetabulum to the ilium and the ischium.

Indications and contraindications for your technique—At present, the cage is indicated as follows:

- Revision arthroplasty with large acetabular floor or roof defects
- Acetabular destruction by metastases
- Acetabular fractures, when immediate weight bearing is desired

- Following Girdlestone Contraindications: Contraindications for this procedure are Paprosky type I and II acetabular bone defects.

Learning curve and how to manage complications: This procedure has a steep learning curve and should only be undertaken by experienced surgeons who practice in centres with high-volume surgery.

Level of evidence concerning the superiority of this method against others: Level III evidence.

32.8 Case Title: Acetabular Revision (Chronic Pelvic Dissociation)

Volodymyr Filippenko, Stanislav Bondarenko, and Volodymyr Mezentsev

32.8.1 Demographics

Age: 50
Sex: Female
BMI: 37.4

32.8.2 Relevant Past Medical History

Principal pathologies: Aseptic instability of left cemented acetabular cup with protrusion into the pelvis

Previous surgical procedures: Cemented primary THA fifteen years before the index procedure, revision THA nine years later due to cup instability

Medication: Analgesics and NSAIDs, antibiotics, and anticoagulants

Other: Grade I hypertension and obesity

History of presenting complaint: Five years after the revision procedure secondary to cup instability, the patient dislocated the prosthetic head and presented with left groin pain, limping, muscle hypertrophy, and leg length discrepancy with pelvic obliquity. The pain was moderate, worst with ambulation, and relieved with rest. There was difficulty with weight bearing on the affected limb, and she ambulates with the aid of crutches. There was no history of fever, anorexia, nausea, weakness, weight loss, and vomiting. She had left leg shorting and limping throughout the period of dislocation and prior to the index procedure.

32.8.3 Clinical Examination

Symptoms: Moderate pain, limping, leg length discrepancy of 67 mm, Trendelenburg gait, pelvic obliquity, two postsurgical scars on the lateral thighs, ipsilateral thigh muscle swelling and pallor, quadriceps muscle hypertrophy, and abductor muscle weakness.

Range of motion: Extension/flexion, 0/0/5; adduction/adduction, 5/0/5; external rotation/internal rotation, 0/0/0.

Specific tests: CBC-T/D: within normal; serum electrolyte, urea, and creatinine (normal); CRP: negative; ESR: 10 mm/h; aspiration: negative; ECG, CT, contrast angiography, and Doppler USS—all within normal limits.

Main disability: Pain, limping, and inability to bear weight.

Scoring: VAS: 5; HHS: 28.

Neurovascular evaluation: The major lower limb nerves (sciatic, femoral and obturator, and superior gluteal) and vessels were intact.

32.8.4 Preoperative Radiological Assessment/Imaging (Figs. 32.24, 32.25, and 32.26)

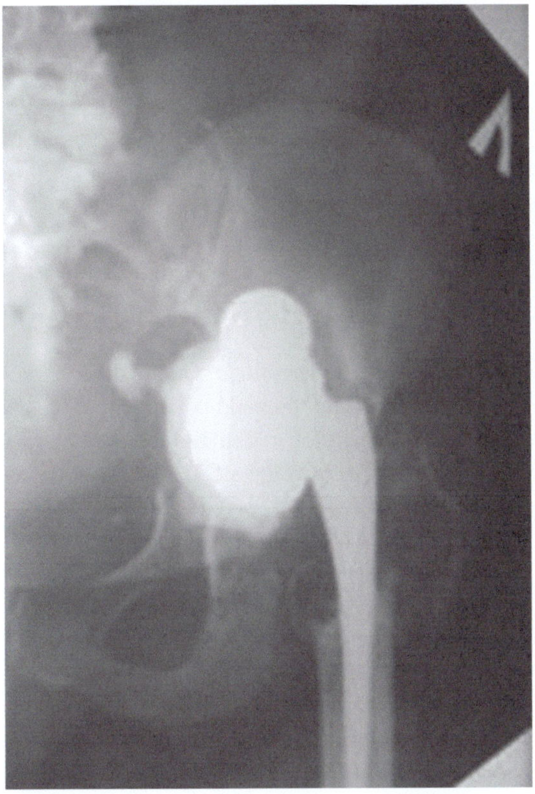

Fig. 32.24 AP X-ray view of the left hip joint showing the migration of the cemented implant into the pelvis, dislocation of the prosthetic femoral head and Paprosky type 3b defects with pelvic discontinuity. Paprosky 3b defect of proximal femur with severe osteolysis

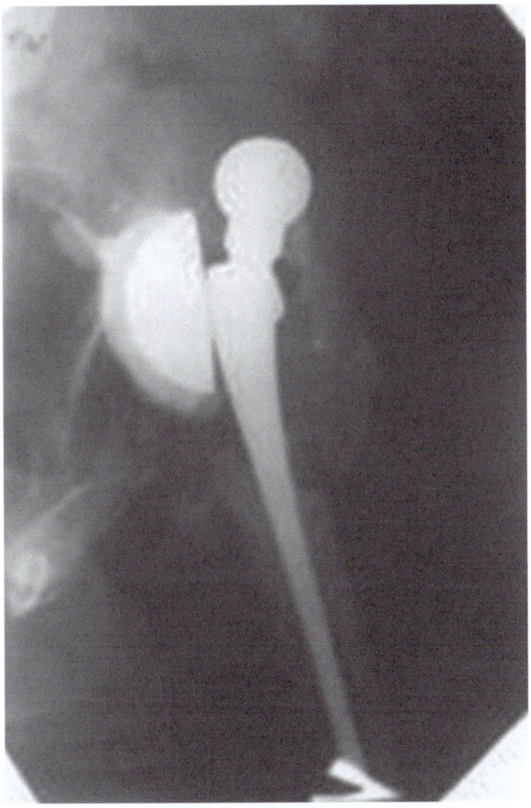

Fig. 32.25 Lateral X-ray view of the left hip joint showing the extent of dislocation (above 6 mm)

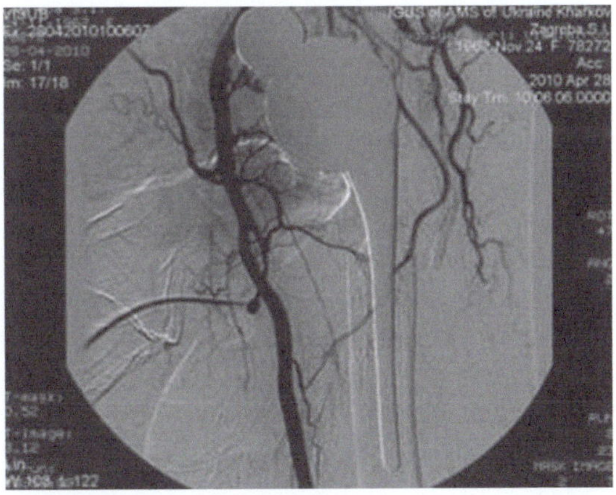

Fig. 32.26 Preoperative angiography scan showing cemented implant migration into pelvis and its proximity to the iliofemoral vessels

32.8.5 Preoperative Planning

Diagnosis: Aseptic instability of left cemented acetabular cup with protrusion into the pelvis with chronic pelvic discontinuity (Figs. 32.24, 32.25 and 32.26).

Possible treatment options: Revision THA with (1) acetabulum reconstruction with reinforcement cage and bone grafting, (2) cementless/cemented cup with posterior ± anterior column plate fixation with bone grafting, (3) cup-cage and acetabular reconstruction, (4) distraction technique with augments, (5) acetabular reconstruction with cemented cup and impaction bone grafting, (6) triflanged components, and (7) combinations of the above.

Chosen treatment method: Two-staged revision—(1) extraction of implant components and (2) reconstruction of acetabular defects with reinforcement cage and bone grafting.

Selection of implants if applicable and rational: Restoration of hip rotation centre, secure mechanical support on ilium and ischium, reliable incorporation of the cancellous graft, mechanical protection for the structural graft, restoration of the bone stock for later revision.

Expected difficulties: The initial difficulty is with the extraction of cup and bone cement from the pelvic cavity which requires retroperitoneal approach with the help of a vascular surgeon to reduce the risk of damage to vessels. The second difficulty is reconstructing severe acetabular bone defect (Paprosky type 3b) with pelvic discontinuity. The third difficulty is reconstruction of Paprosky 3b defect of proximal femur.

Strategies to overcome difficulties: The following strategies were used to overcome difficulties—first we employed the assistance of a vascular surgeon who helped us to mobilize the vessels while extracting the cup and cement. Second, the procedure was carried in two stages to reduce the risk of bleeding and hemodynamic imbalance associated with a prolonged period of anesthesia on the patient. Third, creating conditions for recovery of a bone mass by reconstructing acetabular and femoral bone defects (cavitary, segmental, combined) using cancellous, structural allografts and ceramics.

Templating: Manual templating was done with AP and lateral radiographs using standard templates supplied by manufacturers.

32.8.6 Surgical Note

Patient's position: For extraction of cement cup, the patient was placed supine; for extraction of the stem, the patient was placed laterally; and for revision THA, the patient was positioned laterally.

Type of anesthesia: General anesthesia.

Surgical approach: Retroperitoneal approach for acetabular implant extraction, direct lateral for femoral implant extraction and revision THA.

Main steps: The first stage which is the extraction of the acetabular cup and bone cement begins with incision parallel to the right inguinal ligament. After incision of the skin, subcutaneous tissue, and fat, the aponeurosis of the external oblique muscle is separated; we proceeded between the internal oblique muscle and rectus abdominis toward the transverse acetabular ligament. The acetabulum cup was visualized with fibrosis of the capsule in close proximity to the iliac vessels. After mobilization of vessels, the capsule was resected and the cup and cement extracted. The second stage was the extraction of the uncemented stem from the femur and osteosynthesis of the greater trochanter through a direct lateral approach which was done four weeks after the first stage due to iatrogenic damage to the external iliac artery. After extraction of the femoral implant, an osteolytic bone defect (Paprosky 3b) due to polyethylene wear and granuloma was seen. The index revision THA was performed six months later through direct lateral approach. Paprosky type 3b acetabular defect with separation of the anterior and posterior column (pelvic discontinuity) was visualized intraoperatively. Significant fibrosis and adhesions were excised from the bone tissue until active bleeding was encountered. There was considerable bone tissue remodeling of the defect. Segmental defects were filled with structural allografts from two femoral heads, and cavity defects were filled with morcellized bone grafts. Next was insertion of the Bursch-Schneider cage with the attachment of proximal flange at the ilium and distal flange at the ischium. The proximal flange was held in place with five screws. We inserted cemented cup in the cage. We then proceeded with the insertion of Wagner revision stem and reinforced it with cerclage and cable. The femoral head was reduced into the acetabular cup and satisfactory range of motion was achieved. Three drainages were inserted at the level of the joint capsule, fascia, and subcutaneous fats. The wound was closed in three layers and patient mobilized to intensive care unit (Figs. 32.27 and 32.28).

Reconstruction techniques: The segmental defect of the medial wall of the acetabulum of five cm in diameter was reconstructed using allograft from two femoral heads which were reamed to permit cage insertion. The cavitary defect of the superior wall of the acetabulum was filled by structural allografts from femoral head, and the inferior flange of Bursch-Schneider cage was first attached to the ischium providing the tensile force required to oppose the inferior hemipelvis to the superior flange attached to the ilium with five screws. Part of the osteolytic defects of the proximal femur was resected preserving the quality bone of the greater trochanter with its muscle with cerclage wires. We inserted Wagner revision stem and achieved good mechanical stability in the diaphysis. We then inserted autografts to aid in osseointegration. We then cable the proximal diaphysis as prophylaxis against periprosthetic fracture.

32.8.7 Intraoperative Challenges

Challenges and solutions: The bone defect of acetabulum intraoperatively was greater than what was anticipated preoperatively. We had to use extra allograft to construct the segmental defect of the acetabulum. Traction and dislocation of the limb was difficult due to increased tone of the thigh muscles to overcome this challenge.

Unanticipated problems and solution: There was iatrogenic damage to the external iliac artery during extraction of the femoral implants which was repaired by the vascular surgeon. Due to this complication, the proposed two-staged procedure was extended to three-staged. No other unanticipated problem was encountered in this index case.

Thorough description of decision-making, including the reason for the final decision: Due to the anticipated intrapelvic bleeding, we invited a vascular surgeon who assisted in repairing the vessel damage during cup extraction. We performed the procedure one stage further.

32.8.8 Postoperative Radiographs (Figs. 32. 27 and 32.28)

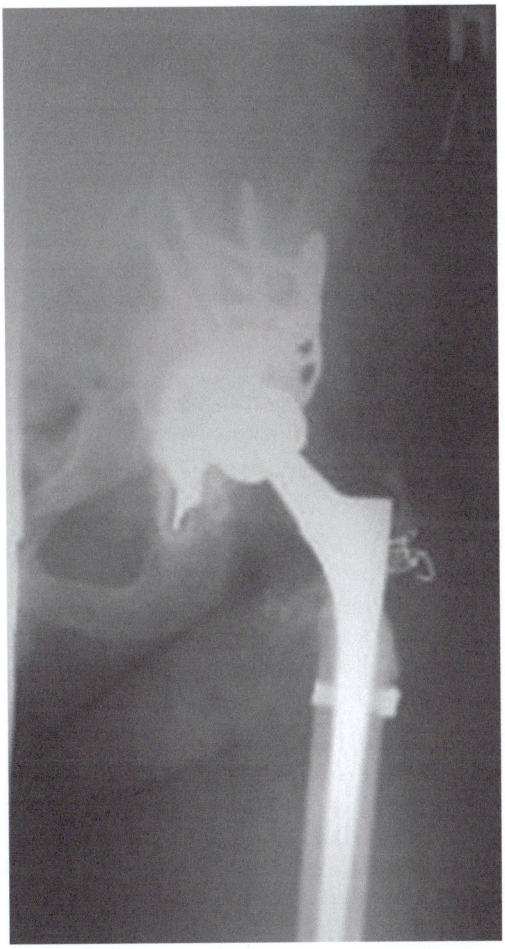

Fig. 32.27 AP postoperative view after revision THA on the left hip with Bursch-Schneider cage and restoration of hip rotation centre

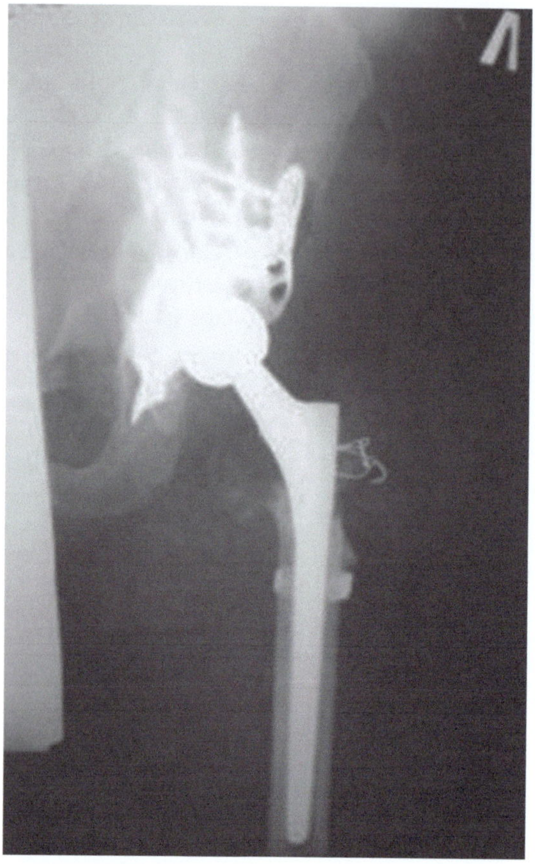

Fig. 32.28 AP view five years after revision THA on the left hip, implant stable, and allograft incorporation with the restoration of bone stock with the healing of pelvic discontinuity. There is osteolysis around the inferior flange

32.8.9 Postoperative Management

Chemoprophylaxis and anticoagulant treatment period: Ceftazidime 1000 mg twice daily for seven days, Clexane 40 mg once daily for 35 days postoperative, celecoxib 200 mg once daily for seven days, one unit of whole blood.

Gait/limb loading until full loading: Patient was on restricted weight bearing with crutches for six months before commencing full weight bearing. During this period there was limited hip flexion and adduction until full weight bearing.

32.8.10 Follow-Up and Complications

There was a postoperative hematoma which was aspirated and covered with antibiotic prophylaxis. Follow-up was at an interval of 3, 6, and 12 months and subsequently yearly.

32.8.11 Discussion [18, 47, 49]

Advantages of the applied method: Restoration of hip rotation centre, secure mechanical support on the ilium and ischium, reliable incorporation of cancellous graft, mechanical protection for structural graft, restoration of bone stock.

Disadvantages of the method: Wide exposure increases neurovascular risks, the potential for decreased abductor function and limp, mechanical construct, dependent on multiple screws for long-term fixation, loosening or breakage at repeated loads. Because it is a two-stage procedure, it requires longer treatment time, more expensive for the patient and labor intensive for the surgeons.

Alternative evidence-based techniques for the case: (1) Cementless/cemented cup with posterior ± anterior column plate fixation with bone grafting, (2) cup-cage and acetabular reconstruction, (3) distraction technique with augments, (4) cemented cup with impaction grafting, and (5) triflanged components.

Why is the chosen technique better for this case? The use of the Burch-Schneider cage enables the surgeon to achieve secured fixation of the flanges to the ilium and ischium, and it protects extensive acetabular bone graft by transferring some of the load from the acetabulum to the ilium and the ischium.

Indications and contraindications for your technique—At present, the cage is indicated as follows: revision arthroplasty with large acetabular floor or roof defects, acetabular destruction by metastases, and acetabular fractures when immediate weight bearing is desired, following Girdlestone. Contraindications for this procedure are Paprosky type I and II acetabular bone defects.

Learning curve and how to manage complications: This procedure has a steep learning curve and should only be undertaken by experienced surgeons who practice in centres with high-volume surgery.

Level of evidence concerning the superiority of this method against others: Level III evidence.

32.9 Case Title: Acetabular Revision (Chronic Pelvic Dissociation)

Neil P. Sheth, Christopher M. Melnic, and Wayne G. Paprosky

32.9.1 Demographics

Age: 57
Sex: Female
BMI: 34

32.9.2 Relevant Past Medical History

Principal pathologies: Rheumatoid arthritis, sarcoidosis, and hypertension

Previous surgical procedures: Left total hip arthroplasty in 2000 and right hip pinning as a child

Medication: Methotrexate, prednisone, and Hytrin

History of presenting complaint: The patient is a 57-year-old female with a history of rheumatoid arthritis that had a well-functioning hip for fifteen years. Over a period of the past six months, the patient noted worsening left groin pain and slight shortening of the left lower extremity. She presented to the outpatient clinic with these complaints.

32.9.3 Clinical Examination

Symptoms: Left groin pain, shortening of the left lower extremity, and difficulty with weight bearing on the left lower extremity

Specific tests: A preoperative erythrocyte sedimentation rate (ESR) and C-reactive protein (CRP) were obtained. The values were 113 (0–20) and 160 (7.4), respectively. The patient was sent for a preoperative left hip aspiration which showed a WBC count of 100 with 12% segmented neutrophils. The five-day results for aerobic and anaerobic cultures demonstrated no growth. The preoperative suspicion for a periprosthetic infection was very low following the aspiration results.

Main disability: Painful ambulation on the left lower extremity.

Neurovascular evaluation: 4/5 motor strength in the distribution of the L4, L5, and S1 nerve roots and minimal sensation to light touch in the distribution of the superficial and deep peroneal, saphenous, sural, and tibial nerves. There were a 2+ femoral, dorsalis pedis, and posterior tibial artery pulse. The patient has baseline motor and sensory neuropathy due to long-standing sarcoidosis.

32.9.4 Preoperative Radiological Assessment/Imaging (Figs. 32.29, 32.30, and 32.31)

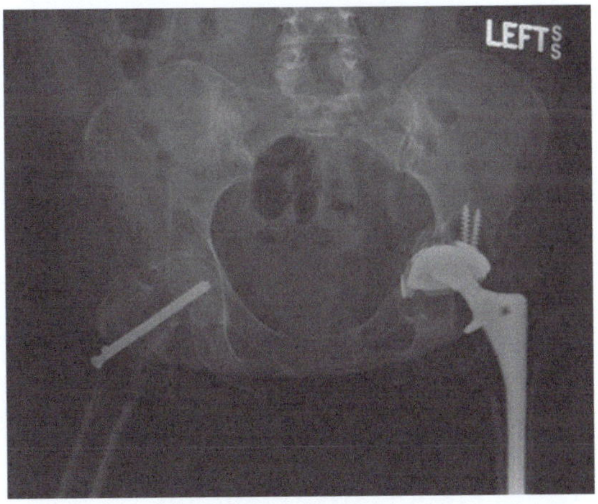

Fig. 32.29 Preoperative AP pelvis X-ray demonstrating a Paprosky 3b (up and in) acetabular defect with the complete wear of the femoral head through the acetabulum liner and metal shell

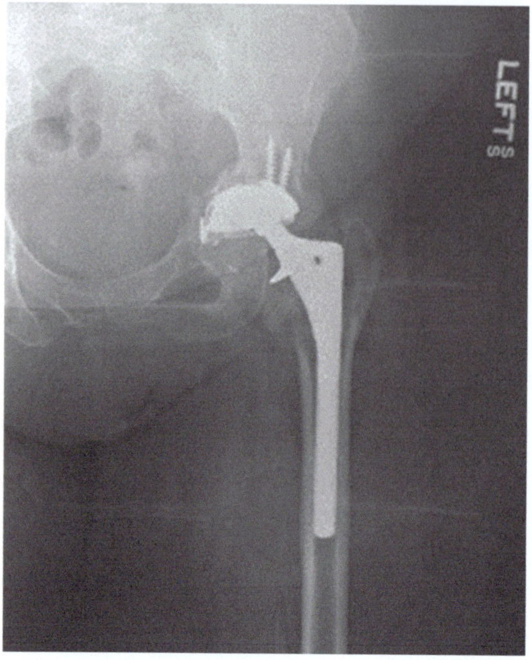

Fig. 32.30 Preoperative AP hip X-ray demonstrating the same pelvic bone loss pattern with a pelvic discontinuity

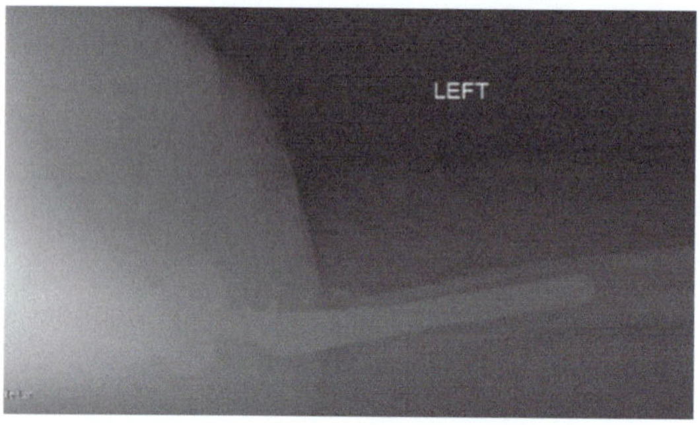

Fig. 32.31 Preoperative cross table lateral depicting malposition (neutral to retroversion) of the acetabular component. The cross table lateral projection can also show the presence of a pelvic discontinuity; however, this is not seen in this radiograph due to the patient's body habitus and obscuring soft tissue shadow

32.9.5 Preoperative Planning

Diagnosis: Aseptic loosening of the left acetabular component with Paprosky 3b acetabular bone loss and associated chronic pelvic discontinuity (Figs. 32.29, 32.30 and 32.31).

Possible treatment options: Ring/cage construct with a cemented liner, acetabular allograft reconstruction with cemented liner, acetabular impaction grafting with a cemented liner, cup-cage construct with a cemented liner, custom triflange acetabular component, acetabular distraction technique with use of a porous metal cup and modular segment.

Chosen treatment method: Acetabular distraction technique with use of a porous metal cup and modular segment.

Selection of implants if applicable and rational: Implants chosen—revision tantalum elliptical shell (Trabecular Metal, Zimmer, Warsaw, IN, USA) and acetabular augments for acetabular reconstruction (Trabecular Metal augments, Zimmer, Warsaw, IN, USA). The use of a tantalum revision shell allows for improved stress distribution to the remaining retroacetabular bone stock, placement of a cemented liner which creates a locked construct with all properly placed screws, fine-tuning of abduction and version by positioning of the cemented liner, and holes to be customized in the tantalum shell with a burr for additional screw fixation.

Expected difficulties: These cases can be challenging when there is an excessive acetabular bone loss in the presence of a chronic pelvic discontinuity. In addition, the residual bone stock is osteoporotic due to long-term prednisone use and a baseline history of rheumatoid arthritis. Also, for this patient, since there is pre-existing sciatic nerve dysfunction, any undue stress on the nerve may result in a complete sciatic nerve palsy.

Strategies to overcome difficulties: Wide surgical exposure with minimal tension on host tissue to diminish the risk of further iatrogenic bone loss. In this setting, the sciatic nerve was not dissected out since access to the posterior column was not necessary.

Templating: Digital templating of the acetabular component was performed to determine a "ball park" size of the component to be used. The revision acetabular shell was templated to a size 58 mm.

32.9.6 Surgical Note

Patient's position: Lateral decubitus.

Type of anesthesia: General anesthesia with an arterial line and Foley catheter placed prior to the start of the procedure.

Surgical approach: A posterolateral approach was utilized for the appropriate exposure.

Main steps:

1. Wide posterolateral surgical exposure.
2. Posterior capsular approach with tagging of the capsule for later repair.
3. Two samples of pseudocapsule should be sent for final microbiology for aerobic and anaerobic culture.
4. Identify the sciatic nerve if visible in the operative field.
5. Following sequential scar excision, dislocate the hip, remove the femoral head, and check the stability of the remaining femoral stem (stem was stable).
6. Placement of acetabular retractors for acetabular exposure (may require additional scar excision for complete exposure).
7. Following adequate acetabular exposure, the acetabular liner and two screws should be removed from the shell.
8. A "cup-out" (Zimmer, Warsaw, IN, USA) osteotome may be required for removal of the acetabular shell to prevent iatrogenic acetabular bone loss.
9. Following acetabular component removal, the acetabulum should be cleared of any fibrous tissue with a Cobb elevator, and the chronic discontinuity should be identified.
10. The superficial portion of the discontinuity should be carefully debrided with a Cobb elevator, making sure not to destabilize the discontinuity by aggressive debridement [now the reconstruction can be performed].

Reconstruction techniques:

(1) The initial step for acetabular reconstruction is to determine the integrity of the anterosuperior (AS) and posteroinferior (PI) columns; in this case, the AS column was intact. (2) An orange slice augment (50 × 10, Zimmer, Warsaw, IN, USA) was secured in place with two screws (length 25 and 30 mm). (3) Following AS column reconstruction, a distractor is placed within the acetabulum to gauge the mobility of the discontinuity—this technique allows for peripheral or lateral acetabular distraction with resultant central or medial compression at the discontinuity. (4) A 2.4 mm K-wire is then placed in host bone over the AS and PI columns, and the distractor is placed over the K-wires. (5) With the acetabulum in a distracted position, a reamer is used on reverse to achieve an interference fit between the AS segment and the host PI column. (6) When the reamer achieves a proper fit between the columns, it will disengage from the reamer handle, and the reamer head can be used as a surrogate acetabular component. (7) In this case, a size 58 reamer was the correct size—a size 58 revision Trabecular Metal shell was used [this shell is elliptical and thus measures 60 mm at the periphery allowing for additional 1 mm peripheral "press fit"]. (8) There is a titanium ring at the edge of the revision shell—this ring is typically removed in order to get access to the periphery of the cup. (9) Once the ring is removed, a metal cutting burr is used to drill additional holes into the cup, specifically at the periphery to allow for screw fixation into the ischium to avoid abduction failure of the final construct ["kickstand screw"]. (10) The chronic discontinuity should be bone grafted with crushed cancellous allograft chips prior to impacting the acetabular component into position with a bone tamp; cement must be placed between the AS segment and the cup for unitization of the construct following bone grafting and prior to cup placement. (11) Following proper positioning of the acetabular shell, the K-wires and distractor are removed. (12) At least four good screws should be placed through the cup into host bone [four screws were placed in this case, but only two screws exhibited good purchase]. (13) An orange slice augment (54 × 15—Zimmer, Warsaw, IN, USA) was placed in the posterosuperior position for supplemental fixation and secured to host bone [two 35 mm screws and a 25 mm screw were used in this case]. (14) Cement should be used to unitize this augment to the acetabular shell, which is done at the same time as cementing the final liner into the shell following trial reduction (Figs. 32.32 and 32.33).

32.9.7 Intraoperative Challenges

Challenges and solutions: The biggest challenge, in this case, is to prevent over-distraction of the acetabulum. Avoiding aggressive debridement of the chronic discontinuity at the beginning of the case decreases the risk of over distraction with use of a distractor.

Unanticipated problems and solution: For this patient, the sciatic nerve was tethered to scar tissue over the posterior wall of the acetabulum. In order to place the PS augment for supplemental fixation, the nerve needed to be dissected out and moved to avoid inadvertent neural injury during placement of the PS augment.

32.9.8 Postoperative Radiographs (Figs. 32.32 and 32.33)

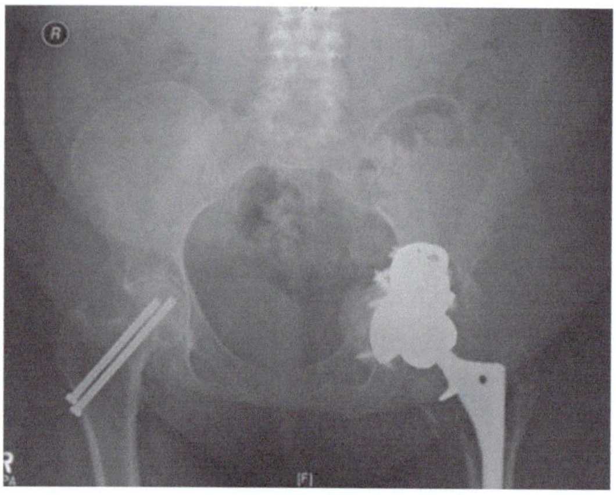

Fig. 32.32 3-month postoperative AP pelvis radiograph following acetabular and augment reconstruction using acetabular distraction technique

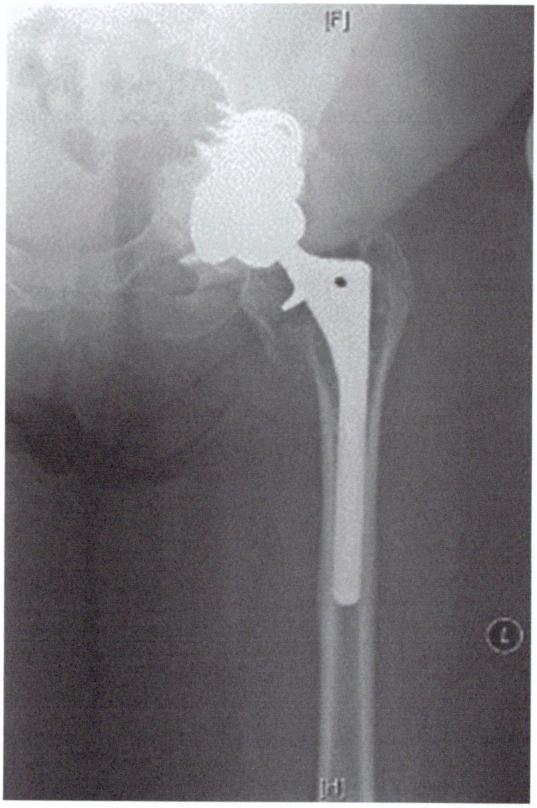

Fig. 32.33 3-month postoperative AP hip radiograph following distraction technique. Bone graft is visible inferomedially which was used to bone graft the discontinuity

32.9.9 Postoperative Management

Chemoprophylaxis and anticoagulant treatment period: The patient was placed on ASA 325 mg po bid × 6 weeks for DVT prophylaxis.

Gait/limb loading until full loading: The patient was made touchdown weight bearing (10%) for six weeks, followed by partial weight bearing (50%) for an additional six weeks. Serial

X-rays were demonstrating no change in component position allowed for weight bearing as tolerated at three months postoperatively.

32.9.10 Follow-Up and Complications

The patient did present with a foot drop on the left lower extremity in the immediate postoperative period. She was given a molded ankle-foot orthosis to maintain a plati-grade foot position for ambulation. Her sensation is intact as per her baseline sensory deficit, and the patient exhibits baseline tibial nerve function with foot plantar flexion. Her neuropathic pain is being treated with gabapentin 300 mg per os three times daily. She has been sent for an electromyography at three months to determine nerve function recovery.

32.9.11 Discussion

Advantages of the applied method: The major advantage to using acetabular distraction technique is the ability to customize and unitize your construct intraoperatively, and it allows for biologic fixation. This technique doesn't require a preoperative CT scan and doesn't require 4–6 weeks for fabrication of a custom implant.

Disadvantages of the method: This method of treatment is technically challenging and may result in over-distraction of the acetabulum. As mentioned above, avoiding aggressive debridement of the discontinuity is critical.

Alternative evidence-based techniques for the case: The treatment of acetabular bone loss in the face of chronic pelvic discontinuity is the most challenging problem to address in the setting of revision total hip arthroplasty. There are several other options which have been supported by the literature. The use of a cup cage has demonstrated favorable clinical results in the short and midterm. The use of a cage allows for bridging of the defect while the cup achieves biologic fixation. Amenabar et al. [33] recently reported 85–93% survivorship of 67 patients that were followed for a mean time of 6.2 years. The use of a custom triflange acetabular component is another technique that has been popularized for the treatment of significant acetabular bone loss and associated chronic pelvic discontinuity. Berasi et al. [38] have recently reported on 23 patients that exhibited 100% survivorship at mean 4.5 years following triflange reconstruction.

Why is the chosen technique better for this case? Acetabular distraction technique was popularized by the senior author, and it is used by two of the authors (NPS and WGP) for all chronic pelvic discontinuities. Longer-term follow-up is needed to determine the true efficacy of this surgical technique.

Indications and contraindications for your technique: The indication for acetabular distraction is an acetabular revision in the face of significant acetabular bone loss with an associated chronic pelvic discontinuity. The contraindications include active infection and history of prior pelvic radiation that has resulted in radiation necrosis.

Learning curve and how to manage complications: The learning curve for this procedure is steep and requires some degree of training prior to its use. We recommend going to observe this procedure performed by an individual experienced in distraction technique.

Level of evidence concerning the superiority of this method against others: There is only one study in the literature regarding this technique for treatment of chronic pelvic discontinuity. Sporer et al. [12] reported on 20 patients that underwent this technique for the treatment of chronic discontinuity. At minimum two-year follow-up, 19 (95%) cases demonstrated radiographic healing of the discontinuity and absence of loosening of the acetabular components.

32.10 Case Title: Acetabular Revision "Chronic Pelvic Dissociation"

Fritz Thorey

32.10.1 Demographics

Age: 51
Sex: Male
BMI: 25.9

32.10.2 Relevant Past Medical History

Principal pathologies: Loosening of the cup

Previous surgical procedures: THA eighteen years before

Medication: Valoron

History of Presenting Complaint: Increasing complaints in the last three years

32.10.3 Clinical Examination

Symptoms: Limping, limited ROM, severe pain

Main disability: Pain

Scoring: VAS for pain: 7; Harris Hip Score: 39 (without section 2 and 3); HOOS: 47.5 (subscales—symp: 50%; pain: 35%; function: 67.7%; sports: 12.5%; QOL: 25%)

32.10.4 Preoperative Radiological Assessment/Imaging (Figs. 32.34 and 32.35)

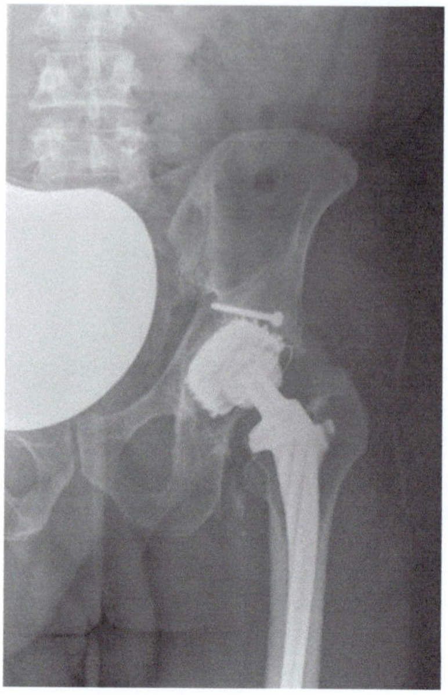

Fig. 32.34 AP view of the left hip showed a beginning of the protrusion of the cup with slight discontinuity of the pelvis

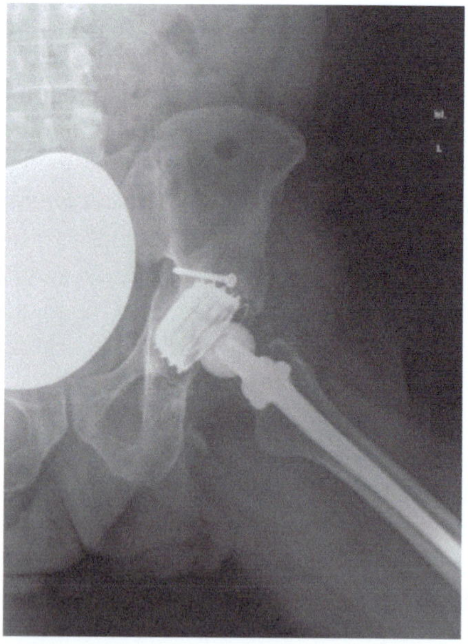

Fig. 32.35 Axial view of the left hip showed the stable stem on the femoral side

32.10.5 Preoperative Planning

Diagnosis: Cup loosening with protrusion (Figs. 32.34 and 32.35)

Possible treatment options: Revision of the cup

Chosen treatment method: Revision of the cup

Selection of implants if applicable and rational: Primary or revision implant

Expected difficulties: The bone defect on the medial side

Strategies to overcome difficulties: Reconstruction of the medial wall with allograft

Templating: Templating of a primary and revision implant with reconstruction of the centre of rotation

32.10.6 Surgical Note

Patient's position: Supine

Type of anesthesia: General anesthesia

Surgical approach: Original approach (lateral transgluteal)

Main steps: Mobilization of the proximal femur, visualization of the cup, removal of the cup, and reconstruction of the bone defect

Reconstruction techniques: Impaction grafting (Figs. 32.36 and 32.37)

32.10.7 Intraoperative Challenges

Challenges and solutions: Bone loss on the medial wall with posteromedial instability

Unanticipated problems and solution: None

Thorough description of decision-making, including the reason for the final decision: Bone loss was reconstructed with impaction grafting and bone block. The anterior and posterior wall at the rim of the acetabulum was stable. Fixation of primary cup was possible.

32.10.8 Postoperative Radiographs (Figs. 32.36 and 32.37)

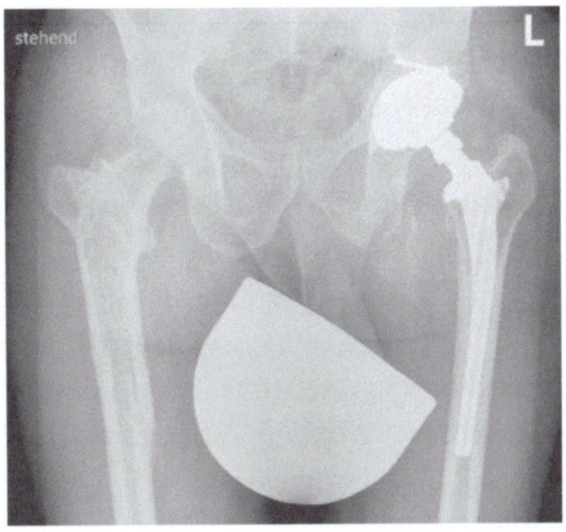

Fig. 32.36 AP pelvic view showed revision with the primary implant and impaction grafting

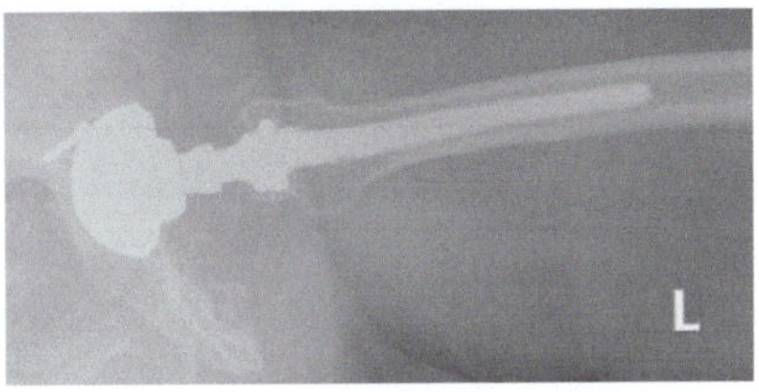

Fig. 32.37 Axial view showed good position of implants

32.10.9 Postoperative Management File

Chemoprophylaxis and anticoagulant treatment period: Xarelto, antibiotics for four weeks

Gait/limb loading until full loading: Weight bearing as tolerated

32.10.10 Follow-Up and Complications

No complications.

Scoring: VAS for pain: 0; Harris Hip Score: 86 (without section 2 and 3).

32.10.11 Discussion [2, 50, 51]

Advantages of the applied method: Reconstruction without using a megaprosthesis or revision cage.

Disadvantages of the method: Perfect stable fixation of the primary implant is mandatory; if there is instability, the implant will fail.

Alternative evidence-based techniques for the case: Revision cage, jumbo cups with trabecular metal.

Why is the chosen technique better for this case? Good body conditions enabled the fixation with the primary implant. For future revisions, there is still a good bone stock.

Indications and contraindications for your technique: Indication for this technique is sufficient stability for a primary cup fixation.

Learning curve and how to manage complications: Longer learning curve.

Level of evidence concerning the superiority of this method against others: Should only be used in cases with sufficient bone conditions to fix a primary implant.

References

1. Abdelnasser MK, Klenke FM, Whitlock P, Khalil AM, Khalifa YE, Ali HM, Siebenrock KA. Management of pelvic discontinuity in revision total hip arthroplasty: a review of the literature. Hip Int. 2015;25(2):120–6.
2. Schwarzkopf R, Ihn HE, Ries MD. Pelvic discontinuity: modern techniques and outcomes for treating pelvic disassociation. Hip Int. 2015;25(4):368–74.
3. Petrie J, Sassoon A, Haidukewych GJ. Pelvic discontinuity: current solutions. Bone Joint J. 2013;95-B(11 Suppl A):109–13.
4. D'Antonio JA, Capello WN, Borden LS, et al. Classification and management of acetabular abnormalities in total hip arthroplasty. Clin Orthop Relat Res. 1989;243:126–37.
5. Gross AE. Revision arthroplasty of the acetabulum with restoration of bone stock. Clin Orthop Relat Res. 1999;369:198–207.
6. Berry DJ, Lewallen DG, Hanssen AD, Cabanela ME. Pelvic discontinuity in revision total hip arthroplasty. J Bone Joint Surg Am. 1999;81(12):1692–702.
7. Wendt MC, Adler MA, Trousdale RT, Mabry TM, Cabanela ME. Effectiveness of false profile radiographs in detection of pelvic discontinuity. J Arthroplasty. 2012;27(7):1408–12.
8. Giori NJ, Sidky AO. Lateral and high-angle oblique radiographs of the pelvis aid in diagnosing pelvic discontinuity after total hip arthroplasty. J Arthroplasty. 2011;26(1):110–2.
9. Chiang PP, Burke DW, Freiberg AA, Rubash HE. Osteolysis of the pelvis: evaluation and treatment. Clin Orthop Relat Res. 2003;417:164–74.
10. Leung S, Naudie D, Kitamura N, Walde T, Engh CA. Computed tomography in the assessment of periacetabular osteolysis. J Bone Joint Surg Am. 2005;87(3):592–7.
11. Bamberg F, Dierks A, Nikolaou K, Reiser MF, Becker CR, Johnson TR. Metal artifact reduction by dual energy computed tomography using monoenergetic extrapolation. Eur Radiol. 2011;21(7):1424–9.
12. Sporer SM, Bottros JJ, Hulst JB, Kancherla VK, Moric M, Paprosky WG. Acetabular distraction: an alternative for severe defects with chronic pelvic discontinuity? Clin Orthop Relat Res. 2012;470(11):3156–63.
13. Stiehl JB, Saluja R, Diener T. Reconstruction of major column defects and pelvic discontinuity in revision total hip arthroplasty. J Arthroplasty. 2000;15(7):849–57.
14. Eggli S, Muller C, Ganz R. Revision surgery in pelvic discontinuity: an analysis of seven patients. Clin Orthop Relat Res. 2002;398:136.
15. Goodman S, Saastamoinen H, Shasha N, et al. Complications of ilioischial reconstruction rings in revision total hip arthroplasty. J Arthroplasty. 2004;19–4:436.
16. Kerboull M, Hamadouche M, Kerboull L. The Kerboull acetabular reinforcement device in major acetabular reconstructions. Clin Orthop Relat Res. 2000;378:155–68.
17. Paprosky WG, Sporer SS, Murphy BP. Addressing severe bone deficiency: what a cage will not do. J Arthroplasty. 2007;22(4 Suppl 1):111–5.
18. Rogers BA, Whittingham-Jones PM, Mitchell PA, Safir OA, Bircher MD, Gross AE. The reconstruction of periprosthetic pelvic discontinuity. J Arthroplasty. 2012;27(8):1499.e1–506.e1.
19. Nicholas A, Beckmann MD. Loosening after acetabular revision: comparison of trabecular metal and reinforcement rings a systematic review. J Arthroplasty. 2014;29:229–35.
20. Rosson J, Schatzker J. The use of reinforcement rings to reconstruct deficient acetabula. J Bone Joint Surg Br. 1992;74–5:716.
21. Gerber A, Pisan M, Zurakowski D, et al. Ganz reinforcement ring for reconstruction of acetabular defects in revision total hip arthroplasty. J Bone Joint Surg Am. 2003;85-A(12):2358.
22. Schlegel UJ, Bitsch RG, Pritsch M, et al. Acetabular reinforcement rings in revision total hip arthroplasty: midterm results in 298 cases. Orthopade. 2008;37–9(904):6.
23. Sporer SM, Paprosky WG. Acetabular revision using a trabecular metal acetabular component for severe acetabular bone loss associated with a pelvic discontinuity. J Arthroplasty. 2006;21–6(Suppl 2):87–90.

24. Unger AS, Lewis RJ, Gruen T. Evaluation of a porous tantalum uncemented acetabular cup in revision total hip arthroplasty: clinical and radiological results of 60 hips. J Arthroplasty. 2005;20–8:1002.
25. Weeden SH, Schmidt RH. The use of tantalum porous metal implants for Paprosky 3A and 3B defects. J Arthroplasty. 2007;22–6(Suppl 2):151.
26. Siegmeth A, Duncan CP, Masri BA, et al. Modular tantalum augments for acetabular defects in revision hip arthroplasty. Clin Orthop Relat Res. 2009;467–1:199.
27. Davies JH, Laflamme GY, Delisle J, et al. Trabecular metal used for major bone loss in acetabular hip revision. J Arthroplasty. 2011;26–8:1245.
28. Flecher X, Sporer S, Paprosky W. Management of severe bone loss in acetabular revision using a trabecular metal shell. J Arthroplasty. 2008;23–7:949.
29. Lingaraj K. The management of severe acetabular bone defects in revision hip arthroplasty using modular porous metal components. J Bone Joint Surg Br. 2009;91-B:1555–60.
30. Del Gaizo DJ. Tantalum augments for paprosky IIIA defects remain stable at midterm follow up. Clin Orthop Relat Res. 2012;470:395–401.
31. Abolghasemian M, Tangsataporn S, Sternheim A, Backstein D, Safir O, Gross AE. Combined trabecular metal acetabular shell and augment for acetabular revision with substantial bone loss: a mid-term review. Bone Joint J. 2013;95-B:166–72.
32. Brown NM, Hellman M, Haughom BH, Shah RP, Sporer SM, Paprosky WG. Acetabular distraction: an alternative approach to pelvic discontinuity in failed total hip replacement. J Bone Joint Surg Br. 2014;96(11):73–7.
33. Amenabar T, Rahman WA, Hetaimish BM, Kuzyk PR, Safir OA, Gross AE. Promising mid-term results with a cup-cage construct for large acetabular defects and pelvic discontinuity. Clin Orthop Relat Res. 2016;474:408–14.
34. Sheth NP, Nelson CL, Springer BD, Fehring TK, Paprosky WG. Acetabular bone loss in revision total hip arthroplasty: evaluation and management. J Am Acad Orthop Surg. 2013;21:128–39.
35. Abolghasemian M, et al. The challenge of pelvic discontinuity cup-cage reconstruction does better than conventional cages in mid-term. Bone Joint J. 2014;96-B:195–200.
36. Kosashvili Y, et al. Acetabular revision using an anti-protrusion (ilio-ischial) cage and trabecular metal acetabular component for severe acetabular bone loss associated with pelvic discontinuity. J Bone Joint Surg Br. 2009;91-B:870–6.
37. Goodman GP, Engh CA Jr. Acetabular Revision. The custom triflange cup. Build it and they will come. Bone Joint J. 2016;98-B(1 Suppl A):68–72.
38. Berasi CC IV, Berend KR, Adams JB, Ruh EL, Lombardi AV Jr. Are custom triflange acetabular components effective for reconstruction of catastrophic bone loss? Clin Orthop Relat Res. 2015;473:528–35.
39. Taunton MJ, Fehring TK, Edwards P, et al. Pelvic discontinuity treated with custom triflange component: a reliable option. Clin Orthop Relat Res. 2012;470:428–34.
40. DeBoer DK, Christie MJ, Brinson MF, Morrison JC. Revision total hip arthroplasty for pelvic discontinuity. J Bone Joint Surg Am. 2007;89-A:835–40.
41. Holt GE, Dennis DA. Use of custom triflanged acetabular components in revision total hip arthroplasty. Clin Orthop Relat Res. 2004;429:209–14.
42. Christie MJ, Barrington SA, Brinson MF, Ruhling ME, DeBoer DK. Bridging massive acetabular defects with the triflange cup: 2- to 9-year results. Clin Orthop Relat Res. 2001;393:216–27.
43. Paprosky W, Sporer S, O'Rourke MR. The treatment of pelvic discontinuity with acetabular cages. Clin Orthop Relat Res. 2006;453(453):183–7.
44. García-Rey E, Madero R, García-Cimbrelo E. THA revisions using impaction allografting with mesh is durable for medial but not lateral acetabular defects. Clin Orthop Relat Res. 2015;473(12):3882–91.
45. Putzer D, Mayr E, Haid C, Reinthaler A, Nogler M. Impaction bone grafting: a laboratory comparison of two methods. J Bone Joint Surg Br. 2011;93(8):1049–53.
46 Coscujuela-Mañá A, Angles F, Tramunt C, Casanova X. Burch-Schneider antiprotrusio cage for acetabular revision: a 5- to 13-year follow-up study. Hip Int. 2010;20(Suppl 7):S112–8.
47 Regis D, Sandri A, Bonetti I, Bortolami O, Bartolozzi P. A minimum of 10- year follow-up of the Burch-Schneider cage and bulk allografts for the revision of pelvic discontinuity. J Arthroplast. 2012;27(6):1057–63.
48 Kawanabe K, Akiyama H, Goto K, Maeno S, Nakamura T. Load dispersion effects of acetabular reinforcement devices used in revision total hip arthroplasty: a simulation study using finite element analysis. J Arthroplast. 2011;26(7):1061–6. doi:10.1016/j.arth.2011.04.019. Epub 2011 Jun 14
49 Korzh NA, Filippenko VA, Mezentsev VA, Bondarenko SE. Reconstruction of acetabular defects in revision total hip arthroplasty. Traumatol Orthop. 2010;9(29):415–7.
50 Blumenfeld TJ. Implant choices, technique, and results in revision acetabular surgery: a review. Hip Int. 2012;22(3):235–47.
51 Pulido L, Rachala SR, Cabanela ME. Cementless acetabular revision: past, present, and future. Revision total hip arthroplasty: the acetabular side using cementless implants. Int Orthop. 2011;35(2):289–98.

Part V

Revision Hip Arthroplasty Femur

Impaction Grafting of the Femur (IGF)

33

Eustathios Kenanidis, Eleftherios Tsiridis, Eduardo García-Cimbrelo, Eduardo García-Rey, Martin Buttaro, Jillian Lee, and William Farrington

33.1 Current Concepts

E. Kenanidis and E. Tsiridis

Impaction grafting technique was initially described for the acetabulum [1, 2]. IGF was first performed with a cemented tapered polished stem and morselized fresh-frozen bone allografts in Exeter, England, in 1987 [3]. Gie and Ling popularised the technique [4] that was refined by the development of specialised instruments from Nijmegen group in Holland [5].

The principal benefit of the technique is that it potentially restores the femoral bone stock as the impacted allograft is incorporated and remodeled by the host skeleton. In the last few years, IGF use was diminished. This was mainly attributed to the ensuing popularity of other less time-consuming surgical techniques [6].

33.1.1 Objective

- The reconstruction of cavitary femoral defects with impacted fresh-frozen morselized bone graft to create a new endosteal surface and neo-medullary canal to host the primary cemented stem [6].
- Initially the densely packed cancellous graft and cement complex support the femoral implant. Subsequently, the graft gradually is vascularized and incorporated contributing to the implant support [7].

33.1.2 Indications

1. Ideally in wide cavitary metaphyseal or diaphyseal bone defects Dorr type 4 (the so-called drain pipe femoral canals) [8, 9].
2. Especially in young patients with less bone stock for two reasons:

E. Kenanidis, M.D., Ph.D., M.Sc. (✉)
Academic Orthopaedic Unit,
Aristotle University Medical School,
Thessaloniki, Greece

E. Tsiridis, M.D., Ph.D., F.A.C.S., F.R.C.S.
Academic Orthopaedic Unit, Papageorgiou General Hospital, Aristotle University Medical School,
Thessaloniki, Greece
e-mail: etsiridis@doctors.org.uk

E. García-Cimbrelo, M.D., Ph.D.
E. García-Rey, M.D., Ph.D.
Hospital Universitario La Paz-Idi Paz,
Madrid, Spain

M. Buttaro, M.D.
Hospital Italiano de Buenos Aires,
Buenos Aires, Argentina
e-mail: martin.buttaro@hospitalitaliano.org.ar

J. Lee, B.H.B., M.B.Ch.B., F.R.A.C.S.
W. Farrington, M.B.B.S., F.R.C.S., F.R.C.S.
North Shore Hospital, Auckland, New Zealand
e-mail: wjfarrington@me.com

E. Tsiridis (ed.), *The Adult Hip - Master Case Series and Techniques*,
https://doi.org/10.1007/978-3-319-64177-5_33

   (a) Most likely they will need an additional reconstructive procedure in their lifetime.
   (b) Better compliance with the rehabilitation process [10].
3. It is also a valuable option when:
   (a) The femur is too wide or damaged to support a fully uncemented cylindrical or tapered device.
   (b) You want to obviate thigh pain appearance using a fully porous-coated stem in a broad (>18 mm) intramedullary canal [10].
   (c) There is not enough cortical bone (4–6 cm) to achieve scratch fit of a porous-coated stem at the isthmus [10].
   (d) The implantation of a long extensively porous-coated femoral stem is impeded from the femoral stem of an ipsilateral TKA [10].
   (e) You need to transfer load proximally revising a previously distally fixated long cementless stem [8].
   (f) You have to manage peri-prosthetic fractures [11]. Although IGF is not the first choice, Tsiridis et al. [11] reported a union rate of 84% in Vancouver B2 and B3 fractures at 4-year follow-up.

33.1.3 Contraindications

1. There are no known absolute contraindications.
2. Perhaps the only unqualified contraindication is a previous peri-prosthetic joint infection. IGF was effective, however, at 92.5% as reconstruction method at the second stage of a two-stage revision of an infected THA [12].
3. It is possibly contraindicated also when:
   (a) There is need of a considerable amount of graft for reconstruction [8].
   (b) The patient will be noncompliant with the rehabilitation program [8].
   (c) The patient is non-fit to tolerate an extended operation.
   (d) The procedure is not designed to be performed carefully.
   (e) The proximal cortical femoral bone loss is near complete and perimetrical. An APC or tumor megaprosthesis or distal fixation with a long stem is then recommended [9].

33.1.4 Preoperative Planning

- The importance of the preoperative planning to diminish the complications has been demonstrated [13].
- Exclude septic loosening by joint aspiration.
- Perform pelvis anteroposterior and lateral X-rays to select size, length, and offset of revision implant and define the site of the distal plug [9].

33.1.5 Surgical Technique [8–10]

- The posterior approach offers better access to the whole femur.
- Remove the stem and all previous cement.
- Debride the intramedullary soft and fibrous tissue and debris.
- Confirm the integrity of the femoral tube; if the femoral canal is not continuous, then convert the segmental defects to contained with a metal mesh or allograft struts or bulk allograft [3, 4].
- Introduce a distal suitable in size, centralizing cement plug into the femoral canal more than two femoral diameters below the most distal cavitary defect or below the distal tip of the implant to be used. An option also is to keep a previous well-fixed plug [10].
- Prepare cancellous bone graft fragments of two different sizes; 7–10 mm in size for the proximal impaction and bone chips of 2–5 mm size for the distal impaction.
- Wash the graft before the impaction to remove the fat and marrow contents and to improve its mechanical properties [14].
- Screw a central guide wire into the plug through which cannulated impactors tamp bone graft distally.
- Introduce and compress the bone allograft into the femoral canal in a retrograde manner using cylindrical packers (tapered rods) of increasing diameters.
- Use bone chips of 2–5 mm size for the distal impaction until the canal is two thirds full and larger chips of 7–10 mm for the proximal femur till the canal is filed up to the metaphysis.
- The impaction must be robust enough to achieve rotational stability but not so vigorous as to fracture the femur.

- Continue the impaction to fill any gap between the dummy prosthesis and the cortical bone; then a trial reduction may be performed.
- Wash with hot water the new endosteum like in preparing for third-generation cementing technique to allow adequate cement penetration, and finally, use pressurized peroxide impregnated swabs.
- Use low-viscosity bone cement, and pressurize it gradually against the neo-endosteum to penetrate the interface.
- A cement mantle ≥2 mm is associated with favourable results [15] as it acts as the distributor of force between the stem and the bone graft.

33.1.6 Rehabilitation

Immediate mobilization with partial weight bearing for six weeks followed by gradual increase of weight bearing for another 6 weeks, as tolerated (total of twelve weeks on crutches) [8]

33.1.7 The Optimal Stem Design

- The best stem design is a subject of ongoing debate [6].
- Initially, the use of a highly polished, collarless, double-tapered cemented stem was supported [3]. The particular design of the Exeter stem was considered to maintain the radial loading of the cement and graft and allow for the controlled subsidence necessary for the implant stabilization [3, 4].
- Several other stem types have been used with this method successfully [16–21]. Leopold et al. [20] demonstrated 92% survivorship at six years for aseptic loosening and 12% failure rate in 29 hips treated with a precoated, collared cemented stem (Harris Precoat stem). Ullmark et al. [18] reported a similar rate of mechanical failure of 4% between two groups of patients treated with impaction bone grafting and either a Lubinus or a Charnley prosthesis. In a large cohort study, Boldt et al. [19] demonstrated survival rate of 97.2% at four years for 181 cemented revisions performed with a Charnley Elite stem and impaction bone grafting.

33.1.8 Advantages

- The only technique that potentially restores the femoral bone stock through the incorporation and remodelling of the impacted morselized bone graft [6]
- It achieves primary stability [22]
- The reconstruction of the center of rotation [9]
- The expectation of good clinical results even in progressed defects when carried out meticulously

33.1.9 Disadvantages

- The likely long-term rehabilitation program until the graft incorporates or remodels
- A time-consuming method [6]
- The risk of disease transmission by the graft [6]
- A technically demanding technique [6, 9, 23]
- The significantly long learning curve [23]

33.1.10 Published Results

Several retrospectives but also prospective cohort studies providing a level of evidence III–IV are presently available [3, 4, 11–13, 16–21, 23–43]. These case series are comprised of 6–1188 patients [25, 35]. They range in mean follow-up from 2 to 17 years. A substantial number of cohorts followed patients for more than ten years [24, 25, 30, 33, 39, 42]. Several favourable studies reported excellent long-term results in independent clinical centres worldwide. The mean survivorship for a revision due to aseptic loosening was consistently reported between 94 and 100% [20, 21, 23–26, 31, 33, 34, 37, 39]. The mean survivorship with endpoint as any femoral revision has been reported from 77 to 96% [13, 20, 23–26, 30, 31, 33, 34, 37, 39–42].

The Swedish arthroplasty registry [25] reported the long-term results of 1180 patients that were treated with IGF with an Exeter stem for revision THA. There were only seventy further revisions, thirty-three reoperations for infection or fracture, thirteen for subsidence, and eleven for aseptic loosening at fifteen years. The cumulative survival rate was 94% at fifteen years.

In another long-term study with a great sample, Lamberton et al. [26] prospectively followed 540 femoral revisions with IGF and a cemented stem at a mean of 6.7 years. The 10-year survival rate was 98.0% with aseptic loosening as the endpoint and 84.2% for reoperation for any reason [26]. In the longest follow-up reported so far, te Stroet et al. [31] supported that the probability of survival at seventeen years of thirty three femoral revisions performed with IGF and the X-change femoral revision system and a cemented polished Exeter stem was 96% for revision for any reason and 100% for revision for aseptic loosening.

The technique also has favorable results for younger patients <55 years with survivorship for any reason at ten years 87% and aseptic loosening 97% [33]. The reported results of the technique seemed to be improved in time.

To our knowledge, no prospective trials are comparing this with other techniques. The long-term outcomes, however, provide sufficient data to predict the long-term results of the IGF technique.

33.1.11 Complications

1. The most commonly reported complications are the peri-prosthetic fractures both intraoperative and postoperative ranging from 0 to 42% [23, 35], the hip dislocation from 0 to 12.5% [21] and the peri-prosthetic infection up to 8.3% [21].
2. The intraoperative femoral fractures are more common than postoperative fractures. These are usually the results of vigorous impaction of the cancellous bone into the compromised femoral bone [8, 16, 44, 45].
3. The postoperative femoral fractures are less likely to occur. They are related to the technique and even more to the poor quality of the bone.
4. The reduction of the incidence of the femoral fractures may be accomplished with:
   (a) The use of cortical struts [41]. They may, however, require extensive stripping of the femur that may adversely affect the blood supply to the bone.
   (b) The use of longer stems [41]. Biomechanical studies demonstrated that compared with a standard stem, a long stem reduces strain at a cortical defect by 31% and a strut graft or plate reduces it by approximately 50% [45].
5. The early subsidence >5 mm of the tapered polished implants is another typical complication that may occur up to 38% in some series [16, 44–48]. It might be related to:
   (a) The cold flow within the cement mantle or to cement mantle fractures
   (b) The insufficient impaction of the allograft and restoration of a cortical tube [6, 49]
   (c) The relatively short stem
   (d) The suboptimal cement mantle [6, 49]
   (e) An unrecognized femoral fracture [6, 49]
   (f) The graft resorption [6, 49]

   It has been associated with pain in the thigh, dislocation of the hip, and revision of the component. A fracture of the femoral stem following suboptimal support from the insufficient proximal bone stock has been reported [50].

33.2 Case Title: Impaction Grafting of the Femur

Eduardo García-Cimbrelo and Eduardo García-Rey

33.2.1 Demographics

Age: 67
Sex: Female
BMI: 34

33.2.2 Relevant Past Medical History

Principal pathologies: Dyslipidemia, high blood pressure

Previous surgical procedures: Uncemented isoelastic total hip replacement at right side on 1989

Medication: Statin, atenolol

History of Presenting Complaint: Groin and thigh pain during daily physical activities

33.2.3 Clinical Examination

Symptoms: Groin and thigh pain during physical activities, difficulty putting on her shoe, use of a cane for short walking distances

Range of motion: Hip flexion 80°, no internal rotation, abduction 10°

Specific tests: Straight leg raising

Main disability: Daily physical activities

Scoring: 2-2 Merle-D'Aubigne and Postel scale

Neurovascular evaluation: Normal

33.2.4 Preoperative Radiological Assessment/Imaging (Fig. 33.1)

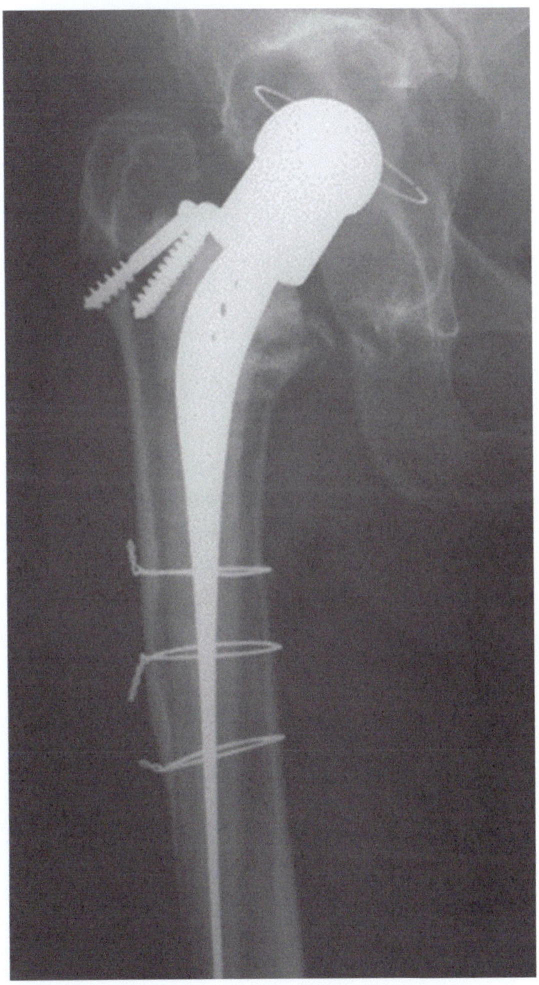

Fig. 33.1 Preoperative radiograph showing large cavitary acetabular and femoral bone defect (Please note the metaphyseal and diaphyseal femoral bone loss)

33.2.5 Preoperative Planning

Diagnosis: Loosened total hip replacement with a large bone defect on both the acetabular and femoral sides (Fig. 33.1)

Possible treatment options: Revision hip surgery to a large uncemented cup and long stem. Impaction bone grafting on both acetabular and femoral sides

Chosen treatment method: Impaction bone grafting

Selection of implants if applicable and rational: Impaction bone grafting with the possible use of meshes on the acetabulum and a cemented cup. Impaction bone grafting and the use of a cemented long stem

Expected difficulties: The extensive bone loss which may be more substantial after the removal of the previous implant

Strategies to overcome difficulties: Bone allograft, four frozen femoral heads, and use of metallic meshes, cemented cup, cemented long stem, and cerclages and wires

33.2.6 Surgical Note

Patient's position: Lateral decubitus

Type of anesthesia: Spinal

Surgical approach: Posterolateral

Main steps: Approach, excision of fibrous tissue, removal of the previous implant with particular attention to the screws close to greater trochanter and the diaphyseal bone loss

Reconstruction techniques: Acetabular impaction bone grafting, according to the Slooff, with the use of a medial metallic mesh before the impaction of the bone chips sized range from 0.7 to 1 cm, and a cemented 28 mm cup. Femoral impaction grafting using smaller bone chips around 0.3 cm morselized by a bone mill and specific instrumentation X-change (Stryker). Introduction of antibiotic-loaded gentamicin cement (Palacos) in a retrograde manner and implantation of a long Exeter stem (Stryker) (Figs. 33.2 and 33.3)

33.2.7 Intraoperative Challenges

Challenges and solutions: The extensive bone defect. The use of a metallic mesh for the medial wall in the acetabulum to convert the uncontained defect to a cavitary defect. The diaphyseal extension of the bone loss in the femur, and the use of intraoperative radiograph

Unanticipated problems and solution: The need for the medial wall mesh in the acetabulum. No complication during surgery in the femur

Thorough description of decision-making, including the reason for the final decision: The planned surgery was performed. No intraoperative fracture was observed.

33.2.8 Postoperative Radiographs (Figs. 33.2 and 33.3)

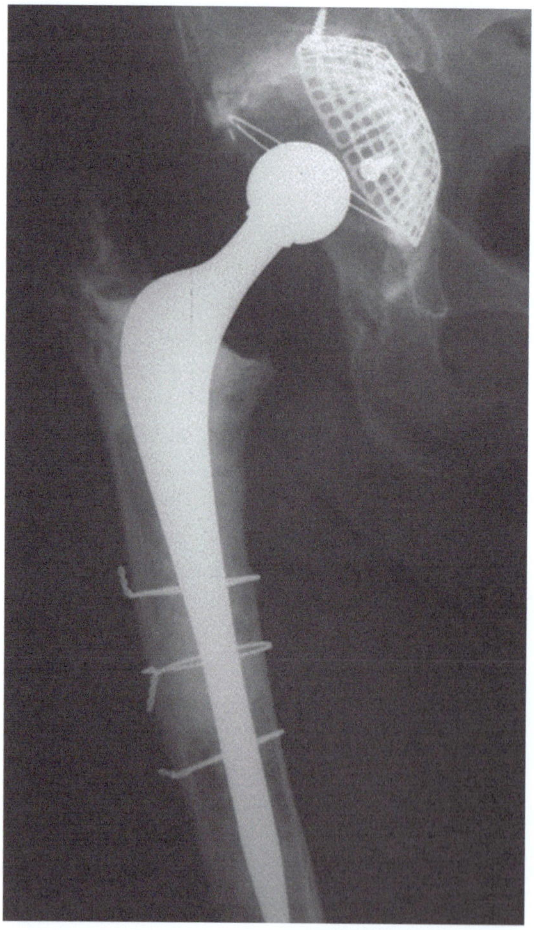

Fig. 33.2 Postoperative radiograph at six months postoperatively. Please note the allograft packing in the acetabulum and femoral sides

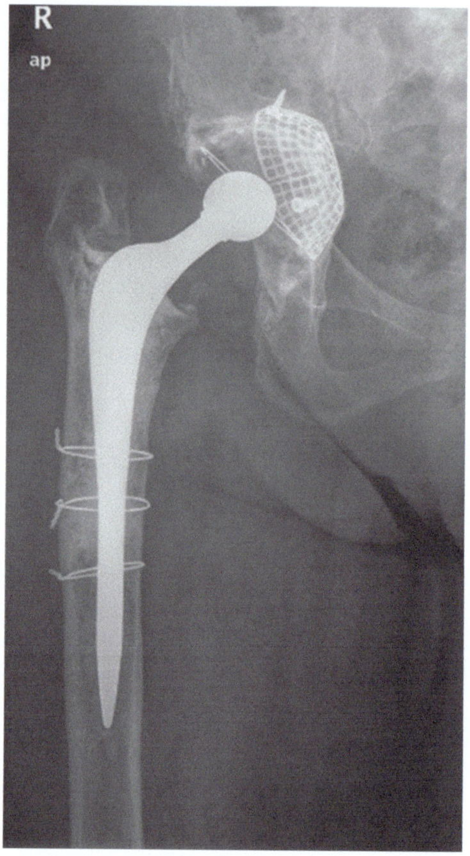

Fig. 33.3 Radiograph at fifteen years postoperatively. Trabecular remodeling can be found

33.2.9 Postoperative Management

Chemoprophylaxis and anticoagulant treatment period: Subcutaneous low-weight heparin during six weeks

Gait/limb loading until full loading: Use of two crutches with toe-touch weight bearing for three months

33.2.10 Follow-Up and Complications

Scoring: 6-5-5 Merle-D'Aubgine and Postel scale

33.2.11 Discussion [23, 43, 51]

Advantages of the applied method: The femoral impaction of the bone restores of the bone stock in complex large bone defects

Disadvantages of the method: The proper allograft packing

Alternative evidence-based techniques for the case: Uncemented long stem, modular tapered fluted stems, composite allograft implants

Why is the chosen technique better for this case? Age and cavitary bone defect

Indications and contraindications for your technique: Indications: the large bone defects, especially in wide femoral canals. The relative young age and physical activity

Learning curve and how to manage complications: Femoral impaction bone grafting can effectively restore the bone stock during revision surgery. Excellent long-term results can be found particularly regarding the aseptic loosening. Trabecular remodeling is frequently observed in radiographs, which may be related to a learning curve during impaction. Complications such as subsidence and peri-prosthetic fractures have been related to this technique; however, the uncemented long stems with modular distal fixation have similar rates. Although improvement in the surgical technique and newer approaches such as the extended trochanteric osteotomy to remove the previous implant may promote excellent results, bone defect is the most important factor that determines the clinical and radiological result. Finally, long stems can be very useful in large defects and even in peri-prosthetic fractures to avoid more complications.

Level of evidence concerning the superiority of this method against others: Restoration of bone stock in large femoral bone defect and similar rates of complications than uncemented long stem

33.3 Case Title: Femoral Impaction Grafting

Martin Buttaro

33.3.1 Demographics

Age: 48
Sex: Female
BMI: 23

33.3.2 Relevant Past Medical History

Principal pathologies: Infected right THA

Previous surgical procedures: Primary and revision right THA

History of Presenting Complaint: Right hip pain, sinus and altered laboratory tests suggesting infection

33.3.3 Clinical Examination

Symptoms: Pain

Range of motion: Severely altered

Main disability: Unable to walk more than 200 m

Scoring: Merle DÁubigne 6 out of 18 points

Neurovascular evaluation: Normal

33.3.4 Preoperative Radiological Assessment/Imaging (Figs. 33.4 and 33.5)

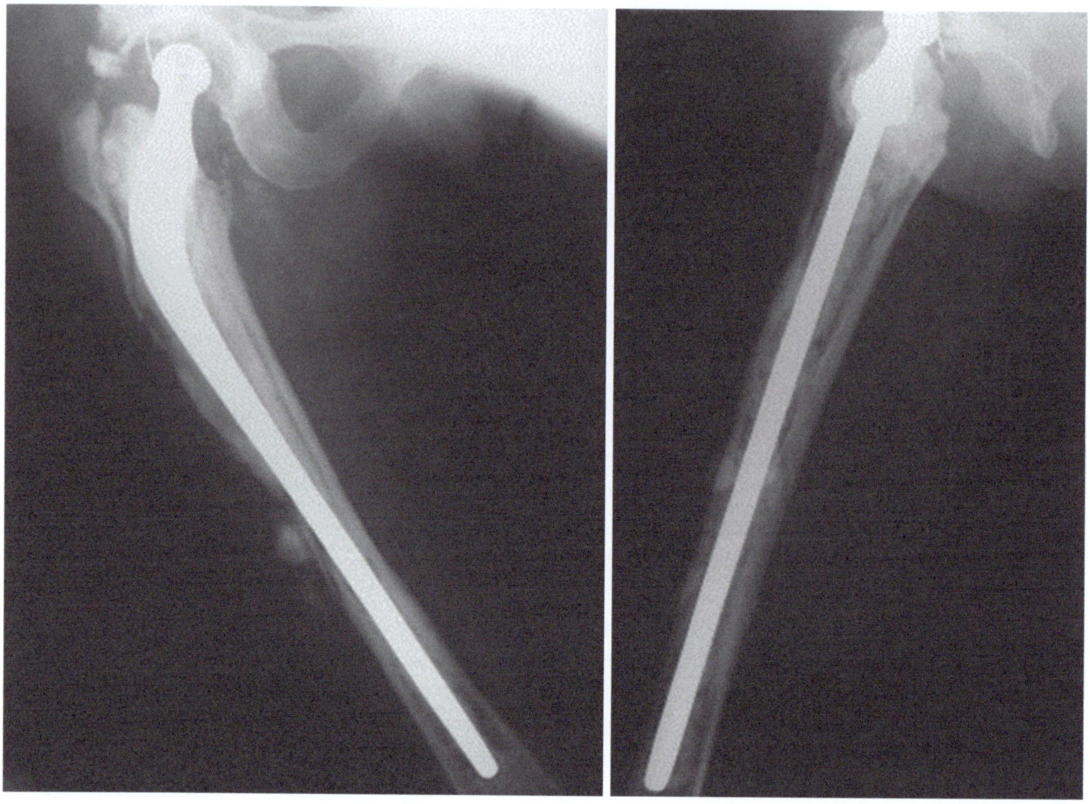

Figs. 33.4 and 33.5 An anteroposterior and lateral right hip and femoral radiograph belonging to a 48-year-old female patient with hip pain, an active sinus, altered laboratory tests, and a methicillin-resistant *Staphylococcus aureus positive culture*

33.3.5 Preoperative Planning

Diagnosis: Infected right THA (Figs. 33.4 and 33.5)

Possible treatment options: Two-stage revision hip surgery

Chosen treatment method: Two-stage revision hip surgery

Selection of implants if applicable and rational: Custom-made cement spacer and hybrid THA for the second stage

Expected difficulties: Femoral bone reconstruction

Strategies to overcome difficulties: Strut allograft and impacted cancellous bone allograft

33.3.6 Surgical Note

Patient's position: Lateral decubitus

Type of anesthesia: Epidural hypotensive

Surgical approach: Posterolateral

Main steps: View attachment (Figs. 33.6, 33.7, and 33.8)

Reconstruction techniques: View attachment (Figs. 33.6, 33.7, and 33.8)

33.3.7 Intraoperative Challenges

Challenges and solutions: View attachment (Figs. 33.6, 33.7 and 33.8)

33.3.8 Postoperative Radiographs (Figs. 33.6, 33.7, and 33.8)

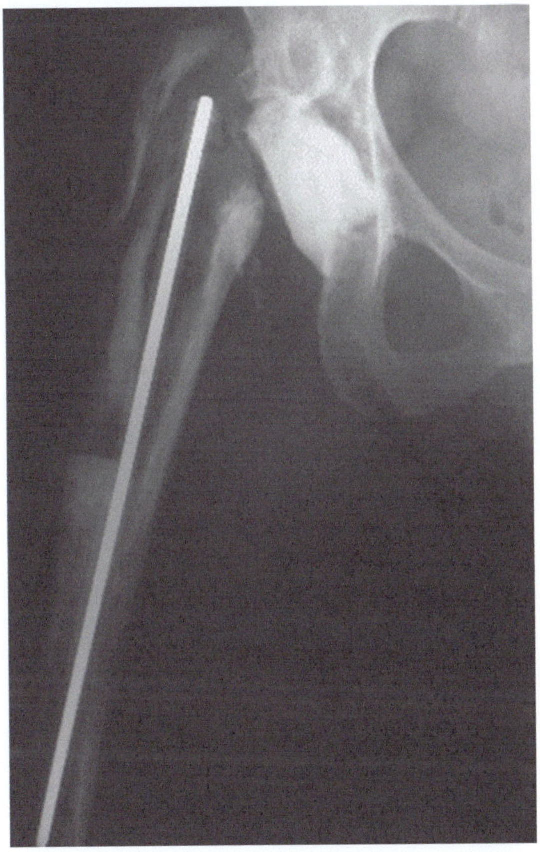

Fig. 33.6 First stage. A dissociated vancomycin-loaded cement spacer was implanted to elute antibiotics locally and to facilitate the second stage. Weight-bearing was not allowed due to the severity of femoral bone compromise

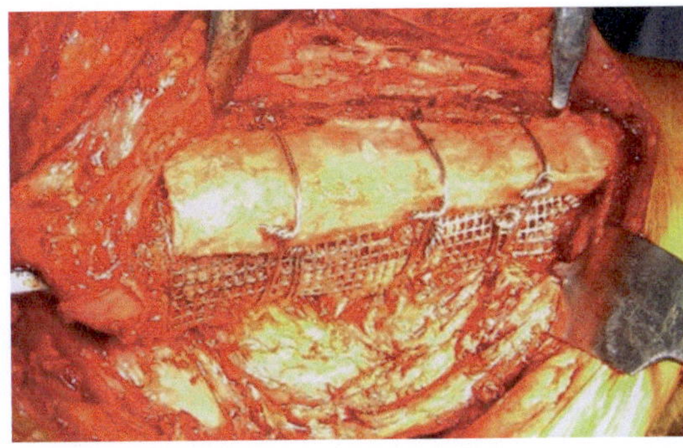

Fig. 33.7 Intraoperative photograph at the second stage, where an intramedullary bone reconstruction was performed with vancomycin-supplemented impacted bone allografts contained by a metal mesh and a lateral strut allograft from a cadaveric tibia for lateral extramedullary stabilization. A standard length polished, taper cemented stem was implanted

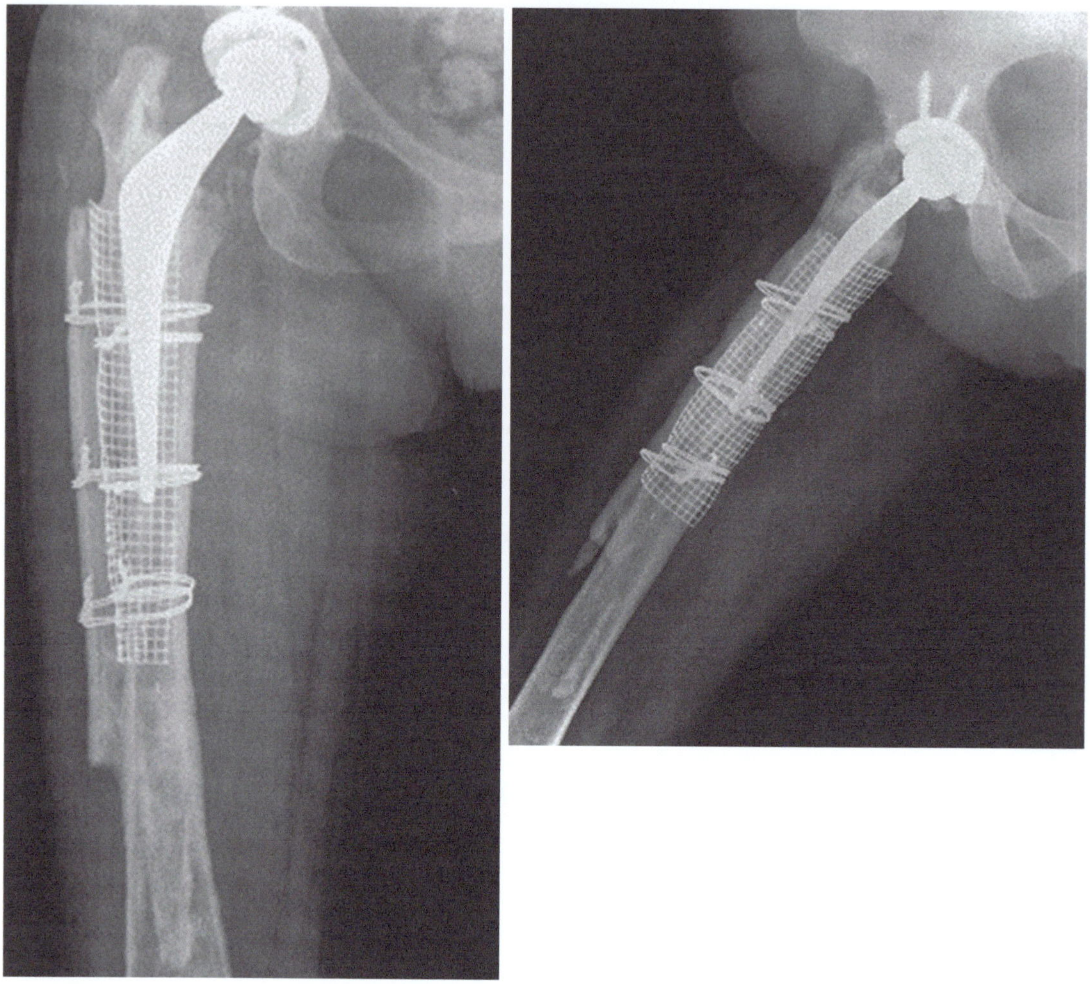

Fig. 33.8 Anteroposterior and lateral right hip and femoral radiograph at 8-year follow-up. Bone allograft strut incorporation without subsidence is observed

33.3.9 Postoperative Management

Chemoprophylaxis and anticoagulant treatment period: Enoxaparin for three weeks

e*Gait/limb loading until full loading*: No weight bearing for forty five days, then partial weight bearing until three months, and then full weight bearing

33.3.10 Follow-Up and Complications

No complications

Scoring: 16 out of 18 points at the Merle DÁubigne scale

33.3.11 Discussion [26, 32, 52]

Advantages of the applied method: Bone reconstruction

Disadvantages of the method: None

Alternative evidence-based techniques for the case: Long cemented tumor prosthesis

Why is the chosen technique better for this case? Recovers bone stock

Indications and contraindications for your technique: Indication: young patients, contraindication: the presence of active infection

Learning curve and how to manage complications: Prolonged learning curve

33.4 Case Title: Cemented Femoral Revision (with Impaction Grafting)

Jillian Lee and William Farrington,

33.4.1 Demographics

Age: 67 years
Sex: Female
BMI: 44

33.4.2 Relevant Past Medical History

Principal pathologies: Obesity, osteoarthritis

Previous surgical procedures: Right total hip arthroplasty 1998, left total knee arthroplasty 2004, umbilical hernia repair 2004, total thyroidectomy 2010, multiple gynecological operations

Medication: Thyroxine, paracetamol, Naprosyn

History of presenting complaint: MB, a 69-year-old female, presented 14 years after a right hybrid total hip arthroplasty (Spectron Reflection) with a 4-month history of progressively worsening hip and thigh pain on weight bearing. No systemic symptoms were present to suggest infection.

33.4.3 Clinical Examination

Symptoms: Groin and thigh pain, worse at night and on weight bearing

Range of motion: Flexion 90 °, FER 30 °, FIR 20 °

Main disability: Unable to ambulate and perform ADLs secondary to weight bearing pain

Scoring if available: Nil available

Neurovascular evaluation: No neurovascular deficit

33.4.4 Preoperative Radiological Assessment/Imaging (Figs. 33.9 and 33.10)

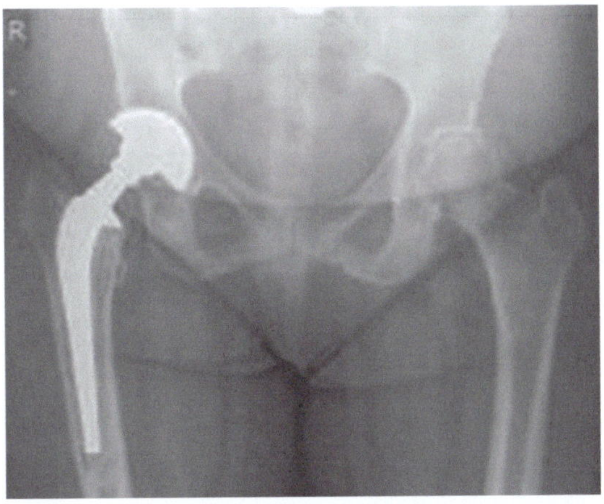

Fig. 33.9 Preoperative AP pelvis radiograph demonstrating loose cement mantle with osteolysis and cortical thinning due to polyethylene wear

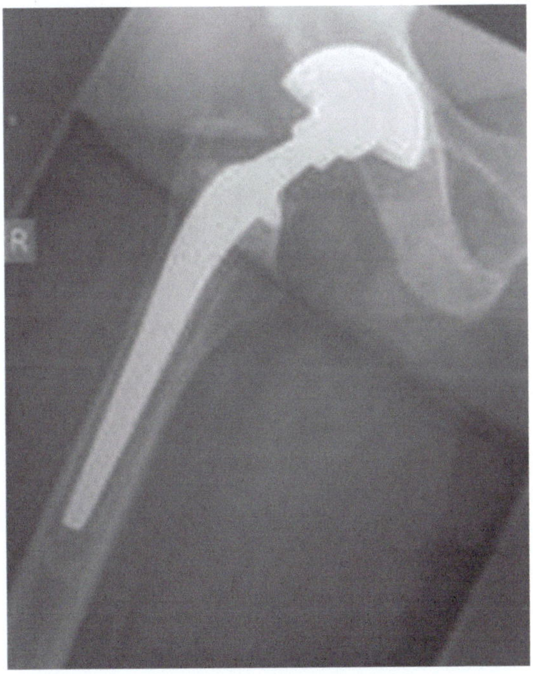

Fig. 33.10 Preoperative right hip radiograph demonstrating loose cement mantle and cortical thinning with polyethylene wear

Other: Preoperative bloods—CRP <3, WCC 3.6, neut 2.1

33.4.5 Preoperative Planning

Diagnosis: Aseptic loosening of cemented femoral stem due to polyethylene wear (Figs. 33.9 and 33.10)

Possible treatment options: Nonsurgical with ongoing serial observation; cemented revision with or without impaction grafting; uncemented femoral revision (modular stem), with or without strut allograft reconstruction

Chosen treatment method: Cemented femoral revision with the use of impaction grafting (and uncemented acetabular revision)

Selection of implants if applicable and rational: Long stem cemented Exeter. The Exeter stem was selected to allow restoration of hip offset and to bypass the femoral lysis at the tip of the previous stem. It has good long-term clinical results with and without impaction grafting.

Expected difficulties: Removal of cement, intraoperative fracture, segmental defects due to cortical breaching while awaiting or during revision surgery

Strategies to overcome difficulties: Appropriate equipment and techniques for femoral cement removal (including long drills, reamers, osteotomes, curettes, distal light source and irrigation tubing (VitalView), intraoperative fluoroscopy, up-to-date X-rays just prior to procedure)

Templating: Calibrated AP pelvis and lateral hip radiographs for pre-op planning. This assists in determining the offset and length of femoral component, bone loss, and femoral anatomy (particularly noting cortical areas at risk of breaching).

33.4.6 Surgical Note

Patient's position: Left lateral

Type of anesthesia: General anesthesia with combined spinal and epidural anesthesia

Surgical approach: Posterior approach (utilizing previous skin incision and approach)

Main steps: Previous incision utilized and extended proximally and distally. Gluteus maximus tendon was released to facilitate exposure. The sciatic nerve was palpated and protected by the short external rotators. The cement at the shoulder of the femoral component was removed prior to the femoral component removal. The stem was loose and easily removed. This allowed space for the acetabular revision. The femoral cement was left in situ until after the acetabulum had been revised to reduce blood loss from the femoral canal. The acetabulum was revised using an explant to remove the uncemented shell. The cancellous bone behind this acetabular component showed evidence of cavitary bone loss and was suitable for a cemented acetabulum. The proximal femoral cement mantle was loose and easily removed. The distal plug and cement mantle were removed using a combination of drills, reamers, osteotomes, and curettes. The femoral bone stock was assessed after cement removal looking at the inside surface of the canal and for any perforations of the cortex. The inside of the canal was sclerotic and thinned but not perforated.

Reconstruction techniques: Impaction grafting was chosen as an adjunct to the cemented stem as the cortical bone was sclerotic, thinned, and expanded but intact. The technique of impaction grafting (IG) was followed as described by the Exeter group using their specifically designed instruments (Stryker). The "X-change canal plug" (specifically designed with a central guidewire screwed in) was inserted to a depth of 230 mm from the tip of the greater trochanter (as determined by preoperative templating), approximately 25 mm distal to the tip of the planned revision stem (205 mm stem length). It's diameter was determined by canal sizers. Impactors were sequentially passed down the canal and a plastic marker placed on the calibration ridges at the level of the greater trochanter. This allowed safe impaction minimizing the risk of a femoral fracture. A fresh-frozen femoral head allograft was suitably prepared by denuding the head of the cartilage and fibrous tissue, nibbled into chips of varying sizes, lavaged in warm saline, and added to 500 mg of vancomycin. This allograft was introduced into the femoral canal in 3–5 mL volumes and was impacted by tamping the impactors to the predetermined level. Sequential addition of graft and impaction built up a distal bone plug above the canal plug by approximately 20 mm. A "phantom" (the cannulated trial stem larger than the definitive stem which allowed for a cement mantle) was then used for impaction of the graft, and a neo-medullary canal was created. Impaction was firm enough to make this rotationally and axially stable. Proximal impaction was performed with specific tamps around the phantom. Once IG was complete, the trial was performed. Third-generation cementing techniques with lavage and suction and retrograde filling and pressurization were used with this construct prior to insertion of a heated long stem (Figs. 33.11 and 33.12).

33.4.7 Intraoperative Challenges

Challenges and solutions: Removal of the existing cement mantle can be time-consuming and difficult. Surgical patience with various techniques and equipment is required to overcome this without resorting to an extended trochanteric osteotomy (ETO). An intraoperative fracture can occur and may require a different construct with fracture fixation (e.g., a long uncemented stem with wiring and strut grafting). Cemented stems with IG have good medium- and long-term result if performed with the correct technique, in cavitary defects, with the fresh-frozen allograft bone. If these prerequisites are not met, the results are disappointing. Weak bone strength can predispose to fracture during impaction. Prophylactic wiring can be a reasonable option with this concern.

Thorough description of decision-making, including the reason for the final decision: This patient was relatively young and had minimal medical comorbidities apart from obesity. She failed to improve with nonsurgical treatment and elected to undergo surgery. We thought her life expectancy was greater than ten years. The results of this technique should give her excellent mid-long-term survival beyond ten years with good hip function. Uncemented femoral revision stems have comparable survival results. However, we decided against using this as our first option due to the relatively high incidence of post-op thigh pain and proximal femur stress shielding. Cemented stem revision can also be performed without impaction grafting of the bone, but the results are not as consistent over the long term and would be better suited to a lower-demand patient with a life expectancy less than ten years.

33.4.8 Postoperative Radiographs (Figs. 33.11 and 33.12)

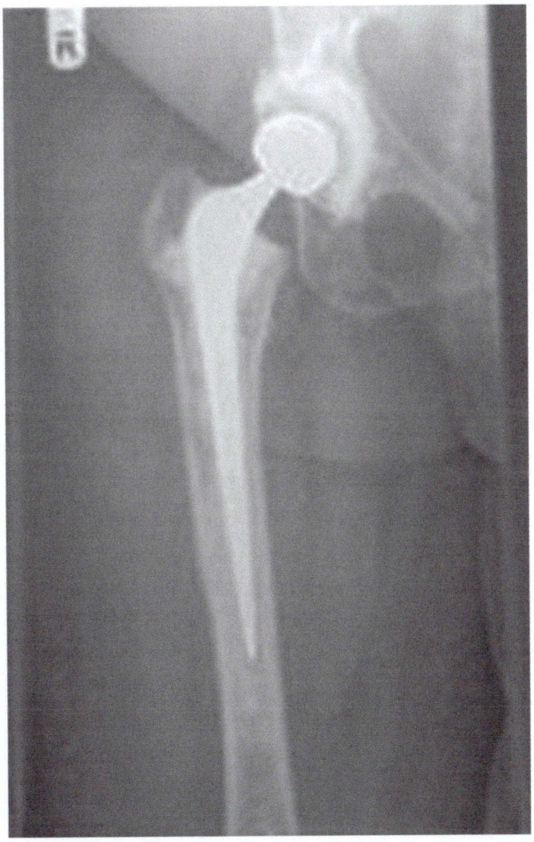

Fig. 33.11 Immediate postoperative AP X-ray after femoral impaction grafting (FIG)

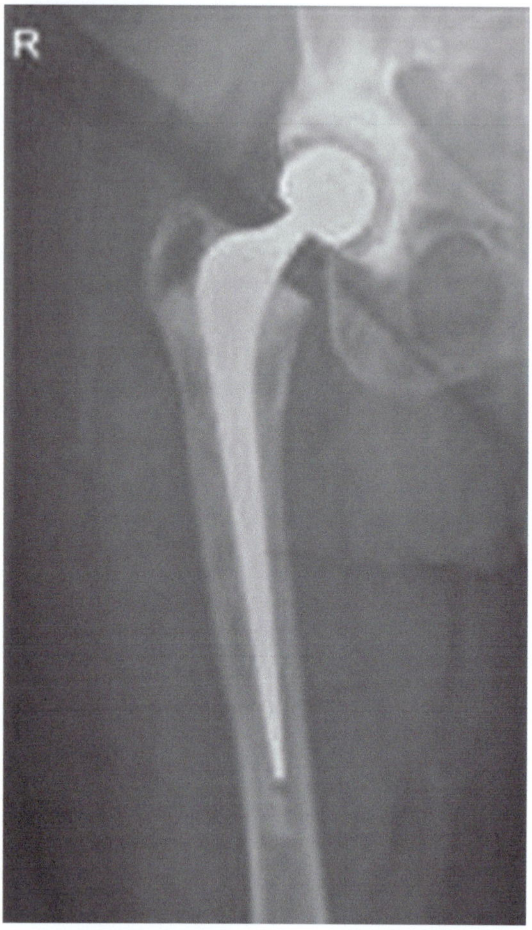

Fig. 33.12 AP X-ray 2 years after FIG demonstrating incorporated graft with minimal stem subsidence

33.4.9 Postoperative Management

Chemoprophylaxis and anticoagulant treatment period: Rivaroxaban 10 mg od was commenced on day 1 post-op and continued for a total of six weeks. Mechanical prophylaxis (foot pumps) was used during the inpatient stay.

Gait/limb loading until full loading: The patient was mobilized with toe-touch weight bearing, commencing postoperative day one, for four weeks. This was followed by four weeks of partial weight bearing before allowing full weight bearing.

33.4.10 Follow-Up and Complications

The patient had a slow postoperative rehabilitation which was multifactorial. She required a 3-week inpatient stay as she lived alone. She had interim care with a family member before returning home six weeks after surgery. She had no post-op complications and remains complication-free to the present day. She lives alone and is independent. She drives and walks unaided and is pain-free.

Scoring: Nil available

33.4.11 Discussion [32, 53–55]

Advantages of the applied method: Cemented femoral stems with impaction grafting in the revision setting have excellent long-term survival. Retrieval studies show this allograft will incorporate within the femoral canal in many areas of the graft. This potentially provides a life-long bond between cement and the bone. The choice of the graft is important: autogenous bone graft is considered the gold standard for bone grafting (as it is osteoconductive and osteoinductive and provides osteogenic cells without the risk of disease transmission). However, it is not possible to obtain sufficient volume of the graft without significant donor-site morbidity, thus the use of femoral head allograft. Residual articular cartilage is removed in its preparation, as inclusion can affect impaction, mechanical stability, and incorporation. We aim for morselized graft between 3 and 5 mm and for the proximal portion, 8–10 mm. This variable size of graft leaves voids which facilitates cement penetration, has sufficient permeability to allow bony ingrowth, and yet provides adequate initial mechanical stability to reduce shear forces and instability of the implant. We lavage the graft with warmed saline before impaction to remove fat and marrow. This improves compatibility by increasing friction and interdigitation. Graft lavage has been shown to reduce stem subsidence in studies of bovine femora and in vivo human femoral impaction grafting. Graft lavage also removes the marrow which reduces the immunological load. Cementing technique is also important: with impaction bone grafting; the ideal amount of cement interdigitation is not known; a balance to achieve remodeling of the bone graft while avoiding stem subsidence with excessive and insufficient cement interdigitation, respectively, needs to be achieved for an optimal result. For primary hip arthroplasty, we know that adequate lavage preparation and the use of a distal plug with a proximal seal (pressurization) reduce the risk of revision by 20%.

Disadvantages of the method: The impaction force and the number of cycles determine the degree of impaction achieved; this can result in intraoperative femoral fracture, in patients with particularly thinned or weakened cortical bone; prophylactic wiring can be used to reduce the risk of femoral fracture. It is time-consuming and is an advanced revision technique which requires considerable attention to detail.

Alternative evidence-based techniques for the case: Use of modular uncemented femoral stem

Why is the chosen technique better for this case? This revision technique would reconstitute her femoral bone stock and has good survival results given her relatively young age and physical demands. When the femoral canal is capacious, and the femoral diameter is >18 mm, there is a high incidence of thigh pain with the use of an uncemented femoral stem. Additionally, there is an increased risk of femoral fracture when inserting a femoral stem to obtain a diaphyseal fit in a thinned diaphyseal cortex, with rates of intraoperative fracture as high as 45% reported. Long cemented stems without IG have good short-medium results, but long-term survival is less predictable. They gain good macro-fit, but bone interdigitation by the cement is less than with IG.

Indications and contraindications for your technique: Indications: sclerotic endosteal surfaces of the femur with little cancellous bone, providing inadequate fixation for a cemented femoral component, intramedullary canal 18 mm or greater, unable to achieve distal press fit with an uncemented stem. Contraindications: Large segmental defects in the femoral canal (small ones can be contained with mesh), proximal femoral deficiency extending below the lesser trochanter, elderly, or medically comorbid patients where bone-stock restoration is not a priority and a prolonged revision procedure is of concern

Learning curve and how to manage complications: Prophylactic cerclage wiring should be performed if the femur is ectatic or weak.

Level of evidence concerning the superiority of this method against others: Retrospective long-term follow-up studies which examine the survivorship of femoral revision utilizing femoral impaction grafting, and uncemented modular stems are available. The 10-year survival for femoral impaction grafting for aseptic loosening is 98% and for all revisions is 84.2%. The 10-year survival for uncemented modular revision stems is reported at 96%. However, high rates of intraoperative fracture/perforation (25–45%) and thigh pain are reported with these implants.

References

1. Hastings DE, Parker SM. Protrusio acetabuli in rheumatoid arthritis. Clin Orthop Relat Res. 1975;108:76–83.
2. Slooff TJ, Huiskes R, van Horn J, Lemmens AJ. Bone grafting in total hip replacement for acetabular protrusion. Acta Orthop Scand. 1984;55:593–6.
3. Gie GA, Linder L, Ling RS, et al. Impacted cancellous allografts and cement for revision total hip arthroplasty. J Bone Joint Surg Br. 1993;75-B: 14–21.
4. Gie GA, Linder L, Ling RS, et al. Contained morselized allograft in revision total hip arthroplasty. Surgical technique. Orthop Clin North Am. 1993;24:717–25.
5. Slooff TJ, Buma P, Schreurs BW, et al. Acetabular and femoral reconstruction with impacted graft and cement. Clin Orthop Relat Res. 1996;324:108–15.
6. Oakes DA, Cabanela ME. Impaction bone grafting for revision hip arthroplasty: biology and clinical applications. J Am Acad Orthop Surg. 2006;14:620–8.
7. Ling RS, Timperley AJ, Linder L. Histology of cancellous impaction grafting in the femur: a case report. J Bone Joint Surg Br. 1993;75:693–6.
8. Gehrke T, Gebauer M, Kendoff D. Femoral stem impaction grafting: extending the role of cement. Bone Joint J. 2013;95-B(Suppl A):92–4.
9. Heyligers IC, Schreurs BW, van Haaren EH. Femoral revision with impaction bone grafting and a cemented polished tapered stem. Oper Orthop Traumatol. 2014;26:156–61.
10. Scanelli JA, Brown TE. Femoral impaction grafting. World J Orthop. 2013;4(1):7–11.
11. Tsiridis E, Narvani AA, Haddad FS, Timperley JA, Gie GA. Impaction femoral allografting and cemented revision for periprosthetic femoral fractures. J Bone Joint Surg Br. 2004;86:1124–32.
12. English H, Timperly AJ, Dunlop D, Gie G. Impaction grafting of the femur in two-stage revision for infected total hip replacement. J Bone Joint Surg Br. 2002;84:700–5.
13. Leone WA Jr, Naughton M, Gratto-Cox G, Luland CM, Kilgore JE, Hill GE. The effect of preoperative planning and impaction grafting surgical technique on intraoperative and postoperative complication rate for femoral revision patients with moderate to severe

bone loss mean 4.7-year results. J Arthroplasty. 2008;23(3):383–94.
14. Dunlop DG, Brewster NT, Madabhushi SPG, Usmani AS, Pankaj P, Howie CR. Techniques to improve the shear strength of impacted bone graft: the effect of particle size and washing of the graft. J Bone Joint Surg Am. 2003;85:639–46.
15. Francés A, Moro E, Cebrian JL, et al. Reconstruction of bone defects with impacted allograft in femoral stem revision surgery. Int Orthop. 2007;31:457–64.
16. Knight JL, Helming C. Collarless polished tapered impaction grafting of the femur during revision total hip arthroplasty: pitfalls of the surgical technique and follow-up in 31 cases. J Arthroplasty. 2000;15:159–65.
17. Piccaluga F, González Della Valle A, Encinas Fernández JC, Pusso R. Revision of the femoral prosthesis with impaction allografting and a Charnley stem. A 2- to 12-year follow-up. J Bone Joint Surg Br. 2002;84:544–9.
18. Ullmark G, Hallin G, Nilsson O. Impacted corticocancellous allografts and cement for femoral revision of total hip arthroplasty using Lubinus and Charnley prostheses. J Arthroplasty. 2002;17:325–34.
19. Boldt JG, Dilawari P, Agarwal S, Drabu KJ. Revision total hip arthroplasty using impaction bone grafting with cemented nonpolished stems and Charnley cups. J Arthroplasty. 2001;16:943–52.
20. Leopold SS, Berger RA, Rosenburg AG, Jacobs JJ, Quigley LR, Galante JO. Impaction allografting with cement for revision of the femoral component. A minimum four-year follow-up study with use of a precoated femoral stem. J Bone Joint Surg Am. 1999;81:1080–92.
21. Krupp RJ, Malkani AL, Crawford CH, Capello WN, Feinberg JR, Baker D. Impaction grafting for femoral component revision using a non-polished bead-blasted chrome cobalt stem—average 8 1/2–year follow-up. J Arthroplasty. 2006;21(8):1180–6.
22. Malkani AL, Voor MJ, Fee KA, Bates CS. Femoral component revision using impacted morsellised cancellous graft: a biomechanical study of implant stability. J Bone Joint Surg Br. 1996;78:973–8.
23. García-Rey E, Cruz-Pardos A, Madero R. The evolution of the technique of impaction bone grafting in femoral revision surgery has improved clinical outcome a prospective mid-term study. J Arthroplasty. 2015;30:95–100.
24. Ten Have BL, Brouwer RW, van Biezen FC, Verhaar JA. Femoral revision surgery with impaction bone grafting: 31 hips followed prospectively for ten to 15 years. J Bone Joint Surg Br. 2012;94-B:615–8.
25. Ornstein E, Linder L, Ranstam J, et al. Femoral impaction bone grafting with the Exeter stem: - the Swedish experience: survivorship analysis of 1305 revisions performed between 1989 and 2002. J Bone Joint Surg Br. 2009;91-B:441–6.
26. Lamberton TD, Kenny PJ, Whitehouse SL, Timperley AJ, Gie GA. Femoral impaction grafting in revision total hip arthroplasty: a follow-up of 540 hips. J Arthroplasty. 2011;26:1154–60.
27. Kamath AF, Voleti PB, Kim TWB, Garino JP, Lee GC. Impaction bone grafting with proximal and distal femoral arthroplasty. J Arthroplasty. 2011;26(8):1520–6.
28. Oshima S, Yasunaga Y, Yamasaki T, Yoshida T, Hori J, Ochi M. Midterm results of femoral impaction bone grafting with an allograft combined with hydroxyapatite in revision total hip arthroplasty. J Arthroplasty. 2012;27(3):470–6.
29. Meding JB, Ritter MA, Keating EM, Faris PM. Impaction bone-grafting before insertion of a femoral stem with cement in revision total hip arthroplasty: a minimum two-year followup study. J Bone Joint Surg Am. 1997;79:1834–41.
30. Schreurs BW, Arts JJ, Verdonschot N, Buma P, Slooff TJ, Gardeniers JW. Femoral component revision with use of impaction bone-grafting and a cemented polished stem. J Bone Joint Surg Am. 2005;87: 2499–507.
31. te Stroet MA, Gardeniers JW, Verdonschot N, et al. Femoral component revision with use of impaction bone-grafting and a cemented polished stem: a concise followup, at fifteen to twenty years, of a previous report. J Bone Joint Surg Am. 2012;94(3):1731–4.
32. te Stroet MA, Rijnen WH, Gardeniers JW, van Kampen A, Schreurs BW. The outcome of femoral component revision arthroplasty with impaction allograft bone grafting and a cemented polished Exeter stem A Prospective Cohort Study Of 208 Revision arthroplasties with a mean follow-up of 10 years. Bone Joint J. 2015;5:771–9.
33. te Stroet MAJ, Rijnen WHC, Gardeniers JWM, van Kampen A, Willem Schreurs B. Satisfying outcomes scores and survivorship achieved with impaction grafting for revision THA in young patients. Clin Orthop Relat Res. 2015;473:3867–75.
34. te Stroet MAJ, Rijnen WHC, Gardeniers JWM, Willem Schreurs B, Hannink G. Predictors of unsuccessful outcome in cemented femoral revisions using bone impaction grafting; Cox regression analysis of 208 cases. Hip Int. 2016;26(5):444–50.
35. Flugsrud GB, Øvre S, Grøgaard B, Nordsletten L. Cemented femoral impaction bone grafting for severe osteolysis in revision hip arthroplasty Good results at 4-year follow-up of 10 patients. Arch Orthop Trauma Surg. 2000;120:386–9.
36. Donald R. Gore Impaction bone grafting for total hip revision. Int Orthop. 2002;26:162–5.
37. Iwase T, Otsuka H, Katayama N, Fujita H. Impaction bone grafting for femoral revision hip arthroplasty with Exeter Universal stem in Japan. Arch Orthop Trauma Surg. 2012;132:1487–94.
38. Takigami I, Otsuka H, Yamamoto K, Iwase T, Fujita H, Matsuda S, Akiyama H. Proximal femoral reconstruction with impaction bone grafting and circumferential metal mesh. J Orthop Sci. 2015;20:331–9.
39. Garvin KL, Konigsberg BS, Ommen ND, Lyden ER. What is the long-term survival of impaction allografting of the femur? Clin Orthop Relat Res. 2013;471(12):3901–11.

40. Cabanela ME. Trousdale RT, Berry DJ: impaction cancellous graft plus cement in hip revision. Clin Orthop Relat Res. 2003;417:175–82.
41. Halliday BR, English HW, Timperly AJ, Gie GA, Ling RS. Femoral impaction grafting with cement in revision total hip replacement: evolution of the technique and results. J Bone Joint Surg Br. 2003;85:809–17.
42. Wraighte PJ, Howard PW. Femoral impaction bone allografting with an Exeter cemented collarless, polished, tapered stem in revision hip replacement: a mean follow-up of 10.5 years. J Bone Joint Surg Br. 2008;90(8):1000–4.
43. Sierra RJ, Charity J, Tsiridis E, Timperley JA, Gie GA. The use of long cemented stems for femoral impaction grafting in revision total hip arthroplasty. J Bone Joint Surg Am. 2008;90:1330–6.
44. Sculco PK, Abdel MP, David G. Lewallen Management of femoral bone loss in revision total hip arthroplasty. Hip Int. 2015;25(4):380–7.
45. Masterson EL, Masri BA, Duncan CP. The cement mantle in the Exeter impaction allografting technique. A cause for concern. J Arthroplasty. 1997;12(7):759–64.
46. Barker R. Biomechanical testing of impaction bone grafting in a femoral model [thesis]. Wales: Cardiff University; 2004.
47. Franzen H, Toksvig-Larsen S, Lidgren L, Onnerfalt R. Early migration of femoral components revised with impacted cancellous allografts and cement. A preliminary report of five patients. J Bone Joint Surg Br. 1995;77(6):862–4.
48. Eldridge JD, Smith EJ, Hubble MJ, Whitehouse SL, Learmonth ID. Massive early subsidence following femoral impaction grafting. J Arthroplasty. 1997;12:535–40.
49. Gokhale S, Soliman A, Dantas JP, Richardson JB, Cook F, Kuiper JH, et al. Variables affecting initial stability of impaction grafting for hip revision. Clin Orthop Relat Res. 2005;432:174–80.
50. Buttaro M, Comba F, Zanotti G, Piccaluga F. Fracture of the C-Stem cemented femoral component in revision hip surgery using bone impaction grafting technique: report of 9 cases. Hip Int. 2015;25(2):184–7.
51. García-Cimbrelo E, García-Rey E, Cruz-Pardos A. The extent of the bone defect affects the outcome of femoral reconstruction in revision surgery. J Bone Joint Surg Br. 2011;93(11):1457–64.
52. Buttaro MA, Costantini J, Comba F, Piccaluga F. The use of femoral struts and impacted cancellous bone allograft in patients with severe femoral bone loss who undergo revision total hip replacement: a three- to nine-year follow-up. J Bone Joint Surg Br. 2012;94(2):167–72.
53. Koster G, Walde TA, Willert HG. Five- to 10-year results using a noncemented modular revision stem without bone grafting. J Arthroplasty. 2008;23(7):964–70.
54. Malkani AL, Lewallen DG, Cabanela ME, Wallrichs SL. Femoral component revision using an uncemented, proximally coated, long-stem prosthesis. J Arthroplasty. 1996;11(4):411–8.
55. Thomsen PB, Jensen NJ, Kampmann J, Baek HT. Revision hip arthroplasty with an extensively porous-coated stem – excellent long-term results also in severe femoral bone loss. Hip Int. 2013;23(4):352–8.

34 Cemented Femoral Revision

Eustathios Kenanidis, Eleftherios Tsiridis, Mohammad Shahid, and Andrew R. J. Manktelow

34.1 Current Concepts

E. Kenanidis and E. Tsiridis

Primary revision of the femoral component of a THA with the use of cement without bone graft reconstruction is less frequently used because it has been associated with early mechanical failure due to aseptic loosening[1, 2]. Indeed the initial reports of cemented femoral revision showed disappointing long-term survival results [3–7]. The results, in fact, depend on multiple parameters as the number of prior revisions, cementing technique quality, residual bone stock, etc. [1]. More recent studies, however, using newer cementing techniques and proper patient selection demonstrated improvement of the results [8–10].

E. Kenanidis, M.D., Ph.D., M.Sc. (✉)
Academic Orthopaedic Unit, Aristotle University Medical School, Thessaloniki, Greece
e-mail: stathiskenanidis@gmail.com

E. Tsiridis, M.D., Ph.D., F.A.C.S., F.R.C.S.
Papageorgiou General Hospital, Pavlos Melas, Greece

Aristotle University Medical School, Thessaloniki, Greece
e-mail: etsiridis@doctors.org.uk

M. Shahid, B.Sc., M.B.B.S., F.R.C.S.
Worcestershire Acute Hospitals NHS Trust, Worcester, UK
e-mail: shahidm99@doctors.org.uk

A.R.J. Manktelow, B.Sc., M.B.B.S., F.R.C.S.
Nottingham University Hospitals NHS Trust, Nottingham, UK
e-mail: a.mank@btinternet.com

34.1.1 Indications

There is no definite indication for cemented revision THA. This technique remains a reasonable option for the first-time revision, for selected patients especially for older and less active patients with adequate bone stock who are managed with modern cementing techniques [2].

34.1.2 Contraindications

Sepsis is the only absolute contraindication. Certain factors, however, are considered predictive of failure.

1. Poor bone quality [1, 9–12]
   Several authors supported that pronounced bone defects are correlated with worse results following cemented revision. Haydon et al. [2] found that poor bone quality (Mallory type IIIA or higher) is related to increased risk for revision for aseptic loosening. Bardou-Jacquet et al. [1] showed that the grade III and IV femurs, according to the bone loss grading system of SOFCOT 99, had a significantly higher risk ($p = 0.0001$) of having type C or type D cementation according to the Barrack classification and subsequently worse results.

E. Tsiridis (ed.), *The Adult Hip - Master Case Series and Techniques*,
https://doi.org/10.1007/978-3-319-64177-5_34

2. Young patient [2, 9, 10, 13, 14]
   The younger patient age has repeatedly been correlated with significantly increased risk of re-revision following cemented revision THA. Stromberg et al. [10] reported 85% survival rate for 57 cemented femoral revisions in patients <55 years old at 7-year follow-up. Haydon et al. [2] supported that more than 60-year-old patients had greater femoral stem survival and less pain than younger patients ($p < 0.05$). The 10-year survival rate for aseptic loosening and any reason for patients 60 years of age or older was significantly better than that for younger patients (96 vs. 83%, $p = 0.044$) and (93 vs. 71%; $p = 0.003$), respectively.
3. Poor cement mantle quality [1, 9, 11, 14–16]
   Poor cement mantle quality and early generation cementing technique are considered negative predictive factors of the stem durability. Risk of loosening following cemented revision THA was also related to a cement mantle extended more than 2 mm, around the revision stem [14]. Haydon et al. [2] supported that the 10-year survival rate for aseptic loosening for hips that had been treated with third-generation cementing techniques was significantly better than that for hips that had been treated with second-generation techniques (94 vs. 85%, $p = 0.049$). The same was also true comparing the second- and first-generation techniques for re-revision due to aseptic loosening and for any reason. Type D cementation on the Barrack scale is a risk factor for significant radiographic loosening compared to A, B or C cementations in cemented revision THA. Bardou-Jacquet et al. [1] demonstrated that the survival rate was significantly better for revisions with type A or B cementations on the Barrack scale than for type C or D (96 vs. 70%, $p = 0.0016$).
4. Standard stems
   Hultmark et al. [9] showed that standard stems increased the risk of re-revision significantly following cemented revision THA compared to long stem revision ($p = 0.002$).
5. Male gender has also been considered a significant risk factor for failure.

34.1.3 Advantages [17]

1. Allows immediate full weight bearing, with no concerns regarding subsidence during the establishment of bone ongrowth; it achieves immediate rigid fixation enhancing rehabilitation and avoiding the comorbidities due to restricted mobilization.
2. The surgeon can revise a well-fixed stem through a cement-within-cement stem exchange, which simplifies the procedure by reducing operating time and blood loss (especially for collarless double-taper stems [17]).
3. Less thigh pain experienced compared to cementless [18].
4. Low cost compared to cementless [17].
5. May overcome issues with the use of cementless stems including the risk of intraoperative fracture, postoperative subsidence and loosening of undersized stems, stress shielding and the occasional need for osteotomy or modularity to achieve fixation of longer stems [17].

34.1.4 Published Results

Several papers providing level IV evidence are presently available [1–17, 19–26]. These are retrospective and prospective case series of 43 to 399 patients with a mean follow-up from 6 up to 20 years. It is difficult to compare the results of these studies because of the lack of consistency of several parameters such as the cementing technique, the design of the stems, the bone quality, etc.

The cemented revision THA without bone graft augmentation was proved to be a viable reconstructive technique with good to excellent intermediate- and long-term outcomes for selected patients. The reported prosthesis survival for any reason ranged from 72 to 98% [1–17, 19–26]. There were favourable results in older than 60-year-old patients with moderate but not severe bone loss and newer cementing techniques [1, 2, 9–16].

The initial reports demonstrated disappointing results. Hunter et al. [6] published a 22% rate of excision arthroplasty for 140 femoral revision arthroplasties that had been performed with cement. Engelbrecht et al. [7] later reported that 31% of 138 cemented femoral revisions had radiographic evidence of loosening at a mean of 7.4 years. Gramkow et al. [22] showed an overall 10-year survival of the femoral component of 77.9% and supported the use of the technique in elderly patients with only minor bone loss.

Later reports were more encouraging. In one of the greatest sample size reported, Raut et al. [25] evaluated prospectively 399 mechanical stem failures treated with cemented femoral revisions. The clinical survivorship of the revised stem was 93.9% at ten years, whereas radiographic survivorship was 91.5% at ten years. Haydon et al. [2] reported significant improvement of the quality of life of 129 cemented femoral revisions at a mean of 10-year follow-up. The 10-year survival rate was 91% with re-revision of the femoral component due to aseptic loosening and 71% with mechanical failure as the end point. Trumm et al. [19] supported that the cemented femoral revision using improved cementing techniques is a durable option in revision hip surgery. There was 7.5% rerevision rate for aseptic femoral loosening for a consecutive series of 83 cemented revisions at a minimum of 20 years [19]. Bardou-Jacquet et al. [1] showed the need for a new good-quality cement technique and a sufficient bone stock to achieve good results; in this study, there was 90% survival rate of a series of 80 cemented primary femoral stems for a mean of 10-year follow-up.

Davis et al. [16] reported also disappointing midterm results of cemented revision THA of a previous failed uncemented THA. There was 72% survival rate with revision for aseptic loosening and 67% with mechanical failure as the end point at six years. The high rate of loosening, during the first postoperative decade, was attributed to the little intramedullary cancellous bone left following bone removal at the time of the primary implantation of the stem and bone loss due to failure of the uncemented implant.

34.1.5 Complications

The most common complications reported include femoral shaft fractures and perforations, deep infection, dislocation and aseptic loosening.

34.2 Case Title: Cemented Revision THA (Cemented Femoral Revision for Paprosky Type 2 Defect)

E. Kenanidis and E. Tsiridis

34.2.1 Demographics

Age: 63
Sex: Female
BMI: 23

34.2.2 Relevant Past Medical History

Principal pathologies: Pain, inability to walk.

Previous surgical procedures: Bilateral THAs abroad less than ten years back, poor cementing technique, early loosening and osteolysis.

Medication: Antihypertensives.

History of presenting complaint: Pain, inability to walk, instability, short limp.

34.2.3 Clinical Examination

Symptoms: Pain, instability, short limp.

Range of motion: Overall limited due to pain. Flexion: 70; extension: 0; rotation, abduction and adduction limited due to pain.

Specific tests: Unable to perform due to pain.

Main disability: Pain, inability to walk on the left hip.

Scoring if available: HHS<70.

Neurovascular evaluation: Intact.

34.2.4 Preoperative Radiological Assessment/Imaging (Fig. 34.1)

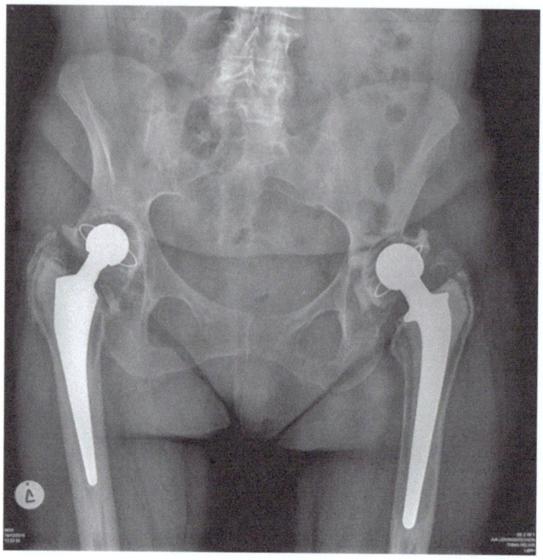

Fig. 34.1 Bilateral cemented THAs. On the right side, there is a loose acetabular component, but the stem is reasonably fixed; however, there is loosening and osteolysis in Gruen zones 1, 6, 7. The left THA has loose socket and stem

34.2.5 Preoperative Planning

Diagnosis: Complete loosening of the left THA planned for revision upon exclusion of infection (Fig. 34.1).

Possible treatment options: Revision THA cemented, uncemented, hybrid.

Chosen treatment method: Uncemented acetabular cup 54 mm/36 mm (DePuy). Exeter long cemented stem, 37.5 mm offset, 205 mm long, size 2 (Stryker).

Selection of implants if applicable and rational: Uncemented revision socket with grid blasted metal mesh outer surface. The stem was revised to a cemented long Exeter stem.

Expected difficulties: Protect femur from a periprosthetic fracture.

Strategies to overcome difficulties: Cerclage wiring before revising the stem. Infection exclusion performed ten days prior to the surgery. Biochemical markers of infection (WBC, ESR, CRP) were normal. Indium-111 WBC bone scan was negative. Hip aspiration under fluoroscopy performed ten days before surgery, and the sample was left in advanced culture for ten days to grow microorganisms.

Templating: Done.

34.2.6 Surgical Note

With the patient in the lateral decubitus position and general anaesthesia, the hip was approached using the posterior approach. The hip was dislocated easily, and six samples were taken both from bone and soft tissues to confirm asepsis. The femoral component approached from the top of the femur, taking down the cement from the shoulder of the prosthesis. Prior to any action taken, cerclage wiring of the femur was performed to protect it from hoop stresses during removal of the stem or insertion of the new one. The stem was then removed easily, leaving however behind the cement mantle. The latter was mobilized using curved osteotomes all around and then removed from the top in large fragments. The cement plague was then pierced with flexible reamers, and the canal was fired from debris. Thorough washing and excision of the fibrous tissue revealed bleeding bone all around the femoral canal. Attention was then turned to the socket. Removing the cemented implant was easy, as it was already terribly loose. The gap left behind was Paprosky 2A and was easily reconstructable using a large/jumbo uncemented revision socket with screws. Reaming was then commenced, removing the scar tissue and exposing the viable bone. The acetabulum was shaped to accommodate a shell size 54 mm (DePuy revision mutlihole) ×36 mm. There was good coverage and tight fitting of the shell. The femur was then approached again; the canal was solid Paprosky type 2 and the cortical bone sufficient to accommodate a cemented revision. The canal washed thoroughly again removing the blood and debris, and a third-generation cementing technique was used to insert a long revision stem 37.5 mm offset 205 mm long size 2 (Stryker). The leg length and the stability of the hip were tested prior to cementation. Stem implantation and a 36 mm ceramic head provided good stability and length to the joint

(Fig. 34.2). The sciatic nerve was observed to be free of tension and the joint was closed over a suction drain.

34.2.7 Intraoperative Challenges

Challenges and solutions: Removing the stem safely by applying protective wires and socket reaming without damaging the walls.

Unanticipated problems and solution: None.

Thorough description of decision making, including the reason for the final decision: Cemented stem revision is rarely now performed considering the full range of uncemented implants available. Occasionally, however, if the femoral canal is adequate, i.e., Paprosky type 2, then cemented long stem revision may be employed with or without impaction grafting. In our case, we had good bone stock available for cementation, and the final decision was based on feasibility and cost.

34.2.8 Postoperative Radiographs (Fig. 34.2)

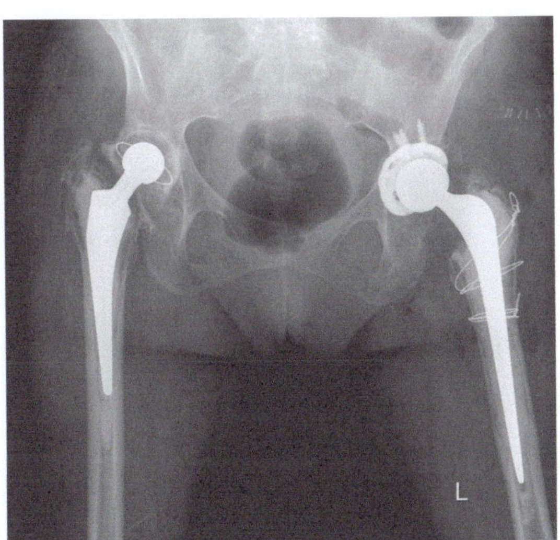

Fig. 34.2 Proper cementing technique and well-aligned stem bypassing the distal end of the previous stem by at least 50 mm. The acetabular component is very well fitted and stable with screws

34.2.9 Postoperative Management

Chemoprophylaxis and anticoagulant treatment period: Vancomycin 500 mg 1 × 2 for 2 days, cefuroxime 750 mg 1 × 3 for 2 days, tinzaparin 1 × 1 for 35 days.

Gait/limb loading until full loading: Partial weight bearing for four weeks and then as tolerated.

34.2.10 Follow-Up and Complications

There were no postoperative complications.

Scoring: HHS: 90

34.3 Case Title: Complex Long Cemented Stem Revision for a Loose Cemented Stem above a Stemmed Knee Replacement and with Previous Fracture Malunion

M. Shahid and A.R.J. Manktelow

34.3.1 Demographics

Age: 67
Sex: F
BMI: 23

34.3.2 Relevant Past Medical History

Principal pathologies: Loose cemented femoral component. Ipsilateral stemmed knee replacement and with a previous fracture malunion.

Previous surgical procedures: Left THR (Cemented) 2007, complex right primary TKR (2004), right THR (Cemented 1998—Charnley monoblock stem)

Medication: Calcichew.

History of presenting complaint: a 67-year-old female who had a right total hip replacement presented with right anterior thigh pain for the last six months. There was no history of any recent trauma or systemic features. She uses two sticks indoors and a scooter outside. She had a previous right stemmed total knee replacement in 2004. She sustained a subsequent periprosthetic fracture, managed conservatively at another hospital. The patient was unclear regarding the circumstances surrounding the management of her fracture.

34.3.3 Clinical Examination

Symptoms: She walked with an antalgic gait.

Range of motion: Right hip—90 passive flexion with limited internal and external rotation. Right knee was in 15 ° of valgus with a range of motion between 0 and 75 °.

Specific tests: Normal inflammatory markers.

Main disability: Pain and reduced mobility.

Neurovascular evaluation: No distal neurovascular deficit.

34.3.4 Preoperative Radiological Assessment/Imaging (Figs. 34.3, 34.4, 34.5, 34.6, and 34.7)

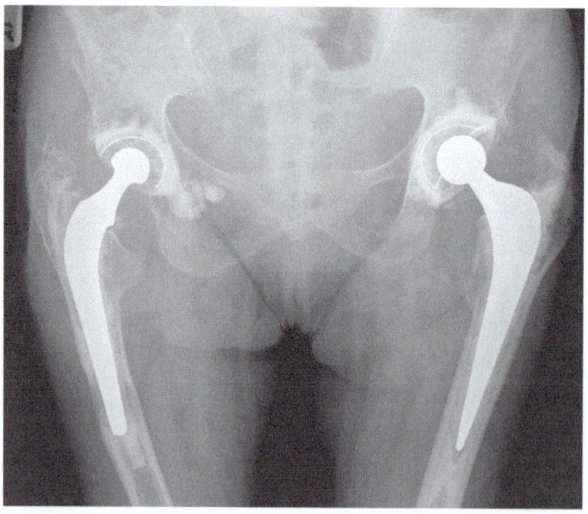

Fig. 34.3 AP pelvis—right hip shows acetabular lucency in Charnley zones 1 and 2. In the right femur, there is subsidence of the monoblock Charnley stem. There are lucencies in Gruen zones 1, 3, 5, 7 with significant bone deficiency and scalloping at the tip of the stem, raising concern regarding possible impending fracture

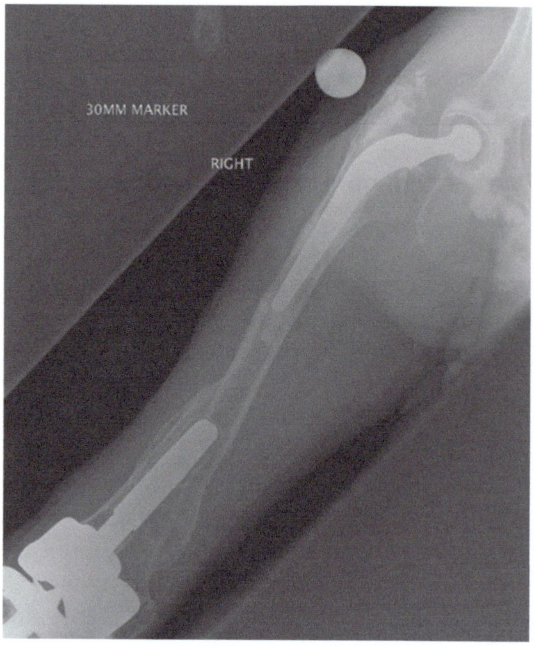

Fig. 34.4 Lateral femur. Show lucencies in zones 8, 10 and 12. The area of malunion is noted above the stem of the knee replacement. Functionally, a 'double lumen' has been created distally below the loose femoral stem

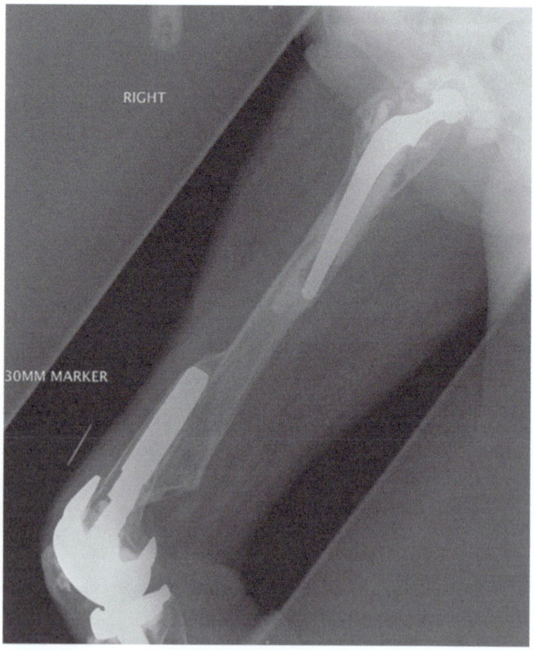

Fig. 34.5 Lateral femur. Show lucencies in zones 8, 10 and 12. The area of malunion is noted above the stem of the knee replacement. Functionally, a 'double lumen' has been created distally below the loose femoral stem

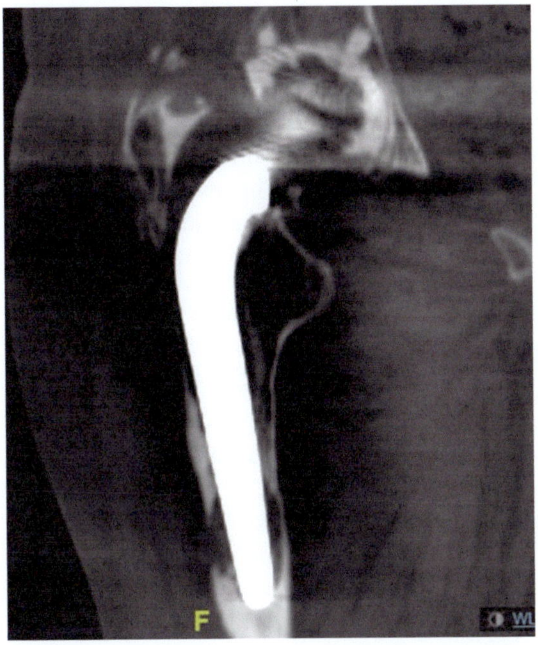

Fig. 34.6 CT is demonstrating endosteal scalloping in the distal stem

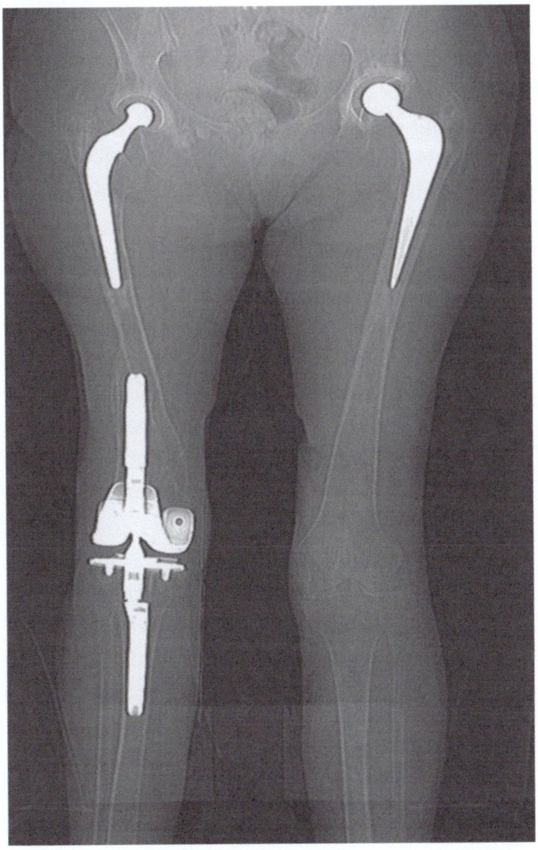

Fig. 34.7 CT scout view is demonstrating the malalignment and 'double lumen' of the femur

34.3.5 Preoperative Planning

Diagnosis: Osteolysis surrounding symptomatic aseptic loosening of the right femoral component with an impending periprosthetic fracture. Distal malunion, complication potential reconstructive options (Figs. 34.3, 34.4, 34.5, 34.6, and 34.7).

Chosen treatment method: Revision of the acetabulum with an uncemented socket and a long cemented stem revision of the femoral component, spanning the two areas of concern.

Selection of implants if applicable and rational: It is often essential to obtain the operation note for the index procedure as part of the preoperative planning. However, in this case, both components were to be revised. In this case, the components used were monoblock Charnley stem with a stainless steel 22.25 mm head. Cemented high-density polyethylene cup (HDP). Acetabulum: With regard to acetabular reconstruction, in addition to our standard instrumentation, we ensured the TMARS (Trabecular Metal Acetabular Revision System—Zimmer Biomet) was available. This system comprises a fully porous trabecular metal ™ revision shell, TM augments and buttresses, with the availability of the 'cup cage' construct. While we did not anticipate concern, following classification of the preoperative radiograph, the system provides a full inventory of options to deal with any unexpected bone loss found at surgery. Femur: On the femoral side, the long cemented stems (Elite 205/220/240) were made available. This would allow a long stem femoral revision. An uncemented modular femoral revision system (ZMR—Zimmer) was also available in this case. The OSCAR (Orthosonics System for Cement Arthroplasty Revision) cement removal system was available in theatre as was the Midas Rex Burr alongside our standard inventory of cement removal instruments. A headlight was also used to improve visualization for femoral cement removal.

Expected difficulties: Acetabular side—the imaging did not demonstrate significant bone loss (Paprosky 1). The revision was planned to provide a better bearing surface, improved alignment and a larger head to enhance stability. Femur—the presence of the stemmed knee replacement and distal malunion was problematic. There is a risk of a periprosthetic fracture from the stress riser and the lytic area at the tip of the existing implant. It was planned that the new stem should both bypass this area but also span the malunion distally. Looking at the CT scan, this appeared feasible as there was a 'double femoral lumen' distally (Fig. 34.7). We also had the option of applying a strut graft to bridge this tenuous region if necessary. There was a concern with uncemented femoral revision regarding identifying a safe area to achieve fixation. Similarly, bone quality was poor, and we were keen to span the most distal malunion to reduce the chance of subsequent inter-prosthetic fracture.

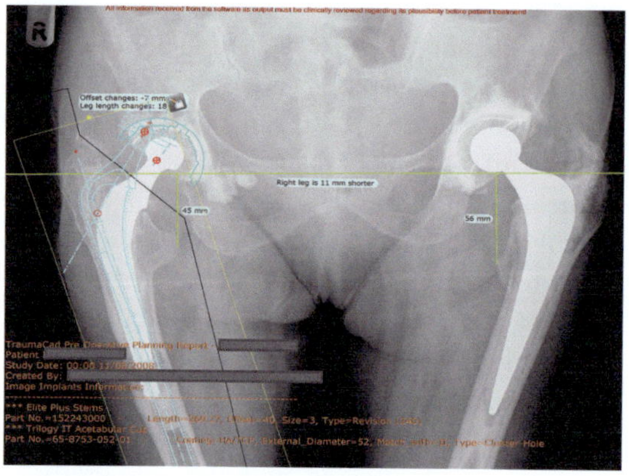

Fig. 34.8 AP template using the Elite 240 stem

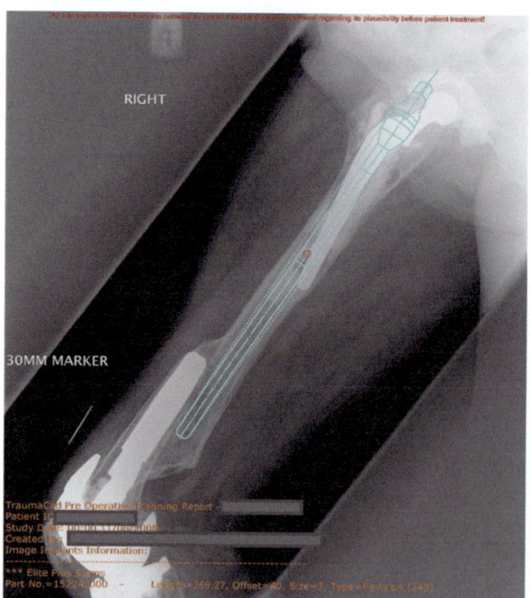

Fig. 34.9 Lateral showing feasibility of stem going down the 'double lumen', bypassing the area of concern distally

Templating: Using the TraumaCad® (Brainlab) system, we templated the acetabulum using the Trilogy IT Acetabular Cup and also the femoral side using the long stem Charnley Elite cemented stem (Figs. 34.8 and 34.9).

34.3.6 Surgical Note

Patient's position: Patient was in the lateral position with pelvis positioned carefully and securely supported.

Type of anaesthesia: Spinal using heavy Marcaine and diamorphine. Antibiotics and tranexamic acid (1 g) were given at induction (flucloxacillin 2 g and gentamicin 200 mg).

Surgical approach: Posterior approach through the old incision.

Main steps: The existing scar was used and extended proximally and distally. The fascia lata was incised. The sciatic nerve was identified and protected. An aspiration of the hip joint was performed. The piriformis was incised, and then this, along with the short external rotators and capsule, was elevated as a single flap. The gluteus maximus insertion was incised to improve access and to prevent undue tension on the sciatic nerve. The hip was dislocated. The femoral component was loose. A high-speed burr was used to remove cement from the shoulder of the implant. The loose stem was removed. The socket was exposed with a circumferential release and with the femur transposed supero-anteriorly. Soft tissue samples were sent for microbiology. The existing cup was worn and was removed. A small curved osteotome was used in between the bone-cement interface. It is important not to remove the socket from the cement mantle before it is fully released as you do not want to remove any remaining acetabular bone with well-fixed cement. Then the cement itself was cleared, with hand instruments and under direct vision, to reduce the possibility of additional bone loss. There was a minimal bone loss. Careful debridement of all membranous debris was performed. Small cement plugs in the acetabulum were removed.

Acetabular reconstruction: The acetabular defect was classified as Paprosky 2A. The acetabulum was reamed sequentially at the desired hip centre. Reamer size was progressively increased towards the anteroposterior dimensions of the acetabulum. As anterior and posterior contact is approached, care must be taken not to lose bone unnecessarily. In this case, we were able to ream sequentially until AP and SI dimensions were identical, but there was an antero-superior defect. We eventually reamed to 50 mm, and a size 52 mm Trilogy IT Cup was implanted with three screws to enhance stability. Using the alignment rod, we oriented it with 25° anteversion and 45° inclination. A 32 mm highly cross-linked polyethylene cup with a lipped liner was inserted with care taken to ensure locking mechanism was soundly engaged.

Femoral reconstruction: Attention was now turned to the femur. All the cement and the distal cement plug were removed using a combination of the OSCAR system, specialized hand instruments and flexible reamers. The canal was lavaged to remove any debris**.** A trial reduction was done using the Elite 240 stem. Great care was taken to ensure the stem passed safely into the 'double lumen' distally. Intraoperative imaging was done to ensure the stem did not breach the cortex. This was trialled with a 32 mm +3 head which gave it the most stability and restored the biomechanics. A 26 mm Hardinge restrictor was then inserted distally to the length of the femur to prevent cement extrusion distally into the posterior aspect of the knee. Again, the trial stem was reinserted to ensure it went down easily. We then prepared the femoral canal with a brush and by washing with normal saline using pulsatile lavage. Cement was mixed and introduced using a long nozzle, with four mixes of refrigerated cement, mixed simultaneously in two cement guns. The cement was introduced relatively early in this challenging case in a retrograde manner. Good pressurization was achieved despite the complexity. The long cemented stem was then inserted carefully and steadily, using the trials to rehearse the correct required alignment at the optimal height and version. After trialling with various head options, the 32 mm +3 metal head was the most stable and restored the biomechanics of hip. It is important to achieve sound soft tissue repair when closing the soft tissues. The short external rotators were attached with numerous 1 Vicryl sutures. A drain was placed just underneath the fascia lata, which was closed with a PDS suture. Deep and superficial fat was closed with 1 and 2–0 Vicryl, respectively. Clips and a pressure dressing were applied (Figs. 34.10 and 34.11).

34.3.7 Intraoperative Challenges

Challenges and solutions: In this particularly challenging case, the major concern was with removing the residual cement carefully without causing a femoral perforation or fracture which would have complicated this case yet further. Removal of the cement can be challenging especially the distal plug. Care must be taken when using hand instruments, reamers and indeed the OSCAR system. A head light can help to ensure all cement is cleared without femoral damage. To ensure that the stem went down the correct lumen, we used intraoperative fluoroscopy to confirm correct alignment and adequate bypass of the two areas of concern in the femur. In this

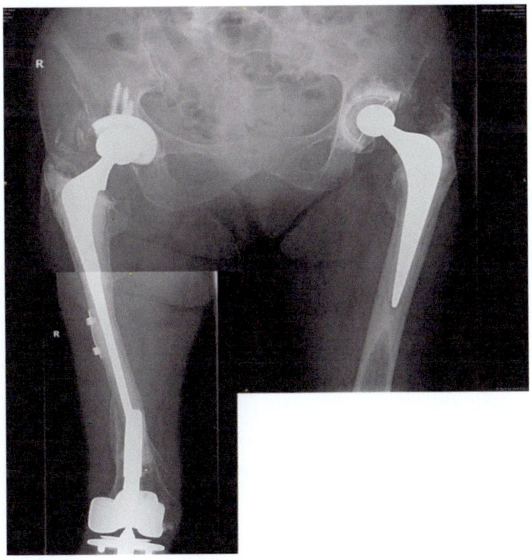

Fig. 34.10 Postoperative AP radiograph showing how the long cemented stem component has successfully bypassed the areas of lysis and malunion. Sound cement fixation has been achieved with no cement extravasation

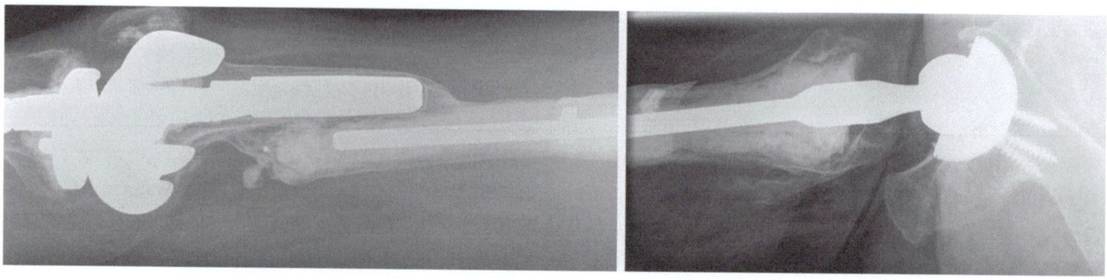

Fig. 34.11 Postoperative lateral radiograph is showing the stem going down the 'double lumen' and overlapping the stem of the femoral knee component. The cement restrictor can be seen distally at the tip of the posterior lumen preventing cement escape. Sound cement pressurization is seen in both AP and lateral projections

case, we determined that the stem should overlap the stem of the femoral knee component to minimize the risk of inter-prosthetic fracture. In fact, the existence of the 'double lumen' caused by the previous fracture malunion was advantageous as we could overlap the femoral stem from the knee replacement. There was an additional concern to ensure the cement didn't extravasate distally, potentially into the popliteal fossa. The distal cement plug was screened in position as distally as was possible as can be seen from the postoperative radiographs.

34.3.8 Postoperative Radiographs (Figs. 34.10 and 34.11)

34.3.9 Postoperative Management

Chemoprophylaxis and anticoagulant treatment period: Low molecular weight heparin for four weeks. We do not use mechanical thromboprophylaxis.

Patient was mobilized: Weight bearing as tolerated on crutches for six weeks.

34.3.10 Follow-Up and Complications

No postoperative complications were reported. All the microbiology samples were negative for infection. The surgery was performed four years prior to writing this report. The patient continues to mobilize soundly with no pain, clinical or radiological concern.

34.3.11 Discussion

Revision of the femoral component, with the removal of any surrounding cement, can be a challenging part of revision hip arthroplasty. The first step is to classify the possible femoral deficiency. The two most commonly used classification systems are the Paprosky and the American Academy of Orthopaedic Surgeons (AAOS) systems. We would advocate the use of the Paprosky system as it correlates well with surgical complexity and can be used as a guide for likely reconstruction. In this scenario, the femoral defect was classified as an IIIB defect, with metaphyseal and diaphyseal damage with likely uncemented fixation available only at the isthmus. Surgical options for femoral revision aim to achieve implant stability while restoring hip biomechanics with the accurate restoration of leg length, version and offset. Fixation options include cementless fixation, with modular, non-modular or distally locked prosthesis, or cemented fixation, with or without impaction grafting. In this case, the particular challenge is related to the need to bypass the defect at the distal end of the existing loose stem, with poor bone quality, while also bypassing the distal femoral malunion, to reduce the chances of an intra-prosthetic fracture through an area of stress concentration.

Cementless fixation: There are many different concepts in uncemented fixation. The surgical decision regarding which is chosen will be based on the femoral defect classification, the surgeon's experience and training and of course any intraoperative concern. Proximally loading porous stems are used most commonly with a minimal metaphyseal bone loss (Paprosky I or II). With a more severe bone loss, proximal fixation becomes a more significant challenge. With Paprosky IIIA and IIIB defects, fixation is typically achieved more distally in the diaphysis. This can be achieved in a number of ways. Previously, fully coated porous-coated monoblock stems were used most commonly. The distal porous-coated stem bypassed the damaged femoral bone. With worsening bone loss, longer stems are available, ensuring at least a 4–5 cm segment of distal 'scratch fit' and ingrowth. Results with this have been favourable, with one study looking at 905 femoral revisions performed with these stems over 26 years demonstrating a rerevision rate of 2.2% with a 1.3% incidence of aseptic loosening [27]. More recently, modular stems have been introduced. With varied lengths of straight and curved stems, these can provide either cylindrical or indeed conical 'taper' fixation distally. Multiple proximal bodies and neck options are available, again with different lengths and offsets and with a wide variability in version, which facilitates excellent restoration of hip biomechanics. While there have been concerns with modular stem failures, there are also more recent designs with strengthened modular junctions. This, coupled with simple, versatile instrumentation, has led to these devices becoming the most commonly used in femoral revision. Distal locked stems, primarily developed in Europe, in the late 1980s, can be considered and provide additional initial stability of the uncemented stem within the damaged femur to facilitate subsequent ingrowth. After a proximal bone loss is restored, removal of the distal screws can be considered, transferring the load back to the proximal femur. Problems with cementless reconstruction include intraoperative fracture, failure of fixation, particularly with poor surrounding bone quality, loosening of undersized stems, subsidence and stress shielding. There are also rehabilitation issues with the need to protect weight bear. Moreover, the modular nature of some of these stems can introduce the risk of corrosion and stem fracture [17]. In this particular case, we had concerns about how and where to achieve fixation with an uncemented stem with intraoperative fracture—a major risk with the patient's bone quality. We were also keen to bypass the stem within the malunited distal femur to reduce the chance of intra-prosthetic fracture. This we felt would have been a major challenge with uncemented fixation.

Cemented fixation: Early use of cemented fixation in femoral revision reported high rates of re-revision, probably as a result of poor stem design, first-generation cementing techniques, concomitant use of cemented acetabular cups and an over-reliance on a standard femoral length component [4, 20]. Femoral revision can be performed in association with femoral impaction bone grafting (FIG). This is a technique which aims to recreate stable cement fixation of the femoral stem and restore bone stock. Milled allograft bone is impacted into a deficient femur. A collarless polished tapered stem is then cemented into the new canal. A study looked at 540 cases of FIG. Survivorship at 10 years was 98% for aseptic loosening and 84% for all other causes of revision [28]. Long stemmed cemented femoral components can be used without bone grafting, and good results have been reported. Perhaps the primary indications have been in the presence of poor bone quality, in lower demand, more elderly patients with type IIIB and type IV defects. Attention to detail in achieving a good bone-cement interdigitation and fixation is crucial to obtain good outcomes. In this case, we felt there were benefits in selecting a long cemented stem reconstruction as detailed above. The long cemented stem has the advantage of ease to which we could adjust the height and version of the implant. Immediate postoperative weight bearing is also permitted with these stems; once solid bone-cement interface fixation has been achieved, there is less concern regarding subsidence. The patients also experience less thigh pain and the stems are cheaper. The long cemented stems need very careful and a fastidious surgical technique. The femoral endosteal surface must be clean and dry prior to cementing. It is imperative to use a distal cement restrictor and proximal pressurization to achieve solid integration at the compromised bone-cement interface. Similarly, particularly in the more elderly patient, care must be taken with pressurization of the cement to reduce the chances of a hypotensive systemic response. One study demonstrated a 98% 9-year survival of long cemented stem revision for aseptic loosening [20]. This was mirrored by a recent study which showed a survival at 14 years of 97% for long stem revision of cemented collarless double-taper stems [17]. Cemented hip replacements are not without their problems. Bone-cement implantation syndrome (BCIS) is characterized by a number of clinical features including hypoxia, hypotension, cardiac arrhythmias, increased pulmonary vascular resistance and cardiac arrest. It can occur during femoral reaming, acetabular or femoral cement implantation, insertion of the prosthesis or joint reduction. The pathophysiology of BCIS is not fully understood. Several mechanisms have been proposed including the formation of emboli during cementing and prosthesis insertion [29]. The use of a long stem femoral component increases the likelihood of developing BCIS [30]. This needs to be considered when deciding on the method of implant fixation. In summary, this was a particularly complicated case that illustrates the versatility of long cemented stem femoral fixation to achieve our goals against the specific challenges, in this case, of poor bone biology, lytic defects and a distal malunion introducing concern with possible intra-prosthetic fracture. As with everything in hip surgery, careful planning, an appreciation of the potential concerns and an understanding of the various options, when combined with fastidious planning and attention to detail in surgery, can maximize the chance of a successful outcome.

References

1. Bardou-Jacquet J, Souillac V, Mouton A, Chauveaux D. Primary aseptic revision of the femoral component of a cemented total hip arthroplasty using a cemented technique without bone graft. Orthop Traumatol Surg Res. 2009;95(4):243–8.
2. Haydon CM, Mehin R, Burnett S, Rorabeck CH, Bourne RB, McCalden RW, MacDonald SJ. Revision total hip arthroplasty with use of a cemented femoral component. Results at a mean of ten years. J Bone Joint Surg Am. 2004;86-A(6):1179–85.
3. Amstutz HC, Ma SM, Jinnah RH, Mai L. Revision of aseptic loose total hip arthroplasties. Clin Orthop. 1982;170:21–33.
4. Pellicci PM, Wilson PD Jr, Sledge CB, Salvati EA, Ranawat CS, Poss R, Callaghan JJ. Long-term results of revision total hip replacement. A follow- up report. J Bone Joint Surg Am. 1985;67:513–6.
5. Kavanagh BF, Ilstrup DM, Fitzgerald RH Jr. Revision total hip arthroplasty. J Bone Joint Surg Am. 1985;67:517–26.
6. Hunter GA, Welsh RP, Cameron HU, Bailey WH. The results of revision of total hip arthroplasty. J Bone Joint Surg Br. 1979;61:419–21.
7. Engelbrecht DJ, Weber FA, Sweet MB, Jakim I. Long-term results of revision total hip arthroplasty. J Bone Joint Surg Br. 1990;72:41–5.
8. Rubash HE, Harris WH. Revision of nonseptic, loose, cemented femoral com- ponents using modern cementing techniques. J Arthroplast. 1988;3:241–8.
9. Hultmark P, Kärrholm J, Strömberg C, et al. Cemented first-time revisions of the femoral component: prospective 7 to 13 years' follow-up using second-generation and third-generation technique. J Arthroplast. 2000;15:551–61.
10. Stromberg CN, Herberts P. Cemented revision total hip arthroplasties in patients younger than 55 years old. A multicenter evaluation of second- generation cementing technique. J Arthroplast. 1996;11:489–99.
11. Ito H, Tanino H, Yamanaka Y, et al. Cemented calcar replacement femoral compo- nent in revision hybrid total hip arthroplasty. J Arthroplast. 2011;26:236–43.
12. Garcia-Cimbrelo E, Munuera L, Diez-Vazquez V. Long-term results of aseptic cemented Charnley revisions. J Arthroplast. 1995;10:121–31.
13. Herberts P, Ahnfelt L, Malchau H, Stromberg C, Andersson GB. Multicenter clinical trials and their value in assessing total joint arthroplasty. Clin Orthop. 1989;249:48–55.
14. Retpen JB, Jensen JS. Risk factors for recurrent aseptic loosening of the femoral component after cemented revision. J Arthroplasty. 1993;8:471–8.
15. Eisler T, Svensson O, Iyer V, Wejkner B, Schmalholz A, Larsson H, Elmstedt E. Revision total hip arthroplasty using third-generation cementing technique. J Arthroplast. 2000;15:974–81.

16. Davis CM 3rd, Berry DJ, Harmsen WS. Cemented revision of failed uncemented femoral components of total hip arthroplasty. J Bone Joint Surg Am. 2003;85-A(7):1264–9.
17. Solomon LB, Costi K, Kosuge D, Cordier T, McGee MA, Howie DW. Revision total hip arthroplasty using cemented collarless double-taper femoral components at a meanfollow-up of 13 years (8 to 20): an update. Bone Joint J. 2015;97-B(8):1038–45.
18. Barrack RL, Paprosky W, Butler RA, et al. Patients' perception of pain after total hip arthroplasty. J Arthroplast. 2000;15:590–6.
19. Trumm BN, Callaghan JJ, George CA, et al. Minimum 20-year follow-up results of revision total hip arthroplasty with improved cementing technique. J Arthroplast. 2014;29:236–41.
20. Howie DW, Wimhurst JA, McGee MA, Carbone TA, Badaruddin BS. Revision total hip replacement using cemented collarless double-taper femoral components. J Bone Joint Surg (Br). 2007;89-B:879–86.
21. Katz RP, Callaghan JJ, Sullivan PM, Johnston RC. Long-term results of revision total hip arthroplasty with improved cementing technique. J Bone Joint Surg (Br). 1997;79:322–6.
22. Gramkow J, Jensen TH, Varmarken JE, Retpen JB. Long-term results after cemented revision of the femoral component in total hip arthroplasty. J Arthroplast. 2001;16:777–83.
23. Callaghan JJ, Salvati EA, Pellicci PM, Wilson PD Jr, Ranawat CS. Results of revision for mechanical failure after cemented total hip replacement, 1979 to 1982. A two to five-year follow-up. J Bone Joint Surg Am. 1985;67(7):1074–85.
24. Estok DM 2nd, Harris WH. Long-term results of cemented femoral revision surgery using second-generation techniques. An average 11.7-year follow-up evaluation. Clin Orthop Relat Res. 1994;299:190–202.
25. Raut VV, Siney PD, Wroblewski BM. Outcome of revision for mechanical stem failure using the cemented Charnley's stem. A study of 399 cases. J Arthroplast. 1996;11:405–10.
26. Raut VV, Siney PD, Wroblewski BM. Revision for aseptic stem loosening using the cemented Charnley prosthesis. A review of 351 hips. J Bone Joint Surg Br. 1995;77(1):23–7.
27. Hamilton WG, Cashen DV, Ho H, Hopper RH Jr, Engh C. Extensively porous-coated stems for femoral revision: a choice for all seasons. J Arthroplasty. 2007;22(4 Suppl 1):106–10.
28 Lamberton TD, Kenny PJ, Whitehouse SL, Timperley AJ, Gie GA. Femoral impaction grafting in revision total hip arthroplasty: a follow-up of 540 hips. J Arthroplasty. 2011;26(8):1154–60.
29 Donaldson AJ, Thomson HE, Harper NJ, Kenny NW. Bone cement implantation syndrome. Br J Anaesth. 2009;102(1):12–22
30 Herrenbruck T, Erickson EW, Damron TA, Heiner J. Adverse clinical events during cemented long-stem femoral arthroplasty, Clin Orthop Relat Res, 2002, vol. 395 (pg. 154-63)

Cement in Cement (CiC) Femoral Revision

35

Eustathios Kenanidis, Eleftherios Tsiridis, Mohammad Shahid, and Andrew R. J. Manktelow

35.1 Current Concepts

E. Kenanidis and E. Tsiridis

The removal of the cement mantle in the revision of cemented femoral implants is technically challenging [1]. During cement removal, numerous significant complications may occur like substantial bleeding, perforation of the femoral cortex and fracture of the femur [2, 3]. The removal of the cement is time consuming, thus increasing the risk of medical complications both intra- and postoperatively [2, 4, 5].

Several authors in the past have published their experience of leaving the solid cement mantle in place and re-cementing a new stem into the femoral canal [6–8]. Currently, CiC technique has attracted more interest following several biomechanical studies [9–11] that support the bonding between the old and the new cement and case series that provide a good medium- to long-term results [5, 6, 12, 13].

35.1.1 Objective

The CiC technique provides an option for revision of a well-fixed cemented stem. An intact cement mantle without residual cracks is a prerequisite to performing this procedure. The aim of the method is to minimize the risk of cement removal during revision THA and to contribute long-term femoral stem stability.

35.1.2 Indications

The indications of the technique are not clear so far. The following have been proposed [1, 4, 12]:

1. The removal of the femoral stem to gain access and facilitate the acetabular revision [12]
2. The exchange of a monoblock stem with a damaged or incompatible taper [12, 14]
3. The revision of a malpositioned stem for the treatment of recurrent instability or leg length discrepancy [12, 15, 16]
4. The conversion of a well-fixed cemented hemiarthroplasty to THA [12, 14]

E. Kenanidis, M.D., Ph.D., M.Sc. (✉)
Academic Orthopaedic Unit,
Aristotle University Medical School,
Thessaloniki, Greece

E. Tsiridis, M.D., Ph.D., F.A.C.S., F.R.C.S. (✉)
Academic Orthopaedic Unit, Papageorgiou General Hospital, Aristotle University Medical School,
Thessaloniki, Greece
e-mail: etsiridis@doctors.org.uk

M. Shahid, B.Sc., M.B.B.S., F.R.C.S.
Worcestershire Acute Hospitals NHS Trust,
Worcester, UK
e-mail: shahidm99@doctors.org.uk

A.R.J. Manktelow, B.Sc., M.B.B.S., F.R.C.S.
Nottingham University Hospitals NHS Trust,
Nottingham, UK
e-mail: a.mank@btinternet.com

E. Tsiridis (ed.), *The Adult Hip - Master Case Series and Techniques*,
https://doi.org/10.1007/978-3-319-64177-5_35

5. The adjustment of the femoral offset
6. The revision of a broken cemented stem with an intact cement mantle

35.1.3 Requirements and Contraindications

- A non-intact femoral cement mantle with residual cracks (preoperative and intraoperative inspection) or radiolucencies in the proximal cement mantle (especially in Gruen zones 1 and 7) are considered contraindications [14, 15].
- Septic revision is another contraindication [15, 17].
- The collarless, polished, straight-tapered stems are more appropriate for the CiC technique; they are easily knocked out of the cement mantle, without damage to the mantle. Matted or pre-coated finishes are not ideal as they are difficult to remove [3, 18].
- The most standard cemented stems, or revision stems are not also ideal for the technique as they are too long to fit in the existing cement mantle; they need distal drilling and removing of the distal cement mantle and plug which is prone to complications.
- In most cases, we use a stem with the same offset as the stem that has been removed but with a slimmer body. The Exeter Short Revision Stem simplifies cement in cement revision, without the need for distal reaming or drilling. An advantage of the latter stem is that despite being short, it still has a 44 mm offset; however, it is slimmer both distally and front to back than a standard 44 mm stem of a similar size.

35.1.4 The Surgical Procedure [1, 2]

- To our opinion, the posterior approach is the most versatile for the handling of the femur.
- Clear the proximal cement above the shoulder of the prosthesis with revision chisels or a speed burr.
- Remove the prosthesis by 'tapping it out'; this is easier for a collarless, polished, tapered stem.
- Recut the femoral neck 2–3 mm below the existing cut if necessary to inspect the cement–bone interface of the proximal mantle.
- If any crack in the cement is visible beyond the first two cm of the mantle (or beyond the lesser trochanter), all cement must be removed, and an alternate revision procedure must be performed [14].
- If the mantle is broad enough to accommodate the revision stem, then the inner surface should not be burred away or roughened. Roughening of the inner surface does not affect the bonding between the old and the new cement mantles [11]. On the contrary, it may weaken the mantle and lead to cement–bone dissociation.
- To alter, however, stem version or allow a wider revision stem to get into the old mantle, much cement may have to be burred away proximally to enable the stem to rotate within the mantle.
- Remove the distal cement plug and the old cement stopper in case a longer stem will be used. This is challenging however but not unusual in the revision setting. The latter procedure may require visualization of the long drills or reamer tips utilizing the C-arm fluoroscopy to make sure the reaming is concentric. It is not unusual for the tip of the reamer or the drill to move against the bare softer lateral cortex bouncing back against the hard solid cement plug. Drilling through the cement plug with a long thin drill may allow for a guide wire to be inserted over which flexible reamers can be attached to concentrically ream the canal and the distal plug until it is removed [5].
- The 'short-stem revision' is an alternative method that employs a shorter than the original stem ignoring the distal cement plug. Medium-term results are available only in small case series [5].
- Clean the cement mantle thoroughly using pulsed lavage and dried as for the proper cementing technique [11].
- Prepare and insert PMMA cement when still in a low state of viscosity in a retrograde fashion and pressurized against the old cement mantle. The pressurization of the cement is necessary for the new cement to fill all the gaps and fissures and to penetrate the exposed bone.

Polymerization with the existing cement mantle will occur providing a very solid bond [11].
- Insert the femoral component following maximal cement pressurization.

35.1.5 Advantages

1. A more straightforward technique as there is no need to remove the entire cement mantle [4]
2. A less time-consuming procedure that decreases perioperative morbidity, mortality and cost [2, 12, 14]
3. The preservation of the bone stock and reduction of the blood loss [12]
4. Earlier postoperative full weight-bearing mobilization [12]
5. Excellent exposure to the acetabulum due to the removal of the femoral component during the acetabular revisions [18]
6. Lower risk of femur fracture or cortical perforation and need for femoral osteotomies to access the distal cement
7. Can be used in certain types of periprosthetic fractures (Vancouver B2 with well-fixed cement and loose stem) [1, 19]

35.1.6 Disadvantages

1. Improper method for the femoral revisions with compromised cement mantle.
2. Difficult correction of the alignment of the new prosthesis [20]. Modifying the version of the existing mantle is necessary to rasp or burr out some of the inner surface of the old mantle. The latter has the risk of damage the old cement mantle proximally or to debond the cement–bone interface, leading to an inadequate or loose mantle and construct failure [11]. There is also increased risk for varus placement of the stem [3].
3. Contamination by blood and marrow fat, despite modern lavage techniques of the cement–cement interface, may act as a stress riser, facilitating the formation of fatigue cracks in the cement [11].
4. Disappointing results of the method in case of septic revision [21].
5. Possible short-stem fracture and failure of the technique [22].

35.1.7 Biomechanical Aspects

Several biomechanical studies have assessed the strength of the interface of the new and prepolymerized cements [7, 9–11, 21, 23]. Although these studies are valuable, they cannot be considered as conclusive as they have a lot of limitations. They lack a realistic three-dimensional model and testing under cyclic loading, and they cannot reproduce in vitro a cement mantle of 10–15 years [2].

Greenwald et al. [7] demonstrated that the early introduction of the new cement increased the availability of the free monomer, promoting polymerization with the existing cement mantle and maximizing shear strength. Although he supported that rasping the surface of the old cement strengthened the bond between the new and old cement, this was controverted in more recent studies [11]. Rudol et al. [11] reported that roughening of the primary mantle was not as crucial as it has been previously thought. The shear strength of the cement–cement interface was found higher than that of the cement–bone interface in all cases of tested human femora [21]. Li et al. [9] proved that the effect of interface contamination with blood and marrow weakened the strength of the cement bond.

35.1.8 Review of Clinical Publications

The clinical research is supportive of the cement in cement technique. Few, however, case series (level IV evidence) are presently available of 10–175 patients [3–5, 8, 12–16, 24, 25]. They range in follow-up from a mean of 1.8 to 12 years. The studies showed acceptable survival rates for aseptic revision of 95–100% and 82–100% for revision for any reason. In one of the longest follow-up studies, Duncan et al. [4] reported 100% survival rate for aseptic loosening and 92% for any reason at a mean follow-up of 8 years for 136 patients treated with CiC technique. Similar results were also reported from Hubble et al. [12]

for a group of 175 patients followed at a mean of 5 years. Te Stroet et al. [5] showed the mid-term survival of 24 Exeter short stems (125 mm) used for the CiC technique in revision THA. He reported 100% survival at a mean of 6 years for aseptic loosening but 82% for revision for any reason. Seventeen percent of femoral components were removed for septic loosening at a mean of 2.4 years [5].

The majority of these clinical studies contained small sample sizes. To our knowledge, there are no prospective trials comparing custom CiC revision to other forms for revision femoral arthroplasty. The outcomes do not provide sufficient data to predict the long-term results of the CiC reconstructive technique. We certainly need a larger cohort of patients for a longer length of time and an expertise-based prospective randomized controlled trial with paired comparison groups.

35.1.9 Complications

- The rates of complications in the studies varied [3–5, 8, 12–16, 24, 25].
- Aseptic loosening, stem subsidence, femoral perforation, periprosthetic fractures, septic revision, heterotopic ossification, varus stem position and stem fractures are the most commonly reported [3–5, 8, 12–16, 24, 25].
- Duncan et al. [4] reported that the subsidence seen when components were inserted with distal centralizers had been the same as that seen after implantation of a primary cemented femoral component. The subsidence was significantly more for the cases where a new centralizer was used compared to an old one. The clinical significance of this observation was disputed as no stems were loosened in this study.
- Goto et al. [15] reported the greatest percentage of perioperative fractures using CiC technique. Twenty-one percent of patients suffered perioperative fractures mainly of the greater trochanter and the proximal femur.
- Although sepsis was randomly reported in the majority of studies, te Stroet et al. [5] demonstrated 21% of septic stem loosening.

35.2 Case Title: Re-revision Cement in Cement THA with a Long Exeter Stem and PLAD

E. Kenanidis and E. Tsiridis

The preoperative radiograph (Fig. 35.1) demonstrates a loose cemented stem and socket. Blade plate was used distally for a previous distal

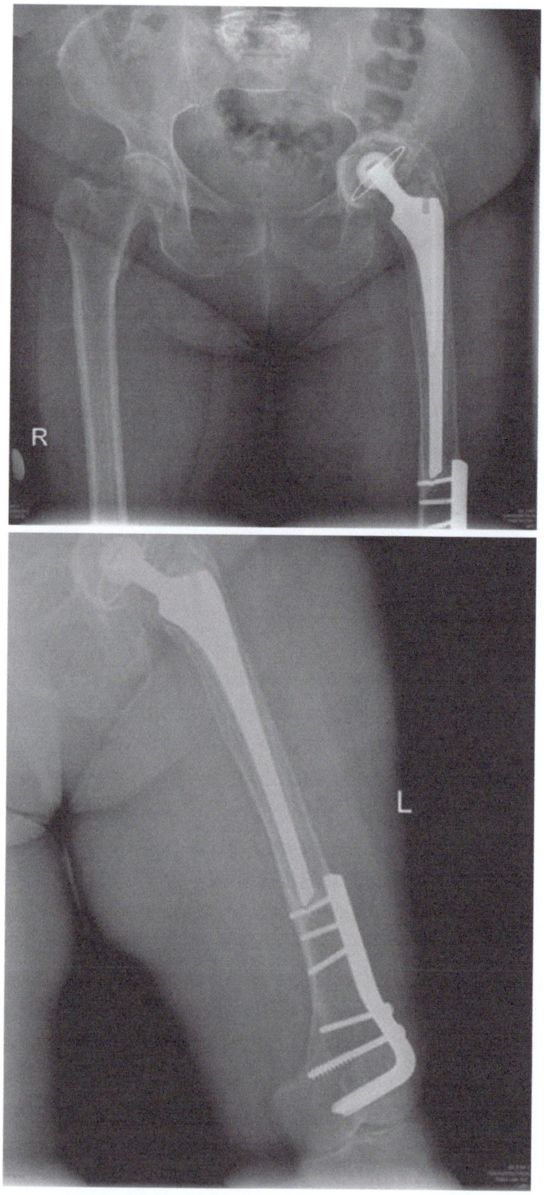

Fig. 35.1 Preoperative AP and lateral radiograph depict a loose cemented stem and socket and a blade plate for a previous distal femoral fracture

femoral fracture. The stem, in particular, has subsided into the canal and the cement mantle causing fracture of the cement in places and breakage of the top screw of the blade plate. Revision of the socket to a cemented implant was combined with a PLAD device to protect against dislocation. The stem was revised to a long Exeter stem by re-cementing the femoral canal and reaching the upper half of the blade plate (Fig. 35.2).

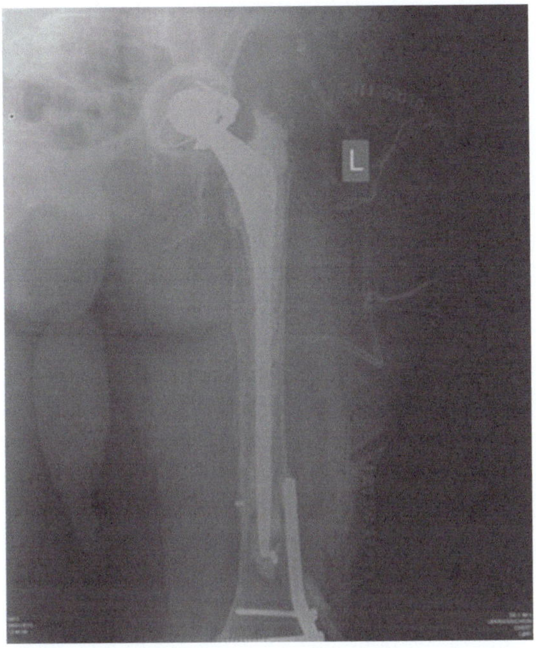

Fig. 35.2 Postoperative x-ray of the first day demonstrating the cemented revision socket with a PLAD and femoral re-cementation with the long Exeter stem

35.3 Case Title: Femoral Revision Using a 'Cement in Cement' Technique

M. Shahid and A.R.J. Manktelow

35.3.1 Demographics

Age: 77
Sex: F

35.3.2 Relevant Past Medical History

Principal pathologies: HTN, hypothyroidism, CVA, epilepsy

Previous surgical procedures: Right THR 1994, right TKR June 2009

Medication: Furosemide, thyroxine, atenolol, omeprazole, sodium valproate

History of presenting complaint: This 77-year-old relatively frail lady presented with right hip pain and the feeling that the hip was about to 'give way'. These symptoms had worsened over the previous six months. Before this, she could mobilize with a stick; however at the time of presentation, she had become wheelchair bound. The index operation was done in 1994 without any immediate complications.

35.3.3 Clinical Examination

Symptoms: Unable to bear weight on the right. Recurrent subluxation of the right hip.

Range of motion: Difficult to assess as patient was in a wheelchair and considerable pain.

Specific tests: CRP <5, WCC 5.3.

Main disability: Instability and pain

Neurovascular evaluation: No distal neurovascular deficit.

35.3.4 Preoperative Radiological Assessment/Imaging (Figs. 35.3 and 35.4)

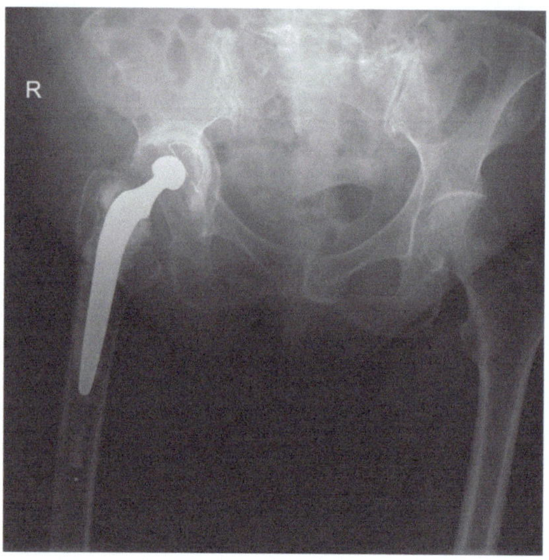

Fig. 35.3 AP radiograph showing proximal migration of the hip centre with associated ischial lysis, 'teardrop' lysis and medial migration, disrupting Kohler's line, making this a Paprosky type IIIB defect

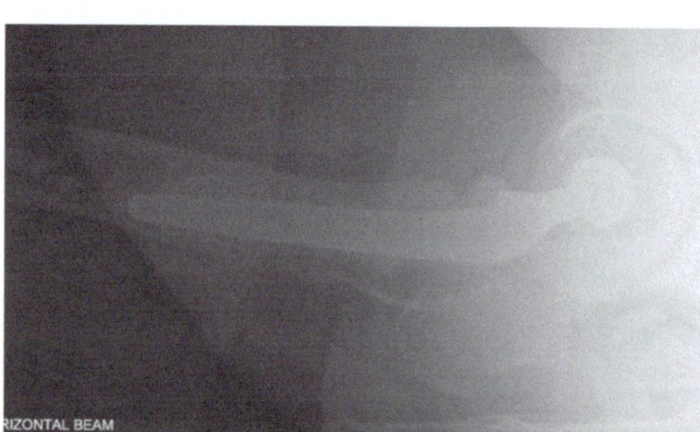

Fig. 35.4 Horizontal beam lateral showing a loose cup and stem

35.3.5 Preoperative Planning

Diagnosis: Right hip aseptic loosening and instability with associated acetabular bone loss (Figs. 35.3 and 35.4).

Chosen treatment method: Acetabular reconstruction with augmentation and femoral 'cement in cement' revision.

Selection of implants if applicable and rational: It is often helpful to obtain the operation note for the index procedure as part of the preoperative planning. This is less important in this case as both components require revision. In this case, the components were a monoblock Charnley stem with a 22.25 mm head and a cemented high-density polyethylene cup (HDPE).

Acetabulum: With regard to acetabular reconstruction, in addition to our standard instrumentation, we ensured the TMARS (Trabecular Metal Acetabular Revision System—Zimmer Biomet) was available. This system comprises a fully porous trabecular metal ™ revision shell, TM augments and buttresses, with the availability of the 'cup cage' construct. This provides the full inventory of options to deal with the bone loss predicted via the classification of the defect as well as any unexpected bone loss at surgery. A femoral head was ordered to use as allograft if required. The aim was to reconstruct the acetabulum with a hemispherical uncemented socket, with or without anteromedial trabecular metal augments.

Femur: On the femoral side, Exeter 44 stems, sizes 0, 1 and 2 stems alongside the 'short' 44 offset 125-mm Exeter stems, were arranged. This would allow a 'cement in cement' femoral revision. An uncemented modular femoral revision system (ARCOS—Zimmer Biomet) in this case was available. The OSCAR cement removal system was available in theatre as was the Midas Rex Burr. This would allow the cement mantle to be freshened or indeed removed if bone stock or the residual cement mantle was unsuitable for a 'cement in cement' revision. Similarly, equipment to do an extended trochanteric osteotomy (ETO), on the femoral side, was available if required.

Expected difficulties: (1) Potentially complex acetabular reconstruction. (2) Possibly poor femoral bone quality. (3) Loose femoral cement preventing any option for a 'cement in cement' femoral revision. (4) Potential for an intraoperative femoral fracture.

Strategies to overcome difficulties: (1) The versatility of the TMARS system to deal with more bone loss than anticipated. (2–4) An uncemented modular femoral revision system was available.

Templating: Using the TraumaCad® (Brainlab) system, we templated the acetabulum using the TMARS system and also the femoral side using both the ARCOS and Exeter systems (Figs. 35.5 and 35.6).

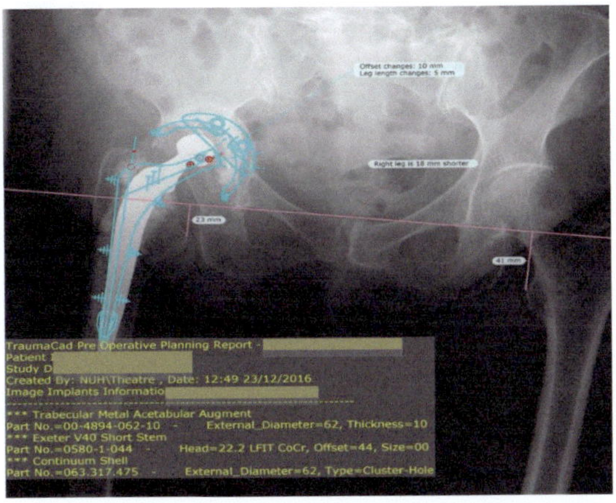

Fig. 35.5 Templating using the short Exeter 125 mm revision stem and the TMARS system, utilizing a 60 mm uncemented cup with peripheral rim contact/support and with trabecular metal augments positioned anteromedially to reconstitute integrity of the acetabulum

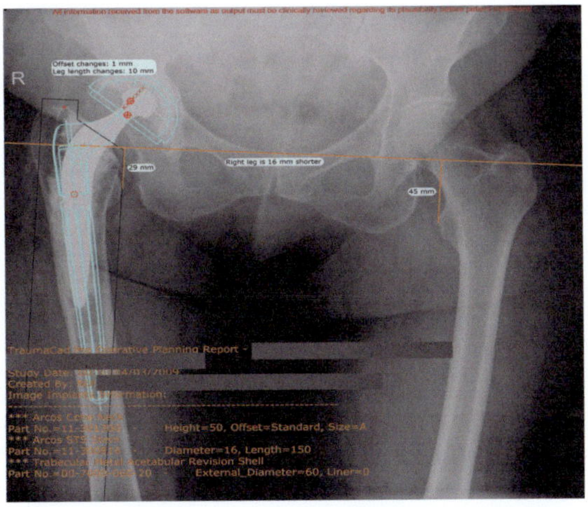

Fig. 35.6 Further templating showing an uncemented hemispherical socket and the ARCOS modular femoral revision system

35.3.6 Surgical Note

Patient's position: Patient was in the lateral position with pelvis positioned carefully and securely supported.

Type of anaesthesia: Spinal using heavy Marcaine and diamorphine. Antibiotics and tranexamic acid (1 g) were given at induction (flucloxacillin 2 g and gentamicin 200 mg).

Surgical approach: Posterior approach through the old incision.

Main steps: The existing scar was used and extended proximally and distally. The fascia lata was incised. The sciatic nerve was identified and protected. An aspiration of the hip joint was performed. The piriformis was incised, and then this, along with the short external rotators and capsule, was elevated as a single flap. The gluteus maximus insertion was incised to improve access and to prevent undue tension on the sciatic nerve. The hip was dislocated. The femoral component was reviewed. The stem was loose, so revision was mandatory. It also allowed us better acetabular exposure. A high-speed burr was used to remove cement from the shoulder of the implant. As this was a monoblock stem, it was removed from within the cement mantle. Some axial blows onto a 'punch' positioned beneath the femoral head were applied, and the stem was successfully extricated (an alternative method is shown when removing a modular femoral cement from within the cement mantle in Fig. 35.7). The cement mantle was then thoroughly examined. A scalpel blade was used to assess the cement–bone interface to ensure that the integrity was maintained (Fig. 35.8). The femoral canal was then packed with a 'mastoid' swab to keep it dry and prevent any debris from falling into the canal while working on the acetabulum (Fig. 35.9).

The socket was exposed with circumferential soft tissue release and with the femur transposed supero-anteriorly. Soft tissue samples were sent for microbiology. The existing polyethylene cup was loose. The component was removed initially using small curved osteotomes to loosen the implant–cement interface. Then the cement itself was cleared, with hand instruments and under direct vision, to reduce the possibility of

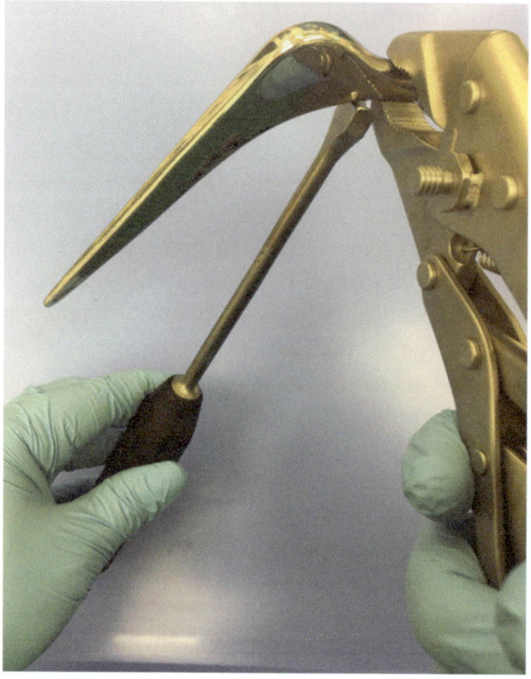

Fig. 35.7 When removing a modular cemented femoral component, a mole wrench can be secured beneath the trunnion, to support the neck of the implant. Then a punch is used to remove the stem impacting on the wrench 'jammed' beneath the trunnion

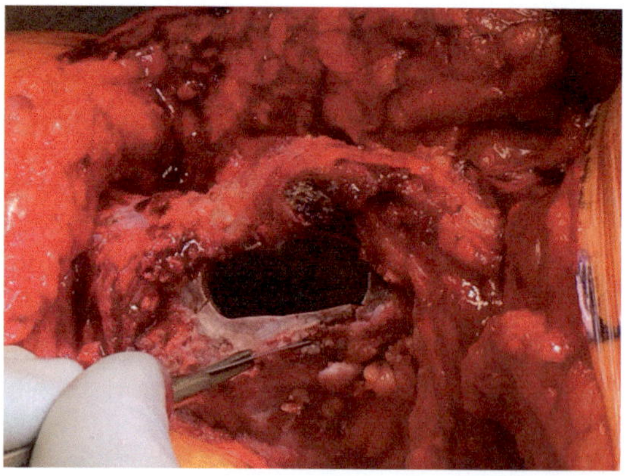

Fig. 35.8 A scalpel blade is used to check the cement–bone interface integrity

additional bone loss. Careful debridement of all membranous debris was performed. Small cement plugs in the acetabulum were removed,

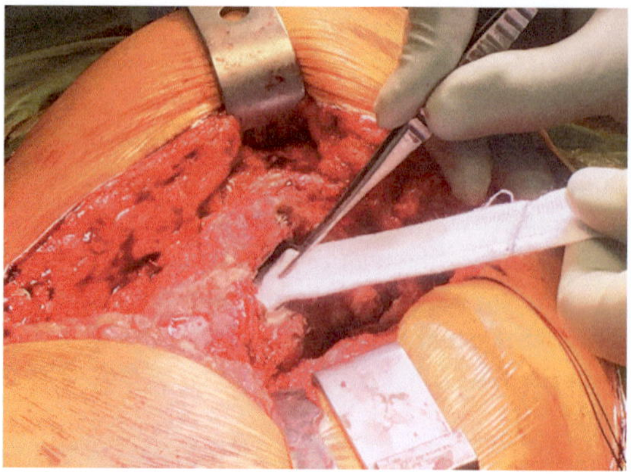

Fig. 35.9 A mastoid swab is inserted to protect the cement mantle to ensure no debris falls into the canal

again being careful to avoid additional bone loss.

Acetabular reconstruction: The acetabulum was reamed sequentially at the desired hip centre. Reamer size was progressively increased towards peripheral dimensions of the acetabulum. Care must be taken when reaming to not lose bone unnecessarily. In this case, we were able to ream sequentially until AP and SI dimensions were identical with some superior bone contact; however there remained an anterosuperior defect. We eventually reamed to 60 mm, and a trial for a 60 mm cup provided some peripheral contact. Two augments (62 × 10 mm and 58 × 10 mm) were then used both to reconstruct the anterosuperior defect and to reconstitute structural support for the hemispherical socket at the desired hip centre. We subsequently implanted the augments, with sound 'press fit' with a size 60 mm Trabecular Metal-Backed Modular Continuum 'Multi-hole' Cup (Zimmer Biomet). Four screws were inserted, with good 'hold', to enhance stability and facilitate early ingrowth. Using the alignment rod, we oriented the socket with 25° anteversion and at 45° inclination**.** A 36 mm highly crossed-linked polyethylene liner with a 15° postero-superior lip was inserted, with care taken to ensure the locking mechanism was engaged.

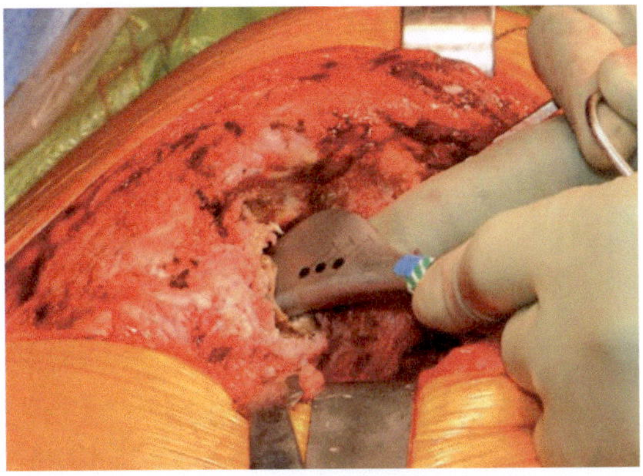

Fig. 35.10 The use of the 125 mm Exeter cement in cement revision stem allows the surgeon a degree of versatility regarding leg length and version to facilitate an accurate biomechanical reconstruction

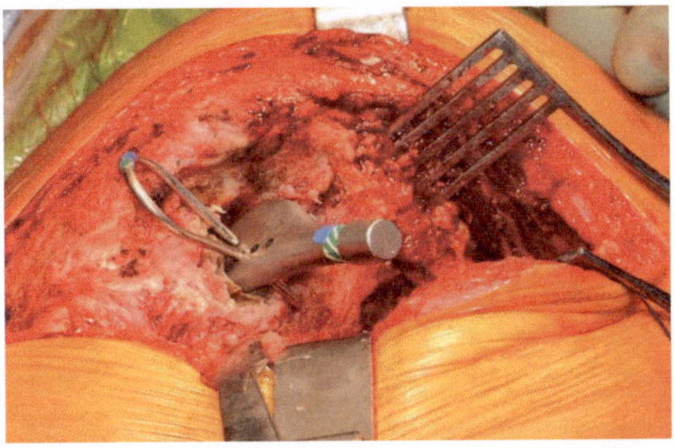

Fig. 35.11 The distal cement mantle can be modified, without disrupting the intact cement interface, with a burr or the specifically designed canal 'reamer'. A trial stem is shown, inserted with a pin, to identify the correct length and to stabilize the trial within the femur at that depth, to allow a trial reduction to be performed

Femoral reconstruction: Attention was now turned to the femur. The mastoid swab was removed from the canal. The cement mantle was scrutinised using a headlight shone down into the canal. The mantle was intact. The canal was lavaged to remove any debris. A trial reduction was done using the short 125 mm long, 44 mm offset Exeter stem, both to assess and identify length and version required and to ensure the stem would pass into the mantle readily (Figs. 35.10 and 35.11). Some surgeons prefer not to use a centralizer in this circumstance as it can prevent the actual stem going down the canal fully. The position of the stem, regarding length and version, after a satisfactory trail, was marked. We then prepared the cement mantle by washing with normal saline and drying with a clean mastoid swab. Cement was mixed and introduced early in a low viscosity state in a retrograde manner using a narrow nozzle. The stem was then inserted and positioned at the predetermined optimal height and correct version (Fig. 35.12).

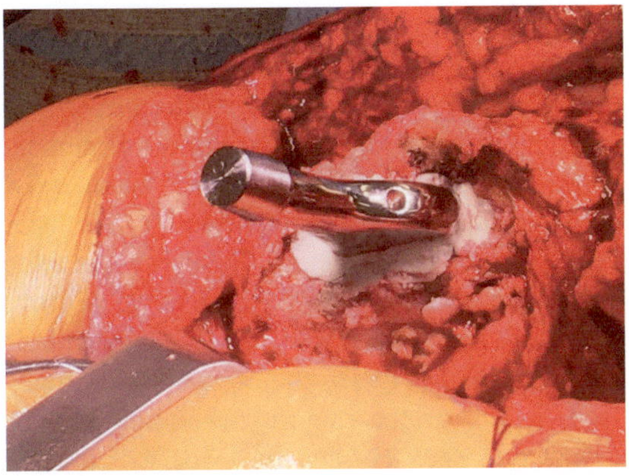

Fig. 35.12 The new cement in cement revision stem is shown after implantation

After trialling with various head options, the 36 mm 0 ceramic head (Biolox Delta, Stryker Orthopaedics) was the most stable and restored the biomechanics of hip. It is crucial to achieving sound soft tissue repair when closing the soft tissues. The short external rotators were attached with numerous Vicryl sutures. A drain was placed just underneath the fascia lata, which was closed with a PDS suture. Deep and superficial fat was closed with 1 and 2–0 Vicryl, respectively. Clips and a pressure dressing were applied.

35.3.7 Intraoperative Challenges

Challenges and solutions: Removal of the existing stem can be a challenge. A high-speed burr is used to remove all of the cement to clear the shoulder of the implant. A mole wrench can be used to support the neck of the implant to prevent torsional injury to the femur or cement mantle and subsequent fracture. Some axial blows are applied to the underneath of the taper of the stem using a punch. The cement mantle must then be thoroughly examined to remove any loose proximal fragments. A scalpel blade can be passed between the cement–bone interfaces to ensure the integrity is maintained. A new 2 mm neck cut can be made to trim any damaged bone at the neck and facilitate assessment of the cement–bone interface. The 'cement in cement' technique has been described and results published when the cement–bone interface is intact above the level of the lesser trochanter. The femoral canal is then packed with a mastoid swab to keep it dry and prevent any debris falling into while working on the acetabulum. To allow adjustment of the stem, the orientation and the internal geometry of the cement mantle can be modified using a high-speed burr, to remove some proximal cement. Similarly, it is possible to remove some of the distal cement to ensure there is room for a new centralizer. The stem is 'trialled' to ensure it fits into the canal and to achieve accurate biomechanical reconstruction. This is then removed, and the canal is lavaged and dried with a mastoid swab before cementing takes place. A cement gun with a narrow nozzle should be used in a retrograde fashion when the cement is of low viscosity. Pressurization is not as important as we are not aiming to fill the cement–bone interface.

35.3.8 Postoperative Radiographs (Figs. 35.13 and 35.14)

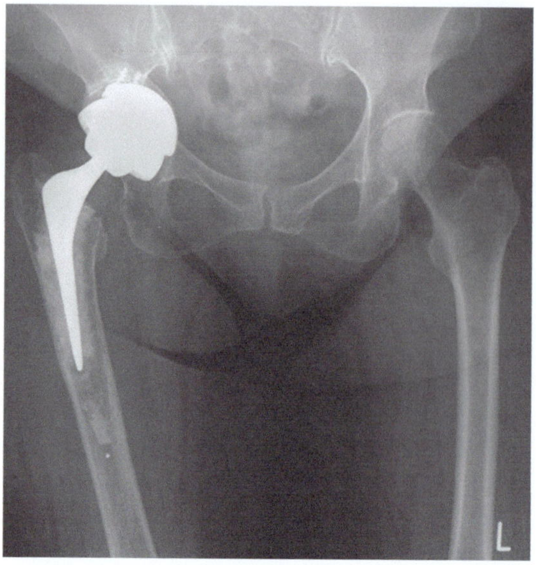

Fig. 35.13 AP pelvis post-surgery. Post acetabular reconstruction, the hip centre of rotation is restored. Whilst there is supero-inferior host bone contact, with the acetabular revision component, structural support has been enhanced with two TM augments. On the femoral side, a 'cement in cement' revision has facilitated accurate restoration of leg length and offset

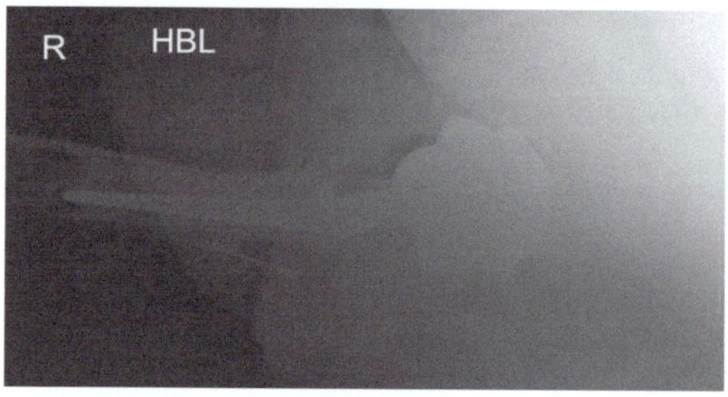

Fig. 35.14 Cross table lateral showing post-op reconstruction

35.3.9 Postoperative Management

Chemoprophylaxis and anticoagulant treatment period: Low molecular weight heparin for four weeks. We do not use mechanical thromboprophylaxis.

Gait/limb loading until full loading: 50% partial weight bearing for four weeks, and then weight bearing is tolerated. Postoperative radiographs were satisfactory (Figs. 35.13 and 35.14).

35.3.10 Follow-Up and Complications

No postoperative complications were reported. The surgery was performed six years before writing this report. The patient continues to mobilize comfortably, albeit with one stick for balance and support and with no clinical or radiological concern.

35.3.11 Discussion

The fixation of primary components for a cemented total hip replacement relies on the creation of a sound mechanical interlock between cement and the host bone. For this to be successful, a cavity lined by strong cancellous bone is created, and any blood and debris is removed. The cement is then 'pressurized' into that cancellous bone. At the time of any subsequent revision, the removal and exchange of the femoral component may be required. Reasons for this include better access to the acetabulum, adjustment of the femoral component position and, of course, most commonly loosening of the stem with or without cement–bone interface loosening. The removal of the cement mantle in a femoral revision can be a time-consuming process, with the potential for increased blood loss and with the risk of femoral perforation, fracture and the resulting loss of bone stock. To minimize these risks, there is the potential option to use a short cemented revision stem, re-cemented into the existing and intact cement mantle. As such, cementing the new prosthesis into the existing mantle allows a more straightforward revision of the femoral stem. This restores bone, permits early weight bearing and therefore enhances patient recovery [26].

A group from Cleveland challenged the rationale behind the necessity of removing a 'well-fixed' femoral cement mantle. They suggested cementing a new component into the existing well-fixed cement mantle. They found that when the old cement was prepared, by drying and rasping, the shear strength of subsequent cemented fixation was achieved that was 94% of that of a single block of cement [7].

The strength of the new cement is due to the formation of polymer chains across the PMMA interface between the old and new cement. This has been shown to have similar tensile and shear strength than a solid block of cement [26]. The Exeter group has been performing cement in cement revisions since 1989 for cases where the cement mantle appears well-fixed clinically and radiologically, down to the level of, but not extending below, the lesser trochanter. The main indications for this technique include improving access to the acetabulum during complex revision, exchanging a monoblock stem with a damaged head or a modular stem with a damaged or incompatible taper, version problems of the stem, leg length inequality, fractured implant and, in some circumstances, infection and periprosthetic fractures [4]. The selection criteria for this technique are that the existing cement mantle should be well-fixed to the host bone and of sound quality to support the new implant. Exclusion criteria include loose cement distal to the lesser trochanter and a loss of host bone or soft tissue 'membrane' in the cement–bone interface, indicating loosening at that interface. Results published in the literature have been favourable using this technique. One study reviewed 136 hips that had a 'cement in cement' revision. 5–15-year follow-up was reported at which time none needed re-revision for aseptic loosening [4]. These results were mirrored by an antipodean group who showed no femoral re-revisions at 12-year follow-up [24]. A recent review article collated a number of studies, encompassing 465 patients, and showed a femoral revision rate for aseptic loosening of 0.6% (3 of 465) [7].

It is imperative that the femoral canal is not contaminated with debris or blood and is dry before re-cementing. It has been shown that blood at the cement–cement interface reduced shear strength by 34% [7], and a drop in shear and tensile strength of over 80% in there was blood or marrow interposed [9]. In the case described, the 'cement in cement' technique was very useful. It allowed better exposure of the acetabulum to facilitate reconstruction, then the reimplantation of a new stem in a more favourable orientation, with a new modular trunnion, with a straightforward technique providing scope for reduced intraoperative time, blood loss and possible complications. In conclusion, 'cement in cement' fixation at the time of femoral revision is a well-established and evidence-based technique. Where a well-fixed existing cement mantle is present, above the level of the lesser trochanter, there is no need or requirement to remove this cement. In many circumstances, a 'cement in cement' revision is a viable option. This technique facilitates acetabular exposure and allows improvement in stem orientation. Studies have shown excellent results to make this a helpful part of a revision surgeon's armamentarium.

Referevnces

1. Holt G, Hook S, Hubble M. Revision total hip arthroplasty: the femoral side using cemented implants. Int Orthop. 2011;35:267–73.
2. Keeling P, Prendergast PJ, Lennon AB, Kenny PJ. Cement-in-cement revision hip arthroplasty: an analysis of clinical and biomechanical literature. Arch Orthop Trauma Surg. 2008;128:1193–9.
3. Marcos L, Buttaro M, Comba F, Piccaluga F. Femoral cement within cement technique in carefully selected aseptic revision arthroplasties. Int Orthop. 2009;33(3):633–7.
4. Duncan WW, Hubble MJW, Howell JR, et al. Revision of the cemented femoral stem using a cement-in-cement technique: a five- to 15-year review. J Bone Joint Surg Br. 2009;91(5):577.
5. te Stroet MAJ, Moret-Wever SG, de Kam DCJ, Gardeniers JWM, Schreurs BW. Cement-in-cement femoral revisions using a specially designed polished short revision stem; 24 consecutive stems followed for five to seven years. Hip Int. 2014;24(5):428–33.
6. Eftekhar NS, Demarest RJ. Principles of total hip arthroplasty. St Louis: Mosby; 1978.
7. Greenwald AS, Narten NC, Wilde AH. Points in the technique of recementing in the revision of an implant arthroplasty. J Bone Joint Surg Br. 1978;60-B:107–10.
8. McCallum JD 3rd, Hozack WJ. Recementing a femoral component into a stable cement mantle using ultrasonic tools. Clin Orthop. 1995;319:232–7.
9. Li PL, Ingle PJ, Dowell JK. Cement-within-cement revision hip arthroplasty; should it be done? A biomechanical study. J Bone Joint Surg Br. 1996;78:809–11.
10. Weinrauch P, Bell C, Wilson L, Goss B, Lutton C, Crawford R. Shear properties of bilaminar polymethylmethacrylate cement mantles in revision hip joint arthroplasty. J Arthroplasty. 2007;22:394–403.
11. Rudol G, Wilcox R, Jin Z, Tsiridis E. The effect of surface finish and interstitial fluid on the cement-in-cement interface in revision surgery of the hip. J Bone Joint Surg Br. 2011 Feb;93(2):188–93.
12. Hubble M, Patten A, Duncan W, Howell J, Timperley AJ, Gie G. Cement in cement femoral revision with the Exeter hip. J Bone Joint Surg Br. 2006;88-B(Supp)
13. Stefanovich-Lawbuary NS, Parry MC, Whitehouse MR, Blom AW. Cement in cement revision of the femoral component using a collarless triple taper: a midterm clinical and radiographic assessment. J Arthroplasty. 2014;29:2002–6.
14. Quinlan JF, O'Shea K, Doyle F, et al. In-cement technique for revision hip arthroplasty. J Bone Joint Surg Br. 2006;88(6):730.
15. Goto K, Kawanabe K, Akiyama H, Morimoto T, Nakamura T. Clinical and radiological evaluation of revision hip arthroplasty using the cement-incement technique. J Bone Joint Surg Br. 2008;90-B:1013–8.
16. Lieberman JR, Moeckel BH, Evans BG, et al. Cement-within-cement revision hip arthroplasty. J Bone Joint Surg Br. 1993;75(6):869.
17. Morley JR, Blake SM, Hubble MJ, et al. Preservation of the original femoral cement mantle during the management of infected cemented total hip replacement by two-stage revision. J Bone Joint Surg Br. 2012;94-B:322–7.
18. Nabors ED, Liebelt R, Mattingly DA, Bierbaum BE. Removal and reinsertion of cemented femoral components during acetabular revision. J Arthroplasty. 1996;11:146–52.
19. Briant-Evans TW, Veeramootoo D, Tsiridis E, Hubble MJW. Cement-in-cement stem revision for Vancouver type B peri-prosthetic femoral fractures after total hip arthroplasty. 3 year follow up of 23 cases. Acta Orthop. 2009;80(5):548–52.

20. Berstock JR, Torrie PAG, Smith JRA, Webb JC, Baker RP. Stem compatibility for cement-in-cement femoral revision: an in vitro study. Hip Int. 2014;24(5):434–41.
21. Leijtens B, Sadeghi N, Schreurs BW, Rijnen WH. Cement-within-cement revision of infected total hip replacement; disappointing results in 10 retrospective Cases. Hip Int. 2016;26(1):67–72.
22. O'Neill GK, Maheshwari R, Willis C, Meek D, Patil S. Fracture of an Exeter 'cement in cement' revision stem: a case report. Hip Int. 2011;21(5):627–9.
23. Rosenstein A, MacDonald W, Iliadis A, McLardy-Smith P. Revision of cemented Wxation and cement–bone interface strength. Proc Inst Mech Eng H. 1992;206:47–9.
24. Mandziak DG, Howie DW, Neale SD, MA MG. Cement-within-cement stem exchange using the collarless polished double-taper stem. J Arthroplasty. 2007;22(7):1000–6.
25. Holland JP, Weber FA. Cement within cement revision hip arthroplasty. A minimum 5 year follow- up study. Hip Int. 1998;8(3):129.
26. Westerman RW, Howell J. Fixation in femoral revision: the role of cement. Orthop Trauma. 2015;29(2): 131–9.

36 Uncemented Femoral Revision: Cylindrical Extensively Porous-Coated and Titanium Fluted Tapered Femoral Stems

Eustathios Kenanidis, Eleftherios Tsiridis, Stanislav Bondarenko, Volodymyr Filippenko, Volodymyr Mezentsev, Rashid Tikhilov, Alexey Denisov, Igor Shubnyakov, M. Ollivier, S. Parratte, X. Flecher, J.-N. Argenson, Sérgio Gonçalves, Thiago Aguiar, Pedro Dantas, Lionel E. Lazaro, Lazaros A. Poultsides, Micheal B. Cross, P.J. Boscainos, S. Patil, D. Meek, Libor Nečas, Marek Rovňák, Ivan De Martino, Peter K. Sculco, and Thomas P. Sculco

E. Kenanidis, M.D., Ph.D., M.Sc. (✉)
Academic Orthopaedic Unit, Aristotle University Medical School, Thessaloniki, Greece

E. Tsiridis, M.D., Ph.D., F.A.C.S., F.R.C.S. (✉)
Academic Orthopaedic Unit, Papageorgiou General Hospital, Aristotle University Medical School, Thessaloniki, Greece
e-mail: etsiridis@doctors.org.uk

S. Bondarenko, M.D., Ph.D. · V. Filippenko, M.D. · V. Mezentsev, M.D., Ph.D.
Department of Joint Pathology, Sytenko Institute of Spine and Joint Pathology, Kharkiv, Ukraine

R. Tikhilov, M.D., Ph.D. · A. Denisov, M.D., Ph.D. · I. Shubnyakov, M.D., Ph.D.
Vreden Russian Research Institute of Traumatology and Orthopedics, Saint Petersburg, Russia

M. Ollivier, M.D., Ph.D. · S. Parratte, M.D., Ph.D. · J.-N. Argenson, M.D., Ph.D.
Department of Orthopaedics and Traumatology, The Institute for Locomotion, Aix-Marseille University, Marseille, France
e-mail: jean-noel.argenson@ap-hm.fr

X. Flecher, M.D., Ph.D.
Department of Orthopaedics and Traumatology Unit, Hospital Nord, Marseille, France

Aix Marseille Univ, APHM, CNRS, ISM, Sainte-Marguerite Hospital, Institute for Locomotion, Marseille, France

S. Gonçalves, M.D., M.Sc. · T. Aguiar, M.D. · P. Dantas, M.D.
Hospital Curry Cabral, Lisbon, Portugal

L. E. Lazaro · L. A. Poultsides · M. B. Cross
I. De Martino, M.D. · P. K. Sculco, M.D.
T. P. Sculco, M.D.
Hospital for Special Surgery and Weill Cornell Medical College, New York, NY, USA
e-mail: LazaroL@hss.edu; PoultsidesL@hss.edu; CrossM@hss.edu; demartinoi@hss.edu; tpstkr@aol.com

P. J. Boscainos, M.D., F.R.C.S. · S. Patil, F.R.C.S. · D. Meek, B.Sc., M.D., F.R.C.S.
Department of Orthopaedic Surgery, Queen Elizabeth University Hospital, Glasgow, Scotland, UK
e-mail: p.boscainos@dundee.ac.uk; rmdmeek@doctors.org.uk

L. Nečas, M.D., Ph.D. · M. Rovňák, M.D.
Jessenius Faculty of Medicine, Comenius University in Bratislava, Martin, Slovakia
e-mail: necas@unm.sk

E. Tsiridis (ed.), *The Adult Hip - Master Case Series and Techniques*,
https://doi.org/10.1007/978-3-319-64177-5_36

36.1 Current Concepts

E. Kenanidis and E. Tsiridis

The aseptic loosening, infection, instability, periprosthetic fracture and component malposition are the major indications for femoral revision that is often complicated by bone loss [1]. A thorough preoperative evaluation including complete history, clinical examination and radiographic evaluation is critical for decision-making concerning the surgical approach, the femoral component removal and the reconstruction method [1].

The purpose of the femoral reconstruction is to achieve axial and rotational stability of the implant and restoration of hip biomechanics [2]. Historically uncemented revision arthroplasty demonstrated better results than cemented, and it is preferred when it is possible [3, 4]. During the last years, however, cemented femoral revision proved its efficacy in type I and II defects too.

36.1.1 Femoral Bone Loss Classification

The type of femoral bone loss is crucial for the choice of reconstruction. There are several classification systems, the most known of them, however, are the Paprosky [5] and AAOS classification [6].

1. Paprosky classification [5]

   This classification is more useful and offers a more objective assessment. It is based on [1, 5]:
   (a) The location of femoral bone loss (metaphyseal or diaphyseal)
   (b) The degree of the remaining support of the proximal femur (i.e. the degree of cancellous bone loss)
   (c) The amount of isthmus remaining for diaphyseal fixation

There are four types [1, 5]:

Type I: Minimal proximal metaphyseal bone loss:

- The proximal metaphysis and diaphysis are intact.
- There is no proximal remodelling.
- Treatment options are standard length cemented or uncemented implants.

Type II: Moderate to severe proximal metaphyseal bone loss:

- This is the most common type [1]
- The proximal metaphysis is absent.
- The diaphysis is intact.
- There is slight proximal remodelling.
- Treatment options are extensively porous-coated implants or cemented implants.

Type III: Metadiaphyseal bone defects. It has two subtypes.

Type IIIA: Severe proximal metaphyseal bone loss with partly intact diaphysis:

- The proximal metaphysis is absent.
- The diaphysis has >4 cm of isthmus for distal fixation.
- There is significant proximal remodelling.
- Treatment options include extensively porous-coated implants if the femoral medullary diameter <19 mm or modular tapered stem if the diameter >19 mm.

Type IIIB: Severe proximal metaphyseal bone loss with partly intact diaphysis:

- The proximal metaphysis is absent.
- The diaphysis has <4 cm of isthmus for distal fixation.
- There is significant proximal remodelling.
- Treatment options include (1) modular tapered stem (corundumized tapered stems with splines/flutes around the tapered stem that confer rotational stability of the implant with only 1–2 cm of diaphyseal bone contact [1]), and (2) impaction bone grafting.

Type IV: Complete loss of metaphyseal and diaphyseal bone:

- Biological fixation is usually impossible.
- The proximal metaphysis is absent.
- The diaphysis has no bone stock too.
- There is slight proximal remodelling.
- Treatment options [1, 2]: (1) allograft-prosthetic composite (APC), (2) a long

cemented stem, (3) impaction grafting with a long cemented femoral component and (4) proximal femoral replacement.

36.1.2 Cylindrical Extensively Porous-Coated Femoral Stems

These stems remain the gold standard for most femoral revisions THA [7–10]. They are cylindrical stems made of cobalt-chrome; its porous coating consists of sintered beads that provide the initial friction interference fit and an ongrowth surface for eventual biologic fixation [2].

This reconstruction method bypasses the bone deficiency completely and obtains stability through distal diaphyseal fixation (minimum 5–7 cm) [9]. It provides [7]:

1. Initial axial stability with several cms of diaphyseal scratch (frictional scratch fit)
2. Rotational stability through three-point collar contact in metaphysis and diaphysis (no use in ETO)

36.1.2.1 Indications of Use/ Prerequisites

- Type I and II Paprosky femoral defects [1]
- Type III Paprosky femoral defects with medullary canal <19 mm [11]
- 5–7 cm of remaining diaphyseal bone for distal fixation [7, 9]

36.1.2.2 Contraindications

- Acute infection [7]
- Less than 5–7 cm of distal diaphyseal cortical supporting bone [7]
- Type III Paprosky femoral defects with medullary canal >19 mm [11]

36.1.2.3 Preoperative Planning [7]

- Take full AP and lateral X-rays.
- Template accurately to select the shortest stem that bypasses the deficiency and has 5–7 cm of distal fixation and the diameter for endosteal contact [9].
- Template the combination of the seating level and neck-head segment required to restore the leg length and appropriate hip offset.
- Determine that the stem fits well the proximal femur and canal in the AP X-ray.
- Determine also that the stem fits well in the lateral X-ray; if not, there is possibility of anterior femoral perforation, and a bowed stem may be needed [9, 10].

36.1.2.4 Surgical Technique

- You will need an adequate exposure to remove the existing implant and cement, and properly prepare the femur for the new stem implant; this is critical because osseointegration is the ultimate goal [1, 9].
- Remember that following a previous failure, the femur tends to have varus and extension remodelling [1].
- In any case that there is considerable bony deformity or any obstruction to the direct access for cement removal or reaming, ETO is favoured [1, 9].
- Ream precisely and carefully to ensure maximum contact between the bone and porous coating on the prosthesis and to avoid femoral fracture and perforation; if any doubt exists, take intraoperative radiographs [1, 9].
- Prepare the femur 0.5 mm undersized. An implant 0.5 mm larger than the last reamer is chosen [10].
- Insert the stem steadily in the femur; there must be a steady progression of insertion with each tap on the component. If the stem does not progress with impaction, remove it, and prepare the canal line to line to avoid femoral fracture [7, 9].
- Establish the desired version carefully and early in the impaction process to prevent a fracture because the stem achieves increasing rotational stability as it further enters the canal [9]. Especially for bowed stems, there is a limited independent adjustment of the femoral anteversion and increase the rate of postoperative instability [7, 8].
- For the majority of revisions. a standard 6-in. stem in the majority of femoral revisions (Paprosky types I and II) is usually needed [10].

36.1.2.5 Postoperative Care

- Partial weight bearing for six weeks followed by full depending on the fixation

- In case of fracture or ETO used at least six weeks no weight bearing

36.1.2.6 Advantages

- Follow the same uncemented principles as in other primary techniques that are familiar to all surgeons [9]
- Feasible to the majority of femoral revisions [1, 7]
- Good long-term results in the majority of studies [7–9, 11–25]

36.1.2.7 Disadvantages

- No use in the type III defects with canals >19 mm in diameter and type IV defects [11].
- Bypass of the defect will produce proximal stress shielding and no encouragement of regeneration of proximal bone stock [7, 9].
- Need for greater exposure or ETO.
- Increased risk of complications as femoral fracture, perforations and stem fracture [7–9, 11–25].

36.1.2.8 Reported Results

Several cohort studies are available [7–9, 11–25]. These case series are comprised of 35–905 patients. They range in mean follow-up from 3.3 to 15 years. A substantial number of cohorts follow patients for more than ten years [7–9, 12–14, 17, 19, 22]. The reported survival rate ranged from 89 to 100% in these studies. Several favourable studies reported excellent long-term results in independent clinical centres worldwide (>90% after ten years) [7–9, 11–25]. These studies do provide sufficient data to predict the long-term outcomes of the technique.

Paprosky et al. [12] reported the follow-up of 170 patients that were treated with extensively coated cementless revision femoral components. At a mean of 13.2 years, survival rate greater than 95% was reported. The overall mechanical failure rate was 4.1%. The stress shielding was greatest in patients with stems larger than 16.5 mm and osteoporotic bone (Dorr type C). Nine percent of the patients had significant thigh pain. Weeden et al. [13] reported the results of 170 revisions with at a mean of 14.2 years postoperatively; half of them were type IIIA. The overall mechanical failure rate was 4.1%. There was a high rate of failure (21%) with worsening bone loss (type IIIB), and the intraoperative fracture rate was 8.8%.

Sporer et al. [11] demonstrated that the efficacy of fully coated uncemented porous stems in femoral revision of type III defects is dependent of the femoral canal diameter. He found no mechanical failure at IIIB type of failure with femoral canal diameter <19 mm but 18% mechanical failure in IIIB with canal >19 mm and 38% in type IV femoral defects. The authors supported no use of the technique in these types.

In one of the greatest series, Engh et al. [7] showed 95.8% survival rate for 777 femoral revisions with these implants. In another study, Engh et al. [8] also reported that the survival of ≥190 mm fully porous-coated stems in 34 patients with extensive bone loss was 89% at ten years. Hamilton et al. [14] reported 95.9% survival rate for 905 revisions at ten years, whether Thomsen [19] published 18 years cumulative survival, free of re-revision for any reason of 94.4% and aseptic loosening 97.6%.

Egan et al. [16] demonstrated three categories of intraoperative complications, eccentric reaming, femoral perforation and femoral fracture in the revision arthroplasty of 135 patients with fully porous-coated stems. The stem length and diameter and the host bone quality affected the complication rate. Femoral perforations and fractures were more common with stems longer than 200 mm, diameter ≥ 18 mm and poorer-quality host bone.

Garcia Cimbrelo et al. [17] reported excellent survival rate 96.9% at ten years in 114 femoral revisions with fully coated uncemented stems; although the clinical relevance is uncertain, progressive stress shielding of the lateral cortex and thickening of the medial one were noticed, which was greater in patients with ETO and stems <25 cm.

36.1.2.9 Complications

1. Postoperative dislocation/instability
   This is attributed to the LLD or inappropriate anteversion of the stem following revision THA [7, 21].
2. Intraoperative fracture
   This is one of the most common complications following forceful impaction of a too large or too long stem. It is prevented by the precise surgical technique, the use of intraoperative radiographs and experience [7, 8, 19]. Egan et al. [16] in his series reported 20% intraoperative fracture due to the increasing femoral diameter, length and poor bone quality.

3. Femoral perforation
   This complication can be prevented by obtaining intraoperative radiographs. It involves anterior perforations usually resulting from drilling too far down a curved femur with a straight drill or lateral perforations caused by the incomplete cement removal [7, 19].
4. Stress shielding
   It is associated with the bypass of a femoral defect with a long uncemented stem [19]. Its clinical relevance, however, is debated. Garcia Cimbrelo et al. [17] in his series demonstrated a progressive stress shielding that was not related to survival. Fukui et al. [22] did not also correlate stress shielding with ten-years survival.
5. Stem fracture
   Busch et al. [18] in a series of 219 patients reported 2.3% stem fracture. The factors associated with fracture of the stem were the poor proximal bone support (type III–IV; $p = 0.001$), a BMI >30; ($p = 0.014$), a smaller diameter of the stem (<13.5 mm; $p = 0.007$) and the use of an ETO ($p = 0.028$).
6. Non-union of the trochanteric osteotomy site.
7. Thigh pain [12, 21].

36.1.3 Titanium Fluted Tapered Stems (TFTS)

The use of this type of femoral reconstruction is steadily increasing in the setting of advanced bone loss [1]. TFTS have the same principle as the extensively porous-coated stems. In case of limited proximal bone, the stem bypasses the bone deficiency and achieves diaphyseal fixation for primary stability [2, 26, 27].

They provide axial and rotational stability. The distal fixation is guaranteed by the taper, with a conical wedge geometry impacted into a matching conically milled diaphysis, while rotational stability is provided by longitudinal ridges, the flutes that engage endosteal bone [2]. Compared with the extensively porous-coated stems that usually need 5–7 cm of diaphyseal fixation, the tapered stems may gain axial and rotational stability over a smaller distance and may favour osseointegration in more compromised diaphyseal bone [1, 2].

There are two types of uncemented taper conical stems:

1. Non-modular
2. Modular

Good midterm clinical results and excellent survivorship have been reported for both types [28, 29]. Non-modular TFTS also have long-term results [30]. To achieve however these results, a good surgical technique is mandatory. They have also been widely and effectively used for the management of periprosthetic fractures [31–35]. In contrast with extensively coated stems that are strongly associated with stress shielding, tapered fluted stems prevent or even augment the proximal bone stock [36–38]. Titanium alloy has a stiffness closer to that of cortical bone than cobalt-chrome. The conical design produces a more even load transfer to the surrounding bone which prevents bone resorption and even contributes to the reconstitution of femoral bone stock. Rodriguez et al. [26] reported bony reconstitution in 75% of 71 femoral revisions with tapered fluted stems; the remaining 21% showed diaphyseal stress shielding.

TFTS are contraindicated in case of severe damage of the isthmus (Paprosky Type IV), infection or the presence of distal femoral stems (i.e., due to previous TKA) [1, 2].

36.1.4 Non-modular Monoblock Tapered Stems

The principle of use of this type of TFTS requires the bypass of the diaphyseal femoral deficiency by at least six cm of distal fixation [1, 2]. Monoblock titanium tapered stems are straight and engage the diaphysis with three-point fixation [2]. The initial stability is diaphyseal:

1. The axial stability is achieved through the conical wedge geometry impacted into a matching tapered cone that is prepared in the femoral canal [2].
2. The rotational stability is reached through the cutting flutes that engaged the endosteal bone [2].

Compared with modular tapered fluted stems the non-modular TFTS:

1. They have difficulties in the proper component position and the restoration of hip biomechanics [1].
2. Due to the inexistence of the modular junction, however, they are not related to the increased risk of stem fracture, fretting corrosion, metallosis and resultant osteolysis [39].

The Wagner stem was the first titanium monoblock tapered stem reported in 1987 [40]. It has eight longitudinal ridges, a 2° taper rough finish surface made of grit-blasted titanium that promotes bone ongrowth and long-term biologic fixation [2]. Kirk et al. [41] demonstrated superior axial and torsional load resistance compared to cylindrical stems.

A recent systematic review [42] of the non-modular tapered titanium fluted stems demonstrated excellent long-term survival rates of 92–98% of the Wagner SL stem at 9- to 16-year follow-up [30, 36, 37, 42, 43]. There was a restoration of the proximal femur in 63–97% [30, 36, 42, 43].

36.1.4.1 Complications

There are no reported fractures of non-modular fluted tapered stems [42]. The main complications are:

1. Subsidence
2. Dislocation
3. Intraoperative fractures

The incidence of these complications usually ranged from 2 to 5% [42]. A subsidence of >10 mm, however, may be the reason for instability with some requiring re-revision. It is attributed possibly to the learning curve of the technique, accurate sizing, new stem design with a 2° taper and inability to make leg length adjustments [2, 30, 43–45]. Isacson et al. [45] reported 12% subsidence greater than 20 mm and 52% subsidence <5 mm in forty three hips revised with Wagner stem; there were also nine dislocations. Gutierrez del Alamo et al. also published eleven dislocations with subsidence out of seventy nine revised femurs with this stem [37].

Intraoperative femoral fractures are considered less common in TFTS than in cylindrical extensively porous-coated stems. They usually involve the greater trochanter or osteotomy fragment and do not affect the implant choice or clinical outcome. Mantelos et al. [43], however, reported 15.8% of intraoperative fractures in his series of ninety five revisions with the Wagner stem.

36.1.5 Titanium Modular Fluted Tapered Stems (TMFT)

The modular fluted tapered stems maintain the fluted tapered design but also demonstrate proximal modularity. TMFT have two parts, a distal tapered fluted part and a proximal modular body [46]. This seems favourable as it deals with the two main problems of fixation separately.

The fluted tapered part of the construct is used for the distal fixation (initial fixation, axial and rotational) [1]. Their stability is achieved through implant wedging into the remaining diaphysis to obtain circumferential contact with the endosteal bone. Further axial loading results in subsequent endosteal engagement, greater stem-diaphyseal diametric mismatch and a resultant increase in circumferential compression of the implant, providing the initial axial and rotational stability [1, 2]. The appropriate oversizing of the implant helps to achieve the initial femoral endosteal-stem diametric mismatch and is crucial for the primary implant axial stability. The longer stems particularly have a 3° anterior taper to accommodate the femoral bow and provide more canal fillings and reduce subsidence [2].

The proximal part gives more options to restore the length, offset and version [1]. This theoretical benefit of the modular tapered stems restores the hip biomechanics and gives possibly better outcomes and stability [1, 2]. Modularity, however, is related to risk of stem fracture at the Morse taper, fretting corrosion, metallosis and resultant osteolysis [1, 28, 42, 47].

They are used for moderate to severe bone loss (types IIIA/IIIB and IV) to achieve lasting fixation [1]. When the femoral canal, however, exceeds the diameter of the largest tapered implant (31 mm) or the implant-cortical contact area is less than 2 cm other techniques as impaction grafting, APC or PFR are more effective [2]. They can also be used in periprosthetic fractures or varus remodelling where there are difficulties in monoblock stem introduction [33].

36.1.5.1 Published Results

Several retrospectives and prospective cohort studies of TMFT stems demonstrate excellent results at short to midterm follow-up in revision THA even with severe femoral bone loss [26–28, 46, 48–59]. The sample size of studies ranges from 18 to 136 patients with a mean follow-up ranging from one to ten years. Consistent good results for overall survival 85–97%, with the majority of them >90%, are reported [26, 27, 46, 48–59]. In one of the longest follow-up studies, Rodriguez et al. [26] retrospectively reviewed seventy femoral revisions for major bone loss (greater than IIIA) with TMFT. Survival for any reason was 88.55% and for aseptic 98.4%.There are also two comparative functional studies [27, 49] favouring titanium modular tapered stems against extensively porous-coated stems and a retrospective comparative between the tapered and cylindrical fluted stems favouring the tapered [48].Richards et al. [27] reported superior quality of life in patients with tapered, fluted, modular titanium femoral components compared with extensively porous-coated cylindrical non-modular cobalt-chrome stems in revision arthroplasty; TMFT stems were used in cases with a more severe femoral bone loss. Patients treated with TMFT stems had better clinical outcome scores, fewer intraoperative fractures and better restoration of the proximal femoral host bone. Garbuz et al. [49] also compared 220 TMFT and CNCC stems and demonstrated better quality of life for TMFT patients; this was attributed to the restored hip biomechanics with TMFT following the modularity and reduced stiffness of titanium. The revision THA study group [48] retrospectively compared titanium modular tapered stems versus cylindrical modular in the management of Paprosky III and IV defects and found that the failure rate for component osseointegration was 1.6% in the tapered and 15.9% in the cylindrical group ($p < 0.01$). The femoral component re-revision rate for any reason was 4.9% in the tapered and 22.7% in the cylindrical group ($p = 0.013$) at a mean of 5-year follow-up.

36.1.5.2 Complications

The most commonly reported complications are the following:

1. Dislocation
   Despite the obvious advantages in the use of modularity, the rate of instability in different studies ranges from 3 to19% [50, 52–54, 56, 57, 59] which is comparable to other studies with non-modular tapered stems or cylindrical stems. Amanatullah et al. [52] reported 19% dislocation rate in 92 patients treated with TMFT for severe bone loss (type III/IV) at a mean of 6.4 years postoperatively. Other simultaneous existing factors as the multiply operated patient with possible abductor deficiency, severe bone deficiencies and subsequently compromised soft tissue make it unclear if a modular stem decreases the risk of dislocation. Comparative studies are needed.
2. Intraoperative femoral fractures
   These are considered to be less frequent than in cylindrical extensively porous-coated stems [34, 43]. Usually it involves the greater trochanter or osteotomy fragment and does not affect the implant choice or clinical outcome. The usual reported rate of fractures is between 3 and 6% [50, 56]; in certain studies, however, the rate is also high [54, 59]. Wang et al. [59] reported 17% intraoperative fracture rate for fifty eight femoral revisions with TMFT.
3. Stress shielding
   It is less common because titanium alloy has stiffness closer to that of the cortical bone than cobalt-chrome 34. The conical design produces a more even load transfer to the surrounding bone which prevents bone resorption and even contributes to reconstitution of femoral bone

stock. In TMFT stems stress shielding can occur in longer follow-up and for large diameter stems [26, 52]. Rodriguez et al. [26] reported a 21% rate of stress shielding in TMFT stems with a mean 10-year follow-up and only in stems larger than 18 mm in diameter. Amanatullah et al. [52] reported 22% rate of stress shielding on ninety two patients with a single TMFT design at a mean of 6.4 years postoperatively.

4. Subsidence
   It was considered to be a less common complication with TMFT [50, 54, 60] than monoblock tapered stems. Rodriguez et al. [26] published 2.8% of >5 mm subsidence and supported that this was attributed to the intraoperative use of C-arm, the particular stem design with 3-degree bow and the surface roughness of the stem. Recently, however, Tangsataporn et al. [55] reported significant subsidence (>10 mm) in 14% of stems with 6% requiring revision due to subsidence at one year. This complication occurred most often in the overweight patients >80 kg and those with the minimal isthmic support with less than two cm of stem-cortex contact.
5. Fracture/failure at the modular junction
   This is a serious complication of modularity resulting of fretting corrosion, wear debris generation and ultimately fracture of the stem. In earlier designs of TFMT, reports of junction fracture ranged from 1 to 18% [26, 42, 47, 56]. Increased fracture rates were considered the result of small diameter taper junction in one design, which has since been modified. Van Houwelingen et al. [28] reported also 18% fractures (5/27, ZMR design, Zimmer Warsaw) that was correlated to increased BMI, ETO and small stem diameters (this junction has been modified, ZMR extra-large (XL)).

36.2 Case Title: Re-revision Left Femoral Implant. Failed Monolithic Fully Coated Straight Stem Through Breakage of the Stem and Periprosthetic Femoral Fracture. Re-revision to a Modular Anatomically Conical Fully Coated Stem for a Paprosky 3B Femur

E. Kenanidis and E. Tsiridis

36.2.1 Demographics

Age: 48
Sex: Male
BMI: 35

36.2.2 Relevant Past Medical History

Principal pathologies: Diabetes type II, obesity and failure of revision surgery performed five years back due to a recent fall

Previous surgical procedures: Left hip THA (twenty one years ago) for DDH Hartofylakidis type I, failure of the prosthesis and revision five years back to a monolithic fully coated stem and a tantalum coated socket and ceramic head (Figs. 36.1 and 36.2)

Medication: Metformin

History of presenting complaint: Pain from implant loosening and fracture. Patient unable to walk, shortened limb by 2 cm

36.2.3 Clinical Examination

Symptoms: Pain and shortening due to periprosthetic fracture

Range of motion: Unable to check ROM due to fracture

Main disability: Shortening fracture, implant failure and needing revision

Scoring if available: HHS<70

Neurovascular evaluation: Intact

36.2.4 Preoperative Radiological Assessment/Imaging (Figs. 36.1, 36.2, and 36.3)

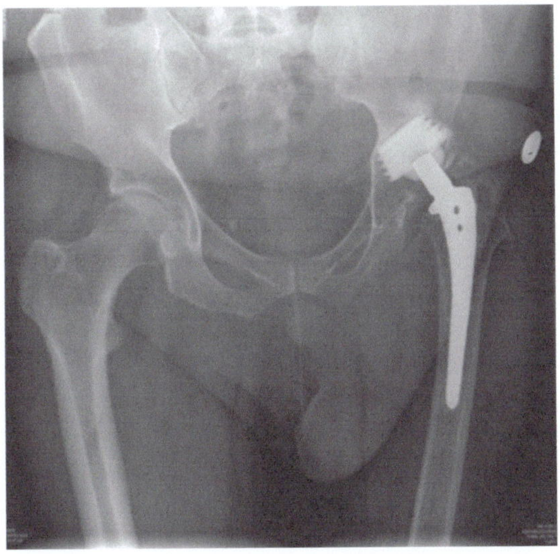

Fig. 36.1 AP pelvic x-ray demonstrating a loose acetabular implant with extensive erosion of the socket almost reaching the sacroiliac joint on the left. This is a screw type of socket design with a ceramic on polyethylene articulation. There is an extensive bone loss below the bottom of the acetabular component reaching the teardrop area and the ischium. There is significant weakening and sclerosis of the inner plate of the acetabulum with mild protrusion deformity. The taper of this prosthesis is not compatible with the current designs; thus, a revision of the stem was deemed necessary. The original radiographic evaluation shows a stem that was very well fitted with a scalloping at the tip of prosthesis indicating extensive osseointegration of the cortical bone to the metal. This is usually the most difficult part of the operation, i.e. to mobilize the distal end of such prosthesis. In addition, the prosthesis proximally is roughly designed with metal scalloping and edges as well as two round holes proximally for bone integration. Such prostheses integrate very well with the bone, and it is very challenging to be removed. Observing the contralateral side, this is a typical Dorr A type femur that may explain the size selection. It is important to know, however, that small stem may fail under a load of a tall overweight male

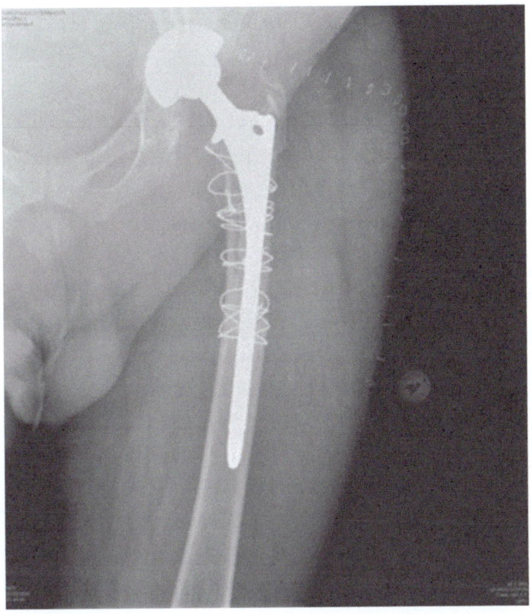

Fig. 36.2 Long ETO to remove the implant turning the femur to a Paprosky 3A and cerclage wires to reconstruct it. Index revision succeeded through a well-fitted acetabular tantalum coated shell with poly and ceramic bearings. The stem was a solid monolithic AML stem (DePuy) fitting well the diaphysis (Dorr A) however looking small in the radiograph

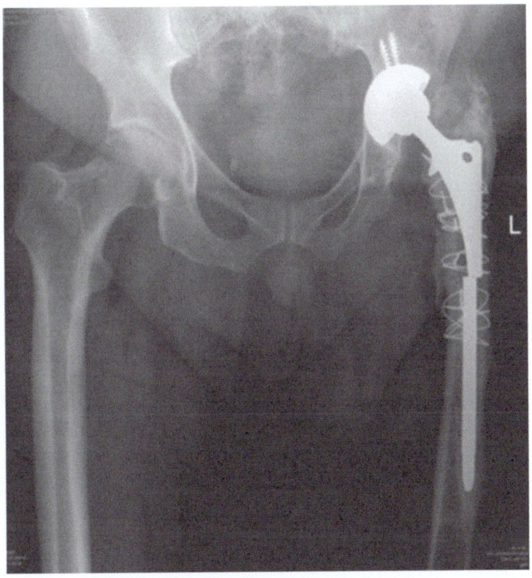

Fig. 36.3 Five years post-op failure of the implant via breakage of stem and a periprosthetic fracture. Evidence of lateral wall scalloping due to chronic cantilevering of the stem into the femur. ETO has healed well

36.2.5 Preoperative Planning

Diagnosis: Re-revision. Removing the broken implant may be a challenge, but the fracture side will work as a ready window to push it upwards. Bowing of the femur is, however, a problem. The distal stem fragment appears to be loose (Fig. 36.3).

Possible treatment options: Uncemented modular stem with the conical bowed distal end is indicated to secure fit into the diaphysis.

Chosen treatment method: Cone conical fluted anatomical modular stem fully grit-blasted surface—"Wagner type" distal end (Restoration Revision Stem Stryker).

Selection of implants if applicable and rational: Better stability and version flexibility proximally to compensate for the Paprosky 3B bone distortion.

Expected difficulties: Straitening the femur may cause a further fracture. Fitting the new stem with some extra cortical reaming. The original femur was type Dorr A with a long and narrow diaphysis.

Strategies to overcome difficulties: Prepare for an intraoperative periprosthetic fracture.

Templating: Modular restoration: cone body 21/132/STD offset conical distal stem 195 mm, bowed.

36.2.6 Surgical Note

With the patient in lateral decubitus position and an extensive posterior approach through the old scar, the hip was exposed. Care was taken to recognize the sciatic nerve starting from the insertion of the gluteus maximus to the back of the femur and going north to the quadratus femoris muscle chasing up the nerve to the top of the greater trochanter. Freeing the sciatic nerve from adhesions and tagging it using elastic vascular bands helped us to approach the hip and the fracture site safely. The incision chased the fracture, and from that point onwards, the femur was approached both proximally and distal at the mid-diaphysis. Exposure of the joint was easy as well dislocating the hip. The proximal fragment of the stem came out with some effort as the bowing of the proximal femur prohibited its dislocation. The distal fragment of the stem came out from the fracture site with no difficulty. The femur was then reduced using wires over a 4.5 mm broad locking plate to create a tube for the reaming. Reaming was a challenge as the old stem had created a calcified truck leading to the lateral cortex especially close to the tip. To overcome this problem, a window was opened distally to directly visualize the mal-trucking. The endosteum reamed carefully, and a speed burr was used to ease down the scalloping of the lateral track. The canal was patent, and the distal flexible reamer went in easily reaming against the wall as planned for good fitting. Reaming followed gradually up to bone-rattling against the reamer at 21 mm diameter and a 195 mm bowed distal conical stem of 22 mm inserted tightly bypassing the fracture site by at least two ipsilateral femoral diameters. The end of the conical stem was left to attach the proximal reamer for the cone over a reaming pole. Reaming proximally reached size 21 mm, and a cone 21 mm/132 was tightly inserted and impacted. The stay screw over the top positioned to adjust the predetermined anteversion calculated during a trial reduction. A STD standard ceramic 36 mm head was attached, and the reduction was easy.

36.2.7 Intraoperative Challenges

Challenges and solutions: The major challenge was reaming up to a large-sized stem to avoid failure of the implant again. In addition, straitening the femoral canal was difficult, and a bowed stem helped to do so. An important point at this stage was to calculate properly the direction of the bowing to avoid damaging the femur. Usually the bowing is aiming towards the lateral cortex, and hammering the distal conical stem in; one must maintain the bowing of the stem towards this direction. Another challenge was to sufficiently bypass the distal fracture site that was achieved by careful evaluation of the total length of the implant using adding up the distal stem and the cone length. The stem worked as an intramedullary nail and secured the fracture site not needing the plate on top.

Unanticipated problems and solution: Periprosthetic intraoperative distal femoral fracture. During relocation of the femur, an unanticipated fracture of the distal femur occurred going down to the flare of the distal femur. Part of the fracture was around the already existing stem in situ; thus, distal plating was only necessary with some overlap with the stem. Unicortical and bicortical locking screws were applied above and below to secure the fracture from propagating further (Fig. 36.4).

Thorough description of decision-making, including the reason for the final decision: Being ready for an intraoperative fracture is important during a re-revision procedure. Locking plates are essential as they can rely on unicortical screws locked onto the plate.

36.2.8 Postoperative Radiographs (Fig. 36.4)

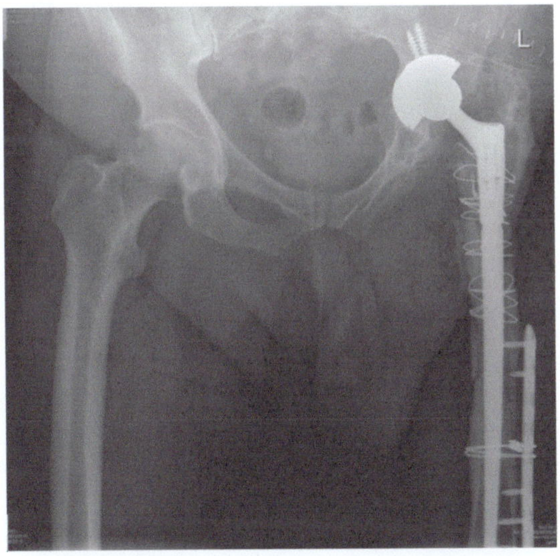

Fig. 36.4 Well-fitted stem into the femoral canal which is now straight. Periprosthetic fracture fixed with a plate and a cable around the plate to maintain reduction. Good alignment and leg length

36.2.9 Postoperative Management

Chemoprophylaxis and anticoagulant treatment period: Vancomycin 500 mg (one dose preoperatively and two doses postoperatively), cefuroxime 1.5 g 1 × 3 for five days, tinzaparin for the days of hospitalization and then rivaroxaban 10 mg for thirty days.

Gait/limb loading until full loading: Partial weight bearing for two months and then assisted full weight bearing with one cane for four months until the fracture site was healed.

36.2.10 Follow-Up and Complications

Scoring: HHS: 85

36.3 Case Title: Femoral Revision "Monolithic Stems"

Stanislav Bondarenko, Volodymyr Filippenko, and Volodymyr Mezentsev

36.3.1 Demographics

Age: 62
Sex: Male
BMI: 31.6

36.3.2 Relevant Past Medical History

Principal pathologies: Fracture of handmade cement spacer following extraction of the implant due to infected THA.

Previous surgical procedures: (1) Primary uncemented arthroplasty five years prior to index procedure. (2) Acetabular cup revision two years after primary arthroplasty. (3) Extraction of implants and handmade spacer 2.5 years after cup revision.

Medication: Analgesics and NSAID's, antibiotics and anticoagulants.

Other: Comorbidities—coronary heart disease, stage 2 hypertension and peptic ulcer disease.

History of presenting complaint: Patient was apparently in good condition until 2.5 years after cup revision when he presented with right thigh pain, swelling, redness and discharging fistula (Fig. 36.5). The pain was moderate, worst with movement and relieved by rest. There was associated limping and difficulty in ambulation. There was no history of fever, nausea, vomiting or anorexia. A swab was taken from the sinus tract and sent for microscopy, culture and sensitivity. *Staphylococcus aureus* was isolated from the culture; the implant was extracted, and a handmade cement spacer was inserted (Fig. 36.6). The patient was advised to return in eight weeks for removal of cement spacer and to undergo definitive revision surgery. However, patient defaulted, and he was lost to follow-up. He returned six months later with right thigh pain, limping and difficulty in ambulation due to fracture of the spacer.

36.3.3 Clinical Examination

Symptoms: Right thigh pain, limping, Trendelenburg gait, hypertrophy of thigh and gluteus muscles and leg length discrepancy of 35 mm.

Range of motion: Extension/flexion—0/10/60; abduction/adduction—10/0/10; and external rotation/internal rotation—20/0/10.

Specific tests: ESR: 10mm/h; CRP: negative; CBC-T/D: normal; aspiration: negative; serum electrolyte, urea and creatinine, within normal limit; ECG, symptoms suggestive of CAD; Doppler USS, normal.

Main disability: Pain, limping and partial weight bearing.

Scoring: VAS: 6; HHS: 34.

Neurovascular evaluation: All major lower limb nerves—sciatic, femoral and obturator nerves were intact.

36.3.4 Preoperative Radiological Assessment/Imaging (Figs. 36.5, 36.6, and 36.7)

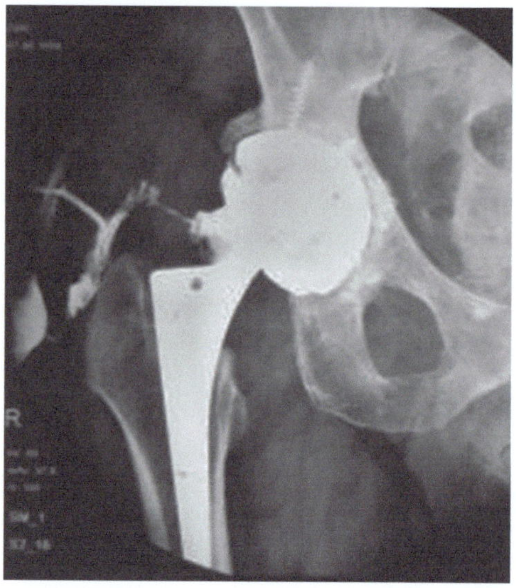

Fig. 36.5 AP X-ray view of right hip showing uncemented implant with osteolysis around the cup and stable fixation of the stem. There is a communicating fistula from the joint capsule to the skin

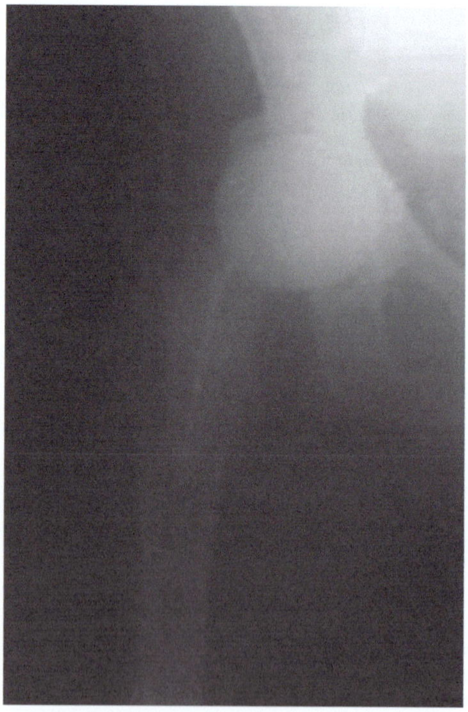

Fig. 36.6 AP X-ray view of right hip showing handmade cemented spacer

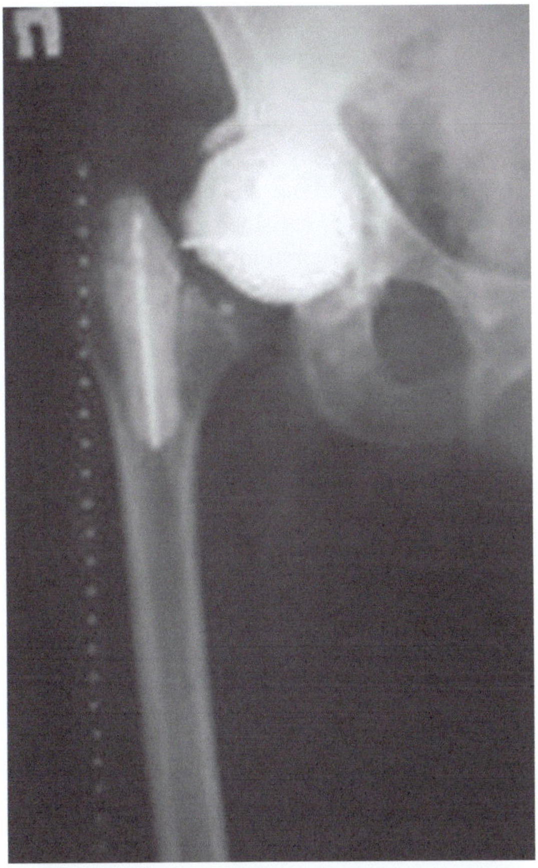

Fig. 36.7 AP X-ray view showing the fracture of the spacer, dislocation of the proximal part of the femur and superior migration about 35 mm and type II Paprosky defect of the femur

36.3.5 Preoperative Planning

Diagnosis: Fracture of handmade cement spacer following extraction of the implant due to infected THA (Fig. 36.7).

Possible treatment options: (1) Monobloc conically tapered with longitudinally raised splines revision stem with bone grafting. (2) Uncemented extensively porous-coated primary long stem prosthesis or porous-coated/grit-blasted combination with bone grafting. (3) Rectangular tapered primary stem with bone grafting.

Chosen treatment method: Monobloc conically tapered with longitudinally raised splines revision stem with bone grafting.

Selection of implants if applicable and rational: This stem provides reliable restoration of bone stock and secures uncemented fixation in the remaining distal, well-preserved femur. It provides rotation stability of the implant in the femoral canal.

Expected difficulties: Difficulty with extracting the cement spacers and mobilization of the proximal femur due to severe fibrosis and contractures of hip motion muscles. There was also severe difficulty in reducing the prosthetic head into the cup due to increase tone of the large thigh muscles.

Strategies to overcome difficulties: Initially, adductor tenotomy was done to facilitate mobilization and to aid reduction of the femur into the prosthetic cup. Secondly, an extensive incision was carried out to adequately excise soft fibrotic tissues and heterotopic ossification.

Templating: Manual templating was done using AP and lateral radiographs. This is supplied by the implant manufacturers.

36.3.6 Surgical Note

Patient's position: Patient was positioned laterally.

Type of anaesthesia: Spinal.

Surgical approach: Extensive direct lateral approach.

Main steps: The first step was the right adductor tenotomy. An extensive incision about 20 cm on the lateral side was carried down to the right hip joint. Aspirates of the joint fluid were sent for microscopy, culture and sensitivity. Fibrous tissues were excised, and the proximal part of the femur was mobilized to remove the cement spacer followed by that of the acetabulum. This, however, is a difficult stage, and adequate instrumentation must be available. Bone grafting of cavitary defects of the acetabulum was done with morsellized cancellous allografts. We then proceeded to insert antiprotrusio ring with four screws. The cemented polyethylene cup was inserted. The femoral canal was reamed and broached with extreme care to prevent iatrogenic fracture. After satisfactory reaming, a trial stem was inserted, and a trial reduction was done before proceeding to insert a monoblock Wagner revision stem. After stable fixation of the stem to the diaphyseal bone, we performed bone grafting of metaphyseal part of the femur. The femoral head was inserted and reduced into the acetabular cup, and satisfactory range of motion was achieved. Three drainages were inserted at the level of the joint capsule, fascia and subcutaneous fats. The wound was closed in three layers and patient mobilized to intensive care unit (Figs. 36.8 and 36.9).

Reconstruction techniques: The anterior and medial defects of the proximal femur were filled with spongy blocks allografts between the cortex and stem. Bone grafting of cavitary defects of the acetabulum was done with morsellized cancellous allografts.

36.3.7 Intraoperative Challenges

Challenges and solutions: Due to the extensive nature of the procedure and the need for extraction of cement spacer which poses significant difficulty during surgery, adequate preoperative planning and required instrumentations for removal of the spacer were made available in the operation room. Also, devices for osteosynthesis like cerclage and cables should be ordered and made available at the time of surgery. There was extensive bleeding after removal of fibrous tissues. The patient was later transfused after the procedure.

Unanticipated problems and solution: There was no unanticipated problem in this index case because we planned of the procedure and ensured that the required instruments, materials and personnel were available.

Thorough description of decision-making, including the reason for the final decision: It was easy for us to diagnose periprosthetic joint infection base on the proposed criteria, and our index case met such criteria like established sinus tract infection; isolation of *Staphylococcus aureus* pathogen in culture; elevated CRP, ESR and PMN%; and elevated synovial leukocyte count. The gold standard for the treatment of PJI is a two-stage procedure, and this index case was no exception. The coexistence of Paprosky 2 femoral defect informed our choice of using Wagner monoblock tapered revision stem. This stem provides reliable restoration of bone stock and secures uncemented fixation in the remaining distal, well-preserved femur.

36.3.8 Postoperative Radiographs (Figs. 36.8 and 36.9)

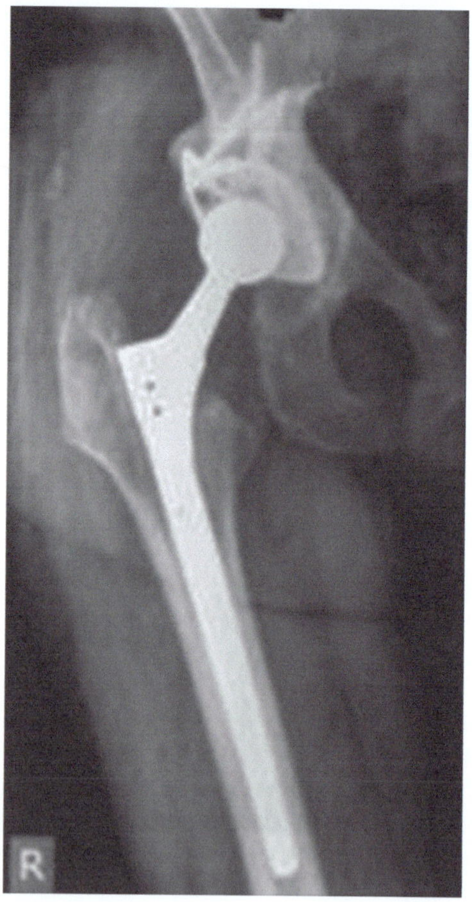

Fig. 36.8 AP view five years after two-stage revision THA on the right hip with Wagner revision stem showing stable implant position and osseointegration of the stem

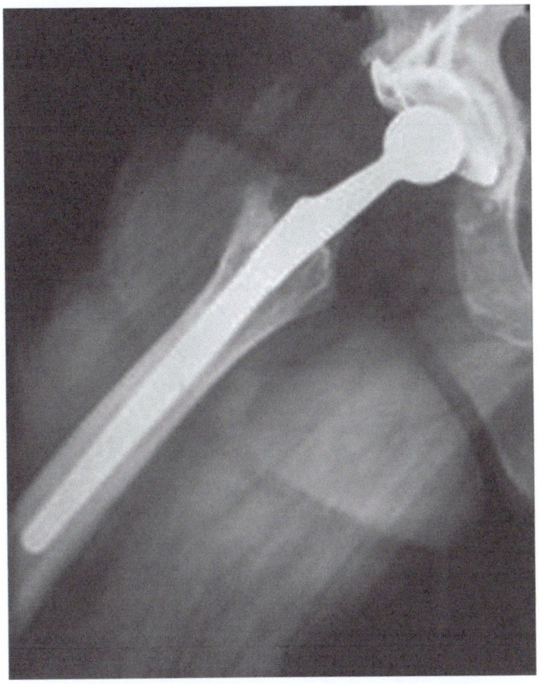

Fig. 36.9 Lateral view five years after two-stage revision THA the on right hip with Wagner revision stem showing stable implant position and osseointegration of the stem

36.3.9 Postoperative Management

Chemoprophylaxis and anticoagulant treatment period: Ceftazidime 1000 mg twice daily for seven days, Clexane 40 mg once daily for thirty five days postoperative, celecoxib 200 mg once daily for seven days and one unit of whole blood.

Gait/limb loading until full loading: The patient was on restricted weight bearing with crutches for six months before commencing full weight bearing. During this period, there was limited hip flexion and adduction until full weight bearing.

36.3.10 Follow-Up and Complications

There were no postoperative complications for this case; the patient was followed up at an interval of 3, 6 and 12 months and subsequently yearly.

36.3.11 Discussion [29, 30, 42]

Advantages of the applied method: Restoration of hip rotation centre and leg length. The stem length coupled with the secure fit of the taper design and the torsional resistant provides for firm fixation to the biological bone. The fixation region of the previous implant is bridged, and it provides mechanical stability. It also aids in the restoration of bone stock.

Disadvantages of the method: Dislocation is a common complication of this design as documented by several articles due to inadequate offset. Wide exposure increases neurovascular risks, the potential for decreased abductor function and limp. Because it is a two-stage procedure, it requires longer treatment time, is more expensive for the patient and is labour intensive for the surgeons.

Alternative evidence-based techniques for the case: (1) Uncemented extensively porous-coated primary long stem prosthesis or porous-coated/grit-blasted combination with bone grafting. (2) Rectangular tapered primary stem with bone grafting. (3) Cemented revision stem.

Why is the chosen technique better for this case? This stem provides reliable restoration of the bone stock and secures uncemented fixation in the remaining distal, well-preserved femur. It provides rotation stability of the implant in the femoral canal.

Indications and contraindications for your technique: Indications—femoral defects and Paprosky types II and III. Contraindications: Femoral defects and Paprosky type IV.

Learning curve and how to manage complications: This procedure has a steep learning curve and should only be undertaken by experienced surgeons who practice in centres with high-volume surgery.

Level of evidence concerning the superiority of this method against others: Level III evidence.

36.4 Case Title: Femoral Revision "Uncemented Monolithic Stems"

Volodymyr Filippenko, Stanislav Bondarenko, and Volodymyr Mezentsev

36.4.1 Demographics

Age: 67
Sex: Male
BMI: 29.7

36.4.2 Relevant Past Medical History

Principal pathologies: Protrusion of the head of the implant of the right hip joint following hemiarthroplasty (Figs. 36.10 and 36.11).

Previous surgical procedures: Primary uncemented hemiarthroplasty five years prior to index procedure.

Medication: Analgesics and NSAIDs, antibiotics and anticoagulants.

Other: Comorbidities—coronary heart disease, stage 2 hypertension and peripheral vascular diseases.

History of presenting complaint: Patient was apparently in good health until four years after hemiarthroplasty when he complained from right groin pain. The pain was moderate initially and later became severe, associated with difficulty in ambulation, limping and shorting of the right lower extremity. There was a marked limitation of movement of the right hip joint with difficulty in the abducting limb. There was no history of fever, anorexia, weight loss or vomiting.

36.4.3 Clinical Examination

Symptoms: Severe groin pain, limping, Trendelenburg gait, atrophy of thigh and gluteus muscles and leg length discrepancy of 40 mm.

Range of motion: Extension/flexion, 0/10/30; abduction/adduction, 0/0/0; and external rotation/internal rotation, 0/0/0.

Specific tests: ESR: 15 mm/h; CRP: negative; CBC T/D: normal; CRP: normal; aspiration: negative; serum electrolyte, urea and creatinine, within normal limit; ECG, symptoms suggestive of CAD; and Doppler USS, normal.

Main disability: Pain, limping and partial weight bearing.

Scoring if available: VAS, 8; HHS, 26.

Neurovascular evaluation: All major lower limb nerves: sciatic, femoral, obturator and superior gluteal nerves were intact.

36.4.4 Preoperative Radiological Assessment/Imaging (Figs. 36.10 and 36.11)

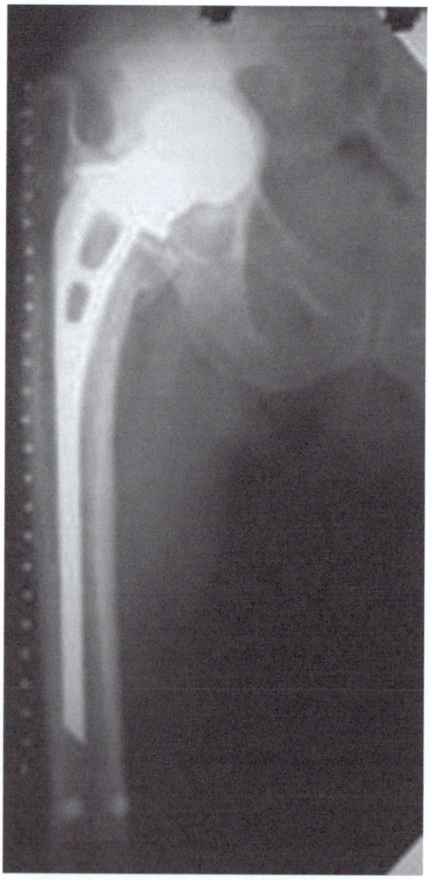

Fig. 36.10 AP X-ray view of the right hip showing the uncemented monoblock hemiprosthesis with protrusion and Paprosky type IIC defect of the acetabulum

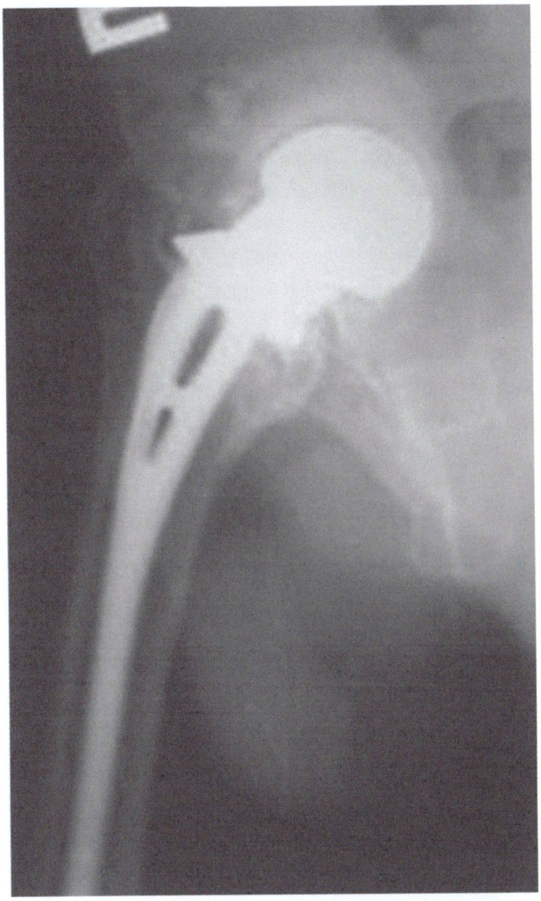

Fig. 36.11 Lateral X-ray view of the right hip showing the uncemented monoblock hemiprosthesis with protrusion and Paprosky type IIC defect of the acetabulum

36.4.5 Preoperative Planning

Diagnosis: Protrusion of the head of implant of the right hip joint following hemiarthroplasty (Figs. 36.10 and 36.11).

Possible treatment options: (1) Monobloc conically tapered with longitudinally raised splines revision stem with bone grafting. (2) Extended trochanteric osteotomy with modular revision stem and bone grafting. (3) Cemented revision stem.

Chosen treatment method: Monobloc conically tapered with longitudinally raised splines revision stem with bone grafting.

Selection of implants if applicable and rational: This stem provides reliable restoration of the bone stock and secures the uncemented fixation in the remaining distal, well-preserved femur. It provides rotation stability of the implant in the femoral canal.

Expected difficulties: Difficult with dislocation because of the endoprosthesis monolithic nature and protrusio. Also, the large diameter of the prosthetic head and extensive osteophytes and fibrous tissues post a significant challenge. The increased risk of periprosthetic fracture during dislocation was another intraoperative issue. Another significant challenge was the difficulty in extracting the femoral stem without osteotomy. This was achieved with the use of narrow and flexible osteotomes.

Strategies to overcome difficulties: Initially, adductor tenotomy was done to facilitate mobilization and to aid reduction of the femur into the prosthetic acetabulum. Secondly, an extensive incision was done to adequately excise the soft fibrotic tissues and heterotopic ossifications. The type of approach used helped facilitate this extensive procedure. Excessive care was taken in handling the osteoporotic proximal femur during dislocation and relocation in order to reduce the risk of intraoperative fracture.

Templating: Manual templating was done with AP and lateral radiographs using standard templates supplied by manufacturers.

36.4.6 Surgical Note

Patient's position: Patient is positioned laterally.

Type of anaesthesia: Spinal.

Surgical approach: Extensive direct lateral approach.

Main steps: The first step was right adductor tenotomy. An extensive incision about 20 cm on the lateral side was carried down to the right hip joint. Aspirates of the joint fluid were sent for microscopy, culture and sensitivity. Fibrous tissues were excised, proximal part of the femur was mobilized, osteophytes were removed and part abductor muscles and iliopsoas were incised from their attachments at the greater and lesser trochanters. We then dislocated the hip joint and extracted the femoral implant with the aid of flexible osteotomes. The acetabulum was reamed, and Paprosky type IIC cavitary defect of the acetabulum was reconstructed with morsellized bone grafts and granules of calcium-phosphate ceramics. We then inserted trabecular metal shell with two screws. The femoral canal was reamed and broached with extreme care, and Paprosky type II was identified. After satisfactory reaming, a trial stem was inserted, and a trial reduction was done before proceeding to insert a monoblock Wagner revision stem. After stable fixation of the stem to the diaphyseal bone, we performed bone grafting of metaphyseal part of the femur. The femoral head was inserted and reduced into the acetabular cup, and satisfactory range of motion was achieved. Three drainages were inserted at the level of the joint capsule, fascia and subcutaneous fats. The wound was closed in three layers and patient mobilized to intensive care unit (Figs. 36.12 and 36.13).

Reconstruction techniques: The anterior and medial defects of the proximal femur were filled with spongy blocks allografts between the cortex and stem. The cavitary defect of the medial wall of the acetabulum was reconstructed with morsellized cancellous allograft and granules of calcium-phosphate ceramic in a ratio 1:2 and was impacted into the defect.

36.4.7 Intraoperative Challenges

Challenges and solutions: Due to the extensive nature of the procedure and the need to extract a well-fixed monoblock with long stem, hemiprosthesis posed significant difficulty during surgery. Adequate preoperative planning and required instrumentations for the removal of implants were made available in the operation room. Also, devices for osteosynthesis like cerclage and cables should be made available in cases of intraoperative fractures of the femur during dislocation and extraction of the prosthesis. There was extensive bleeding after removal of fibrous tissues. The patient was managed with haematinics postoperatively.

Unanticipated problems and solution: The was no unanticipated problem in this index case because we planned of the procedure and ensured that the required instruments, materials and personnel were available.

Thorough description of decision-making, including the reason for the final decision: The design features of the primary implant (monoblock with long stem hemiprosthesis) also with the coexistence of Paprosky 2 femoral defect after removal informed our choice of using Wagner monoblock tapered revision stem. This stem provides reliable restoration of bone stock and secures uncemented fixation in the remaining distal, well- preserved femur. Due to Paprosky type IIC defect of the medial wall of the acetabulum, we used uncemented primary TM cup with allograft and ceramic reconstruction of the defect.

36.4.8 Postoperative Radiographs (Figs. 36.12 and 36.13)

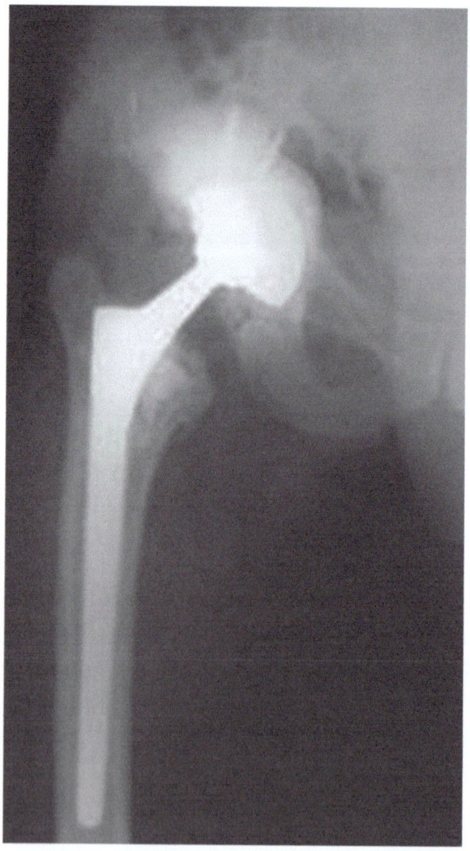

Fig. 36.12 AP view six years post-revision THA on the right hip with Wagner revision stem showing the stable implant position and the osseointegration of the stem

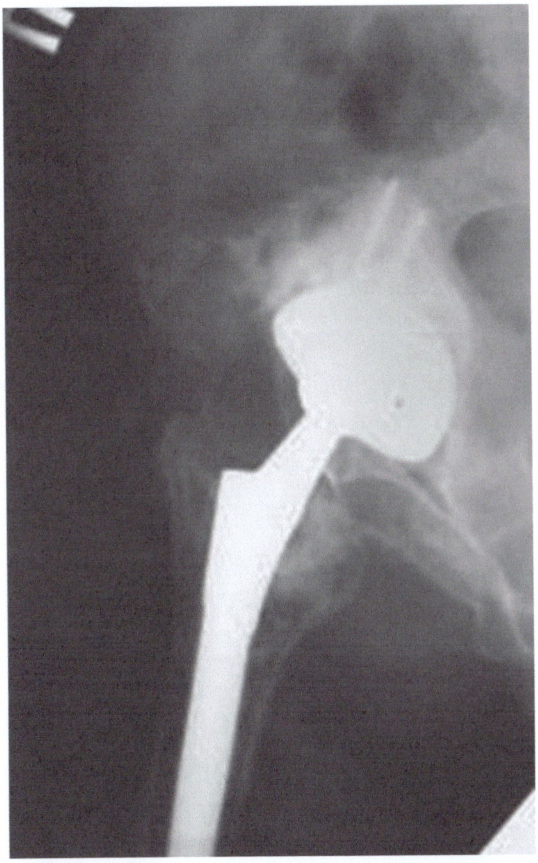

Fig. 36.13 Lateral view six years post revision showing similar features as in Fig. 36.10

36.4.9 Postoperative Managements

Chemoprophylaxis and anticoagulant treatment period: Ceftazidime 1000 mg twice daily for seven days, Clexane 40 mg once daily for thirty five days postoperative and celecoxib 200 mg once daily for seven days.

Gait/limb loading until full loading: Patient was on restricted weight bearing with crutches for three months before commencing full weight bearing. During this period, there was limited hip flexion and adduction until full weight bearing.

36.4.10 Follow-Up and Complications

There were no postoperative complications for this case; the patient was followed up at an interval of 3,6 and 12 months and subsequently yearly.

36.4.11 Discussion [29, 30, 42]

Advantages of the applied method: Restoration of hip rotation centre and leg length. The stem length coupled with the secure fit of the taper design and torsional resistance provides for firm fixation to the biological bone. The fixation region of the previous implant is bridged, and it provides mechanical stability. It also aids in the restoration of bone stock.

Disadvantages of the method: Dislocation is a common complication of this design as documented by several articles due to inadequate offset. Wide exposure increases neurovascular risks, the potential for decreased abductor function and limp.

Alternative evidence-based techniques for the case: (1) Extended trochanteric osteotomy with modular revision stem and bone grafting. (2) Cemented revision stem.

Why is the chosen technique better for this case? This stem provides reliable restoration of bone stock and secures uncemented fixation in the remaining distal, well-preserved femur. It provides rotation stability of the implant in the femoral canal.

Indications and contraindications for your technique: Indications—proximal femoral defects of Paprosky types II and III. Contraindications: Proximal femoral defects of Paprosky type IV.

Learning curve and how to manage complications: This procedure has a steep learning curve and should only be undertaken by experienced surgeons who practice in centres with high-volume surgery.

Level of evidence concerning the superiority of this method against others: Level III evidence.

36.5 Case Title: Revision Arthroplasty with Implantation of the Monolithic Femoral Component and the Use of Massive Allografts

Rashid Tikhilov, Alexey Denisov, and Igor Shubnyakov

36.5.1 Demographics

Age: 27
Sex: Female
BMI: 28

36.5.2 Relevant Past Medical History

Principal pathologies: Post-traumatic osteoarthritis

Previous surgical procedures: 2001: osteosynthesis of the femur using intramedullary nail. April 2002: extraction of the intramedullary nail of the left femur and plate osteosynthesis. August 2002: arthroplasty of the left hip joint. November 2002: lengthening of the left femur with plate fixation. 2005: plate fracture—extraction of the plate and osteosynthesis of the femur using intramedullary nails. 2007: complication—fistula of the left thigh and osteosynthesis of the femur using intramedullary nail with bone cement. 2008: complication—recurrent infection, the extraction and revision surgery of the endoprosthesis using the cement spacer (Figs. 36.14 and 36.15)

Medication: NSAID, chondroprotective drugs

Other: Walking with crutches

36.5.3 Clinical Examination

Symptoms: Inability to rely on the lower limb

Range of motion: Flexion 100^0/extension 0^0, external rotation 5^0/internal rotation 5^0 and abduction 30^0/adduction 10^0

Specific tests: A positive Trendelenburg sign

Main disability: Unable to move without additional support

Scoring if available: Harris Hip Score: 37 points

Neurovascular evaluation: Without pathology

36.5.4 Preoperative Radiological Assessment/Imaging (Figs. 36.14 and 36.15)

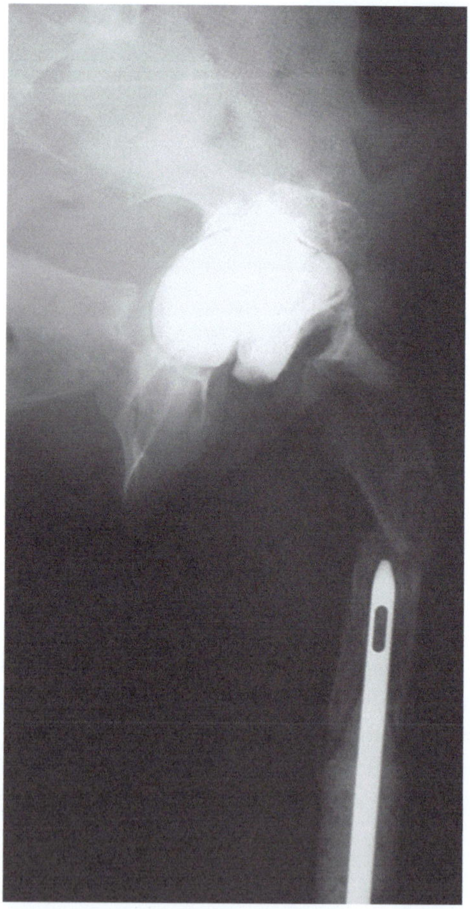

Fig. 36.14 Anteroposterior X-Ray of the left hip joint—periprosthetic infection, contrast in sinus tract and subtrochanteric deformity of the femur block spacer of the left hip

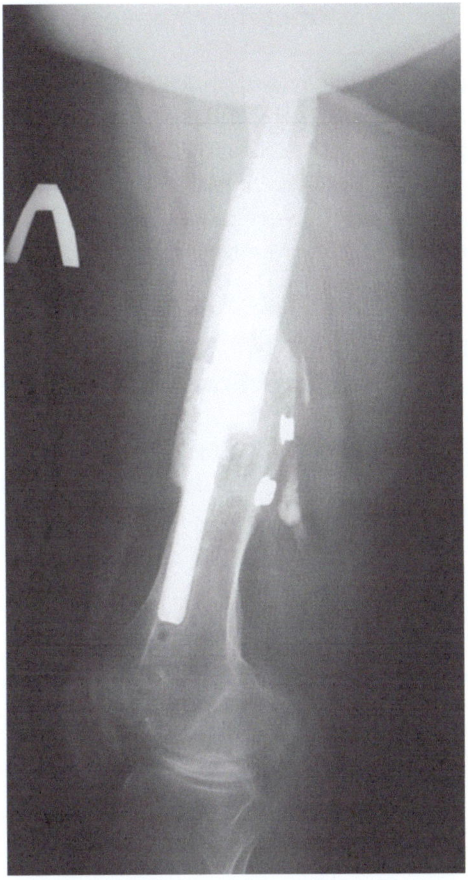

Fig. 36.15 Anteroposterior X-ray of the left distal femur: Defect of the femoral shaft—cemented spacer and intramedullary nail

36.5.5 Preoperative Planning

Diagnosis: Spacer of the left hip joint with a defect of the proximal femur, type IIB Paprosky defect (Figs. 36.14 and 36.15).

Possible treatment options: Femoral osteotomy at the CORA level

Chosen treatment method: Revision arthroplasty with femoral osteotomy and application of structural allografts.

Selection of implants if applicable and rational: Due to significant bone deficit and severe deformity, the only option is the implantation of a femoral revision component.

Expected difficulties: Achievement of a stable structure.

Strategies to overcome difficulties: The use of the femoral revision component.

Templating: Selecting the optimal size of the acetabular and femoral components.

36.5.6 Surgical Note

Patient's position: Lateral position

Type of anaesthesia: General anaesthesia.

Surgical approach: Extended anterolateral approach with excision of the old scar.

Main steps: Removal of the spacer. Osteotomy of the greater trochanter at the CORA level. Mobilization of the greater trochanter. Implantation of the acetabular component (Zimmer TMT) and the femoral component (Wagner Revision) of the hip endoprosthesis. Placement of the femoral head. Reduction of the prosthesis (Figs. 36.16 and 36.17)

Reconstruction techniques: The distal and proximal fragments of the femur and structural allograft reamed with a special device.

36.5.7 Intraoperative Challenges

Challenges and solutions: The correct positioning and the reliable fixation of all the fragments of the femur and implantation of the femoral component with the use of allograft

Unanticipated problems and solution: No

Thorough description of decision-making, including the reason for the final decision: Due to severe bone defects and the need to restore the integrity of the femur, the use of a standard femoral stem was impossible. This could only be achieved through revision components.

36.5.8 Postoperative Radiographs (Figs. 36.16 and 36.17)

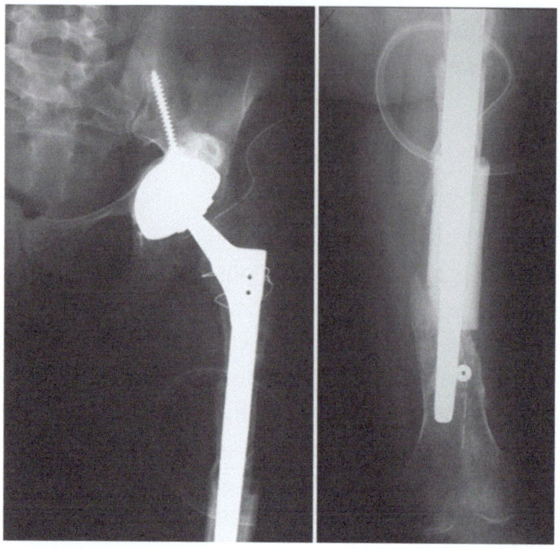

Fig. 36.16 Anteroposterior X-ray of the left hip postoperatively

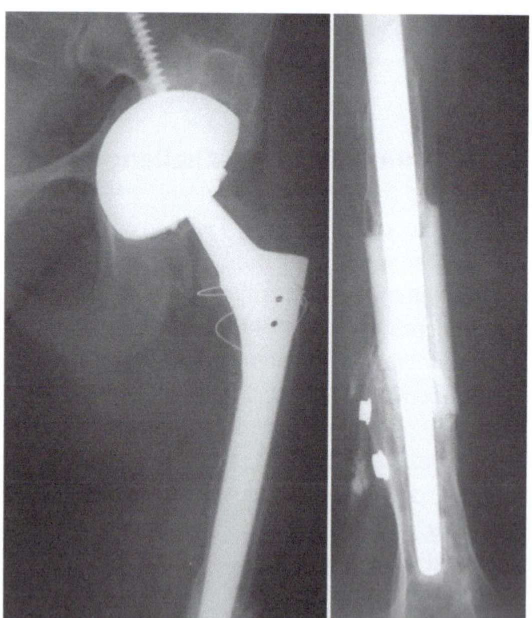

Fig. 36.17 Anteroposterior X-ray of the left hip at the seven-postoperative year

36.5.9 Postoperative Management

Chemoprophylaxis and anticoagulant treatment period: Vancomycin 1.0–2 a day №10, t. Ciprofloxacin 0.5–2 a day №21, LMWHs

Gait/limb loading until full loading: Walking with crutches for three months without the support of the operated limb

36.5.10 Follow-Up and Complications

There were no complications.

Scoring: Harris Hip Score—84 points after 7 years

36.5.11 Discussion [61–64]

Advantages of the applied method: The opportunity to restore the integrity of the limbs and the femoral axis, therefore achieving high structural stability.

Disadvantages of the method: There are technical difficulties with the implantation of the revision monolithic femoral component due to needing to model the proximal and distal parts separately. Limited of choices for the offset.

Alternative evidence-based techniques for the case: (1) Use of a modular femoral component. (2) In the presence of a type II Paprosky defect, it is advisable to use in the revision femoral component. (3) The use of the femoral component with distal locking for the prevention of rotational instability.

Why is the chosen technique better for this case? The experience of our clinic allows us to recommend the use of these types of implants when considered defects.

Indications and Contraindications for Your Technique: Indications—revision of a total hip prosthesis where extensive bone resorption has caused considerable widening of the medullary cavity with grave cortical bone thinning. Revision of an unstable total hip prosthesis after fractures or cortical bone defects in the prosthetic bed. Extensive comminuted fractures in the proximal third of the femur in elderly patients for whom the indication for a prosthesis exists but in whom a standard total hip prosthesis cannot be anchored. Deformations or osseous cicatrisation on the proximal third of the femur after fractures or osteotomies where preparation of the prosthesis seat with rasps is not possible, but careful conical reaming of the proximal medullary cavity can be carried out without any problem to fit the shorter revision stem, unless the still shorter cone prosthesis is indicated. Deformations of the proximal third of the femur for which a corrective osteotomy has to be performed at the same time as fitting a prosthesis. Here the revision stem can be used as a medullary pin to stabilize the osteotomy. Contraindications: Severe atrophy of the femur diaphysis, which rules out a reliable fixation of the revision prosthesis. The implantation of the revision prosthesis requires both extreme care in dealing with the damaged bone and the surrounding tissues and a stable implant fixation; it is only under such conditions that good bone reconstruction and secure prosthetic fixation can be expected. This makes high technical demands on the surgeon; therefore the revision prosthesis is only for use by the experienced specialist.

Learning curve and how to manage complications: This type of a procedure can only be performed by experienced surgeons.

Level of evidence concerning the superiority of this method against *others*: Expert opinion.

36.6 Case Title: Femoral Revision Using a Custom Tapered Stem

M. Ollivier, S. Parratte, X. Flecher, and J.-N. Argenson

36.6.1 Demographics

Age: 30
Sex: Male
BMI: 24

36.6.2 Relevant Past Medical History

Principal pathologies: Bilateral Legg-Perthes-Calve disease.

Previous surgical procedures: Bilateral THA, periprosthetic join infection of the left THA.

Medication: Pain killer, antibiotics.

History of Presenting Complaint: At five years after the left THA, the patient started to suffer again from his left hip. The THA was painful for more than two months at the first orthopaedic evaluation. A chronic THA infection (*Staphylococcus aureus* Methi-S) was diagnosed after hip aspiration (Figs. 36.18 and 36.19). A two-stage THA exchange was planned to treat the periprosthetic infection (Fig. 36.20). We present here the strategy that was decided for the reimplantation procedure.

36.6.3 Clinical Examination

Symptoms: Groin pain, unable to walk without crutches

Range of motion: 0° extension, 100° flexion, 25° ER , 15° IR

Main disability: Unable to walk

Scoring: Harris Hip Score, 35

36.6.4 Preoperative Radiological Assessment/Imaging (Figs. 36.18, 36.19, and 36.20)

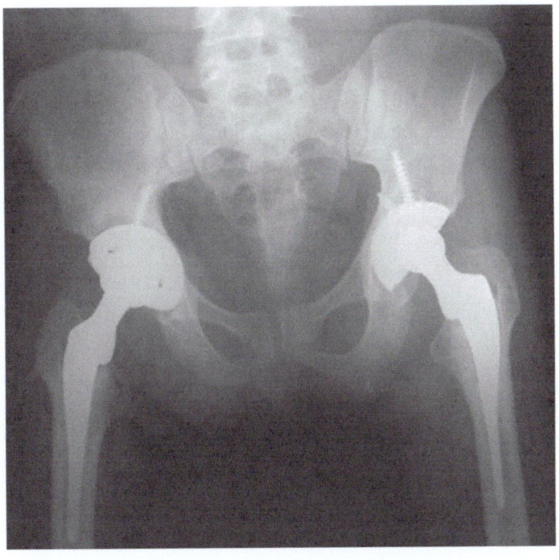

Fig. 36.18 AP pelvic X-ray showing bilateral custom THAs at 5-year follow-up from the left operation

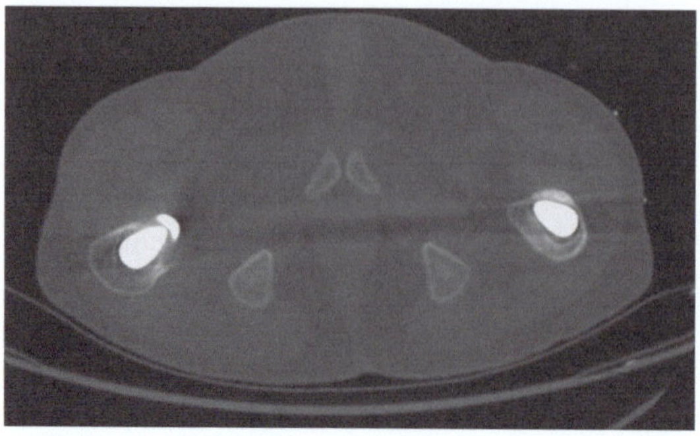

Fig. 36.19 CT scan showing radiolucencies surrounding the femoral component

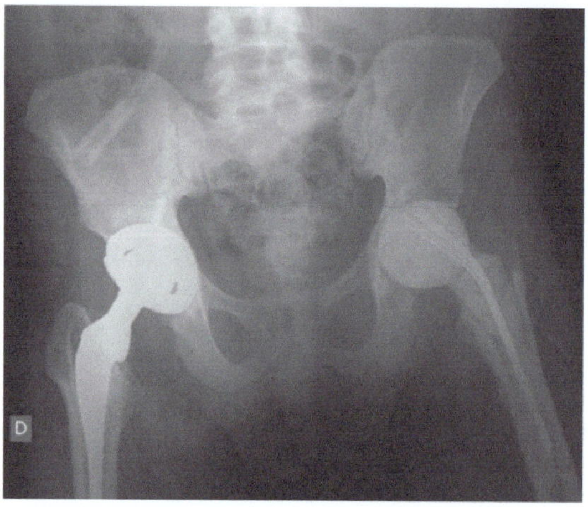

Fig. 36.20 Postoperative AP X-ray—THA resection replaced with an articulated antibiotic-loaded cement spacer

36.6.5 Preoperative Planning

Diagnosis: Periprosthetic deep infection of the left THA (Figs. 36.19 and 36.20).

Possible treatment options: Suppressive antibiotic therapy, one-stage exchange and two-stage exchange.

Chosen treatment method: Two-stage exchange.

Selection of implants if applicable and rational: The rationale for the reimplantation procedure was due to (1) The patient's age: uncemented fixation. (2) The metaphyseal and diaphyseal femoral anatomy: anatomical stem. (3) The shape of the femoral canal: custom (3D CT scan-based) femoral stem. To correct leg length inequality (1 cm) and optimize femoral offset, a "varus-long" neck stem was designed.

Expected difficulties: First stage—the approach and the removal of the periarticular scar tissue, cement and all uncemented implants. Moulded antiobiotic-loaded spacer using a k-wire to avoid fracture at the neck level. Second stage: same approach, antibiotic-loaded spacer removal, debridement and acetabular cup implantation. Femoral stem implantation (thin femoral canal).

Strategies to overcome difficulties: Extensive Watson-Jones approach. Multihole acetabular shell. Custom-made femoral stem.

Templating: A preoperative CT scan was done to design an individual custom femoral stem (Fig. 36.19).

36.6.6 Surgical Note

Patient's position: Supine position.

Type of anaesthesia: General anaesthesia.

Surgical approach: Watson-Jones extended approach.

Main steps: With the patient in supine position, a classic WJ approach was performed and gave us access to the capsule and the antibiotic-loaded cement spacer. The capsule and the periarticular scar tissue were resected. The acetabulum was reamed to permit the implantation of a multihole acetabular shell. A custom-designed file was used to prepare the femoral canal at the exact size of the definite implant. The femoral stem was then implanted into the femur (Figs. 36.21 and 36.22).

36.6.7 Intraoperative Challenges

Challenges and solutions: Spacer removal: the antibiotic-loaded spacer was extracted easily. Acetabular cup implantation: due to previous cup implantation and revision, only a small bony anterior column was left. To enhance primary press-fit stability, two screws were placed at the upper part of the shell. Finally, during hip testing, we found a leg length inequality (5 mm), and we then decided to increase femoral neck-head length using an extra-long neck-head junction.

36.6.8 Postoperative Radiographs (Figs. 36.21 and 36.22)

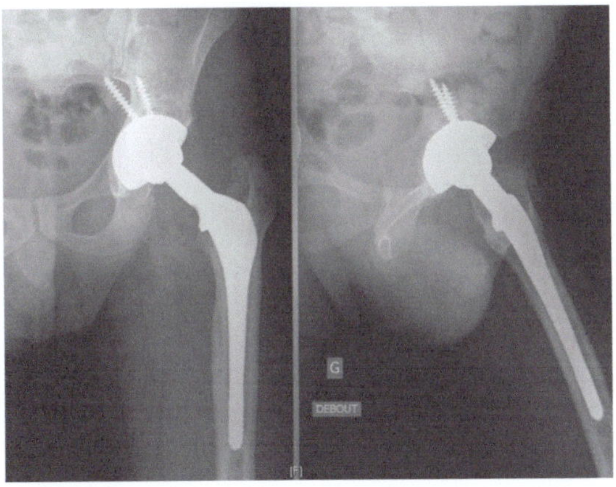

Fig. 36.21 Postoperative AP and lateral X-rays of the first month showing the revision femoral stem implanted

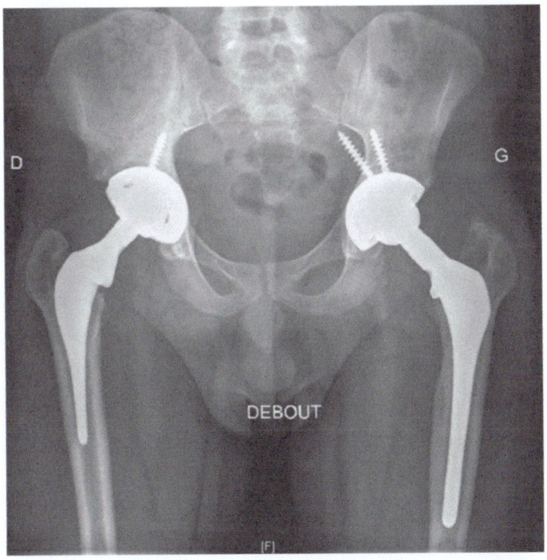

Fig. 36.22 Last follow-up anteroposterior pelvic X-ray at three years postoperatively, showing the good integration of the implants, no sign of loosening and no radiolucencies

36.6.9 Postoperative Management

Chemoprophylaxis and anticoagulant treatment period: Low weight heparin for 35 days

Gait/limb loading until full loading: Full weight bearing starting the first postoperative day

36.6.10 Follow-Up and Complications

Scoring: Harris Hip Score at three years is 94.

36.6.11 Discussion [65–67]

Advantages of the applied method: Bone sparing technique with a minimal cortical and cancellous bone loss (custom 3D-designed file). The perfect compromise between metaphyseal-diaphyseal stem fixation and anatomical reconstruction. The monobloc implant is decreasing the risk of implant failure.

Disadvantages of the method: Preoperative CT scan. Cost of the femoral implant.

Alternative evidence-based techniques for the case: Metaphyseal and/or neck modularity.

Why is the chosen technique better for this case? Using a classic quadrangular or anatomic stem would imply substantial canal bone resection to fit the thin femoral canal to the size of the final implant. The use of modular implant would have conducted to extra-long/varus neck implantation which is very often involved in prosthetic fractures.

Indications and contraindications for your technique: Indication—revision with sufficient bone quality/amount. Revision of uncemented short or anatomic stem.

Learning curve and how to manage complications: The preparation of the femoral canal might be difficult. The CT scan provides information regarding the density of the femoral cortices. It is thus essential to prepare the femoral canal correctly using a curette before using the custom file (reproducing exactly the femoral stem shape) to avoid any risk of intraoperative fracture.

Level of evidence concerning the superiority of this method against others: (1) Bone sparing technique. (2) Perfect compromise between bone implantation/stability and anatomical reconstruction (femoral offset, neck shaft angle). (3) Monoblock implant decreasing the risk of stem fracture and tribo-corrosion.

36.7 Case Title: Femoral Revision Using a Cementless Tapered Stem for a Type II Paprosky Defect

Sérgio Gonçalves, Thiago Aguiar, and Pedro Dantas

36.7.1 Demographics

Age: 65
Sex: Female
BMI: 28.3

36.7.2 Relevant Past Medical History

Principal pathologies: Gastroesophageal reflux disease, left hip tuberculous arthropathy at the age of fifteen years.

Previous surgical procedures: Left hip drainage and debridement at the age of fifteen years, ipsilateral total hip replacement (THR) in 1982 aged 42. The Watson-Jones approach was used in the primary arthroplasty, and there were no healing problems.

Medication: Omeprazole.

History of presenting complaint: The patient was referred to our institution presenting with progressive left hip and thigh pain, limitation of the walking distance. These symptoms worsened in the last five years.

36.7.3 Clinical Examination

Symptoms: Pain aggravated by walking, radiating from the groin to the thigh and worsened by hip flexion and attempted internal rotation. Log roll in internal rotation produces thigh pain.

Range of motion: Left hip—flexion 70°, extension 0°, abduction 45°, adduction 10°, internal rotation 0° and external rotation 15°. Flexion and rotations were painful.

Specific tests: Left lower limb shortening of 1 cm. Positive left Trendelenburg test.

Main disability: Pain and limited walking distance.

Scoring: Preoperative Harris Hip Score: 42.

Neurovascular evaluation: No changes.

36.7.4 Preoperative Radiological Assessment/Imaging

Other: Blood leukocyte count and differential were normal, C- reactive protein 0.41 mg/dL and erythrocyte sedimentation rate 10 mm/h.

36.7.5 Preoperative Planning

Diagnosis: Aseptic loosening of a Charnley-Muller THR resulting in a type IIC acetabular defect (we will ignore it for simplicity, as the purpose of this case is to address the femoral revision) and a type II femoral defect according to Paprosky classification (23 years after implantation) (Figs. 36.23, 36.24 and 36.25).

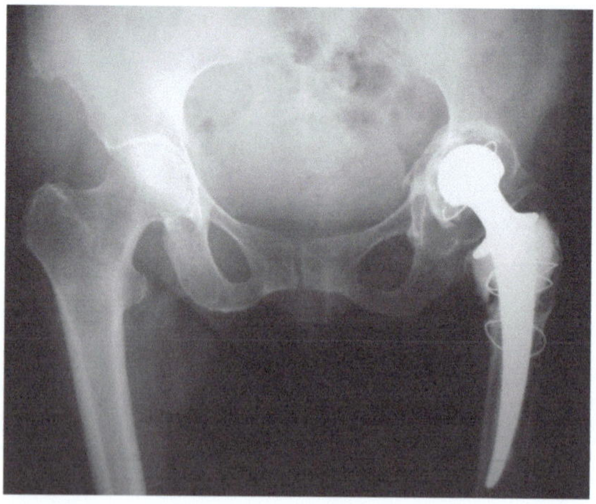

Fig. 36.23 AP Pelvic x-ray. Charnley-Muller left total hip arthroplasty. Loose cup with supero-medial migration (Paprosky type IIC acetabular defect). Cemented femoral stem with extensive metaphyseal bone loss and cortical thinning but intact femoral diaphysis (Paprosky type II femoral defect). A metaphyseal femoral fracture is visible

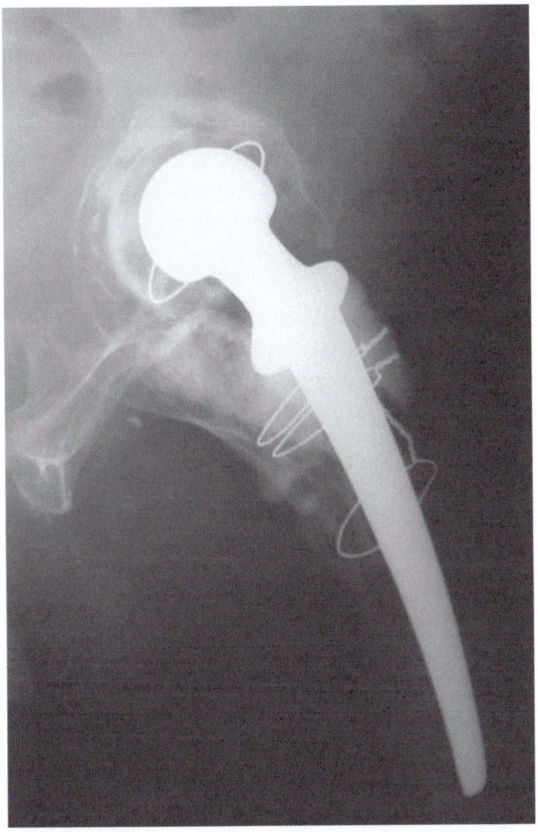

Fig. 36.24 Lateral hip x-ray. The greater trochanter is loose and tilted posteriorly. No significant diaphyseal bone loss and a good working length (>4 cm) are present

Possible treatment options: Cemented femoral revision. Uncemented femoral revision: proximally porous-coated, modular stem; extensively porous-coated, cylindrical stem; and tapered fluted modular stem.

Chosen treatment method: Femoral revision using an uncemented tapered fluted modular stem, with proximal strut allograft and cerclage wire fixation.

Selection of implants if applicable and rational: An uncemented femoral stem was chosen because it's difficult to achieve adequate cement interdigitation into the host bone in the revision setting. Diaphyseal fixation employing the tapered fluted implant design allows adequate stability despite a frail metaphyseal segment [68]; the modularity of the implant will facilitate the restoration of limb length, version and offset. Greater trochanter fracture management can be done either with the use of cerclage wires or a

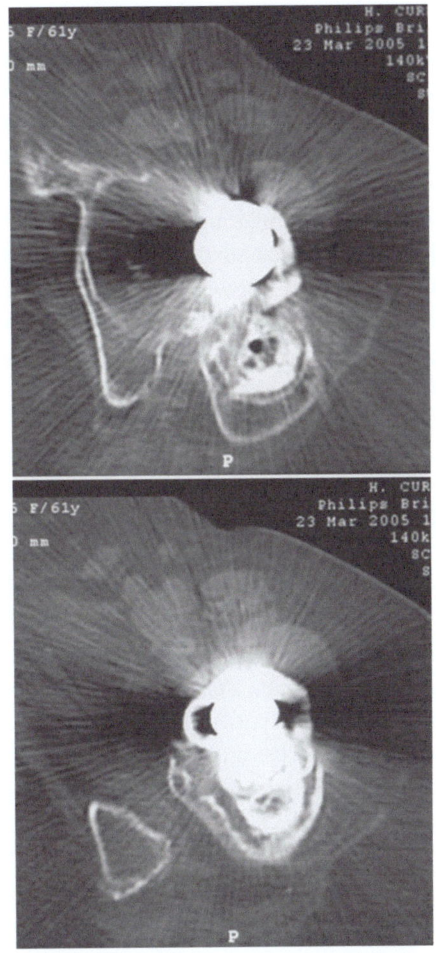

Fig. 36.25 Axial CT scan. The extent of the femoral metaphyseal bone loss is visible; there is a wide gap between the cement mantle and cortical bone. The greater trochanter is loose and posteriorly deviated

trochanteric plate. A strut allograft was planned to reinforce the proximal femur.

Expected difficulties: a) Removing the implants and cement mantle without further compromising bone stock b) trochanteric non-union which needs stabilization c) achieving adequate diaphyseal scratch fit avoiding three-point fixation which could result in undersizing and later subsidence of the stem and d) intraoperative femoral fracture from component oversizing or malalignment.

Strategies to overcome difficulties: Having cement removal specific instrumentation is fundamental; identify and catalogue THR components from previous interventions, and obtain specific instrumentation to aid with removal; an extended trochanteric osteotomy may be required should difficulty arise; working through the metaphyseal fracture may help in the removal of the distal cement mantle; preoperative planning will help to estimate implant sizing and length thus decreasing intraoperative fracture or postoperative subsidence risk.

Templating: Templating is performed to evaluate the diameter necessary to achieve adequate fit in the diaphyseal region and to estimate the length needed to bypass any bony defects or stress risers. The size of the metaphyseal component which would result in limb length equality and offset restoration is also estimated.

36.7.6 Surgical Note

Patient's position: Lateral decubitus.

Type of anaesthesia: Combined general and epidural anaesthesia.

Surgical approach: Posterolateral approach.

Main steps: The patient positioning is carried out under the direct surgeon supervision to ensure that adequate references are available for implant positioning and decision-making. Intraoperative fluoroscopy is positioned and tested so that a correct and complete field of view is possible and easily reproduced. Prophylactic antibiotic therapy was administered after microbacteriological samples are collected (three samples) and a biopsy for pathology. The loose components were successfully removed without significant additional bone loss utilizing the endofemoral approach and the trochanteric fracture line.

Reconstruction techniques: Acetabular reconstruction with morsellized allograft and a hemispherical cementless cup with screws was performed, cement and debris were removed, and the femoral canal preparation was initiated. Care was taken to choose the correct entry point close to the greater trochanter in the metaphyseal area which can be difficult due to the lack of references, and good exposure is crucial. The rreamers were advanced incrementally in diameter and depth until a good segment of the femur was prepared into a wedge (~4 cm), and a prophylactic cerclage wire was applied prior to reaming in the distal femoral segment. An 18/140 mm distal and 55 mm proximal components were assembled for final insertion after fluoroscopic confirmation of a good fit and height restoration with the trial implants. Additional cerclage wires were used for the final fixation of the trochanteric region, and a medial strut allograft was applied to reinforce the proximal femur (Figs. 36.26 and 36.27).

36.7.7 Intraoperative Challenges

Challenges and solutions: Uncemented press-fit preparation and final implantation can lead to intraoperative fractures; prophylactically application of cerclage wires can avoid the propagation of such fractures. Obtaining a stable trochanteric osteosynthesis can be especially difficult due to the small size of the fragment, cortical thinning and abductor muscles pull. Cerclage wires and trochanteric plate are reliable options for the greater trochanter fixation.

Thorough description of decision-making, including the reason for the final decision: Diaphyseal fixation with a tapered fluted implant permitted adequate distal fixation despite a frail metaphyseal segment. The tapered design ensures press-fit fixation (wedge effect) and primary stability.

36.7.8 Postoperative Radiographs (Figs. 36.26 and 36.27)

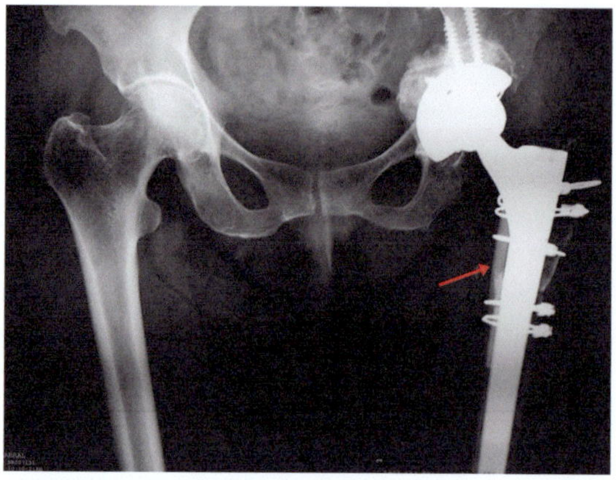

Fig. 36.26 AP Hip x-ray. Early postoperative roentgenogram where adequate restoration of the hip centre of rotation is visible. Acetabular and femoral allograft is still patent. The red arrow points the structural allograft.

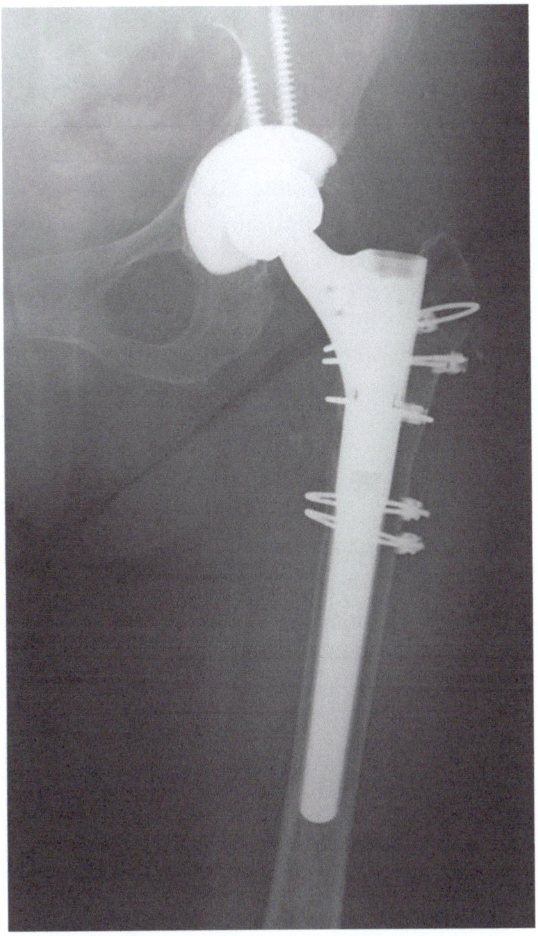

Fig. 36.27 AP Left Hip x-ray. A 10-year follow-up demonstrating well-fixed femoral implant with metaphyseal medial bone regeneration. The greater trochanter has healed in place. The structural allograft was reabsorbed

36.7.9 Postoperative Management

Chemoprophylaxis and anticoagulant treatment period: Low molecular weight heparin was administered for thirty days.

Gait/limb loading until full loading: Partial weight bearing was assisted by crutches for eight weeks with progression to full weight bearing at twelve weeks.

36.7.10 Follow-Up and Complications

The structural allograft used to reinforce the proximal femur was reabsorbed.

Scoring: Postoperative Harris Hip Score: 83.

36.7.11 Discussion

Advantages of the applied method: Uncemented revision techniques are preferred because it's difficult to achieve adequate interdigitation of cement into host bone that has thin cortices and poor cancellous bone. Usually, an extensive metaphyseal bone loss is also present, and distal femoral fixation bypasses it. Tapered implant design creates secure fixation with less area of contact needed for fixation compared to a cylindrical stem. A finned stem has a better rotational stability than circular cross-sectioned stems. Modularity is crucial as it allows for a staged creation of the final implant and better coupling with bone defects and patient morphology (leg length, offset, version). Good clinical outcomes are to be expected with 5-year survival rates of 98% of the implanted stems [69]. Proximal metaphyseal reconstruction is useful as it can provide additional proximal fixation, restores muscular vector forces indispensable for stability and provides bone stock for future procedures if needed.

Disadvantages of the method: Uncemented implants carry a higher risk of intraoperative fractures due to the press-fit effect necessary for achieving primary stability. This primary stability can be undermined by failing to properly size the final implants resulting in subsidence and poor fixation leading to fibrous ingrowth. A size mismatch between intraoperative trials and final implants exists and can lead to errors in achieving adequate fit and centre of rotation restoration. The femoral bow can be a problem when longer stems are used and has to be assessed preoperatively because of the risk of anterior cortical penetration. Modular implants require several coupling joints, which are fragility areas that can result in structural failure and wear.

Alternative evidence-based techniques for the case: Extensively porous-coated, cylindrical stems have also demonstrated good outcomes when dealing with type II Paprosky femoral defects [70].

Why is the chosen technique better for this case? Given the extensive metaphyseal bone loss with an associated greater trochanter fracture, proximal fixation was very precarious, and a distal fixation technique was a better option. The tapered design with a wedge fixation offers the possibility of choosing a shorter stem in comparison to a cylindrical stem. Metaphyseal reconstruction enhances stability by restoring the abductor muscle vector, contributes to a solid osseointegration of the implants and restores bone stock.

Indications and contraindications for your technique: Indicated in the metaphyseal bone loss with a segment of femoral diaphysis (>4 cm) that can be prepared into a wedge for press-fit fixation. If the femur is curved in the frontal plane, a femoral osteotomy is advisable for the implantation of a straight stem. Contraindicated when femoral sagittal bowing is significant or extensive femoral diaphysis bone loss is present; in these cases, diaphyseal screw fixation or allograft composite reconstruction techniques can be used.

Learning curve and how to manage complications: The use of uncemented techniques has become widespread, and the principles of their application are transversal to several implants thus softening the learning curve. The critical use of preoperative templating and planning, adequate exposure and intraoperative fluoroscopic control are the mainstay for avoiding complications.

Level of evidence concerning the superiority of this method against others: Level of evidence 3 (retrospective cohort study or case-control study).

36.8 Case Title: Managing Large Femoral Defects in Revision Total Hip Arthroplasty

Lionel E. Lazaro, Lazaros A. Poultsides, and Micheal B. Cross

36.8.1 Demographics

Age: 70
Sex: Male
BMI: 37.4

36.8.2 Relevant Past Medical History

Principal pathologies: Diabetes mellitus, Type II, hypercholesterolemia, obesity, depression, hypertension, PTSD (post-traumatic stress disorder), asthma and diabetic neuropathy.

Previous surgical procedures: Left total hip arthroplasty 1998.

Medication: Naproxen sodium, tramadol, aspirin 81, atorvastatin, insulin, linagliptin, metformin and sertraline.

History of presenting complaint: Patient is being followed for polyethylene wear and osteolysis over the years. He now presents with worsening left thigh pain that limits his ability to ambulate, needing to depend on assistive device daily. At this point, he is unable to bear weight on the left lower extremity because of pain.

36.8.3 Clinical Examination

Symptoms: Left thigh pain exacerbated by bearing weight

Range of motion: Range of motion is limited secondary to pain

Main disability: Inability to bear weight and ambulate

Neurovascular evaluation: Full motor and sensory exam distally, capillary refill <2 s and 2+ pulses DP/TP

36.8.4 Preoperative Radiological Assessment/Imaging (Figs. 36.28, 36.29, and 36.30)

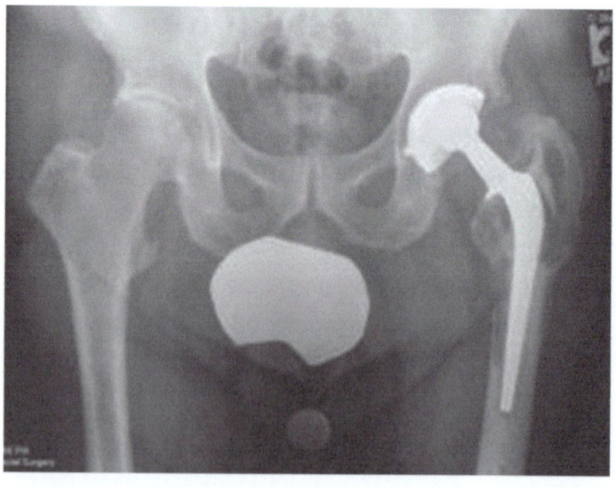

Fig. 36.28 Anterior-posterior view of pelvis revealed extensive osteolysis around the femoral component, greater medially extending into Gruen zones 6 and 7. No acute osseous abnormality or periprosthetic fractures. There is also an eccentric position of the femoral head, suggestive of polyethylene wear

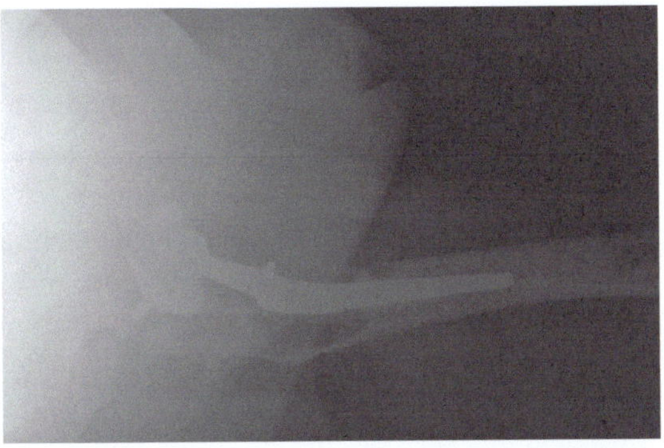

Fig. 36.29 Cross-table lateral view of the left femur revealed extensive osteolysis around the femoral component. No acute osseous abnormality or periprosthetic fracture

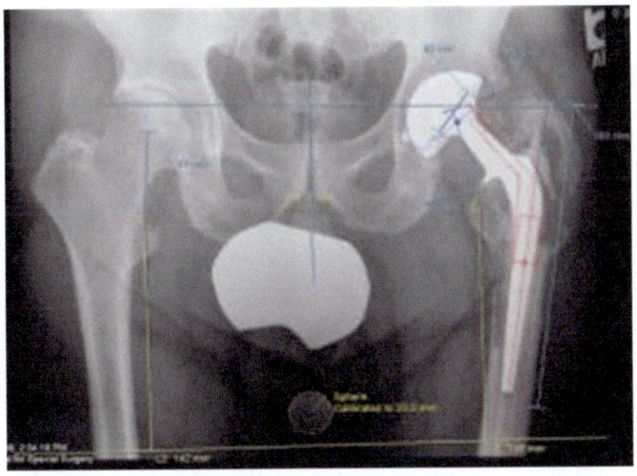

Fig. 36.30 Anterior-posterior view demonstrating preoperative surgical planning using computerized system

36.8.5 Preoperative Planning

Diagnosis: The difficulties in revision total hip replacement (THR) are to assess the available bone stock/bone quality and determine the appropriate implant to achieve stable and reliable fixation. The Paprosky classification categorizes the extent of the femoral bone loss and helps to decide preoperatively on what type of implant to use based on the type of bone defect. With minimal bone defect at the metaphyseal and diaphyseal area (type I and type II femoral bone defects), a modular tapered stem is not necessary. Nevertheless, those cases with a greater diaphyseal bone loss (type IIIB and type IV femoral bone defects), modular tapered stems may be employed with favourable outcomes. In some cases, remodelling of the proximal femur leads to alteration of the lesser trochanter and/or varus remodelling increasing the difficulty in assessing and applying the appropriate version. A modular tapered stem provides the adaptability to accommodate the proper femoral version and minimize instability of the hip joint. In periprosthetic fractures (Vancouver B2 and B3), where the implant is not supported by the proximal femur, a modular tapered stem can be beneficial. This patient had an extensive metadiaphyseal bone loss with 2–4 cm of intact cortical bone in the diaphysis (Paprosky IIIB) (Figs. 36.28 and 36.29).

Possible treatment options: With this large femoral defect (Paprosky IIIB), the options are impaction bone grafting, mainly indicated for large canals and thin cortices (Paprosky IIIb and IV defects); allograft-prosthetic composite, mainly indicated for large metadiaphyseal bone defect in young patients and a nonsupportive diaphysis (Paprosky IV); and fully porous, cylindrical or modular tapered stems, indicated for compromised metaphysis and diaphysis (Paprosky III).

Chosen treatment method: Fluted tapered modular stem.

Selection of implants if applicable and rational: Controlling femoral version and length is paramount during hip revisions. With a massive proximal bone loss, a modular tapered fluted stem provides the advantages of correctly controlling femoral version and length. With a diaphyseal bone loss, the splines of the taper provide rotational control in a short segment of bone, while the taper design provides axial stability. Modular tapered stems only require two centimetres of diaphyseal contact to obtain stability. Allowing the proximal body trial to spin on a well-fixed distal segment, while performing a trial reduction, facilitates the application of appropriate anteversion. This improves intraoperative stability and decreases the dislocation risk. Nevertheless, implant fracture and corrosion at modular junctions may still occur with modular implants and should not be used for all femoral revisions.

Strategies to overcome difficulties: One of the difficulties is to achieve stable fixation with the known poor bone quality. Splines on the taper allow for rotational control, while the taper engaged in the diaphysis allows axial stability. The distal taper is placed first to establish distal diaphyseal fixation. With massive proximal bone defect, the anatomical landmarks are not available and accurate; judgement of version, offset and length becomes a challenge. Once you know exactly where the taper engages the diaphysis, the proximal body then allows for independent control of version, offset and length. A stable distal tapered stem accurately restores length. Additionally, during trial reduction, the proximal body trial spins on a well-fixed distal segment and allows for appropriate judgement of anteversion improving intraoperative stability and decreasing the dislocation risk. The end goal is to minimize leg length discrepancies while also increasing stability. Femoral remodelling into varus and retroversion usually develops with a loose stem, and the distorted lesser trochanteric anatomy further complicates the ability to judge femoral version with a monoblock stem. In severe varus remodelling, the distal curved portion of the stem can be inserted independently of the version of the proximal body. Modularity prevents anteversion mismatch that would occur with a monoblock stem and decreases the risk of femoral cortex perforation or erroneously anteverting the stem. Disadvantages of using a modular stem include corrosion at the modular tapers and implant fracture. However, there are lower rates of fractured implants with newer designs. Further, currently, there are few reports of severe corrosion of modular revision implants. Maybe you can mention that Wagner type stems are monoblock and allow for version control due to the presence of splines.

Templating: For templating we prefer to use an electronic computerized system (Fig. 36.30).

36.8.6 Surgical Note

Patient's position: Lateral decubitus.

Type of anaesthesia: Combined spinal epidural anaesthesia.

Surgical approach: Posterolateral approach to the hip.

Main steps: A skin incision was made based on his previous scar and extending distally. After placement of the Charnley retractor, we created a full-thickness peel off the posterior femur. We placed an Aufranc retractor underneath the medius to protect it and then carried our peel superiorly onto the acetabulum. We exposed the implant and carried our peel down distally 18 cm from the tip of the lesser trochanter including a release of the gluteus maximus tendon. This allowed for sufficient exposure for our planned osteotomy. We released portions of the lateralis posteriorly which allowed us to gain visualization to the bone distally. We then placed one cable distal to our planned osteotomy site and tightened it. We took care to keep the hip located during this procedure. We then made our trochanteric osteotomy using a combination of micro sagittal saw and osteotome. We made our incision through the posterior cortex the full length of the femur down to the planned osteotomy site at 18 cm. We then made the horizontal cut going around anteriorly. We then began the anterior portion of the cut from its distal edge going up approximately 3–4 cm and then turned our attention back to the hip joint. The hip was dislocated, and we used the Midas to remove portions of the overgrown bone around the shoulder of the implant. We removed the implant and then completed our osteotomy with a large saw through the posterior cut scoring the anterior surface. Once the osteotomy was done, we were able to visualize the femoral canal to begin our femoral component revision. We used a quarter inch osteotome to remove the cement mantle along the edge of the osteotomy site. We then used a 3.2 drill bit and drilled down through the bone plug and used the cement back slap screws to engage the mantle and knocked the entire plug out including the restrictor. We then reamed with the distal reamers for the restoration modular set up until we had good scratch fit. We then impacted the final distal stem into place and then trialled proximal bodies until we found the correct diameter. We placed a trial head and reduced it into the acetabulum and found it to be very stable. We then removed this proximal body. We turned attention to the acetabulum. Portions of the hypertrophic capsule were removed. We were able to remove the liner without difficulty and cleaned off the inner shell. We then impacted and found the cup to be stable and impacted a liner with the lip posterior superior in place and then opened and impacted the final trial body to the distal stem with the appropriate version. We then placed the final head which was a + 2.5 mm and performed a final reduction. We then secured the osteotomy in its appropriate position and placed three cables circumferentially to hold it down. We took it through a range of motion and found the entire femur to move as a unit. We thoroughly irrigated the area and performed some soft tissue closure posteriorly with the capsule to the abductor mechanism. We then closed the iliotibial band and the subcutaneous tissues in layers with interrupted stitches. The skin was closed with staples. An Owens dressing was placed over this and a hip spica (Figs. 36.31 and 36.32).

36.8.7 Intraoperative Challenges

Challenges and solutions: Extended trochanteric osteotomy was performed to remove the osteolytic area in the medial calcar safely.

Thorough description of decision-making, including the reason for the final decision: With the amount of osteolysis and bone loss, extraction of the components and cement can *lead* to fractures and further compromise of the available bone stock for fixation. The extended trochanteric osteotomy was performed to remove the osteolytic area in the medial calcar safely. Fixation of the implant was obtained distally in the available diaphyseal bone, by engaging the splines of the modular tapered fluted stem to the diaphyseal bone. After achieving a well-fixed distal segment, version and length is then judge and adjusted using the proximal body trial.

36.8.8 Postoperative Radiographs (Figs. 36.31 and 36.32)

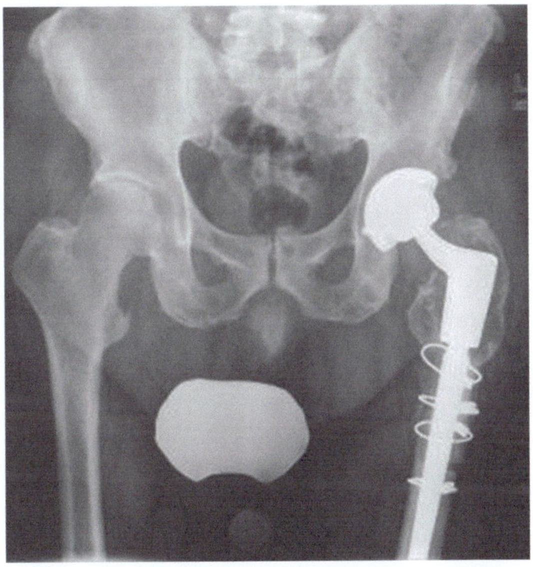

Fig. 36.31 Anteroposterior view of the pelvis demonstrates the final reconstruction twelve weeks after revision surgery. No hardware failure is noted, and the good fit was obtained distally. The length and offset were restored

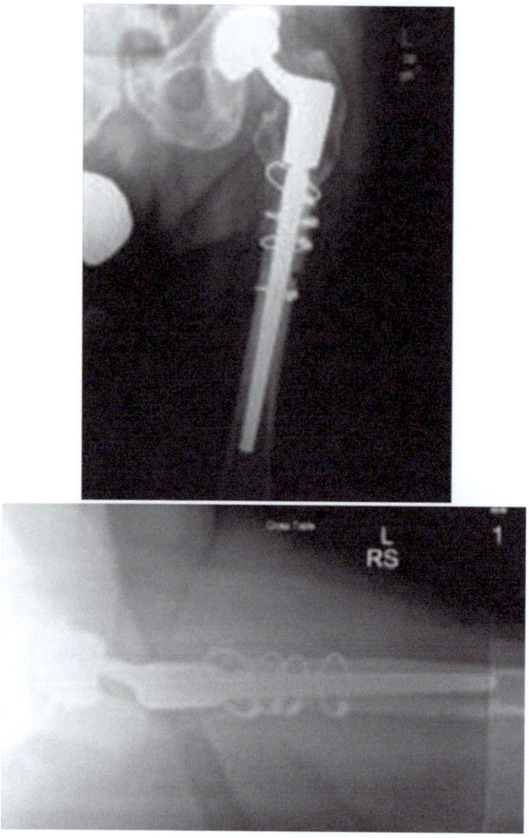

Fig. 36.32 Anteroposterior view and cross-table lateral demonstrates the final reconstruction twelve weeks after revision surgery

36.8.9 Postoperative Management

Chemoprophylaxis and anticoagulant treatment period: Coumadin for six weeks

Gait/limb loading until full loading: Toe-touch weight bearing for six weeks

36.8.10 Follow-Up and Complications

No reported complication

36.8.11 Discussion

Advantages of the applied method: A modular tapered stem provides the advantage of allowing intraoperative control of femoral version and length and maximizing stability. These stems are beneficial for those cases with a severe bone loss (Paprosky type IIIB and type IV), an altered lesser trochanter anatomy and a periprosthetic fracture. To gain stability with modular tapered stems, a minimum of two centimetres of diaphyseal contact is needed. Appropriate anteversion is easier to obtain when the proximal body spins on a well-fixed distal segment improving postoperative stability.

Disadvantages of the method: However, implant fracture and corrosion at the modular junctions can still occur, and modular stems should not be used as a routine for all femoral revisions.

Alternative evidence-based techniques for the case: Impaction bone grafting, mainly indicated for large canals and thin cortices (Paprosky IIIb and IV defects); allograft-prosthetic composite, mainly indicated for large metadiaphyseal bone defect and a nonsupportive diaphysis (Paprosky IV); and monoblock or modular stems, indicated for compromised metaphysis and diaphysis (Paprosky III).

Indications and contraindications for your technique: Revision total hip arthroplasties in patients with massive femoral deficiency (Paprosky IIIb and IV).

Learning curve and how to manage complications: The learning curve may have an effect on the postoperative subsidence of a tapered stem. Undersizing the implant is the most frequent cause.

Level of evidence concerning the superiority of this method against others: Monoblock femoral component has demonstrated to have a higher rate of failure when used in the setting of severe proximal femoral bone deficiency (Paprosky IIIb and IV) [11, 15, 71]. Fluted, tapered modular stems have demonstrated a high rate of osseointegration with excellent survival rate (97%) at twelve years [52]. Despite the advances of modular systems, mean subsidence of 2–9 mm has been reported, and instability continues to be a significant drawback (19%) [60, 72]. Additionally, failure at the modular junction is a known complication of this implants. In the presence of extensive proximal femoral deficiency (Paprosky IIIb and IV), a fluted modular tapered stem can achieve reliable distal fixation while allowing the control of both leg length and axial stability. These implants have the potential to achieve long-term biologic fixation, despite extensive bone deficiency [47], and have outperformed non-modular implant when treating massive proximal femur deficiency.

36.9 Case Title: Revision Femoral Arthroplasty Following Extended Trochanteric Osteotomy Using an Uncemented Modular Tapered Prosthesis

P.J. Boscainos, S. Patil, and D. Meek

With numbers of revision hip arthroplasty rising, there is an increased interest in surgical techniques that can provide safe access in the femoral canal, by minimizing bone loss. The extended trochanteric osteotomy (ETO) technique has provided such an option for revision of both cemented and uncemented femoral stems. This chapter will cover two examples, one with an uncemented and one with a cemented stem, as well as the indications, limitations and complications of ETO.

36.9.1 Revision of an Uncemented Stem Utilizing an Extended Trochanteric Osteotomy Approach

A 90-year-old female patient was transferred by ambulance to the accident and emergency department reporting right hip and thigh pain and inability to move the hip, following a mechanical fall. The patient had a history of a right hip Austin Moore hemiarthroplasty for femoral neck fracture performed 24 years prior to presentation. The past medical history included hypertension, atrial fibrillation and chronic kidney disease stage 3. The patient was on antihypertensive and warfarin.

Clinically there was the inability for the patient to stand or bear weight, absent active range of movement of the right hip and knee joints, secondary to pain and no lower limb neurovascular deficit. Plain radiographs showed a periprosthetic right femoral fracture (type Vancouver B2) around an Austin Moore hemiarthroplasty prosthesis with femoral shaft comminution. In Gruen zones 1 and 7, there were radiolucent lines, increasing the probability of loosening along with the disruption of bone-prosthesis interface at the fracture site. Also, there was a proximal migration of the prosthesis into the ilium (Fig. 36.33a–c). Following the diagnosis, warfarin was stopped, and surgery was scheduled when the INR had reached 1.5 or less.

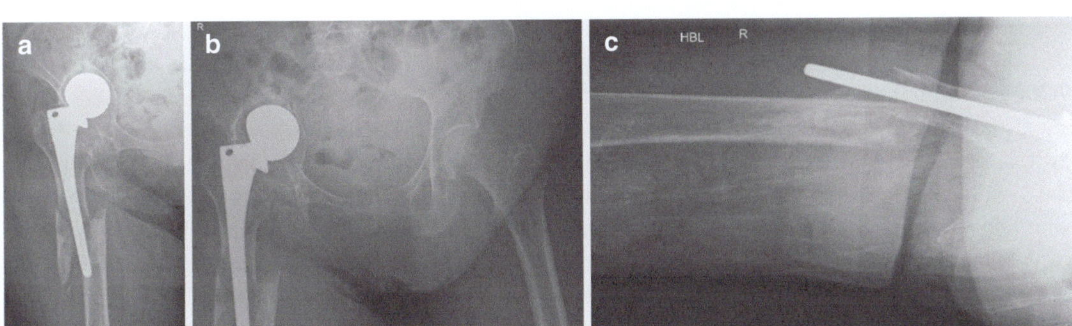

Fig. 36.33 A 90-year-old female patient admitted with a periprosthetic right femoral fracture around a right Austin Moore hemiarthroplasty performed 24 years before. (**a**) Radiographic anteroposterior view of the right hip and femur, showing the periprosthetic fracture of the right femur and proximal migration of the prosthesis into the ilium. (**b**) Radiographic anteroposterior view of the pelvis. (**c**) Radiographic lateral view of the right hip femur

The management options of a periprosthetic femoral fracture depend on the fixation of the prosthesis and the available femoral bone stock. In addition, access to the acetabulum should also be considered during preoperative planning. In this case, the proximal migration and gross protrusion of the prosthesis made access to the acetabulum, for the removal of the monoblock prosthesis and reconstruction, an additional consideration. The weak femoral cortices risked the possibility of further fractures during manipulation. The option of open reduction and internal fixation of such a fracture, in this case, would not be applicable, given the prosthesis loosening, weakness of cortices and need to mobilize this elderly patient quickly postoperatively. An ETO was chosen as the surgical approach to address all the issues discussed and minimize risk. As a reconstruction option for the acetabulum, impaction grafting of morsellized bone allograft and a cemented cup was selected. For the femoral side, a modular titanium stem was chosen to allow both distal and proximal femoral loading, as well as to address any possible dimension mismatch between the femoral diaphysis and the proximal metaphysis. The fracture and ETO were reduced with and held with a polymer cerclage system.

36.9.2 Surgical Technique

Under general anaesthesia and with the patient in the lateral decubitus position, a posterior approach with release of the gluteus maximus tendon and an ETO was performed. For the ETO, a Stryker (Kalamazoo, MI, USA) sagittal sawblade (25 mm width, 0.97 mm thickness) was used. With the leg in internal rotation, the posterolateral femoral cortex was osteotomized lateral to the linea aspera. The sawblade was passed through the prosthesis-bone interface in a posterior to anterior direction towards the anterior femoral cortex. The anterior aspect of the ETO was performed from a distal to proximal direction. The aim is for approximately one-third of the femoral circumference, with the greater trochanter, gluteus medius and vastus lateralis attached, to be reflected anteriorly. The vastus lateralis was reflected anteriorly from intermuscular septum; only as much is required to perform the posterior and distal aspects of the osteotomy and was not stripped off the femur to expose the anterior aspect of the osteotomy. As a result, some of the blood supply to the ETO fragment is retained. The distal end of the ETO was completed using the same sawblade. The ETO fragment with its muscular attachments was reflected anteriorly using wide osteotomes and held with a Hohmann retractor. At this stage removal of the anterior pseudocapsule increased exposure and reduced tension on the ETO fragment. With the ETO complete, the prosthesis was mobilized using osteotomes and a 5 mm high-speed burr. The stem was removed from the acetabular protrusion position with care to avoid any acetabular fractures. Multiple specimens of acetabular and femoral membrane were sent for microbiology. The protruded acetabulum was reamed to healthy cancellous bone margins. A femoral head allograft was used to prepare morsellized bone. The morsellized bone was washed, dried and augmented with Osteoset T bone graft substitute (Wright Medical Technologies, Arlington, TN, USA). The allograft bone was impacted into the defect. Palacos R + G bone cement (Heraeus Medical, Wehrheim, Germany) and a 32 mm internal diameter Marathon flanged cross-linked polyethylene cup (DePuy, Warsaw, IN, USA) were used to reconstruct the acetabulum. Prior to preparation of the femur a Supercable (Kinamed, Camarillo, CA, USA) prophylactic cerclage was placed at the femoral diaphysis distal to the osteotomy. The distal femur was reamed to prepare for a modular tapered titanium Reclaim stem (DePuy, Warsaw, IN, USA). With the distal reamer in place, a trial proximal shaft and neck were assembled, the estimated anteversion dialled in and a trial reduction showed good stability. The trials were removed, and the definitive distal stem was inserted at the same insertion depth with satisfactory press fit. The proximal body was inserted and secured at the same version. A further reduction showed good stability. With the hip dislocated, the proximal femur was reconstructed around the stem with a further four cerclage wires.

A particular challenge with this patient was the deficient femoral bone stock in the presence of a periprosthetic fracture. In such cases, it is useful to have available a proximal femoral

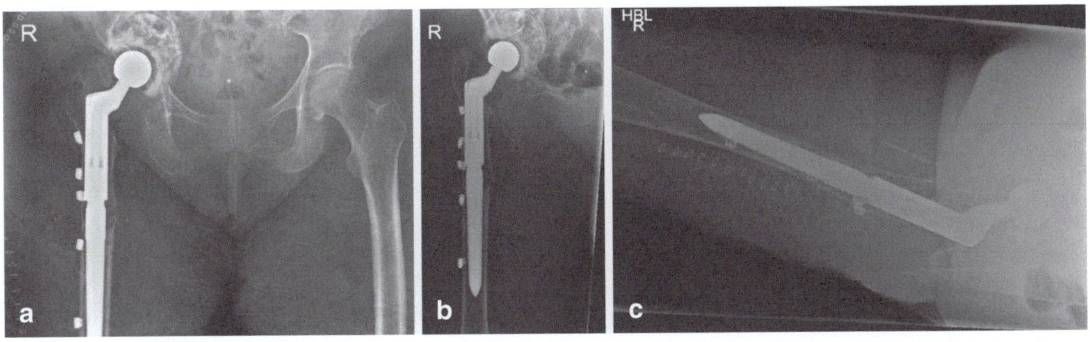

Fig. 36.34 Postoperative radiographs of the patient in Fig. 36.34. (**a**) Radiographic anteroposterior view of the pelvis, showing the acetabular reconstruction with morsellized cancellous allograft and a cemented cup. On the femoral side, an extended trochanteric osteotomy was performed to remove the prosthesis, and the reconstruction was made using a titanium modular prosthesis with a metal femoral head. The osteotomy was closed using a polymer cerclage system. (**b**) Radiographic anteroposterior view of the right hip and femur. (**c**) Radiographic lateral view of the right hip and femur

replacement system or a proximal femoral allograft, to address the possibility of the proximal femur being severely comminuted or lytic and thus not reconstructable in a way to allow proximal loading. Also, the protrusion of the acetabulum posed an additional challenge. Given the age and osteoporosis of the patient as well as the protrusion, metal augmentation and a press-fit uncemented cup were considered an additional fracture risk. Postoperative radiographs confirmed the adequate reconstruction of the acetabulum and femur, the femoral alignment and the leg lengths (Fig. 36.34a–c).

Postoperatively, the patient received a low molecular weight heparin subcutaneous injection once daily until discharge, followed by aspirin for a total of 35 days from surgery. She was allowed to weight bear as tolerated and advised to avoid active abduction for six weeks. Microbiology samples did not yield any growth. The patient developed medical complications, which included acute kidney injury and cholecystitis, and were managed conservatively.

36.9.3 Revision of a Cemented Stem Utilizing an Extended Trochanteric Osteotomy Approach

An 84-year-old male patient was admitted for elective revision of a loose Charnley cemented right total hip replacement that was performed eighteen years ago for primary osteoarthritis. The past medical history included hypertension, ischaemic heart disease for which the patient had undergone coronary artery bypass graft and aortic valve replacement, chronic kidney disease stage 3 and oesophageal hernia repair. The patient was on antihypertensives, nitrazepam, aspirin, simvastatin and omeprazole.

The patient had reported increasing right hip pain over a period of 1 month without a history of injury. He had severe difficulty rising from a chair and inability getting out of bed unaided. He reported side-effects to opiate analgesia and could not use non-steroidal anti-inflammatory drugs. Clinically there was right hip and thigh pain with restricted range of movement of the right hip due to pain. The left hip range of motion was also found restricted. There was no lower limb neurovascular deficit. There was no evidence in the history, clinical examination and serology to indicate septic loosening. Plain radiographs showed eccentric polyethylene wear of the cemented acetabular component. There were areas of osteolysis and radiolucent lines in multiple Gruen zones, along with femoral stem subsidence. Bone cement appeared to have surpassed the femoral cement restrictor. Also, there was heterotopic ossification over the right greater trochanter and osteoarthritis of the left hip (Fig. 36.35a–c).

The management options of a loose cemented hip arthroplasty depend on the bone stock, the

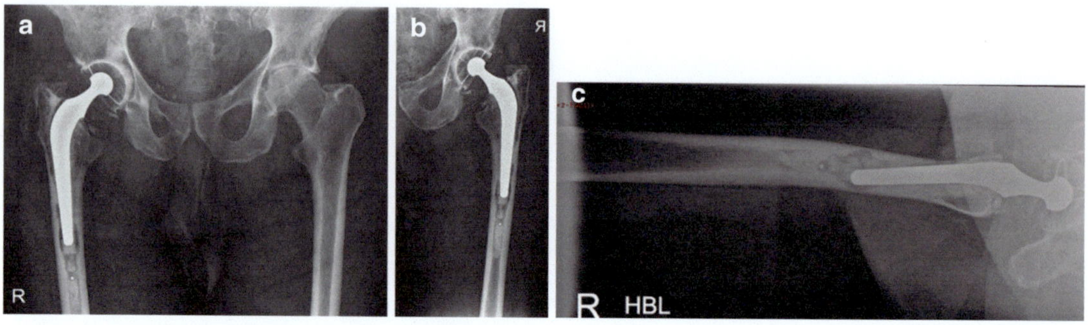

Fig. 36.35 An 84-year-old male patient admitted for revision of a painful, loose, cemented Charnley right total hip replacement performed eighteen years before. (**a**) Radiographic anteroposterior view of the pelvis, showing eccentric polyethylene wear of the cemented acetabular component, areas of osteolysis and radiolucent lines in multiple Gruen zones with femoral stem subsidence. Bone cement appears to have surpassed the femoral cement restrictor. Also, there is heterotopic ossification over the greater trochanter. (**b**) Radiographic anteroposterior view of the right hip and femur, showing the extent of the bone cement escaping beyond the femoral cement restrictor well into the femoral diaphysis. (**c**) Radiographic lateral view of the right hip femur, showing further lysis around the tip of the femoral stem and cement fragmentation. The tip of the stem has been in contact with the posterior femoral cortex, and there is almost full cortical thickness lysis in that area

presence and the location of osteolytic defects as well as any concomitant bone deformity. In addition, in this case, the extrusion of the femoral bone cement distal to the restrictor within the femoral diaphysis is an important consideration in the decision of technique applied. Lytic areas in the femur need to be bypassed or grafted. Although femoral impaction grafting has been reported in patients of similar age to this patient, the distal cement extrusion was a deciding factor for performing an ETO. In addition, femoral impaction grafting carries a risk of stem subsidence as well as intraoperative femoral fracture, which in this case was considered to be increased due to patient's age and osteolysis. Furthermore, an ETO approach is more expedient in reaching the distal cement and more successful in removing it in its totality.

36.9.4 Surgical Technique

Under general and spinal anaesthesia and with the patient in the lateral decubitus position, a posterior approach was performed. The hip was dislocated, and the femoral stem was removed from the femur, following decompression of the shoulder of the femoral prosthesis and the use of an extraction slap hammer. The cemented polyethylene liner was worn and loose. The cement was removed, and the acetabulum reamed to the healthy cancellous bone. Palacos R&G bone cement (Heraeus Medical, Wehrheim, Germany) and a 32 mm internal diameter Marathon flanged cross-linked polyethylene cup (DePuy, Warsaw, IN, USA) were used to reconstruct the acetabulum. The femoral stem was superimposed on the femur and used as a guide for the distal length of the ETO. The surgical technique for the ETO is described in detail in the previous case. The cement mantle was fully removed using a 5 mm high-speed burr, and the Moreland cemented hip revision instrumentation (DePuy, Warsaw, IN, USA). Following the removal of the distal cement and restrictor, the femoral reconstruction was similar to the previous case. Contouring of the ETO fragment to fit the revision stem and close the osteotomy window was performed using a high-speed burr.

The first challenge of this case was to remove the femoral component without risking the integrity of the greater trochanter. To address this in a situation of a composite beam round back femoral stem design, the proximal cement was removed with osteotomes and then the stem removed with an extraction slap hammer. Removal of the femoral stem allowed for adequate visualization of the acetabulum to allow reconstruction. An ETO early on in the surgery may achieve safe removal of the stem but increases blood loss and risks a femoral fracture during manipulation. The removal of the distal femoral cement was more expedient with an

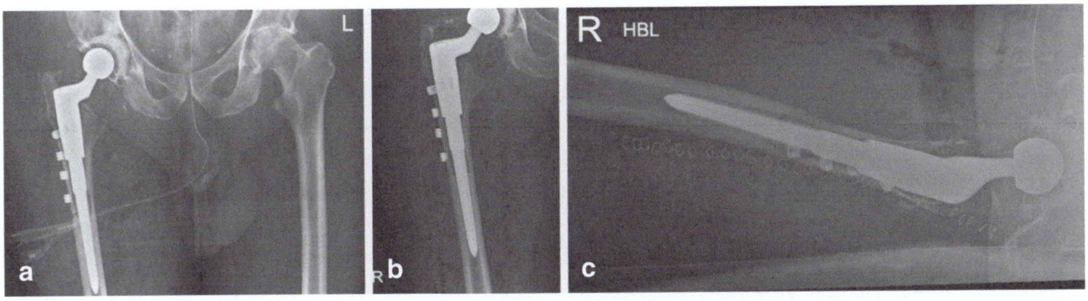

Fig. 36.36 Postoperative radiographs of the patient in Fig. 36.35. (**a**) Radiographic anteroposterior view of the pelvis, showing the acetabular reconstruction a cemented cup. The cement-bone interface from the index procedure was clinically and radiographically stable and has been maintained, utilizing a cement-in-cement technique. On the femoral side, an extended trochanteric osteotomy was performed to remove the prosthesis and the distally reaching cement plug. The reconstruction was made using a titanium modular prosthesis with a metal femoral head. The osteotomy was closed using a polymer cerclage system. (**b**) Anteroposterior view of the right hip and femur. (**c**) Radiographic lateral view of the right hip femur

ETO. Reaching and removing the distal cement completely from the top of the femur can be very challenging and increases the risk of a fracture or femoral cortex penetration. Postoperative radiographs confirmed the adequate reconstruction of the acetabulum and femur, the femoral alignment and the leg lengths (Fig. 36.36a–c).

The postoperative thromboprophylaxis and rehabilitation management was as in the previous case. All culture samples did not yield any growth. The patient developed medical complications (gastrointestinal bleeding and a chest infection) that were managed conservatively.

36.9.5 Discussion [50, 73–76]

The most common indication for ETO by far is the aseptic loosening of the femoral prosthesis. The choice of an ETO carries several advantages. It is a controlled approach to the femoral canal to remove a well-fixed femoral stem and, if present, distal cement and restrictor. By maintaining the abductor and vastus lateralis attachments, the myo-osseous flap retains its blood supply and, with the aid of reduction and fixation, its' mechanical stability, both of which increase the healing potential. ETO union rates between 91 and 98% have been reported in the literature. The wide exposure also allows excellent visualization and access to the acetabulum for either component removal or complex reconstruction. In cases of varus femoral deformity, the osteotomy can also be extended medially and facilitate correction following reconstruction. With an ETO the time required to remove the femoral stem and cement mantle is reduced, and the process is more controlled. There is less risk of a femoral fracture or cortical perforation during this stage of surgery.

Smaller series have reported on the use of ETO as part of two-stage revision for management of prosthetic joint infection. Even in cases where the ETO fragment is only fixed during the second-stage procedure, union rates are over 90%, although noted to occur approximately a month later compared to primary fixation at the first-stage procedure. In those studies, infection and patient outcomes were also very satisfactory.

More recently the use of ETO as an approach to access and manage periprosthetic fractures has been described. The periprosthetic fracture can be used as part of the osteotomy to allow access to the femoral canal for implant removal and revision reconstruction. In such circumstances, a slight variation in the original ETO surgical technique has been described, where the proximal end of the posterior aspect of the osteotomy is performed between the gluteus medius anteriorly and the external rotators posteriorly.

Careful preoperative planning for an ETO is important. The main goals are to create an adequate window of visualization to safely remove the prosthesis and cement while at the same time have an approximately 4–6 cm in the area of intact bone at the isthmus to allow for press-fit fixation of an uncemented stem. To achieve this, templating on both the anteroposterior and lateral planes is required. In situations where there is a femoral deformity, a bypassing uncemented femoral stem risks femoral cortex perforation or a fracture. The ETO lends itself well to correct any varus femoral deformity that may have occurred as part of the femoral component loosening process, osteolysis and bone remodelling under loading. In such a situation, the length of the ETO should take into account the centre of rotation of the deformity to allow for safe stem and cement extraction, as well as deformity correction, by extension of the distal aspect of the osteotomy to the medial cortex. The ETO as an approach has also been used in complex primary THR, where there is a femoral deformity. Such cases have included subtrochanteric malunion, developmental and fibrous dysplasia.

Technical considerations during the planning of an ETO in revision hip surgery are the type of implant, the degree of fixation at the implant-bone interface or the cement-bone interface and the length of the required osteotomy. Polished tapered cemented stems are removed easily in most cases. Precoated cemented stems, or composite beam designs are not removed easily and require an ETO. In such cases, the level of osteotomy is determined by the extent of precoating or the extent of the well-fixed bone cement. Uncemented stems are more difficult to remove, and such a procedure is associated with a higher incidence of intraoperative periprosthetic fractures. In such circumstances, the level of osteotomy is determined by the stem length as well as the intact diaphyseal bone to allow adequate fixation of the revision stem. Flexible osteotomes and Gigli saws through the ETO are useful in disrupting the prosthesis-bone interface of a well-fixed uncemented stem. For long curved stems or broken stems, the osteotomy length is determined by the position of the stem curve or stem fracture. The curved stem can be sectioned with a diamond tip high-speed burr and the distal aspect removed using hollow trephine reamers.

A further issue that has attracted attention is that of fixation of the ETO fragment. It is widely accepted that a secure fixation of the ETO fragment improves patient outcomes. There is a debate on whether cable fixation is superior to wires with a number of biomechanical and cadaveric studies favouring cable fixation. The number of cables required is largely determined by the length of the osteotomy. Nonmetallic cables have an additional advantage of reducing the risks of fraying and third-body wear. It is important that all cables are passed directly on the femur, under the vastus lateralis, so that there is no vascular compromise on the fragment that could affect healing. Close apposition of the ETO fragment is important to achieve healing, and frequently contouring of the fragment is required to close the osteotomy over the revision implant.

Alternative approaches that have been described for revision of the femoral prosthesis are those of removing the femoral canal contents (stem and or cement) from the femoral neck osteotomy site, a posterior longitudinal femoral split and a trochanteric slide osteotomy. While removing a tapered cemented prosthesis from the proximal osteotomy may be relatively straightforward in most cases, removing a well-fixed cement mantle and the distal cement plug is time-consuming and risks femoral cortical perforation and/or fracture, thus negating the potential advantage of an intact femoral cortex. In a situation of a distally well-fixed uncemented stem, this approach carries the same challenges as with a well-fixed cement mantle. A posterior longitudinal split has been described in a few case series as an alternative for femoral stem extraction. This technique has similar difficulties with the removal of the cement mantle or a well-fixed uncemented stem from the femoral neck osteotomy. A trochanteric slide osteotomy, while it allows for good acetabular exposure, provides little advantage in facilitating the removal of the femoral canal contents.

An important issue to address in revision surgery of the femur is that of bone loss. Bone loss may exist preoperatively or may result from the surgical intervention to remove the femoral prosthesis and any residual cement. Other challenges faced during revision surgery may be those of femoral bone deformity (usually in varus) and mismatch of the proximal metaphyseal and diaphyseal dimensions. The host bone is more fragile and sclerotic compared to the bone in a primary setting. Sclerotic bone does not allow for bone-cement interdigitation, thus reducing the shear strength of the bone-cement interface. In the presence of full-thickness cortical defects, bone cement cannot be pressurized adequately. Also, cement may escape through the ETO increasing the risk of non-union. A described alternative, especially in younger patients, is that of femoral bone impaction grafting and a cemented stem within the impacted allograft morsellized bone bed. A small number of studies have advocated this technique, particularly in Paprosky 4 femoral defects. Femoral impaction grafting is time-consuming and technical and inherently carries the risks of an intraoperative femoral fracture and postoperative femoral stem subsidence. For these reasons, an uncemented femoral revision option was considered more favourable in the cases discussed. A fully porous-coated implant carries the risks of proximal stress shielding and postoperative thigh pain. In cases where revision of an ingrown fully porous-coated stem is required, this adds increased technical complexity and possible compromise to the femoral bone stock. Furthermore, the dimensions of fully porous-coated cylindrical stems cannot always address the anatomical variation that may exist between the dimensions of the proximal femoral metaphysis and the diaphysis of an osteolytic femur. Also such a stem may not be able to negotiate femoral bowing. Such stems rely in distal fixation that may lead to pain, implant failure, fracture or fixation failure. Apart from the advantage of a Young's modulus closer to that of cortical bone, a modular titanium prosthesis can address the difference in proximal metaphyseal and diaphyseal anatomy. Adjustments can be made to ensure both distal and proximal press-fit loading of the host bone, as well as adjustments to ensure appropriate leg lengths and offset. Conical tapered modular stems have the advantage of utilizing a limited sector of the diaphyseal femur (usually 4–6 cm) for press fit. This allows for the use of shorter stems reserving bone for future surgery but also allowing for a small degree of subsidence. Limitations in using modular prostheses in revision situations are a very osteoporotic femur that does not allow proximal and distal stem press-fit, curved femur without isthmus or destroyed isthmus.

Complications that have been described with an ETO approach are fractures, osteotomy non-union, osteotomy fragment migration and stem subsidence. Intraoperative fractures may occur either at the osteotomy fragment or the remaining femur. These are dependent on surgical technique, bone stock and use of hardware. Underreaming for either a straight or bowed stem can be a fracture risk, even without an ETO. The use of prophylactic wiring distal to the osteotomy and prior to femoral canal preparation to prevent fractures has been advocated by several authors. The release of the anterior hip pseudocapsule and scar tissue reduces the tension on the osteotomy fragment and may reduce the risk of fracture on the fragment. If this occurs, a claw plate to secure the trochanter may be required. The distal aspect of the osteotomy has been shown to be a stress riser, and several authors have advocated rounding the edges of the distal aspect, but fractures may still occur, and this hypothesis is not widely accepted. Non-union may occur to 1–3% of cases. This may relate to the number of previous procedures, devascularization of the osteotomy fragment during the approach and poor fixation. Implant failure and subsidence may occur when the proximal bone is not supportive to the stem. Some authors have advocated that the use of a supportive femoral strut allograft on the anterior aspect of the femur is useful in such circumstances, but this is not widely accepted. When using a modular stem in the mechanical environment of an ETO without supportive proximal bone, it is important to choose one without a track record of junction failures between the proximal body and distal stem. Cable fixation failures following an ETO have been widely reported. The concerns associated with such a failure are that of third-body generation and wear of the bearing or fraying. In our cases we have been using nylon cables to mitigate that possibility. Iatrogenic vascular injury cases have also been reported, mainly associated with the passing of cerclage wires, but these are uncommon.

The extended trochanteric osteotomy technique has provided significant advantages of controlled access, reduced risk of removing the femoral canal contents, reliable healing rates and improved patient outcomes. As such, it is a very useful surgical approach in the armamentarium of the revision hip surgeon.

36.10 Case Title: Breakage of Femoral Stem

Libor Nečas and Marek Rovňák

36.10.1 Demographics

Age: 82
Sex: Female
BMI: 34.67

36.10.2 Relevant Past Medical History

Principal pathologies: Arterial hypertension, ischemic cardiac disease and gastroesophageal reflux

Previous surgical procedures: Right hip replacement 2009, left hip replacement 2010 and operation of the spine 2013

Medication: Urapidil, omeprazole, calcium channel blockers, isosorbide mononitrate, betablockers, acetylsalicylic acid, furosemide, hydrochlorothiazide and ACE-inhibitors

Other: Food allergy

History of presenting complaint: This is a patient that received a cemented right replacement in 2009 and cemented left hip replacement in 2010. She had a history of fall on left hip in 2011; subsequently she felt pain in the left hip during walking. She was checked in the surgical ambulance in the field without X-ray, and she was sent home, after the check. She came in our orthopaedic ambulance in August 2013, where there was verified breakage of the stem in medial third with the loosening of the proximal half.

36.10.3 Clinical Examination

Symptoms: Severe pain by standing on the left extremity; unable to weight bear; shortening of the left extremity, 2 cm; and slight extra-rotation of the left extremity

Range of motion: S 0–0–60, F 10–0–10, R 10–0–5

Main disability: Unable to full weight bear

Scoring: WOMAC 29.2%, HHS 24

Neurovascular evaluation: Without any neurovascular deficit

36.10.4 Preoperative Radiological Assessment/Imaging (Figs. 36.37 and 36.38)

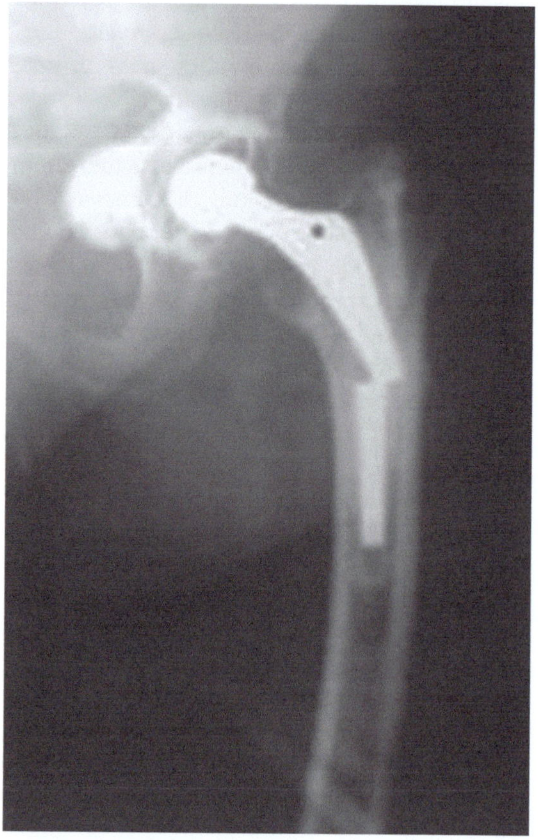

Fig. 36.37 X-ray of the left hip with breakage of the femoral stem 2013

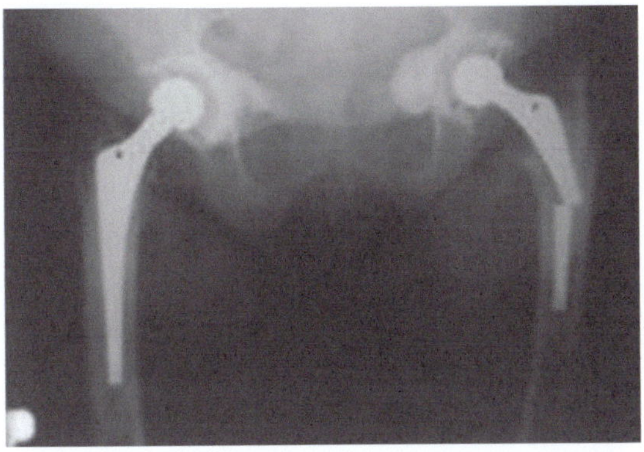

Fig. 36.38 Comparison with contralateral site with the same stem implanted one year before

36.10.5 Preoperative Planning

Diagnosis: Fatigue fracture of femoral stem (Figs. 36.37 and 36.38)

Possible treatment options: Anterograde reaming and removal of the stem, transfemoral approach, bone window and retrograde removal of the fractured stem

Chosen treatment method: Anterograde removal of the stem and modular revision stem

Expected difficulties: Extraction of the distal part of the stem

36.10.6 Surgical Note

Patient's position: Supine position

Type of anaesthesia: General anaesthesia

Surgical approach: Transgluteal

Main steps: Removal of the proximal segment, removal of the distal segment and bone cement

Reconstruction techniques: Anterograde reaming and modular stem

36.10.7 Postoperative Radiographs (Figs. 36.39 and 36.40)

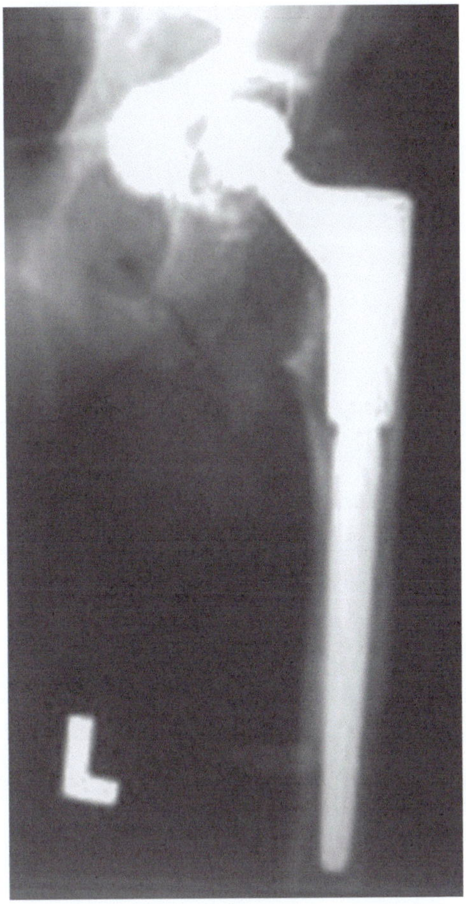

Fig. 36.39 Postoperative X-ray with revision stem

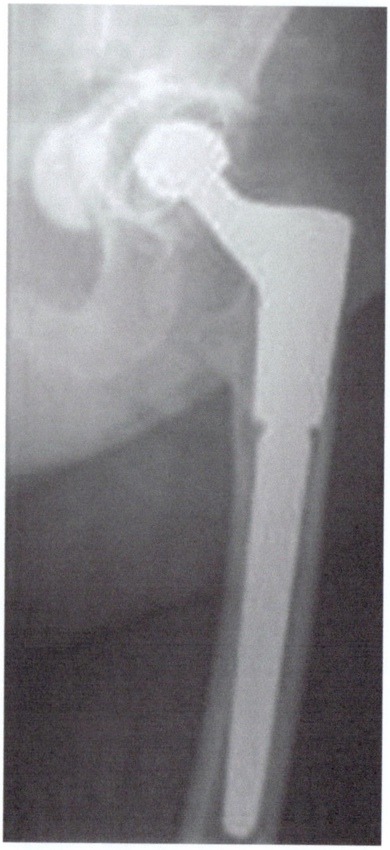

Fig. 36.40 AP femur and hip X-ray two years postoperatively

36.10.8 Postoperative Management

Chemoprophylaxis and anticoagulant treatment period: Cefazolin 2–1-g intravenously with first dose two h preoperatively, Enoxaparin sol. Inj. 0.4 mL/4000 anti-Xa IU subcutaneously thirty days

Gait/limb loading until full loading: three months

36.10.9 Follow-Up and Complications

Scoring: three months postoperatively—HHS 79, WOMAC 75%, six months postoperatively HHS 79 WOMAC 66.7%, one-year postoperatively HHS 81, WOMAC 63.5%

36.11 Case Title: Femoral Revision "Monolithic Stem"

Ivan De Martino, Peter K. Sculco, and Thomas P. Sculco

36.11.1 Demographics

Age: 95
Sex: Female
BMI: 18.3

36.11.2 Relevant Past Medical History

Principal pathologies: Coronary artery disease (CAD), mitral valve regurgitation, chronic systolic congestive heart failure due to CAD, bradycardia, chronic obstructive pulmonary disease, left lower extremity deep vein thrombosis and osteoporosis.

Previous surgical procedures: Open reduction and internal fixation (cephalomedullary nail) for intertrochanteric fracture of the right femur in September 2015, permanent pacemaker in 2003, coronary artery stents in 2006, percutaneous mitral valve repair in 2012 and inferior vena cava filter in November 2015.

Medication: Acetaminophen, tiotropium inhalation powder, beclomethasone dipropionate HFA inhalation aerosol, metoprolol succinate extended-release, rivaroxaban, acetylsalicylic acid, furosemide, calcium and vitamin D.

Other: Stage 1 sacral ulcer.

History of Presenting Complaint: A 95-year-old female who underwent an ORIF (cephalomedullary nail) for an intertrochanteric fracture of right femur approximatively six weeks before the presentation at our office. During the last two weeks, she had increasing pain and limitation of the function of her right hip which was exacerbated during physical therapy sessions. She denies any falls or trauma. States was able to still participate in physical therapy despite the pain.

36.11.3 Clinical Examination

Symptoms: Increasing pain in her right hip that is exacerbated with weight-bearing and is currently wheelchair bound.

Range of motion: Motion is limited by pain.

Specific tests: On supine examination, she had pain with any motion of the right leg. She is currently unable to bear weight on the right side.

Main disability: Unable to bear weight on right leg due to pain.

Neurovascular evaluation: Sensation is intact to light touch, she has 5/5 neuromuscular strength throughout and she has palpable dorsal pedal pulses, less than a 3-s capillary refill.

36.11.4 Preoperative Radiological Assessment/Imaging (Figs. 36.41 and 36.42)

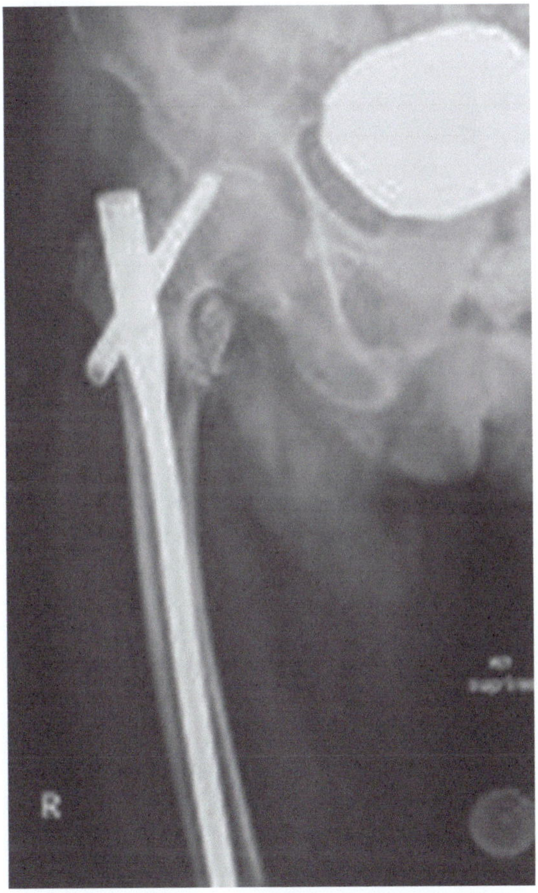

Fig. 36.41 Anteroposterior radiograph of the right hip at the time of initial consultation for right hip pain two months after cephalomedullary nail for intertrochanteric fracture showing blade cut-out and catastrophic failure

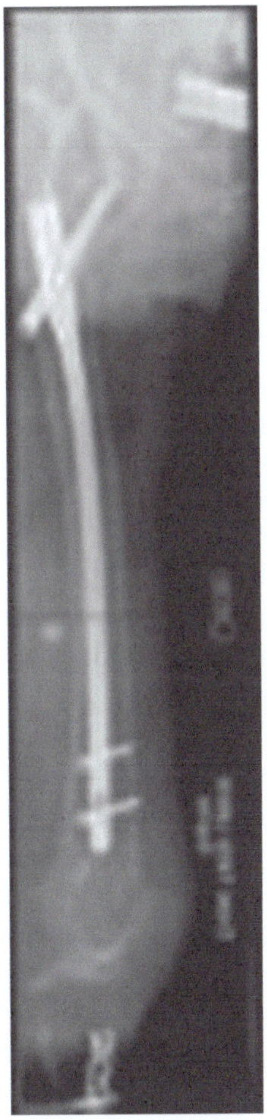

Fig. 36.42 Lateral radiograph of the right hip at the time of initial consultation for right hip pain two months after cephalomedullary nail for intertrochanteric fracture showing blade cut-out and catastrophic failure

36.11.5 Preoperative Planning

Diagnosis: Right hip cephalomedullary nail cut-out and mechanical failure (Figs. 36.41 and 36.42).

Possible treatment options: Revision with monolithic tapered fluted femoral stem, revision with modular tapered fluted femoral stem, revision with extensively porous-coated femoral stem and revision with calcar-replacing cemented stem.

Chosen treatment method: Monolithic fluted tapered stem.

Selection of implants if applicable and rational: Wagner SL revision femoral stem (Zimmer

Biomet) 19 × 190 mm, cobalt-chrome femoral head 28 mm −3 and dual mobility acetabular component.

Expected difficulties: Intraoperative fracture, postoperative hip dislocation secondary to abductor dysfunction, cephalomedullary nail removal and cortical perforation risk due to the neocortex around the cephalomedullary nail.

Strategies to overcome difficulties: Hip dislocation before nail removal to reduce the risk of stress riser fracture. C-arm fluoroscopy to assist with screw and nail localization as needed, appropriate extraction instruments and universal nail extraction set for nail removal. The use of high-speed burr to identify the blade or screws if there is bone overgrowth. The use of a dual mobility cup to reduce the risk of dislocation due to abductor insufficiency.

Templating: Since the lesser trochanter was fractured, the tip of the greater trochanter was utilized for leg length recreation. The contralateral hip was used as a guide to assess the position of the femoral head in relation to the greater trochanter. In addition, the contralateral hip was used as a general guide for appropriate offset recreation. Once the acetabulum was templated, the centre of rotation was determined. The distal length of the prosthesis was chosen based on a sufficient anchorage in cortical bone. The diameter of the conical distal stem was established in the region of the femoral cortices that allowed for at least three cm of diaphyseal fixation.

36.11.6 Surgical Note

Patient's position: Left lateral decubitus position with bony prominences padded.

Type of anaesthesia: Spinal-epidural with sedation.

Surgical approach: Posterolateral approach.

Main steps: Exposure and removal of the cephalomedullary nail. Placement of the acetabular component. Reaming of the diaphysis of the femur into a tapered shape using the appropriate reamers to the depth established by preoperative templating. Trial reduction with the provisional femoral stem to adjust leg length, offset and anteversion as needed for stability. Impaction of the monolithic stem into to the prepared distal femur to the previously determined depth level. Placing the definitive femoral head (Figs. 36.43 and 36.44).

Reconstruction techniques: A prophylactic cable was used around the proximal femur to prevent initiation and propagation of iatrogenic fracture during canal reaming.

36.11.7 Intraoperative Challenges

Challenges and solutions: (1) Cephalomedullary nail removal. The two distal screws were removed utilizing the previous skin incision. The standard posterolateral approach to the hip was performed. The hip was dislocated with a bone hook and the top of the nail unlocked. The nail was extracted with company-specific instrumentation. (2) The presence of neocortex was addressed with a high-speed burr and was used to open the diaphyseal canal and avoid perforation of the lateral cortex. Avoiding intraoperative fracture of osteoporotic bone was achieved with the use of a prophylactic cable, manual reaming of the diaphysis, and the use of a tapered titanium stem rather than a cylindrical cobalt-chrome stem.

Thorough description of decision-making, including the reason for the final decision: A fluted tapered stem was selected to bypass the area of proximal femoral bone loss and achieve fixation is diaphyseal bone. The fluted design promoted rotational stability in the setting of metaphyseal deficiency. In addition, a monolithic stem was chosen because the tip of the greater trochanter was intact and could be utilized to restore leg length reliably. Prior to femoral preparation, a prophylactic cable was placed 1 cm below the starting point of the intact femur. This cable allows for more aggressive reaming and implant insertion while minimizing the risk of intraoperative fracture.

36.11.8 Postoperative Radiographs (Figs. 36.43 and 36.44)

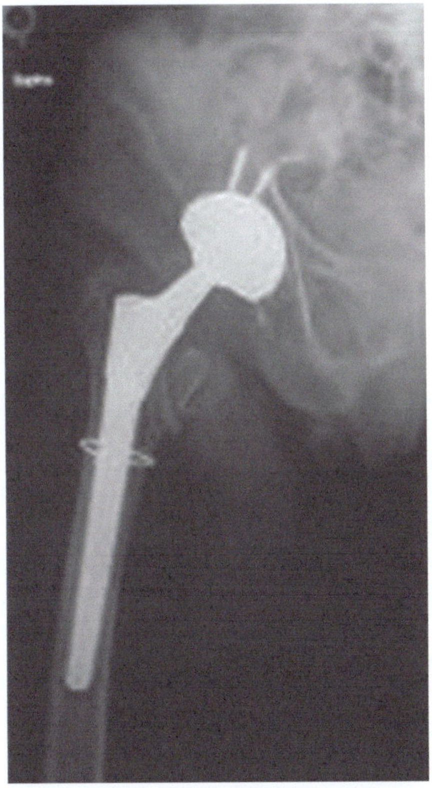

Fig. 36.43 Anteroposterior radiograph of the right hip six weeks after the revision with a monolithic tapered fluted stem

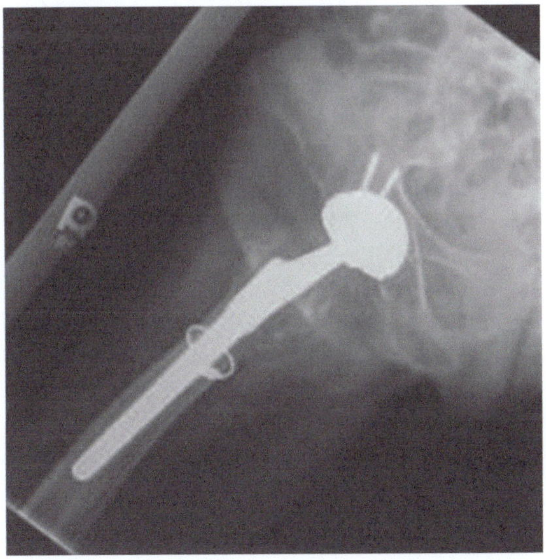

Fig. 36.44 Frog-leg lateral radiograph of the right hip six weeks after the revision with a monolithic tapered fluted stem

36.11.9 Postoperative Management

Chemoprophylaxis and anticoagulant treatment period: Warfarin for six weeks.

Gait/limb loading until full loading: WBAT in the immediate postoperative period with a walker.

36.11.10 Follow-Up and Complications

There were no postoperative complications.

36.11.11 Discussion [27, 77, 78]

Advantages of the applied method: Monolithic fluted tapered stem allows surgeons to establish stable diaphyseal fixation.

Disadvantages of the method: The major disadvantage for this type of implant is stem subsidence that can lead to instability and leg shortening. Early subsidence has been attributed to the component undersizing.

Alternative evidence-based techniques for the case: Calcar-replacing cemented femoral stem and modular fluted tapered cementless stem have been used with satisfactory results.

Why is the chosen technique better for this case? The chosen technique provides reliable diaphyseal fixation. The use of a monolithic stem is an efficient way to achieve diaphyseal fixation while using the tip of the greater trochanter as a guide for leg length restoration.

Indications and contraindications for your technique: Indication for the use of monolithic fluted tapered stem varies according to the surgeon's philosophy and the amount of femoral bone loss. Indications for this technique include situations where the proximal femur is damaged, and diaphyseal fixation is necessary. A monolithic fluted tapered titanium stem is advantageous when the tip of the greater trochanter is intact and can be used during preparation of the femoral canal for accurate leg length restoration. Contraindications for this technique are when diaphyseal diameter or offset recreation cannot be achieved with the use of a monolithic stem. Situations where both the greater trochanter and lesser trochanter are deficient make use of a monolithic stem more challenging. Some surgeons use these stems for the majority of femoral revisions, while others use these stems for severe diaphyseal bone loss including Paprosky types IIIA and IIIB femora, where proximal bone is deficient and cannot support stems that rely on proximal fit and fill. These stems are also particularly valuable for treating Vancouver types B1 and B2 periprosthetic fractures. These stems are contraindicated when the diaphyseal bone loss is extensive (Paprosky type IV), and a stable fixation of the implant cannot be achieved. However, some surgeons have had success in this scenario with these stems.

Learning curve and how to manage complications: During the learning curve, it is possible to undersize the femoral component. Manual reaming is recommended for this monolithic stem, and the surgeon should be familiar with the different feedback between manual versus power reaming.

Level of evidence concerning the superiority of this method against others: Monolithic tapered fluted stems have demonstrated excellent long-term results in several studies. Titanium fluted tapered stems have a lower rate of intraoperative fracture compared to cobalt-chrome stems which are advisable in cases of osteoporotic bone where diaphyseal fixation is required.

36.12 Case Title: Femoral Revision "Modular Stem"

Ivan De Martino, Peter K. Sculco, and Thomas P. Sculco

36.12.1 Demographics

Age: 77
Sex: Male
BMI: 40.9

36.12.2 Relevant Past Medical History

Principal pathologies: Coronary artery disease, type 2 diabetes mellitus, hypertension, high cholesterol, orthostatic hypotension and obstructive sleep apnoea.

Previous surgical procedures: Right total hip arthroplasty in 2003, left total hip arthroplasty 2015, coronary artery bypass grafting in 2013 and cholecystectomy in 2000.

Medication: Acetaminophen, metformin Hcl, diltiazem, rosuvastatin, metoprolol tartrate and acetylsalicylic acid.

History of presenting complaint: A 77-year-old gentleman presented to the office twelve years after from an uncomplicated right metal-on-metal total hip arthroplasty with a modular femoral stem. During the last six months, he had increasing pain in his right leg with weight-bearing activity and limitation of function. He is currently unable to ambulate without a crutch due to pain.

36.12.3 Clinical Examination

Symptoms: He walks with a slow severe right-sided antalgic gait with a crutch.

Range of motion: Hip range of motion is limited by pain.

Specific tests: On supine examination, he had markedly positive Stinchfield test on the right side with significant thigh pain with rotation of the leg. Negative Stinchfield test on the left side.

Main disability: worsening severe pain with weight bearing and significant pain with basic activities of daily living.

Neurovascular evaluation: Sensation is intact to light touch. He has 5/5 neuromuscular strength throughout, and he has palpable dorsal pedal pulses, less than a 3-s capillary refill.

36.12.4 Preoperative Radiological Assessment/Imaging (Figs. 36.45, 36.46, and 36.47)

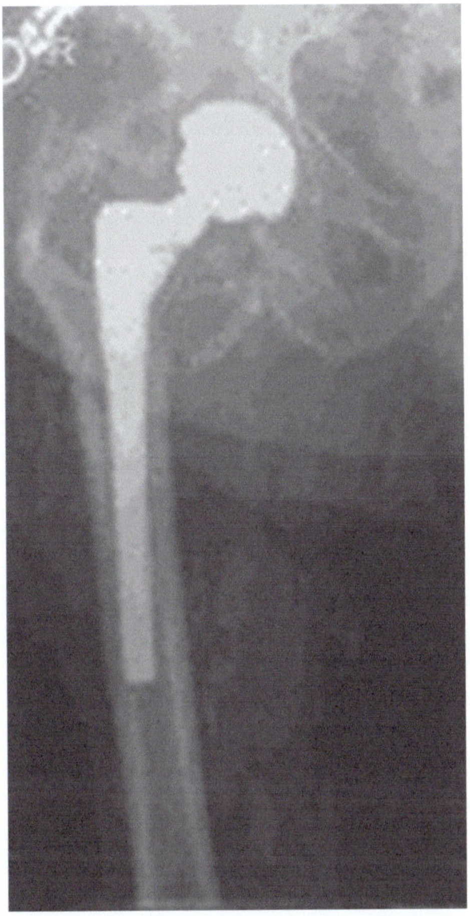

Fig. 36.45 Anteroposterior (AP) radiograph of the right hip at the time of initial consultation for right hip pain twelve years after total hip arthroplasty. A metal-on-metal bearing surface with massive osteolysis around the femoral stem. AP radiograph shows hazy but diffuse retroacetabular lysis. Booker III/IV heterotopic ossification involving the abductor mechanism and extending to the superolateral acetabulum. Medial calcar and lesser trochanter osteolytic resorption with associated fragment displacement

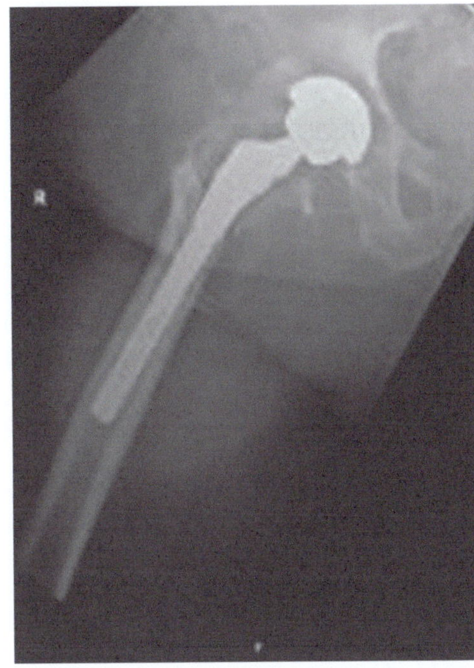

Fig. 36.46 Frog-leg lateral radiograph of the right hip at the time of initial consultation for right hip pain, twelve years after total hip arthroplasty. A metal-on-metal bearing surface with massive osteolysis around the femoral stem and mild bone lysis around the acetabular cup (medial wall)

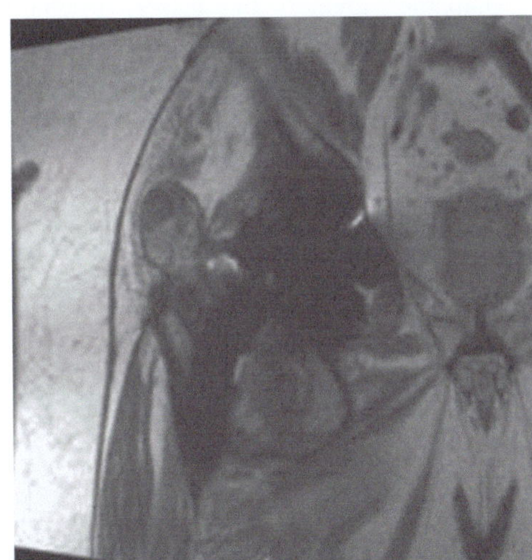

Fig. 36.47 Sagittal magnetic resonance imaging sequence (MAVRIC) showing prominent synovial expansion with intermediate and low signal intensity debris and heterogeneous signal in the trochanteric region, proximal femur, pubis, ischium and ilium suggestive of extensive osteolysis and wear-related disease. Interestingly, there is no fluid collection or evidence of pseudotumor to suggest an adverse reaction to metallic debris

36.12.5 Preoperative Planning

Diagnosis: Likely aseptic loosening of femoral and acetabular components with massive osteolysis without evidence of ARMD. Femoral bone loss was classified as Paprosky type IIIA (Figs. 36.45, 36.46 and 36.47).

Possible treatment options: Revision with modular tapered fluted femoral stem, revision with monolithic tapered fluted femoral stem and revision with extensively porous-coated femoral stem.

Chosen treatment method: Modular fluted tapered stem.

Selection of implants if applicable and rational: Restoration modular revision femoral stem (Stryker), conical distal stem 17 × 155 mm, proximal cone body 25 mm +0132 o, 32 mm + 4 ceramic femoral head and constrained cemented all-polyethylene component.

Expected difficulties: Femoral stem removal, metaphyseal (S-ROM) sleeve removal; avoid perforation of the lateral cortex due to varus stem position and the presence of lateral pedestal. Accurate restoration of leg length equality without palpable greater or lesser trochanter. Achieving intraoperative stability and reducing the risk of postoperative dislocation second to abductor dysfunction, obesity and revision surgery.

Strategies to overcome difficulties: Extensile posterolateral approach, the use of a pencil tip burr to remove remaining bone around the metaphyseal sleeve, and carefully open the distal femur with a bullet-tipped reamer to penetrate the pedestal. Utilizing identifiable femoral landmark to access distance to femoral head centre and utilize this intraoperatively for accurate leg length restoration. The use of modular proximal body to allow for intraoperative leg length, offset and version adjustments based on intraoperatively trialling. The use of a constrained liner to decrease the risk of postoperative dislocation.

Templating: Since we didn't have either the greater trochanter nor, the lesser trochanter, we used the distance between the centre of rotation and the most proximal part of the medial femur as a reference to assess preoperative leg length discrepancy. Once the acetabulum was templated, the centre of rotation was determined. The distal length of the prosthesis was chosen based on a sufficient anchorage in good cortical bone (two canal diameters below the tip of the existing implant in this case). The proximal cone body length and offset were chosen based on the templated femoral head centre of rotation.

36.12.6 Surgical Note

Patient's position: Left lateral decubitus position with bony prominences padded.

Type of anaesthesia: Combined spinal/epidural anaesthesia.

Surgical approach: Posterolateral approach utilizing the previous surgical incision.

Main steps: Exposure and removal of the previous femoral stem. Reaming of the diaphysis of the femur into a tapered shape using the appropriate reamers to the depth established by preoperative templating. Impaction of the distal portion of the stem into to the prepared distal femur to the previously determined depth level. Reaming the proximal cone body. Trial reduction with adjustments made for leg length, offset and anteversion as needed for stability. Placing the definitive proximal body component and femoral head (Figs. 36.48 and 36.49).

Reconstruction techniques: A prophylactic cable was used around the proximal femur to prevent fracture.

36.12.7 Intraoperative Challenges

Challenges and solutions: (1) Surgical exposure. Patient BMI was greater than 40. Required extension of the original surgical incision. A massive amount of osteolytic debris and disruption of the proximal femur. The greater and lesser trochanter was not present with only a soft tissue sleeve with abductor and vastus lateralis attachments remaining. A large amount of heterotopic ossification in the abductor musculature made the osteolytic and scar debris difficult to mobilize. (2) The metaphyseal sleeve was fixed only on the lateral and distal section. A pencil tip burr was utilized around the sleeve to facilitate its removal. (3) The presence of lateral pedestal. A pencil tip burr in combination with an AO bullet-tipped reamer inserted manually was used to open the diaphyseal canal and to avoid perforation of the lateral cortex.

Thorough description of decision-making, including the reason for the final decision: A modular fluted tapered stem addressed several of the reconstruction challenges in this case. First off, the proximal femur and unsupported secondary to extensive osteolysis. A diaphyseal engaging stem that bypassed this proximal femoral bone loss was best suited for this reconstruction. Since the metaphysis is completely unsupported, a tapered stem design instead of a cylindrical stem was chosen. Fluted stem designs have increased rotational stability compared to cylindrical stems. Cylindrical stems gain rotational stability with three-point contact in the metaphysis. In this case, without metaphyseal support, a cylindrical stem may lack the rotational stability required for initial implant stability. There was no identifiable greater or lesser trochanter making it difficult to template leg length restoration. For the posterior approach, the two most common methods for leg length is using the tip of the greater trochanter or measuring the lesser trochanter to femoral head centre distance. In this case, on the preoperative radiograph, the distance from the most proximal portion of the intact femur to the centre of the prosthetic femoral head was measured. Intraoperatively, the same location on the femur was identified, and the goal of the reconstruction was to re-establish this preoperatively measured distance. Since anatomic femoral landmarks were not present, the use of a modular system allows for adjustments in leg length and offset. Prior to femoral preparation, a prophylactic cable was placed 1 cm below the starting point of the intact femur. This cable allows for more aggressive reaming and implant insertion while minimizing the risk of intraoperative fracture.

36.12.8 Postoperative Radiographs (Figs. 36.48 and 36.49)

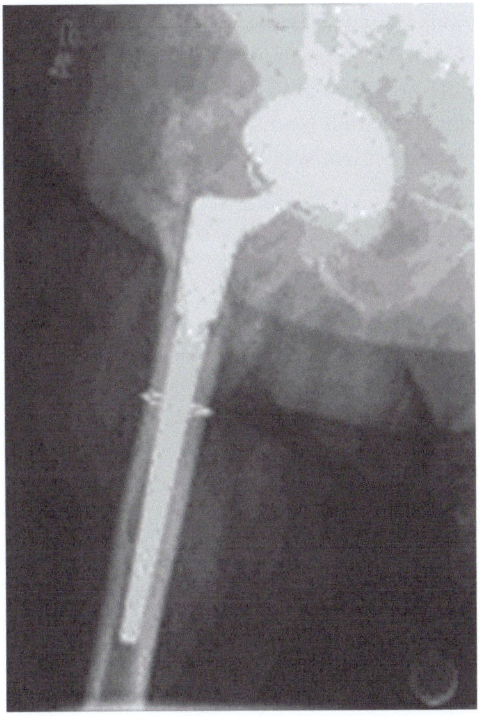

Fig. 36.48 Anteroposterior radiograph of the right hip six weeks after the revision with a modular tapered fluted stem. Standing AP radiographs demonstrate no subsidence of the femoral component. No migration or change in orientation of the acetabular component. Excellent cortical contact with the diaphyseal fluted tapered stem

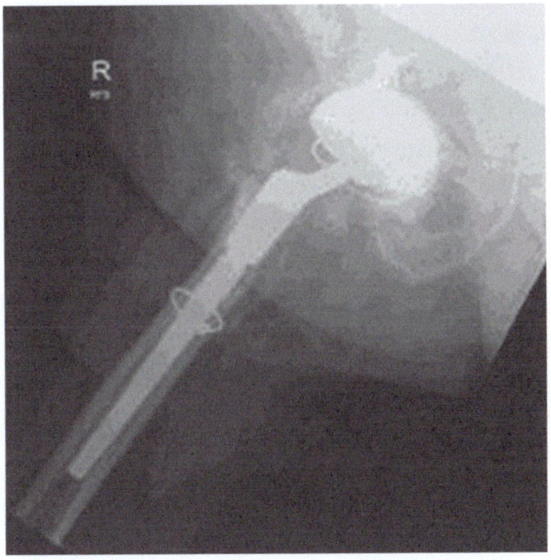

Fig. 36.49 Frog-leg lateral radiograph of the right hip six weeks after the revision with a modular tapered fluted stem also demonstrating excellent endosteal contact with the proximal femur

36.12.9 Postoperative Management

Chemoprophylaxis and anticoagulant treatment period: Warfarin for six weeks.

Gait/limb loading until full loading: Toe touch for the first six weeks followed by partial weight bearing for four weeks. At ten weeks postoperatively the patient was WBAT without an assistive device.

36.12.10 Follow-Up and Complications

The patient tolerated the procedure well without complication.

36.12.11 Discussion [28, 77, 78]

Advantages of the applied method: Modular fluted tapered stem allows surgeons to establish stable diaphyseal fixation while independently attaining leg length, offset and version.

Disadvantages of the method: The major disadvantage for this type of implant is an unsupported taper junction that can be weakened by repetitive stresses with a consequent fatigue fracture at the modular taper junction. Another disadvantage is stem subsidence that can lead to instability and leg shortening. Early subsidence has been attributed to component undersizing.

Alternative evidence-based techniques for the case: Extensively porous-coated femoral stems have been used with satisfactory results.

Why is the chosen technique better for this case? Increased rotational stability with diaphyseal fixation alone due to cutting flutes. Intraoperative flexibility to better restore leg length, offset and version.

Indications and contraindications for your technique: Indication for the use of modular fluted tapered stems varies according to the surgeon's philosophy and the amount of femoral bone loss. Some surgeons use these stems for the majority of femoral revisions, while others use these stems for severe metaphyseal and diaphyseal bone loss including Paprosky types IIIA and IIIB femora. These stems are also particularly valuable for treating Vancouver types B1 and B2 periprosthetic fractures. These stems are contraindicated when the diaphyseal bone loss does not provide 2 cm of implant-host bone contact or if the ectatic femoral canal is larger than the largest-sized tapered stem (31 mm). Surgeons have used these stems in Paprosky type IV femurs with good result demonstrating the efficacy of this reconstruction method.

Learning curve and how to manage complications: Early in the learning curve, the tendency is to undersize the stems due to concerns of intraoperative fracture and avoiding excessive bone removal. Undersized stems increase the risk of subsidence and leg length inequality. Cortical perforation can occur during re-establishment of the femoral canal. Using a canal finder by hand can help identify the true femoral canal. If the reamer is not passing smoothly within the canal, an intraoperative radiograph should be obtained to confirm that the reamer is safely within the femoral canal. In addition, with the use of longer stems, the anterior bow of the femur needs to be assessed, and anterior cortical perforation can occur, particularly if a non-bowed stem is utilized.

Level of evidence concerning the superiority of this method against others: Modular tapered fluted stems have been shown excellent long-term clinical results with a low rate of aseptic loosening. In addition, titanium stems decrease stress shielding and promote proximal bone stock reconstitutions, particularly in the setting of periprosthetic fracture. While these stems allow for better restoration of leg length, offset and version, dislocation rates between these modular stems and cylindrical stems are similar. Recent report has demonstrated superior functional results in patients treated with modular stems which may be secondary to more accurate restoration of hip biomechanics.

References

1. Sheth NP, Nelson CL, Paprosky WG. Femoral bone loss revision total hip arthroplasty: evaluation and management. J Am Acad Orthop Surg. 2013;21:601–12.

2. Sculco PK, Abdel MP, Lewallen DG. Management of femoral bone loss in revision total hip arthroplasty. Hip Int. 2015;25(4):380–7.
3. Kavanagh BF, Ilstrup DM, Fitzgerald RH Jr. Revision total hip arthroplasty. J Bone Joint Surg Am. 1985;67(4):517–26.
4. Pellicci PM, Wilson PD Jr, Sledge CB, et al. Long-term results of revision total hip replacement: a follow-up report. J Bone Joint Surg Am. 1985;67(4):513–6.
5. Paprosky WG, Aribindi R. Hip replacement: treatment of femoral bone loss using distal bypass fixation. Instr Course Lect. 2000;49:119–30.
6. D'Antonio J, McCarthy JC, Bargar WL, et al. Classification of femoral abnormalities in total hip arthroplasty. ClinOrthopRelat Res. 1993;296:133–9.
7. Engh CA Jr, Hopper RH Jr, Engh CA Sr. Distal ingrowth components. ClinOrthopRelat Res. 2004;420:135–41.
8. Engh CA Jr, Ellis TJ, Koralewicz LM, McAuley JP, Engh CA Sr. Extensively porous-coated femoral revision for severe femoral bone loss: minimum 10-year follow-up. J Arthroplasty. 2002;17(8):955–60.
9. McAuley JP, Engh CA Jr. Femoral fixation in the face of considerable bone loss: cylindrical and extensively coated femoral components. Clin Orthop Relat Res. 2004;429:215–21.
10. Sporer SM, Paprosky WG. Cementless femoral revision: the role of monoblock versus modular stems. Curr Orthop. 2006;20:171–8.
11. Sporer SM, Paprosky WG. Revision total hip arthroplasty: the limits of fully coated stems. Clin Orthop Relat Res. 2003;417:203–9.
12. Paprosky WG, Greidanus NV, Antoniou J. Minimum 10-year results of extensively porous-coated stems in revision hip arthroplasty. Clin Orthop Relat Res. 1999;369:230–42.
13. Weeden SH, Paprosky WG. Minimal 11-year follow-up of extensively porous coated stems in femoral revision total hip arthroplasty. J Arthroplasty. 2002;17(4 suppl 1):134–7.
14. Hamilton WG, Cashen DV, Ho H, Hopper RH Jr, Engh CA. Extensively porous-coated stems for femoral revision: a choice for all seasons. J Arthroplasty. 2007;22(4 Suppl 1):106–10.
15. Paprosky WG, Weeden SH. Extensively porous-coated stems in femoral revision arthroplasty. Orthopedics. 2001;24(9):871–2.
16. Egan KJ, Di Cesare PE. Intraoperative complications of revision hip arthroplasty using a fully porous-coated straight cobalt chrome femoral stem. J Arthroplasty. 1995;10(Suppl):S45–51.
17. Garcia-Cimbrelo E, Garcia-Rey E, Cruz-Pardos A, Madero R. Stress-shielding of the proximal femur using an extensively porous-coated femoral component without allograft in revision surgery: a 5- to 17-year follow-up study. J Bone Joint Surg Br. 2010;92(10):1363–9.
18. Busch CA, Charles MN, Haydon CM, Bourne RB, Rorabeck CH, Macdonald SJ, et al. Fractures of distally-fixed femoral stems after revision arthroplasty. J Bone Joint Surg Br. 2005;87(10):1333–6.
19. Thomsen PB, Jensen NJ, Kampmann J, Bæk Hansen T. Revision hip arthroplasty with an extensively porous-coated stem - excellent long-term results also in severe femoral bone stock loss. Hip Int. 2013;23(4):352–8.
20. Chung LH, Wu PK, Chen CF, Chen WM, Chen TH, Liu CL. Extensively porous-coated stems for femoral revision: reliable choice for stem revision in Paprosky femoral type III defects. Orthopedics. 2012;35(7):e1017–21.
21. Jayakumar P, Malik AK, Islam SU, Haddad FS. Revision hip arthroplasty using an extensively porous coated stem: medium term results. Hip Int. 2011 Mar-Apr;21(2):129–35.
22. Fukui K, Kaneuji A, Sugimori T, Ichiseki T, Matsumoto T. Bone remodeling after a mean of 10 years in diaphyseal cortical defects repaired with femoral revision using bypass fixation of extensively porous-coated stems with high stiffness. Eur J OrthopSurgTraumatol. 2015 May;25(4):741–7.
23. Hamilton WG, McAuley JP, Tabaraee E, Engh CA Sr. The outcome of rerevision of an extensively porous-coated stem with another extensively porous-coated stem. J Arthroplasty. 2008 Feb;23(2):170–4.
24. Crawford CH 3rd, Malkani AL, Incavo SJ, Morris HB, Krupp RJ, Baker D. Femoral component revision using an extensively hydroxyapatite-coated stem. J Arthroplasty. 2004 Jan;19(1):8–13.
25. Moreland JR, Bernstein ML. Femoral revision hip arthroplasty with uncemented, porous-coated stems. Clin Orthop Relat Res. 1995;319:141–50.
26. Rodriguez JA, Deshmukh AJ, Robinson J, et al. Reproducible fixation with a tapered, fluted, modular, titanium stem in revision hip arthroplasty at 8-15 years follow-up. J Arthroplasty. 2014;29(9 Suppl):214–8.
27. Richards CJ, Duncan CP, Masri BA, Garbuz DS. Femoral revision hip arthroplasty: a comparison of two stem designs. Clin Orthop Relat Res. 2010;468(2):491–6.
28. Van Houwelingen AP, Duncan CP, Masri BA, Greidanus NV, Garbuz DS. High survival of modular tapered stems for proximal femoral bone defects at 5 to 10 years follow up. Clin Orthop Relat Res. 2013;471(2):454–62.
29. Regis D, Sandri A, Bonetti I. Long-term results of femoral revision with the Wagner Self-locking stem. Surg Technol Int. 2013;23:243–50.
30. Regis D, Sandri A, Bonetti I, Braggion M, Bartolozzi P. Femoral revision with the Wagner tapered stem: a ten- to 15-year follow-up study. J Bone Joint Surg Br. 2011;93(10):1320–6.
31. Ko PS, Lam JJ, Tio MK, Lee OB, Ip FK. Distal fixation with Wagner revision stem in treating Vancouver type B2 periprosthetic femur fractures in geriatric patients. J Arthroplasty. 2003;18:446–52.
32. Weber M, Hempfing A, Orler R, Ganz R. Femoral revision using the Wagner stem: results at 2-9 years. Int Orthop. 2002;26:36–9.
33. Abdel MP, Lewallen DG, Berry DJ. Periprosthetic femur fractures treated with modular fluted, tapered stems. Clin Orthop Relat Res. 2014;472:599–603.

34. Munro JT, Masri BA, Garbuz DS, Duncan CP. Tapered fluted modular titanium stems in the management of Vancouver B2 and B3 peri-prosthetic fractures. Bone Joint J. 2013;95-B(suppl A):17–20.
35. Munro JT, Garbuz DS, Masri BA, Duncan CP. Tapered fluted titanium stems in the management of Vancouver B2 and B3 periprosthetic femoral fractures. Clin Orthop Relat Res. 2014;472:590–8.
36. Böhm P, Bischel O. Femoral revision with the Wagner SL revision stem: evaluation of one hundred and twenty-nine revisions followed for a mean of 4.8 years. J Bone Joint Surg Am. 2001;83-A:1023–31.
37. Gutiérrez Del Alamo J, Garcia-Cimbrelo E, Castellanos V, Gil-Garay E. Radiographic bone regeneration and clinical outcome with the Wagner SL revision stem: a 5-year to 12-year follow-up study. J Arthroplasty. 2007;22:515–24.
38. Boisgard S, Moreau PE, Tixier H, Levai JP. Bone reconstruction, leg length discrepancy, and dislocation rate in 52 Wagner revision total hip arthroplasties at 44- month follow-up. Rev Chir Orthop Reparatrice Appar Mot. 2001;87:147–54. (In French)
39. Konan S, Garbuz DS, Masri BA, Duncan CP. HIP arthroplasty: avoiding and managing problems Modular tapered titanium stems in revision arthroplasty of the hip the risk and causes of stem fracture. Bone Joint J. 2016;98-B(1 Suppl A):50–3.
40. Wagner H, Wagner M. Cone prosthesis for the hip joint. Arch Orthop Trauma Surg. 2000;120(1–2):88–95.
41. Kirk KL, Potter BK, Lehman RA Jr, Xenos JS. Effect of distal stem geometry on interface motion in uncemented revision total hip prostheses. Am J Orthop (Belle Mead NJ). 2007;36(10):545–9.
42. Konan S, Garbuz DS, Masri BA, Duncan CP. Non-modular tapered fluted titanium stems in hip revision surgery: gaining attention. Bone Joint J. 2014;96-B(Suppl A):56–9.
43. Mantelos G, Koulouvaris P, Kotsovolos H, Xenakis T. Consistent new bone formation in 95 revisions: average 9-year follow-up. Orthopedics. 2008;31(7):654.
44. Grünig R, Morscher E, Ochsner PE. Three-to 7-year results with the uncemented SL femoral revision prosthesis. Arch Orthop Trauma Surg. 1997;116(4):187–97.
45. Isacson J, Stark A, Wallensten R. The Wagner revision prosthesis consistently restores femoral bone structure. Int Orthop. 2000;24(3):139.
46. Kang MN, Huddleston JI, Hwang K, Imrie S, Goodman SB. Early outcome of a modular femoral component in revision total hip arthroplasty. J Arthroplasty. 2008;23(2):220–5.
47. Lakstein D, Eliaz N, Levi O, et al. Fracture of cementless femoral stems at the midstem junction in modular revision hip arthroplasty systems. J Bone Joint Surg Am. 2011;93-A:57–65.
48. Revision Total Hip Arthroplasty Study Group. A comparison of modular tapered versus modular cylindrical stems for complex femoral revisions. J Arthroplasty. 2013;28(8 Suppl):71–3.
49. Garbuz DS, Toms A, Masri BA, Duncan CP. Improved outcome in femoral revision arthroplasty with tapered fluted modular titanium stems. Clin Orthop Relat Res. 2006;453:199–202.
50. Park YS, Moon YW, Lim SJ. Revision total hip arthroplasty using a fluted and tapered modular distal fixation stem with and without extended trochanteric osteotomy. J Arthroplasty. 2007;22(7):993–9.
51. Palumbo BT, Morrison KL, Baumgarten AS, Stein MI, Haidukewych GJ, Bernasek TL. Results of revision total hip arthroplasty with modular, titanium-tapered femoral stems in severe proximal metaphyseal and diaphyseal bone loss. J Arthroplasty. 2013;28(4):690–4.
52. Amanatullah DF, Howard JL, Siman H, Trousdale RT, Mabry TM, Berry DJ. Revision total hip arthroplasty in patients with extensive proximal femoral bone loss using a fluted tapered modular femoral component. Bone Joint J. 2015;97(3):312–7.
53. Dzaja I, Lyons MC, McCalden RW, Naudie DD, Howard JL. Revision hip arthroplasty using a modular revision hip system in cases of severe bone loss. J Arthroplasty. 2014;29(8):1594–7.
54. McInnis DP, Horne G, Devane PA. Femoral revision with a fluted, tapered, modular stem seventy patients followed for a mean of 3.9 years. J Arthroplasty. 2006;21(3):372–80.
55. Tangsataporn S, Safir OA, Vincent AD, Abdelbary H, Gross AE, Kuzyk PR. Risk factors for subsidence of a modular tapered femoral stem used for revision total hip arthroplasty. J Arthroplasty. 2015;30(6): 1030–4.
56. Ovesen O, Emmeluth C, Hofbauer C, Overgaard S. Revision total hip arthroplasty using a modular tapered stem with distal fixation: good short-term results in 125 revisions. J Arthroplasty. 2010;25(3):348–54.
57. Fink B, Urbansky K, Schuster P. Mid term results with the curved modular tapered, fluted titanium Revitan stem in revision hip replacement. Bone Joint J. 2014;96-B:889–95.
58. Hoberg M, Konrads C, Engelien J, Oschmann D, Holder M, Walcher M, Rudert M. Outcome of a modular tapered uncemented titanium femoral stem in revision hip arthroplasty. Int Orthop. 2015;39:1709–13.
59. Wang L, Dai Z, Wen T, Li M, Hu Y. Three to seven year follow-up of a tapered modular femoral prosthesis in revision total hip arthroplasty. Arch Orthop Trauma Surg. 2013;133:275–81.
60. Kwong LM, Miller AJ, Lubinus P. A modular distal fixation option for proximal bone loss in revision total hip arthroplasty: a 2- to 6-year follow-up study. J Arthroplasty. 2003;18(3 Suppl 1):94–7.
61. Marx A, Beier A, Jung L, Lohmann CH, Halder AM. Peri-prosthetic femoral fractures treated with the uncemented Wagner revision stem. Hip Int. 2012;22(3):286–91.

62. Singh SP, Bhalodiya HP. Results of Wagner SL revision stem with impaction bone grafting in revision total hip arthroplasty. Indian J Orthop. 2013;47(4):357–63.
63. Baktır A, Karaaslan F, Gencer K, Karaoğlu S. Femoral revision using the Wagner SL revision stem: a single-surgeon experience featuring 11-19 years of follow-up. J Arthroplast. 2015;30(5):827–34.
64. Steno B, Necas L, Melisik M, Almasi J. Minimally invasive hollow trephine technique is recommended for revision of broken uncemented and extensively porous-coated monolithic femoral stems: a review of three cases. Eklem Hastalik Cerrahisiss. 2014;25(2):112–6.
65. Flecher X, Buord JM, Blanc G, Sainsou B, Argenson JN. A technique for decision-making in cementless femoral revision hip arthroplasty. Hip Int. 2013;23(1):60–5. doi:10.5301/HIP.2013.10723.
66. Flecher X, Pearce O, Parratte S, AUbaniac JM, Argenson JN. Custom cementless stem improves hip function in young patients at 15-year followup. Clin Orthop Relat Res. 2010;468(3):747–55. doi:10.1007/s11999-009-1045-x. Epub 2009 Aug 19
67. Kop AM, Keogh C, Swarts E. Proximal component modularity in THA-at what cost ? An implant retrieval study. Clin Orthop Relat Res. 2012;470(7):1885–94. doi:10.1007/s11999-011-2155-9.
68. Rodriguez JA, Deshmukh AJ, Klauser WU, Rasquinha VJ, Lubinus P, Ranawat CS. Patterns of osseointegration and remodeling in femoral revision with bone loss using modular, tapered, fluted, titanium stems. J Arthroplast. 2011;26(8):1409–17.
69. Weiss RJ, Beckman MO, Enocson A, Schmalholz A, Stark A. Minimum 5-year follow-up of a cementless, modular, tapered stem in hip revision arthroplasty. J Arthroplast. 2011;26(1):16–23.
70. Lakstein D, Backstein D, Safir O, Kosashvili Y, Gross AE. Revision total hip arthroplasty with a porous-coated modular stem: 5–10 years followup. Clin Orthop Relat Res. 2010;468(5):1310–5.
71. Sporer SM, Paprosky WG. Femoral fixation in the face of considerable bone loss: the use of modular stems. Clin Orthop Relat Res. 2004;429:227–31.
72. Klauser W, Bangert Y, Lubinus P, Kendoff D. Medium-term follow-up of a modular tapered non-cemented titanium stem in revision total hip arthroplasty: a single-surgeon experience. J Arthroplast. 2013;28(1):84–9.
73. Levine BR, Della Valle CJ, Lewis P, Berger RA, Sporer SM, Paprosky W. Extended trochanteric osteotomy for the treatment of vancouver B2/B3 periprosthetic fractures of the femur. J Arthroplast. 2008;23:527–33.
74. Lim SJ, Moon YW, Park YS. Is extended trochanteric osteotomy safe for use in 2-stage revision of periprosthetic hip infection? J Arthroplast. 2011;26:1067–71.
75. Mardones R, Gonzalez C, Cabanela ME, Trousdale RT, Berry DJ. Extended femoral osteotomy for revision of hip arthroplasty: results and complications. J Arthroplasty. 2005;20:79–83.
76. Miner TM, Momberger NG, Chong D, Paprosky WL. The extended trochanteric osteotomy in revision hip arthroplasty: a critical review of 166 cases at mean 3-year, 9-month follow-up. J Arthroplast. 2001;16:S188–94.
77. Pui CM, Bostrom MP, Westrich GH, Della Valle CJ, Macaulay W, Mont MA, Padgett DE. Increased complication rate following conversion total hip arthroplasty after cephalomedullary fixation for intertrochanteric hip fractures: a multi-center study. J Arthroplast. 2013;28(8 Suppl):45–7.
78. Sandiford NA, Duncan CP, Garbuz DS, Masri BA. Tapered, fluted titanium stems in revision total hip arthroplasty: role and results in contemporary practice. Instr Course Lect. 2015;64:359–66.

37 Total Femoral Replacement (TFR)

Eustathios Kenanidis, Eleftherios Tsiridis, Adolph V. Lombardi Jr, Andrew B. Richardson, and Michael Müller

37.1 Current Concepts

E. Kenanidis and E. Tsiridis

TFR is an established treatment method in oncologic reconstruction [1]. Additionally, TFR has also been used in the non-oncologic setting, as a salvage option for the management of extensive femoral bone loss in revision THA [2]. When performed in specialized centres, TFR can restore the femoral integrity, control pain, and allow the patients to continue ambulation, albeit at a compromised level; this is considered to be superior to the alternative, which is amputation or hip disarticulation. Careful patient selection, excellent surgical technique, a complete rehabilitation program, and the immediate management of postoperative complications are crucial to ensure optimal long-term outcomes in this challenging patient population [3].

37.1.1 Indications

The non-oncologic indications of TFA are not clear [3]. The non-oncologic patient should be carefully evaluated and selected. The specific reconstructive needs and functional expectations of the patient must be prudently assessed to ensure achievement. One must also take into account that the surgical alternatives to this procedure include hip disarticulation and above-knee amputation. Possible indications of TFR for the non-oncologic patient that needs revision THA are the following:

1. Extensive bone loss following multiple revision surgeries [4]
2. Extreme reduction of femoral bone stock following repeated surgical debridement in the setting of periprosthetic joint infection [5]
3. Extensively comminuted periprosthetic fractures [6]
4. Simultaneous management of multiple concurrent ipsilateral orthopedic issues in the

E. Kenanidis, M.D., Ph.D., M.Sc. (✉)
Academic Orthopaedic Unit, Aristotle University Medical School, Thessaloniki, Greece
e-mail: stathiskenanidis@gmail.com

E. Tsiridis, M.D., Ph.D., F.A.C.S., F.R.C.S. (✉)
Papageorgiou General Hospital, Pavlos Melas, Greece

Aristotle University Medical School, Thessaloniki, Greece
e-mail: etsiridis@doctors.org.uk

A.V. Lombardi Jr, M.D., F.A.C.S.
Joint Implant Surgeons, Inc., New Albany, OH, USA

Department of Orthopaedics, The Ohio State University Wexner Medical Center, Columbus, OH, USA

Mount Carmel Health System, Columbus, OH, USA
e-mail: LombardiAV@joint-surgeons.com

A.B. Richardson, M.D.
Joint Implant Surgeons, Inc., New Albany, OH, USA
e-mail: RichardsonAB@joint-surgeons.com

M. Müller, P.D., Dr.
Department of Traumatology and Reconstructive Surgery, Charité Universitätsmedizin Berlin, Berlin, Germany
e-mail: Michael.Mueller@charite.de

E. Tsiridis (ed.), *The Adult Hip - Master Case Series and Techniques*,
https://doi.org/10.1007/978-3-319-64177-5_37

context of the so-called shattered femur (e.g., the coexistence of severe knee or hip osteoarthritis) [7]

37.1.2 Preoperative Evaluation and Surgical Technique [3]

- Carefully evaluate these patients that frequently have multiple comorbidities.
- The expected extensive dissection predisposes to a greater volume of blood loss; take care to minimize the blood loss having technological advancements as the intraoperative blood salvage and the bipolar sealing device [8, 9].
- You are advised to have all the possible implant options readily available at the time of surgery [7].
- Choose a surgical approach following consideration of the preexisting surgical scars to ensure optimal wound closure. An inadequate preoperative planning predisposes to insufficient wound healing and may lead to secondary periprosthetic infection [10].
- Minimize the risk of postoperative dislocation. Choose implants that allow some customizability of the proximal femoral version and also constrained liner; the majority of TFR systems, however, are fixed with limited control of the proximal femoral version [11].
- Evaluate and optimize the patellofemoral tracking distally before the wound closure; rotate the tibial component externally, make lateral retinacular release with or without reefing, and imbricate the vastus medialis [7].
- Reattach the soft tissue adequately to the implant and particularly the hip abductor muscle group with sutures through holes on prostheses [4].
- Use a custom-molded polypropylene brace to limit flexion and adduction for up to 6 weeks postoperatively [12].

37.1.3 Advantages [3]

1. The salvage of the limb
2. The achievement of immediate fixation that permits early mobilization

37.1.4 Disadvantages

1. A technical complex procedure [3]
2. The significantly longer operating time than the most other revision THAs [3]
3. The increased risk of postoperative complications (instability and deep infection) [2, 4, 7, 11]
4. The greater postoperative volume of blood loss [3, 7]

37.1.5 Published Results

Limited studies are reporting short- to midterm results of patients undergoing revision THA with TFA. These are usually retrospective cohort studies with mixed or not, oncologic and non-oncologic patients [2, 4, 6, 7, 11, 13–16]. We certainly need larger patient prospective series of non-oncologic revision arthroplasty patients treated with TFA to better understand the functional outcomes and complications of the procedure. Nonneoplastic cohort studies [2, 4, 6, 7, 11, 13] have small to moderate sample size ranging from 14 to 100 patients and a mean age of patients from 65 to 75 years old; the mean follow-up ranges from 58 to 90 months. The total survivorship of the implants was reported to be 65–70%; this was not however answered in all studies. Revision rate for all reasons ranged between 21 and 36% [2, 4, 6, 7, 11, 13]. The most frequent complications were deep infection, hip dislocation, and mechanical failure.

In the largest sample ever reported, Friesecke et al. [13] evaluated 100 consecutive TFRs that had been implanted for aseptic revision arthroplasty. The mean age of patients was 68 years old. In the 77 patients, the indication for TFR was a complication of THA including the loosening of a long-stem THA (22/100), the management of severe knee osteoarthritis in the presence of existing long-stem THA (30/100), and the periprosthetic fractures (21/100). Other indications were complications of TKA, diaphyseal femoral fractures between existing THA and TKA, etc. In patients followed up for a mean period of 5 years, 68% of them had no complications. The total reported revision rate was 21%; the main complications were the deep infection (12%), the dislocation (6%), and the failure of the prosthesis (3%). Similar results were reported by Lombardi et al. [7] that retrospectively evaluated 75 patients with end-stage prosthetic disease at a mean of 42 months postoperatively. Complication rate was 30.7%; again infection 11%, hip dislocation 7%, and tibial component loosening were the main complications. In the longest follow-up, Fountain et al. [4] reported the results of 14 patients that had undergone TFA after complications of revision arthroplasty surgery. In 88% of them, the indication for TFA was a reconstruction after chronic sepsis; all were treated with a two-stage revision procedure. A third of patients achieved almost 75% of improvement in function at an average follow-up of 7.5 years. The revision rate reached 35.7% with the dislocation (5/14) and the infection (3/14) to be the most frequent complications. In a recent study, Amanatullah et al. [11] reviewed retrospectively 20 patients treated with TFA for complications of THA. Half of them suffered from deep sepsis; periprosthetic fractures and aseptic loosening were also preoperative reasons. Amanatullah reported a total implant survival rate of 70% at five years. The revision rate was 30%; the overall infection rate was 35%, and five patients had postoperative instability.

37.1.6 Complications

The main postoperative complications in revision THA treated with TFA are the deep periprosthetic infection and hip instability [2, 4, 6, 7, 11, 13].

There are multiple predisposing factors for postoperative infection in these patients as the extensive surgical dissection, the large metal surface area, the prolonged operative time, multiple patient comorbidities, and repeated hospitalization for past surgical procedure including prior revision arthroplasty for periprosthetic infection [2, 4, 6, 7, 11, 13]. The inadequacy of the initial antibiotic therapy, the total drug resistance, or a lack of thorough surgical debridement (secondary to retained cement or implant hardware) are further reasons. A two-stage revision arthroplasty with cement spacer placement seems to be the main treatment option [12].

The postoperative hip instability is another frequent complication of TFR revision. Meticulous attention to the surgical technique including preservation of the greater trochanter via the Wagner-type transtrochanteric osteotomy wrapped around the implant with wires or cables, the component positioning, the soft tissue tensioning, the use of large diameter femoral heads and constrained acetabular liners when necessary is of paramount importance [2, 4, 6, 7, 11, 13].

Other less possible complications include limb length discrepancy, mechanical failure of the prosthesis, acetabular or tibial component loosening, and patellar complications (e.g., patellar maltracking).

37.2 Case Title: Total Femoral Replacement for Salvage of End-Stage Prosthetic Disease

Adolph V. Lombardi Jr and Andrew B. Richardson

37.2.1 Demographics

Age: 80 years old
Sex: Female
BMI: 37.2

37.2.2 Relevant Past Medical History

Principal pathologies: Previous Vancouver B1 periprosthetic femur fracture status post open reduction internal fixation (ORIF) with a distal femoral locking plate, now with a failure of fixation and loss of reduction. Associated pathologies include severe osteoporosis and tricompartmental osteoarthritis of the ipsilateral knee.

Previous surgical procedures: Right hip hemiarthroplasty 1993, Right total hip arthroplasty 1995, Cholecystectomy 1986, Right cataract extraction 2008, Total abdominal hysterectomy 2010, hemorrhoidectomy, right hip revision 2010, and ORIF Right periprosthetic femur fracture 2011.

Medication: Losartan 100 mg p.o. daily, Miralax 17 mg p.o. daily p.r.n, fish oil 1000 mg p.o. daily, trazodone 25 mg p.o. daily pm, Lortab 5/325 mg Q4H p.r.n pain, Ecotrin 81 mg p.o. daily, Colace 100 mg p.o. daily, and ibuprofen 200 mg p.o. Q8H p.r.n pain.

History of presenting complaint: An 80-year-old female status post revision total hip arthroplasty with a long-stem prosthesis with constrained acetabular liner who sustained a Vancouver B1 periprosthetic femoral fracture one year following the revision. She was treated with open reduction and internal fixation (ORIF) with a distal femoral locking plate using cerclage cables to bypass the distal stem. Three years post-op, the patient presented with new onset thigh pain and inability to bear weight on the right lower extremity after a low energy fall at home. Imaging demonstrated that the patient had refractured the distal femur at the level of her previous fracture with a failure of fixation and displacement of the distal fragment. Prior to her initial fracture, she had been evaluated and treated nonsurgically for tricompartmental osteoarthritis (OA) of the ipsilateral knee.

37.2.3 Clinical Examination

Symptoms: Pain in the right thigh with any motion of the extremity. Before the initial fracture, she was noted to have global pain in the right knee worse with activity.

Range of motion: At presentation, the patient's exam was limited by pain. Prior to the injury, the patient's exam was as follows: right hip: flexion is 95°, abduction is 25°, internal rotation is 27°, external rotation is 45°, and adduction is 20°. There is no fixed deformity of the right hip present. Right knee: ROM: 0–105, no flexion contracture or extension lag present, tibiofemoral alignment: 5° valgus, anteroposterior stability: <5 mm, mediolateral stability: <5°. Activity: sedentary. She is unable to ascend or descend stairs and requires the use of a walker at all times for ambulation.

Specific tests: A complete radiographic evaluation should be obtained including anteroposterior and lateral views of the femur, hip, knee, and pelvis. Standing long leg alignment films should also be obtained preoperatively if possible.

Main disability: Pain limiting function and resulting in immobilization.

Scoring if available: Unavailable at the time of presentation. Prior to sustaining the fracture: Harris Hip Score: 62.5; Knee Society Clinical Rating System: 91.

Neurovascular evaluation: Patient has a full neurovascular function with appropriate motor control.

37.2.4 Preoperative Radiological Assessment/Imaging (Figs. 37.1, 37.2, and 37.3)

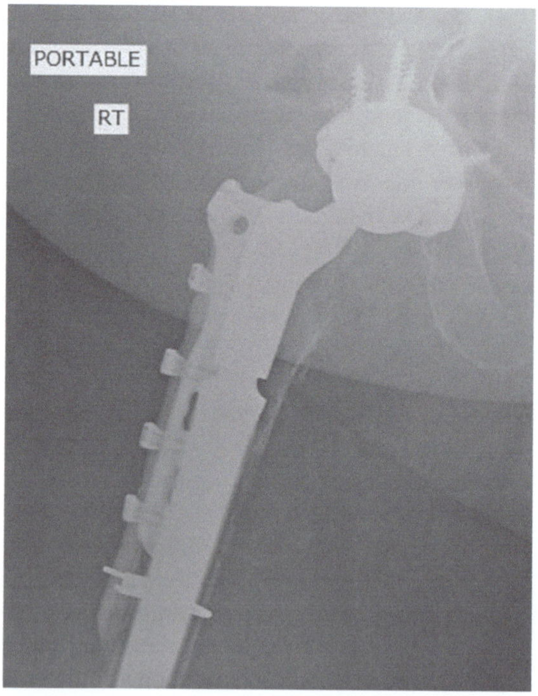

Fig. 37.1 AP right hip—Demonstrates a long-stem constrained total hip arthroplasty status post-op previous revision

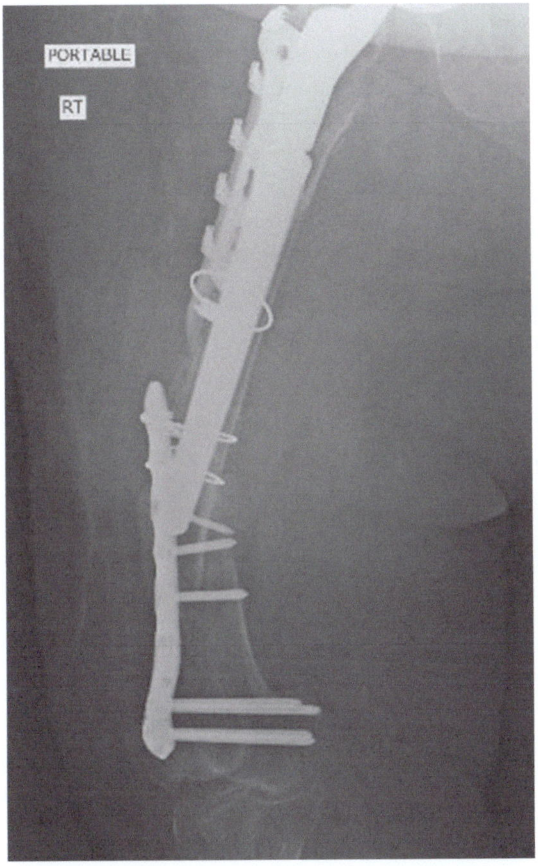

Fig. 37.2 AP distal femur—Demonstrates a Vancouver B1 periprosthetic distal femur fracture at the site of the previous fracture with fracture displacement and failure of fixation

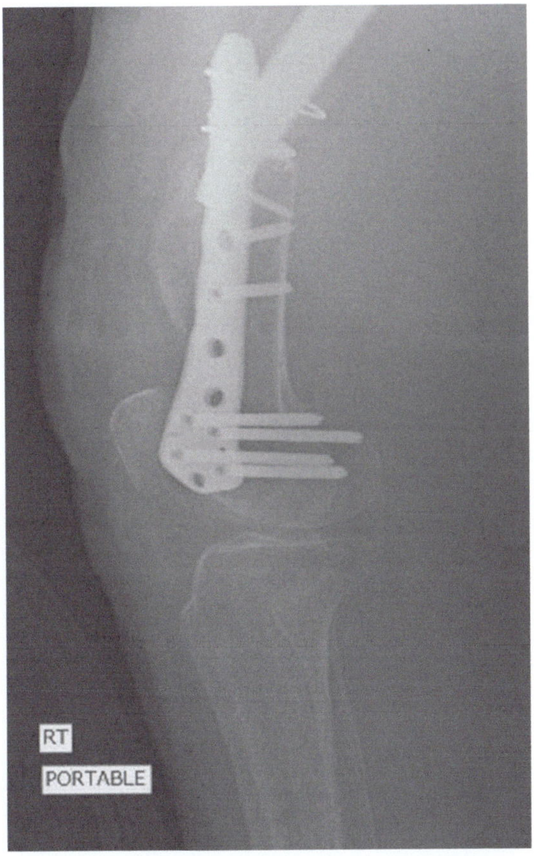

Fig. 37.3 Lateral femur—Demonstrates a Vancouver B1 periprosthetic distal femur fracture at the site of the previous fracture with fracture displacement and failure of fixation

37.2.5 Preoperative Planning

Diagnosis: Recurrent Vancouver B1 periprosthetic femur fracture status post previous ORIF likely secondary to persistent non-union of the fracture site in the setting of previous long-stem revision constrained total hip arthroplasty, severe osteoporosis, and end-stage OA of the ipsilateral knee (Figs. 37.1, 37.2 and 37.3).

Possible treatment options: Given the patient's advanced age and comorbidities, as well as her inability to mobilize secondary to pain, non-operative management is not an option in this setting. Surgical treatment options include revision ORIF with distal femoral locking plate with bone grafting and possible staged right total knee arthroplasty versus total femoral arthroplasty versus above-knee amputation or hip disarticulation.

Chosen treatment method: The total femoral arthroplasty (TFA) was chosen in setting given the patient's poor bone stock, low probability of healing, and concomitant right knee arthritis. TFA has been shown to be a viable salvage option in the setting of significant bone loss and/or poor bone stock in the setting periprosthetic fracture of the femur [6, 17].

Selection of implants if applicable and rational: Modular mega-endoprosthesis with rotating hinge knee and constrained acetabular liner. Modularity of the endoprosthesis allows for fine intraoperative adjustments, mainly to limb length and hip stability. The acetabular constraint is required for hip stability secondary to loss of the abductor complex.

Expected difficulties: Proper soft tissue management and dissection through significant scarring in the multiply operated patient; abductor muscle deficiency secondary to loss of attachment to the greater trochanter resulting in hip instability and, proper determination of limb length.

Strategies to overcome difficulties: A thorough understanding of the relevant anatomy coupled with meticulous dissection to ensure that the dissection is carried out in the proper anatomic planes, taking care to protect the neurovascular structures during the approach to excision of the femur. During the dissection of the proximal femur, it is vital to preserve as much of the abductor complex in continuity with the vastus lateralis as possible to preserve a soft tissue sleeve that can be repaired to the proximal aspect of the total femur construct. Additionally, utilization of a constrained acetabular liner is mandatory to maintain the proper stability of the hip joint. Limb length can be assessed and properly determined preoperatively with a standing long leg alignment plain radiograph in those patients who can bear weight on the affected limb. Proper limb length can additionally be assessed intraoperatively with a comparison to the contralateral limb and by restoring appropriate soft tissue tension.

37.2.6 Surgical Note

Patient's position: Right semi-lateral decubitus with the limp prepped to well below the knee. The position of the patient should be such that access to both the hip and knee is facilitated. The contralateral limb should be positioned so that an intraoperative comparison of limb length can be made.

Type of anesthesia: General anesthesia combined with a single-shot spinal anesthetic.

Surgical approach: The author's favored surgical approach that involves an extensile exposure of the acetabulum and entire femur through an extended direct lateral (Hardinge) approach and a separate, standard medial parapatellar approach to the knee. This approach is utilized in the setting of failed total hip and/or knee arthroplasty with poor remaining bone stock where previous incisions dictate the surgical approach. In cases where previous incisions do not exist (i.e., oncologic cases), a single extended anterolateral approach down to the lateral aspect of the tibial tuberosity is often used. In this case, the patient had previously undergone a direct lateral approach to the femur during the previous hip surgeries and an anterior midline approach with a lateral parapatellar arthrotomy during fixation of her previous fracture. Therefore, a direct lateral approach to the proximal femur was extended distally, and an anterior midline approach with a medial parapatellar arthrotomy was used to facilitate preparation of the proximal tibia.

Main steps: Patient was prepped and draped in the standard sterile fashion. The skin was incised at the hip incorporating the previous surgical incision. Dissection was carried down to underlying tensor fascia lata, which was then incised along the line of the incision. The vastus lateralis was elevated in continuity with the anterior inferior fibers of the gluteus medius and minimus, allowing exposure of the femoral head and neck to remove the constrained ring and dislocate the femur. Once the hip was dislocated, the proximal femur was skeletonized to the level of the fracture site. The knee was then flexed, and an anterior midline incision was made utilizing the previous surgical incision, and a medial parapatellar arthrotomy was performed. The dissection was then carried proximally, skeletonizing the distal femur and allowing the entire femur to be extracted. Following removal of the femur, the proximal tibia was prepared. The periacetabular scar tissue was removed, and the acetabular liner was removed. The acetabular component was inspected and found to be well-fixed. If any suspicion of component loosening exists, the implant should be revised. Trial implants were then place to determine the appropriate leg length. The patella was then resected to obtain a smooth, flat face surface and prepared for the patellar resurfacing implant. The final components were then placed starting with the tibial and patellar component which were cemented in place. The acetabular liner was placed into the acetabular cup. Once these components were in place, the modular total femoral endoprosthesis was constructed on the back table. The final implants were then placed and final stability of the construct was confirmed (Figs. 37.4 and 37.5).

Reconstruction techniques: Total femoral replacement using a modular mega-endoprosthesis.

37.2.7 Intraoperative Challenges

Challenges and solutions: No specific challenges were encountered intraoperatively. Meticulous dissection was carried out to skeletonize the femur and ensure the neurovascular structures were protected. Limb length was assessed clinically intraoperatively by comparing to the contralateral limb. No standing long leg alignment films were obtained preoperatively due to the patient's inability to stand for the film.

Unanticipated problems and solution: No unanticipated problems were encountered.

Thorough description of decision making, including the reason for the final decision: The patient in this case presented with a refracture of a Vancouver B1 distal femoral fracture around a long-stem revision total hip prosthesis secondary to nonunion. The patient's relevant comorbid conditions included end-stage OA of the ipsilateral knee, significant osteoporosis, and previous nonunion of the fracture site. Management of periprosthetic femoral fractures can be extremely challenging. These patients often require revision of the components and/or internal fixation. There is a relatively high rate of significant postoperative complications following revision arthroplasty and internal fixation for periprosthetic fractures. Complications requiring additional surgery have been reported in 10–33% of patients following fixation of these fractures [6]. Non-oncologic TFA has been reported to have good outcomes for the management of periprosthetic femur fractures [6, 17]. Implant 10-year survival rate has been reported to be as high as 86%; improved functional outcomes have also been reported following TFA with reported improvement in Harris Hip scores from a preop value of 30.2 to a post-op value of 65.3 [6, 11]. Given this evidence in addition to the patient's comorbid conditions and previous failure of internal fixation, total femoral arthroplasty was chosen for this patient.

37.2.8 Postoperative Radiographs (Figs. 37.4 and 37.5)

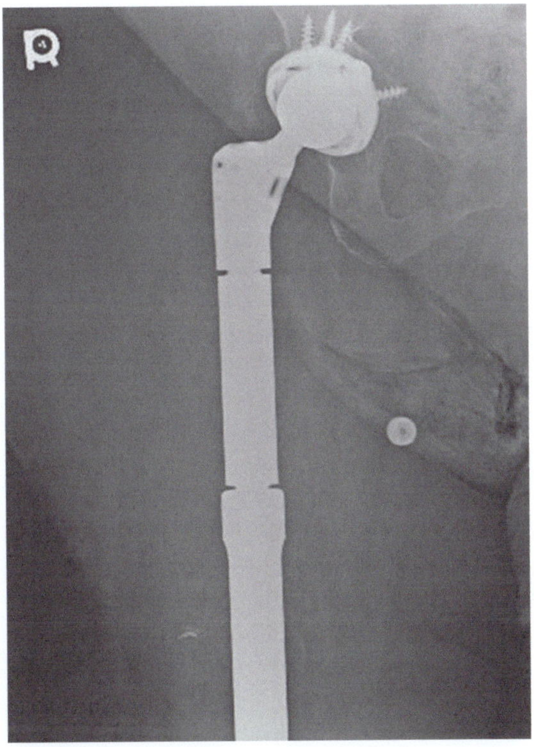

Fig. 37.4 AP Hip—Appropriate placement and alignment of the TFA component. The component is well-fixed without evidence of failure or migration

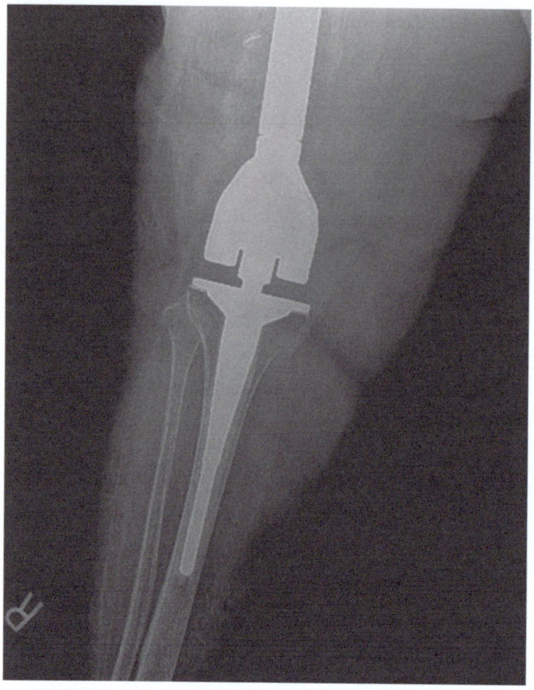

Fig. 37.5 AP Knee—Appropriate placement and alignment of the TFA component. The component is well without evidence of failure or migration

37.2.9 Postoperative Management

Chemoprophylaxis and anticoagulant treatment period: Chemoprophylaxis against deep- venous thrombosis was prescribed according to the ACCP 2012 CHEST guidelines. This patient did not have medical predisposition to DVT and was subsequently maintained on a regimen of aspirin 325 mg BID and bilateral lower extremity sequential compression devices.

Gait/limb loading until full loading: Patient was made immediate weight bearing as tolerated and started gait training and limb strengthening exercises with physical therapy immediately post-op.

37.2.10 Follow-Up and Complications

No complications were encountered postoperatively.

Scoring: Harris Hip Score: 61.5.

37.2.11 Discussion

Advantages of the applied method: Non-oncologic TFA for limb salvage following failed arthroplasty or periprosthetic fracture in the setting of a poor femoral bone stock has several advantages. Patients are able to bear wear as tolerated immediately in postoperative period allowing for early mobilization and avoidance of complications associated with prolonged immobilization (pneumonia, DVT, PE, etc.). The risks of non-union or failure of fixation associated with internal fixation are nonexistent. There is evidence demonstrating that patients receive significant pain relief and a significant improvement in postoperative function with an improvement in Harris Hip scores reported from a preop value of 30.2 to a post-op value of 65.3, and a majority of patients are able to maintain ambulatory status, albeit the majority of patients do require the use of a walker [6, 11, 17]. Further, implant 10-year survival rate has been reported to be as high as 86% [6, 11].

Disadvantages of the method: While there are significant advantages to TFA, there are significant drawbacks to this method. The 10-year mortality rate has been reported to be 58% [6]; this may be in part attributable to the high number of comorbid medical conditions typically seen in this patient population. Complication rates are also high following TFA. Dislocation and infection are the most common complications reported. Dislocation has been reported from 5 to 25% [6, 11, 17], while the rate of new infection following TFA has been reported 10–25% [6, 11, 17].

Alternative evidence-based techniques for the case: Alternative techniques for failed total hip and/or knee arthroplasty in the setting of poor femoral bone stock are limited. Surgical alternatives include revision arthroplasty with impaction grafting, massive allografts, strut grafting, or a combination of all of these techniques. In the setting of periprosthetic femur fracture, surgical alternatives include ORIF with or without bone grafting. In both settings, above-knee amputation or hip disarticulation remain viable alternatives.

All of these techniques are associated with high complication and failure rates.

Why is the chosen technique better for this case? TFA was the best solution in this case for several reasons. (1) The patient had already failed to internal fixation of the periprosthetic femur fracture. (2) There was poor bone stock both proximally around a well-fixed long-stem revision THA prosthesis and distally around the distal femoral locking plate. (3) TFA allowed for immediate weight bearing and mobilization minimizing the risks of immobilization. (4) The patient had known end-stage OA of the ipsilateral knee. TFA addressed both the current issue of periprosthetic fracture and the issue of the ipsilateral OA. (5) Non-oncologic TFA in the setting of failed arthroplasty and/or periprosthetic fracture is associated with good long-term survivability and functional outcomes.

Indications and contraindications for your technique: Indications for non-oncologic TFA are limited but include failed total hip and/or total knee arthroplasty due to mechanical (aseptic loosening or fracture) or following periprosthetic infection in association with poor femoral bone stock that is not amenable to revision arthroplasty. No specific contraindications have been described, but each patient must be carefully selected based on preoperative functional level, comorbid status, and postoperative expectations with the understanding that the TFA is associated with a high-level of postoperative complication and mortality.

Learning curve and how to manage complications: There is a significant learning curve associated with this procedure. Care should be taken to maintain a meticulous dissection protecting the soft tissue envelope and ensure that the neurovascular structures are protected during the procedure. While associated with good survivability and functional outcomes, complications are relatively common following this procedure. Dislocation and infection remain the most common complication following TFA. Constrained liners are recommended in all cases, but dislocation can still occur. Management of infection and recurrent dislocation can be difficult to manage and may ultimately result in hip disarticulation.

Level of evidence concerning the superiority of this method against others: Several studies support the use of TFA for salvage of end-stage prosthetic disease. However, the use of TFA remains limited, and all reports are retrospective case series (Level IV evidence).

37.3 Case Title: "Total Femoral Replacement"

Michael Müller

37.3.1 Demographics

Age: 52
Sex: Female
BMI: 40.9

37.3.2 Relevant Past Medical History

Principal pathologies: Aseptic stem loosening with subsidence and perforation into the knee joint, severe femoral bone loss—Paprosky Type IV, abductor insufficiency caused by lacking of the proximal femur, immobilization (wheelchair).

Previous surgical procedures: Status post multiple correction osteotomies of the femur and knee joints during childhood and adolescence, primary total hip arthroplasty 1998 caused by dysplastic arthritis of the right hip. The revision total hip arthroplasty 2004 caused by aseptic loosening. Primary total knee arthroplasty 2000 of the right knee.

Medication: Opiate long-term medication.

Others: Dysmelia from birth caused by thalidomide, obesity, hip dysplasia arthritis of the left side.

History of presenting complaint: The patient presented to the outpatient department with increasing pain in the right hip joint, thigh, and also in the knee joint. She complains about growing painful restrictions in flexing the knee. In the last four years, she is mobilized in a wheelchair only, caused by increased abductor weakness and thigh pain, not able to walk; only transfer movements from bed to chair are possible. She had one revision surgery before due to aseptic loosening. Primary THA was performed for the reason of dysplastic arthritis, and a total knee arthroplasty was performed for the reason of a valgus knee arthritis. She was born without arms which were caused by thalidomide.

37.3.3 Clinical Examination

Symptoms: Pain in the right femur, thigh, and knee joint, restrictions in ROM of the knee. Clear abductor insufficiency and clear restrictions on flexion and extension of the knee and, painful movements of the left hip. Increasing leg length discrepancy over the last year with a current leg length discrepancy of more than 5 cm of the right leg.

Range of motion: HIP (right): extension/flexion 0/0/100; abduction/adduction 30/0/20 external rotation/internal rotation 35/0/10; knee (right), extension/flexion 0/25/45.

Specific tests: Tenderness in Scarpa's triangle, pain provocation upon femoral rotation, tenderness over thigh upon palpation.

Main disability: Won't be able to walk, clear restrictions in knee flexion and extension, abductor weakness of the right hip.

Neurovascular evaluation: No peripheral neurovascular deficits.

37.3.4 Preoperative Radiological Assessment/Imaging (Figs. 37.6 and 37.7)

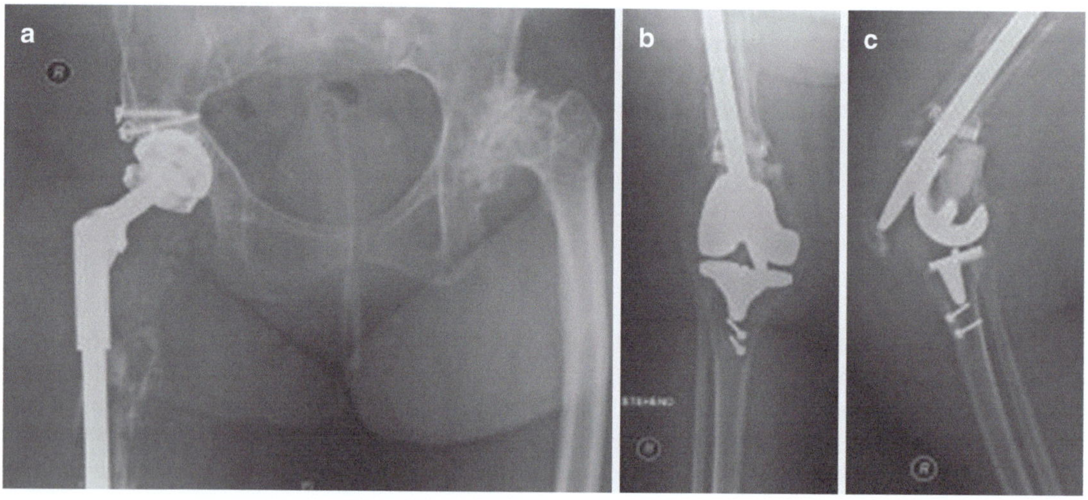

Fig. 37.6 (**a**) AP pelvic radiograph, (**b**) AP Knee, (**c**) Knee lateral

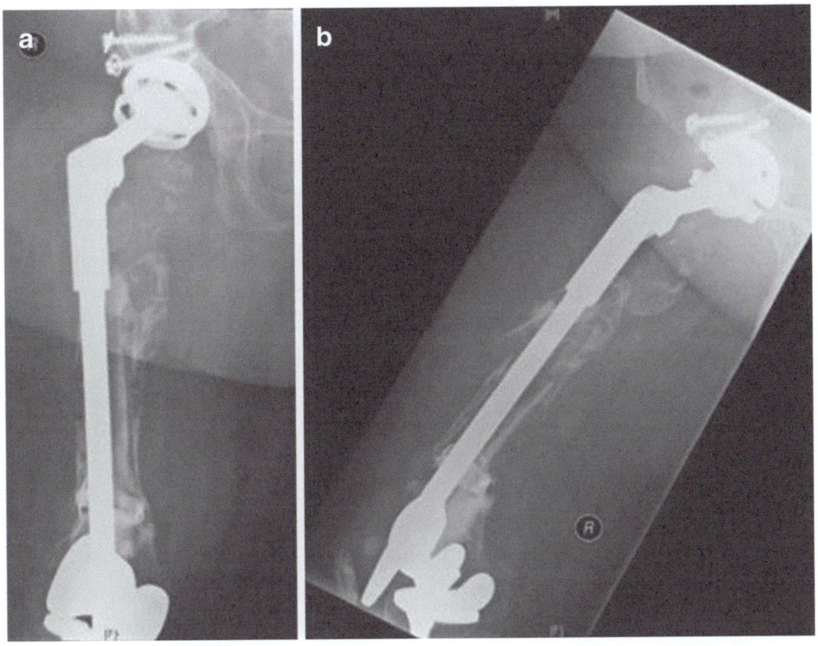

Fig. 37.7 (**a**) AP radiograph of the femur, (**b**) lateral radiograph of the femur

37.3.5 Preoperative Planning

Diagnosis: Aseptic stem loosening with subsidence into the knee joint, severe femoral bone loss with a Paprosky Type IV defect, abductor insufficiency (Figs. 37.6 and 37.7).

Possible treatment options: (1) Revision THA with total femur replacement and tripolar cup to reduce the risk of postoperative dislocation. (2) Amputation/exarticulation.

Chosen treatment method: Total femur replacement.

Selection of implants if applicable and rational: Caused by the severe bone loss of the total femur and the perforated knee joint, the decision for a total femur replacement was made.

Expected difficulties: To reconstruct a stable joint with a correct leg length considering the abductor insufficiency with a higher risk of instability and dislocation. To remove the femur including the old prosthesis with the risk of additional damage to the knee joint (extensor mechanism) and the risk of bleeding from perforantes arteries. Considering the risk of damage to the neurovascular structures in general. A loosed cup with limitation in refixation of a revision cup.

Strategies to overcome difficulties: Good preoperative templating of the size of the prosthesis using the non-affected contralateral site. Using a tripolar cup to reduce the risk of instability. Providing enough blood products, using tranexamic acid and a cell saver to minimize the risk of higher blood loss.

37.3.6 Surgical Note

Patient's position: Lateral decubitus surgical position.

Type of anesthesia: General anesthesia.

Surgical approach: Lateral approach to the hip, femur and knee joint. For the preparation of the femoral bone, a subvastus approach was used to preserve the lateral vastus muscle.

Main steps: Long skin incision from above the greater trochanter to the lateral side of the knee joint was made. After subcutaneous preparation and splitting the iliotibial band, the hip joint was exposed through an anterolateral approach. Then, the total femur was carefully prepared from ventral and posterior side starting from cranial under a full bleeding control. After the complete preparation and mobilization, the femur could be removed including the migrated stem and femoral knee arthroplasty component. The extensor mechanism of the knee joint was spared. Then, the hip joint was exposed, and the liner of the cup was removed. The cup was tested for stability and was judged as well-fixed. A tripolar cup was cemented into the preexisting cup considering the correct position. After that, the proximal tibia was prepared, and the tibial component, as well as the cement, removed without bone loss. After preparation, a new tibia component in the optimal size was implanted considering correct rotation. Afterwards, the femoral component trials were assembled and connected to the tibia and cup, and the proper length of the femur was estimated. Following the ex-situ montage, the original femur component was connected to the knee and relocated to the hip joint. By using a connection tube, the soft tissue including muscle and tendons were fixated to the total femur replacement (Fig. 37.8).

37.3.7 Intraoperative Challenges

Challenges and solutions: Reconstruction of a stable joint biomechanics with correct leg lengths considering the abductor insufficiency with a high-risk of instability and dislocation of the hip joint in such cases. Another challenge is the removing of the femur including the old prosthesis. Additional damage to the knee joint should be avoided, and the risk of bleeding from perforantes arteries should be considered. Respect the risk of damage to neurovascular structures during surgery. Reduce the operation time to a minimum concerning the higher risk of infection which correlates to operation time.

Unanticipated problems and solution: Loose cup with poor bone stock of the acetabulum.

Thorough description of decision making, including the reason for the final decision: The severe femoral bone defect of Paprosky type IV with perforated knee joint caused by femoral component perforation.

37.3.8 Postoperative Radiographs (Fig. 37.8)

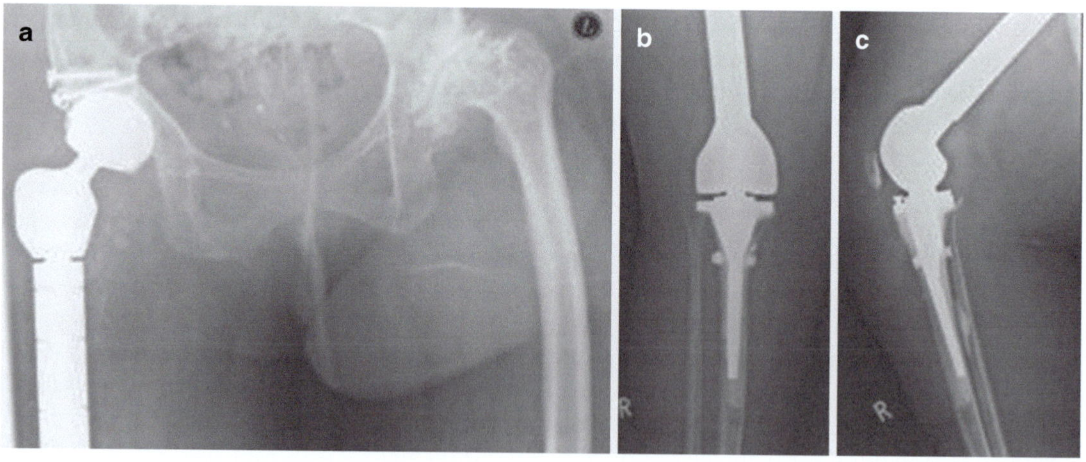

Fig. 37.8 (**a**) AP pelvic radiograph, (**b**) AP knee, (**c**) Knee lateral 2

37.3.9 Postoperative Management

Chemoprophylaxis and anticoagulant treatment period: A perioperative dose of cephalosporin was administered and a second after three hours of surgical time. Until the final results of intraoperative microbiology probes were available, a prolonged antibiotic therapy with a combination of ampicillin and sulbactam was administered to the patient (up to the 10th postoperative day). Postoperative anticoagulative treatment was performed with a weight-based dosage of low-molecular-weight heparin.

Gait/limb loading until full loading: The patient was mobilized from the second postoperative day. A weight bearing of the right leg was not possible caused by the dysmelia.

37.3.10 Follow-Up and Complications

Due to a postoperative hypotension and anemia, the patient was observed for one night at our postanesthesia care unit. A second surgery was necessary after two weeks on the height of the distal wound caused by a seroma.

37.3.11 Discussion [18–20]

Advantages of the applied method: A well fixated, stable joint with correct biomechanics and leg length is possible.

Disadvantages of the method: Artificial femur with a higher rate of periprosthetic joint infection.

Alternative evidence-based techniques for the case: There exists no adequate alternative except the amputation of the leg.

Why is the chosen technique is better for this case? A faster postoperative mobilization is possible, and the leg can be preserved.

Indications and contraindications for your technique: Existing infection or other life-threatening diseases.

Learning curve and how to manage complications: The implantation of a total femur is only for very well-experienced orthopedic surgeons with excellent knowledge of the revision total joint replacement. Main complications which have to be considered are instability and infection.

Level of evidence concerning the superiority of this method against others: There is no clear answer because in patients with an inferior bone stock without any fixation possibility into the femur, the total femur replacement is—beside amputation or exarticulation—the only meaningful method without any alternative.

References

1. Sewell MD, Spiegelberg BG, Hanna SA, Aston WJ, Bartlett W, Blunn GW, David LA, Cannon SR, Briggs TW. Total femoral endoprosthetic replacement following excision of bone tumors. J Bone Joint Surg Br. 2009;91:1513–20.
2. Berend KR, Lombardi AV, Mallory TH, Adams JB, Dodds KL. Total femoral arthroplasty for salvage of end-stage prosthetic disease. Clin Orthop Relat Res. 2004;427:162–70.
3. Ramanathan D, Siqueira MBP, Klika AK, Higuera CA, Barsoum WK, Joyce MJ. Current concepts in total femoral replacement. World J Orthop. 2015;6(11):919–26.
4. Fountain JR, Dalby-Ball J, Carroll FA, Stockley I. The use of total femoral arthroplasty as a limb salvage procedure: the Sheffield experience. J Arthroplasty. 2007;22:663–9.
5. Sherman SL, Cunneen KP, Walcott-Sapp S, Brause B, Westrich GH. Custom total femur spacer and second-stage total femur arthroplasty as a novel approach to infection and periprosthetic fracture. J Arthroplasty. 2008;23:781–6.
6. Clement ND, MacDonald D, Ahmed I, Patton JT, Howie CR. Total femoral replacement for salvage of periprosthetic fractures. Orthopedics. 2014;37:e789–95.
7. Lombardi AV, Berend KR. The shattered femur: radical solution options. J Arthroplasty. 2006;21:107–11.
8. Ashworth A, Klein AA. Cell salvage as part of a blood conservation strategy in anesthesia. Br J Anaesth. 2010;105:401–16.
9. Kaibori M, Matsui K, Ishizaki M, Sakaguchi T, Matsushima H, Matsui Y, Kwon AH. A prospective randomized controlled trial of hemostasis with a bipolar sealer during hepatic transection for liver resection. Surgery. 2013;154:1046–52.
10. Nerubay J, Katznelson A, Tichler T, Rubinstein Z, Morag B, Bubis JJ. Total femoral replacement. Clin Orthop Relat Res. 1988;229:143–8.

11. Amanatullah DF, Trousdale RT, Hanssen AD, Lewallen DG, Taunton MJ. Non-oncologic total femoral arthroplasty: retrospective review. J Arthroplasty. 2014;29:2013–5.
12. Hwang JS, Beebe KS, Patterson FR, Benevenia J. Infected total femoral replacements: evaluation of limb loss risk factors. Orthopedics. 2011;34:e736–40.
13. Friesecke C, Plutat J, Block A. Revision arthroplasty with use of a total femur prosthesis. J Bone Joint Surg Am. 2005;87:2693–701.
14. Mankin HJ, Hornicek FJ, Harris M. Total femur replacement procedures in tumor treatment. Clin Orthop Relat Res. 2005;438:60–4.
15. Steinbrink K, Engelbrecht E, Fenelon GC. The total femoral prosthesis. A preliminary report. J Bone Joint Surg Br. 1982;64:305–12.
16. Ward WG, Dorey F, Eckardt JJ. Total femoral endoprosthetic reconstruction. Clin Orthop Relat Res. 1995;316:195–2.
17. McLean AL, Patton JT, Moran M. Femoral replacement for salvage of periprosthetic fracture around a total hip replacement. Injury. 2012;43(7):1166–9. doi:10.1016/j.injury.2012.03.024. Epub 2012 Apr 27
18. Sheth NP, Melnic CM, Rozell JC, Paprosky WG. Management of severe femoral bone loss in revision total hip arthroplasty. Orthop Clin North Am. 2015;46(3):329–42, ix. doi:10.1016/j.ocl.2015.02.002. Epub 2015 Apr 11
19. Bianchi L, Galante C, Zagra L. The management of femoral bone stock in THA revision: indications and techniques. Hip Int. 2014;24(Suppl 10):S37–43. doi:10.5301/hipint.5000174.
20. Mayle RE Jr, Paprosky WG. Massive bone loss: allograft-prosthetic composites and beyond. J Bone Joint Surg Br. 2012;94(11 Suppl A):61–4. doi:10.1302/0301-620X.94B11.30791.

38 Proximal Femoral Replacement

Eustathios Kenanidis, Eleftherios Tsiridis, Anthony Viste, Michael J. Taunton, Mathew P. Abdel, Valeriy Murilev, Yaroslav Rukin, Rashid Tikhilov, and Georgi I. Wassilew

E. Kenanidis, M.D., Ph.D., M.Sc. (✉)
Academic Orthopaedic Unit, Aristotle University Medical School, Thessaloniki, Greece

E. Tsiridis, M.D., Ph.D., F.A.C.S., F.R.C.S.
Papageorgiou General Hospital, Pavlos Melas, Greece

Aristotle University Medical School, Thessaloniki, Greece
e-mail: etsiridis@doctors.org.uk

A. Viste, M.D., Ph.D.
Hospices Civils de Lyon, CHU Lyon Sud, Lyon, France

Service de Chirurgie Orthopédique et Traumatologique, Lyon, France

M.J. Taunton, M.D. · M.P. Abdel, M.D.
Department of Orthopaedic Surgery, Mayo Clinic College of Medicine, Mayo Clinic, Rochester, MN, USA
e-mail: Taunton.Michael@mayo.edu; Abdel.Matthew@mayo.edu

V. Murilev, M.D., Ph.D.
Head Adult Hip and Knee Reconstruction, Department of Botkin Hospital, Moscow, Russia

Y. Rukin, M.D., Ph.D.
Head Adult Hip and Knee Reconstruction, Department of First Sechenov Medical University, Moscow, Russia

R. Tikhilov, M.D., Ph.D.
Vreden Russian Research Institute of Traumatology and Orthopedics, Sankt-Petersburg, Russia

G.I. Wassilew, M.D.
Center for Musculoskeletal Surgery, Orthopaedic Department, Charité-Universitätsmedizin Berlin, Berlin, Germany
e-mail: Georgi.Wassilew@charite.de

38.1 Current Concepts

E. Kenanidis and E. Tsiridis

PFA is an established treatment method for the management of bone loss following oncological resection [1]. PFA is also rarely used for non-neoplastic conditions with a massive femoral bone loss [2]. The main reasons for major proximal femoral segmental defects or massive bone loss following THA are septic and aseptic loosening, periprosthetic fractures and multiple previous failed reconstructive procedures [3]. Possible treatment options for these patients include:

1. Cementless fixation with a modular tapered fluted stem
2. Long cemented or press-fit revision stems
3. Impaction allografting [3]
4. Allograft-prosthetic composites [4]
5. Proximal femoral replacement with a megaprosthesis [2]
6. Resection arthroplasty

The exact role of PFR in revision THA remains unclear, but indeed, the indications for the use of megaprostheses are narrow [2]. The megaprostheses are usually reserved for elderly or sedentary patients with a massive proximal femoral bone loss that cannot be repaired by other reconstructive procedures [2, 5]. The new generation PFR implants are modular, with length resection versatility to

E. Tsiridis (ed.), *The Adult Hip - Master Case Series and Techniques*, https://doi.org/10.1007/978-3-319-64177-5_38

restore limb length and soft tissue tension [5]. The use of trabecular metal or improved coatings promotes osseointegration of the retained proximal host bone to the prosthesis and more secure soft tissue reattachment [6].

38.1.1 Indications [5–7]

1. Massive proximal femoral defects.
2. Older patients.
3. Metaphyseal and diaphyseal bone defects that extend below the lesser trochanter, but sufficient distal femoral length is left for secure fixation of the stem of the megaprosthesis. In cases where diaphyseal fixation of a femoral stem is precluded, total femoral replacement with prosthetic replacement of the knee is performed.

38.1.2 Preoperative Evaluation and Planning [5]

- Assessment of the medical comorbidities especially for elderly patients.
- Full clinical examination including the range of hip motion, the motor and sensory function and the vascular status of the lower limb and specific tests for the hip and limb length discrepancy.
- Exclude infection with serological tests, bone scan and joint aspiration [1].
- Full anteroposterior and lateral X-rays of the entire femur to assess the femoral deformity, evaluate the bone stock, and estimate the size of the megaprosthesis. Radiographs may underestimate the amount of bone loss, mainly if osteolysis is present.
- CT scan with 3D reconstruction to assess periprosthetic osteolysis.
- MRI to evaluate the medullary canal and the soft tissues around the hip joint.
- The accurate preoperative templating of the megaprosthesis is mandatory; the surgeon should also have a variety of prosthetic sizes, acetabular cups and rings, constrained liners, etc. [1] and instruments to remove the existing hardware [2].
- Inspect the surgical wounds and use a previous skin incision to avoid skin flap necrosis [2].
- You may need large amounts of blood transfusion.

38.1.3 Surgical Technique [1, 8]

- Use an anterolateral or posterolateral approach with trochanteric slide osteotomy.
- Expose adequately and carefully handle the soft tissue.
- Dissect the abductors through their tendinous attachments and retract them to expose the joint and acetabulum.
- Preserve the vastus lateralis to cover of the prosthesis.
- Remove the pseudo-capsule and the scar to expose the prosthesis.
- Perform a thorough capsulectomy, dislocate the hip and debride meticulously.
- Take deep tissue specimens for frozen section and cultures.
- Examine the stability and the orientation of the cup intraoperatively carefully. If it is unstable or malpositioned, go for an acetabular revision. If not, leave it in place and exchange the liner.
- Choose the type of acetabular liner after reconstruction of the femur. Using constrained liners for intraoperative instability may be necessary.
- Remove the previous implant; to make it possible, you may need a vertical osteotomy to split the proximal femur if the femur is intact.
- Preserve the soft tissue attachments.
- Preserve the maximum possible length of the distal femur for the optimal stability of the megaprosthesis. The distal osteotomy must be sparing.
- Prepare the femoral canal with reamers for intramedullary stem fixation.
- Insert the trial components and make a trial reduction to assess stability and soft tissue tension of the joint and the limb length.
- Place a polyethylene cement restrictor 2 cm beyond the tip of the stem, insert 3rd generation cement and introduce the stem of the megaprosthesis with axial pressure to avoid varus position.
- Reduce the hip and repair the posterior capsule, short rotators and abductors using sutures passing through the holes of the prosthesis.
- The patient is mobilized postoperatively with a hip abduction brace to reduce the risk of

dislocation rate and with partial weight bearing for 12 weeks for adequate soft tissue healing.

38.1.4 Advantages [2, 5, 7, 9]

1. No need for allograft use and no risk of disease transmission
2. No problems of graft resorption, healing and fracture
3. Relative easy reconstruction
4. No adverse effect of chemotherapy or irradiation to the implants

38.1.5 Disadvantages [2, 8, 10]

1. Healing difficulties of the abductor apparatus to the prosthesis
2. High risk of complications such as dislocation and infection

38.1.6 Outcomes

There are few studies on the use of PFA in non-neoplastic conditions with massive bone loss [1, 6, 11–24]. These are usually retrospective cohorts with small to medium patients' samples demonstrating short- to midterm follow-up of the patients. The vast majority of the patient samples are heterogeneous concerning the preoperative reason of bone loss; this made the analysis difficult. It was hard to conclude the studies where patients due to aseptic or septic loosening or fractures have been managed together. In addition, the use of first-generation monobloc implants fixed with first-generation cementing techniques may not wholly reflect the modern practice [7].

In a recent systematic review, Korim et al. [7] found fourteen studies concerning the use of PFA in non-neoplastic conditions with a massive bone loss caused by fractures, aseptic loosening and septic loosening. The management of a total of 356 patients were reported with a mean of 3.8 years follow-up. Studies had a low methodological profile as only three of them used preoperative and postoperative scores. In almost half of them (43.5%) primary, secondary or periprosthetic fractures were the reason for PFA. Aseptic loosening (36%) and infection (17.1%) were other reasons. In 75% of the patients, the fixation was cemented; 15.7% of them used a constrained liner primarily. There was a failure rate for any reason of 23.9% over a mean of 3.8 years. The most common cause of failure was the dislocation (15.7%); other reasons were the infection (7.6%), the aseptic loosening (2.5%) and the component fractures (0.5%).The PFA implant retention rate was 83%. Instability and aseptic loosening were significantly more common in the pre-2000 studies compared to the post-2000 studies.

Haentjens et al. [20] in a homogenous study, evaluated nineteen patients with a mean age of 78 years suffering from aseptic loosening treated with first generation monobloc implants. At a mean follow-up of five years, they demonstrated dislocation and infection rate of 37 and 11%, respectively. The patients reported good score results, but all needed a crutch or other walking aid for ambulation. PFA was a viable salvage option for cases of bone loss secondary to loosening. The high dislocation rate may be secondary to the use of a monobloc implant and the lower use of dual-mobility sockets and constrained liners.

Mclean et al. [18] demonstrated short-term results of twenty periprosthetic fractures treated with PFA (15/20) and total femoral replacement (5/20). There were three postoperative dislocations, two postoperative infections and a fracture of the distal stem at 48 months postoperatively. Klein et al. [24] also reported the short-term results of 21 patients with a mean age of 78.3 years and Vancouver type B3 fractures treated with PFA. At a mean of 3.2 years, all patients except one were able to walk independently with minimal or no pain. PFA for periprosthetic fractures remains a viable option in the elderly patients. However, the reoperation rate is high, and dislocation remains a common problem.

In five heterogeneous studies [7], 61 patients with infected hip arthroplasties were treated with PFA. The overall clearance of infection averaged 78.9% (30/38) from 56 to 92%. This low-infection clearance was attributed to the previous multiple surgeries with compromised soft tissues and the resistance of organisms.

38.1.7 Complications

- The main complications of PFA for failed THA are instability, aseptic loosening, periprosthetic fracture, infection and leg-length discrepancy [1, 6, 11–24].
- The instability was the most common complication ranging from 0 to 43% [4, 22]. This was mainly attributed to the older age of patients, multiple previous operations with compromised soft tissue envelope, inability to achieve secure repair of the abductors and secure fixation of the prosthesis to the remaining host bone and inappropriate soft tissue tension [2, 5, 8, 24].
- The rate of aseptic loosening of the acetabular and femoral components after the proximal femoral replacement for failed THA is relatively high ranging from 0[6] to 8[15]%. Failures are often multifactorial and include poor cement technique, undersized broaches, increased stem offset, decreased stem length, rough stem surface and circular stem cross section.

38.2 Case Title: Proximal Femoral Replacement in Revision Total Hip Arthroplasty

A. Viste, M.J. Taunton, and M.P. Abdel

38.2.1 Demographics

Age: 79 years
Sex: Male
BMI: 37 kg/m^2

38.2.2 Relevant Past Medical History

Principal pathologies: Type 2 diabetes mellitus.

Previous surgical procedures: 1974, primary left THA (status post pelvic fracture in the 1960s); 1993, revision left THA; 1973, primary right THA; 1992, revision right THA due to femoral component fracture; 1996, re-revision right THA due to femoral loosening and multiple lumbar spine surgeries in 2005 and 2006.

Medication: Humalog, Lantus, Metformin.

History of presenting complaint: Right distal thigh pain for the past six months.

38.2.3 Clinical Examination

Symptoms: Pain in the right thigh towards the knee.

Range of motion: 0–90° of flexion, 5° of internal rotation, 10° of external rotation, 10° of abduction, 5° of adduction.

Specific tests: No pain with log rolling of the hip; negative Stinchfield's test.

Main disability: Walking.

Neurovascular evaluation: Neurovascularly intact right lower extremity.

38.2.4 Preoperative Radiological Assessment/Imaging (Figs. 38.1, 38.2, and 38.3)

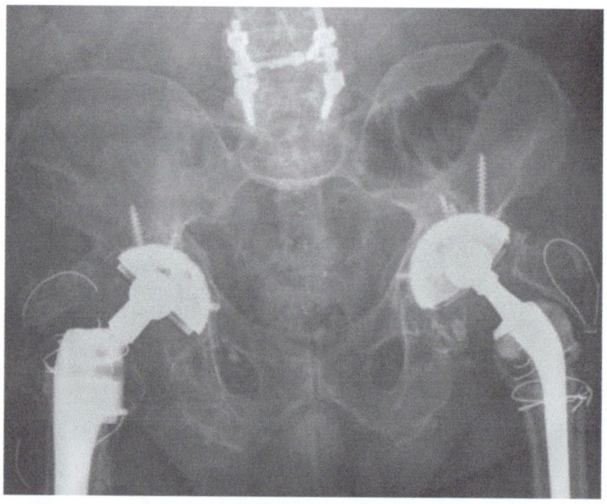

Fig. 38.1 AP pelvic radiograph: Reveals bilateral revision THAs, prior instrumented lumbar fusion, un-united bilateral greater trochanters, a loose cemented femoral component on the right and massive bone loss

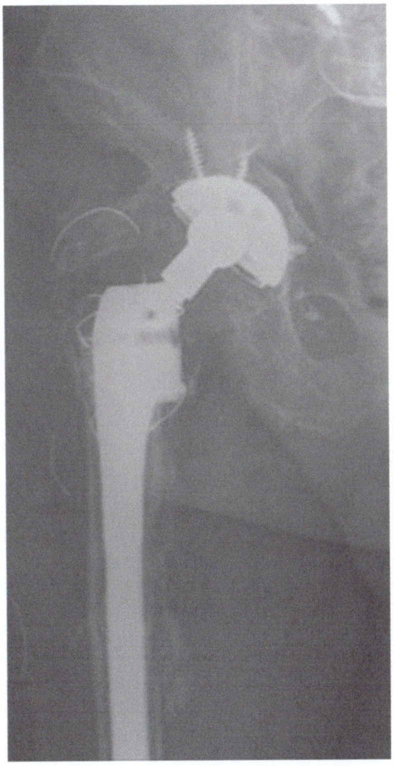

Fig. 38.2 AP right hip: Reveals un-united right greater trochanter with a loose cemented femoral component and massive bone loss

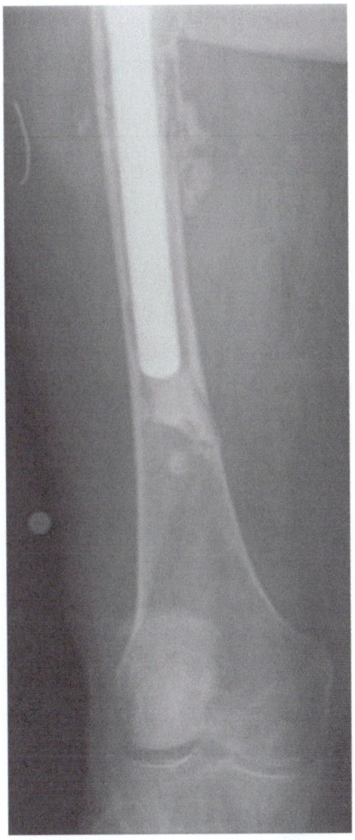

Fig. 38.3 Distal AP of the right femur: Reveals the distal extent of loose cemented femoral stem and bone loss

38.2.5 Preoperative Planning

Diagnosis: Loose cemented femoral component with massive proximal femoral bone loss and un-united greater trochanter (Figs. 38.1, 38.2 and 38.3).

Possible treatment options: Allograft-prosthetic composite (APC), proximal femoral replacement, total femoral replacement.

Chosen treatment method: Revision THA with proximal femoral replacement and constrained liner.

Selection of implants if applicable and rational: Long cemented stem with proximal femoral replacement selected due to remaining bone and massive proximal bone loss, ability to modulate limb length and version and ability to have immediate axial and rotational stability.

Expected difficulties: Massive proximal femoral bone loss, un-united greater trochanter increases risk of postoperative instability, minimal remaining distal bone uncemented fixation.

Strategies to overcome difficulties: Transfemoral approach, prepared for APC and total femoral replacement, constrained liners available for stability.

Templating: Templating is essential to determine limb lengths as well as diameter and length of stem and proximal femoral replacement.

38.2.6 Surgical Note

Patient's position: Lateral decubitus.

Type of anaesthesia: General endotracheal anaesthesia and psoas block.

Surgical approach: Transfemoral approach.

Main steps: Bony transfemoral approach, stem and remaining cement removed with use of back-biting gouges and ultrasound device, acetabular component tested for stability and optimal position by removing screws and replacing with new screws, implantation of the new cemented stem to bypass poor bone quality and quantity, proximal modularity is used to dial in version and length, constrained liner is used given lack of abductors and greater trochanter.

Reconstruction techniques: Long curved cemented stem with proximal femoral component, three cables around transfemoral osteotomy, three sutures in the un-united greater trochanter and in the proximal femoral component holes (Figs. 38.4 and 38.5).

38.2.7 Intraoperative Challenges

Challenges and solutions: Poor bone quantity proximally and poor bone quality distally, removal of cement, un-united trochanter.

Unanticipated problems and solution: None.

Thorough description of decision making, including the reason for the final decision: See above.

38.2.8 Postoperative Radiographs (Figs. 38.4 and 38.5)

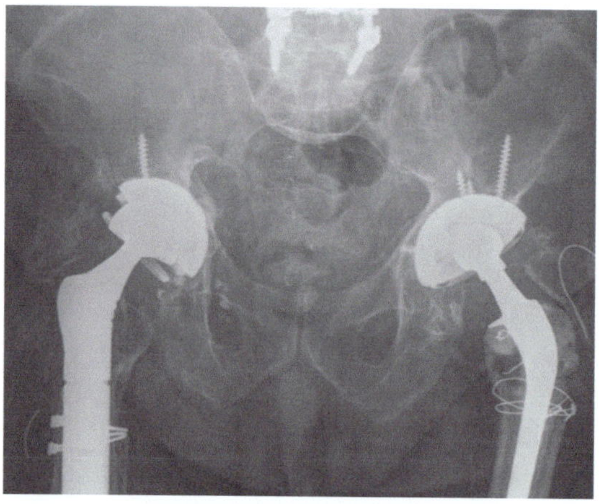

Fig. 38.4 AP pelvis radiograph: Reveals well-fixed and well-aligned cemented proximal femoral replacement with constrained liner

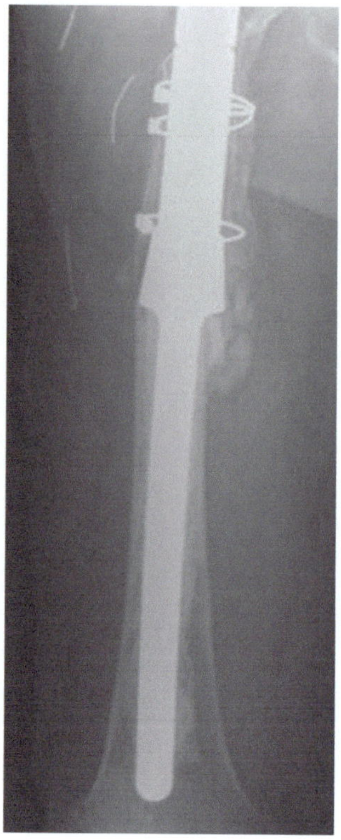

Fig. 38.5 AP of right femur: Reveals distal fixation of cemented proximal femoral replacement into remaining host bone

38.2.9 Postoperative Management

Chemoprophylaxis and anticoagulant treatment period: Low-molecular-weight heparin for fourteen days followed by aspirin for four weeks, mechanical compression devices and encouraged ambulation.

Gait/limb loading until full loading: Weight bearing as tolerated.

38.2.10 Follow-Up and Complications

There were no complications.

38.2.11 Discussion [25–27]

Advantages of the applied method: Immediate fixation, able to modulate version and length, bypass proximal defect, expeditious.

Disadvantages of the method: No biologic fixation distally and high risk of instability without greater trochanter.

Alternative evidence-based techniques for the case: APC, total femoral replacement.

Why is the chosen technique better for this case? Immediate fixation, able to modulate version and length, bypass proximal defect, expeditious, maintains native knee joint.

Indications and contraindications for your technique: Massive proximal femoral loss.

Learning curve and how to manage complications: Requires a skilled revision hip surgeon.

38.3 Case Title: Proximal Femoral Replacement for Re-revision of a Failed THA for Congenital Hip Dysplasia

Valeriy Murilev, Yaroslav Rukin, and Rashid Tikhilov

38.3.1 Demographics

Age: 66 years
Sex: Female
BMI: 38.6

38.3.2 Relevant Past Medical History

Principal pathologies: Congenital dislocation of the left hip.

Previous surgical procedures: The left femur diaphysis osteotomy was performed in 1975. The left femoral head was removed in April 1996. The total hip replacement on the left side with Protek endoprosthesis was performed in May 1996. Since 2005, pain in the left hip was returned. The revision hip arthroplasty with Biomet endoprosthesis was performed in March 2008. The dislocation of the implant occurred in February 2009. In April 2009, an acetabular component revision was performed with a Burch/Schneider ring. Recurrent dislocation happened in February 2010. The re-osteotomy of the femur diaphysis without reduction of the hip dislocation was performed in March 2010. Since March 2011, there was fever up to 39 ° with the appearance of the fistula. In our hospital in March 2011, we performed the component removal with implantation of an articulating antibiotic-loaded cement spacer. After two weeks, the spacer migrated from the femoral canal with infection recurrence. We performed the spacer exchange in April 2011. After one year, there were no signs of the infection in the left hip (Figs. 38.6, 38.7 and 38.8).

Medication: NSAIDs.

38.3.3 Clinical Examination

Symptoms: Permanent pain in the left hip, shortening of the left lower limb to 8 cm, walking with two crutches.

Range of motion: Minimal range of active movements. Passive movements: flexion 30°, extension abs., abduction 15°, adduction abs., rotation within 10°.

Specific tests: Hb 103 g/L, WBC 4.4 × 10.9, CRP 3.3 mg/dL, ESR 23mm/h.

Main disability: Walking with two crutches, disability to walk up the stairs, disability to work.

Scoring: HHS 26,175.

Neurovascular evaluation: There were no neurovascular problems.

38.3.4 Preoperative Radiological Assessment/Imaging (Figs. 38.6, 38.7, and 38.8)

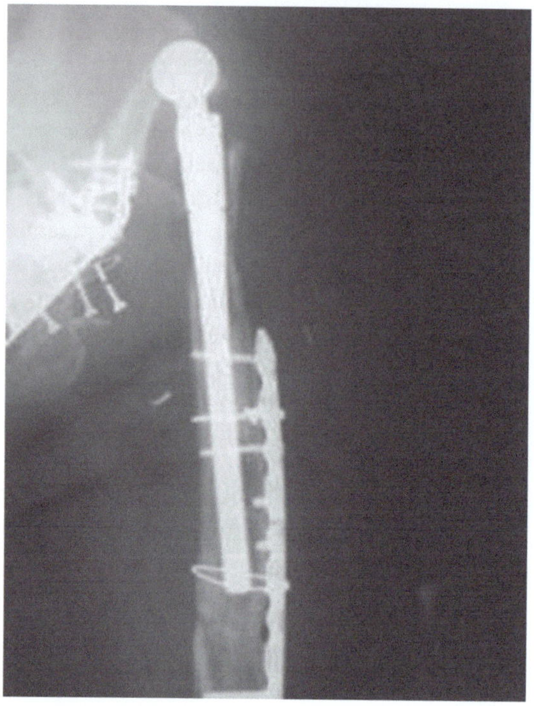

Fig. 38.6 March 2011. Unreduced dislocation of the hip. Deep periprosthetic infection

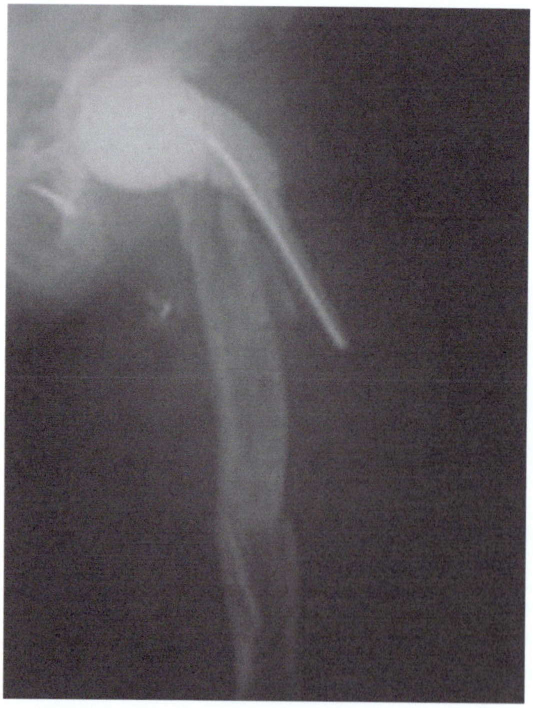

Fig. 38.7 March 2011. Migration of the articulating spacer

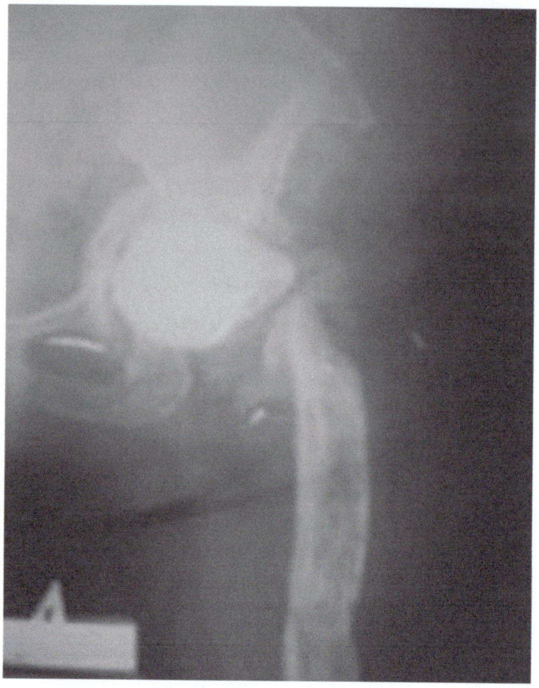

Fig. 38.8 January 2012. Non-articulating spacer

38.3.5 Preoperative Planning

Diagnosis: Non-articulating spacer of the left hip. Paprosky IIIB acetabular defects, Paprosky IV femoral defects (Figs. 38.6, 38.7 and 38.8).

Possible treatment options: Conservative treatment, revision hip arthroplasty.

Chosen treatment method: Revision hip arthroplasty.

Selection of implants if applicable and rational: Trabecular metal shell with augments, Mutars Implantcast Femoral stem with cemented fixation, constrained polyethylene-metal bearing.

Expected difficulties: Deficiency of the anterior column and the medial wall of the acetabulum, absence of intact cortical bone in the femoral isthmus, absence of the metaphysis of the femur, high risk of the dislocation, difficulties with the restoration of leg length, substantial blood loss.

Strategies to overcome difficulties: To use buttress augment to fill the defect of anterior column, to use cemented fixation of the stem, to use constrained bearing, to restore limb length to ensure the stability of the endoprosthesis, to use cell-saver.

Templating: Determine the approximate size of the cup and the stem, the position of buttress augment, the position of the hip centre of rotation.

38.3.6 Surgical Note

Patient's position: Lateral position.

Type of anaesthesia: Endotracheal anaesthesia with epidural catheter.

Surgical approach: Lateral approach.

Main steps: Surgical approach, removal of the spacer and scars, taking microbiological samples, reaming of the acetabulum, fixation of the buttress augment, implantation of the cup (connection cup and another augment by cement), reaming of the femur, use of trial femoral components, connection of modular femoral component, implantation of modular femoral component by cement, trial reduction of endoprosthesis, final reduction of endoprosthesis with constrained bearing, drain and wound closure.

Reconstruction techniques: After reaming, the right posterior buttress augment was fixed to the anterior column with four screws. Following a trial cup, we decided to add another augment to the TM cup before its implantation. Then we impacted the acetabular shell using bone cement between this shell and the buttress. We achieved enough stability with three screws (Figs. 38.9 and 38.10) .

38.3.7 Intraoperative Challenges

Challenges and solutions: Implantation of Mutars Implantcast Femoral stem with cemented fixation.

Unanticipated problems and solution: Difficulties to restore muscle balance.

Thorough description of decision making, including the reason for the final decision: Due to restore the integrity of the femur standard installation designs possible. It is advisable to only use revision constructions.

38.3.8 Postoperative Radiographs (Figs. 38.9 and 38.10)

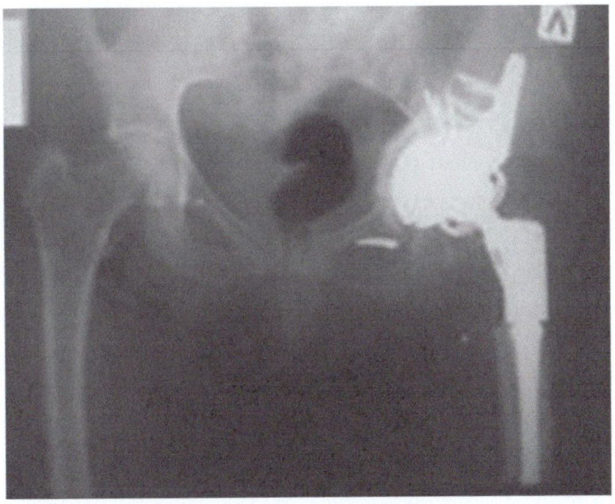

Fig. 38.9 January 2012. Two days after the operation

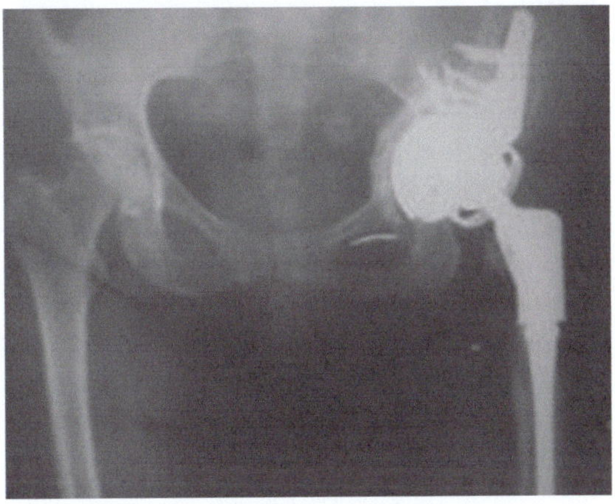

Fig. 38.10 June 2014. Two years after the operation

38.3.9 Postoperative Management

Chemoprophylaxis and anticoagulant treatment period: Dabigatran etexilate 220 mg per os for five weeks after operation and ciprofloxacin 0.4–2 for a day.

Gait/limb loading until full loading: Walking with two crutches for two months after surgery.

38.3.10 Follow-Up and Complications

There were no postoperative complications.

Scoring: HHS 71,475 at two years after the operation.

38.3.11 Discussion [28–30]

Advantages of the applied method: Trabecular metal has the initial strength fixation and excellent potential for bone ingrowth. Using the augment allowed to fill the defect of the posterior column and to achieve the initial stability of the cup. We had no supporting isthmus of the femur and chose the cemented fixation of the hip. Constrained liner was the excellent method of preventing dislocation of the hip.

Disadvantages of the method: Constrained bearing has the high risk of prosthesis loosening.

Alternative evidence-based techniques for the case: Bone grafting of the acetabular and femoral defects, use of dual-mobility for preventing dislocation.

Why is the chosen technique better for this case? Massive bone grafting has the higher risk of periprosthetic infection and loosening. Trabecular metal surfaces have an excellent initial stability and a potential to ingrowth. Trabecular metal surfaces may have antibacterial activity.

Indications and contraindications for your technique: Indication: Difficult cases of primary and revision hip replacement with acetabular and (or) femoral defects. Contraindications: Untreated periprosthetic infection, severe osteoporosis and a total absence of supporting bone.

Learning curve and how to manage complications: It can only be performed by experienced surgeons.

Level of evidence concerning the superiority of this method against others: Long-term survival of the implant (2 years) is the main advantage of the method.

38.4 Case Title: Proximal Femoral Replacement

Georgi I. Wassilew

38.4.1 Demographics

Age: 32
Sex: Female
BMI: 30

38.4.2 Relevant Past Medical History

Principal pathologies: Girdlestone resection arthroplasty of the left hip after removal of a total hip arthroplasty because of periprosthetic joint infection with *Enterococcus faecalis* and fistula.

Previous surgical procedures: Implantation of a primary total hip arthroplasty of the left hip in 2004 with two postoperative wound revisions. Additionally, there is a history of THA instability with three dislocations, all of which were treated by closed reduction.

Medication: L-Thyroxin.

Others: Hashimoto thyroiditis.

History of presenting complaint: The patient presented to the emergency department with a progressive erythema of the left hip. Fever or shivering was negated. Upon clinical inspection, a 4 by 3 cm large erythema was presented in line with the previous approach over the greater trochanter. The paraclinical signs of infection (CRP and ESR) were both elevated. Due to the clinical suspicion of periprosthetic joint infection, the patient was admitted for further investigation and surgical intervention. A preoperative hip aspiration yielded a dry tap. However, a MARS-MRI revealed an abscess formation around the left hip, so that the indication was given to proceed with surgical intervention (Fig. 38.11). Because of the unknown causative bacterial species, due to the dry tap, and critical soft tissue situation, the indication for a two-staged septic THA revision was made. To ensure a complete removal of all foreign objects during the surgical interval, we do not employ spacers in our department. During the Girdlestone resection, the greater trochanter presented as an avital, very thin osseous fragment and was lacking perfusion, so that a resection was performed. The proximal femur was entirely osteolytic. In the intraoperative microbiological samples, a polymicrobial infection with *Staphylococcus epidermidis* and *Enterococcus faecalis* was identified. After a course of i.v. and oral antibiotics for 6 weeks and a complete resolution of the clinical signs of infection, the THA reimplantation was performed.

38.4.3 Clinical Examination

Symptoms: Four by three-centimetre large erythema with colour over the previous approach over the greater trochanter. The patient was pain-free; however, there was a history of instability with three previous dislocations. All dislocations were treated by closed reduction.

Range of motion: Extension/flexion 0/0/120, abduction/adduction 30/0/20, internal rotation/external rotation 20/0/40.

Specific tests: Dry tap upon hip aspiration. The patient had a deficiency of the abductors and was Trendelenburg positive on the left side.

Main disability: The chief complaints of the patient were a progressive abductor insufficiency and progressive swelling over the previous approach over the greater trochanter.

38.4.4 Preoperative Radiological Assessment/Imaging (Figs. 38.11, 38.12, and 38.13)

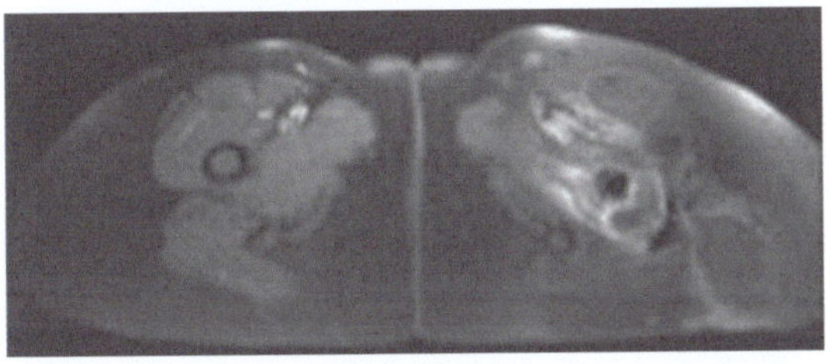

Fig. 38.11 MR image showing a pronounced abscess formation around the left hip extending towards the lateral thigh into the subcutaneous tissue

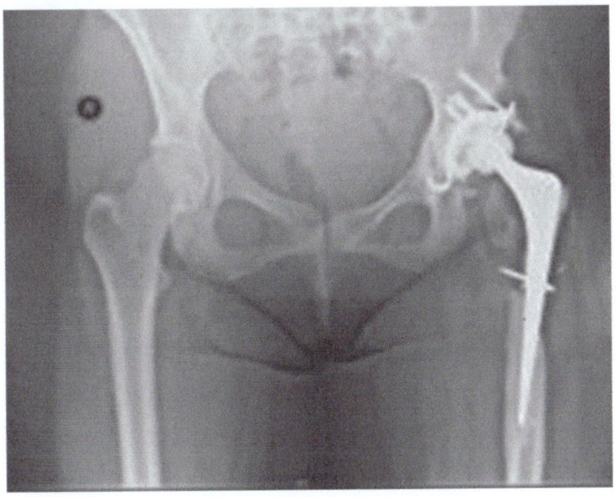

Fig. 38.12 AP pelvis radiograph showing a massive osteolysis and structural deficiency of the proximal femur

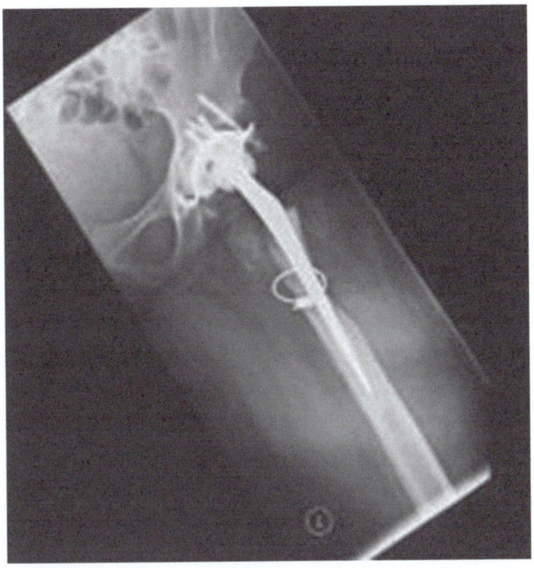

Fig. 38.13 Frog-leg lateral radiograph of the left hip showing an osteolysis of the proximal femur with dislocation of both the greater and lesser trochanter

38.4.5 Preoperative Planning

Diagnosis: Girdlestone's resection arthroplasty with a bone stock deficiency of the proximal femur and an oval defect of the acetabulum with a deficient anterior rim (Figs. 38.12, 38.13 and 38.14).

Possible treatment options: One-stage septic THA exchange, permanent Girdlestone's resection arthroplasty, two-stage septic THA exchange with or without a spacer.

Chosen treatment method: Reinforcement ring, tripolar cup and proximal femoral replacement.

Expected difficulties: One challenge is the stable fixation of the acetabular component in the presence of a deficient anterior rim. Secondly, due to the preoperative abductor insufficiency, obtaining a stable THA can be challenging.

Strategies to overcome difficulties: To reduce the risk of THA instability with subsequent luxation, the use of a tripolar cup was chosen.

38.4.6 Surgical Note

Patient's position: Lateral decubitus position.

Type of anaesthesia: General anaesthesia.

Surgical approach: Direct lateral approach.

Main steps: After exposure of the hip joint, a thorough debridement is performed. The osseous defect is filled with allogenic bone grafting. After placement of the reinforcement ring and screw fixation, a tripolar cup is cemented into the reinforcement ring. Next, the proximal femur is exposed and also thoroughly debrided. The proximal femoral replacement is implanted, and a Goretex membrane placed circumferentially around and attached to the femoral implant. The ball is pressed into the inlay, and the THA is repositioned. Finally, the musculature of the proximal femur is reattached to Goretex membrane, and the wound is closed (Fig. 38.15).

38.4.7 Intraoperative Challenges

Challenges and solutions: The stable fixation of the acetabular component is critical since the patient is young with a high level of activity and since the tripolar cup places higher stress on the acetabular fixation. Secondly, the refixation of the abductors to the prosthesis is crucial for the postoperative function.

Unanticipated problems and solution: None.

Thorough description of decision making, including the reason for the final decision: Due to the oval defect of the acetabulum and a segmental defect of the anterior rim, a reconstruction using a reinforcement ring and impaction bone grafting was chosen. To reduce the risk of THA dislocation in the presence of an abductor deficiency, a tripolar cup was selected. To allow for a reattachment of the pelvic trochanteric musculature in the presence of a 10 cm long defect of the proximal femur, a proximal femoral replacement including a Goretex membrane was utilized.

38.4.8 Postoperative Radiographs (Figs. 38.14 and 38.15)

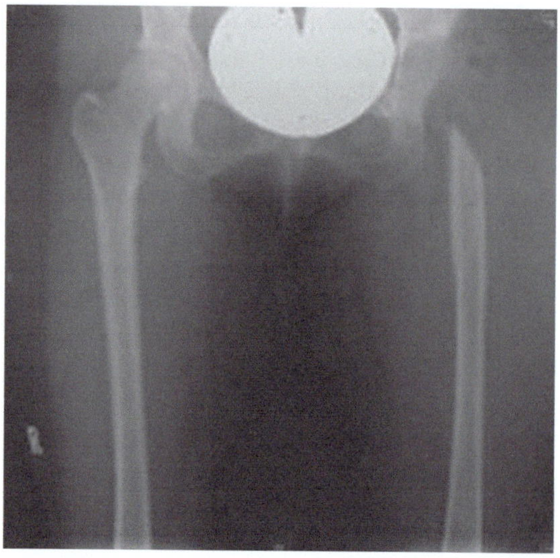

Fig. 38.14 AP pelvis radiograph of the Girdlestone's resection arthroplasty prior to THA reimplantation

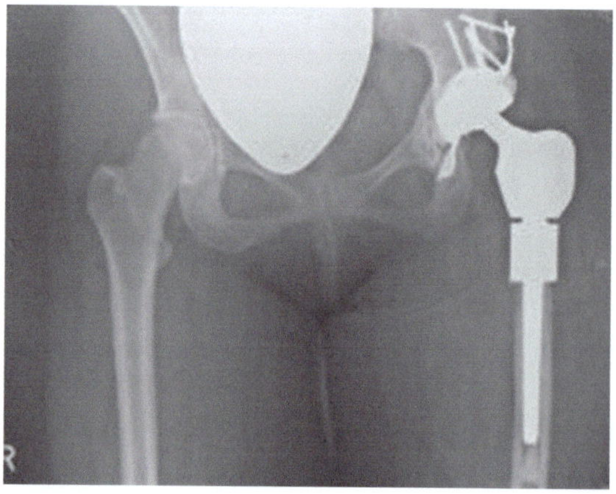

Fig. 38.15 AP radiograph of the pelvis after THA reimplantation

38.4.9 Postoperative Management

Chemoprophylaxis and anticoagulant treatment period: A perioperative chemoprophylaxis was performed with 1 g of Vancomycin and 5 g Fosfomycin 1 and 2 h before skin incision. This intravenous chemoprophylaxis was continued postoperatively until the results of the intraoperative cultures were received. Prior to discharge the chemoprophylaxis was given orally and continued until completion of the sixth postoperative week with a combination of Cotrimoxazole, Rifampicin and Amoxicillin. Amoxicillin was continued until the completion of the sixth postoperative week. Postoperative anticoagulative treatment was performed with weight-based dosage of low-molecular-weight heparin.

Gait/limb loading until full loading: Protective weight bearing in a three-point gait pattern on forearm crutches for six weeks. Afterwards, a transition to full weight bearing as tolerated is commenced.

38.4.10 Follow-Up and Complications

Despite the continuous intraoperative i.v. application of tranexamic acid (TXA), there was a postoperative anaemia. This was mainly attributed to the large wound area and the extended operation time. The patient received a postoperative transfusion of red cell concentrates (RCC).

38.4.11 Discussion [31, 32]

Advantages of the applied method: The advantage of the chosen method is the possibility of reattachment of the musculature to the implant. Secondly, the risk of THA luxation is reduced because of the utilization of a tripolar cup. A secure fixation of the acetabular component is achieved through the use of a reinforcement ring in the case of a deficient anterior acetabular wall. Because of the impaction bone grafting underneath the reinforcement ring, there is a chance of improving the host bone stock in the case of graft integration.

Disadvantages of the method: The disadvantage of the chosen method is that an osseous integration of the reinforcement ring is not possible and that increased wear rates are reported for tripolar cups.

Alternative evidence-based techniques for the case: An alternative reconstruction method for the acetabular defect is the use of a trabecular metal cup-cage construct. This also allows for a stable fixation of the acetabular component in the current defect situation. However, the smallest available cage size is for 56 mm cups. In this case, this size is too large for the acetabulum of the patient. Additionally, a long cemented stem could be used to reconstruct the femoral defect.

Why is the chosen technique is better for this case? The use of a small diameter reinforcement ring allows for retention of the remaining acetabular wall, and in the case of graft, integration can lead to an improvement of the host bone stock for future revisions.

Indications and contraindications for your technique: The indications for the use of a reinforcement cage are large defects of the acetabular floor or roof. Contraindications for the use of a reinforcement ring are a deficient posterior acetabular wall.

Learning curve and how to manage complications: The insertion of the reinforcement cage in the ischium can be challenging if the exposure is not adequate. Secondly, the reinforcement cage as well as the superior flange must sit flush against the posterior acetabular wall and the ilium. This placement requires a certain learning curve.

References

1. Sim FH, Chao EY. Hip salvage by proximal femoral replacement. J Bone Joint Surg Am. 1981;63:1228–39.
2. Parvizi J, Sim FH. Proximal femoral replacements with megaprostheses. Clin Orthop Relat Res. 2004;420:169–75.
3. Boldt JG, Dilawari P, Agarwal S, Drabu KJ. Revision total hip arthroplasty using impaction bone grafting with cemented nonpolished stems and charnley cups. J Arthroplasty. 2001;16:943–52.
4. Donati D, Giacomini S, Gozzi E, Mercuri M. Proximal femur reconstruction by an allograft prosthesis composite. Clin Orthop Relat Res. 2002;394:192–200.
5. Savvidou OD, Mavrogenis AF, Sakellariou V, Christogiannis I, Vottis C, Christodoulou M, Vlasis K, Papagelopoulos PJ. Salvage of failed total hip arthroplasty with proximal femoral replacement. Orthopedics. 2014 Oct;37(10):691–8.

6. Parvizi J, Tarity TD, Slenker N, et al. Proximal femoral replacement in patients with non-neoplastic conditions. J Bone Joint Surg Am. 2007;89:1036.
7. Korim MT, Esler CNA, Ashford RU. Systematic review of proximal femoral arthroplasty for non-neoplastic conditions. J Arthroplasty. 2014;29:2117–21.
8. Parvizi J, Bender B, Sim F. Revision total hip arthroplasty with femoral bone loss: proximal femoral replacement. In: Wiesel SW, editor. Operative techniques in orthopaedic surgery. Philadelphia, PA: Lippincott Williams & Wilkins; 2011. p. 823–30.
9. Allan DG, Lavoie GJ, McDonald S, Oakeshott R, Gross AE. Proximal femoral allografts in revision hip arthroplasty. J Bone Joint Surg Br. 1991;73:235–40.
10. Rasouli MR, Porat MD, Hozack WJ, et al. Proximal femoral replacement and allograft prosthesis composite in the treatment of periprosthetic fractures with significant proximal bone loss. Orthop Surg. 2012;4:203.
11. Al-Taki MM, Masri BA, Duncan CP, et al. Quality of life following proximal femoral replacement using a modular system in revision THA. Clin Orthop Relat Res. 2011;469:470.
12. Gebert C, Wessling M, Götze C, et al. The modular universal tumour and revision system (MUTARS®) in endoprosthetic revision surgery. Int Orthop. 2010;34:1261.
13. Colman M, Choi L, Chen A, et al. Proximal femoral replacement in the management of acute periprosthetic fractures of the hip: a competing risks survival analysis. J Arthroplasty. 2014;29(2):422–7.
14. Dean BJF, Matthews JJ, Price A, et al. Modular endoprosthetic replacement for failed internal fixation of the proximal femur following trauma. Int Orthop. 2012;36:731.
15. Malkani AL, Settecerri JJ, Sim FH, et al. Long-term results of proximal femoral replacement for non-neoplastic disorders. J Bone Joint Surg Br. 1995;77:351.
16. Bertani A, Helix M, Louis ML, et al. Total hip arthroplasty in severe segmental femoral bone loss situations: use of a reconstruction modular stem design (JVC IX). Retrospective study of 23 cases. Orthop Traumatol Surg Res. 2009;95:491.
17. Sewell MD, Hanna SA, Carrington RW, et al. Modular proximal femoral replacement in salvage hip surgery for non-neoplastic conditions. Acta Orthop Belg. 2010;76:493.
18. McLean AL, Patton JT, Moran M. Femoral replacement for salvage of periprosthetic fracture around a total hip replacement. Injury. 2012;43:1166.
19. Lundh F, Sayed-Noor AS, Brosjö O, et al. Megaprosthetic reconstruction for periprosthetic or highly comminuted fractures of the hip and knee. Eur J Orthop Surg Traumatol. 2014;24(4):553.
20. Haentjens P, De Boeck H, Opdecam P. Proximal femoral replacement prosthesis for salvage of failed hip arthroplasty: complications in a 2-11 year follow-up study in 19 elderly patients. Acta Orthop Scand. 1996;67:37.
21. Schoenfeld AJ, Leeson MC, Vrabec GA, et al. Outcomes of modular proximal femoral replacement in the treatment of complex proximal femoral fractures: a case series. Int J Surg. 2008;6:140.
22. Shih S-T, Wang J-W, Hsu C-C. Proximal femoral megaprosthesis for failed total hip arthroplasty. Chang Gung Med J. 2007;30(1):73.
23. Johnsson R, Carlsson A, Kisch K, Moritz U, Zetterström R, Persson BM. Function following mega total hip arthroplasty compared with conventional total hip arthroplasty and healthy matched controls. Clin Orthop Relat Res. 1985;192:159–67.
24. Klein GR, Parvizi J, Rapuri V, et al. Proximal femoral replacement for the treatment of periprosthetic fractures. J Bone Joint Surg Am. 2005;87(8):1777–81.
25. Sculco PK, Abdel MP, Lewallen DG. Management of femoral bone loss in revision total hip arthroplasty. Hip Int. 2015;25(4):380–7.
26. Amanatullah DF, Siman H, Pallante GD, Haber DB, Sierra RJ, Trousdale RT. Revision total hip arthroplasty after removal of a fractured well-fixed extensively porous-coated femoral component using a trephine. Bone Joint J. 2015;97-B(9):1192–6.
27. Amanatullah DF, Trousdale RT, Hanssen AD, Lewallen DG, Taunton MJ. Non-oncologic total femoral arthroplasty: retrospective review. J Arthroplasty. 2014;29(10):2013–5.
28. Deirmengian GK, Zmistowski B, O'Neil JT, Hozack WJ. Management of acetabular bone loss in revision total hip arthroplasty. J Bone Joint Surg Am. 2011;93(19):1842–52.
29. Hartman CW, Garvin KL. Femoral fixation in revision total hip arthroplasty. J Bone Joint Surg Am. 2011;93(24):2310–22.
30. Issack PS. Use of porous tantalum for acetabular reconstruction in revision hip arthroplasty. J Bone Joint Surg Am. 2013;95(21):1981–7.
31. Wegrzyn J, Tebaa E, Jacquel A, Carret JP, Béjui-Hugues J, Pibarot V. Can dual mobility cups prevent dislocation in all situations after revision total hip arthroplasty? J Arthroplasty. 2015;30(4):631–40. doi:10.1016/j.arth.2014.10.034. Epub 2014 Nov 10
32. Grazioli A, Ek ET, Rüdiger HA. Biomechanical concept and clinical outcome of dual mobility cups. Int Orthop. 2012;36(12):2411–8. doi:10.1007/s00264-012-1678-3. Epub 2012 Oct 17

39 Periprosthetic Femoral Fractures (PFFs)

Eustathios Kenanidis, Eleftherios Tsiridis, Libor Nečas, Marek Rovňák, Martin Buttaro, John A. Scolaro, Ran Schwarzkopf, Joseph M. Statz, Cameron K. Ledford, and Robert T. Trousdale

39.1 Current Concepts

E. Kenanidis and E. Tsiridis

The prevalence of femoral periprosthetic fractures is steadily increasing following the continuous rise of patients undergoing primary and revision THA [1, 2]. Periprosthetic fractures were the third most common reason for revision THA following aseptic loosening and dislocation in Sweden [3, 4]. In the vast majority of patients, these fractures present with minimal or even no history of trauma [1, 5, 6]. More than 85% of them result from low-energy trauma and only 15% from high-energy trauma [7, 8]. Mortality following periprosthetic fractures is highly similar to hip fractures in some studies [2, 3]; more aggressive treatment of these with revision THA has been proposed to reduce mortality due to faster mobilization [8, 9].

PFFs can be classified as intraoperative and postoperative [10]. In a recent systematic review [11], the incidence of PFFs after primary THA was lower than after revision THA both for intra- and postoperative PFFs. The incidence of intraoperative PFFs ranged from 0.1 to 27.8% and of postoperative from 0.07 to 18% [11]. PFFs are more frequent in uncemented than cemented both in primary and revision THA [12].

Risk factors for intraoperative PFFs are osteoporosis, rheumatoid arthritis, the femoral preparation and the surgical technique used to insert the rasp or the femoral component, the use of press-fit cementless stems [3, 5], and revision THA [11, 13]. In case of postoperative PFFs, significant risk factors are the following: advanced age [7], female gender [5],

E. Kenanidis, M.D., Ph.D., M.Sc. (✉)
Academic Orthopaedic Unit,
Aristotle University Medical School,
Thessaloniki, Greece
e-mail: stathiskenanidis@gmail.com

E. Tsiridis, M.D., Ph.D., F.A.C.S., F.R.C.S. (✉)
Papageorgiou General Hospital, Pavlos Melas, Greece

Aristotle University Medical School, Thessaloniki, Greece
e-mail: etsiridis@doctors.org.uk

L. Nečas, M.D., Ph.D. · M. Rovňák, M.D.
Jessenius Faculty of Medicine, Comenius University in Bratislava, Martin, Slovakia

Slovac Republic and Orthopaedic Clinic,
University Hospital Martin, Martin, Slovakia
e-mail: necas@unm.sk

M. Buttaro, M.D.
Hospital Italiano de Buenos Aires,
Buenos Aires, Argentina
e-mail: martin.buttaro@hospitalitaliano.org.ar

J.A. Scolaro, M.D.
University of California Irvine, Orange, CA, USA

R. Schwarzkopf, M.D., M.Sc.
Department of Orthopaedic Surgery,
NYU Langone Health Orthopaedic Hospital,
Hospital for Joint Diseases, New York, NY, USA

J.M. Statz, M.D. · C.K. Ledford, M.D.
R.T. Trousdale, M.D.
Mayo Clinic, Rochester, MN, USA
e-mail: Statz.Joseph@mayo.edu;
Ledford.Cameron@mayo.edu; trousdale.robert@mayo.edu

E. Tsiridis (ed.), *The Adult Hip - Master Case Series and Techniques*,
https://doi.org/10.1007/978-3-319-64177-5_39

post-traumatic osteoarthritis, osteoporosis [14] and rheumatoid arthritis, Paget's disease [5, 8], proximal femoral deformities, a previous surgery of the affected hip, the implant type (cementless stems and press fit), technical errors such as cortical perforation, low-energy trauma, malposition of the stem [14], and revision THA [11].

39.1.1 Classification

Numerous classifications for PFFs have been proposed [15]. The so-called Vancouver classification (VC), however, has proved to be quite practical due to its reliability, high validity, and its established treatment algorithm [16–19]. Vancouver classification is based on the (1) location of the fracture, (2) stability of the stem, and (3) bone loss.

Vancouver classification recognizes the following types of postoperative PFFs:

Type A: PFF in the trochanteric region or the proximal metaphysis:

AL: Lesser trochanteric fractures

AG: Greater trochanteric fractures

Type B: PFF around or just distal to the stem:

B1: The stem in situ is considered stable, and there is adequate bone stock.

B2: The stem is loose, and there is satisfactory bone stock.

B3: The stem is loose, and there is severe bone loss or severe comminution.

Type C: PFF is well below the tip of the stem

The main fault of VC is the reliability to estimate the stem stability preoperatively and distinguish between type B1 and type B2 fractures [8].

A modification of Vancouver classification is used for the intraoperative PFFs. These are classified into three types [15]:

Type A: Proximal metaphyseal fractures not extending into the diaphysis

Type B: Diaphyseal fractures not extending into the very distal diaphysis

Type C: Distal metaphyseal fractures extending beyond the longest revision stem

For each intraoperative PFF type, there are also three subtypes:

Type 1: Simple cortical perforations

Type 2: Nondisplaced linear cracks

Type 3: Displaced and unstable fractures

39.1.2 Preoperative Evaluation

1. Patient's history
   (a) Take a thorough history focused on the premorbid functional status and symptoms that may be suggestive of loosening before the injury [5]. The reported thigh femoral pain before fracture that was experienced with initiation of ambulation or rising from a chair was indicative sign of femoral stem loosening whereas groin pain for acetabular loosening [8].
   (b) Find previous medical records to clarify preexisting pain, LLD, and the implants used at surgery.
2. Exclude infection
   (a) The rate of joint infection in periprosthetic fractures has been reported up to 11% [20]; one has to exclude infection preoperatively.
   (b) CRP and ESR are not reliable for diagnosis due to the inflammation related to the fracture. Chevillotte et al. [20] found a false-positive rate for infection of 43% for CRP level and 31% for ESR in 204 periprosthetic hip fracture patients.
   (c) On suspicion of occult infection [5]:
      (i) Proceed to an image-guided aspiration for Gram stain and culture.
      (ii) Sent intraoperative tissue samples for frozen section.
      (iii) If infection is proved, then follow two-stage management.
   (d) At no suspicion, proceed with the procedure and send intraoperative frozen section only when intraoperative findings are suspicious.
3. Radiographic evaluation
   (a) Take full-length AP and lateral X-rays to classify the fracture and diagnose loosening or not of the prosthesis [8].
   (b) Compare with previous X-rays and try to find signs of loosening including a subsidence >10 mm, varus tilt, a fracture of the cement mantle [5, 8], and a complete or progressive continuous radiolucencies around the prosthesis interfaces (bone-metal or bone-cement-metal) [21].

(c) Evaluate also the cup. Katzer et al. [22] reported >60% loosening of the cup in a study of 900 THAs.
(d) Be aware that the sensitivity of the radiologic evaluation for the stability of the stem reaches 80% [16–19]. The misclassification of B1 and B2 fractures is the main reason for the greater reported failure of B fractures. Lindhall et al. [4] in a study from the Swedish registry reported 30% reoperation rate for B1 PFF treated with ORIF and only 18.5% for B2 treated with revision arthroplasty.
(e) The determination of the proper fixation of the stem is critical [13] for the management of PFFs. Whenever stability is in doubt, proceed to intraoperative dynamic testing with fluoroscopy or arthrotomy and dislocation especially for those patients with symptoms before fracture [8].
(f) If the distal aspect of the stem is exposed at the fracture site, a possible test is to generate a shear force along the longitudinal axis between the implant and bone or cement proximally (pointed reduction forceps on the femur and a Kocher forceps grasping the stem tip) [5].

39.1.3 Management

A. Intraoperative PFFs

A1: It is usual in revision setting but seldom compromises the implant stability. It is managed with bone autografting or can be ignored and observed [4].

A2: It occurs during the canal preparation or stem insertion. If the stem is stable, cerclage or cable wire fixation may prevent further fracture propagation [6, 15].

A3: Calcar fractures that compromise the medial metaphysis and the proximal fixation are managed with diaphyseal-fitting uncemented revision stems [15]. Greater trochanter fractures are reattached with wire, cable, or claw plates [5].

B1: It is made by the surgeon during stem removal or accidentally during canal preparation. Cerclage wiring before stem insertion is proposed to prevent crack propagation and autograft. Bypass the perforation with a long stem by at least two femoral diameters [15, 23].

B2: It is usually the result of hoop stresses from broaching or insertion of an uncemented stem. If it is recognized intraoperatively, then protect the femur with cerclage wires or cables and bypass the fracture with a longer stem. If this is not possible, use a supplement fixation with a cortical strut or a plate and screws [15, 24]. If a stable fracture will be recognized postoperatively, then proceed with observation and protected weight bearing for up to twelve weeks.

B3: It usually occurs in revision during femoral dislocation or vigorous canal preparation, femoral cement removal, or insertion of the prosthesis. Stabilize the fracture before implanting the stem with cerclage wires or cable, and bypass the fracture with a longer stem for two cortical diameters. Augment the bone stock with double cortical strut grafts placed perpendicular to each other (anterior and lateral cortex) or combine of strut and plate [15].

C1: Treat with strut grafting or autograft these small defects to avoid a stress riser that could potentially lead to postoperative fracture.

C2: Long spiral fractures with inherent stability are treated with cerclage cabling alone +/− strut allograft. For unstable fractures use strut graft and plates.

C3: Treat with ORIF using locking or standard plates depending on the bone quality. If the fracture goes up to the tip of the stem, then the plate should overlap the stem sufficiently to prevent a stress riser between the two implants [15].

B. Postoperative PFFs

1. *Non-operative treatment*

There are limited indications for non-operative treatment. It is associated with a high rate of severe complications as the loss of reduction, malunion and nonunion, pseudarthrosis, long hospital admission, delayed mobilization, and high mortality [15].

The indications for non-operative treatment are:

(a) Unfit patients to undergo a long-lasting surgical procedure
(b) Stable greater trochanter fractures

2. *Surgical treatment*

   (a) *General principles*

   The restoration of anatomical alignment and length, the stability of the prosthesis, the maintenance or enhancement of the bone stock, the early mobilization, and the fracture union are the aims of surgical treatment [15]. Many methods have been proposed, mainly fixation and reconstruction techniques. During the last years, there is a tendency for revision techniques than ORIF even in elderly to ensure stability and earlier mobilization of the patient [5, 13, 21].

   There are difficulties, however, in comparing different treatment options. Much of the existing literature is difficult to integrate because of retrospective methods, inconsistent classification, poorly defined outcomes, and series that mix results of hip and knee arthroplasty cases [5].

A-type fractures

These are fractures of the greater (AG) or lesser (AL) trochanter and are associated with osteolysis-related avulsion fractures [5, 10, 21]. The mainstay of the treatment is to address the underlying osteolysis, typically with polyethylene liner exchange.

AG

1. These are usually stable fractures that are treated conservatively with 6–12 weeks protection weight bearing and hip abduction. Indications for surgical treatment are [25]:
   (a) Painful nonunion
   (b) Abduction instability and weakness
   (c) Proximal migration >2 cm
2. In the presence of a stable prosthesis and lytic lesions, proceed with polyethylene liner exchange, proximal femoral impaction autografting, and internal fixation of the greater trochanter (tension band with wires, heavy nonabsorbable braided suture, or plates) [21]. When the osteolysis goes distally, or the stem is unstable, go for revision of the stem.

AL

These are unusual fractures. They are mainly avulsion fractures by iliopsoas and are treated symptomatically. It is supported that their incidence rises with the increasing use of anatomical and tapered cementless stems [15]. Only in case of a large posteromedial fragment with loss of medial support that makes the stability of the stem questionable revise with a distal diaphyseal fixation revision stem (the pseudo-AL type).

B-type fractures

Fractures around a well-fixed stem are managed with internal fixation, whereas fractures with femoral stem loosening require revision arthroplasty; those with poor bone stock must also be augmented with a bone graft [8, 21]. The classification, however, of the stability of a stem is often tricky even intraoperatively; this misclassification is considered the main reason of higher reported rate of failure for the osteosynthesis of fractures around a well-fixed stem compared with the revision of fractures around a loose stem [8]. Unrecognized pathology of fractures with osteolysis or weakening of bone stock, difficult fracture patterns, or cemented stems may also be reasons for worse outcomes [8].

B1

General considerations for the treatment of these fractures are:

(a) Exclude infection preoperatively.
(b) Confirm the stability of the implant pro- or intraoperatively if in doubt.
(c) Have adequate preoperative planning.
(d) Minimize the soft tissue trauma to obtain reduction and apply the plate [5]. Preserve the blood supply to the fracture fragments and the surrounding soft tissues using less invasive surgery [5].
(e) Avoid too rigid fixation to enhance callus formation [26]. The relative stability can be useful, particularly in the setting of comminuted fractures [5].

(f) Leave three or four screw holes empty at the fracture site to avoid local stresses and effectively increase the working length [1].
(g) Insert screw heads in the empty holes to reduce the risk for plate fracture at these points of weakness [27].
(h) Use the appropriate implants with sufficient length. Bypass the fracture distally by at least two cortical diameters [28].
(i) Bicortical screws are less likely to pull out and provide better rotational stability; although not proved [8], they can jeopardize the stability of the stem or the integrity of the cement mantle when aimed proximally [27].
(j) Use locking plates especially in the osteopenic bone with the option to place also non-locked screws.
(k) Use cables as an adjunctive stabilization technique [8].
(l) In the short oblique or transverse fractures, consider about double plating.
(m) Augment the poor bone stock with cortical strut allograft secured with cables.
(n) Span the femoral stem of an ipsilateral TKA to avoid a stress riser.

Controversy exists for the best surgical option of these fractures. The available literature is mostly comprised of small- to medium-sized case series and does not offer a consensus [8]. The use of three common constructs is supported: plate-cable systems, locking plates for osteoporotic bone, and compression plates. Single or double plating and strut allograft are used in most cases. None of them is considered superior to the others [8].

1. *Plate-cable systems*
   Several studies reported a variable efficacy in the treatment of B1 PFFs [28–38]; the rate of failure ranged from 0 to 66%. The results were better for studies of more than fifteen patients from large-volume centers and in cases where the proximal fixation was performed with screws and cables and not cables alone; proximal bicortical screws have been found to give better rotational stability [38]. Plate-cable constructs with proximal unicortical screws alone or screws with cables provide biomechanical superiority compared to proximal cables alone [8].
   Tsiridis et al. [35] reported the results of treatment of 3 B1 out of 16 PFFs with ORIF with the Dall-Miles plate. In two of the three patients, nonunion occurred. The authors recommended supplemental fixation with long-stem revision or strut allograft, depending on the stability of the reconstruction. Several other surgeons reported that the reason for failure of the plate-cable system was the varus malpositioning of the stem [32, 34].
2. *Locking plates*
   During the last decade, a large number of studies reported the use of locking compression plates for the treatment of B1 PFFs [28, 39–49]. These plates are particularly suitable for fixation in patients with osteoporosis and poor bone quality [8] and placed with minimally invasive surgery. In a recent systematic review, Dehghan et al. [50] reported that 36% of B1 PFFs were treated with locking plates; the reported failure rate ranged from 0 to 50%, but it was lesser for the studies where more than twenty patients were treated [28, 39–49]. The reported high rate of nonunion and hardware complications with locking plates was attributed to an overreliance of the surgeons on the locking plate, the inadequate fracture reduction and to the selection bias as they were used in more difficult cases, as those with severe osteoporosis [50]. The newer designs of locking plates having the possibility to combine locked and non-locked screws and screw placement at oblique angles are more promising [51]. Buttaro et al. [44] reported fourteen consecutive B1 PFFs treated with ORIF and a locking compression plate; in five of them, strut allografts were also used. Union of eight PFFs was reported at an average of 5.4 months; there were three plate fractures and three plate pullouts; in five of them, no strut allograft was used.
3. *Dynamic compression plates*
   Fewer studies have addressed the efficacy of dynamic compression plates in these fractures. They are effective in the [52–55] treatment of simple fracture patterns (transverse or short oblique) with no comminution [8]. Sen

et al. [52] reported 83% union rate at an average of seven months for twelve PFFs treated with dynamic compression plates. Ricci et al. [53] also reported a high union rate (100%) at twelve months for 41 PFFs managed with ORIF and dynamic compression plates. Tsiridis et al. [55] reported also one out of six B1 PFFs nonunion with this type of management.

4. *Strut allografts*

   Cortical onlay strut allografts act as biological bone plates, serving both a mechanical and a biological function [56–61]. They provide support [39], restore potentially the bone stock [39], and increase the cortical strength [5]. They can be used with or without a plate based on the stability of the stem. It is supported that the plates protect the strut till it is incorporated and offer better fixation than strut alone [61]. Tsiridis et al. [60] supported that the allograft/plate constructs should bypass any cortical defect by two cortical diameters and that the construct should be staggered distally to avoid stress risers. A major disadvantage of allograft use is the need for complete muscle stripping of the medial and anterior cortex [5, 39] that may interfere with blood supply. So their use is opposed to minimal invasion surgery. Possible complications related to their use are graft infection, viral disease transmission, and graft availability. It is recommended that short oblique or transverse fractures with comminution and poor bone stock need strut allograft [8]. In a recent systematic review, Moore et al. [61] performed a systematic review of fractures treated with or without an allograft strut using various fixation techniques. In 37 manuscripts including 682 fractures, the union rate was comparable for Vancouver B1 fractures managed with or without an allograft strut (90.7% vs. 91.5%). Time to the union (4.4 vs. 6.6 months) and deep infection (3.8% vs. 8.3%) were increased with the use of allograft struts but remained unaffected by plate type or the use of cerclage. They supported that allograft struts should be used cautiously during the operative treatment of Vancouver B1 factures.

B2

The diagnosis of a loose stem necessitates the revision of the femoral stem [13]. When there is adequate bone stock as in B2 PFF, the basic principles of reconstruction are the following [13]:

1. Removal the loose device, the cement, and the biomembrane
2. Reconstruction of the host femoral shaft
3. Implantation of a long-stemmed prosthesis that bypasses the most distal fracture line by at least two femoral diameters to obtain stable distal fixation

The main treatment options are [13]:

1. Monoblock extensively porous-coated uncemented prostheses
2. Modular stems
3. Extramedullary fixation methods (cables, plates, and/or struts) for rotational stability

1. *Monoblock extensively porous-coated stems*

   These implants achieve distal diaphyseal fixation; at least 4–6 cm of interference fit is recommended for optimal stability [62]. There are two geometric types of stems, straight and bowed [13]. The straight stems achieve three-point fixation in a bowed femur; they demonstrate an increased risk of anterior distal cortical perforation. The bowed stem may be needed when the stems surpass a length of 8 in. The main limitation of their use is the disability to change the anteversion of the prosthesis. Haidukewych et al. [21] supported that this stem is appropriate when the distal femoral fragment has parallel endosteal cortices with ≥5 cm of tubular diaphysis (usually with a diameter of <18 mm). Several studies [62–64] reported excellent results with these stems. Garcia Rey et al. [63] reported the union of twenty B2 and 13 B3 PFFs and no thigh pain at eight years postoperatively; more than one cm of subsidence was reported in almost half of the patients. Subsidence and other intraoperative and postoperative complications of these stems tend to make them the second chance following the modular stems in many centers [21].

2. *Modular fluted tapered stems*

   There are two types of fluted tapered stems: modular that is most often used and also monoblock tapered stems (i.e., Wagner-type stems). These stems have certain advantages compared to previous ones [65]:

1. Allow diaphyseal fixation (with 4 cm interference fit)
2. Give rotational stability through their splines
3. Have reduced risk of anterior perforation
4. Have independent control of component anteversion, length, and offset and of the distal diameter

It is supported that a fluted, grit-blasted, titanium, tapered modular stem can be used effectively when the distal diaphysis has divergent endosteal morphology, <5 cm of the parallel endosteal cortex, or large endosteal diameters (typically >18 mm) [21]. These stems are available in widths of ≤30 mm and can be useful in large femoral intramedullary canals [21].

The modular stems are comprised of a distal component that engages the diaphysis and a modular proximal component that mates via a Morse taper; there are concerns about the durability of the modular junction of such stems [21]. Another usual complication is the subsidence managed with proper sizing of these implants [65].

They have better-reported outcomes regarding intraoperative fracture rate, modularity, immediate stability, stress shielding, and thigh pain and seem to be preferred than extensively porous-coated non-modular stems [65–68]. Abdel et al. [67] reported 98% radiographic union of twenty five B2 and nineteen B3 PFFs with 4.5 years follow-up; 11% of the patients had reoperation for instability. Munro et al. [65] also demonstrated 98% union rate for thirty eight B2 and seventeen B3 PFFs.

3. *Long-stem cemented prosthesis*
   They are also used in rare circumstances when the likelihood of biologic fixation is low (e.g., postradiation therapy, severe osteoporosis, severe femoral bone loss) [21].
4. *Cement-in-cement revision*
   This type of revision with a long stem is considered an option in elderly with many comorbidities and unstable B2 PFF, with a stable cement mantle [69, 70].

B3

B3 PFF has a loose implant and poor bone quality with a deficient and unsupportive proximal femur. This is usually the result of a multiple-revised hip, with repeated devascularization from canal reaming, multiple cable applications, and prior osteotomies [13]. The treatment principles are focused on the implant stability, the fracture healing, and the bone stock management.

The femoral fixation in the diaphysis is mandatory. A long-stem revision hip arthroplasty usually with a modular tapered stem is used with very good results [71]; this stem requires 4–6 cm of interference fit and has splines for rotational stability. In more severe cases, an allograft-prosthetic composite revision, proximal femoral replacement with megaprosthesis, or impaction grafting may be needed [5]. In low-demand patients, a distally locked stem with host proximal femur remnants around the new construct and constrained acetabular liners to improve joint stability may be used as a salvage procedure.

In case of little comminution, a standard surgical management is followed, with reduction of the fragments and then implantation of the stem; in severe, however, comminution and bone loss, first implant a distally fixed revision prosthesis, and try to reduce the remnants of bone around the proximal stem with cables or wires. In cases of severe proximal femoral deformity, the extended trochanteric osteotomy may be needed to allow the stem inserted into the distal femoral part [72].

1. *Impaction grafting*
   This rarely used technique is described for type B2 and B3 PFFs [13, 73]. It can be used in severely ectatic bone and simple fracture patterns. The metaphyseal bone defects may be large, but contained (Paprosky II and III), and usually a stem diameter of 17 mm and above is used with good results.

   Oblique or spiral fracture patterns are reduced with cables and augmented with circumferential wire mesh at least two cortical diameters above and below the fracture site. The canal is then reamed and reformed with impaction of corticocancellous bone. A cemented prosthesis is then placed at least two cortical diameters below the fracture [13].

To achieve good proximal stability, two thirds of the circumference of the bone needs to be present. Strut graft augmentation of the posteromedial calcar region with or without mesh is used to enhance stability. Subsidence of the stem with consequent loosening and implant instability remains a concern.

Lee et al. [73] demonstrated good results of impaction grafting technique in seven patients with a mean age of 64 years. All patients suffered a PFF with severe bone loss and a loose implant. At a mean of 56 months postoperatively, all fractures have been healed, and no subsidence was mentioned.

2. *Allograft prosthesis composite* (*APC*)
   This technically demanding technique involves the cementation of the proximal portion of a long stem into an allograft and then the distal stem into the host distal femur. The femur and reciprocally the allograft are prepared with step cut to optimize fixation. The fracture is enhanced with the remaining proximal host bone and any soft tissue attachments as vascularized autograft and cerclage cables [13].

   The technique is time-consuming, expensive due to allografts, and falling out of favor [13]. A high rate of complication has been reported as allograft nonunion, graft resorption, and disease transmission [74, 75].

   Maury et al. [74] reported 16% rerevision of twenty five B3 PFFs treated with APC method at five years postoperatively. The majority of patients reported no or mild pain and were able to walk, half of them with a walking aid. Haddad et al. [75] demonstrated the results of forty fully cemented APC in revision THA. There were 10% early revisions, junctional (8%) and trochanteric nonunions (46%), and in 17.5% full resorption of the graft.
3. *Tumor megaprosthesis*
   This is another reconstruction technique with distally locked salvage prostheses for the management of severe proximal bone loss (often compromising the trochanter) in revision THA. It can be used with constrained acetabular revision, in elderly low-demand patients with limited life expectancy and bone loss [13]. It is less time-consuming. Following removal of the prosthesis and debridement, the femur is cut transversely as proximally as possible, and a usually cemented stem is implanted in the prepared canal. Anteversion is controlled by the orientation of the implant and the offset and LLD with modularity.

   There is limited literature with small sample size and limited follow-up. McLean et al. [76] reported the results of twenty patients treated with proximal or total femur tumor prosthesis for salvage of a periprosthetic femoral fracture with bone loss. At a mean of four years follow-up, no implant was loose, but there were six major complications, three dislocations, two infections, and a postoperative fracture.

C type

In these fractures the stem is stable, and the use of standard internal fixation techniques is usually appropriate [77]. It is supported that the fracture can be treated with a plate and screws only if the fracture allows for four bicortical screws distal to stem and it is at least two cm distal to the stem [78]. When the fracture line is close to the tip of the stem, a longer plate that bypasses the tip of the stem proximally is needed, to avoid a stress riser between the two implants.

39.2 Case Title: Long Cemented THA Revision for a Periprosthetic Femoral Fracture Around a Cemented Hemiarthroplasty

E. Kenanidis and E. Tsiridis

A very frail 92-year-old female Caucasian sustained a PFF due to loosening of a cemented bipolar hemiarthroplasty. She has also a weak cement mantle, very fragile bone, missing lesser trochanter, and a gamma nail on the left side for an intertrochanteric fracture.

Removing the stem is potentially easy; however, removing the cement mantle is challenging. Reduction of the fracture and simultaneously protection of the lateral femoral cortex were achieved using a broad 4.5 mm DCP plate attached to the bone with cables and cerclage wires. The femur thus turned to a continuous tube, and a revision to a long stem was then feasible. For the socket, a constrained cemented socket (Stryker) was elected for stability due to age and revision. For the femur, a cemented long-stem 205-mm-long and 44 mm offset Exeter was used bypassing the most distal fracture line by at least two ipsilateral femoral diameters. The plate was deemed necessary to stay for extra femoral reduction stability and to protect the frail lateral cortex. No screws were used to avoid fragmenting the cement mantle (Fig. 39.1).

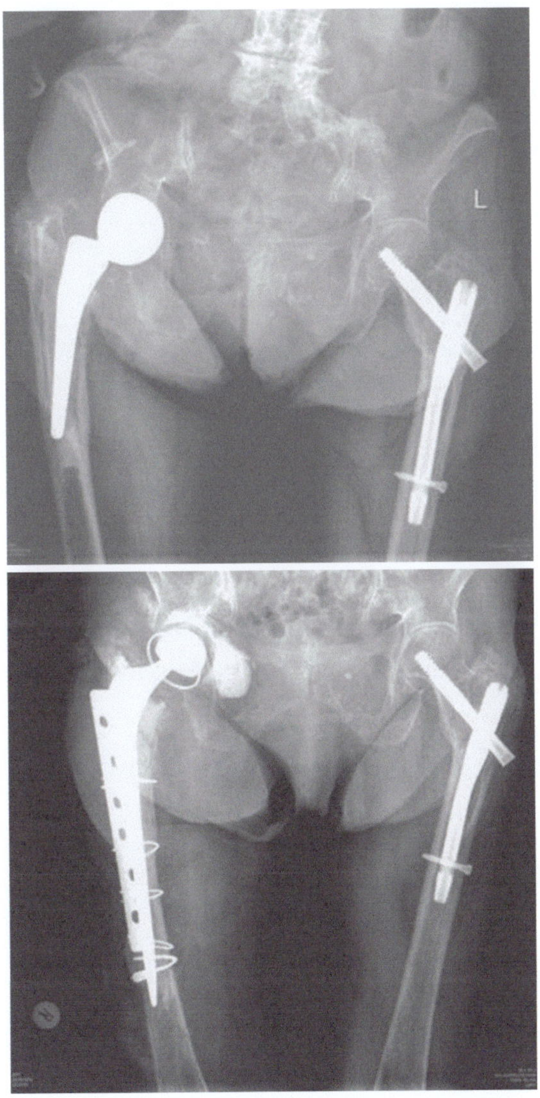

Fig. 39.1 (**a**) Preoperative pelvic x-ray of the right PFF (**b**) Postoperative pelvic x-ray showing the reconstruction with a DCP plate and a long Exeter stem

39.3 Case Title: Repeated Periprosthetic Fracture

Libor Nečas and Marek Rovňák

39.3.1 Demographics

Age: 71
Sex: Female
BMI: 22.6

39.3.2 Relevant Past Medical History

Principal pathologies: Arterial hypertension, osteoporosis

Previous surgical procedures: Right hip replacement 2004, left hip replacement 2008, periprosthetic fracture on the right side 2012

Medication: ACE inhibitors, calcium, vitamin D

History of presenting complaint: The patient experienced a hybrid right hip replacement in 2004. In 2012 after a direct fall on the right hip deserved periprosthetic fracture VC type B1 (Fig. 39.2), which was stabilized by 12 holes LCP periprosthetic plate (Fig. 39.3); in 2013 while walking, she felt crack and pain in the right hip, and later on, the X-ray verified a fracture of the plate in the level of the previous fracture (Fig. 39.4).

39.3.3 Clinical Examination

Symptoms: Swelling and palpation tenderness in the middle thigh, severe pain by standing on the right extremity, unable to weight bearing

Range of motion: S 0-0-70, F 20-0-10, R10-0-0

Main disability: Unable to stand and walk on the extremity

Neurovascular evaluation: Without any neurovascular deficit

39.3.4 Preoperative Radiological Assessment/Imaging (Figs. 39.2, 39.3, and 39.4)

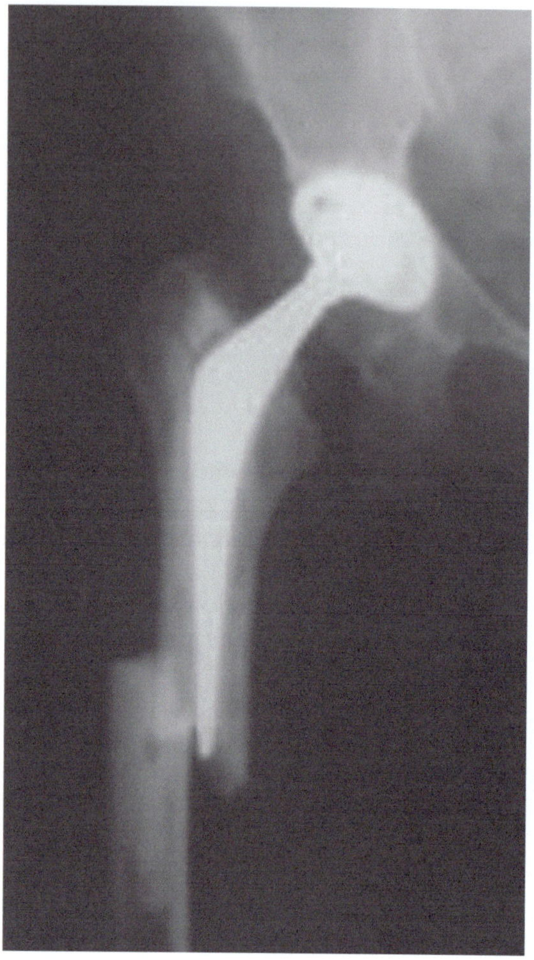

Fig. 39.2 Periprosthetic fracture type B1 after direct fall in 2012

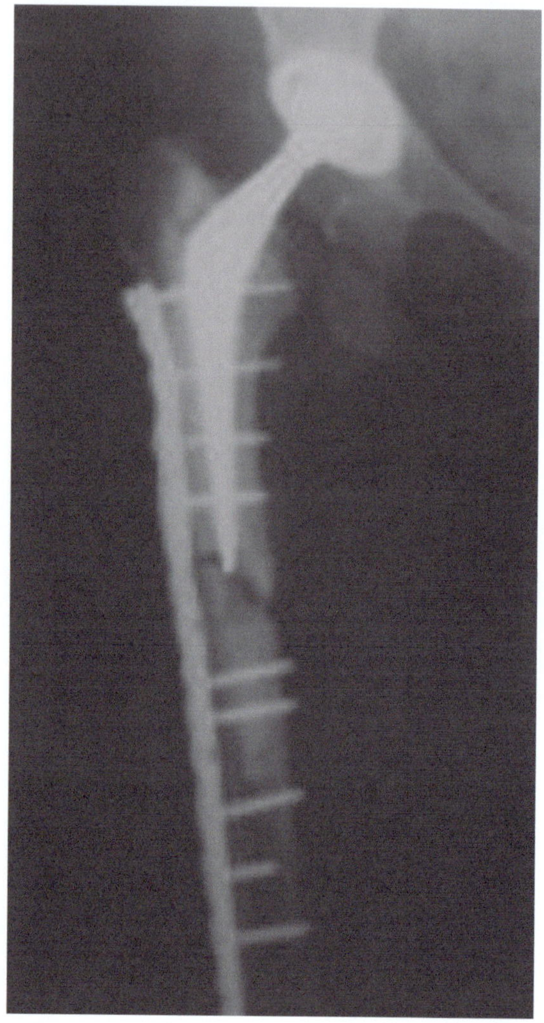

Fig. 39.3 Osteosynthesis by a periprosthetic plate in 2013

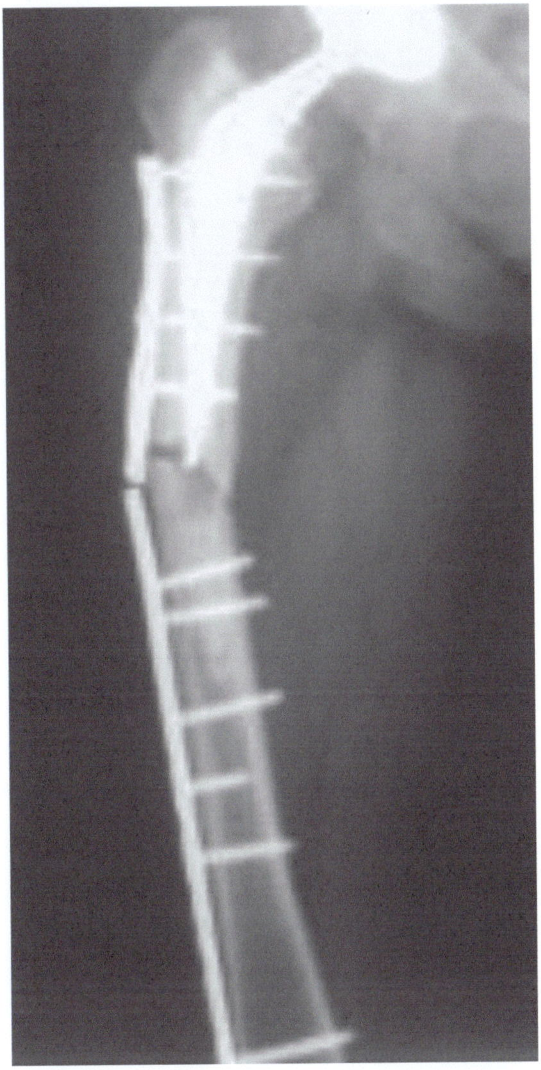

Fig. 39.4 Fracture of the plate with the same periprosthetic fracture in 2013

39.3.5 Preoperative Planning

Diagnosis: Fatigue fracture of the plate due to the lack of support and inadequate reposition (Fig. 39.4)

Possible treatment options: New plate and bone grafting, long revision stem

Chosen treatment method: Long modular revision stem

Selection of implants if applicable and rational: Modular stem with titanium band

Expected difficulties: Due to the bone-cement loosening breakage of the proximal segment of the femur

Strategies to overcome difficulties: Cerclage of the proximal bone segment

39.3.6 Surgical Note

Patient's position: Supine position

Type of anesthesia: General anesthesia

Surgical approach: Transgluteal

Main steps: Removal of the plate, protection of distal fragment for good anchorage of the revision stem (Figs. 39.5 and 39.6)

39.3.7 Intraoperative Challenges

Challenges and solutions: Bone quality

39.3.8 Postoperative Radiographs (Figs. 39.5 and 39.6)

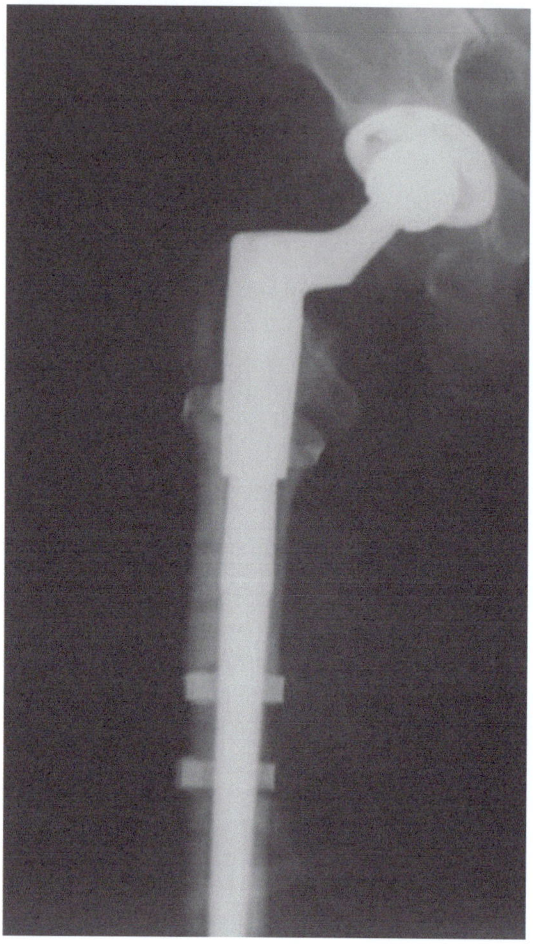

Fig. 39.5 Postoperative X-ray with revision stem

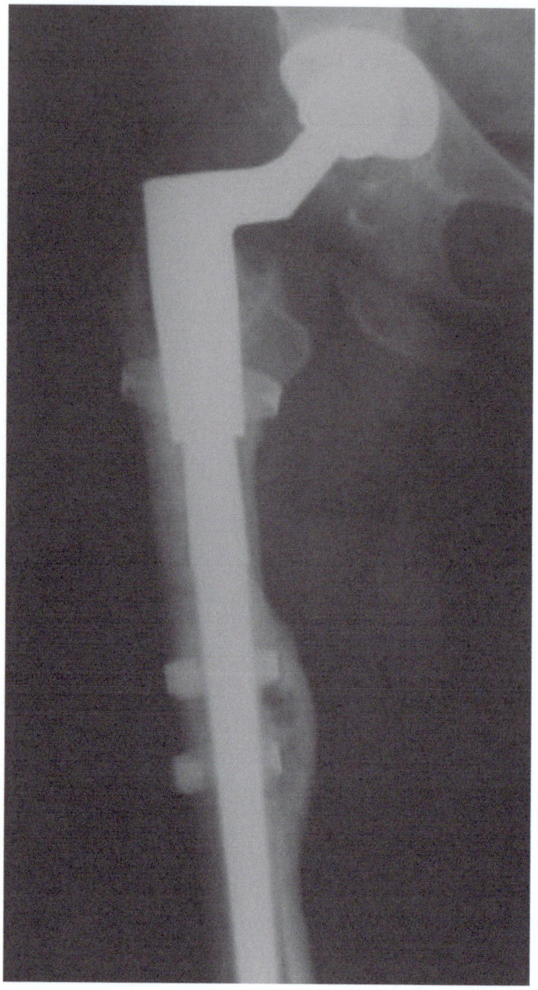

Fig. 39.6 X-ray 6 months after operation with obvious callus formation

39.3.9 Postoperative Management

Chemoprophylaxis and anticoagulant treatment period: Vancomycin 2 × 1 g intravenously with first dose 12 h preoperatively, nadroparin sol. inj. 0.6 mL/5.7 kIU subcutaneously for 45 days

Gait/limb loading until full loading: six months

39.3.10 Follow-Up and Complications

Scoring: three months postoperatively HHS 65, WOMAC 87.5%; six months postoperatively HHS 76, WOMAC 84.4%; one year postoperatively HHS 100, WOMAC 92.7%

39.3.11 Discussion

Advantages of the applied method: The usage of the titanium tapes secured the proximal segment to the revision stem.

Disadvantages of the method: Extensive approach

Alternative evidence-based techniques for the case: Proximal femoral segment replacement with the tumor-type stem

Why is the chosen technique better for this case? Preserving the bone stock

39.4 Case Title: Periprosthetic Femoral Fracture

Martin Buttaro

39.4.1 Demographics

Age: 63
Sex: Male
BMI: 21

39.4.2 Relevant Past Medical History

Principal pathologies: Periprosthetic hip fracture

Previous surgical procedures: Right THA 23 years ago

History of Presenting Complaint: Right hip pain

39.4.3 Clinical Examination

Symptoms: Pain
Range of motion: Severely altered
Main disability: Unable to walk
Scoring: Merle DÁubigne 5 out of 18 points
Neurovascular evaluation: Normal

39.4.4 Preoperative Radiological Assessment/Imaging (Figs. 39.7 and 39.8)

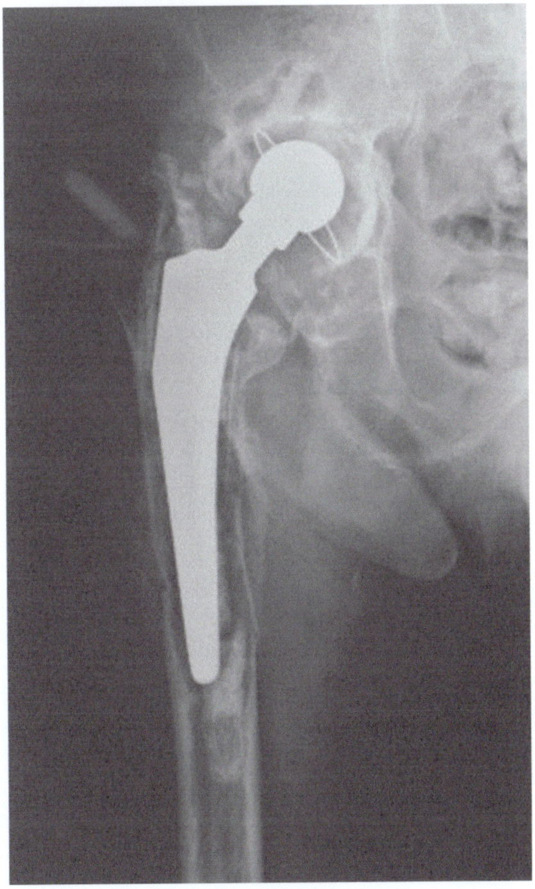

Fig. 39.7 Anteroposterior right hip radiograph showing a Vancouver B3 periprosthetic fracture in a 63-year-old male patient

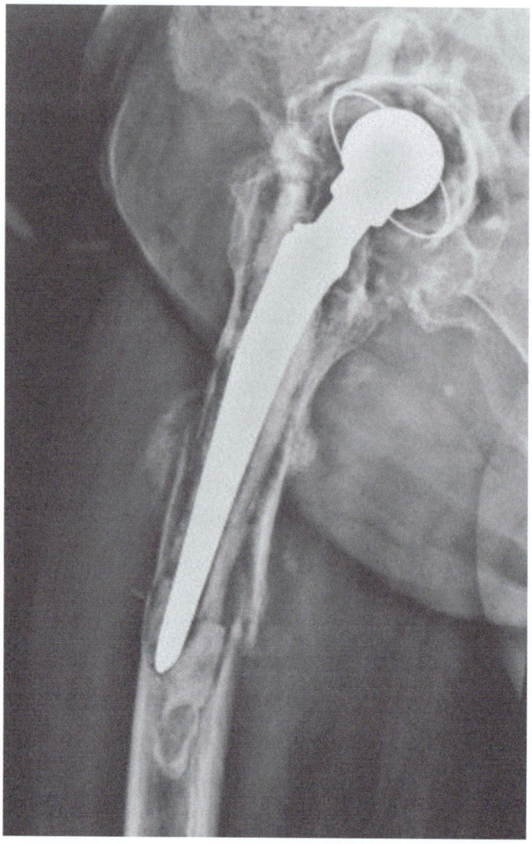

Fig. 39.8 Lateral right hip radiograph showing a Vancouver B3 periprosthetic fracture in a 63-year-old male patient

39.4.5 Preoperative Planning

Diagnosis: Vancouver B3 periprosthetic right hip fracture (Figs. 39.7 and 39.8)

Possible treatment options: Impaction grafting with cemented long stem vs. distal fixation with an uncemented long stem

Chosen treatment method: Impaction grafting with cemented long stem

Selection of implants if applicable and rational: Cemented long polished tapered stem

Expected difficulties: Bone reconstruction

Strategies to overcome difficulties: Transfemoral osteotomy

39.4.6 Surgical Note

Patient's position: Lateral decubitus
Type of anesthesia: Epidural hypotensive
Surgical approach: Posterolateral
Main steps: See attachment.

Reconstruction techniques: Impaction grafting and metal mesh containment of bone allografts (Figs. 39.9, 39.10 and 39.11)

39.4.7 Postoperative Radiographs (Figs. 39.9, 39.10, and 39.11)

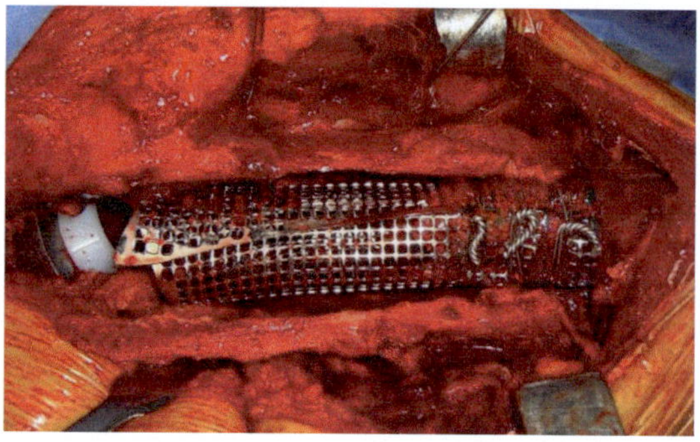

Fig. 39.9 An intraoperative photograph depicting the femoral reconstruction through a transfemoral approach with a circumferential metal mesh, impacted bone allograft, and a long polished taper cemented stem

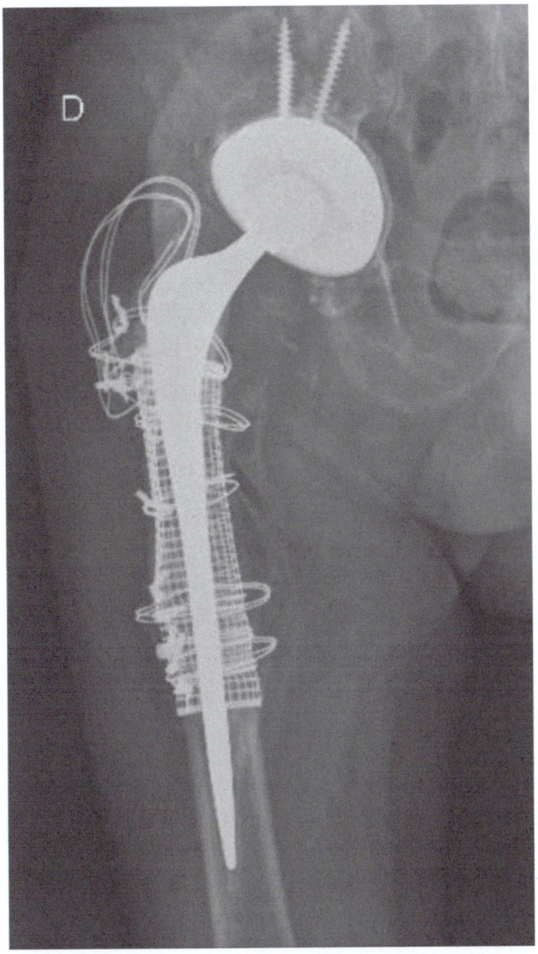

Fig. 39.10 Anteroposterior right hip radiographs showing follow-up at six years. Note the amount of bone that has developed in the medial and lateral aspect of the femur

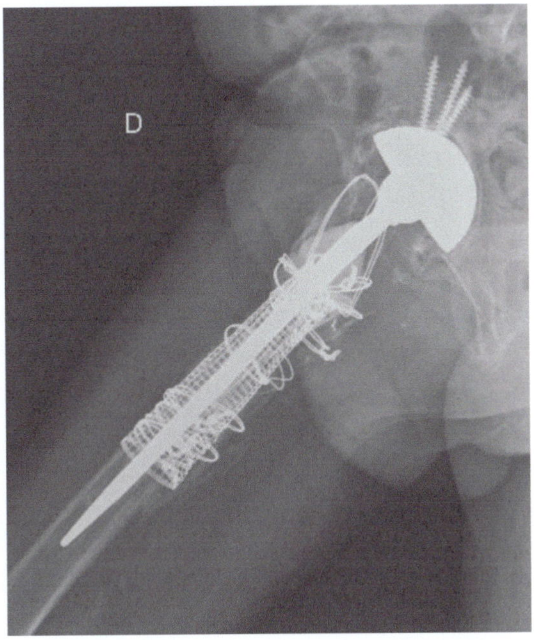

Fig. 39.11 Lateral right hip radiographs showing follow-up at six years. Note the amount of bone that has developed in the medial and lateral aspect of the femur

39.4.8 Postoperative Management

Chemoprophylaxis and anticoagulant treatment period: Enoxaparin for three weeks

Gait/limb loading until full loading: 45 days of partial weight bearing with a walker and 45 days with a cane with full weight bearing

39.4.9 Follow-Up and Complications

There was no complication.

Scoring: 16 out of 18 points using the Merle DÁubigne score

39.4.10 Discussion [79–81]

Advantages of the applied method: Bone reconstruction, economic solution

Disadvantages of the method: Technically more demanding than a distal uncemented fixation

Why is the chosen technique better for this case? Due to economic reasons, this was the chosen alternative.

Indications and contraindications for your technique: Young patients and active infection

Learning curve and how to manage complications: Steep learning curve

39.5 Case Title: Acute Periprosthetic Femoral Shaft Fracture Following THA

John A. Scolaro and Ran Schwarzkopf

39.5.1 Demographics

Age: 70
Sex: Female
BMI: 23.2, short stature 150 cm height

39.5.2 Relevant Past Medical History

Principal pathologies: Breast cancer, multiple hereditary exostosis (MHE), depression

Previous surgical procedures: Caesarean section, lymph node biopsy, lumpectomy

Medication: Sertraline, tramadol

History of presenting complaint: This patient is a 70-year-old female who underwent a primary left total hip arthroplasty for osteoarthritis. The patient worked with physical therapy on postoperative day #1 and was discharged on postoperative day #2 to her home after clearing all needed goals. On postoperative day #3, while climbing out of the bathtub, she heard a "crack" in her left leg with immediate onset of pain and inability to bear weight. The patient was seen in the office the following day for radiographic and clinical evaluation.

39.5.3 Clinical Examination

Symptoms: Left leg pain
Main disability: Pain in the mid-thigh

Neurovascular evaluation: Left hip surgical wound—clean, dry, and intact with staples in place. Left lower extremity—warm and well-perfused foot with a palpable dorsalis pedis pulse. Intact sensation to light touch in the L2–S2 dermatomal distribution with intact 5/5 strength in the quadriceps, hamstrings, extensor hallucis longus, flexor hallucis longus, tibialis anterior, as well as gastrosoleus complex.

39.5.4 Preoperative Radiological Assessment/Imaging (Figs. 39.12, 39.13, and 39.14)

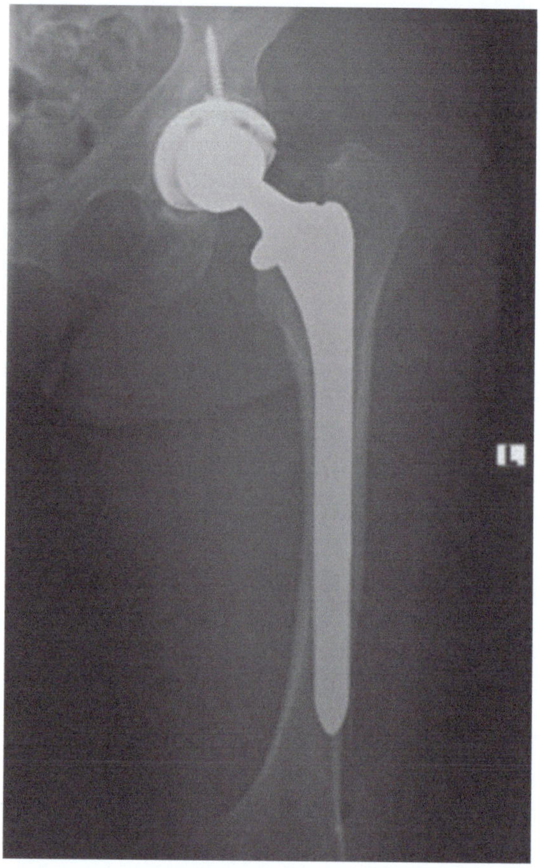

Fig. 39.12 Anteroposterior (AP) radiograph of the left hip taken on postoperative day #4 demonstrating a long-stem fully coated total hip prosthesis in place. The distal aspect of the stem is noted to have broached the anterior-lateral femoral cortex

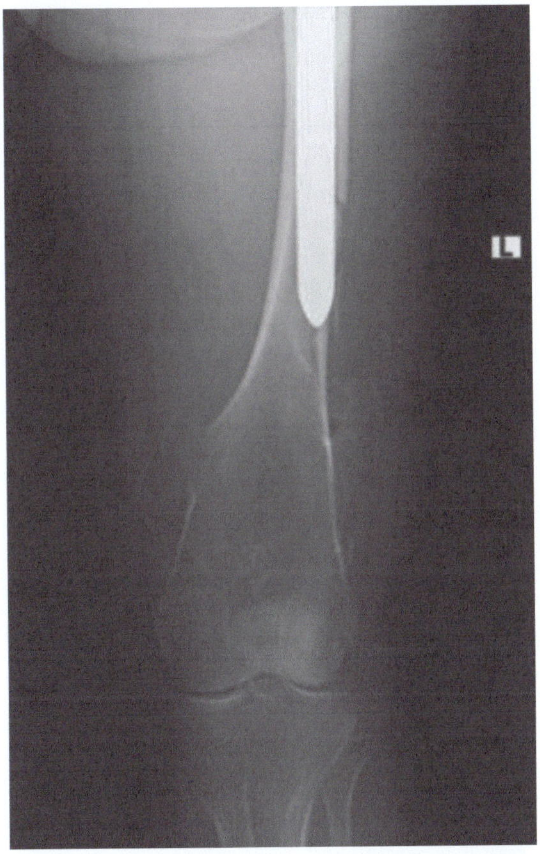

Fig. 39.13 AP radiograph of the distal femur showing the distal portion of the femoral stem as well as the characteristic metaphyseal morphology of a patient with MHE as well as both medial and lateral distal femoral osseous exostoses

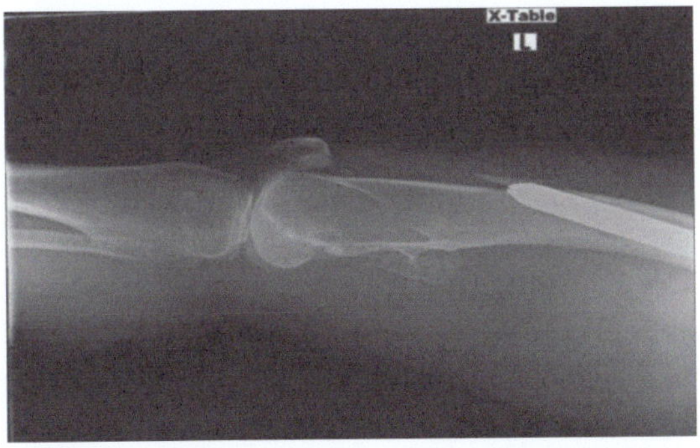

Fig. 39.14 Lateral radiograph of the distal femur demonstrating the anterior-lateral cortical breach of the femoral stem, abnormal morphology of the distal femur due to her MHE, as well as the radius of curvature mismatch between the femoral stem and the patient's femur

39.5.5 Preoperative Planning

Diagnosis: Acute Vancouver B2 periprosthetic femur fracture (Figs. 39.12, 39.13 and 39.14)

Possible treatment options: Open reduction and internal fixation (ORIF) of fracture with plate and screw device, revision of femoral prosthesis to longer tapered or bowed stem implant with or without ORIF of fracture, revision of femoral prosthesis to shorter stem implant, and ORIF of fracture

Chosen treatment method: ORIF of femoral fracture with allograft and revision of femoral stem to a shorter press-fit prosthesis

Selection of implants if applicable and rational: Smith and Nephew Echelon size 16, 150 mm high offset femoral stem. Smith and Nephew Oxinium 36 mm, +4, 12/14 taper femoral head. Synthes 9 hole 2.7 mm dynamic compression plate (DCP), Zimmer 324 mm NCB periprosthetic proximal femoral locking plate, 15 cm femoral strut allograft

Expected difficulties: The anticipated difficulties of this case were (1) revision of a long-stem prosthesis to a different prosthesis to accommodate the patient's unique femoral radius of curvature and short stature, (2) revising the femoral prosthesis with provisional fracture fixation, (3) plate fixation in the setting of abnormal femoral morphology and exostoses, (4) proximal plate fixation around a press-fit implant, and (5) addressing the anterolateral cortical defect that had resulted from the femoral stem breach.

Strategies to overcome difficulties: Preoperatively the plan was to remove the implanted prosthesis and then perform provisional fixation of the femoral fracture that would allow for trial and placement of a new femoral stem. Fracture fixation would be modified to account for the patient's geometry and then change or supplement fracture fixation as needed.

Templating: The preoperative X-rays were reviewed, and templating was completed to evaluate proper implant length selection for the revision procedure; both AP and lateral images were used for templating. The approximate length of the patient's femur was obtained from the preoperative full-length femoral radiographs, and multiple plates within this range were available at the time of surgery.

39.5.6 Surgical Note

Patient's position: Lateral decubitus

Type of anesthesia: General endotracheal

Surgical approach: Hip: posterior. Leg: direct lateral with elevation of vastus lateralis

Main steps: The hip was exposed using the previous posterior surgical approach, and the femoral stem was removed. The skin incision was extended distally along the lateral aspect of the leg, and the remainder of the femur was exposed. A large lateral exostosis was resected to accommodate the plate. The fracture was reduced and provisionally fixed with two plates with unicortical screws. A shorter fully coated press-fit stem was trialled and placed. Finally, additional proximal and distal points of fixation were placed in the plate to complete stable fixation of the fracture and protect the entire femur.

Reconstruction techniques: The original acetabular component was secured and positioned well and did not require revision. Stem and head options that were compatible with the cup were made available. Different press-fit stem options were available due to the femoral curvature and reduced length options. The metaphysis and proximal diaphysis were intact and would provide adequate fixation; thus a fully coated 150 mm stem was utilized (Figs. 39.15 and 39.16).

39.5.7 Intraoperative Challenges

Challenges and solutions: (1) The long fully coated femoral stem was removed and changed to a press-fit femoral stem of shorter length to accommodate the patient's proximal femoral geometry. (2) The femoral fracture was reduced, clamped, and provisionally fixed with a short posterior plate and long lateral periprosthetic femoral plate using unicortical screws and cerclage wires. (3) The plate was bent distally to accommodate the patient's distal femoral geometry as well as removing a large lateral exostosis. (4) A provisional unicortical screw was converted to a bicortical screw placed into the lesser trochanter, and a second cerclage wire was added to secure the proximal aspect of the plate. (5) The anterolateral cortical defect was covered with a contoured femoral strut allograft and held to the plate and bone via cerclage wires.

Unanticipated problems and solution: (1) Intraoperatively the fracture at the tip of the stem was noted to spiral both posteriorly and proximally toward the subtrochanteric region. This fracture was reduced, clamped, and provisionally held with a 2.7 mm DCP plate using unicortical screws. (2) Provisional fixation of the proximal aspect of the plate was inadequate with unicortical screws alone, some of which prevented proper stem trialing and placement; cerclage cables were used for additional fixation. (3) The lateral distal femoral exostoses prevented proper plate application; an osteotome was used to osteotomize two exostoses and provide a suitable surface for the plate. Good proximal fixation of the stem was established.

Thorough description of decision-making, including the reason for the final decision: The initially placed femoral stem required conversion to a shorter prosthesis to accommodate the patients femoral geometry and avoid risk of propagating the diaphyseal femoral fracture. Anatomic fracture reduction and stable provisional fixation restored the proximal femoral morphology to correctly size and place a new femoral stem. A plate was used that spanned the entire length of the femur to avoid any stress risers and protect the entire bone. Finally, an allograft strut was used to provide additional support in the area of the anterolateral femoral cortical defect and give perpendicular support to the lateral plate along the anterior tension side of the femur. Due to the severe deformity of the femur especially on the sagittal plane, a longer stem that bypasses the fracture site would not be possible.

39.5.8 Postoperative Radiographs (Figs. 39.15 and 39.16)

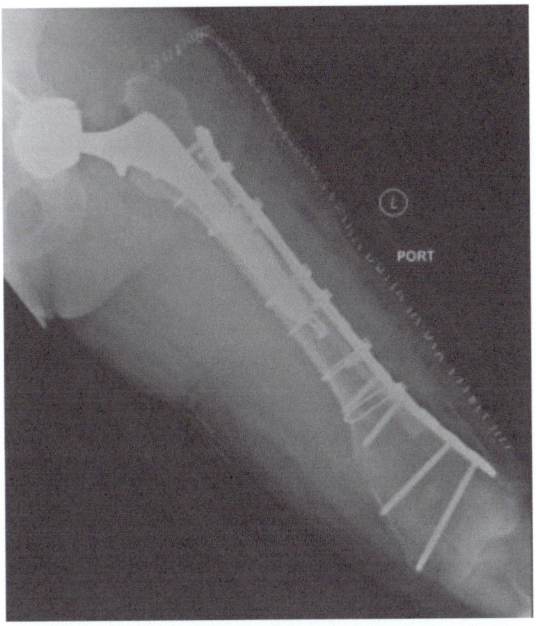

Fig. 39.15 AP radiograph taken immediately following surgery showing a shorter femoral prosthesis in place with a contoured periprosthetic lateral femoral locking plate, provisional posterior DCP, and femoral strut allograft

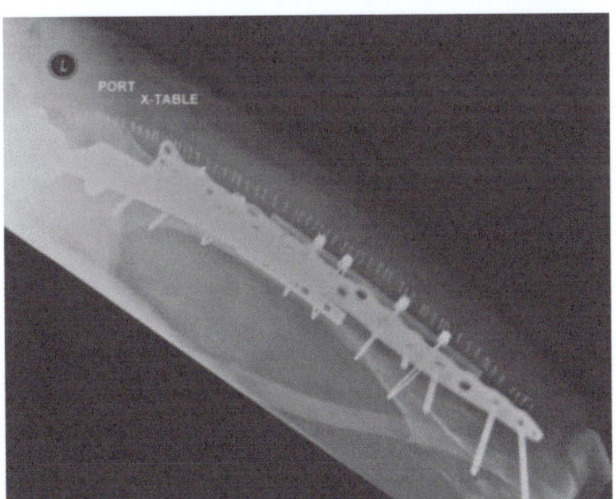

Fig. 39.16 Lateral postoperative radiograph demonstrating fixation components as described in Fig. 39.14

39.5.9 Postoperative Management

Chemoprophylaxis and anticoagulant treatment period: Low-dose Coumadin – three weeks followed by ASA 325 daily for three more weeks

Gait/limb loading until full loading: Foot flat weight bearing for six weeks, and then advanced to partial weight bearing for six more weeks. At the three months follow-up after evaluation of radiographs, the patient was advanced to full weight bearing.

39.5.10 Follow-Up and Complications

None, the patient healed uneventfully with excellent function at the last follow-up, having returned to all desired activities.

39.5.11 Discussion [82–84]

Advantages of the applied method: Stable fracture fixation and implantation of stable prosthesis allowing for early mobilization and range of motion

Disadvantages of the method: Second procedure, large incision and increased soft tissue stripping of the femur with an increased risk of surgical and periprosthetic infection

Alternative evidence-based techniques for the case: None

Why is the chosen technique better for this case? Anatomic and stable fracture fixation and placement of a stable arthroplasty implant are the ideal treatment modality for this periprosthetic fracture case.

Indications and contraindications for your technique: The indication for surgery, in this case, was an acute displaced fracture of the femur following total hip arthroplasty. Contraindications to immediate intervention would be any medical condition that caused the patient to be unfit for surgery.

Learning curve and how to manage complications: Acute fracture of the femur following total hip arthroplasty is an uncommon occurrence, and the surgeon must be prepared to address this situation with the appropriate intervention. Perioperative periprosthetic fractures with fully coated femoral stems have been reported in the literature in the past. In this case, the fracture was likely related to the mismatch of the patient's femoral radius of curvature and the implanted stem. Unlike most Vancouver B2 fractures, where a longer stem prosthesis must be used, this case required a shorter prosthesis to properly fit the femoral morphology.

Level of evidence concerning the superiority of this method against others: This is a unique case that has not been described or studied in the literature.

39.6 Case Title: Periprosthetic Femur Fracture

Joseph M. Statz, Cameron K. Ledford, and Robert T. Trousdale

39.6.1 Demographics

Age: 90
Sex: Female
BMI: 29

39.6.2 Relevant Past Medical History

Principal pathologies: Hypertension, gastroesophageal reflux disease, hypothyroidism

Previous surgical procedures: Right primary total hip arthroplasty twenty five years ago

Medication: Levothyroxine, simvastatin, Tylenol

History of presenting complaint: A 90-year-old female underwent right THA 15 years previously sustained a low-energy mechanical fall at home. There was an immediate pain in her right hip with the inability to ambulate. No other injuries were identified.

39.6.3 Clinical Examination

Symptoms: Pain in right hip with inability to bear weight

Range of motion: Right lower extremity shortened and externally rotated; range of motion limited due to pain

Main disability: Bed rest due to right hip pain/fracture

Neurovascular evaluation: Intact including motor and sensory function with palpable distal pulses

39.6.4 Preoperative Radiological Assessment/Imaging (Figs. 39.17 and 39.18)

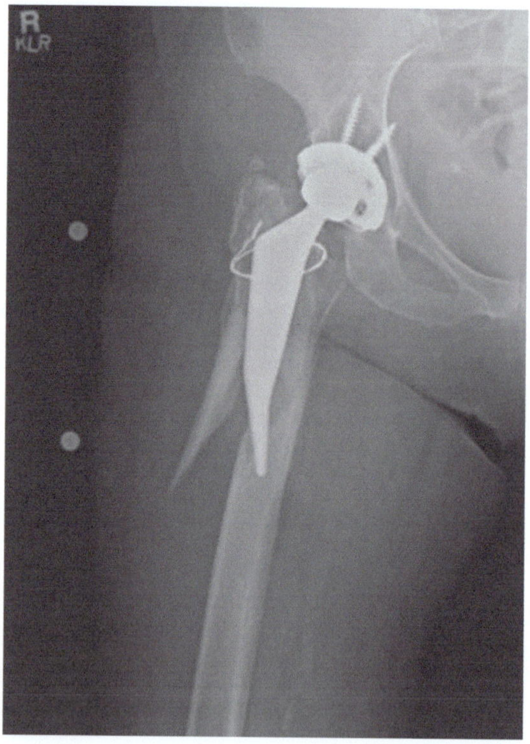

Fig. 39.17 AP hip radiograph demonstrating right THA with spiral periprosthetic femur fracture at the level of the implant and stem subsidence indicating loosening of the implant

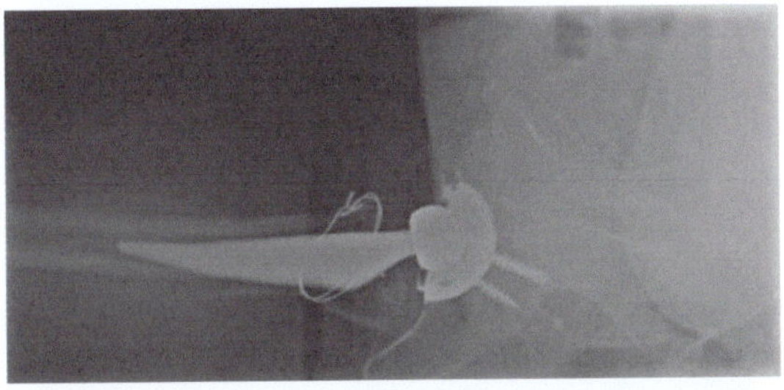

Fig. 39.18 Cross-table lateral radiograph further demonstrating fracture pattern, stem subsidence, and thick cortices indicating reasonable proximal bone stock

39.6.5 Preoperative Planning

Diagnosis: Right periprosthetic femur fracture at the level of the stem, component subsidence and loosening, good proximal bone stock (Vancouver classification, B2) (Figs. 39.17 and 39.18)

Possible treatment options: Revision of femoral component to: monoblock or modular fluted tapered stem; monoblock extensively porous-coated cylindrical stem; long cemented stem with fracture reduction (and possible cortical strut allografts); resection arthroplasty; or non-operative treatment with traction and bedrest Chosen treatment method: Revision THA with extensively porous-coated cylindrical stem performed through a transfemoral osteotomy Selection of implants if applicable and rational: Extensively porous-coated cylindrical stem for excellent fracture healing, stability, component positioning, and bony ongrowth. Expected difficulties: Exposure and stem preparation; implantation of the stem to the correct depth and version to restore hip biomechanics; fixation of fracture fragments.

Strategies to overcome difficulties: utilizing the existing fracture pattern and incorporating fracture into the planned osteotomy will aid in exposure and closure, reaming to solid diaphyseal chatter and to the exact depth required to restore leg lengths, implanting stem with careful attention to anteversion, and cable/wire fixation of osteotomy and fracture site

Templating: Templating to a stem size that fills the diaphyseal femoral canal obtains satisfactory distal fixation and restores leg length and offset.

39.6.6 Surgical Note

Patient's position: Lateral decubitus position on the pegboard

Type of anesthesia: General endotracheal anesthesia

Surgical approach: Lateral approach to the hip with a transfemoral osteotomy incorporating the existing fracture lines

Main steps: (1) Direct lateral transfemoral osteotomy utilizing the fracture line was performed for exposure. (2) The loose stem was easily extracted. (3) The cup was assessed to be well fixed and was retained. New highly cross-linked polyethylene insert implanted into the existing shell. (4) Distal femur was reamed with a flexible reamer until some good cortical contact was made distally, and then a straight, rigid reamer was utilized until solid cortical chatter was obtained. (5) Trial stem and head placed, hip reduced, and intraoperative radiographs were taken to show excellent diaphyseal fit with at least four cm of an interference fit. (6) New cup liner was placed followed by an excellent range of motion and soft tissue tension testing with the femoral trial component. (7) Implantation of the final femoral component was performed, carefully maintaining correct anteversion during insertion. (8) The transfemoral osteotomy was closed using double Luque (smooth) wires to secure the osteotomized shaft to the implant, and single Luque wires were used to reduce the trochanteric split and reduce the trochanter down to the distal bone. (9) Repeated intraoperative radiograph showed acceptable osteotomy reduction and component position (Figs. 39.19 and 39.20).

Reconstruction techniques: Transfemoral osteotomy; implanting an extensively porous-coated femoral stem; appropriately reaming the femoral diaphysis; obtaining excellent length, stability, and anteversion; smooth wire reduction of the osteotomy and fractured femur.

39.6.7 Intraoperative Challenges

Challenges and solutions: Challenge: difficult exposure. Solution: incorporating the fracture pattern into the extended osteotomy. Challenge: difficulty in seating the implant correctly to restore leg lengths. Solution: careful preoperative planning/templating and meticulous intraoperative reaming to ensure the component will seat exactly where it should to restore leg length and stability. Challenge: monoblock stem does not allow for adjustment of anteversion after seating. Solution: pay meticulous attention to anteversion during preparation and implantation. Challenge: femoral bow preventing the use of a straight stem. Solution: utilize a bowed stem in femurs requiring a stem longer than eight inches.

Unanticipated problems and solution: Problem: extension of the fracture intraoperatively. Solution: use of a longer stem with diaphyseal extension two cortical diameters past the most distal extent of the fracture and wire or cable reduction of the fragments to the stem.

Thorough description of decision-making, including the reason for the final decision: Periprosthetic fractures of the proximal femur are treated based upon fracture pattern, implant stability, and bone stock. In this case, the surgeon must plan to revise with an implant that provides fracture stability and attains initial and long-term fixation. The extensively porous-coated femoral prosthesis achieves excellent fixation in the intact diaphyseal femur distal to the fracture site while simultaneously affording the fracture fragments to heal and grow onto the porous stem. Furthermore, the implant can effectively restore limb length, version, and joint stability.

39.6.8 Postoperative Radiographs

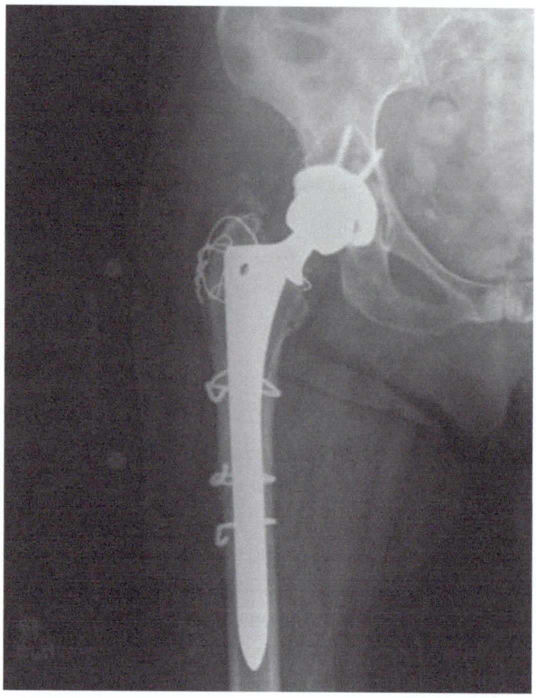

Fig. 39.19 Postoperative AP right hip radiograph demonstrating a well-fixed extensively porous-coated stem placed through a transfemoral osteotomy that was closed around the stem with multiple smooth wires

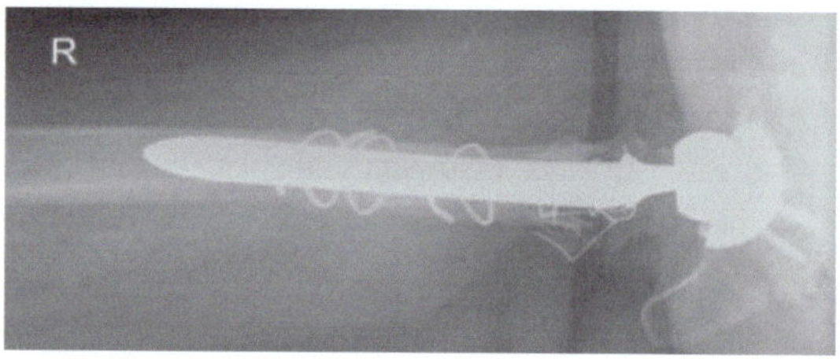

Fig. 39.20 Postoperative lateral right hip radiograph redemonstrating well-fixed extensively porous-coated stem placed through a now-healed transfemoral osteotomy and fracture

39.6.9 Postoperative Management

Chemoprophylaxis and anticoagulant treatment period: Mechanical compressive devices during inpatient hospitalization with low-molecular-weight heparin subcutaneously for ten days followed by five weeks of aspirin 325 mg twice daily

Gait/limb loading until full loading: Toe-touch weight bearing with a maximum of 30 pounds on operative extremity for six weeks followed by progression to weight bearing as tolerated after that.

39.6.10 Follow-Up and Complications

There was no complication.

39.6.11 Discussion

Advantages of the applied method: Utilization of an extensively porous-coated femoral stem for treatment of a Vancouver type B2 periprosthetic fracture is the traditional and viable option. This implant can obtain stability in distal diaphyseal bone through interference fit and allow for simultaneous fracture fixation with the use of smooth wires to secure the fracture fragments to the stem. The construct will reconstitute a functional total hip with excellent long-term survival rates of 95.9% [62].

Disadvantages of the method: It may be difficult to consistently obtain a full four cm of interference fit distally due to the cylindrical geometry of the implant and a potential lack of bone stock. This can also lead to difficulty in obtaining correct leg lengths and anteversion. Some studies have found a 52% rate of subsidence greater than 1 cm after utilization of this implant [63].

Alternative evidence-based techniques for the case: A more recent alternative technique is the utilization of the modular fluted, tapered stems. Such implants have excellent intermediate-term outcomes with 98% survival reported at a mean of 4.5 years [67]. These are also thought to be easier to fine-tune as the modularity allows one to adjust anteversion and leg length after the stem is seated in the diaphyseal bone. Additionally, less than four cm of interference fit is thought to be acceptable with the use of this type of implant.

Why is the chosen technique better for this case? The extensively porous-coated femoral stem is a reliable option particularly for the Vancouver type B2 periprosthetic fracture, though modular tapered stems have become more commonly used and dependable implant for femoral reconstruction [67]. Nonetheless, this device consistently achieves diaphyseal fixation with at least 4–6 cm interference fit, which is recommended for optimal stability of the implant.

Indications and contraindications for your technique: Indications: revision total hip arthroplasty, particularly for periprosthetic fractures along the length of a loose femoral stem with (Vancouver B2) or without (B3) supportive femoral bone stock. Contraindications: periprosthetic fracture well below level of implant (Vancouver C, treat with open reduction internal fixation with plate) or extensive meta-diaphyseal bone loss with nonsupportive diaphysis

Learning curve and how to manage complications: The principles of reconstruction require the removal of the loose device and or cement, implantation of the long-stemmed prosthesis, and reconstruction of the host femur. In the presence of a simple fracture pattern, it may be preferable to reduce and fix the fracture before implantation. Otherwise, the best strategy is to implant a distally fixed revision prosthesis first, utilizing the fracture site as the exposure window. The extended trochanteric osteotomy of the proximal fracture fragment is useful when there has been varus remodeling of the femur. Often, the proximal host bone will need to be reshaped/debulked to be reduced around the proximal implant. *Complications inherent to this advanced reconstruction include*: intraoperative fracture (greater trochanter or anterior perforation of the distal implant), subsidence, and infection [62]. Intraoperative fracture rates may be reduced with careful exposure (use of osteotomy as needed) and intraoperative radiographs to assure that the distal implant remains within the intramedullary canal. Assurance of a tight 4–6 cm distal interference fit will limit the amount of postoperative subsidence. Acute infection may be treated with debridement, liner exchange, and removal of fixation wires if the fracture site is healed, whereas the surgeon and patient may decide to utilize suppression in the face of chronic infection.

Level of evidence concerning the superiority of this method against others: Level IV

References

1. Marsland D, Mears SC. A review of periprosthetic femoral fractures associated with total hip arthroplasty. Geriatr Orthop Surg Rehabil. 2012;3:107–20.
2. Bhattacharyya T, Chang D, Meigs JB, et al. Mortality after periprosthetic fracture of the femur. J Bone Joint Surg Am. 2007;89:2658–62.
3. Lindahl H, Malchau H, Herberts P, et al. Periprosthetic femoral fractures classification and demographics of 1049 periprosthetic femoral fractures from the Swedish national hip arthroplasty register. J Arthroplasty. 2005;20:857–65.
4. Lindahl H, Malchau H, Odın A, Garellick G. Risk factors for failure after treatment of a periprosthetic fracture of the femur. J Bone Joint Surg Br. 2006;88:26–30.
5. Pike J, Davidson D, Garbuz D, Duncan CP, O'Brien PJ, Masri BA. Principles of treatment for periprosthetic femoral shaft fractures around well-fixed total hip arthroplasty. J Am Acad Orthop Surg. 2009;17:677–88.
6. Masri BA, Meek RM, Duncan CP. Periprosthetic fractures evaluation and treatment. Clin Orthop Relat Res. 2004;420:80–95.
7. Moreta J, Aguirre U, de Ugarte OS, et al. Functional and radiological outcome of periprosthetic femoral fractures after hip arthroplasty. Injury. 2015;46:292–8.
8. Fleischman AN, Chen AF. Periprosthetic fractures around the femoral stem: overcoming challenges and avoiding pitfalls. Ann Transl Med. 2015;3(16):234.
9. Langenhan R, Trobisch P, Ricart P, et al. Aggressive surgical treatment of periprosthetic femur fractures can reduce mortality: comparison of open reduction and internal fixation versus a modular prosthesis nail. J Orthop Trauma. 2012;26:80–5.
10. Tsiridis E, Pavlou G, Venkatesh R, Bobak P, Gie G. Periprosthetic femoral fractures around hip arthroplasty: current concepts in their management. Hip Int. 2009; 19(2):75–86.
11. Sidler-Maier CC, Waddell JP. Incidence and predisposing factors of periprosthetic proximal femoral fractures: a literature review. Int Orthop. 2015;39:1673–82.
12. Berry DJ. Epidemiology: hip and knee. Orthop Clin North Am. 1999;30:183–90.
13. Shah RP, Sheth NP, Gray C, Alosh H, Garino JP. Periprosthetic fractures around loose femoral components. J Am Acad Orthop Surg. 2014;22:482–90.
14. Franklin J, Malchau H. Risk factors for periprosthetic femoral fracture. Injury. 2007;38:655–60.
15. Rayan F. Fares Haddad Periprosthetic femoral fractures in total hip arthroplasty – a review. Hip Int. 2010;20(04):418–26.
16. Brady OH, Garbuz DS, Masri BA, et al. The reliability and validity of the Vancouver classification of femoral fractures after hip replacement. J Arthroplasty. 2000;15:59–62.
17. Brady OH, Garbuz DS, Masri BA, Duncan CP. Classification of the hip. Orthop Clin North Am. 1999;30:215–20.
18. Naqvi GA, Baig SA, Awan N. Interobserver and intraobserver reliability and validity of the Vancouver classification system of periprosthetic femoral fractures after hip arthroplasty. J Arthroplasty. 2012;27:1047–50.
19. Rayan F, Dodd M, Haddad FS. European validation of the Vancouver classification of periprosthetic proximal femoral fractures. J Bone Joint Surg Br. 2008;90:1576–9.
20. Chevillotte CJ, Ali MH, Trousdale RT, et al. Inflammatory laboratory markers in periprosthetic hip fractures. J Arthroplasty. 2009;24:722–7.
21. Haidukewych GJ, Langford J, Liporace FA. Revision for periprosthetic fractures of the hip and knee. Instr Course Lect. 2013;62:333–40.
22. Katzer A, Ince A, Wodtke J, et al. Component exchange in treatment of periprosthetic femoral fractures. J Arthroplasty. 2006;21:572–9.
23. Larson JE, Chao EY, Fitzgerald RH. Bypassing femoral cortical defects with cemented intramedullary stems. J Orthop Res. 1991;9:414–21.
24. Haddad FS, Duncan CP. Cortical onlay allograft struts in the treatment of periprosthetic femoral fractures. Instr Course Lect. 2003;52:291–300.
25. Pritchett JW. Fracture of the greater trochanter after hip replacement. Clin Orthop Relat Res. 2001;390:221–6.
26. Moazen M, Jones AC, Jin Z, et al. Periprosthetic fracture fixation of the femur following total hip arthroplasty: a review of biomechanical testing. Clin Biomech. 2011;26:13–22.
27. Graham SM, Moazen M, Leonidou A, et al. Locking plate fixation for Vancouver B1 periprosthetic femoral fractures: a critical analysis of 135 cases. J Orthop Sci. 2013;18:426–36.
28. Moloney GB, Westrick ER, Siska PA, et al. Treatment of periprosthetic femur fractures around a well-fixed hip arthroplasty implant: span the whole bone. Arch Orthop Trauma Surg. 2014;134:9–14.

29. Lever JP, Zdero R, Nousiainen MT, et al. The biomechanical analysis of three plating fixation systems for periprosthetic femoral fracture near the tip of a total hip arthroplasty. J Orthop Surg Res. 2010;5:45.
30. Shah N, McCabe J. Dall-Miles cable and plate system for periprosthetic femoral fracture. Eur J Orthop Surg Traumatol. 2002;12:137–9.
31. Beals RK, Tower SS. Periprosthetic fractures of the femur. An analysis of 93 fractures. Clin Orthop Relat Res. 1996;327:238–46.
32. Sandhu R, Avramidis K, Johnson-Nurse C. Dall-Miles cable and plate fixation system in the treatment of periprosthetic femoral fractures: a review of 20 cases. J Orthop Surg. 2005;13:259–66.
33. Spina M, Rocca G, Canella A, et al. Causes of failure in periprosthetic fractures of the hip at 1- to 14-year followup. Injury. 2014;45(Suppl 6):S85–92.
34. Tadross TS, Nanu AM, Buchanan MJ, et al. Dall-Miles plating for periprosthetic B1 fractures of the femur. J Arthroplasty. 2000;15:47–51.
35. Tsiridis E, Haddad FS, Gie GA. Dall-Miles plates for periprosthetic femoral fractures. A critical review of 16 cases. Injury. 2003;34:107–10.
36. Venu KM, Koka R, Garikipati R, et al. Dall-Miles cable and plate fixation for the treatment of periprosthetic femoral fractures-analysis of results in 13 cases. Injury. 2001;32:395–400.
37. Dargan D, Jenkinson MJ, Acton JD. A retrospective review of the Dall-Miles plate for periprosthetic femoral fractures: twenty-seven cases and a review of the literature. Injury. 2014;45:1958–63.
38. Ricci WM. Periprosthetic femur fractures. J Orthop Trauma. 2015;29:130–7.
39. Bryant GK, Morshed S, Agel J, et al. Isolated locked compression plating for Vancouver type B1 periprosthetic femoral fractures. Injury. 2009;40:1180–6.
40. Chakravarthy J, Bansal R, Cooper J. Locking plate osteosynthesis for Vancouver type B1 and type C periprosthetic fractures of femur: a report on 12 patients. Injury. 2007;38:725–33.
41. Ebraheim NA, Gomez C, Ramineni SK, et al. Fixation of periprosthetic femoral shaft fractures adjacent to a wellfixed femoral stem with reversed distal femoral locking plate. J Trauma. 2009;66:1152–7.
42. Froberg L, Troelsen A, Brix M. Periprosthetic Vancouver type B1 and C fractures treated by locking-plate osteosynthesis: fracture union and reoperations in 60 consecutive fractures. Acta Orthop. 2012;83:648–52.
43. Xue H, Tu Y, Cai M, et al. Locking compression plate and cerclage band for type B1 periprosthetic femoral fractures preliminary results at average 30-month follow-up. J Arthroplasty. 2011;26:467–71.e1.
44. Buttaro MA, Farfalli G, Paredes Núñez M, et al. Locking compression plate fixation of Vancouver type-B1 periprosthetic femoral fractures. J Bone Joint Surg Am. 2007;89:1964–9.
45. Müller M, Kääb M, Tohtz S, et al. Periprosthetic femoral fractures: outcome after treatment with LISS internal fixation or stem replacement in 36 patients. Acta Orthop Belg. 2009;75:776–83.
46. Laurer HL, Wutzler S, Possner S, et al. Outcome after operative treatment of Vancouver type B1 and C periprosthetic femoral fractures: open reduction and internal fixation versus revision arthroplasty. Arch Orthop Trauma Surg. 2011;131:983–9.
47. Kobbe P, Klemm R, Reilmann H, et al. Less invasive stabilisation system (LISS) for the treatment of periprosthetic femoral fractures: a 3-year follow-up. Injury. 2008;39:472–9.
48. Füchtmeier B, Galler M, Müller F. Mid-term results of 121 periprosthetic femoral fractures: increased failure and mortality within but not after one postoperative year. J Arthroplasty. 2015;30:669–74.
49. White RR. Fixation of periprosthetic femur fractures around total hip implants without the use of cables or struts. Tech Orthop. 2013;28:218–24.
50. Dehghan N, McKee MD, Nauth A, et al. Surgical fixation of Vancouver type B1 periprosthetic femur fractures: a systematic review. J Orthop Trauma. 2014;28:721–7.
51. Meiners J, Faschingbauer M, Voigt C, et al. Polyaxial locked implants in the treatment of type vancouver B1 periprosthetic fractures of the femur: retrospective clinical examination in 58 cases with review of the literature. Eur J Trauma Emerg Surg. 2010;36:53–9.
52. Sen R, Prasad P, Kumar S, Nagi O. Periprosthetic femoral fractures around well fixed implants: a simple method of fixation using LC-DCP with trochanteric purchase. Acta Orthop Belg. 2007;73:200–6.
53. Ricci WM, Bolhofner BR, Loftus T, Cox C, Mitchell S, Borrelli J Jr. Indirect reduction and plate fixation, without grafting, for periprosthetic femoral shaft fractures about a stable intramedullary implant. J Bone Joint Surg Am. 2005;87:2240–5.
54. Mukundan C, Rayan F, Kheir E, et al. Management of late periprosthetic femur fractures: a retrospective cohort of 72 patients. Int Orthop. 2010;34:485–9.
55. Tsiridis E, Narvani AA, Timperley JA, Gie GA. Dynamic compression plates for Vancouver type B periprosthetic femoral fractures: a 3-year follow-up of 18 cases. Acta Orthop. 2005;76:531–7.
56. Haddad FS, Duncan CP, Berry DJ, Lewallen DG, Gross AE, Chandler HP. Periprosthetic femoral fractures around well-fixed implants: use of cortical onlay allografts with or without a plate. J Bone Joint Surg Am. 2002;84:945–50.
57. Head WC, Malinin TI. Results of onlay allografts. Clin Orthop Relat Res. 2000;371:108–12.
58. Emerson RHJ. Basic science of onlay allografts: a review. Instr Course Lect. 2000;49:97–102.
59. Pak JH, Paprosky WG, Jablonsky WS, et al. Femoral strut allografts in cementless revision total hip arthroplasty. Clin Orthop Relat Res. 1993;295:172–8.
60. Tsiridis E, Spence G, Gamie Z, et al. Grafting for periprosthetic femoral fractures: strut, impaction or femoral replacement. Injury. 2007;38:688–97.
61. Moore RE, Baldwin K, Austin MS, et al. A systematic review of open reduction and internal fixation of periprosthetic femur fractures with or without allograft strut, cerclage, and locked plates. J Arthroplasty. 2014;29:872–6.

62. Weeden SH, Paprosky WG. Minimal 11-year follow-up of extensively porous-coated stems in femoral revision total hip arthroplasty. J Arthroplasty. 2002;17(4 Suppl 1):134–7.
63. García-Rey E, García-Cimbrelo E, Cruz-Pardos A, Madero R. Increase of cortical bone after a cementless long stem in periprosthetic fractures. Clin Orthop Relat Res. 2013;471(12):3912–21.
64. OνShea K, Quinlan JF, Kutty S, et al. The use of uncemented extensively porous-coated femoral components in the management of Vancouver type B2 and B3 periprosthetic femoral fractures. J Bone Joint Surg Br. 2005;87(12):1617–21.
65. Munro JT, Garbuz DS, Masri BA, Duncan CP. Tapered fluted titanium stems in the management of Vancouver B2 and B3 periprosthetic femoral fractures. Clin Orthop Relat Res. 2014;472(2):590–8.
66. Mulay S, Hassan T, Birtwistle S, et al. Management of types B2 and B3 femoral periprosthetic fractures by a tapered, fluted and distally fixed stem. J Arthroplasty. 2005;20(6):751–6.
67. Abdel MP, Lewallen DG, Berry DJ. Periprosthetic femur fractures treated with modular fluted, tapered stems. Clin Orthop Relat Res. 2014;472(2):599–603.
68. Srinivasan A, Jung E, Levine BR. Modularity of the femoral component in total hip arthroplasty. J Am Acad Orthop Surg. 2012;20(4):214–22.
69. Briant-Evans TW, Veeramootoo D, Tsiridis E, Hubble MJW. Cement-in-cement stem revision for Vancouver type B peri-prosthetic femoral fractures after total hip arthroplasty. 3 year follow up of 23 cases. Acta Orthop. 2009;80(5):548–52.
70. Holt G, Hook S, Hubble M. Revision total hip arthroplasty: the femoral side using cemented implants. Int Orthop. 2011;35:267–73.
71. Berry DJ. Treatment of Vancouver B3 periprosthetic femur fractures with a fluted tapered stem. Clin Orthop Relat Res. 2003;417:224–31.
72. Levine BR, Della Valle CJ, Lewis P, Berger RA, Sporer SM, Paprosky W. Extended trochanteric osteotomy for the treatment of vancouver B2/B3 periprosthetic fractures of the femur. J Arthroplasty. 2008;23(4):527–33.
73. Lee GC, Nelson CL, Virmani S, Manikonda K, Israelite CL, Garino JP. Management of periprosthetic femur fractures with severe bone loss using impaction bone grafting technique. J Arthroplasty. 2010;25(3):405–9.
74. Maury AC, Pressman A, Cayen B, Zalzal P, Backstein D, Gross A. Proximal femoral allograft treatment of Vancouver type-B3 periprosthetic femoral fractures after total hip arthroplasty. J Bone Joint Surg Am. 2006;88(5):953–8.
75. Haddad FS, Garbuz DS, Masri BA, Duncan CP. Structural proximal femoral allografts for failed total hip replacements: a minimum review of five years. J Bone Joint Surg Br. 2000;82(6):830–6.
76. McLean AL, Patton JT, Moran M. Femoral replacement for salvage of Periprosthetic fracture around a total hip replacement. Injury. 2012;43(7):1166–9.
77. Abdel MP, Cottino U, Mabry TM. Management of periprosthetic femoral fractures following total hip arthroplasty: a review. Int Orthop. 2015;39:2005–10.
78. Corten K, Vanrykel F, Bellemans J, Frederix PR, Simon JP, Broos PL. An algorithm for the surgical treatment of periprosthetic fractures of the femur around a well-fixed femoral component. J Bone Joint Surg Br. 2009;91:1424–30.
79. Youssef B, Pavlou G, Shah N, Macheras G, Tsiridis E. Impaction bone grafting for periprosthetic fractures around a total hip arthroplasty. Injury. 2014;45(11):1674–80. https://doi.org/10.1016/j.injury.2014.07.028. Epub 2014 Aug 15. Review
80. Te Stroet MA, Bronsema E, Rijnen WH, Gardeniers JW, Schreurs BW. The use of a long stem cemented femoral component in revision total hip replacement: a follow-up study of five to 16 years. Bone Joint J. 2014;96-B(9):1207–13. https://doi.org/10.1302/0301-620X.96B9.33304.
81. Dearden PM, Bobak PP, Giannoudis PV. Impaction bone grafting and cemented stem revision in periprosthetic hip fractures: a novel surgical technique. Hip Int. 2014;24(2):210–2.
82. Mitchell PA, Greidanus NV, Masri BA, Garbuz DS, Duncan CP. The prevention of periprosthetic fractures of the femur during and after total hip arthroplasty. Instr Course Lect. 2003;52:301–8. Review
83. Vaishya R, Swami S, Vijay V, Vaish A. Bilateral total hip arthroplasty in a young man with hereditary multiple exostoses. BMJ Case Rep. 2015;2015. pii: bcr2014207853. https://doi.org/10.1136/bcr-2014-207.853.
84. Bonnin MP, Neto CC, Aitsiselmi T, Murphy CG, Bossard N, Roche S. Increased incidence of femoral fractures in small femurs and women undergoing uncemented total hip arthroplasty - why? Bone Joint J. 2015;97-B(6):741–8. https://doi.org/10.1302/0301-620X.97B6.35022.033.052.

Management of Leg Length Discrepancy after THA

40

Eustathios Kenanidis, Eleftherios Tsiridis, and Viktor Janz

40.1 Case Title: Revision THA for Clinically Symptomatic Leg Length Discrepancy Using Impaction Grafting and Cemented Stem

E. Kenanidis and E. Tsiridis

40.1.1 Demographics

Age: 66
Sex: Female
BMI: 25

40.1.2 Relevant Past Medical History

Principal pathologies: Asthma, hiatus hernia, arterial hypertension, dyslipidaemia

Previous surgical procedures: Right AMIS uncemented THA, 8-month history of pain and limping, calcification removal of the breast (2003)

Medication: Atenolol, simvastatin, omeprazole

History of presenting complaint: Leg length discrepancy, limping back and thigh pain

40.1.3 Clinical Examination

Range of motion: Tight range painful arch 0–90 limitation to adduction

Specific tests: LLD 3 cm

Main disability: Unable to walk straight, back pain, unable to climb stairs, knee pain and sense of instability

Scoring: HHS 85 due to pain

Neurovascular evaluation: Normal

E. Kenanidis, M.D., Ph.D., M.Sc. (✉)
Academic Orthopaedic Unit, Aristotle University Medical School, Thessaloniki, Greece
e-mail: stathiskenanidis@gmail.com

E. Tsiridis, M.D., Ph.D., F.A.C.S., F.R.C.S.
Papageorgiou General Hospital, Pavlos Melas, Greece

Aristotle University Medical School, Thessaloniki, Greece
e-mail: etsiridis@doctors.org.uk

V. Janz, M.D.
Center for Musculoskeletal Surgery, Orthopaedic Department, Charité-Universitätsmedizin Berlin, Berlin, Germany
e-mail: Viktor.Janz@charite.de

E. Tsiridis (ed.), *The Adult Hip - Master Case Series and Techniques*,
https://doi.org/10.1007/978-3-319-64177-5_40

40.1.4 Preoperative Radiological Assessment/Imaging (Fig. 40.1)

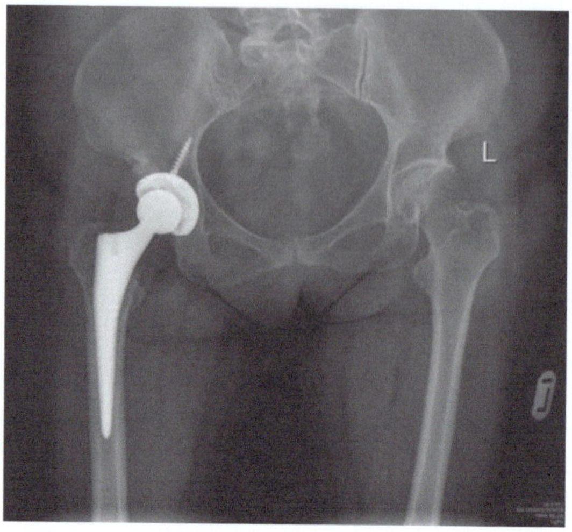

Fig. 40.1 Obvious and measurable LLD minimum of 3 cm. Tight, good fit of the stem into the femoral canal. Stem is a titanium spray-coated anatomical design

40.1.5 Preoperative Planning

Diagnosis: LLD 3 cm (Fig. 40.1).

Possible treatment options: Stem removal and cemented or uncemented replacement shortening.

Chosen treatment method: Cemented hip stem EXETER 35.5 mm offset, Stryker femoral head 28 mm.

Expected difficulties: Removing the implant may require ETO.

Strategies to overcome difficulties: Part of the preoperative planning was to exclude infection and loosening. A surgical tap of the hip joint performed before surgery and the culture of the fluid obtained revealed no microorganisms. Also, a Tc-99m MDP bone scan demonstrated no loosening of the components which reinforced our strategy for ETO for removal of the stem.

40.1.6 Surgical Note

With the patient in the lateral decubitus position, a posterior approach was performed. The hip was exposed and dislocated easily. The proximal femur was then exposed to assess the stem in situ. The stem was found very well fixed to the surrounding bone. Attempts were made to break the implant-bone interface from the top using flexible thin osteotomes and thin K-wires, but the bone was not strong enough to withstand those efforts and in places we experience perforation of the cortex. The decision was then made to remove the implant using an extended trochanteric osteotomy. The ETO was performed in a standard manner using the oscillating saw with a small but long blade. Breaking out the osteotomy component was very difficult as the osseointegration was very strong in places. The inner surface of the implant was also detached from the femur with great difficulty and by using a Gigli saw. The vigorous removal of the implant resulted in significant bone loss especially on the lateral and the anterior cortex. The decision was made to proceed with impaction grafting of the proximal femur and cemented stem to adjust for the LLD. The osteotomy was recovered using cerclage wires and a femoral mesh to support the deficient anterolateral aspect of the proximal femur for the subsequent impaction grafting. The impaction grafting was performed using the standard protocol. Morselized bone allograft (two femoral heads) washed several times to remove fat was inserted distally and impacted using the distal impactors over the guiding pole. Phantom stems were then used to create the proximal neo-endosteum using larger cheeps of bone allograft of at least 2 cm each. Vigorous impaction and third-generation cementing were followed by a 37.5 mm offset stem insertion at the appropriate depth to compensate for the LLD (Fig. 40.2).

40.1.7 Postoperative Radiographs (Fig. 40.2)

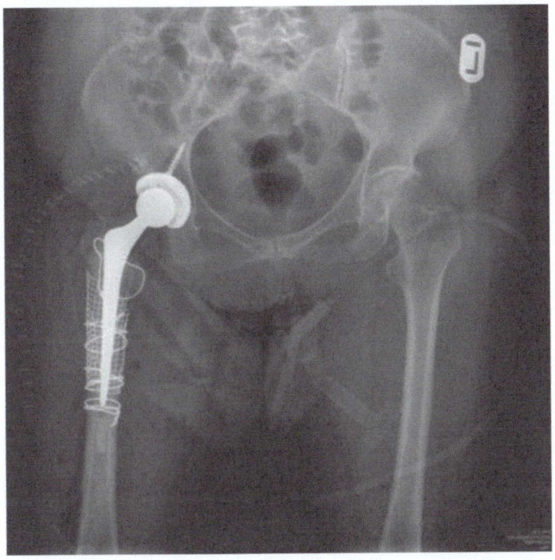

Fig. 40.2 ETO recovered with cerclage wires and metal mesh to compensate for the anterolateral bone loss. Impaction grafting revision cemented standard stem

40.1.8 Postoperative Management

Chemoprophylaxis and anticoagulant treatment period: Cefuroxime 1.5 g (one dose preoperatively and two doses postoperatively), vancomycin 500 mg (one dose preoperatively and two doses postoperatively), enoxaparin sodium 1 × 1 for 35 days

Gait/limb loading until full loading: Partial weight bearing for eight weeks. At eight weeks walking with one aid on the contralateral side for another month. Full weight bearing without a walking aid at four months postoperatively

40.2 Case Title: Hip Revision for Leg Length Discrepancy

Viktor Janz

40.2.1 Demographics

Age: 63
Sex: Female
BMI: 20.9

40.2.2 Relevant Past Medical History

Principal pathologies: Aseptic stem loosening with resulting stem subsidence and leg length shortening of −2 cm.

Previous surgical procedures: 2003 ORIF after a medial femoral neck fracture, proximal femoral osteotomy because of avascular necrosis of the femoral head, postoperative pseudarthrosis of the proximal femur with resulting conversion to total hip arthroplasty (2004).

Medication: NSAID as needed.

Other: Tinnitus.

History of presenting complaint: After conversion to a THA in an external clinic, the patient presented to our outpatient department with pain in the proximal femur radiating to the right knee. The pain had primarily occurred in October and was progressive. Additionally, the patient had noticed a shortening of the right leg of −2 cm and reported a progressive abductor insufficiency.

40.2.3 Clinical Examination

Symptoms: Progressive pain in the right groin, radiating along the ventral proximal femur and the right knee. Progressive abductor insufficiency

Range of motion: Extension/flexion 0/0/100 (right), 0/0/120 (left); abduction/adduction 40/0/20 (right), 40/0/20 (left); external rotation/internal rotation 30/0/10 (right), 40/0/20 (right)

Specific tests: Tenderness in Scarpa's triangle, pain provocation upon femoral rotation, tenderness over femoral shaft upon palpation

Main disability: Pain upon weight bearing in the proximal femur

Neurovascular evaluation: No peripheral neurovascular deficits

40.2.4 Preoperative Radiological Assessment/Imaging (Figs. 40.3, 40.4, and 40.5)

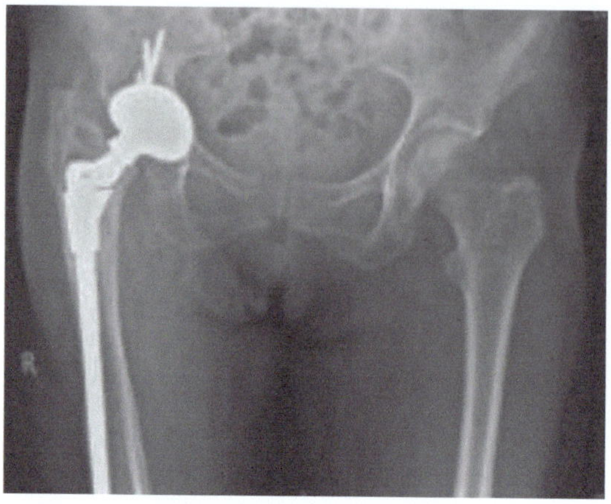

Fig. 40.3 AP pelvic radiograph

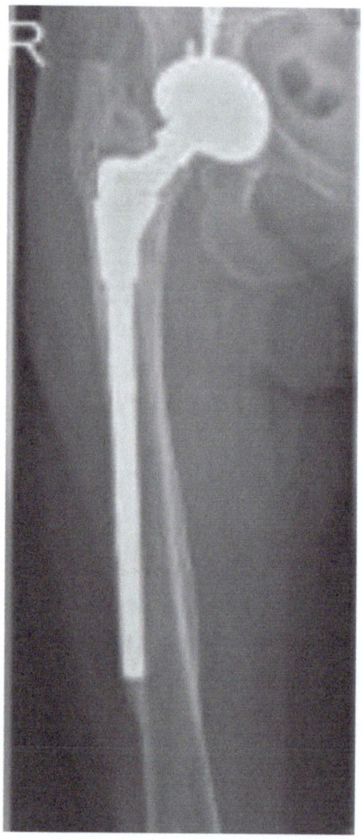

Fig. 40.4 AP radiograph of the proximal femur

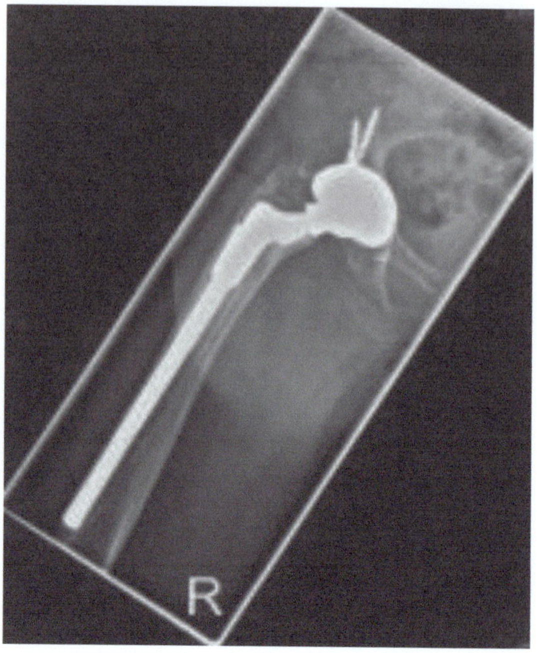

Fig. 40.5 Axial radiograph of the proximal femur

40.2.5 Preoperative Planning

Diagnosis: Aseptic stem loosening with resulting stem subsidence (Figs. 40.3, 40.4, and 40.5).

Possible treatment options: One stage stem exchange with a cementless modular fluted tapered stem, stem exchange to a long cemented stem or isolated ball and liner exchange to a longer neck length.

Chosen treatment method: Stem exchange for a cementless modular tapered fluted stem.

Selection of implants if applicable and rational: The decision for a cementless modular, tapered fluted stem was made because of the intraoperative flexibility offered by the modularity of the implant allowing for a precise reconstruction of the leg length and the lower risk of embolic complications in comparison to a cemented fixation.

Expected difficulties: There is a risk of perforation of the femoral shaft or trochanteric fracture during the retrograde removal of the in situ stem. Since the in situ stem has passed the femoral isthmus, the new revision stem is at risk for a postoperative stem subsidence in the case of implant undersizing. Additionally, since the intramedullary canal has been widened and displaced by the loose in situ stem, care must be taken to position the new revision stem in the anatomical intramedullary femoral canal. If the new stem is not centred in the intramedullary canal, there is a risk of femoral perforation with the tip of the new revision stem.

Strategies to overcome difficulties: During removal of the in situ stem, extreme caution should be taken to avoid a trochanteric fracture. The shoulder of the in situ stem must be meticulously cleared so that the implant shoulder does not stress the greater trochanter upon retrograde removal.

40.2.6 Surgical Note

Patient's position: Supine position.

Type of anaesthesia: General anaesthesia.

Surgical approach: Minimally invasive anterolateral approach.

Main steps: After exposure of the hip joint and soft tissue release to gain exposure to the proximal femur, the soft tissue covering the shoulder of the in situ stem must be completely removed. Additionally, any ossification must also be removed to allow for a retrograde removal of the in situ stem without placing stress on the greater trochanter. After a complete exposure of the proximal stem, the shoulder has been achieved, the osseous-implant interface of the metaphyseal portion of the in situ stem was loosened with Lambotte osteotomes. Utilizing a universal femoral stem extractor, a retrograde removal of the stem was possible. To ensure that the new stem is placed properly in the intramedullary canal and reduces the risk of perforation, the femur should be reamed under fluoroscopic control using intramedullary guide wires. After completion of the femoral reaming, the distal component is inserted and impacted. A proximal component of appropriate height is selected to properly restore the leg length; a trial reduction is performed. After verification of the proper height and orientation of the proximal component, the final proximal component is assembled and fixed (Figs. 40.6, and 40.7).

Reconstruction techniques: The loose and varus misaligned stem was replaced with a modular fluted tapered stem of greater length and larger diameter. This allows for a reconstruction of proper leg length.

40.2.7 Intraoperative Challenges

Challenges and solutions: It can be challenging to place the new stem straight into the femoral canal without being misguided into the varus malalignment of the previous stem.

Unanticipated problems and solution: No unanticipated problems were encountered.

Thorough description of decision-making, including the reason for the final decision: After removal of the in situ stem, a guide wire is inserted into the intramedullary canal. The reamer is inserted into the femoral canal, and the correct position is verified by fluoroscopy. After verification of the correct position, reaming is commenced. This procedure is repeated until the desired diameter is achieved. If the reamer is misled to an off-axis position despite the intramedullary guide wire, then the obstruction can be removed with a long, straight chisel. After removal of the obstruction, reaming can be commenced in the previously described fashion.

40.2.8 Postoperative Radiographs (Figs. 40.6 and 40.7)

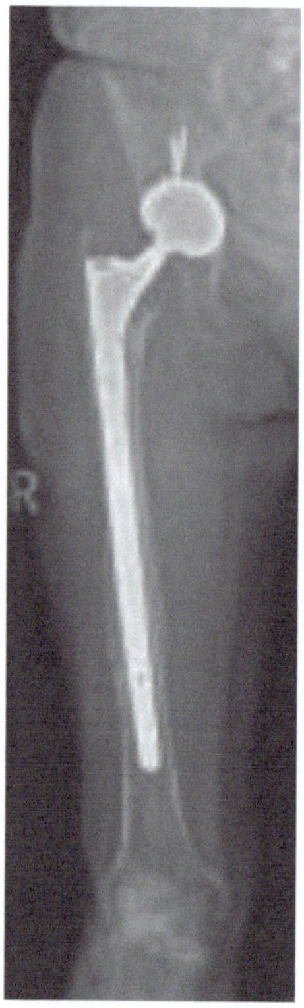

Fig. 40.6 Proximal femur AP radiograph

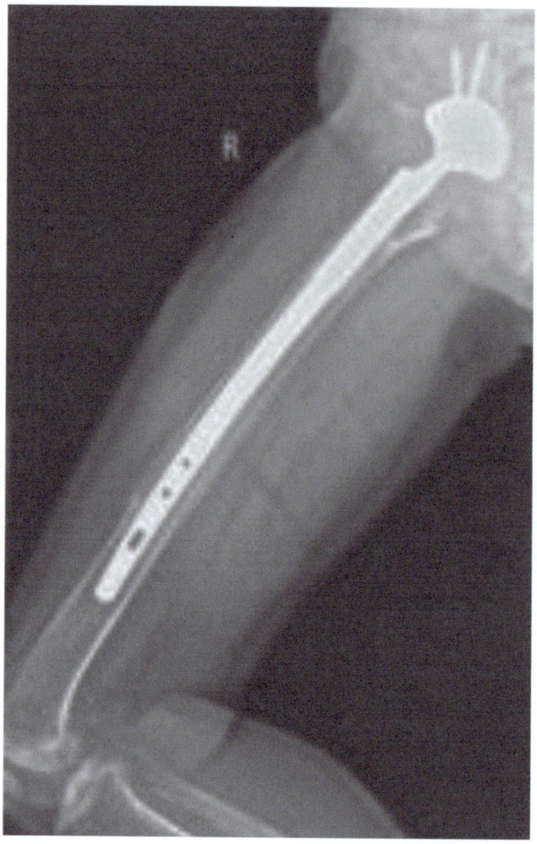

Fig. 40.7 Axial radiograph of the proximal femur

40.2.9 Postoperative Management

Chemoprophylaxis and anticoagulant treatment period: A perioperative dose of cephalosporin was administered. Postoperative anticoagulative treatment was performed with a weight-based dosage of low molecular weight heparin.

Gait/limb loading until full loading: The patient was mobilized from the first postoperative day with protective weight bearing on the right leg. The protective weight bearing was continued until the end of the sixth postoperative week.

40.2.10 Follow-Up and Complications

Due to a postoperative hypotension and anaemia, the patient was observed for one night at our post-anaesthesia care unit.

40.2.11 Discussion

Advantages of the applied method: The advantage of using a modular fluted tapered stem is that the modularity allows for intraoperative adaptation to allow for a correct reconstruction of the leg length.

Disadvantages of the method: The disadvantage of using a modular fluted tapered stem is that there is a risk of varus alignment or femoral fracture during stem implantation. Secondarily, there is a risk of stem subsidence. Thirdly, there is an increased risk of fracture in an osteoporotic bone, due to the long fixation distance of the chosen implant.

Alternative evidence-based techniques for the case: An alternative treatment would be a cemented fixation of the femoral component. This fixation type has a higher risk of embolic complications or cement-associated hypotension. Also, there are reports of an increased rate of loosening at midterm follow-up for cemented revision of failed uncemented femoral components [1].

Why is the chosen technique better for this case? The lower risk of embolic complications and the intraoperative flexibility offered by the modularity of the implant are the decisive factors that made us choose a modular fluted tapered stem.

Indications and contraindications for your technique: Contraindications for the use of a modular fluted tapered stem are extensive diaphyseal osseous defects, which compromise the press-fit fixation.

Learning curve and how to manage complications: When using modular tapered fluted stems initially, there can be a learning curve for finding the correct sizing of the distal component.

Level of evidence concerning the superiority of this method against others: The reported survival rate for modular fluted tapered cementless stems in revision THA is excellent with a reported survival rate of 96% at a follow-up of 7.5 years [2].

References

1. Davis CM 3rd, Berry DJ, Harmsen WS. Cemented revision of failed uncemented femoral components of total hip arthroplasty. J Bone Joint Surg Am. 2003;85-A(7):1264–9.
2. Fink B, Urbansky K, Schuster P. Mid term results with the curved modular tapered, fluted titanium Revitan stem in revision hip replacement. Bone Joint J. 2014; 96-B(7):889–95. doi:10.1302/0301-620X.96B7.33280.

Part VI

Navigation and VR Software in Joint Reconstruction

41 Psychomotor Surgical Training in Virtual Reality

George Papagiannakis, Panos Trahanias, Eustathios Kenanidis, and Eleftherios Tsiridis

41.1 Introduction

Surgical training has evolved considerably from the traditional apprenticeship of the first surgeons to a complexly structured training programe with multiple assessments. As trainee numbers increase, opportunities to develop procedural and technical skills become increasingly limited. Furthermore, the introduction of the European Working Time Directive across Europe [1] and the 40 h per week limit introduced by the Accreditation Council for Graduate Medical Education in the United States of America [2] have led to a reduction in training hours available during the designated training period. Working time restrictions and a drive towards senior-led care demand that proficiency is gained in a shorter period while requiring a greater skill set than that in the past.

Innovation has meant that there are more occasions where surgical intervention may be indicated. The latter is coupled with an aging population more expectant of treatment, has resulted in greater demand for surgery than ever before, leading to a conflict between service provision and training. The resulting conflict between service delivery and training has necessitated the development of alternative methods to compensate for the reduction in 'hands-on', psychomotor experience.

In the same period, there has been a significant development of novel techniques requiring current trainees to master a greater array of specialist skills, despite having less time in which to do so. Many different solutions including e-Learning, simulation and compulsory fellowship training programs have been proposed to maximize learning opportunities within existing resource constraints.

Simulation training provides the opportunity to develop surgical skills in a controlled environment while minimising risks to patient safety, operating theatre usage and financial expenditure [3]. Many options for simulation exist within orthopaedics from cadaveric or prosthetic models to arthroscopic simulators, advanced virtual reality and three-dimensional software tools. There are limitations to this form of training, but it has significant potential for trainees to achieve competence in procedures before real-life practice. The evidence for its direct transferability to oper-

G. Papagiannakis · P. Trahanias
Department of Computer Science, University of Crete, Crete, Greece

Computational Vision and Robotics Laboratory, Institute of Computer Science, Foundation for Research & Technology—Hellas (FORTH), Science and Technology Park of Crete, Crete, Greece

E. Kenanidis, M.D., Ph.D., M.Sc.
Academic Orthopaedic Unit, Aristotle University Medical School, Thessaloniki, Greece

E. Tsiridis, M.D., Ph.D., F.A.C.S., F.R.C.S. (✉)
Academic Orthopaedic Unit, Papageorgiou General Hospital, Aristotle University Medical School, Thessaloniki, Greece
e-mail: etsiridis@doctors.org.uk

E. Tsiridis (ed.), *The Adult Hip - Master Case Series and Techniques*,
https://doi.org/10.1007/978-3-319-64177-5_41

ating theatre performance is limited, but there are obvious benefits such as increasing trainee confidence and familiarity with equipment. With progressively improving methods of simulation available, it is likely to become more important in the ongoing and future training and assessment of surgeons.

Simulation in medicine can be broadly defined as 'any technology or process that recreates a contextual background in a way that allows a learner to experience mistakes and receive feedback in a safe environment' [4]. This definition is always evolving due to advances in technology, which allow increasingly complex situations to be modelled and tested. Simulation aims to recreate the experience of patient care without compromising patient safety. The ability to modify a case allows trainees to experience novel and often important situations that may not be commonly experienced in clinical practice. The advantages of a VR-based simulation, recent serious games and gamification approaches for interactive learning events extend beyond mere technical and procedural skills. Simulation allows trainees to engage with a multidisciplinary team, focus on individual and group-based cognitive skills including problem-solving, decision-making and team behavior skills in realistic, reactive virtual environment and have a unique hands-on experience.

41.2 Previous Work

Cadaver models were historically used as part of surgical training. In recent decades, significant progress has been made in developing new and varied simulation-based techniques to provide virtual training [5] in a safe and modifiable environment [6–8]. The simulation improves trainee confidence and understanding of techniques while also allowing practice and development of specific technical skills [9].

The current 3D simulation of surgical procedures is mostly confined to a non-operator interaction of static, noninteractive image or video-based examples that can teach the customer several steps of a process, and very few examples of gamified, VR approaches have been showcased [10]. Surgery, however, in real life is not predictable for two reasons: First, human anatomy is unique per individual, and surgery replication can never be 100% due to surgeon- or patient-related factors. The latter parameters make the current 3D simulations not realistic enough to the most trainees and definitely of no use for the specialist surgeons. As an example we can say that the current, cognitive-only virtual simulations are equivalent to a linear, video manual for a flying simulation for a pilot, lucking, however, any degree of immersive reality or ability to follow and react to different scenarios according to user hand actions (psychomotor). We aim to increase 3D realism but most importantly to provide natural, gesture-based interaction between the consumer surgeon and the virtual patient.

A few companies are recently targeting products that are indirectly competing with our system. They are broadly classified into two categories:

1. Cognitive VR/AR and medical simulation:
   (a) Touch Surgery (https://www.touchsurgery.com/focuses) on a tablet-based, interactive gamified simulation of various medical procedures, using touch-based cognitive metaphors. It is not an immersive solution or natural, hand-based, psychomotor interaction.
   (b) SURGEVRY (http://www.surgevry.com/#root) focuses on immersive, 360, stereoscopic videos, experienced first person by the trainee. However, this is not an interactive VR application (video-based).
   (c) Surgical Theater (http://www.surgicaltheater.net) focuses on an immersive VR flythrough of 3D MRI data, with no natural interaction or gamification options.
   (d) VR Med (http://www.vr-med.com) is a recently developed start-up that seems to

promote simulation-based medical applications without however specifying or describing any related products or services.

(e) VRMedApp (http://vrmedapp.com) is another newly created start-up utilising recent advances in VR HMDs. However, no product is yet developed, and the company primarily focuses on well-being medical applications, such as pain management and rehabilitation.

(f) SimX (http://simxar.com) is a recently aquired start-up utilising recent Meta-AR HMDs for first-aid, cognitive medical training in AR.

(g) Augmedix (http://www.augmedix.com) allows for hands-free medical charting whilst interacting with patients, utilizing Google Glasses in monocular AR.

(h) Osso VR (http://www.ossovr.net) is a very recent start-up that aims to tackle medical surgical simulation using the Oculus Touch controllers that allow hand manipulation of objects, without finger tracking. The company has just appeared online with a concept video and no other product information or demo.

2. Education and medical simulation using custom, expensive h/w:
   (a) Surgical Science (http://www.surgical-science.com/products/employs) is a 3D navigation system and desktop-based educational simulation of specific operations. However, it does not focus on orthopaedic surgeries at all or VR gamification and natural interaction.
   (b) SimSurgery (http://www.simsurgery.com/ectopic-pregnancy.html) provides haptic-based navigation and desktop-based medical simulations, without any VR gamification solution.
   (c) Intuitive Surgical (http://www.intuitive-surgical.com/products/skills_simulator/provides) is their custom h/w, desktop 3D simulation for specific surgery types, without providing VR gamification/interaction.
   (d) SimPORTAL (http://www.simportal.umn.edu/surgery.htm) is a solution from the University of Minnesota for medical students to be trained using desktop 3D simulation systems in particular medical procedures. However, no VR gamification with natural interaction is provided or any applications related to orthopaedic surgeries.

Our system dramatically capitalises on previously developed and assessed, state-of-the-art technologies, which are owned by ovidVR. Such technologies regard enhanced character interpolation animation, gamification, sensor fusion and tracking algorithms that endow the relevant product with essential, unprecedented characteristics [11–14].

41.3 Methodology and Results

The presented ovidVR system offers to surgeons the unique opportunity to perform with their hands, realistically, 'as if they are Present in the operating theatre' as many demanding operations as necessary to master the different techniques. At the same time, manufacturers such as artificial joint makers will have a complete VR simulation customised to their joint implant. All in all, we aim at establishing VR psychomotor medical simulation as a key component of medical training and continuing assessment throughout a surgeon's or physician's career, in a similar manner to the mandatory nature of flight simulators to modern pilots.

A beta product version currently exists, integrating our advanced VR simulation and tracking technologies. Figure 41.1 below illustrates a snapshot from the ovidVR system in operation. The named product is a novel, gamified, VR-based, interactive 3D medical simulation training s/w. It requires standard h/w (PCs, lap-

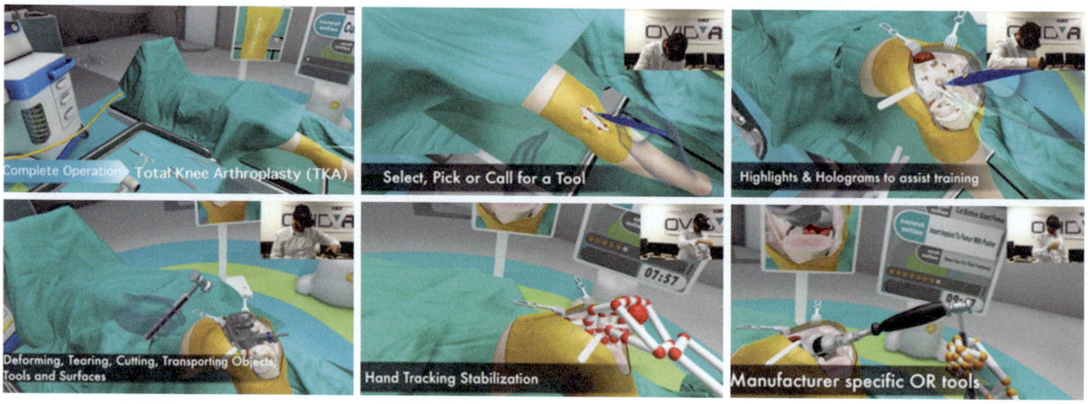

Fig. 41.1 The ovidVR psychomotor VR simulation system (Figure created by the authors)

tops) irrelevant of the operating system. For optimal user experience, a commodity VR head-mounted display (HMD) should be employed along with the latest HMD motion or other hand sensors. The open architecture supports all current and forthcoming VR HMDs and standard 3D content generation pipelines.

It is not a question of whether VR will enter the medical training space, but when ovidVR is exceptionally positioned to pioneer and has a recipe for succeeding; all it needs is investment support to monetarize on its technology and business plans, delivering unprecedented impact to the healthcare and VR ecosystems.

References

1. Association of Surgeons of Great Britain and Ireland. The Impact of EWTD on Delivery of Surgical Services: A Consensus Statement; 2008.
2. Philbert I, Friedmann P, Williams WT, SCGME Work Group on Resident Duty Hours. Accreditation Council for Graduate Medical Education: new requirements for resident duty hours. JAMA. 2002;288:1112–4.
3. Aggarwal R, Mytton OT, Derbrew M, Hananel D, Heydenburg M, Issenberg B, MacAulay C, Mancini ME, Morimoto T, Soper N, Ziv A, Reznick R. Training and simulation for patient safety. Qual Saf Health Care. 2010;19(Suppl 2):i34–43.
4. Gaba DM. The future vision of simulation in health care. Qual Saf Health Care. 2004;13(Suppl 1): i2–i10.
5. Wiet GJ, Stredney D, Kerwin T, Hittle B, Kang DR. Simulation for training in resource-restricted countries: using a scalable temporal bone surgical simulator. Int J Med Educ. 2016;7:293–4. https://doi.org/10.5116/ijme.57c1.4c8a.
6. Frank RM, Erickson B, Frank JM, Bush-Joseph CA, Bach BR, Cole BJ, Romero AA, Provencher MT, Verma NN. Utility of modern arthroscopic simulator training models. Arthroscopy. 2014;30(1):121–33.
7. Tay C, Khajuria A, Gupte C. Simulation training: a systematic review of simulation in arthroscopy and proposal of a new competency-based training framework. Int J Surg. 2014;12(6):626–33.
8. Dawe SR, Pena GN, Windsor JA, Broeders JAJL, Cregan PC, Hewett PJ, Maddern GJ. Systematic review of skills transfer after surgical simulation-based training. Br J Surg. 2014;101(9):1063–76.
9. Sabri H, Cowan B, Kapralos B, Porte M, Backstein D, Dubrowskie A. Serious games for knee replacement surgery procedure education and training. Procedia Soc Behav Sci. 2010;2(2):3483–8. https://doi.org/10.1016/j.sbspro.2010.03.539.
10. de Ribaupierre S, Kapralos B, Haji F, Stroulia E, Dubrowski A, Eagleson R. Healthcare training enhancement through virtual reality and serious games. In: Virtual, augmented reality and serious games for healthcare 1, vol. 68. Berlin, Heidelberg: Springer; 2014. p. 9–27. https://doi.org/10.1007/978-3-642-54816-1_2.
11. Sigalas M, Baltzakis H, Trahanias P. Gesture recognition based on arm tracking for human-robot interaction. Intelligent Robots and Systems (IROS), 2010 IEEE/RSJ international conference, pp. 5424–5429 2010.
12. Sigalas M, Pateraki M, Trahanias P. Robust articulated upper body pose tracking under severe occlusions. International conference. Intelligent Robots and Systems, IROS2014, pp. 4104–4111, Chicago, 2014.
13. Papagiannakis G. Geometric algebra rotors for skinned character animation blending. Technical Brief, ACM SIG-GRAPH ASIA 2013, Hong Kong, November 2013, 2013.
14. Papagiannakis G, Papanikolaou P, Greassidou E, Trahanias PE. glGA: an OpenGL geometric application framework for a modern, shader-based computer graphics curriculum. Eurographics'14 (Education Papers Track). 2014, pp. 9–16.

MIX
Papier aus verantwortungsvollen Quellen
Paper from responsible sources
FSC® C105338

If you have any concerns about our products,
you can contact us on
ProductSafety@springernature.com

In case Publisher is established outside the EU,
the EU authorized representative is:
Springer Nature Customer Service Center GmbH
Europaplatz 3, 69115 Heidelberg, Germany

Printed by Libri Plureos GmbH
in Hamburg, Germany